D0586192

A General Textbook
of Nursing

Dedicated to
Students of Nursing

THE AUTHOR

Member of the General Nursing Council for England and Wales, formerly Examiner in Nursing to the Council. For many years Senior Nursing Tutor, The Middlesex Hospital, Examiner in Fever Nursing and Epidemiology for the Diploma in Nursing, London University, and in General Nursing, Leeds University. State Registered General and Fever Nursing, State Registered Sister Tutor. State Certified Midwife. Teacher's Certificate Chartered Society Physiotherapy.

other books by the author

★

MEDICAL AND NURSING DICTIONARY AND ENCYCLOPAEDIA

A TEXTBOOK OF ORTHOPAEDIC NURSING

ANATOMY AND PHYSIOLOGY FOR NURSES

FEVERS AND FEVER NURSING

A COMPLETE HANDBOOK OF HYGIENE IN QUESTIONS AND ANSWERS

INSTRUMENTS, APPLIANCES AND THEATRE TECHNIQUE

A GENERAL TEXTBOOK OF NURSING

a comprehensive guide

---

by

EVELYN PEARCE

ELEVENTH EDITION

FABER AND FABER LTD
24 Russell Square
London
1950

First published in 1937
Second edition, October 1938
Third edition, October 1939
Fourth edition, September 1940
Fifth edition, June 1941
Sixth edition, January 1942
Seventh edition, September 1942
Eighth edition, April 1943
Ninth edition, 1945
Reprinted 1945, 1946 and 1947
Tenth edition, 1949
Eleventh edition, 1950
By Faber and Faber, Limited
Printed in Great Britain by
Purnell & Sons, Ltd.
Paulton, Somerset and London

Preface to the Tenth Edition

In preparing the *Tenth Edition* of my book the work has been completely revised. Unhappily the available paper supplies do not yet permit of the re-insertion of the illustrations in the text. They are placed in groups where it has been most convenient to include them.

Details of treatments now rarely used have been omitted, such treatments as hot air baths, wet packs, etc., but the illustrations have been retained as a guide where required.

New material includes a section (5) on communicable diseases, a short chapter (27) on diseases and disorders of metabolism, a short chapter (46) on the care of patients after thoracic surgical operations, and a list of the abbreviations of terms used in prescriptions is included as an additional appendix.

I should like to take this opportunity of expressing my thanks for the letters of encouragement I have received and for many helpful suggestions as to alterations and additions to the book. All of these have been most carefully considered and many have been adopted. In particular I thank the Sisters of the Middlesex Hospital for their valuable help.

I am grateful to the publishers for the interest they have taken in this book and the care and attention they have given to it in its passage through the press.

February, 1949.

This *Eleventh Edition* follows so closely on the tenth that the inclusion of several new notes only has been necessary. In particular, mention is made of the new antibiotics, aureomycin and chloromycetin which already give promise of revolutionizing the treatment of enteric and typhus fevers.

EVELYN C. PEARCE

1950.

Preface to the First Edition

In writing this book for nurses it has been my endeavour to provide one which is sufficiently comprehensive to enable the student to find in it the introduction to nursing she needs on entering hospital, a useful book of reference as she works in one department of the hospital or other and the information she requires in order to pass the Hospital and State Examinations in the different branches of nursing subjects included in the curriculum.

The information I have been able to give is largely derived from personal experience in the care of the sick and in the teaching of nurses. I desire to express my gratitude to my teachers first of all, then to those whose books and articles I have read and also to many friends who have helped me by advice and kind criticism. I should like to thank them all individually, but space does not permit. Will they please accept my thanks for helping me to help others?

I have the greatest pleasure in expressing my gratitude to Sister Marjorie Wenger for help in arranging the illustrations, to Mr. B. D. H. Watters for his able photography and to C. W. Stewart of Messrs. Faber and Faber for his co-operation and assistance. I acknowledge also my indebtedness to Miss G. E. Davies, the Registrar of the General Nursing Council, for permission to make use of State Examination question papers.

EVELYN C. PEARCE

March 31st, 1937

Contents

Section 1. General and Special Nursing Measures and Procedures

Section 2. The Feeding of Adult Patients and Infants. Elementary Dietetics

Section 3. The Administration of Drugs and Medicines. Elementary Materia Medica. Poisons and Poisoning

Section 4. Medical Conditions and Diseases and their Treatment and Nursing

Section 1

General and Special Nursing Measures and Procedures

Introductory

This book is dedicated to students of nursing. Professional nursing only dates from the establishment of the Nightingale School in 1860, so that nursing as we know it is not yet 100 years old. Nursing is described as a science, an art and a vocation. The vocational aspect is of greatest importance because it begins with the high qualities and ideals of service the student brings to nursing and, rightly guided and well practised, these develop a *love of nursing* without which no one can be a good nurse.

THE HOSPITAL

The hospital is a place to which the sick come for investigation, treatment and cure. Doctors and nurses learn their arts in hospital and have opportunities to develop their ideals of service. As medicine becomes more and more specialized so the hospital team becomes more numerous, and treatment unfortunately often slightly more impersonal. The corridors of any great hospital seem like a railway terminus, people are being interviewed, directed and helped; messengers are passing to and fro, and there is a constant stream of people coming and going to and from some place or other.

THE PATIENT

When relatives bring a patient into hospital, they wonder how he will be received, and whether he can be cured or relieved. The patient too feels a stranger. He has come from the most comfortable room his home could provide, where he was surrounded by loving care, to lie in bed in a ward with others. He realizes he may be helpless, and that he will be in the hands of strangers to do their bidding, he fears they may not understand him and his needs, he feels that if ever he needed support it is now; and he is alone.

He does not yet know that he will probably be visited by a dozen or more doctors, some interested in his history, home conditions, onset of illness, others in the condition of his teeth, hearing, sight, blood, body fluids, diet, muscle reactions and so on. But in the midst of all this will be *the nurse*, the one stable influence upon which the patient can always depend.

THE NURSE

The nurse who receives the patient can by kindness and sympathy dispel most of his fears. She can make it clear by her interest and devotion that the hospital is there for his benefit. A nurse who develops the gift of making a patient feel at home, and free from fear, inspires confidence, and provides that atmosphere of serenity and security which is so important for the relaxation of mind and body necessary for recovery.

The doctor is the director of the hospital team but the nurse (the ward sister) is the *captain of the team*. She is first of all the *hostess* and as hostess she will see to the care and comfort of her patient which will include seeing that he is not lonely, and that he has some interesting occupation. She is entirely responsible for the welfare of her patients, no matter to whom she may delegate certain duties. She it is who forms a link or liaison between the patient and the numerous specialists who may attend to him; the nurse must of necessity, if she is to take her full part in the health team, develop the attitude of mind that sees the patient as an individual, a person—body, mind and soul. In addition to co-ordinating his treatments, she will console him, explain what is taking place, and so on, and she may even have to protect him.

Florence Nightingale taught, 'The very alphabet of a nurse is to be able to read every change which comes over a patient's face, note every alteration of attitude, and every change of voice, without causing him the exertion of saying what he feels.' She taught the importance of respecting confidences and never answering questions about a patient except to those who have a right to ask, the need for the nurse to have great devotion to duty, and respect for her own calling because 'God's precious gift of life is often placed in her hands'.

The Nurse as Teacher. The nurse is a teacher of health in relation to her own patients whom she gets to know well and can help and guide in making the best use of the experience of illness and recovery. She is also the teacher in the hospital and must endeavour so to inspire and guide each individual that everyone is interested in health and realizes to the full the part he or she can take in the health team. People like working in hospital, they feel it is good to be there because everyone is helping others. The sister in charge of ward or department who is capable of leadership, of giving and stimulating loyalty to good team work, will keep everyone interested, and on their toes to give the best service possible. This teaching function is well worth developing for it can result in everyone doing most satisfying and satisfactory work, and its ramifications by instructing, in the laws of healthy living, the entire community into which every member of the hospital team penetrates, are innumerable.

THE CANDIDATE TO NURSING

The student, attracted to nursing, has the wellbeing of her fellow men at heart; she wants to help others; she knows that nursing is not an easy life and is prepared for this. She will find that illness gives rise to abnormality, that patients can be trying and nursing duties are not always pleasant. But all these difficulties are surmountable if she always remembers that she set out to help her patients—the sick.

The candidate to nursing has embarked upon the noblest and highest service one human being can do for another. She has set out to become the *vital link* in the great chain of health workers, the link between them and the patient, always helpful, never discouraged, realizing the therapeutic value of a well-timed smile, giving generously those small services done to the lowliest which possess an eternal value, providing the life-giving forces prescribed by medical science. To quote Florence Nightingale again, 'The physician prescribes for supplying the vital force, but the nurse supplies it'.

TRADITION

Tradition depends on men and women, it is 'the handing down of opinions or practices to posterity unwritten'. Whether the hospital in which a nurse trains is under the state or independent, whether the building is modern or out of date, the standard of work, the tradition, depends on the workers within those walls and upon the ideals they cherish.

The lady with the lamp following the tradition of a long line of Christian workers, having in mind the teaching contained in the parable of the Good Samaritan, was inspired to serve others. In this same spirit students of nursing will keep the lamp of their vocation bright and clear, temper their skilled work with gentleness, cheerfulness and thoughtful understanding, serve in the spirit which asks *not* What do you want? but What can I do for you? How can I help you?

THE FLORENCE NIGHTINGALE PLEDGE

Do you promise to live a pure life and practise your profession faithfully?
I solemnly pledge myself before God, and in the presence of this assembly to pass my life in purity and to practise my profession faithfully.

Will you abstain from whatever that is hurtful?
I will abstain from whatever is deleterious and mischievous and will not take or knowingly administer any harmful drug.

Will you try and elevate the standard of your profession?
I will do all in my power to elevate the standard of my profession and will hold in confidence all personal matter committed to my keeping and all family affairs coming to my knowledge in the practice of my calling.

Will you promise to be loyal to the physician and his work?
With loyalty will I endeavour to aid the physician in his work and devote myself to the welfare of those committed to my care.

Chapter 1

Reception and Admission of a Patient

The reception and admission of a patient—Observations to be made on a patient's condition—Examination of a patient—Discharge and transfer of patients

A junior probationer may quite early in her career be accosted at the doorway of her ward by a patient and his friends on his arrival at the hospital. He is not to know that she is not a very senior official, even the sister of the ward; she must therefore be prepared to meet him with smiling courteous dignity, receiving him like a hostess, listening carefully to the questions he may put to her, and answering them with tactful consideration; then, inviting the patient and his friends to be seated while she informs the sister of the ward, who she may correctly say is prepared to receive and is expecting this patient, leaving him for a moment contentedly seated and waiting to be received by the sister who expects him.

The nurse responsible for admitting the patient walks towards him with alacrity, pleased to see the patient for whom she has prepared the bed and whom she is expecting. She rapidly glances down the card he presents and gives him a smile of reassurance, calls him by name which she has learnt from the card, notes the diagnosis, and makes a rapid survey of the condition of the patient, by which she is enabled to determine whether he may remain seated for a few moments, or whether he should be put to bed immediately.

The *admission card* contains particulars of the name, age, address of the patient, and his occupation, the name of the physician or surgeon under whom he is to be admitted, the name and address of the patient's private doctor, the diagnosis of his condition, including remarks on this, which may possibly have been made when the patient was examined in the casualty department before being sent to the ward. The nurse makes a mental note of these and, observing the address, notices whether it is local or some distance away, and immediately inquires the sort of journey he had and when he last had anything to eat. As already stated, the condition of the patient will indicate whether he is to be put to bed immediately or not: for example, if he is a surgical case for operation next day he might have his temperature taken, then be given some food and afterwards be bathed in the bathroom before getting into bed; on the other hand, if the patient is at all ill or in pain, or suffering from any uncomfortable symptoms, he should be put to bed at once. In this case it is usual to ask the relatives to wait until the patient is in bed; in some hospitals the relatives take the patient's clothes away with them. They may go to the bedside and speak to the patient before leaving.

There are certain questions which it is practically always advisable to ask the relatives. Make sure that the address on the admission slip is *where they are staying*; ask whether they are at home all day, or out at business; in the latter case get the business address, the hours they will be there and the telephone number. Then ask the name of the nearest police station, informing them that this is required in case untoward symptoms should occur with rapidity, when the police will undertake to deliver a message day or night, in the event of there being no telephone in the house. If the patient is a junior and has come in for operation, get their signed permission for this. It is also advisable to ask questions of the relatives which could not reasonably be put to the patient; for example, if the patient is being admitted to the eye department, the condition of his mental health is of vital importance, as he will be subjected to mental strain owing to the necessity of lying still with his eyes covered and being made so helpless that he has to be fed. In most cases it is a very good plan to find out if the patient is occasionally subject to attacks of any kind, such as vomiting, depression or fits, and also whether he has ever had a nervous breakdown.

It will be very reassuring to the relatives if the nurse asks for little intimate details about the patient, such as the position he likes to sleep in, how many pillows he is used to, whether he likes to sleep in sheets or blankets, how he sleeps, whether he is troubled by having to pass urine in the night, whether he likes a cup of tea when he wakes, and the condition of his appetite, including any special likes or dislikes. She might also ask the religion of the patient, and whether any minister has been visiting him, explaining, if so, that such visits can be continued, at the same time informing the relatives that if the patient wishes he can be visited by the attending chaplain of whatever denomination he belongs to.

She should tell the relatives which are the visiting days, give them the necessary cards of admission, and ask them to inquire later on in the day as to the patient's comfort, giving them the hospital telephone number. They might also be informed of any little delicacies they may bring the patient. If the hospital does not provide clothing and towels for the patient, the relatives should be informed as to what is necessary; if, however, this information was included when the patient was written for, the nurse should see that the necessary articles have been brought. These usually include personal bed attire, at least two sets of bath and face towels; toilet accessories—soap, flannel, sponge, toothbrush and paste, brush and comb. If the relatives are to take the *patient's clothes* home (see below) the nurse should go carefully through these and make a list of any articles that are retained for his use whilst in hospital.

The house doctor should be notified of every admission as soon as practicable, giving him the diagnosis, time of admission, temperature, pulse and respiration rate, and any urgent special symptoms noticed.

The bed card should be made out, and the temperature, pulse and respiration rate charted; if possible a specimen of urine should be obtained and tested and the specimen kept until the house doctor has made his first visit, in case he wishes to inspect it.

Patient's clothing. If the patient is well enough when he is admitted, the nurse should check his belongings over with him, unless this is done with his relatives. If they are taken home she should get a receipt for them. Should the patient be brought in unaccompanied by any friend or relative, and be in a state in which he is not fit to be troubled, or for any other reason is unable to check his own belongings, the nurse should make a list of these, inspect them for cleanliness, and the presence of vermin, in which case they might have to be disinfected and washed. She should then fold them carefully and put them away in a cupboard, labelling the parcel with the name of the patient, the name of the ward and the date, unless separate locked receptacles are provided for the use of patients.

Money and valuables are separately listed and taken to a special department or given into the custody of the ward sister with the exception of the patient's watch and a little pocket money which he may wish to keep in his locker for the purchase of newspapers, stamps and so on.

Infection. In admitting a patient it is very important that the nurse should find out whether he has been in contact with any infection. It is a good plan to ask whether there are any other ill persons in the house from which he has come and, if so, the nature of their illness. It is also important to find out if the patient is suffering from a sore throat or headache, which might indicate the onset of an infectious disease.

In taking the history—and by this is meant the history of a present illness—the following points have to be considered:

Present complaints, i.e. of what symptoms the patient is complaining.

How the illness began, and whether the patient has been in bed all the time; and whether he has been completely in bed, or getting up for sanitary purposes. Questions regarding the condition of his *appetite*, *bowels* and *urine*; the quantity and character of the *sleep* he usually obtains.

Having heard and recorded the complaints of the patient, the nurse observes which organs are particularly affected, and in taking the subsequent history she might begin by asking him questions regarding the different systems involved. For example, if the patient complains of coughing and pain in the chest, she would next make inquiries regarding the character of the cough, whether paroxysmal, whether the patient coughs more first thing in the morning, or after exertion, or after eating. The existence of any expectoration, character of it, including the colour and quantity, whether it is difficult to bring up, and if it has an unpleasant taste. She might also inquire whether there is any pain in the chest, asking the patient to indicate the position of this.

Having asked questions on the points about which a patient has complained, the nurse should then proceed to discover any other symptoms and, in order to elicit fairly accurate and comprehensive information, she might consider the different systems of the body, taking them each in turn and running through them in the following manner. At the same time she should avoid putting her questions in such a way as to suggest that the patient had any particular symptom.

Nervous system. Headache, drowsiness, sleeplessness, any wanderings of the mind or delirium, fits or twitchings, pain, hyperaesthesia or anaesthesia and any other sensory symptoms such as tingling and profuse sweatings.

Respiratory system. Cough, sputum, breathlessness, and blood-spitting.

Circulatory system. Palpitation, pain over the heart, swelling of the ankles or other parts of the body, attacks of faintness or fatigue, coldness of extremities, pallor or blueness, any sense of fullness in the neck, pulsation or throbbing of the blood vessels.

Alimentary system. Loss of appetite, nausea, dryness of mouth, bad taste in the mouth, dirty tongue, any indigestion, flatulence, vomiting, diarrhoea, constipation or abdominal pain. Sometimes dimness of vision, black spots before the eyes, headache, skin irritation or jaundice may accompany digestive disturbances.

Renal system. Character of urine, regarding quantity, whether scanty or copious, the colour and any deposit. Any difficulty in passing urine, including any pain on passing it, having to get up in the night to pass urine, frequent micturition during the day, the presence of any blood in the urine and whether there is any offensive odour. She should also inquire whether there is any pain in the loins, or over the bladder, whether the ankles swell at night or whether the patient wakens with puffiness of the face or under the eyes. Symptoms such as those of nausea or headache may frequently accompany renal disorder.

Past illnesses. The nature of any other illnesses the patient has had, any operations he has undergone, or accidents he has sustained should next be ascertained.

In admitting women patients, the nurse should inquire regarding the regularity of menstruation, its character, including the number of diapers used, any discomfort experienced, and whether this is sufficient to incapacitate the patient; also the presence of any vaginal discharge; and she should obtain a brief outline of the history of any pregnancies, abortions or miscarriages.

In admitting a child, all particulars must be obtained from those who bring him and, in order to do this effectively, the nurse should make it her business to receive the full confidence of the person who may be, and probably is, the mother of the child.

History of birth. It may be possible for the nurse to say, 'What a lovely baby—did he have a normal birth' and having thus gained the mother's heart she will hear the full story of this and can then interpose questions which will elicit any history of abnormality at the time of birth.

Breast fed. Whether this was found satisfactory, how long it was possible, the nature of the weaning; or, if the child had to be artificially fed, the type of food used and the results obtained.

Normal childhood. Whether the child had any infectious diseases; if so, at what age, and whether he was nursed in hospital or at home, and any complications which occurred.

Convulsions. Without actually mentioning this terrifying word, the nurse in a casual way may say, 'I suppose the child has never had any fits when teething', and this again will elicit the history as to whether the eruption of the teeth was normal or irregular.

School life. The health when at school, and the regularity of attendance —irregularity of attendance usually means defective health, either mental or physical.

Appetite, condition of *bowels*, and *sleep*, particularly whether the child sleeps all night; particulars of any *night fears* or *bedwetting*.

The *history of the present illness* will next be elicited on the lines indicated in the case of an adult.

It is usual to ask if the child has been vaccinated and christened. In the event of the latter having been omitted, find out the wishes of the parents should the child become suddenly very dangerously ill.

If the child is being admitted for operation, consent for the operation should be obtained from the parents.

The admission bed. The empty beds in a ward are usually made up ready for use so that patients can be admitted without delay. In many hospitals the wards take it in turn to be ready for taking in emergency cases. In other hospitals emergency cases are admitted to any ward at any time. It is, therefore, advisable to have a certain number of beds ready for the reception of cases in an emergency. The top bedclothes are neatly rolled to the side of the bed farthest away from the door, and two bath blankets are placed in position on the bed well covering the bottom sheet and the pillow. Toilet requisites, including soap, flannels and towels, and personal bed clothing are placed ready on the locker.

When a patient is expected, and the nature of the case is known, certain other articles might be required, such as fracture boards and bed-cradles, in case of fracture; bedblocks, in case of bleeding; bedrest and oxygen in case of dyspnoea; carbon dioxide and oxygen in case of coal gas poisoning and so on.

OBSERVATIONS OF A PATIENT'S CONDITION

Nursing observations are necessary from the moment a patient enters a ward until his discharge. The keenness and interest which a probationer displays when she first enters the hospital should never be permitted to lapse into routine. She should always be on the look-out for something new and she will never be disappointed. She must realize that, quite apart from the value of her observations in the subsequent treatment of the patient, this is one of the ways she has of learning her profession. A nurse must teach herself and, when she does this, she will find her contemporaries and seniors ever ready to help her. She must never behave as a passenger in her hospital, but always be an energetic member of the crew.

For example, whenever a patient is bathed something new can be learnt. It is a mistake to try and be too clever, especially at the beginning, or to think 'I can't make observations because I do not know how to classify them'. The best observations are made by people who are content to be simple and will therefore record accurately what they *see*, *hear*, *feel* and *smell*. When a patient is admitted it is important to notice his general attitude, postures and gait; his mental expression, whether cheerful or depressed, whether he appears comfortable or in pain, looks warm or cold —he may be trembling or shivering, clean or dirty, fat or thin; the colour of his skin should be noted. In this way, before getting him into bed a general impression of the type of person one is called upon to deal with can be formed. Again, what can be heard—is the patient crying, groaning or sighing? What is the character of his breathing, is it loud, wheezy, soft or shallow, and is he coughing or hawking? Any odour from the mouth, body or clothing should be noted.

Very important observations may be made whilst the patient is being put or helped into bed. In most hospitals patients, in whatever condition they may be admitted, have their first bath in bed and in no circumstances are they permitted to go to the bathroom. This enables the following observations to be made: The *condition of the hair*, whether lank and damp, dull or bright, and the presence of nits or lice; the hair should be separated in order to ascertain the condition of the scalp.

The *expression of the face*, particularly whether drawn as in pain; the condition of the *eyes*, any discharge from them; whether the pupils are uneven, normal size; whether the sclera are white, or too bluish white which indicates anaemia; are they jaundiced or bloodshot? whether the eyes are sunken or prominent; is there any squint, ptosis, or other abnormality of the eyelids, such as oedema, ulcers, deformed eyelashes? does the patient wear an artificial eye?

The *nose*, whether it moves in breathing, indicating dyspnoea, whether pinched and blue, the presence of beads of perspiration on it, whether the edges of the nostrils are sore, or covered with crusts, and the presence of any herpes round the nose and lips.

The *lips*, their colour, whether steady or trembling, whether dry or moist, the presence of any sores, cracks or sordes.

The *mouth* is carefully inspected when it is cleaned; but at this point the nurse might ask the patient to open his mouth, in order to get a general impression of the condition of his teeth, and to put out his tongue so that she may notice whether it is dry or moist, red or grey, furred, cracked or oedematous, whether it is marked by the impression of the teeth round its margins, and whether it is steady or trembling. She should also notice the odour of the breath.

The *colour of the cheeks* should be observed as to whether a malar flush is present, whether the capillaries are prominent in this region and, in this case, whether they appear red or bluish, whether both sides of the face are even in contour and the presence of any facial paralysis.

The presence of any rash. (See types of skin lesions, p. 449.)

By this time the patient will have settled down in bed and the next thing to notice is the position which he adopts, whether he lies limply on his back, taking no apparent interest in his surroundings, or is raising himself on his pillows, apparently anxious as to what is to happen next; which side he is lying on, whether he objects to facing the light, and whether his knees are curled up, which would indicate either that he was extremely cold or perhaps in abdominal pain. Notice also where he places his arms, particularly if he raises them above his head, which would indicate an attempt to assist the movements of the chest in breathing. Then notice any pulsation of the veins, or any enlargement of the thyroid or lymphatic glands in the neck, and note whether the patient moves his head easily or not.

The *skin* of the trunk and limbs should be inspected for the presence of any rash, abrasion, wounds, scars or lumps. The colour should be noted and the general condition of the skin, as to whether it is dry and harsh, normally soft and flexible, or abnormally wet and sticky. The nurse should feel the limbs, and notice whether they are hot, cold, limp, firm, whether there is any tremor, whether both sides of the body are equally developed, and whether the muscles feel limp and wasted, normally firm, or whether they are abnormally spastic and rigid. She should be on the look-out all the time for any indication of twitching or convulsion, either local or general, and she should investigate every part, particularly the abdomen, and the back, each side of the vertebral column, for the presence of tender spots. She should note whether there is any odour from the patient's body.

The *conditions of hands and feet* are deserving of special observation, since much can be learnt from them. The development will perhaps suggest the type of work, and in some cases be a guide to the temperament of the individual, as to whether he is energetic or lethargic. The age of the patient is often indicated by his hands, and by this is meant the physiological age rather than the actual age in years. The ends of the fingers and toes should be observed for the presence of clubbing, and the nails as regards colour, character, particularly whether cracked and brittle or deformed—the state of these is often an indication of the amount of interest the patient takes in his personal appearance.

During the procedure of getting the patient into bed, the nurse should also notice the condition of the special senses, whether these are perfect. She should discover the presence of any hyperaesthesia, and anaesthesia of any part of the body. She should observe his mode of speech, and by talking to him a little about his condition she may elicit very valuable information (see also mode of taking a history, p. 22) such as the condition of his appetite, his likes and dislikes in regard to food. She should find out when he last had his bowels open and any specially troublesome symptoms he may be suffering from, such as coughing, vomiting or insomnia.

By the time the patient is undressed and comfortably settled in bed the nurse will have discovered what type of drink he would like—provided of course that he is allowed one—but she should take his temperature, pulse and respiration before this is given.

EXAMINATION OF A PATIENT

A nurse should have some knowledge of the routine examination of a patient so that she may be able to anticipate the wishes of the doctor whom she is assisting.

The physical examination is carried out as follows:

By inspection. The light must be good, the room warm and the patient comfortable, and not unduly exposed. Inspection provides information regarding the general condition of the patient's body, state of nutrition, any deformities, rashes, injuries, irregularities or other marks, the colour and character of the skin, the state of the eyes, whether bloodshot or jaundiced, presence of pallor or cyanosis, and also any distressing symptoms such as dyspnoea, restlessness, twitchings or tic.

Palpation. By touching and handling different parts of the body, alterations and variations in development are found. For example, in diseases of the lungs, palpation would discover that there was less movement on one side of the chest than on the other. Palpation of a tumour would provide information regarding its character and size.

Percussion. By tapping an area of the body over different organs, the note obtained will suggest the presence of air, when this is *resonant*; and of some fluid or other cause of solidity when the note obtained is *dull*.

Auscultation. This means listening to the sounds of the heart and lungs either directly by placing the ear against the surface of the body (in this case the nurse should provide the doctor with a towel on which to place his ear), or he may listen by means of a stethoscope. It is very important that friction rub between clothing should not be permitted to take place during auscultation.

Preparation of the patient for any definite form of examination. The patient should be told of the nature of the examination unless he is too ill, or for some reason incapable of taking any interest in the matter: for example, a patient who is in an exceedingly toxic state will be quite oblivious to anything that may be happening. The following points should be taken into consideration:

The light should be good, whether it be artificial or natural. The patient should be placed in such a position that shadow does not fall on the part under examination.

Absolute quiet is essential—the patient should not talk and the nurses should move as quietly as possible. The bedclothes should be handled quietly and gently, as even the rustling of these may make it difficult for the doctor to detect the sound he is listening for, or the note he is trying to elicit in percussion.

The bed and personal clothing should be conveniently arranged so that different parts of the body can be exposed with comparative ease, without undue movement and unnecessary exposure of the patient's body, as the examination progresses. For examination of the chest the bedclothes might be folded down to the level of the patient's waist. The personal clothing could either be removed, or the jacket or gown merely held out of the way so that the clothing does not come in contact with the doctor's hands, or with his stethoscope, as the examination proceeds.

Only one part of the patient's body—that which is under examination—should be exposed at a time, covering the parts finished with from time to time. Whenever possible it is a good plan to have the patient's shoulders draped with a blanket, shawl or jacket which can be easily drawn round him, and as easily removed when required.

For examination of the chest the patient may be lying in the semi-recumbent position or sitting. If he is sitting, support should be supplied for the lower part of the back so that his lumbar region does not ache. As separate sides of the chest are examined the nurse should turn the patient's head from side to side so that he does not breathe directly into the doctor's face.

When the *back of the chest* is to be examined, the personal clothing should either be removed or drawn well up to the root of the neck, and well forward on each side, so that the area of the axillae is clearly visible. The patient may sit up leaning forward, or lie forward on one side in a semi-prone position. When the former posture is used, draw the pillows down to the small of the back as the patient sits, to give support here; and support the patient from the front by putting one arm across his chest, unless the doctor prefers that he should lean forward—in this case see that the patient's arms are resting on his knees in front of him, and not held stiffly at his sides.

Examination of the abdomen. It is important that the bladder be empty, otherwise the patient is inconvenienced by anxiety about this. The patient should lie on his back quite straight and flat with his arms down by the sides of his body. The doctor may require his knees to be either straight or slightly flexed; in the latter case a soft knee pillow may be provided. The shoulders and chest should be protected by a small jacket, or by a blanket folded round, shawl fashion. The bedclothes should be folded down to below the pubes as the patient lies ready. The lower part of the trunk may be covered by a blanket, or in warm weather merely by a sheet; either can easily be moved about during the examination. It is a good plan to tuck one of the blankets, which has been folded down, under the patient's buttocks; this prevents the clothes slipping, and gives a sense of confidence that exposure will be avoided, for which the patient will be exceedingly grateful.

When the *pubic region* is included in the examination it is usual to place a towel over the folded bedclothes, as the nurse will find it easier to manipulate this small article during the doctor's movements.

If a woman patient is undergoing abdominal examination, and students are present at the bedside, a towel might be provided with which to shield her face, in order to avoid embarrassment.

Examination of the legs and feet. For examination of this portion of the body, the bedclothes should be untucked at the sides and bottom of the bed, and turned up to above the knees, leaving one sheet or blanket over the legs. Only the leg to be examined ought to be exposed. If both are to be examined the sheet can be turned back on to the other bedclothes, or pleated up in folds to lie between the legs, so that it can be in readiness to cover one leg when one is finished with.

EXAMINATION OF THE DIFFERENT CAVITIES OF THE BODY

Examination of the mouth and throat (see fig. 1, p. 33). The nurse should supply a good light, a warm tongue spatula, a receiver in which to place it when soiled, a towel to put under the patient's chin, and a mouth-wash to be used afterwards. Swabs and culture glasses should be at hand in case these are needed.

If a nurse is examining the throat, in order to be able to report upon its condition, she should ask the patient to open his mouth, and observe the condition of his *tongue*, whether it is clean or furred; the presence of any cracks or fissures, and whether the patient moves it easily or not. The *teeth and gums* should be observed regarding their colour, whether they are healthy or pale and spongy, and the presence of any sordes on the teeth. The *condition of the lips* should be inspected to see whether these are cracked or fissured; whether there are any little ulcers or sores on the inside of the lips; the presence of herpes, and the colour of the lips should also be noted.

In order to *inspect the throat*, the nurse should ask the patient to put his tongue out and say 'ah'. This will permit examination of the upper part of the pharynx. She should then take a spatula, place it gently on the tongue, as the tongue lies in the mouth, not protruded. She should place the spatula about halfway along the tongue and press gently, and again ask the patient to say 'ah', when the soft palate and uvula, the posterior pharyngeal wall and tonsil area can be seen. She will notice whether these tissues are pale, injected or congested, whether there is any exudate or any membrane, whether any deposit is present in the follicles of the tonsils, or whether the whole area is covered with an exudate.

As the mouth and throat are examined, the odour of the breath should be noted.

Examination of the rectum (see fig. 2, p. 33). For a rectal examination performed in bed, a lubricant, antiseptic lotion, gloves, swabs and towels are all that will be required. Should a specimen be taken, cotton wool applicators and sterile test tubes will be needed in addition. For a more extensive rectal examination a proctoscope and light will be needed (see also sigmoidoscopy, p. 172).

The patient should be prepared by having the bladder and rectum empty. The external parts should be quite clean and protected by towels. The patient may lie on his back, in a semi-recumbent position, or in the left lateral or the Sims's semi-prone position for simple examination. For more extensive examination in which a proctoscope is used the surgeon may prefer to have the patient kneeling on the bed, leaning forward resting on his head with his arms hanging by his side, which is a modification of the knee-chest position and one used solely for this form of examination.

Examination of the vagina. This examination is usually performed with the patient in bed, except in the theatre where the lithotomy position would be used. When in bed, the examination will be performed with the patient in the left lateral position, in the Sims's semi-prone, or the dorsal recumbent position. In some instances two of these positions are used. The patient lying in the left lateral position has the vagina examined and is then turned on to her back for *bimanual examination* in which the anterior abdominal wall is palpated with the examiner's free hand at the same time. In preparing patients for these various positions, the bedclothes should be folded to below the level of the knees, leaving only one sheet or blanket covering the patient. The bedgown must be well rolled up, and if the patient feels cold, or the weather is cold, long warm stockings should be worn.

In the preparation of the patient the bladder and rectum should be empty, and the external genitals and perineum recently washed.

The *articles required* (see fig. 174, p. 521) for this examination include gloves, antiseptic lotion, a lubricant, swabs and towels, and some form of vaginal speculum, either Fergusson's, Sims's or Cusco's. It is important that the nurse should see that these are sterile and are delivered warm, by having them ready in a basin of warm water. Swabs and sterile test tubes and culture glasses may be needed.

In a few instances and particularly when the examination is performed in the lithotomy position, tenaculum and uterine forceps, Playfair's probe and a uterine sound may be required in addition.

For examination of the ear, nose and throat see p. 734, and for examination of the eye, p. 750.

DISCHARGE AND TRANSFER OF PATIENTS

The discharge of a patient, either to his home or to some other hospital or to an institution, is a very important undertaking. Everything therefore should be done to make his departure easy and as free from anxiety as possible, and he should also be given an opportunity to express his opinion as to whether he has been comfortable during his time in hospital and whether there is anything he would like to say regarding this. To secure that the answer to such inquiry may be made as freely as possible, it is usual in some hospitals for a member of the secretarial staff or one of the almoners or, in their absence, the officer who is in charge of the hospital or one of his or her subordinates, to visit the patient for this special purpose.

A day or two before the date of discharge the relatives or friends are informed that they may come for the patient at a given time on a stated day and, if they have taken his clothes home, they are asked to bring them when they come.

The ward sister sees that the patient is ready to go home, that he is recently bathed, that his head is clean and that he has safely in his own custody, if he is capable of this, any articles of his own which he has been using and, at the last minute, any valuables which have been kept safely locked up for him. It is her duty to see that the patient clearly understands the nature of any treatment which is to be carried out at home—she will also supply the relatives with details about this—and that he knows whether he is to come up to the hospital to be seen again and, if so, that he is quite clear about the date and time of this visit.

When the friends arrive and the patient is ready dressed, the ward sister sees that they are given all the patient's belongings and in most cases either she, or her head nurse, accompanies the patient to the door of the hospital, conducting him downstairs in a lift, assisting him as necessary, providing a wheel chair if required and taking pains to see that he does not carry anything himself—as the patient, especially if a man, will object if a nurse carries his suitcase for example—but he is still a patient and this must be tactfully explained and he must submit. She will then hand him over to the head porter at the door, say good-bye to the patient, and arrange for the porter to obtain a conveyance for the patient if he wishes to have one.

Transfer to another hospital or institution. Should a patient have to be transferred to another hospital, it is usual to inform the relatives of this first; if the transfer has to be made quickly, it must proceed before they may have received the information, but the nurse, whilst making arrangements for it, must try to get into touch with the relatives. If, however, they have not arrived by the time the patient departs, she must see the driver of the ambulance or other person who comes to take the patient away, and obtain the address of the place to which the patient is going, in order to give or send this to the relatives at the earliest opportunity.

As a rule all the patient's belongings will be sent with him—if not, they are given to the relatives when they call and a receipt is obtained.

Transfer to another ward in the same hospital. The management of hospitals varies considerably in the arrangement of this matter. The majority probably require the patient to be discharged and readmitted, should he be transferred from a medical to a surgical ward for example. But should he be transferred from one medical or one surgical unit to another, this is not usually necessary. In the former case, the discharge slip will be made out and sent to the medical officer as before, and the sister will go to the admitting office and have the patient readmitted to the ward to which he is going.

She will then see the sister of this ward, find out when it would be most convenient for her to receive the patient and send him to her, giving at the same time any information she can about his condition and treatment, particularly with regard to the diet the patient is having.

Case sheet. Immediately on the discharge of a patient the ward sister examines the bed card, sees that it is complete, removes any unused sheets and sends it to the department where records are kept; unless the patient has been transferred, in which case she sees that the bed card accompanies the patient to his new ward.

Treatment of the bed and other appurtenances, after discharge of a patient. Immediately after the discharge of a patient the ward sister arranges that the nurse who has been in charge of the case, or in her absence another nurse, strips the bed, sends all linen to the laundry, brushes and, if a balcony is available, airs the mattress, pillows and bedding, washes all mackintoshes, and all the utensils used by the patient, turns the locker out, has it washed and scrubbed if necessary and when dry puts clean paper in, and has the bedside chair washed.

The *bedstead* is then carbolized, first placing a sheet on the floor to protect it from drippings; the bed is dried and polished and the bed made up clean.

Fresh charts and bed cards are replaced on the bedboard ready for the use of the next patient; insertion of the visiting cards also will ensure they are ready to be given to the relatives on admission of the patient who is next to occupy this bed.

The **discharge of a patient with a communicable disease,** or one who has been suffering from some infective condition, is rather more complicated. After any infection, however slight, the mattress, pillows, bedding and linen, both the bed linen and patient's personal linen, should all be steam disinfected, and all the utensils which have been used for the patient should be sterilized by boiling or by chemical means. The soap and washcloths should be burnt. The area of the floor around the bed, and between it and the adjacent beds, and wall space behind this area, should be well washed with soap and water. If the patient has been occupying a separate room or small isolation ward, the ward might be closed for formalin fumigation. (For terminal disinfection of patient see p. 465).

REHABILITATION

Rehabilitation is the co-ordination of all the departments of a hospital to one common end, which is their *raison d'être*—the care, cure, welfare and return to full health and normal occupation of the individual who presents himself, for the time being, as a patient.

A scheme of medical rehabilitation should include, in addition to the medical, surgical and nursing resources of the hospital, the work of the almoners, research departments and laboratories where disease can be studied and aids to diagnosis provided, physiotherapy, radiotherapy, occupational therapy, hospital library, education, recreational facilities, canteen, follow up and after care, with vocational training in special cases.

Nurses should be specially interested in rehabilitation, as they are in the first line of advance and can do more than others to bring to the patient just that help which he needs exactly when he needs it most. Hospital treatment is only a stage in recovery and rehabilitation begins when the patient is admitted. In taking the history of his illness the nurse gains some knowledge of his background, learns what his occupation is, realizes where the aim of all treatment lies for him, and henceforth she sees him where he wants to be—fully restored to health and back at his normal occupation. All her work is then directed towards this end.

Social medicine is the term used to describe a study of the patient's background and environment. It is important to find out whether the conditions under which the patient has been living have contributed to his illness. This study is made in order to effect improvement in a known set of circumstances so that they shall not continue to be a source of breakdown in health, and to create good social conditions.

The *hospital almoner* is specially trained to help with a patient's personal and domestic difficulties, study his environment and see how improvement can be carried into effect. Nurse and almoner should work hand in hand or as one sister aptly expressed it 'hand in glove'. The actual treatment a patient receives in hospital is infinitesimal in comparison with his welfare and happiness in the details of his entire life, and he cannot derive the benefit which should accrue from treatment unless he has the freedom from worry and anxiety which is the basis of relaxation of mind and body.

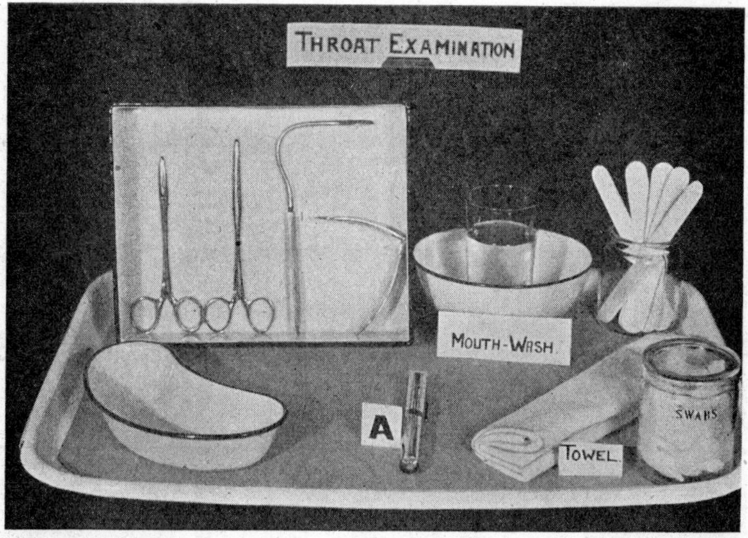

FIG. 1.—*see page* 28. (A) Electric torch. The instruments shown are two types of tongue depressor, and two pairs of forceps for swabbing the throat, if necessary.

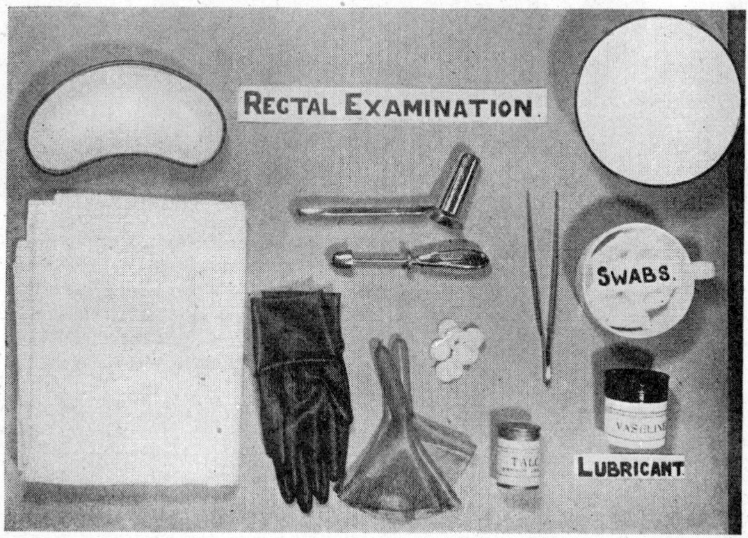

FIG. 2.—*see page* 28. A proctoscope is shown in the middle of the picture; a lubricant is supplied for this. The doctor may need gloves or a finger stall. The drawsheet at the left is for covering the buttocks when the bedclothes are folded back. An enamel bowl is supplied for used swabs and a receiver for soiled gloves or finger stall.

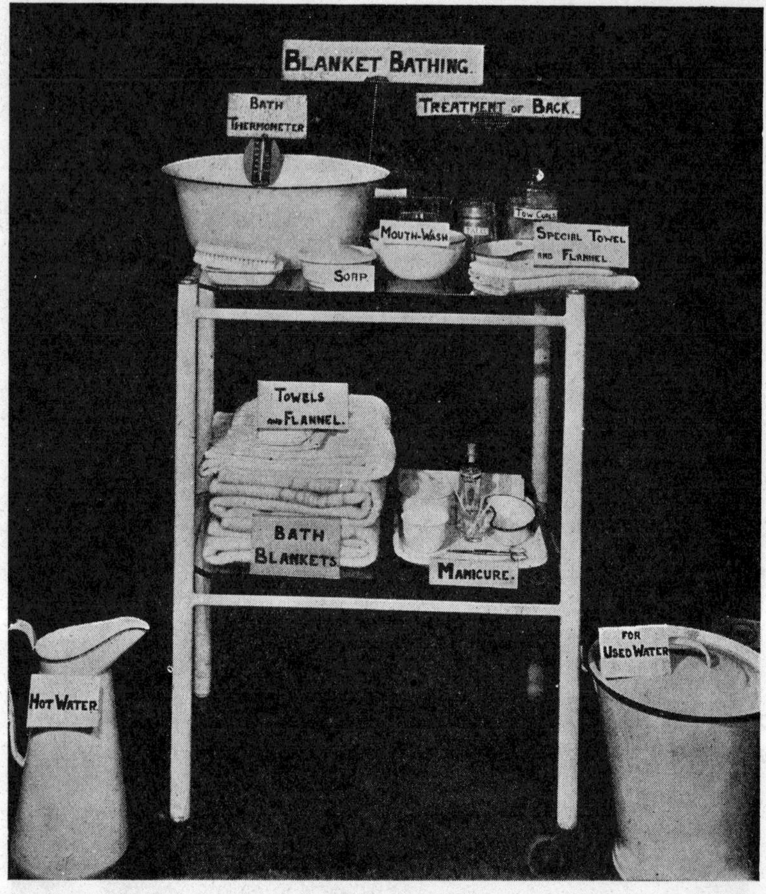

FIG. 3.—*see page* 55. The articles required include those for washing the patient: warmed bath blankets, bath, face and back towel, and two washing cloths. Tow for the initial swabbing of genitals. Soap, nail-brush, nail scissors and a receiver for nail parings and used swabs. Powder for body creases and back. All articles required for bathing, cleansing of the mouth, attention to the nails and treatment of pressure points should be prepared. Clean warm clothing for the patient should be ready to hand.

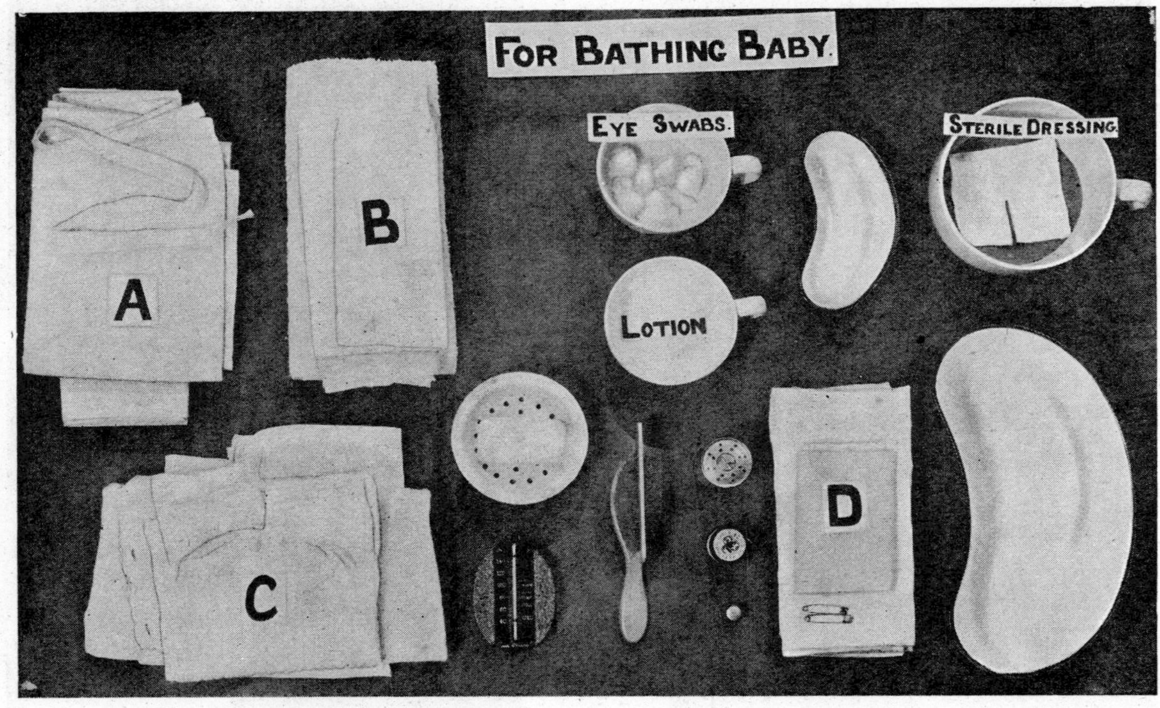

FIG. 4.—*see page* 57. (A) Mackintosh apron and flannel apron. (B) bath towels, and soft washed gauze for drying baby's body and face. (C) vest and gown. (D) napkin and safety pins, and binder with needle and cotton. Other articles shown include: eye swabs, a weak solution of boracic for the eyes and nose, sterile powder and dressing for the cord if it has not separated and bath thermometer, soap and brush and comb.

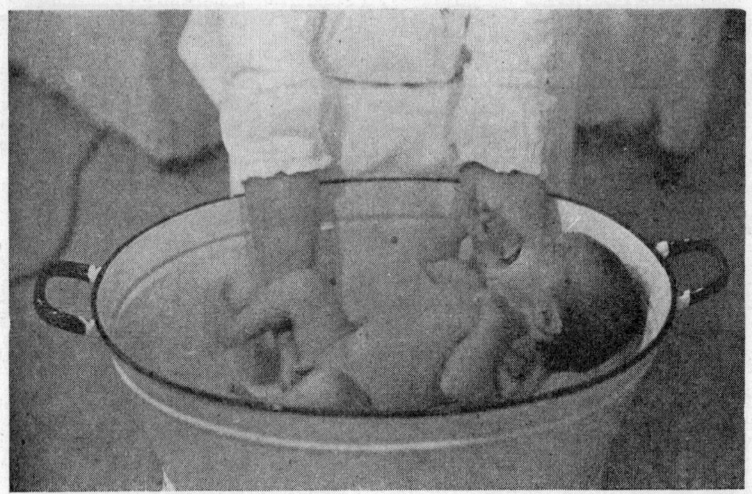

FIG. 5.—*see page* 57. The position of the Nurse's hands when lowering baby into his bath.

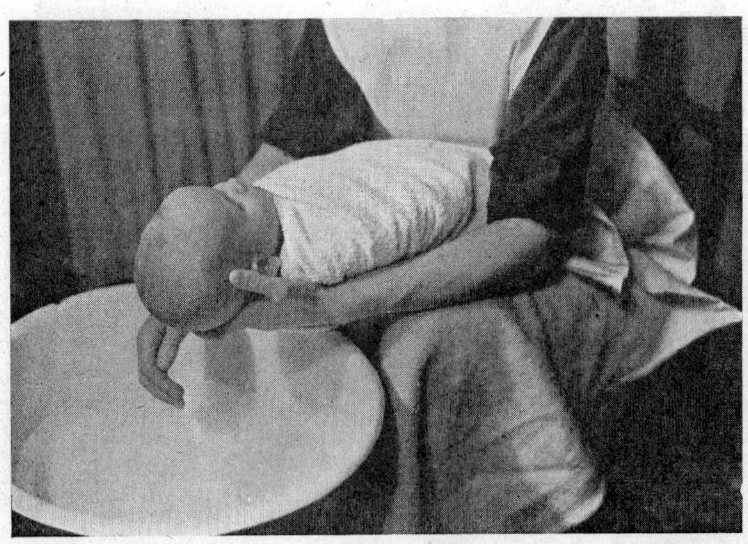

FIG. 6.—*see page* 57. Method of holding a baby when washing the head.

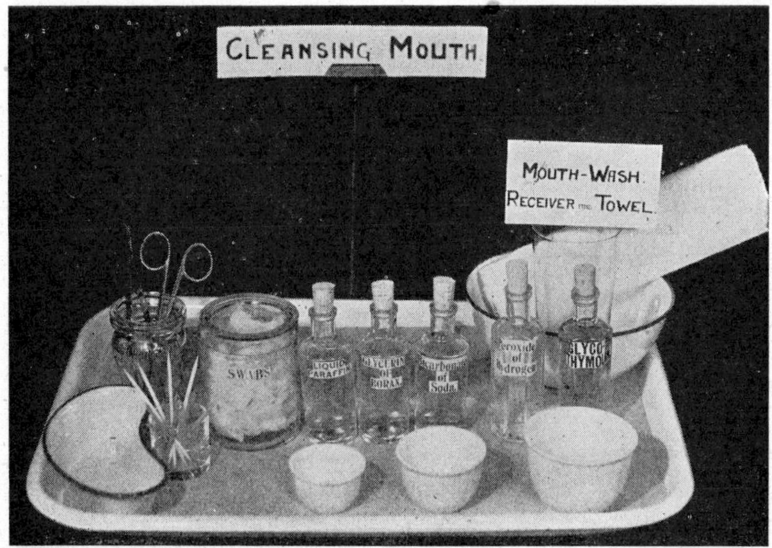

FIG. 7.—*see page* 58. Two pairs of forceps are supplied, artery forceps or dressing forceps to hold the swabs when cleansing the mouth, and dissecting forceps to remove the used swab so that it is not handled by the fingers. Orange sticks are used to remove particles from between the teeth. A choice of lubricant and antiseptic is provided in this example.

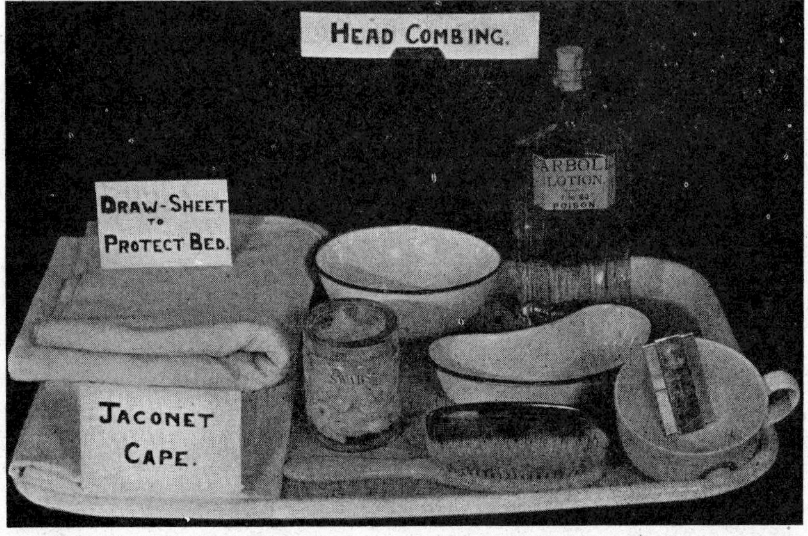

FIG. 8.—*see page* 60. The small toothcomb is used wet when combing a head for the removal of lice. In this example carbolic lotion 1/80 is employed. Dry wool swabs are provided for cleaning the comb, removing hair and lice, if any.

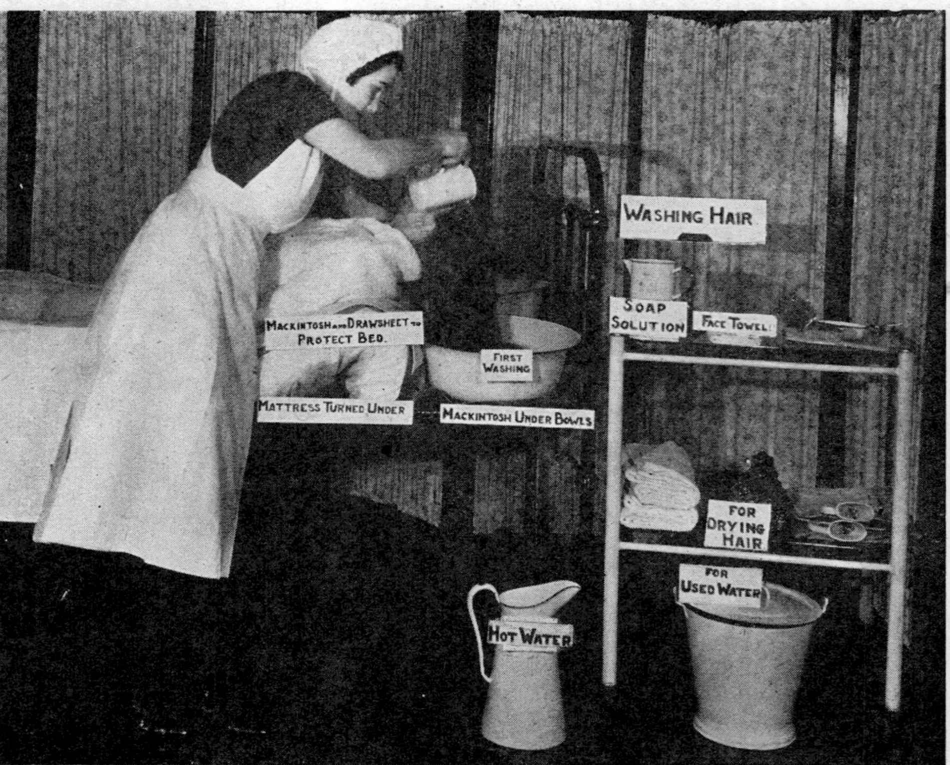

Fig. 9.—*see page* 61.

Washing a Patient's Hair in Bed. The articles required include mackintosh cape, mackintosh sheets, towels to dry hair and electric hair dryer if available, small face towel, prepared soap solution, plenty of water for washing and rinsing, bowls, jugs and pails. The patient's brush and comb will be required to complete the hair dressing when the hair is dry.

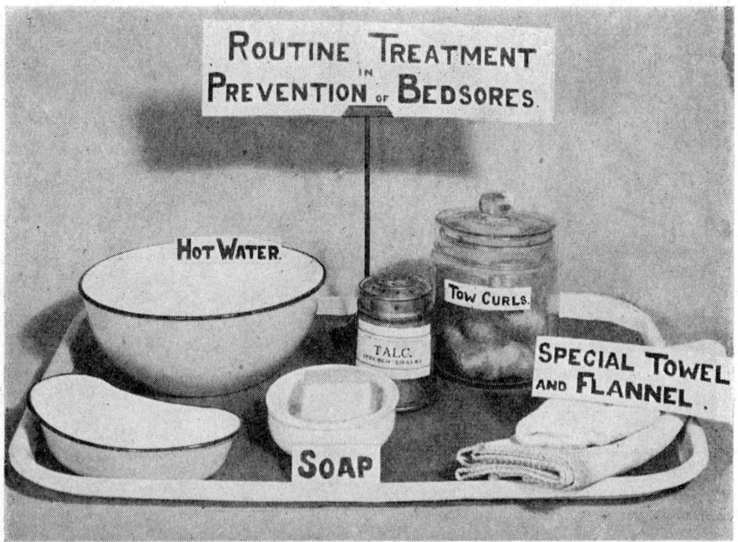

FIG. 10.—*see page* 63. For routine treatment of pressure points either soft tow or a washing cloth kept solely for this purpose should be supplied for washing the skin.

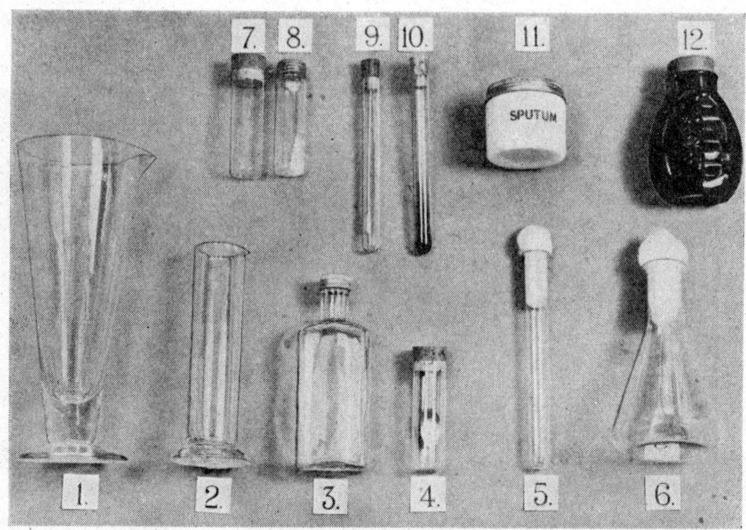

FIG. 11.—*see page* 77. RECEPTACLES FOR COLLECTION OF SPECIMENS. 1 and 2—urine specimen glasses; 3—flask for catheter specimen of urine; 4—for faeces; 5 and 6—sterile test tube and flask for blood, fluid, stomach contents, etc.; 7 and 8—sterile bottles for specimens of blood (one containing potassium oxalate); 9—sterile swab; 10—glass containing culture media; 11—for specimen of sputum; 12—pocket sputum flask.

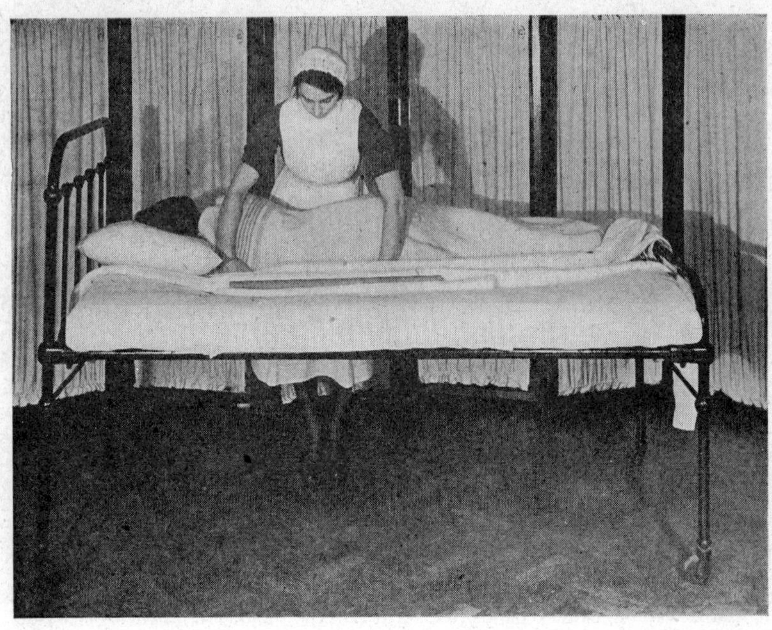

FIG. 12.—*see page* 86. CHANGING THE BOTTOM SHEET WHEN THE PATIENT MAY BE TURNED ON TO ONE OR BOTH SIDES. The short mackintosh and drawsheet are being changed at the same time.

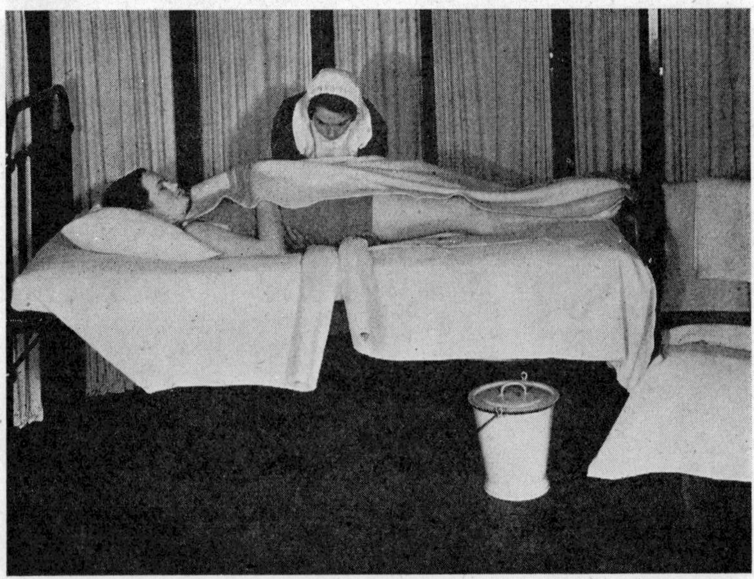

FIG. 13.—*see page* 86. CHANGING THE BOTTOM SHEET WHEN THE PATIENT CAN BE LIFTED BUT MAY NOT BE TURNED ON HIS SIDE. The short mackintosh and drawsheet have been removed.

Chapter 2

Temperature, Pulse and Respiration

Temperature: The variations of temperature in health and disease—Methods of taking the body temperature—Notes on the febrile state—The stages of a rigor. Pulse: The variations of the pulse in health and disease—Abnormal pulses—Blood pressure Respiration: Variations of respiration in health and disease—Abnormal respirations—Dyspnoea and cyanosis

The **normal body temperature** is 98.4° F., having a diurnal range from 97.4° F. to 99° F. The temperature is taken by means of a clinical thermometer, which registers from 95° to 110° on the Fahrenheit scale. It is a self-registering thermometer having a slight constriction in the glass tube immediately above the bulb of mercury which prevents the mercury, which has risen up the glass tube in response to the heat to which it has been subjected, from falling again until it is shaken down.

In health very little variation of temperature occurs. The degree recorded depends on the part of the body in which the temperature is taken. A *rectal* temperature gives the highest reading, probably two degrees higher than the *skin* temperature and one degree higher than a temperature taken in the *mouth.* In conditions of starvation and after exposure to cold and during sleep the temperature is a little lower. It may be slightly increased by muscular activity, by mental excitement or any other form of nervous tension and also by taking a hot bath or sitting closely over a fire or by exposure to an abnormally high, humid atmosphere; but these variations are slight and usually only temporary. The body temperature is higher in the evening than in the morning.

Variation in disease. The temperature is decreased in all conditions which produce dehydration, as in vomiting and diarrhoea, severe haemorrhage, marked toxaemia and in conditions of shock and collapse. It is also depressed in certain conditions of auto-intoxication as in jaundice. The temperature is *increased* in all febrile conditions, of which there are many causes in medicine and surgery, including infective conditions, metabolic disorders, and derangements of the heat-regulating centre such as occur in certain nervous conditions.

It is very important for a nurse to realize that a condition of fever, pyrexia or temperature—all these terms being used synonymously to indicate a rise in temperature—is *protective in function* because the increased temperature is antagonistic to the growth of the organisms causing the disease. It is also thought by some that the increased heat assists in the formation of immunizing bodies.

Degrees of temperature (Fahrenheit scale).
Hyperpyrexia, over 105°.
Pyrexia: High—103° to 105°.
Moderate—101° to 103°.
Low—99° to 101°.

Normal, 98.4° (ranging from 97.4° to 99°).
Subnormal, 95° to 97°.
Collapse, below 95°.

Types of Fever (temperature or pyrexia).

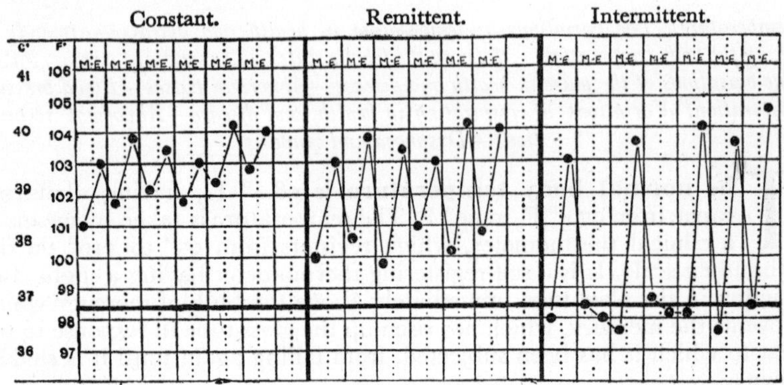

FIG. 14.—TYPES OF PYREXIA.

Constant, when the fever, remaining high, varies not more than two degrees between night and morning.

Remittent, a fever characterized by variations of more than two degrees between night and morning, but which does not reach normal during the 24 hours.

Intermittent. This is also described as *hectic*, or *swinging*, because the range of temperature varies from normal or subnormal to high fever at intervals varying from 24 hours to two or three days, but whatever the duration they occur with a fair amount of regularity.

Irregular. A fever not corresponding to any of the above three groups, but manifesting characteristics of some or all of them at one time or another.

Inverse. In this type the highest range of temperature is recorded in the morning hours, and the lowest in the evening, which is contrary to that found in the normal.

Apyretic. Sometimes a fever, typhoid fever for example, will run its course without any increase in temperature. This is described as an apyretic type.

TAKING THE TEMPERATURE

The articles required are: *a clinical thermometer* standing in a jar with cotton wool at the bottom in order to protect the end of the bulb, the jar being three parts filled with some disinfectant solution, such as 1-20 carbolic, 1-1,000 perchloride of mercury.

A jar containing some either moist or dry *wool swabs* with which to wipe the thermometer after use, a *receiver* in which to place the used swabs. It has been found that wiping the thermometer with wool adequately cleanses it because the surface is shiny and smooth so that germs do not readily adhere to it. If there is a sink handy, the thermometer is held under running cold water for a few seconds after taking it from the patient before wiping it.

The temperature may be taken most conveniently in the mouth, rectum, or on the skin of the axilla, groin or popliteal space. The thermometer should never come in contact with a diseased part.

The mouth. The temperature may be taken in the mouth, except in the case of infants, unconscious, delirious or insane patients, or where keeping the mouth closed would inconvenience the patient as in conditions characterized by cough, dyspnoea, or obstructed nasal breathing.

In taking the temperature in the mouth, the patient is asked to open his mouth, then the thermometer is placed under the tongue, and he is told to close the lips but not the teeth on it. The nurse should then consider whether it is necessary for her to hold the thermometer or not.

The rectum. A special thermometer should be kept for this, and it should have a short blunt bulb. In many hospitals quite distinctive thermometers are used, filled with alcohol instead of mercury, and having a coloured bulb.

Before insertion the thermometer should be lubricated with vaseline for about two inches of its length, care being taken not to lubricate it too heavily lest the lubricant by forming a coating should make an accurate reading difficult. In the case of infants the patient should either be held face downwards on the lap for the insertion of the thermometer; or, if lying in the cot, the legs may be held up with the left hand and the thermometer passed into the rectum with the right. In older children and adults the thermometer can be inserted while the patient is in almost any position. In all cases it is very important that the patient should be held steady while the thermometer is in the rectum, and it should be inserted for quite two inches.

Skin reading. Whether the temperature is taken in the axilla, groin or popliteal space, it is important to see that the skin surfaces are dry, and that the thermometer bulb is closely in contact with two skin surfaces in order to exclude air, since upon this the accurate recording of the temperature largely depends.

After taking the temperature, read the thermometer carefully, make a note of it, then shake the mercury down below 96° F., wipe or wash the thermometer and replace it in the disinfectant.

To shake a thermometer down take hold of it between the thumb and two fingers of one hand, grasping the lower third of the thermometer just above the bulb, hold it away from the body, supinate and extend the forearm and extend wrist, and then sharply pronate and flex the wrist.

The *time required to obtain an accurate reading* varies according to the area where the temperature is taken, and with the type of thermometer used—some thermometers are supposed to record a temperature in half a minute, one minute, two minutes and so on, but to obtain an absolutely accurate reading five minutes should be allowed.

The mercury will rise most rapidly in the rectum because in the interior of the body the surfaces are very close together, and air is excluded. The next quickest record will be obtained in the mouth, and it will take longest when the skin surface is used. It has been found by experience that a thermometer marked to record a temperature in half a minute will usually do so if the patient is suffering from a fairly high degree of fever; but, in cases where there is a low degree of pyrexia, an accurate reading will usually not be obtained under five minutes (see above).

If the nurse is at all in doubt as to the reading she has obtained and thinks it does not conform to what she knows the patient's condition might lead her to expect, she should take the temperature a second time. If she doubts the accuracy of the thermometer, she should use a second one and test the first by placing it in a little water not over 100° F. In a few instances she may have to be on the look-out for the recording of a false temperature either accidentally, or intentionally assisted by the patient. It may be that the patient has recently had a hot drink, or has been smoking, which might alter the temperature of the mouth locally for say half an hour. If a hot-water bottle had been near the axilla or other skin surface used, the same thing might happen there. A skin temperature should not be taken within half an hour of having a bath.

Specially made thermometers are necessary in certain cases. One graduated to register a temperature as low as 85° F. may be needed for accurately recording the temperature of premature babies. On rare occasions a patient acutely ill may run a temperature above 110° F., in which case a special thermometer will have to be used.

NOTES ON THE FEBRILE STATE

The course of a specific disease, characterized by a rise in temperature, is divided into different stages:

(1) Following the incubation period is the stage of *onset* or *invasion* during which the first symptoms appear.

(2) The full development of the disease is described as the *fastigium*, *stage of advance*, or *height of the fever*.

(3) This is followed by *decline* of the symptoms, including the temperature, as the disease passes into the last stage—that of convalescence when the normal is gradually re-established.

Mode of onset and decline of fever. A disease characterized by a rise in temperature may have a *rapid* or a *gradual onset*. In the former a very high temperature is reached in a few hours, frequently being ushered in by an attack of shivering which may be severe enough to be a rigor; in children convulsions more often occur. In the case of a *gradual onset* the temperature rises a little each day until, at the end of several days or a week, it has reached its maximum degree.

Similarly the fever may *decline suddenly* when the temperature falls in a few hours, within 24 at most; this is termination by *crisis*, provided that there is a corresponding, though perhaps not such a complete, drop in the pulse and respiration rate.

It sometimes happens that during the course of a serious febrile disease such as pneumonia the temperature falls but there is no accompanying decrease in pulse and respiration rate and the temperature rises again; this is described as *false crisis*.

Lysis. This is the term used to describe a more *gradual decline* of fever when it takes from 2 to 10 days or longer to return to normal. A *short lysis* such as is seen in scarlet fever occupies about 3 days; a *long lysis*, for example that usually seen in enteric fever, may occupy from 7 to 10 days (see accompanying charts)

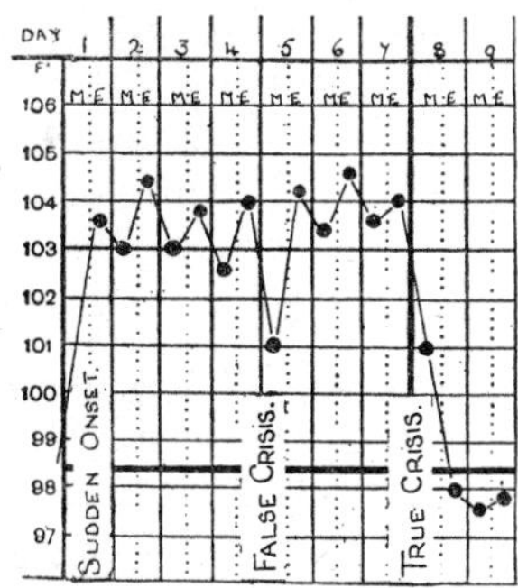

Fig. 15.—Lobar Pneumonia.
Example of abrupt onset and decline by crisis (in an untreated case).

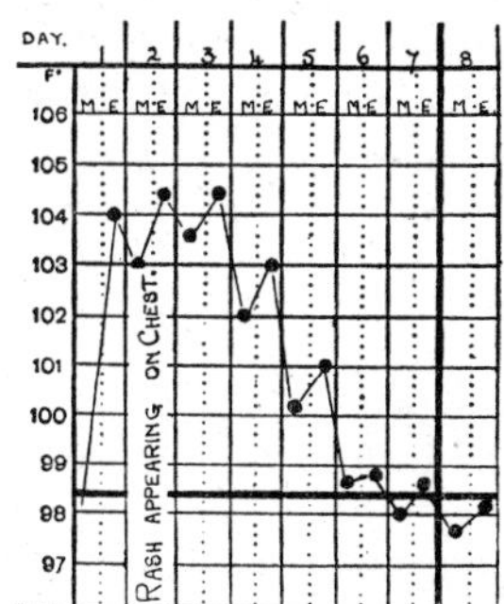

Fig. 16.—Scarlet Fever.
Example of decline of fever by lysis.

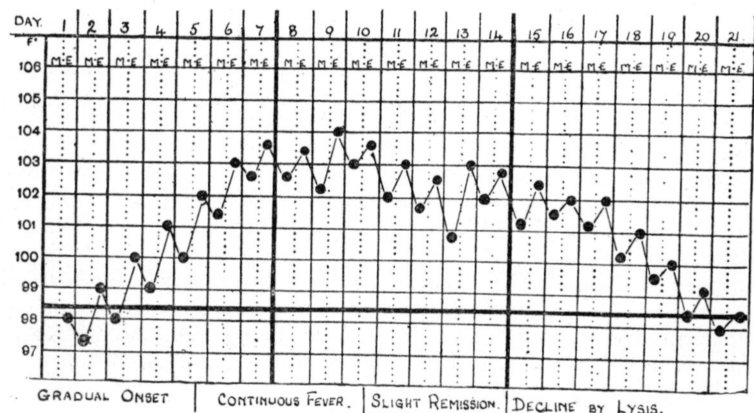

Fig. 17.—Typhoid Fever.
Example of gradual onset of fever.

Symptoms which accompany the febrile state vary with the nature of the disease from which the patient is suffering. They can most conveniently be considered according to the changes produced in the various systems:

Respiratory system.	Increased rate of breathing.
Circulatory ,,	Increased pulse rate, cold extremities.
Alimentary ,,	Dry mouth, dirty tongue, loss of appetite, indigestion, nausea and vomiting, constipation or diarrhoea.
Excretory ,,	Diminished urinary output, high-coloured urine depositing urates on cooling, possibly albuminuria.

Muscular ,, Malaise and fatigue and general aches and pains with weariness.

Nervous ,, Headache, restlessness, maybe irritability and insomnia. The skin may be hot and dry or hot and perspiring. Shivering or rigors, fits, twitchings, convulsions or delirium may occur.

Nursing a febrile case. Probably the most important point to be considered in nursing a patient who has a high temperature is to endeavour to relieve this as much as possible, or at least to provide conditions which will not aggravate it.

It is a mistake often made to pile extra bedclothes on to the bed of a patient so afflicted; instead, bedclothes should be removed, leaving the patient covered with a light blanket and in some cases only a sheet. Personal clothing should be as light as possible, non-irritating, and should not fit too well. Bedsocks and hot-water bottles might be removed.

The *room should be well ventilated*, as warm as is considered necessary according to the condition of the patient, but the windows may be freely opened provided the patient is protected from draughts.

Cooling drinks, given frequently, will help; in addition the fluid will moisten the tissues, and so make the mouth cleaner and the tongue moist instead of dry, relieve the thirst and help rid the body of waste products by providing more fluid to be eliminated by means of the different excretory channels and also render the work of these organs more efficient.

Sponging the hands helps the patient to feel cooler. Apart from the routine washing an occasional sponging of the skin of the whole body will cool and comfort a patient and may induce sleep which, by providing as it does the best form of rest, will aid recovery by increasing the patient's resistance to disease.

In most febrile cases the *diet* should be light but plenty of fluids should be given. The *bowels* should be kept daily acting if possible without the aid of aperient drugs; orange and prune juice being used instead and, if necessary, liquid paraffin. If aperients are ordered it is important to see that they do not purge the patient.

Reduction of a temperature. As stated elsewhere a rise in temperature is one of the protective mechanisms of the body, and drugs are therefore not, as a general rule, used in order to reduce it. It is generally considered inadvisable to permit a patient to sustain a temperature of over 105° F., or in some instances over 103° F., for long at a time, as this leads to great prostration often accompanied by delirium, which lowers the resistance of the patient and retards his recovery. It is therefore customary to order these cases to be sponged with tepid or cold water or to have some other general cold or cool application made to the body (see p. 121) in order to relieve, for a time, the degree of fever present.

A special note is made of the time this treatment was used and of the effect obtained and, in order to note its general effect, the result is charted as shown on the accompanying illustration on p. 124.

RIGOR

A rigor is a severe attack of shivering which may occur at the onset of disease characterized by a rise in temperature, such as pneumonia. It may also arise during the course of infective diseases and conditions. A rigor is marked by three stages which are fairly distinct one from another:

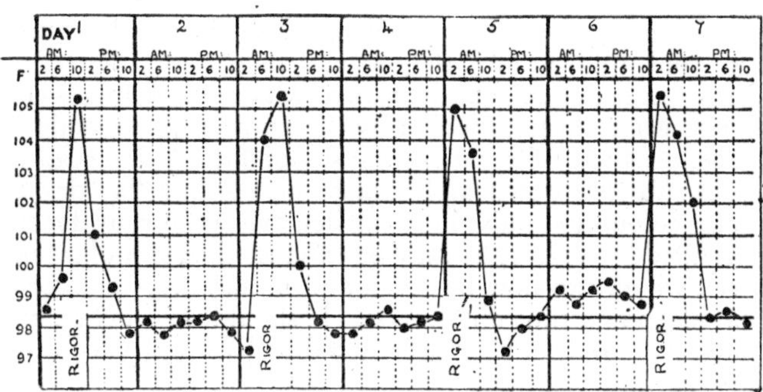

FIG. 18.—EXAMPLE OF RIGORS OCCURRING IN BENIGN TERTIAN MALARIA.

The *first* or *cold stage* in which the patient shivers uncontrollably. The skin is cold, the face pinched and blue and the pulse rapid and small. The temperature is rising rapidly and may reach 104° F. whilst the patient still feels cold.

The *second* or *hot stage* follows immediately. The patient is now uncomfortably hot, his skin hot and dry, and he suffers thirst and headache and tosses about in bed in an agony of restlessness. The pulse becomes full. The temperature may continue to rise.

The *third* or *stage of sweating* sets in. The skin acts, the patient sweats profusely, the temperature falls, the pulse improves and the former acute discomfort abates, though the patient is now conscious of his dripping skin and if not well cared for will get very cold and may collapse.

Nursing. A patient should not be left alone during a rigor. The different stages require appropriate treatment. *During the shivering attack*

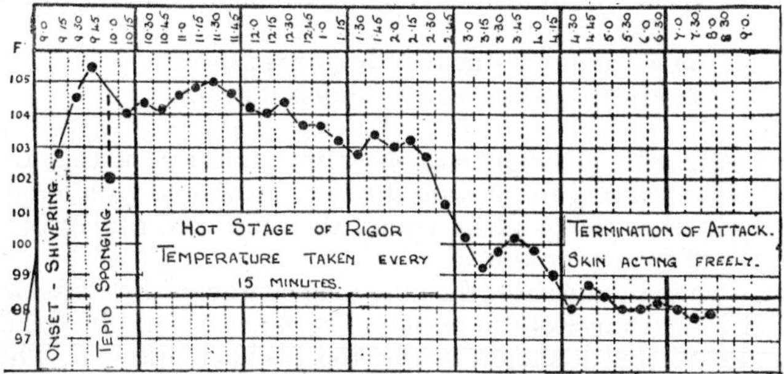

FIG. 19.—METHOD OF RECORDING TEMPERATURE DURING RIGOR.

the patient must be given hot drinks, have hot blankets put around him and his bed maintained at as high a temperature as possible; but as soon as he begins to feel hot this treatment must cease. His temperature is carefully recorded every 10 or 15 minutes throughout the rigor, and should it rise to 105° F. or over it is usual to cool-sponge him. At this stage he is given cool drinks, cool compresses are applied to his forehead or an ice-bag to his head to relieve his sensation of head congestion and the pain he is suffering.

The *first signs of sweating* are carefully watched for, as this must not be retarded by cold applications; they should then cease, the temperature being recorded as before so that the rate at which it is falling is constantly observed. The sweat must be wiped by the nurse at his bedside from the patient's face, neck and chest to prevent discomfort. At intervals as necessary she will rub him down and change his clothing for dry clothing, and watch his colour and pulse most particularly as now, at the end of the suffering entailed by a rigor, he may be exhausted. A stimulant may have been ordered which can now be given and if made very comfortable the patient may sleep and thus obtain rest. He should be watched constantly and his pulse rate and its character noted at least every 15 minutes for some hours.

THE PULSE

The pulse is the heartbeat—conveniently felt at the wrist. Each pulse represents a cardiac cycle. A cardiac cycle includes a period of *systole* or contraction, *diastole* or rest. The pulse may be felt at any point where an artery passes superficially and lies over a bone. It is most conveniently felt at the *radial artery* just below the root of the thumb.

The normal pulse rate varies with age and sex, and with the position of the patient, being more rapid when standing than when sitting and slowest when lying fully relaxed. It is *increased* in conditions of excitement, including anger, fear and anxiety. It is *decreased* during sleep, and to a less extent during rest and relaxation.

Pulse rate. In a newborn infant—140 beats per minute.
At 12 months—120.
From 2 to 5—about 100.
From 5 to 10—about 90.
Adult—from 70 to 80, being five beats quicker in a woman than in a man.
In old age, pulse usually becomes slower.
In extreme old age, it may quicken again.

As a rule the *ratio of the pulse* to the respiration rate is that there are four pulse beats to every respiration. Its ratio compared with temperature suggests that, other things being equal, the pulse will rise 10 beats with every degree of fever over 100° F.

A normal pulse should show the following characteristics. Its *rate* should correspond with the age of the person. The *rhythm* should be regular, the *volume* moderate, and it should not be too easily compressed. The blood vessel should be soft and pliant under the examining finger but not wiry or tortuous.

In taking a pulse the patient's hand and arm should be supported, and the muscles on the anterior aspect relaxed; this may be obtained by flexing elbow and wrist as the limb lies on the bed. If there is no indication to the contrary the arm might be laid across the patient's chest or abdomen. If this is not possible, then it should be supported on a pillow as in the accompanying fig.

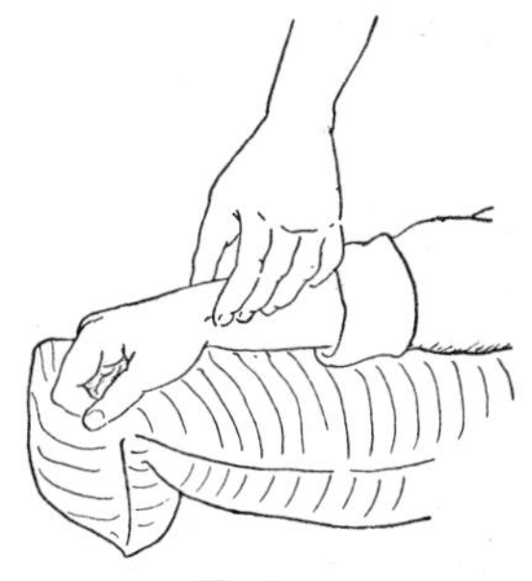

FIG. 20.

Support the hand and flex the wrist when taking the pulse.

The nurse gently places three fingers of one hand on the anterior surface of the forearm, just above the wrist, and feels the pulsation of the radial artery here. She notes the rate, rhythm, volume, tension and degree of compressibility and the condition of the artery. When she is familiar with the general character of the pulse she is feeling, she begins to count, and counts for a minute, taking particular care that she begins to count when the finger of the second-hand of her watch is on a definite figure, usually at the ¼, ½ or full minute mark. If in any doubt as to the accuracy of her findings she begins and counts the number of beats again until she is satisfied.

Should the wrists not be available the pulse may be taken at some other part—the temporal artery being a convenient place.

It is a wise plan, on the admission of every new patient, to take the pulse at both wrists simultaneously, as in some conditions—such as for example an aneurysm of the blood vessels of one side—the pulse would be found to be slightly delayed on the affected side and this might be the first means of detecting the condition.

ABNORMAL PULSES

The pulse may vary in its different characteristics:

Rate. A rapid pulse may be anything up to 140—above that it is difficult to count. A term used to describe any rate above 100 is *tachycardia*, and this state may be continuous or paroxysmal. It may be functional in character or due to organic disease. A slow pulse is described as *bradycardia*. It may be due to the fact that the cardiac contractions are not strong enough to reach the radial artery.

The *cardiac impulse* starts in the sino-auricular node near where the inferior vena cava communicates with the auricle. From here it is transmitted through the auricle to the *bundle of His*, which is a highly specialized neuro-muscular bundle which picks up the auricular impulses and as it were stabilizes them, acting as a *pacemaker* (which it is frequently called), and passing them on to the ventricle. The ventricle contracts in order to force blood into the arteries, and this contraction transmitted along these vessels becomes the *pulse wave*. A second wave, due to closure of the aortic valve, is described as a *dicrotic wave*. In conditions of *heartblock*, which condition may be partial or complete, impulses do not reach the ventricle. If partial, a ventricular beat, and consequently a pulse beat, may be missed at regular or irregular intervals. In complete heartblock, when no impulses pass, the ventricle contracts independently of any control from the auricle, and this results in a very slow pulse, usually below 40, and is always a serious condition.

Variations in rhythm. By rhythm is meant that beats occur at regular intervals and the distance between them is equally regular, and any interference with this results in a state of *arrhythmia.*

A pulse is described as *intermittent,* when beats are missed—for example, every third or fifth beat may be missed, or the pulse may be irregularly intermittent. In taking such a pulse the nurse should count the cardiac impulses by placing her fingers over the apex beat of the heart which she will find a little to the left of the nipple line and just below it, or she might use a stethoscope for this purpose, in order to satisfy herself and enable her to make an accurate report of cardiac beat and pulse beat.

A pulse is *irregular* when the pauses between the beats are of varying lengths. Beats are not missed, they simply run together at one time and are widely separated at another. This condition is seen in cases of *extra systole,* when some of the cardiac contractions occur prematurely, that is, before they are normally due in the cardiac cycle. This is caused by irritability of the muscle. The premature beat occurring before the heart is quite ready for it, is weak in character and unable to transmit the impulse to the arteries.

Auricular fibrillation is a condition in which the auricles, being very irritable, are quivering rather than contracting. The bundle of His deals with this as best it can, but the result is a rapid and irregular pulse.

In *sinus arrhythmia* the pulse is rapid during inspiration and slower during expiration. This is comparatively unimportant and occurs most commonly in children and, if the child is asked to hold his breath, the irregularity will disappear.

Strength. A pulse contraction should be strong enough not to be too easily compressed. This is intimately bound up with the condition of *volume,* that is, the amount of blood in the artery. The pulse is described as full, or large, or small, according to its volume. The *tension* also determines to some extent the degree of compressibility. A high tension pulse is difficult, and a low tension is easy, to compress. Other abnormalities involving these characters include a *thready pulse,* which is one which is rapid and weak and easily compressible; a *running pulse* when in addition the tension is markedly low; and a *wiry pulse* which is the type met with when the arteries are hard, and yet at the same time the pulse is weak and rapid and thready.

Pulsus alternans, which occurs when the contraction of the ventricle varies and results in alternately weak and strong pulse beats, is usually serious.

Another point that the nurse must be very careful to observe when taking the pulse, is the condition of the artery as it lies under her examining finger. Normally it would be soft and pliant. She should note whether it is flabby and lacking in tone, or wiry, hard and tortuous.

Dicrotic pulse. In conditions where prostration has been very marked, or grave toxaemia has been present for a long time, the muscles become toneless; when this happens to the muscles of the blood vessels, the flabbiness permits the dicrotic wave, spoken of on p. 49 to be felt. This is experienced by the nurse as if she were feeling a pulse beat followed by an echo of a beat. She is really feeling a true pulse wave and also the dicrotic wave, present normally, but not normally perceptible. She should therefore take the cardiac contraction rate at the apex beat and compare the two.

Corrigan's pulse. This is named after the doctor who first described it. It is also described as a *collapsing pulse*, and *waterhammer pulse*. It is present in cases of aortic incompetence, where the blood, having been forced into the artery by the ventricular contraction, regurgitates back into the ventricle owing to the non-closure of the aortic valve. In taking this pulse the wave is felt to rise and then immediately recede. It can be more definitely experienced by raising the patient's arm.

BLOOD PRESSURE

Nurses are sometimes required to keep records of a patient's blood pressure. This can only be done by means of a sphygmomanometer.

The normal blood pressure is estimated as being 100 plus the age in years. Systolic pressure is greater than pressure during diastole. In a man of 20 the systolic pressure is estimated as being 120, the diastolic pressure will be fairly constant at about 70.

The pulse of a person with high blood pressure, hyperpiesis or hypertension, is described as hard, full in volume and difficult to compress. That in a person with low blood pressure, or hypopiesis, is low in volume, soft in character and easily compressed by the examining finger.

Persistent hypertension leads to cardiac dilation and results in the pulse which is described as wiry, which means that it is hard but not of large volume—a similar condition in a person with normal blood pressure would give rise to a weak, thready pulse, but in the present instance it is wiry, not thready.

To take a reading the patient lies on a bed or couch with his arm stretched out. The sphygmomanometer is placed beside his arm and on the same level. The sphygmomanometer consists of a mercury manometer and a collapsible bag in a band for encircling the arm or limb used. A pump attached to the bag has a valve which when closed retains the air pumped into the bag, and when open releases it.

This pneumatic band is wound round the arm above the elbow; it is inflated by pumping, the operator palpating the radial artery at the wrist notes the level of the mercury at which the pulse disappears. He then releases slightly the pressure on the arm, places his stethoscope on the radial artery just below or at the bend of the elbow, and inflates the bag until the mercury registers 5 millimetres above the figure noted at the first reading. The flow of blood into the artery is obliterated and the air in the bag is then slowly released until the first sound is heard—this is the *systolic sound* and the level of the mercury at this point gives the systolic pressure. The operator continues to release the pressure, listening carefully, the sound increases in intensity, reaches a maximum and then a first soft sound is heard followed by a second soft sound—this is the *diastolic sound.* The level of the mercury gives the diastolic pressure.

RESPIRATION

Respiration consists of an inspiration, expiration and pause. By means of respiration oxygen is taken round the body, carbon dioxide is collected and excreted. Respiration is involuntarily performed. It is brought about by stimulation of the respiratory centre in the medulla oblongata due to the presence of carbon dioxide in the blood, representing the need of the body for oxygen. The centre thus stimulated causes impulses to be passed out by the phrenic and intercostal nerves to stimulate these muscles, and this results in a rhythmical rise and fall of the chest walls accompanied by descent and ascent of the diaphragm, alternately enlarging and decreasing the size of the chest as air passes in and out.

Normal respiration is rhythmical, quiet, regular and comfortable. The rate varies with age, and sex.

Rate. A newborn infant—40.
At 12 months—30.
From 2 to 5—24 to 28.
An adult—from 16 to 18, slightly quicker in a woman than in a man.

It may be *increased* in a normal person by taking exercise, and by any excitement or emotion. It is *decreased* during rest and sleep and when fatigued.

In abnormal conditions. It is *increased* in most febrile states, in all chest diseases, in many states of toxaemia, and after the administration of drugs which stimulate respiration such as atropine. It is *decreased* in injuries to the brain, in most conditions of coma, and after the administration of hypnotics, particularly opium.

The *ratio* of the respirations and pulse rate is normally 1–4. This alters very considerably in certain chest diseases, particularly in pneumonia, when the ratio may be as low as 1–2; for example, a patient's pulse may be 100 and the respiration rate 50.

In taking the respiration, the nurse should note the rate, character regarding its depth, regularity and rhythm, and any discomfort which may be apparent. She must be careful that the patient is not conscious of what she is doing, and she should try and divert his attention from himself. It is quite easy to count the respiration rate with the hand on the pulse, having a watch or pulsometer in such a position that the movements of the patient's chest might be seen at the same time. She should count for a full minute.

It is also important to notice where the movements occur during respiration. Abdomino-thoracic breathing is the normal. When the diaphragmatic action predominates, the epigastrium will be seen protruding during inspiration. In cases of diaphragmatic paralysis this movement is absent, and, instead of protrusion, recession occurs here. In acute abdominal conditions thoracic movement will predominate, as the abdomen is held rigid; and conversely, in painful conditions of the chest, abdominal movement predominates. The nurse may be of great assistance to the physician by observing and reporting on these points.

Abnormal respirations. The rate may be abnormally quick or slow. As a rule the depth is shallow when the respirations are rapid, and slow respirations are usually deep in character.

The *rhythm* may also vary. *Sighing* is manifested by long, slow inspiration followed by a rapid expiration. It occurs in shock, collapse, and in certain emotional states. *Yawning* indicates a condition of syncope. In pneumonia the pause at the end of expiration is short and terminates in a grunt. In *Cheyne-Stokes's* breathing the rhythm is very irregular. The respiration begins fairly normally and increases in depth and vigour until a maximum is reached, then gradually fades until a period of apnoea occurs, after which the cycle commences again.

Inverse. In this type of breathing which is most frequently met with in children, a pause occurs between inspiration and expiration, instead of, as in the normal, after expiration.

DYSPNOEA

In dyspnoea the breathing is difficult and noisy and in most instances it is painful or at least uncomfortable. The difficulty may affect inspiration or expiration, or both acts may be difficult. In *orthopnoea* the difficulty is usually relieved when the patient sits up. *Apnoea* is a feature of some types of dyspnoea and indicates that there is absence of breathing for a short period.

Causes. Dyspnoea may be due to a variety of causes, including *pressure or obstruction in the respiratory passages* such as a tumour, the membrane present in croup, the presence of blood, mucus or a foreign body, the occurrence of oedema in congestion, for example, of the larynx, and stricture which may follow an injury.

The obstruction may be due to pressure on the trachea or larynx as in hanging by strangling, the presence of a mediastinal tumour, an aneurysm of the aorta or an enlarged thyroid gland. Dyspnoea may also be due to *paralysis of the respiratory muscles*, to *diminished lung capacity* as in emphysema, bronchiectasis and advanced pulmonary tuberculosis; to *cardiac failure* for any cause, most often seen in diseases of the heart and acute lung diseases—pneumonia for example.

Varieties. Whatever the cause may be, certain varieties of dyspnoea are described. The *expiratory grunt* of discomfort met with in pneumonia has already been mentioned. When there is obstruction in the air passages and it is difficult to inspire, breathing is *stridulent*, the passage of air giving rise to shrill whistling and sometimes to crowing sounds.

Stertorous breathing is jerky and snoring in character, and occurs in coma. *Wheezing* and *rattling noises* occur when the air is forced through fluid as in the later stages of bronchitis. (Cheyne-Stokes's and the inverse type of respiration have been mentioned under disorders of rhythm.)

Nursing. Whenever possible, patients suffering with dyspnoea should be propped up in bed in the erect sitting position, taking care to see that they are entirely supported, and that support is provided for the arms and head. The head support should permit of the patient inclining his head to either side if he wishes to do so. Some means should also be provided to enable him to lean forward, such as a bed table on which he can place his arms in order to fix his shoulders when the extraordinary muscles of respiration are used. These include the trapezius and sternomastoid which help to fix the top of the chest and the scaleni and quadratus lumborum which fix the lower part of it.

The patient's wants should be anticipated and he must be spared every possible effort; when fed or given drinks, only small quantities should be allowed at a time; he should be given frequent rests during a meal as eating and swallowing are a great effort in these cases. This is one of the conditions in which it would be most inconvenient to take the patient's temperature in the mouth.

All irritation and excitement must as far as possible be prevented, and in attending to patients with dyspnoea the nurse should be particularly quiet and calm of manner, not hurried or hustled in the least, and she must move him very gently. In anticipating his wants she will not need to ask him any questions—talking is specially difficult for him.

Again, she will see that he does not have many visitors, and those who come should be warned that he finds it difficult and tiring to talk, and only those who can be trusted to sit quietly at his side or who will tell him little interesting items of news, not requiring answers, should be encouraged to visit such a patient.

CYANOSIS

Owing to the defective oxygenation of the blood due either to the existence of cardiac failure, as in heart disease and pneumonia, to interference with the mechanism of respiration either as the result of obstruction in or on the air passages, or to embarrassment of the movements of the chest, many patients with dyspnoea are cyanosed.

Cyanosis may be very marked, the patient being lividly blue; or it may be slight, when perhaps it will first be seen in the lips, at the tips of the ears or the ends of the fingers and toes.

As a rule the presence of cyanosis in diseased conditions indicates congestive heart failure and calls for the administration of oxygen for its immediate relief.

Chapter 3

The Toilet of the Patient

Bathing adult patients and infants—Care of the mouth—Care of the head—Prevention of bedsores—Giving bedpans and urinals

BATHING ADULT PATIENTS AND INFANTS

One of the first nursing duties with which a junior probationer may be confronted is the bathing of a patient either in bed or in the bathroom. She may or may not have been responsible for the care of the patient on admission; but she should be familiar with this procedure and also with the observations of a patient's condition described on pp. 24–5. In many hospitals it is the rule that all new patients must be bathed in bed, and this is insisted on, partly because those who are responsible for the making of hospital rules realize the value of the observation of a patient during the process of bathing—the whole of his body can be observed and handled, thus providing excellent opportunites for an intelligent nurse to make many observations which may be of great value in the diagnosis and subsequent treatment.

It is important to work firmly, steadily and evenly when washing and drying a patient; a light touch is apt to be irritating, a patient likes to feel that he has been washed and he likes to be well dried. If only nurses could be persuaded to do so, it would be an excellent plan if each would submit to be bed-bathed by her other nurse friends, in order to learn what it feels like to be washed by another—how to do it and, furthermore, how not to do it.

During his stay in hospital a patient should be bathed every day, either morning or evening.

Articles required for bathing a patient in bed (see fig. 3, p. 34).

2 bath blankets, warmed if possible.
1 bath towel, 1 face towel and 1 small towel for the back.
2 washing cloths, one for the face, neck, chest and arms, and the other for the abdomen, lower limbs and back.
Tow to be provided for the initial washing of the genitals.
Soap and nailbrush.
Nail scissors, brush and comb, and a receiver to receive the cut nails, and some swabs moist with methylated spirit to clean the edges of the nails.
Water in a basin, comfortably hot, and a jug of boiling water by which it can be heated from time to time unless arrangements can be made to change the water during the washing process.

In addition, articles should be supplied for the toilet of the mouth, and if the patient is helpless articles for mouth cleaning will be needed: if he can help himself, a mug, toothbrush, paste and bowl may be given to him and he may clean his teeth and rinse out his mouth for himself.

Articles for routine attention to the back.

Clean clothing, shirt, pyjamas, bedsocks, which should be warming on a radiator near by.

The nurse should inspect the bed to see whether clean sheets will be required and if necessary supply these.

A receptacle for soiled clothing.

The nurse should inquire if the patient wishes to use a bedpan before the treatment begins, close the windows and screen the bed, placing a chair at the foot of the bed, and removing the top bedclothes, as in making a bed (see p. 86). She then places one of the bath blankets immediately over the patient, rolling the second underneath him, and removes his personal clothing.

The washing is performed in the following order. The face, neck and ears are washed and dried. The chest and arms are next treated and the patient is allowed to swill the soap off his hands by dabbling them in a basin of water which the nurse holds conveniently near him. The lower part of the chest and abdomen and sides of the body are best done by working under the blanket without exposing the patient. The umbilicus must be cleaned and carefully dried.

The lower limbs are washed separately. Then the patient is turned and his back thoroughly washed and dried; the genital region is most easily washed from this aspect; tow well soaked and soaped is used to wipe the parts down first, and then placed in a receiver provided for that purpose as it must be burnt. If the patient is a male, he does this for himself, if possible, and is then handed a well-soaped washing cloth and finally a clean rinsed one. The towel provided for the back is used for drying the genitals. The routine treatment of the back, as described in the prevention of bedsores, is then carried out.

The nails may be attended to during the bath, cutting them, receiving the scraps of nail into a kidney dish, and if necessary cleaning the parts around the nails with small swabs moistened with methylated spirit. The soles of the feet may be very grimy, requiring the use of the nailbrush, in which case the nurse should scrub firmly and not irritate the patient by tickling. The mouth and hair are next attended to before the bed is remade. The patient's clean clothing is put on, the bed made, he is inspected to see that he has not lost heat, and if necessary a hot-water bottle is supplied, a drink is given in most cases, and then the articles used should be cleared away, the windows opened and the screens removed.

Bathing a patient in the bathroom. The room must be prepared first, windows closed, the bath half filled with water, running the cold water in first, then the hot. The water should be well stirred up and tested with a bath thermometer; it should not be hotter than 100° F.; the bath mat should be arranged, the patient's clean clothing and towels placed ready on the radiators, and the soap, washing cloths, nailbrush and towels put comfortably within reach. The key should be removed from the hot-water tap so that the patient cannot turn this on; a bell must be within reach of the patient and it should not be possible for the bathroom to be locked or bolted from the inside, though a screen can be placed round the bath for the comfort of the patient.

The nurse will bathe a female patient, paying attention to the points described in giving a blanket bath. For a male patient an attendant will be required unless the ward sister considers this unnecessary, in which case he bathes himself and, after he has returned to bed, the nurse takes pains to see that he is quite clean, for example, with regard to the umbilicus and his feet particularly.

Bathing a small infant. Quite a number of articles are required for this purpose, as an infant is a very helpless, delicate creature, and its skin and little orifices require special care.

The following articles will be needed in addition to clean baby clothing and napkin (see fig. 4, p. 35). Boracic swabs or sterile wool with boracic lotion for cleaning the eyes, nose and ears. Squares of soft handkerchief linen, and glycerine of borax for the mouth.

A baby bath of water, temperature of 99° F. A mild soap—no wash-cloths need be provided as the nurse uses her hands. Soft towels, one on the nurse's knee, and one with which to dry the baby. Some sisters use powder to ensure proper drying of the skin, though others consider the skin can be adequately dried without the use of powder which tends to cause harshness and cracking.

If the baby is a very tiny infant and is still wearing a binder a needle and thread are required, with which to stitch up the clean binder that will be put on. In this case also, a dressing for the cord will be required. A camelhair brush should be provided for doing the baby's hair.

When everything has been collected, and the bath has been placed before a fire if one is available—the fire being screened so that the rays of heat do not fall direct on the infant's body—the windows of the room should be closed, and the nurse seats herself on a low stool of convenient height, with a screen behind her to exclude draughts if necessary and, wearing a mackintosh and soft flannel apron, takes the baby on her lap and undresses him. Wrapping him in one of the towels, so that his arms are gently restrained, she washes her hands, and first gently swabs the eyes, nose and ears with the wool swabs, and then washes the infant's face with a piece of the soft handkerchief linen, moistened in the boracic lotion, drying it with a second dry piece. She then turns the baby so that its head lies over the bath of water (as in fig. 6, p. 36), and placing her left hand on the back of the shoulders, with thumb and finger separated, she supports the occiput and, holding the infant's head in this position, soaps the top and back of the head with her right hand, and rinses the soap off with the same hand, lifts the baby back on to her lap, and dries the head gently but thoroughly with a soft bath towel.

She then uncovers the baby's body as he lies on her lap, and using both hands soaps the body all over, back, front and sides, arms and legs, passing her hands well into all the crevices. She now places her left hand at the back of the shoulders supporting the occiput as before, and with her right hand under the buttock lifts the baby over the bath and lowers him into the water (as in fig. 5, p. 36). She places the infant in the bath and continues to support his head and shoulders with her left hand in order to keep his head out of the water. She swills water over his body to remove all soap, and lifts him back with the same movements that were used when placing him in the water, placing him on his face on her lap, on one of the bath towels. She folds the towel up over his back and dabs him dry, paying special attention to see that all creases and crevices are thoroughly dry. If the baby clothes are open in front she can place them in position on his back as he lies on her lap, before turning him over to complete the toilet of the skin of the front part of his body. He is then lifted bodily over, clothes and all, and put to lie on his back. In order to keep him quiet and good he may now be given a square of soft linen soaked in glycerine of borax or in sterile water. He sucks this and no further attention will be needed for the mouth of a normally healthy infant.

If the cord has not separated it should then be dressed, and the baby clothes fastened in front. He is then dressed, his napkin fastened, and his toilet is now completed. A tiny infant should be bathed once a day, preferably in the morning. An older infant, in his second year may be bathed twice a day. Premature babies should not be bathed at first, but should be anointed with olive oil.

THE CARE OF THE MOUTH

The care of the mouth is an important measure as most patients who are in the least dehydrated either as a result of a rise in temperature, septicaemia or toxaemia have dry, dirty mouths.

The articles required are best prepared on a small tray (see fig. 7, p. 37) which, if frequent treatments are required for one patient, may be kept covered and left ready for use at the bedside.

A bowl of *antiseptic swabs*.

Artery forceps with which to grip the swabs when using them so that they cannot be swallowed or come off the forceps in the mouth.

Dissecting forceps, for removing the used swabs from the artery forceps.

Lotions. Some substance to dissolve mucus, such as sodium bicarbonate solution, or a solution of borax, is invariably used first. A lubricant, such as glycerine or liquid paraffin with a little lemon juice added, moistens and removes crusts, the lemon juice increasing salivation. An antiseptic lotion such as glycothymoline, with which the mouth will be swabbed after cleansing or, in the case of a patient able to help himself a little, may be used as a mouth-wash.

A *receiver* for the soiled swabs, and one for the mouth-wash.

Orange sticks, with which crusts and particles may easily be removed from between the teeth.

A *soft toothbrush* may sometimes be used by the nurse and will always be used by the patient if he can help himself.

A *small towel*, a piece of jaconet or a square of linen may be provided to put under the patient's chin.

A lotion containing antiseptic in which to place the patient's dentures should also be provided.

Procedure. Having protected the bed if considered necessary, and explained to the patient what is to be done, the mouth should be inspected and the treatment begun in some definite order.

Dentures will be removed first, placed in the basin provided and taken to the sluice room where they may be cleaned in warm water, using a soft nailbrush, replacing them in a little warm water ready for use again.

It is very comforting if the mouth is rinsed or at least swabbed with a liquid preparation before the cleansing by rubbing is commenced. In preparing the swabs, see that they are firmly gripped by the forceps; moisten the lips and tongue with the first solution, clean the teeth with an up and down movement, paying special attention to the insides, using the orange stick to remove particles from between the teeth; the insides of the cheek should receive careful attention, as also the gums, tongue and roof of the mouth, taking care when touching the two last named parts not to make the patient 'gag'. If this should happen, allow him to rinse his mouth out if possible and thus obtain a little rest for fear lest he should be made sick.

Great care must be taken to remove all sordes and crusts very gently as sometimes there is a tendency for parts underneath to bleed. Each swab should only be used once. It should be dipped in the solution and then pressed against the side of the gallipot to prevent its being dripping wet, and the various lotions are used in the order previously indicated. After the treatment the patient should be given a drink, either water or weak lemonade. In the case of a patient on milk feedings, the mouth will be cleaned before the feeding and a small drink of water follow the feeding in order to prevent milky particles from remaining in the mouth, remembering that sordes consist of dry mucus and saliva and decomposing food, which form a favourable collecting ground for micro-organisms.

In cleaning the mouth the nurse should make very careful observation of the condition of the patient's tongue. When thickly furred, it is a good plan to smear it with a little white vaseline or liquid paraffin before cleansing, as this helps to soften it. The same precaution might be taken with regards to the lips if they are very hard and badly cracked.

All swabs and materials used for cleansing a mouth should either be destroyed by burning as in a private house, or treated as other soiled dressings would be in a hospital. The articles used, including forceps, must be washed and resterilized as the tray should always be ready for use.

It seems unnecessary to say that a nurse should be very gentle in handling a patient's mouth. Sometimes when it is very sore it may be better for her to use squares of linen wrapped round her finger instead of swabs on forceps, that is, provided there is no danger that the patient may bite the finger.

In some cases of insane and delirious patients a mouth gag may have to be inserted whilst the mouth is cleaned.

The *nose* should receive attention at the same time as the mouth, as it frequently becomes full of crusts and dried secretion. It is very important to keep the nose clear. It should always be kept free of discharge, and the edges of the mucous membrane could be smeared with a bland ointment whenever it appears at all sore.

Routine cleansing of the mouth in patients who are less seriously ill and able to help themselves forms part of their personal toilet and is usually carried out twice a day; the patient should be propped in a comfortable position, have a towel placed under his chin, and a receiver arranged to collect the fluid from his mouth; the nurse should put some paste or powder on his toothbrush, and hand it to him to use, renewing as necessary.

In cleaning a baby's mouth, it is very important to remember that in the normal baby it does not require cleaning, as the baby should be given enough water to drink to keep the mouth clean. In the case of very ill babies, it may be necessary to make some attempt at cleansing, but rubbing or friction cannot be used.

A rare *complication*, occasionally met in artificially fed babies, is *thrush*, in which small white flakes appear on the mucous surfaces of the mouth.

This will be found to respond to cleanliness, both of the mouth and the utensils used, and does not usually call for any handling by the nurse.

Complications which may occur if the mouth is neglected. The first is the collection of the sordes and crusts on the lips and teeth, cracking of the lips and furring of the tongue, and the occurrence of herpes at the corners of the mouth.

A condition of dirty mouth, which will invariably have an odious taste, unless it has destroyed the sense of taste altogether, leads to nausea and the refusal of food. This in turn lowers the resistance of the patient and interferes with his progress towards recovery. As the mouth communicates with so many other parts of the body infection may spread, for example, to the stomach, giving rise to gastritis; to the lungs, causing inhalation pneumonia; by the passing of infection to the middle ear otitis media may arise; by the posterior nares rhinitis may be set up and infection spreading from this part to the meninges may cause meningitis. Sepsis may travel by Stenson's duct and infect the parotid glands or by way of the local lymphatics and bloodstream giving rise to adenitis and tonsillitis.

CARE OF HEAD AND HAIR

On the admission of every patient a nurse inspects the head to see that it is clean and free from lice.

In routine care of the hair, it is brushed and combed twice a day. In doing this the nurse must avoid giving pain; the hair should be held firmly at the roots and the ends combed first; when all tangles have been removed the hair may be combed from root to end. If hair is badly tangled, moistening it with a little spirit helps and the tangled part should be gently teased with a comb until the individual hairs are loosened and it is free. Long hair should be arranged in two plaits, one each side, so that the patient does not lie on it.

A nurse should notice if the scalp is clean and free from dandruff. Any dandruff that remains after brushing the hair can be removed by rubbing with a little spirit diluted with water. It is of great importance in surgery of the head to keep the scalp quite free from any scurf or scales. If a head is badly covered with dandruff, the application of moist powdered borax well rubbed into the scalp before washing will usually be effective in removing it.

Fine-combing the head for the removal of lice. The following articles should be collected (see fig. 8, p. 37):

Mackintosh cape, to protect the patient's shoulders, and a drawsheet to place over the pillows at the top of the bed.
Dressing comb and fine toothcomb in a receiver containing some antiseptic.
Bowl containing *white wool swabs*, either moist or dry.
Receiver for the soiled swabs.

The head louse, which varies in colour, deposits nits on the hairs which become fixed to them by means of a sticky film; nits will be found near the roots of the hair, particularly in the warm spots at the nape of the neck and behind the ears, and it is therefore advisable, when fine-combing the head, to part the hair and begin at the nape of the neck.

When combing, the comb should be drawn through the hair close to the head; and, in order to prevent any lice or particles of scurf from dropping about, the underneath of the comb should be protected by a moist swab, held in the left hand, as it is drawn out at the ends. Do the parts behind the ears next, and finally when these are clear comb the whole head systematically, working from front to back, taking small strands separately, until every part has been covered.

In *treating* a verminous head it is necessary to destroy both nits and lice. 5% lethane in kerosene is rubbed into the scalp—the head is thoroughly treated, the hair being parted and the preparation rubbed into the scalp. The hair is washed after 10 days.

Alternatively some solution may be employed, either sassafras oil, paraffin, weak lysol, carbolic 1–40 or industrial spirit 7 parts in 3 parts of water. In every case the hair must be well saturated. The one important point is the complete saturation of every hair of the head. The hair is then wound round the head and covered by a compress of a single layer of lint. The fluffy side of the lint should be next to the head, as this helps to entangle the stupefied lice as they attempt to escape from the carbolized head. This is then covered with a piece of jaconet and bandaged on, either using a roller bandage (capeline), or a triangular bandage. The pillow nearest the head should have a jaconet casing whilst this is worn. It is usual to carry out this treatment overnight, and to wash the head first thing in the morning.

Experiments have been made with applications of D.D.T. either liquid or in an emulsion in the treatment of head lice.

NITS

It is always possible to tell how long a head has been verminous by the position of the nits, because these are deposited at the roots of the hair and, as the hair grows about an inch a month the time of infection can easily be calculated. Nits cling firmly to the hair and are difficult to remove—probably the best methods are to moisten the hair with olive oil or wash it with a soap and borax solution and then comb it with *Sacker's nit comb*.

WASHING A PATIENT'S HAIR IN BED

This is not such a formidable task as once upon a time it was, since so many women today have short hair. If the patient can move about at all, it is comparatively easy to wash the head as she leans forward over a basin, or backward with the basin arranged behind her; but when the hair is long, and the patient comparatively helpless, a method which is described below had better be used (see fig. 9, p. 38).

The articles required are: *mackintosh cape* to protect the patient's shoulders and *large mackintoshes* to protect the top of the bed.

Towels, to dry the hair, and a *small face towel* with which the patient can keep water from her face and out of her ears; unless she is helpless, and then it is better to put a little cotton wool into the ears in case of accident.

A large bowl in which to wash the hair.

A pail for dirty water.

A jug of *prepared soap solution* with which to lather the head, and jugs of warm water for washing and rinsing purposes.

Brush and comb with which to complete the toilet of the head.

Method. Unless the top of the bed has a movable back, which can be taken out, and the treatment performed from behind the head of the bed, it is necessary either to draw the mattress down over the foot of the bed, or to roll it under at the top, so that the basin can be placed on the wire mattress. A long mackintosh is used to protect the mattress at the top, and the bowl is placed on it. The pail is placed conveniently at the side of the bed. When all articles are ready, the mackintosh is arranged over the patient's shoulders, and she is drawn to the top of the bed, and her head held over the basin by a hand placed under the occiput. With the other hand the nurse wets the hair with warm water, and then pours small quantities of soap solution over it, rubbing well with her hand or hands to lather the hair and cleanse the scalp. The first lather is rinsed off and the treatment repeated. The second rinsing should be very effective and leave the hair quite free from soap lather. The nurse then presses the hair close to the head from roots to ends in order to squeeze as much water as possible out of it, wrings the ends and coils them up on top of the head, covers it turban fashion with the bath towel, removes the mackintosh from the top of the bed and the mackintosh from the patient's shoulders (replacing this by a bath towel), places the patient comfortably with her head on a mackintosh-covered pillow and clears away the articles she has used. She then proceeds to dry the hair by rubbing with the bath towel until quite dry. Many hospitals supply electric hair dryers for this purpose, but if one of these is not available, or if continued rubbing of the head would be injurious to the patient's condition, very long hair might be spread out behind the patient on a towel over several hot water bottles.

BEDSORES AND TROPHIC SORES

Bedsores may occur while lying long in bed. At first the skin is reddened, the part looks sore and is tender; and as the condition progresses the skin becomes abraded, superficial tissues are destroyed and ulceration results. The surface is now covered with an exudate which, if the condition progresses still further, becomes a serous discharge, and as ulceration deepens, sloughing of the central parts follows and, as a slough is a foreign body, the parts are now surrounded by a zone of inflammation, and take on the characters of any other typical ulcer.

Patients liable to bedsore are those who for any reason may have to lie in bed for a long time, particularly if emaciated, paralysed, incontinent, old, senile, or mental, and those suffering from any nutritional disorders such as certain nervous diseases, heart, lung and kidney disease, and any bedridden cases where nursing attentions are neglected.

Causes. The causes of bedsore may be divided into local causes, and predisposing general causes. The type of patient liable to bedsore suggests the latter group.

Local causes include pressure, which may be merely the weight of the patient's body as it lies on the bed, or else due to the fact that the bed is too hard or too lumpy, or the pressure of the bedclothes too heavy as they rest on the patient's body.

Dampness is a potent source of bedsore—some people go so far as to say that a bedsore cannot arise if the parts are always dry—and moisture may be the result of perspiration, or of the soiling of bedclothes by excreta or discharges.

Friction may be a cause of bedsore, as the skin frequently irritated first becomes reddened and is then rubbed off. This may occur as the patient moves about on the bed, or as he moves his legs up and down under the top bedclothes and thus causes friction over the knees.

Creases and crumbs, or other foreign bodies in the bed, increase pressure locally, they press into the tissues and so cause red marks first, and eventually give rise to soreness.

Parts liable to bedsore. Starting at the top and working downwards over the entire body: the *back of the head* may become sore, particularly in the case of infants and children who continually rub their heads, or who are given to head banging; the *shoulderblades*, which are prominent, particularly in emaciated persons; over the *vertebral spines*, throughout the entire extent of the column and over the *sacrum* and *coccyx* at the end of the column; and the *backs of the heels* as they lie heavily on the bed—all of these protuberant parts of a human body that lies long in bed may become liable to bedsores.

In patients who lie on the side, bedsores might occur over the *great trochanters*, on the *outer aspect of the knees*, *between the knees* and *ankles* as they may rub together when in this position. Soreness *over the knees* has already been mentioned as occurring in persons who restlessly move their legs up and down in bed. The *elbows* are very apt to become sore in people who lie on the back or who lean on their elbows for reading and eating.

Prevention of bedsores. Certain routine local treatment must be applied as often as necessary to all patients who lie in bed, in order to prevent any manifestation of redness on any parts that are subject to pressure. In the majority of hospital patients this treatment is carried out twice a day, and following any attention to the back such as after a surgical dressing in this area, or after sponging a patient.

The *requisites for routine attention to the back* (see fig. 10, p. 39):

A bowl of *water*.

Patient's *soap* and *special washcloth* for back, or a wad of tow may be used.

Dusting powder to dry the parts thoroughly.

Special towel kept for the back which will be laid on the bed during the treatment, and used for drying the genitals.

Method. Thoroughly wash the back, using soap and a pad of tow or the washcloth, and rubbing fairly vigorously; do not dry, but lather the palm of the hand well with soap and rub this into the skin of the back for a few minutes using circular kneading movements, so that the tissues under the skin are moved about without allowing the hand to slip over the skin; then rinse the soap off the skin, as if left on it may cause irritation and roughness, and dry well and then sprinkle powder on the palm of the hand and dab it well over the skin with gentle tapping movements which assist in stimulating the skin, at the same time covering it with powder. Do this until the back is very thoroughly dry.

Special care necessary with patients who are paralysed and incontinent. Every effort must be made to keep incontinent patients from lying on a wet sheet, since if they do the skin of the back will always be sodden and cold, and so, deprived of its blood supply, will rapidly become very sore. In some of these cases the urine is irritating in character and may cause soreness and excoriation of the skin unless contact with it can be adequately prevented. In such circumstances it is advisable to protect the skin by rubbing in a small quantity of ointment, of a greasy nature, such as a mixture of zinc and castor oil; but, when the routine treatment is performed, great care must be taken to wash off all stale ointment, and for this very hot water will be needed and a good soap lather in order to prevent interference with the functions of the skin by blockage of the pores. The routine treatment described above is then carried out, but instead of powdering the skin a small quantity of ointment is well rubbed in. The skin is waterproof and is oiled naturally by its own secretion, *sebum*, and the ointment applied may therefore be regarded as increasing the natural protection of the skin by preventing the urine from soaking in and thus enabling it to run off as water runs off a greasy surface.

In the prevention of bedsores the importance of the conditions which predispose to soreness have to be taken into consideration.

Prevention of Pressure. Pressure is probably the most potent cause of bedsore, and prevention needs imagination and ingenuity on the part of the nurse. A patient who shows any signs of soreness of the back should if possible lie on one or other side alternately for short intervals. If this is not possible then the back must be relieved of its pressure in some other way, such as by the use of woollen ring pads or air and water ring cushions. In applying these the edges of the ring must be bevelled, otherwise the tissues of the back sagging through the hole will become oedematous and sore round the margins. This sagging oedematous mass, deprived of blood supply, is readily injured.

Patients sometimes are nursed on full-size water or air beds, or are supplied with water cushions or pillows from the commencement of their illness. In patients who are suffering from some condition known to devitalize the tissues very markedly, or to result in marked emaciation, such as in the first case, a fractured spine, for example, and in the second instance, serious pulmonary tuberculosis, it is good nursing to supply these articles from the outset, as the treatment of bedsores is primarily preventive.

Moisture. A moist skin soon gets cold, and a cold skin interferes with blood supply to the part, which therefore, easily devitalized, soon becomes sore. It is a comparatively easy matter to keep a patient quite dry. The sheet should be changed often enough, and if possible the patient should be washed and powdered locally after the use of the bedpan. In cases where there is frequency of micturition it may be impracticable to wash each time, but powdering should never be omitted.

Friction. In the use of utensils and appliances all friction should be avoided. For example, a chipped enamel bedpan may be a source of friction, but this should never be used.

Patients who are restless, but in a condition to have matters explained to them, should be told that frequent rubbing gives rise to soreness and is inadvisable. If there is a tendency to rub the knees and ankles together, woollen ring pads might be bandaged over the prominences. The same measures might be taken with patients who insist on moving their legs up and down in the bed and so rubbing the skin off their knees. In patients whose skin is very tender, so that the slightest friction seems to injure it the limbs should be wrapped in cotton wool bandages; but the nurse must remember that these have to be moved daily for careful inspection and washing of the skin. Bedcradles can be used to remove the weight of the bedclothes if these are a source of irritation.

Curative treatment of bedsores. Whilst emphasizing the doctrine that bedsores should never occur, we are nevertheless faced in some instances by the necessity of treating them. Once the skin is abraded, every care must be taken to prevent the entry of micro-organisms—such a wound is therefore treated with all aseptic precautions. During the early stages probably stimulating healing dressings, combined with a lubricant, to prevent the dressing from sticking to the part, may be employed. Examples of such lubricants are liquid paraffin, flavine and tannic acid, as would be employed in the treatment of a burn. When the surface is covered with exudate or discharge, it may be sufficient to clean this off with peroxide of hydrogen, followed by the use of an antiseptic dressing; or more drastic measures may be needed to clean the parts, such as the application of fomentations. Whenever the surface is raw and red, as may be seen in bedsores that occur rapidly, or in others where sloughs have been removed by hot applications, a highly stimulating dressing such as red lotion, containing zinc sulphate, may be used. Frequent change of dressing may help, many of the aniline dyes are very useful in this respect, such as brilliant green and scarlet red—these are antiseptic and stimulating and do not act as irritants. The application of elastoplast is valuable where frequent change of dressings is not required or recommended.

TROPHIC SORES

This condition may be aggravated by any of those described as possible causes of bedsore. But a trophic sore is one which occurs because the nutritional nerves are affected. Such a condition may occur in injuries to the spinal cord, in anterior poliomyelitis and in peripheral nerve lesions, and may also be associated with other diseases of the nervous system and occur under conditions of severe toxaemia.

A trophic sore may begin very much like a bedsore, or it may first appear as a patch of discoloration of the skin, a purpuric patch or a blister.

Prevention and treatment. The precautions described in the preventive treatment of bedsore apply here. Very careful watch should be kept of any patient who could be suspected, by reason of his condition, of a tendency to develop trophic sores, and even the slightest irritation should be avoided. Such a patient for example should never be rolled over to have his sheet or drawsheet changed, he should always be lifted; he should never be placed on an unprotected bedpan, the edge or rim of which must always be covered by wool, though an air cushion might be used for this purpose. Water or air beds should be utilized from the commencement of the illness; no two skin surfaces should ever be permitted to come together; it may be necessary to bandage ring pads on the inner side of the knee and over the inner malleoli, and the heels should be protected in the same way. In many instances it is advisable to bandage the limbs in cotton wool, removing it twice daily and washing and powdering and carefully inspecting the skin.

Trophic sores unfortunately may not always be preventable, they are very difficult to treat, and in many cases improvement occurs only as the nutrition of the part is reorganized by improvement in the patient's condition.

GIVING BEDPANS AND URINALS

In most hospitals the ward is 'closed' at regular stated times for the purposes of the *sanitary round*, by placing a screen in front of the ward door, thus indicating to visitors, including the doctors and clergy, that they may not enter without first inquiring if this could be arranged for them because, during the time the sanitary round is in progress, every patient is being given either a bedpan or a urinal.

It has to be remembered, however, that in very many cases patients will require bedpans in between these stated times. This necessitates screening the bed of the patient. Some probationers think a patient is exacting if he asks for a bedpan at an unusual time, but if she has the right kind of imagination she should realize that many concessions must be made to sick people, and that as a general rule they only ask for these things when driven by necessity. Most people will suffer much discomfort rather than ask, and this discomfort has preceded their request.

Most nurses perform both this and many other similarly unpleasant services most willingly, and if a nurse wants reward she will get it in the relief, gratitude and peace expressed on the face of the patient who may have been summoning all his courage to ask for this vessel at what he fears might be an inconvenient moment.

The nurse's sleeves should be rolled up during the performance of the sanitary round and she should wash and scrub her hands and forearms afterwards.

When **giving a patient a bedpan** it should be warm and dry, and be carried to the bedside under a calico cover; if a round pan is used, it should have its lid and handle cap on in addition. If the patient can help himself, that is, get himself on to the bedpan, the nurse should turn the bedclothes back and slip it under his buttocks from the right side, unless contraindicated, as for example when the patient has a wound on the left side.

To place a patient on a bedpan who is unable to do much to help himself, the nurse should turn the quilt and blanket down to the foot of the bed, leaving the patient covered by a sheet and blanket; and then, standing on the right side of the bed, by placing her left hand under the lower part of the patient's back, raise him sufficiently to slip the bedpan under his buttocks with her right hand. She should then feel that the pan is in a convenient position, neither too high nor too low, and arrange the patient's pillows so that he is propped comfortably on it. In the case of a thin patient the bedpan might have to be padded with brown wool to effect this.

For *helpless patients*, two nurses will be required, one at each side of the bed.

To cleanse the patient. Either toilet paper, moist tow or brown wool swabs may be used for cleaning the patient after the use of the bedpan. If he particularly wishes to do so and is able he may perform this office for himself; otherwise the nurse will do it. If moist swabs are used the patient's skin should either be dried with dry swabs or with the 'back towel' provided for drying these parts. The used swabs are put into a receiver provided for this purpose, as if placed in the bedpan they would have to be picked out by forceps before it could be emptied. If the patient has cleansed himself after the use of the bedpan he should either be given an opportunity to wash his hands, or if this is not convenient—as for instance in a very large ward—he should be given moist swabs on which to wipe his fingers. The contents of all bedpans should be inspected before they are emptied.

To empty a bedpan. After removing the lid and handle, and inspecting the contents and removing any bits of wool or other material which should not be put down a drain, the pan is put into an automatic bedpan flush, which is the ideal method, or alternatively inverted over a rose or upward spray. The pan should then be inspected and if not clean, a mop, which is standing ready in disinfectant, is passed round the inside of the pan and through the handle, the pan again rinsed, the outside dried and it is then put away.

Urinals are usually made of porcelain, glass or enamel. Glass ones are best, since they are easily cleaned, it is easy to see that they are clean, and the character of the urine in them is most easily inspected.

A urinal is taken to the bedside covered by a calico cloth which should have some indication by a distinguishing mark as to which is the inside and which the out.

The cloth should not be left in a prominent position such as the floor, except during the sanitary round when the ward is closed. On other occasions it may be placed on the rail at the head of the bed, below the level of the mattress, or tucked in over the side of the bedstead. In this way the fact that the patient is using a urinal is not evident.

Urinals should be emptied immediately after use and rinsed with cold water, which is most conveniently performed by means of an inverted spray, and they are then placed upside down to drain.

A nurse should always make sure whether a specimen of urine or stool is to be saved. She should observe the character of these in every instance and also any untoward symptoms, such as frequency, variations in quantity and so on. If all urine is being saved, as in a collection of 24-hour specimens (see fig. 11, p. 39), the amount taken from the patient should be charted on the label provided on the bottle on every occasion.

In the routine care of bedpans and urinals, means are taken to keep them clean and quite free from any deposit, such as may be the result of highly concentrated urines depositing urates or phosphates. Some ward sisters have these articles soaked for two hours in a strong disinfectant solution once in 24 hours; others consider that rinsing them with disinfectant after use is sufficient. In maternity and infectious disease wards they should be boiled.

To keep urinals free from deposit, washing with water containing washing soda and using a bottle brush to help remove any deposit may be adequate; in some cases of marked phosphaturia a urinal may become crusted in a very short time.

Chapter 4

Observations of Excreta and Discharges and Collection of Specimens

The characteristics of normal urine and its variations in health and disease—The testing of urine—Characteristics of normal faeces with variations in health and disease—Handling and disposal of sputum and observations—Types of vomit; care of a patient when vomiting—Vaginal discharges, observations and nursing care—The collection of specimens of urine, faeces, sputum and vomit; of pus, fluid and secretions and of blood

THE CHARACTERISTICS OF NORMAL URINE, VARIATIONS IN HEALTH AND DISEASE

The normal characteristics of urine are:
Colour—pale amber.
Odour—aromatic.
Quantity—in the adult—40 to 60 ounces.
Reaction—slightly acid to litmus.
Specific gravity—1,010 to 1,020.

The urine should be clear without deposit—there may be a light flocculent cloud of mucus floating in the centre of the specimen.

Variations in health and disease. The quantity is decreased in health when the amount of fluid taken is limited, or when perspiration is heavy as the result of exercise or excessive clothing and in hot weather. When the quantity is much diminished the colour becomes deeper, the specific gravity higher, and there may be a deposit of urates on cooling.

The *quantity is increased* in opposite conditions, such as when the skin is acting slightly, as in cool weather, in conditions of fear and nervousness, when little exercise is taken, and if the diet should be low, and when the fluid intake is increased. In these circumstances the colour is paler and the specific gravity is lower.

The *normal odour* varies very little during health, and the *variation in the reaction* is also slight—for example, it may be found to be alkaline after a meal rich in carbohydrates.

The characteristics vary more considerably under conditions of disease. The *quantity is decreased* in febrile conditions, heart disease, acute nephritis; in some cases of chronic nephritis, in some surgical diseases of the kidneys; after the administration of certain drugs such as opium and ergot; and in all cases in which fluid is lost to the body as in haemorrhage, vomiting and diarrhoea, and in many conditions of toxaemia, and also when there is marked oedema.

The *quantity is increased* in diabetes, in some disorders of the pituitary gland, in hysteria and other functional nervous conditions, in most cases of chronic nephritis, by the administration of diuretic drugs, such as potassium citrate, digitalis and mercurial diuretics, and when the intake of fluid is increased.

The *colour* varies with the quantity as previously mentioned. *Bile* colours the urine very dark olive green, *blood* renders it smoky or red, *chyle* makes it look milky. *Certain drugs also alter the colour of urine;* in carbolic acid poisoning it is green, the administration of phenolphthalein colours an alkaline urine red; santonin gives a yellow colour.

The *urine is rendered opaque* by the presence of blood, chyle, pus, excessive mucus, and also by phosphates and urates until these have been deposited.

The *deposits* normally seen in urine are *urates*, which may be pink or white; *phosphates*, usually whitish grey, but sometimes slightly tinged by pink; *pus*, which is very dense, lying heavily at the bottom of the glass; *blood* may be present in clots; *particles of uric acid* suggest a sprinkling of cayenne pepper over the specimen glass; *excess of mucus* may form a gelatinous mass.

The *odour* is slightly fishy when decomposition is commencing; when very marked the odour becomes ammoniacal. The presence of acetone bodies gives a scented urine which recalls the smell of newmown hay. The odour of certain drugs such as carbolic may be detected in the urine, and turpentine produces a pungent odour described as being like the scent of violets.

The *reaction* may vary very considerably in disease. A concentrated urine is usually highly acid, and consequently irritating; urine containing phosphates is neutral or alkaline, and urates give an acid urine. As a rule the urine is alkaline in cystitis. Certain drugs are administered to effect alteration in the reaction in the treatment of disease—for example, potassium citrate renders the urine alkaline, and acid sodium phosphate makes it acid.

As a general rule, the specific gravity is low when the quantity is increased and high when decreased; in diabetes mellitus, however, the presence of large quantities of sugar in the urine results in the passing of large quantities with a characteristically high specific gravity.

ABNORMAL CONSTITUENTS OF URINE

The substances for which urine may be chemically examined by a nurse are protein, blood, bile, sugar, acetone bodies, pus, diacetic acid, urates and phosphates, and the quantity of chlorides. In addition, urine may be examined for uric acid, the presence of red blood cells and pus cells, casts and bacteria, and for the quantity of urea, albumin and sugar; but these tests are not usually performed by a nurse, and are therefore not described here.

EXAMINATION OF URINE

1. Ascertain quantity from which specimen is taken.

2. Notice colour and clearness, and presence or absence of deposit.

N.B.—No urine should be stirred before testing.

3. Take the reaction.

Acid urine turns blue litmus paper red and has no effect on red.

Alkaline urine turns red litmus paper blue and has no effect on blue.

Normal urine is acid. It may be alkaline after a meal, especially of vegetable food, in cystitis, and while taking certain drugs, such as citrates, etc., and also from decomposition on exposure to air. If alkaline, it must be made acid by a few drops of dilute acetic acid before testing further.

4. Take the specific gravity.

The temperature of urine should be approximately room temperature.

The normal specific gravity is between 1,010 and 1,020.

A *low specific gravity* may be temporary only or suggests kidney disease.

A *high specific gravity* with pale urine suggests diabetes. See that the urinometer floats and stands clear of the sides of the vessel; read the number with the eye on a level with the surface of the urine.

5. Examine for substances in solution.

These may be:
- Protein (albumin).
- Blood.
- Bile.
- Sugar or glucose.
- Acetone.

N.B.—The finding of one substance does not preclude the presence of another.

A. Tests for Protein.

Boiling test.

The urine should be filtered before testing for protein. Fill a test tube with the urine to about 1 in. from the top. Boil the top of the column of clear urine over a naked flame (see below). Compare any cloud which develops with the lower clear layer. A precipitate or cloud denotes:

1. Proteins

or 2. Phosphates.

Add a few drops of dilute acetic acid. If the precipitate dissolves it is phosphates. If the precipitate does not dissolve it is proteins.

Nitric acid test.

If albumin is suspected it may be tested for by nitric acid without heat when the urine is clear.

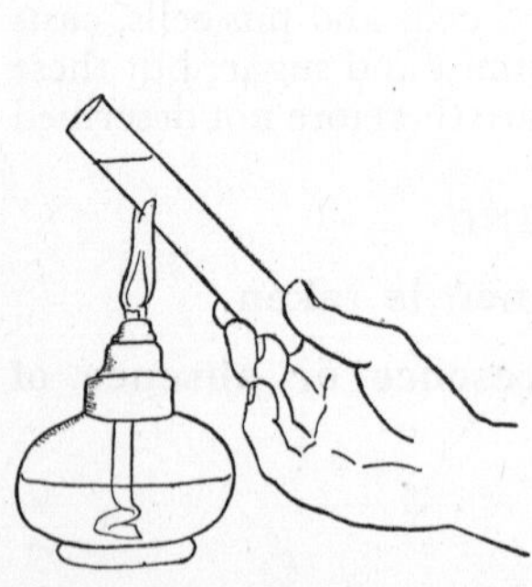

FIG. 21.

Method of holding a test tube when heating the upper part of a column of liquid.

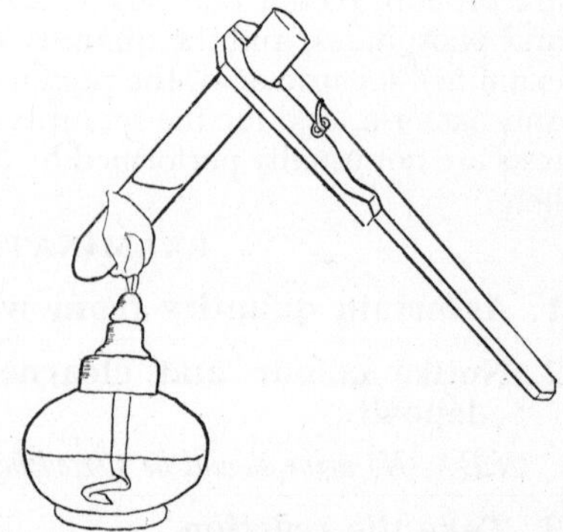

FIG. 22.

A special holder may be employed when boiling a small quantity of fluid in a test tube.

Pour a small quantity of nitric acid into a clean test tube; allow a similar quantity of urine to trickle steadily down the side of the test tube—where the two fluids meet, a layer of coagulated albumin is seen.

Salicyl sulphonic acid test.

This test is useful if only a small quantity of urine is available.

To 1 in. of clear urine in a test tube add a few drops of a saturated solution of salicyl sulphonic acid. If protein is present the liquid in the tube will appear turbid in comparison with the control tube containing the original urine.

The quantity of albumin may be ascertained by Esbach's albuminometer. This is a graduated corked test tube. Filter the urine if not already clear, and if alkaline render slightly acid with dilute nitric acid. If the specific gravity be 1,010 or more, dilute the urine sufficiently to reduce the specific gravity to below that level. Fill the tube with urine up to the mark 'U'. Add the reagent (Esbach's solution of picric acid and citric acid) up to the mark 'R'. The tube is then gently inverted a few times to allow the fluids to mix, and kept standing upright for 24 hours. The albumin is deposited and is read off on the graduated marks, which represent grammes of dried albumin per litre of urine. The percentage of albumin is obtained by dividing by 10. Allowance must be made if the urine has been diluted before the estimation was undertaken.

B. Tests for Blood.

Pour about 1 in. of urine into a test tube, boil and cool. Add ½ in. of glacial acetic acid and mix. Add 1 in. of ether and invert several times. Into another test tube add ½ c.c. of alcoholic guaiac solution and 2–3 c.c. of ozonic ether. Pipette the etheral extract from the first tube into the tube containing the guaiac and ozonic ether. If blood is present a blue colour will develop.

N.B.—If the ethereal extract in the first tube does not separate, add a few drops of water to the contents without shaking. This usually brings about the separation of the ether.

C. Tests for bile.

1. *Bile pigments.*

Fill a test tube ¾ full of urine. Shake vigorously. If the urine contains bile the froth will be coloured yellow.

Bile in the urine always colours the urine suggestively when in any quantity. Let fall a few drops from a pipette on a white tile and beside them a few drops of strong nitric acid; allow them to run together; where the two fluids mix, a passing play of colours, of which one *must* be green, will appear if bile be present.

Iodine test for bile.

Add 0.5 per cent. tincture of iodine drop by drop to the urine. In the presence of bile pigments a dark green colour develops.

2. *Bile salts.*

Hay's test.

Place the urine in a glass beaker. Sprinkle some sublimed flowers of sulphur on the surface of the urine. If bile acids are present, the sulphur sinks sooner or later in accordance with their percentage.

D. Tests for sugar.

Fehling's test.

If the urine be pale, increased in quantity, and of high specific gravity, sugar will be suspected.

A small quantity of freshly made Fehling's solution is poured into a test tube and heated to boiling, and an equal quantity of urine added and heated—an orange red deposit proves the presence of sugar. Instead of Fehling's solution, its component parts may be used separately—the liquor potassae and the urine boiled together and a few drops of sulphate of copper solution added—the result will be the same.

The test fluid and the urine may be boiled in separate test tubes and allowed to flow together down the inclined tubes.

Benedict's test.

Place 5 c.c. of Benedict's reagent in a test tube, and add 8 drops of urine. Boil over a flame for 2 minutes or place in boiling water for 5 minutes.

Some idea of the amount of sugar present may be obtained by allowing the tube to stand for a few minutes.

Greenish liquid without deposit, denotes 0.1 per cent.

Slight yellow deposit with greenish liquid above, 0.2 per cent. An orange deposit with colourless liquid above it, indicates that the urine contains about 2 per cent of sugar.

E. Tests for acetone bodies.

1. *Aceto-acetic acid syn. diacetic acid.*

Ferric chloride test.

Add a few drops of 10 per cent ferric chloride to 1 in. of urine in a test tube. At first a precipitate of ferric phosphate appears. Continue to add ferric chloride and the phosphate will dissolve and a port wine colour is given if diacetic acid is present.

N.B.—The test must be performed on freshly passed urine, because if the urine is allowed to stand the diacetic acid becomes oxidized to acetone which does not give the test.

A positive ferric chloride test shows that a very severe degree of ketosis is present.

Rothera's test.

Into a test tube put 1 in. of urine. To it add about 1 in. of ammonium sulphate *crystals* and shake. Add 2 drops of freshly prepared weak sodium nitro-prusside and about 1 in. of concentrated ammonia. A permanganate colour develops in the presence of diacetic acid.

2. *Acetone.*

Rothera's test. (See above.)

6. Examine Deposit. The deposit may consist of:

Urates.
Phosphates.
Uric Acid.
Mucus.
Red blood cells.
Pus cells.

Urates disappear on heating the urine.

Phosphates may be dissolved by the addition of acetic acid.

Uric acid crystals. These resemble cayenne pepper grains lying at the bottom of the specimen glass. They have a characteristic appearance under the microscope.

Mucus. This appears as a flocculent cloud in most urines and can be seen on the surface of the urine if the specific gravity is high, or at the foot of the column of urine if the specific gravity is low. This is the only satisfactory test for mucus and its presence is of no significance.

Red blood cells. If present in large amount they can be recognized as a red deposit colouring the supernatant fluid reddish brown or yellow.

Pus cells. Pipette about 1 in. of the deposit from the foot of the specimen glass and transfer to a clean test tube. Add 1 in. of strong liquor potassae and stir. If pus is present in large amounts a gelatinous ropy mixture results. (Blood cells and pus cells can be identified under the microscope.)

STOOLS

The normal stool varies in health, according as the individual is an infant, child or adult, and to some extent with the diet. A fluid diet produces soft stools, a dry diet gives a hard stool. A heavy protein diet will make a stool offensive and dry, a milk diet will render it dry and crumbly and pale in colour. Certain vegetables may alter the colour, spinach producing a greenish stool and carrots a reddish colour. Certain drugs taken may produce some effect; astringents, such as tannic acid contained in tea, will decrease the quantity, iron and bismuth will render the stool greyish black; laxatives and purgatives are intended to increase the quantity and the fluidity.

The characteristics of a normal stool are:

Frequency—one or two a day.
Quantity—in the adult about four ounces.
Consistency—soft solid.
Colour—light brown.
Odour—characteristic but inoffensive.

Variations in disease. The *quantity is increased* in intestinal catarrh, diarrhoea, and whenever peristalsis is stimulated. It is *decreased* when peristalsis is sluggish, as in constipation, and in conditions in which fluid is being lost, as in sweating, vomiting and excessive bleeding.

The *consistency* is always in relation to the quantity: increased quantity produces fluidity, decreased quantity renders the stool hard and solid, as water has been excessively absorbed. Very hard stools are described as *scybala*. Gritty particles occur when faecal collections have formed as in diverticulitis. The term 'sheep droppings' is used to describe little hard round knobbly bits of faeces which have probably been passed through a spastic colon. *Ribbonlike* stools are those which have been passed through a constricted colon, which may be due to spastic constipation or may indicate the presence of a sclerotic growth. A soft solid stool may sometimes be grooved as it is pressed past a prominence in the wall of the rectum and usually indicates the presence of an abscess in this region.

Ricewater stools are a special type of fluid stool which has a turbid appearance with little flecks of mucus in it, characteristic of cholera.

The *odour* of the stool is very little changed; sour-smelling stools occur in digestive disorders, and the stools are offensive whenever there is excessive decomposition, tissue destruction as in ulcerative enteritis and typhoid fever, and when the bile is absent as in jaundice.

The *colour* varies rather more considerably. Bile, which normally colours the stool brown, is absent in jaundice, and so the stools are *clay* or *putty coloured*; and it might be noted here that the absence of bile retards peristalsis—thus causing dryness of stool—gives rise to defective digestion of fats so that fat globules may be seen in the stool, and that these stools are also offensive and are the characteristic stools of jaundice.

Green stools suggest digestive disorder and may also be produced by the administration of calomel.

Blood alters the colour of the stool in several ways. The presence of altered blood (melaena) gives a tarry stool. When blood coming from the lower part of the small intestine is well mixed with the stool, but not seriously altered by the digestive juices, the colour is chocolate. Bright red blood indicates bleeding from the large intestine or very rapid bleeding from the lower part of the small intestine. In these two instances clot may be present.

The more common abnormal constituents which are occasionally present are:

Blood as just described.
Mucus, which may be in flakes or shreds, or as epithelial casts.
Pus.
Sloughs, usually indicating separation of ulcers, as in typhoid fever.
Gallstones—little grey particles, usually searched for after an attack of biliary colic.
Undigested food—fat as globules; curds, from undigested milk; and substances as fruit stones, skins, fish bones, etc.
Intestinal Worms.

The stools of an infant. During the early days, *meconium* is passed, which is a dark green fluid; during the first two months of life, the stools are like beaten-up egg in colour and consistency, slightly sour and numbering three to four a day. They then gradually become slightly feculent, and at the age of about six months have become of the consistency of porridge and slightly brown in colour.

SPUTUM

Sputum or expectoration is usually coughed up from the lungs, though in many instances it contains a lot of saliva.

Observations. It is important that a nurse should observe the *amount* of sputum, its *colour*, *odour*, *tenacity*—that is, whether or not it is clinging to the patient's lips, and difficult to spit up. It is important to note the time when most of the expectoration is brought up, whether it is early morning, after a meal or after exertion.

Character. Sputum is described according to its character. It may be *abundant* or *scanty*, *clear* or *opaque*; if opaque it may be *mucoid*, *muco-purulent*, *purulent*, *albuminoid*, *bloodstained* or *rusty*. It may also be *frothy*, *deposited in layers* or *nummular*; *it may resemble prune juice* in colour in gangrene and abscess of the lung, *egg yolk* in jaundice, and *anchovy sauce* in pulmonary abscess complicating dysentery.

Certain diseases have very characteristic sputa. In *pneumonia* it begins by being mucoid, then becomes tenacious and rusty, and later, when the condition is clearing up, it is frequently abundant, mucoid and frothy.

In *bronchiectasis*, the sputum is fetid, having a deposit of pus, a layer of brown fluid on top of this surmounted by froth.

In *pulmonary tuberculosis* the sputum is described as *glairy*, when it looks like sago grains. It is *nummular*, which means that it comes up in coin-shaped masses lying on the bottom of the vessel into which it is expectorated. This occurs when cavities are present. When the disease is advanced, and there is a good deal of destruction of lung tissue, the sputum is greenish-grey and purulent.

In *asthma*, the sputum is scanty, frequently brought up in pellet-shaped masses, described as *Laennec's pearls*.

Precautions in handling sputum. The ordinary sputum cup has a little antiseptic placed at the bottom for the sputum to fall on unless a specimen is required; here again when specimens are needed a sterile flask is invariably provided (see fig. 11, p. 39). Patients who are walking cases carry a *pocket sputum flask*, made of blue glass with a screw top; and this, in order to avoid soiling the pocket, should be provided with a *separate removable calico pocket*. Patients with less copious sputum might be able to manage with handkerchiefs, but in this case *paper handkerchiefs* should be supplied and the nurse in charge should be careful to see that before the patient receives a clean handkerchief he should account for his soiled one which should be burnt.

Disposal of sputum. Non-infectious sputum may be emptied down the sluice or lavatory pan, care being taken to avoid soiling the sides of the basin. *Infectious sputum* and *sputum from all tuberculous persons* should either be rendered innocuous by boiling or disinfection, or it may be disposed of by burning.

VOMIT

The causes of vomiting are numerous, but there are certain observations a nurse will be called upon to make with regard to the manner in which the vomit is expelled and also regarding the character of the matter vomited. In most cases the contents of the stomach are first brought up—food, then gastric juice and later bile-stained fluid.

Food is vomited in gastric and intestinal disorders. In *biliousness* subsequent vomit is green because it contains a good deal of bile. In conditions of *dilatation of the stomach* vomit is usually at first copious, frothy and offensive, and is later followed by copious quantities of fluid which are bile-stained. In *intestinal obstruction* the vomit becomes feculent in odour.

Blood, when vomited, is usually of the colour and consistency of *coffee-grounds*, and acid in reaction; but if it is regurgitated from the duodenum it may be alkaline, and if bleeding is taking place very rapidly it may be bright red because it is unaltered by digestive juices.

Anaesthetic vomit is usually yellowish-green and smells of the anaesthetic.

When corrosive acids or alkalis have been swallowed, as in cases of poisoning, the vomit contains altered blood and frequently casts of the oesophagus and stomach. The vomit is phosphorescent when phosphorus has been taken.

As a rule vomiting implies considerable effort, and is associated with nausea, except in the following instances: in intestinal obstruction it is regurgitant in character, flowing out of the mouth without effort; in pyloric stenosis it is described as projectile since the stomach contents are forcibly ejected; cerebral vomiting is unassociated with the intake of food—it may be projectile in character.

Nursing care. The act of vomiting reflexly stimulates the vagus nerve, and so causes the patient to feel faint and dizzy, and also temporarily lowers the blood pressure and depresses the heat regulating centre. Moreover, it is a very unpleasant symptom, and the patient needs sympathy and tactful nursing attention. The nurse herself may be nauseated as she stands by a patient who vomits, but she must not show this by look or gesture.

During the act of vomiting she should protect the bedclothes, remove the patient's false teeth, hold the basin for him and support his head by placing her hand over his forehead. She should consider whether the patient has any abdominal wound which might be strained and get the patient to support it during the act, since she herself already has her hands full. After the attack she should rinse the patient's mouth out, clean it if necessary, clean his dentures and replace them, note the patient's general condition, the amount of distress and prostration caused, wipe the cold clammy perspiration from his skin, wrap him in a hot blanket, give him a hot-water bottle and, unless contraindicated, give some hot water containing saline or glucose or sodium bicarbonate to sip, disguising the flavour with a little lemon juice if necessary. The nurse must remember that vomiting is one of the sources of dehydration, as it not only removes fluid by the act but also lowers the blood pressure, consequently diminishing the amount of fluid circulating in the tissues of the body.

Vomiting in infants may be due to an acute or a chronic condition, or it may occur as the result of some deformity or malformation, most commonly that associated with pyloric stenosis.

Acute forms of vomiting occur in acute gastro-intestinal disease as in epidemic diarrhoea and vomiting; and at the onset of acute febrile or infectious diseases such as meningitis. The severe vomiting which characterizes congenital pyloric stenosis may also be considered to be acute.

Less acute, or more chronic vomiting is usually due to errors of feeding, which include the swallowing of air, too rapid feeding, during which the infant is not given the rests necessary for him to bring air up, and jumping or jerking the infant about either before or after feeding. The use of unsuitable foods containing either too much sugar or fat or forming too heavy a curd may also be the cause of vomiting. A little unaltered food brought up during or soon after a feeding is described as *posseting*.

Nursing care. It is important that the nurse in charge of an infant who may be vomiting should consider whether the cause be attributable to the food given or to the manner of giving it, and she should take steps to correct what may be wrong.

In making a report on the vomit she should be careful to state whether it contains curds, and of what type these are; and also to note the presence of blood, bile or mucus.

The type of vomiting should be noted, whether *projectile* as in meningitis, or *effortless* as in serious cases of vomiting and diarrhoea, when the vomit dribbles out of the mouth and runs down over the chin.

Ruminating vomiting is a type which occurs in healthy infants; the baby or toddler is seen to make a succession of movements of his jaws and tongue and begin mastication; he gulps and brings fluid, or solid food, in the case of a toddler, into his mouth. It is thought that the cause is a psychological factor, and probably the infant wishes to create a disturbance and receive notice. The treatment is to break the habit by giving thickened feedings, in the case of a tiny baby; and limiting the intake of fluid, particularly not to give water between meals, in the case of an older infant.

The time factor is important in relation to the intake of food, and the nurse should note whether the infant vomits before or after feedings or in between them.

VAGINAL DISCHARGES

A nurse should never imagine that a vaginal discharge is normal. The vagina certainly is moist, but garments should never be stained by its secretions.

Leucorrhoea, which is a white yellowish opaque discharge, is probably the one most commonly seen, and it indicates excessive secretion of the cervical glands and is frequently met with in young women. It is comparatively unimportant, and will usually be found to improve when the standard of general health is raised.

Any inflammatory condition of the genital tract may produce a discharge of *mucus*, a mixture of *mucus and pus*, or *pus*. In *gonorrhoea* the discharge is definitely purulent.

An *offensive vaginal discharge* may be due to a streptococcal infection or to gonorrhoea. The discharge is always offensive in cases of senile vaginitis and endometritis.

In ulcerative conditions of the cervix and uterus such as occur in the late stages of carcinoma, the discharge is *bloodstained and offensive*.

Nursing care. The toilet of the vulva should be frequently attended to in order to prevent excoriation of the surrounding skin by vaginal discharge. Sterile pads should, if possible, be used.

The quantity, colour, odour and general character of the discharge should be noted. In removing the pad, place the palmar aspect of the hand over it, and double and fold it gently on to itself, at the same time wiping in a direction from before backwards; then place it flat on a receiver brought to the bedside for this purpose, covered with a second receiver while carrying it. If the pad is to be kept for the doctor's inspection it may remain in these vessels, but otherwise it should be wrapped in paper and placed in the sanitary bin which will eventually be emptied by the hospital porter. In a private house it might be possible to burn it immediately.

COLLECTION OF SPECIMENS

A nurse will be called upon to collect specimens of the excretions and more rarely of the secretions of the body from time to time. Most commonly specimens of urine, faeces, sputum and vomit will be required.

The examination of such specimens will be necessary for a variety of reasons, particularly in order to arrive at a *diagnosis*, to note the *progress* of the disease, to observe the effect of any special treatment or drug, and, in case of specimens of urine, before the administration of a general anaesthetic.

A specimen required for bacteriological examination may be rendered useless by being carelessly collected. Specimens that have been in contact with disinfectants are of little or no value. All specimens should be handled aseptically in order to avoid contamination. Proper labelling of specimens is as important as careful handling.

Urine. An ordinary specimen—that is, the routine specimen collected either on admission or daily, or twice weekly, in the routine administration of a ward—may be taken first thing in the morning after the patient has had a night's sleep, or last thing at night after the patient has sustained the rigours of the day.

To collect this, the nurse gives the patient a clean bedpan or urinal, and saves 5 ounces of the quantity passed in a clean specimen glass, which should then be covered and labelled with the name of the patient, the ward, and the date on which it was collected. In collecting such a specimen from a female patient warn her that it is required and ask her not to have her bowels moved at the same time if she can avoid this; should she be menstruating the nurse should swab the vulva and place a pad of absorbent wool into the vaginal orifice over which the urine trickles into the bedpan and, with care, mixing of the menstrual flow can be avoided. In this case, however, it is as well to make a note that the woman from whom the specimen was obtained is menstruating.

A *sterile specimen* can only be obtained by means of catheterization and should then be put up in a sterile specimen glass or flask and the word 'sterile' added to the label.

When a *24-hours' specimen* is necessary it is important to ensure that it is collected from the whole 24 hours, neither less nor more. The nurse accordingly gives the patient a vessel, notes the time, writes it down on a label, puts this label on a large clean bottle, usually a winchester holding 4 or 5 pints, and throws that urine away. She then puts all urine collected until the same time next day into that bottle and, for checking purposes, should write on the label the amount obtained, and the time it was passed, each time she adds urine to the bottle. She must inquire whether the whole of the urine collected is to be sent to the laboratory, or whether only a specimen of it is needed—in the latter case she should mix the urine by inverting the bottle several times, then pour out 5 ounces, cover and label as before described, adding to the label the fact that a specimen had been taken from a 24-hours' collection of urine.

To collect a specimen from a baby. In the case of a girl, use a sterile napkin, place a pad of wool in front and below the vulva, and when the baby has passed urine the nurse places this wool in a sterile wringer by means of forceps and squeezes the urine into a clean glass. If the infant is a boy the penis may be placed in a sterile test tube provided the sharp edges of the top are covered by stretching a piece of rubber from the finger of an old surgical glove over it, or by means of wool.

In either case it may be possible to obtain a specimen by 'holding the infant out' over a clean vessel.

Faeces. A sterile specimen glass should be labelled, and the specimen sent to the laboratory as soon as possible after it is passed, the hour it was obtained being added to the information on the label. The specimen should not contain any disinfectant. When collecting it, choose the soft solid portion of the stool, removing this from the bedpan by means of a sterile spatula or scoop specially provided for the purpose; add to the specimen anything that looks abnormal in the stool and take great care not to contaminate the outside of the glass. See that it is securely corked.

Wrap the glass in a piece of clean white paper, or enclose it in an envelope, marked 'faecal specimen'.

If a specimen of faeces is to be examined for the presence of amoeba, the whole stool should be poured into a receptacle warmed by placing it in water at a temperature of 100° F. and sent to the laboratory while still warm from the patient's body.

When a specimen of faeces is needed for examination to detect the presence of *occult blood* it is important for the nurse to see that the diet has not included red meat during the previous 48 hours. She should also warn the patient to try and avoid injuring his gums when cleaning his teeth, and she should also ask him to let her know if by any chance he swallows a little blood from the back of his nose, mouth or throat, as this would render the test useless.

Any abnormal stool should be saved intact for inspection at the doctor's next visit, either in the vessel in which it is received or in a shallow bowl. It should be covered and placed in an air cupboard if one is available.

Sputum. In collecting a specimen of sputum it is best to get this first thing in the morning, before the patient has had his breakfast. He should be told that such a specimen will be required. A small corked specimen glass, ready labelled, is provided standing on a receiver at his bedside, and he is told that he is to expectorate the secretion that comes up from his lungs into this without moving it about in his mouth or collecting a lot of saliva. It is important that saliva should not form the bulk of the specimen so collected.

Vomit. As a general rule vomit is kept in the bowl in which it is received, which should be covered as it is moved about the ward or conveyed to a laboratory for examination.

(See also receptacles for the collection of specimens, fig. 11, p. 39.)

Specimens from the throat are usually collected on sterile cotton swabs and placed in sterile tubes plugged with sterile cotton and taken immediately to the laboratory. Care should be taken to insert the specimen without touching the mouth of the tube. Some specimens are placed directly on to culture media ready in the culture tubes. In taking a swab from the throat, the specimen should be taken from the inflamed area, taking care not to touch any other part of the mouth.

The same precautions apply to specimens taken from the ear, nose and naso-pharynx.

A nurse may be expected to provide for the accommodation of a specimen of blood, cerebrospinal fluid, fluid from one of the serous cavities such as may be obtained on aspiration of the chest or pericardial sac, or of the peritoneum, or specimens from any of the body cavities such as the nose, conjunctival sac, throat or vagina, or the pus or other contents from any wound or abscess.

Specimens of *cerebrospinal fluid*, or *fluid from the serous cavities* are usually collected in sterile test tubes. When handling the tube the nurse must be careful to see that it is not contaminated, and that the rubber bung or cork which is also sterile is replaced as quickly as possible, without touching the sides of the glass.

The label conveying the necessary information should immediately be attached to the specimen.

Pus or fluid from wounds and abscesses may be collected in the same way.

A *specimen of the secretion* from the eye or other mucus-lined cavity is usually taken by means of a sterile swab. This consists of a fine piece of wire or a thin stick with a wisp of absorbent cotton wool wound on to one end; this is placed in a test tube, the free end of the wire being attached to the cork or rubber bung which fits the tube, all of which have been sterilized. The specimen is obtained by gently touching the part affected, so that secretion is received on to the cotton wool; the swab is then immediately replaced in the test tube, putting it in carefully so as to avoid touching the sides of the tube as the swab is replaced. The tube is labelled as necessary and put aside for examination.

Specimens of blood. A nurse will frequently be asked to prepare for the collection of blood for examination, but only rarely will she be expected to collect this.

When a large quantity is required it is obtained from a vein. The *apparatus required* is:

A *spirit lamp* and *sterile test tubes* or *culture tubes.*

Forceps to handle the different parts of the apparatus when fitting it together.

Antiseptic and *swabs* to cleanse the skin.

A *tourniquet* to compress the vein, so that it will stand out prominently and make it easy to insert the needle. This tourniquet may be a piece of rubber tubing, stretched and placed round the arm and held by a pair of Spencer-Wells's artery forceps. Or an inflatable tourniquet may be used, such as that employed with the sphygmomanometer. In some cases the nurse, being adept, compresses the vein by manual pressure.

A *sterile syringe and needle*, of 5 c.c. or 10 c.c. capacity; this may be standing in sterile water or sterile paraffin.

A *small quantity of blood* is usually collected either by means of a Wright's capsule, by a graduated pipette or on a glass slide, and a nurse may be expected to do this.

Wright's capsule (see illustration). The skin is cleansed with a little antiseptic or ether, and jabbed or pricked with a Hagedorn needle, the point of which is sterilized by holding it in the flame of a spirit lamp. After it has cooled blood is drawn, the bent end of the tube is placed in the drop of blood and it passes along up the tube by capillary attraction. When it is three-quarters full remove the tube, gently heat the top part to get the air out, and then seal both ends by heating them in a flame.

Several capillary tubes should be supplied, as sometimes the blood clots just as it enters the tube and then it does not fill. This specimen would be discarded and another attempt made.

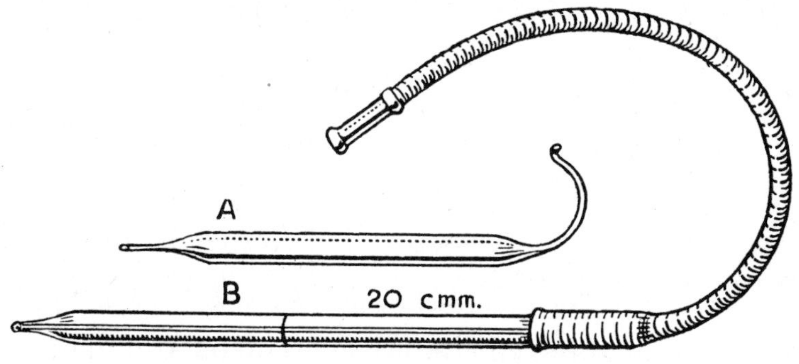

Fig. 23.
(A) Wright's capsule. (B) Graduated pipette.

Glass slide. Blood is obtained in the same way; a drop is received on to a clean slide, and this is smeared to render a thin film of blood available by taking a second slide and wiping it along the first.

A *graduated pipette* is provided when estimating the amount of *haemoglobin* in the blood. The skin is cleansed and dried and a fixed amount of blood is drawn into the pipette. Some means is then employed to liberate the haemoglobin by breaking down the red corpuscles and so liberated the amount can be determined.

SEDIMENTATION RATE

The rate at which the *red blood cells* sink in plasma is increased in cases of tissue breakdown due to infection and toxaemia. The fewer cells present in blood the lower is the surface tension and consequently the sedimentation rate is greater.

Estimation of the sedimentation rate is valuable only as an indication of the progress a patient is making, it is looked upon as a gauge of prognosis and is not used as an aid to diagnosis. The rate is increased in pleural effusion, tuberculosis, in practically all true febrile conditions and in rheumatism. By observation of the sedimentation rate at weekly intervals improvement can be noted.

A number of methods are employed for making this investigation; when Westergren's method is used four cubic centimetres of blood are added to one cubic centimetre of a solution of 3·8 per cent sodium citrate and placed in a vertical glass tube. This tube is graduated from 0 to 200, *after one hour a reading is taken* and the figure on the tube to which the blood cells have sunk in the plasma is noted. As the tube is graduated to 200, this figure is divided by two in order to obtain the percentage. In normal persons the sedimentation rate is from 1 per cent to 10 per cent. In pathological conditions it may be high, e.g. from 30 to 50 per cent.

Chapter 5

The Care of Materials and Appliances Used in Making Beds

Hospital beds and bedding—Removing stains from materials—Care of rubber goods—Making beds: moving patients in bed—Special types of bed—The use of bedblocks, cradles, rests and tables, air and water beds and pillows

THE MATERIALS USED FOR HOSPITAL BEDS AND BEDDING

For general purposes the **ordinary hospital bed** is 26 in. high, 6 ft. 6 in. long and 3 ft. wide. The framework is of enamelled steel or iron, the castors are well made, and so move easily without jarring. The spring mattress is of stout wire, easily cleaned. There are many modifications of this bed, some have a movable back, and this is convenient as it can be moved forward to act as a bedrest or removed when required for washing and dressing the head. Other bedsteads are so planned that by means of levers the top or bottom of the bed can be lowered or raised; another bed is so modified that it can be made to support the patient in Fowler's position, and various other modifications are also supplied by different makers.

The mattresses used are made of horsehair, as this material is non-absorbent and durable, and withstands constant exposure to heat—as in steam disinfection—better than other materials. From time to time as the mattresses lose shape and get thin the horsehair can be washed and picked and new mattresses made up by the addition of some fresh hair. Mattresses are covered by strong bed ticking which lasts a considerable time in spite of frequent brushing and handling. Leather tags should not be used, as these perish when heated.

Care. It is important to protect mattresses from becoming wet and stained, and this is best done by the use of long mackintoshes. They should be brushed at regular frequent intervals to prevent collection of dust in the seams and under the buttons if these are used for the mattressing. As far as possible cotton mattress covers which fit and completely cover the mattresses should be used, and these can be changed every two weeks when in use and also on the discharge of a patient.

To prevent the rusting of the mattress from the wires of the spring, stout covers of sacking or canvas are used; these are tied on to the bedstead by tapes, top and bottom and each side, in order to prevent their slipping or rucking under the mattress.

Pillows are filled with a variety of materials, as some pillows must be firm, while those under the head should be soft and comfortable. Ticks which are impervious to dust are used, and over these a cotton cover is *stitched* which can be removed for washing. In this way the pillow tick, which is expensive, is kept clean, while the cotton cover which is frequently changed looks clean also.

Pillows require inspecting from time to time, as they may get lumpy or thin, and may then require renewing. They should be protected from becoming wet or stained and, when pillows are used in circumstances where such protection is impossible, then mackintosh covers should be provided; these may be loose, tied with tapes or buttoned, but it is better for the covers to be stitched on so that the pillow is thoroughly protected.

Pillowcases may be of linen or cotton material; they should be sufficiently large to fit the pillow loosely, otherwise a comfortable soft pillow compressed by the case it is in will be made hard and uncomfortable. The fastenings supplied, whether tapes, buttons or envelope flaps, should be kept in good condition.

Blankets should be light in weight and large enough to tuck in at the bottom and sides and come well up on to the patient's shoulders. They should not be used doubled, as this only adds to the weight without giving warmth. These are expensive articles and they do not readily stand frequent washing or steam disinfection without shrinkage. Blankets should be protected by the quilt, and by turning the sheet well over at the top, and they should never be exposed to dust. When a blanket is to be used under or next to the patient, thin old ones should be used or non-inflammable blankets of flannelette may be specially provided for this purpose. Thin old blankets should also be provided for blanket bathing.

When in store, blankets should be carefully protected from moth, and should be covered by dust sheets.

Linen. Sheets, drawsheets and pillowcases may be made of linen or cotton material. *Sheets* must be long and wide for the type of bedstead described. Stains should be removed from all linen materials as soon as possible, but bleaching substances should not be used for this as they tend to weaken and rot the material.

Care of linen. Linen must be inspected as it is put away on return from the laundry, all pieces showing tears or thin places being put aside for mending; no torn linen should ever be used on a bed or allowed to remain in use for a moment once it is torn, as the injury will become greater if it is used, and this would constitute a serious extravagance as linen is an expensive item of hospital expenditure.

Condemned linen. Most ward sisters have a book in which they make a list of the linen they consider unfit for further use, and this linen is in due course inspected by one of the administrative sisters, who endorses the book and issues new linen to replace the old. In this way the stock is kept up, and a check is also kept on the length of time linen is usable (and used), the way in which it wears, and the cost it is to the hospital. Probationers should remember this, especially when they are tempted to use some badly torn article as cleaning rags.

Old linen. The linen-room staff which decides upon the condemnation of old worn linen, and the issue of new, whilst using every old piece possible for patching other articles, will still have for disposal much that is too thin and worn for any further use, and this should be available whenever old linen is needed, as in dressing skin cases; old pieces of blanket are available too, and can be utilized for medical fomentations and stupes, etc.

Drawsheets are supplied in a slightly warmer and more readily absorbent material than the ordinary bed sheets, and they may be either single or double. They are called 'drawsheets' because they are long enough to be drawn through from one side of the bed to the other so that the patient may from time to time be given a cool part to lie on. In no circumstances whatever should a damp or soiled drawsheet be drawn through, as if this were done the dirty part would be left tucked under one side of the mattress, which would be unhygienic, while in addition the soiled sheet would probably cause the mattress to be soiled as moisture soaked through it.

Drawsheets are sometimes soiled by excreta, and when this happens they should be soaked in cold water containing some disinfectant, then well scrubbed with a brush and finally, when the stain has been removed as much as possible, sent to the laundry, specially marked 'wet and stained linen'.

A drawsheet should never be hemmed, patched or darned, because the patient's buttocks lie heavily on it and any unevenness or lumpiness of the surface will predispose to bedsoreness.

Mackintoshes. Long mackintoshes are used to cover the mattress, and they should tuck in at the top and bottom of the bed. Short mackintoshes are used under the drawsheet, and these, so that they may be completely covered by the drawsheet, should not be quite as wide as the latter, but in order to keep them taut they must be long enough to tuck in on each side under the mattress.

Mackintoshes are best if 'proofed' both sides.

Quilts. Cotton quilts are used as they are easily washed.

REMOVING STAINS FROM MATERIALS

The materials most commonly stained in hospitals are bed linen and bedding and personal linen. For the removal of such a stain some solvent is used which will either dissolve or remove the substance.

Bloodstains and stains from some forms of excreta contain proteins which are coagulated by the application of heat; so for all stains of this nature, including milk stains, the article should be soaked in cold water for some time and then washed in tepid or hot water. If the staining element contains a good deal of fat, hot water and soap should be used.

When an oily or fatty substance has contaminated an article of clothing, some alkali should be added to the hot water such as soda, soap powder, borax or ammonia. Greasy marks can be removed by petrol, benzine or ether, but these substances are highly inflammable.

Any stains of medicine may be treated by water or methylated spirit as many drugs are soluble in spirit and many more in plain water.

Iodine stains and most of the aniline dyes can be washed out if treated immediately. Stale iodine stains may respond to carbolic lotion 1–20.

Stains of paint or varnish can usually be removed with turpentine or alcohol.

Stains of tea, coffee, and fruit will usually be removed by soaking the material in water, or more quickly by stretching the stained part over a basin and pouring boiling water on to it; if borax can be obtained, this should be applied first and the boiling water poured over it.

If the stains do not respond to this treatment, lemon juice rubbed in may do it, or a little peroxide of hydrogen, but the latter is a bleaching agent and tends to destroy materials. Bleaching in the sun is better.

Inkstains in linen respond most quickly to soaking in milk, or lemon juice may be tried, washing in water and bleaching in the sun.

Stains from scorching can often be removed by bleaching in the sun, slight stains will wash out. If the scorch is noticed as soon as made, rubbing the surface over with a penny is very effective.

The application of some absorptive substance such as salt, starch or borax will prevent any liquid from spreading and thus reduce the ultimate damage to the material.

Bleaching agents are frequently used in rendering linen white, but they require care in use as most of them are destructive to linen.

CARE OF RUBBER GOODS

Rubber goods in use should not be **creased** or **folded**, and they should be protected from friction and injury—pins for example must not be put through them, neither should they come into contact with hot-water bottles, and metal bottles particularly tend to injure mackintoshes.

Mackintosh articles should always be covered by a cotton or linen cover and never in any circumstances should two rubber surfaces be permitted to lie together. Any fluid spilt on them should be wiped off at once. Oil is very injurious.

All mackintosh and rubber goods require to be washed regularly, and some definite order should be made, such as a weekly or at least fortnightly washing for goods in use.

To clean mackintoshes. The best way to remove stains and to cleanse them without injury is as follows:

(1) Soak the mackintoshes in cold water.

(2) Rub each surface well over with soap jelly or soft soap, and then either roll each mackintosh up separately or, better still if treating a number, place them one on the other in a pile and allow them to stand, for say half an hour; though, if a large number are being treated, by the time the last is rubbed over with the soap the first, that is the lowest one of the pile, will be ready for rubbing and rinsing.

(3) Spread each mackintosh on the board provided and rub it well over with tow or a soft cloth, treating both sides.

(4) Then put the mackintosh to soak in warm water in the sink or mackintosh bath. Continue until all the mackintoshes are soaking in the warm water.

(5) Now dry the board and place a cloth on it, and lifting each mackintosh out separately place it on this and dry with a cloth and then place it over the mackintosh roller to dry off completely. When all have been treated, they will be ready for return to the beds or for storage.

Most hospitals are now provided with a specially wide sink, used as a mackintosh bath, and an equally wide board, usually grooved and arranged on a slight incline towards the sink so that water easily runs off it. If this is not provided, it is convenient to use a board placed across a sink or bath for the purpose of cleaning mackintoshes.

To store mackintosh goods. Seeing they are perfectly dry, powder lightly with french chalk and put away either flat or rolled—*not folded*—

taking care to see that two mackintosh surfaces do not lie together but are separated by special cloths, or old linen or paper.

Rubber beds and *cushions* and *rubber hot-water bottles* may be cleaned in exactly the same way as mackintosh sheets, but it is advisable to inflate these very slightly as otherwise when rubbing them there is a tendency for the pressure of the hand to bring strain upon the seams at the sides of the articles, and in time they may crack or weaken here.

The valves of beds and cushions should not be immersed in water as it spoils them and is one of the reasons why they easily get out of order.

When storing these articles they should be slightly inflated, and the precautions taken in the case of mackintosh sheets also used. Rubber goods should not be kept long in storage as they lose their elasticity and tend to harden and crack—those in store should therefore be changed with those in use once a fortnight. If it seems imperative to store some these should be taken out and treated by washing and rubbing, and stretched by hand every two or three weeks in order to help preserve the elasticity.

BEDMAKING

Certain principles have to be considered, and certain points remembered, in making beds: (*a*) in order that the patient's comfort may be enhanced, and (*b*) that due economy may be observed in the use of equipment.

The locker or bedside table should be cleaned and either one wide-backed chair, or two chairs faced back to back, should be arranged two or three feet distant from the bottom of the bed, on which the bedclothes can be neatly laid whilst the bed is being made, so that they will not drag along or touch the floor.

All articles likely to be required should be collected such as the linen, a receptacle for soiled linen, a bedbrush or duster. If the bed is occupied it should be inspected to see what clean linen may be necessary, and also as to whether clean bed attire is needed for the patient, and these should then be provided.

For a helpless patient, two nurses would be required to make the bed; as far as possible one should take the lead and the other follow, so that they work together in harmony: their work should be quietly and quickly performed. The nurses should be opposite one another, at each side of the bed; needless journeys up and down the bedside should be avoided, the whole of the arm from the shoulder should be employed in the necessary movements, which should not be limited to the forearm as this is poor economy of energy and leads to clumsiness of movement. All patting of bedclothes and jarring of the bed should be most carefully avoided. The bedclothes, including the bottom sheet, should be untucked all round before beginning to make or strip a bed.

The **articles required for making a bed** include a *canvas cover* to protect the mattress from ironmould stains caused by contact with the wires of the bed. A cotton cover may be used to protect the mattress from dust; similar *covers for pillows* may be supplied, but in some cases cotton covers are stitched on over the pillow ticking. Cotton material costs much less than bed ticking, and the covers used can easily be removed for washing when soiled.

For hospital patients a long bed mackintosh is provided under the sheet; it protects the mattress from dampness or soiling and may or may not be covered by a thin underblanket. Two sheets will be required; a short mackintosh and drawsheet; one or two blankets—or more, if liked; a day quilt, and a cotton cover for the night time, so that the blankets are not exposed to dust when the day quilt is removed. Several pillows and pillow-cases will be provided.

Other articles that may be needed include: air rings and water pillows to increase comfort for patients who are thin, or who have to lie in any one position for a long time. A bedcradle may be needed to keep the weight of the bedclothes off a painful part. Some form of heat may be needed, either hot-water bottles, or an electric blanket or electric cradle. A bedrest may be needed when the patient has to sit up, a knee pillow when his knees are to be flexed, and a footrest if he is likely to slip down the bed.

The bedclothes should be placed ready on one or two chairs by the bed-side; they should be arranged in the order in which they will be used; linen articles will be folded by the laundry and the folds will make creases; as everything ought to be put on the bed straight, the crease down the centre of a sheet may be used as a guide to straightness.

The bottom bedclothes, long mackintosh and sheet should be taut; the latter should be tucked over the mattress at the top, then pulled taut and tucked in at the bottom of the bed, then across the middle where the patient's buttocks will rest, then at the top and from side to side across the bottom part of the bed which is tightened last. This order of handling the bedclothes is also adhered to when making a bed with a patient in it.

The short mackintosh and drawsheet are supplied to prevent soiling of the bottom sheet by excreta when sanitary utensils have to be used in bed; drawsheets are from 2 to 2½ yards long, this is so that the sheet may be drawn through, from time to time.

A patient's face should never be covered by a sheet whilst making the bed. If the clothes are turned up, they should be folded under his chin and not placed over his face. The bedclothes should not be drawn tightly over the patient's body, nor taut over his feet. They must be comfortable, and the patient should always be able to dorsiflex his feet quite easily and freely and move his legs up and down in bed, and turn over as he wishes.

A patient must always be warned when movement is expected or is about to be carried out; if he is unable to help himself, or this is inad-visable, he should be properly helped and well supported during movement.

Any part of the bed likely to be soiled should be specially protected by a mackintosh and drawsheet, or by a towel lined with jaconet.

In making a bed with a patient in it, the method depends to a great extent on the condition of the patient. Figs. 12 and 13 on p. 40, show stages in the changing of a bottom sheet (*a*) when the patient may be rolled, and (*b*) when he must be lifted. Bedmaking is so essentially practical that detailed instructions of the various methods are not in-cluded.

LIFTING AND MOVING PATIENTS IN BED

Certain principles have to be considered when about to move a patient in his bed: (1) It is essential to have a decided plan, which should be ex-plained to the assistant so that she may thoroughly understand what is about to happen and that any jerky uncomfortable movements may be avoided. The one in charge should give the commands throughout.

(2) The bedclothes should be rearranged so that their weight does not impede movement of the patient. In the majority of cases all top bedclothes are removed as in the making of a bed, and the patient lies beneath one covering blanket.

(3) The nurses should bend from the hips, keeping the back straight; in this way a great effort can be made with the minimum of discomfort.

(4) The arms of the nurses handling the patient should pass fairly well round his body, and in lifting him from the bed should be passed well under the patient, and as far to the other side as possible, in order to give adequate support.

(5) It is essential to have sufficient help. Nurses should never attempt to move a patient who is too heavy for them to lift, as this will give the patient great discomfort, probably mean that he loses confidence in his nurse and, in addition, cause undue and unnecessary strain on the nurse.

SPECIAL TYPES OF BED

Beds may be modified in different ways for the convenience of nursing a variety of cases. Some of the commonest modifications include:

Operation bed. A bed for a patient who has had an anaesthetic (see fig. 36, p. 185). Certain points require consideration in the preparation of this bed: (1) It should be warmed, and this may be carried out by the use of an electric cradle or an electric blanket or by means of hot-water bottles; when the latter are used three should be employed, placed down the middle of the bed. In all cases the appliance used should be covered by the bedclothes, in order to keep the warm air in the bed.

(2) One or two blankets should be provided in which to wrap the patient. These should be warmed and this may be done either by folding them over the hot-water bottles or placing them beneath the electric cradle. The bedclothes that are to cover the patient should be conveniently arranged so that they can easily be removed when the patient is brought back to the ward. The usual order is maintained—i.e. top sheet, blanket and quilt.

(3) The bottom of the bed should be protected by a long bed mackintosh as incontinence may occur while the patient is unconscious. In addition, the part of the bed on which the affected part is to lie should be further protected by a small mackintosh and towel or drawsheet, placed to lie, for example, under an affected leg, shoulder or head.

(4) Any pillows for use in the vicinity of the wound are likely to be soiled and should be provided with mackintosh covers.

(5) A fresh nightdress should be ready at the bed in case of necessity, and screens should be provided. A vomit bowl and towel should be placed at the bedside and swabs with which to wipe the patient's mouth. In cases in which an airway is not used it is advisable to have ready tongue forceps, mouth gag and sponge holders.

(6) Certain other appliances may be required. For example, bedblocks or, as they are sometimes called, shock blocks, for elevation of the foot of the bed in case of shock or collapse. The articles for the administration of a rectal saline or blood transfusion should be at hand. In some cases oxygen may be required and, in others, carbon dioxide may be necessary.

Reception of the patient. When the patient is brought to the ward the nurse should see that there is a clear gangway from the ward door to the bedside. The upper bedclothes, hot-water bottles, or electric cradle should be removed and the patient placed gently on the bed in the position in which he is to lie until he has recovered from the effects of the anaesthetic. In the majority of cases he will be placed on his back; if the abdomen has been the site of operation a pillow may be placed under his knees, and if he is at all restless the knees may be tied together by means of a soft flannel or domette bandage.

The head should be turned to one side in case the patient vomits, as there is danger of inhalation of the vomited material. The towel provided should be tucked round the patient's neck, and under his chin, and spread out on to the bed and so arranged that the patient's cheek rests on it; in this way the bedclothes would be saved should a little vomiting occur before the nurse can reach the bedside.

If one warmed blanket has been provided the patient should be carefully wrapped up in it. If there are two he should be laid on one, which should be brought up at the sides to cover the lower limbs, the top one being tucked in round the patient's body.

Before proceeding to complete the bedmaking, the nurse should notice whether the patient's colour is good, whether his breathing is deep and regular and whether his pulse is satisfactory. She should then arrange the heating apparatus and the hot bedclothes over him. As far as possible a patient recovering from an anaesthetic should be screened from the view of other patients in the ward, but the screens should be so arranged that the nurses passing backwards and forwards up and down the ward can see the patient. If the patient is inclined to vomit or is at all restless the bedside should not be left. In all cases the ward or room in which the patient lies should never be left until he is properly round from the general anaesthetic.

Divided bed. This term is used to describe a bed in which the upper clothing which covers the patient is divided—usually about the middle. It may be used when an examination of the lower part of the abdomen or pelvis is necessary, or when a dressing, or other treatment of this area, has to be carried out: for example, catheterization. It is also used in cases of amputation of the lower limb above the knee, and because of this use it is described by some authorities as an *amputation bed.* It is also conveniently used in preparation of a vapour or hot air bath, where the thermometer is hung from a cradle in the middle of the bed, and when, by means of divided bedclothes, this can more easily be seen.

To prepare. For the purpose of making a divided bed the lower bedclothes are put on as usual, but for making the top of the bed two sheets will be required and two blankets. In some instances specially short blankets are employed, in other instances sisters have been known to use cot blankets, or bath blankets for this purpose.

To arrange the lower half of the top bedclothes, a sheet is placed lengthways over the patient and tucked in at the bottom; one blanket is laid on this, folded over so that it reaches to the level of the patient's pelvis. The upper part of the sheet is folded down over this blanket and the bottom and sides are tucked in. A second sheet is taken, also placed lengthways on the bed, and a blanket is placed on top of this sheet to cover the upper part of the patient's body. The lower part of this sheet is then folded up, over the lower edge of the doubled blanket, and the upper part of the sheet brought down over it to look like an ordinary sheet overlay. This part of the bedclothes is then tucked in at the sides.

It is important to arrange for the bedclothes to overlap from eight to twelve inches where they meet in the middle; unless contraindicated the lower part should overlap the upper part, so that as the patient moves and a little separation of the bedclothes may occur he does not feel that he is exposed to the gaze of persons in the room—this arrangement is also neater. The bedclothes can easily be separated for purposes of examination, inspection or treatment without unduly exposing or uncovering the patient, and this type of bed is particularly useful when treatment to the lower part of the abdomen, perineal area, or upper part of the thighs requires to be frequently repeated. Moreover, the necessity of making the bed each time—which proves not only trying to the patient, but exhausting to the nurse—is obviated.

Should this form of bed be utilized in the case of an amputation of a lower limb above the knee, a small bedcradle should be placed over the stump and the divided bedclothes arranged around the stump but not over it (see next note).

Amputation bed. This is a bed so arranged that the stump is visible to the nurses moving about the ward. It is specially necessary to have this arrangement in cases in which sepsis may occur and so give rise to the complication of secondary haemorrhage. Bleeding from a large vessel may prove rapidly fatal, and in the preparation of an amputation bed, therefore, the first consideration is to provide a tourniquet conveniently near the bedside. It is necessary that every nurse in the ward should know how to use this tourniquet in case of emergency, as in sudden bleeding from an artery as large as one in the leg no time can be wasted seeking for help.

In the preparation of an amputation bed, a long bed mackintosh is necessary for the protection of the mattress, and a short mackintosh covered by a drawsheet or towel should be placed on the bed under and around the area on which the stump is to rest.

Sandbags encased in mackintosh covers should be provided, and laid against the limb in order to prevent its 'jumping', when twitching of the muscles occurs. These sandbags should be recently carbolized and they should be covered with special sterile covers, or wrapped in sterile towels. In addition, a sterile towel should be placed across the limb; the ends of the towel on each side should be secured in position by the weight of the sandbags placed on them. This acts as an additional restraint to involuntary movements of the stump. Some authorities use a long, narrow, lightly filled sandbag placed across the limb above the stump for the same purpose.

For the first twenty-four to forty-eight hours a pillow, which should be covered by a mackintosh and wrapped in a sterile towel, may be provided on which to rest the stump. In the case of a thigh it would lie in an elevated position against this pillow; but its use should be omitted as soon as possible as, if persisted in, flexional deformity tends to occur at the hip joint, which may cause considerable discomfort and pain when it has to be corrected later before the patient can wear an artificial limb.

In making an amputation bed the position of the stump has to be taken into consideration. If, for example, the amputation is above the knee, a divided bed as described above can be employed; but if the foot only has been amputated, at the level of the ankle, the stump may be allowed to lie on a pillow with a bedcradle over it and the bedclothes, arranged as in making up an ordinary bed, can then be turned back on the side on which the affected limb lies and arranged above and around the cradle and covering it, so that the stump is exposed to view. This turning back of the bedclothes allows air to enter the bed and may cause the patient to feel cold, but to prevent this either the good leg should be wrapped in a small blanket or a blanket should be placed next to the patient and wrapped well round him.

Fracture bed. A bed in which a case of fracture is to be nursed, particularly of the spine, pelvis or femur, must provide a firm unyielding surface on which the broken bone is to lie. For this purpose fracture boards may be used; these are boards fitted over the wire mattress and resting on the sides of the bedstead beneath the hair mattress. Either one large lathed board may be used, or several small boards with holes bored in them. In either case sufficient air will reach the mattress.

Several appliances have been in use from time to time in order to provide suitable bed accommodation for fractures. The *Bradford frame* was an early type of this apparatus, and more recently the *Pearson bed* has been used.

Plaster bed. The term 'plaster bed' is used in two connexions—one in which a plaster of paris trough is employed for the patient to lie in, so that he is rendered immovable on the bed—but the connexion in which it is used here indicates the preparation of an ordinary bed in which a patient, who has had plaster of paris applied, is to be placed and nursed.

As in the case of a bed for a fracture, this also requires to be firm and unyielding, particularly when the trunk is encased in plaster or when a plaster spica of the hip has been applied. In both these cases any sagging of the bed before the plaster was completely dry would be likely to cause deformity.

Another point to be considered is that the bed should assist in drying the plaster. Plaster of paris is applied wet. It is not moved until it has set but, even after this, considerable evaporation of moisture must take place before it can be considered satisfactorily dry and hard. Arrangements should therefore be made so that the part encased in plaster is exposed to the air for evaporation and drying. In the case of a trunk in plaster, for example, a divided bed might be utilized, with bedcradles over the patient's trunk, and one or two inlets arranged to allow air to circulate freely around the body. In the case of a leg in plaster, having first wrapped the foot, if exposed, in cotton wool to prevent its getting cold, the bedclothes might be turned back so that the entire limb is exposed, but a blanket should be placed next to the patient so that he is not chilled by this process.

Some authorities require the addition of heat as an aid to the drying of the plaster of paris, and in this case when possible the bed may be drawn up near a fire or radiator; an electric cradle may be placed over it, or hot bottles may be used.

The commonest modification of the hospital bed in a medical ward is the **blanket bed.** In this bed the patient should be lying between blankets; thin old soft blankets are best. The average drawsheet is 36 inches wide, therefore this cannot be used or half of the patient's length will not be lying on blanket. It is usual either to double an ordinary drawsheet, or to have narrow ones—18 inches wide—specially made. An equally narrow strip of mackintosh is used beneath the drawsheet, immediately beneath the buttocks as they rest on the bed. This serves two purposes: (1) the usual protection of the under bedclothes from soiling during the use of sanitary utensils in bed, (2) the provision of a smooth cotton surface rather than a slightly irritating fluffy one.

A patient is nursed between blankets whenever he tends to perspire, as in rheumatism, so that the more absorbent woollen material will not result in chilling him, as would a cotton sheet; and also whenever extra warmth is necessary, as in diseases of the heart and circulation and in renal disease when it is desirable to assist the action of the skin by removing water and other waste matter in order to relieve the work of the diseased kidney.

In a bed for rheumatism, the blankets should be specially soft and absorbent as these patients perspire a great deal. Some form of heat may have to be provided such as hot-water bottles; bedcradles will usually be required to take the weight of the bedclothes from the aching joints and limbs, and pillows and sandbags to support the weight of the limbs in a comfortable position.

In planning a bed for the reception of a case of acute rheumatism, care should be taken to see that it is firm and not liable to be moved by a slight touch, since every movement of the bed causes pain in such cases.

A bed for a renal case should be warm, therefore hot-water bottles may be required. The number of pillows required will depend on whether there is oedema—a patient with swollen legs, and ascites rendering his abdomen large and prominent, will require to be propped up on an inclined plane of pillows, as he will be unable to bend forward with any comfort.

As patients with oedema are readily predisposed to bedsore it may be necessary to supply a water or air bed. An air bed is preferable as it remains fairly warm, warmed by the heat of the patient's body; but the great expanse of water in a large size water bed is difficult to keep warm. It is useful to remove a gallon or two of water each day, replacing it by the addition of the same amount of water at 120° Fahrenheit. The air or water bed should be beneath the bottom blanket.

A bed prepared for a case of heart disease is often described as a heart or cardiac bed. The position in which the patient will be nursed depends entirely on the condition of his heart. In cases of *acute heart disease*, with fair compensation, they are best nursed flat; in this position the greatest rest is obtained. But in cases of *chronic heart disease* in which pulmonary symptoms, including dyspnoea, have developed, or in any case where decompensation is marked, the patient may have to be propped up in order to breathe comfortably.

The bed for a case of chronic disease of the mitral valve will, for example, require a bedrest, and several pillows, to support the patient's back; a ring air pillow to protect the bottom of his back from pressure, a footrest to prevent his slipping down the bed and a bedtable or armrest in case he wishes to lean forward, as he may do when dyspnoea is so marked that the muscles of extraordinary respiration are continually in action, when this position, by fixing the shoulder girdle, makes their movement easier.

THE USE OF BEDBLOCKS, BEDCRADLES, BEDRESTS AND BEDTABLES

Bedblocks are used for raising a bed at one or other end. They are often made of wood, and vary in height from 4 to 24 inches.

The foot of the bed is raised in the treatment of shock; in aiding the arrest of bleeding from the lower limbs, pelvis and abdomen; in the relief of oedema of the lower extremities and the vulva and scrotum and in order to assist in the administration of high colonic lavage or for the purpose of securing that an enema be retained.

The head of the bed is raised in treatment for the relief of bleeding from the head and chest; as an aid in respiration in cases of dyspnoea, when this position assists breathing by causing the diaphragm to be slightly lower. It is also used when drainage from the lower part of the abdomen or the pelvis is necessary.

In putting blocks in position it is advisable to arrange them near the bedposts under which they are to be placed, one or two nurses elevating the end of the bed while another places them in position. The bed should be steadied on the blocks before the weight is released, in order to ensure that the bed is firm. In lifting a bed down from blocks, the same careful handling is necessary; the bed should not be moved quickly, but lowered slowly and deliberately.

Bedcradles are appliances which are provided for the purpose of elevating the weight of the bedclothes from the patient's body. They may be applied over a limb which is painful, or may be used to relieve the body of the weight of the clothes in cases where breathing is difficult, or when the patient is uncomfortable and restless. They are also employed when it is desired to suspend some articles a little distance from some part of the patient's body, as in applying an icebag suspended over the epigastrium in the relief of haematemesis.

Bedcradles may be made of wicker, light wood, wire or fine metal tubing. Wicker ones are light, and when metal cradles are employed care must be taken to see that no hot appliance in the bed comes into contact with the

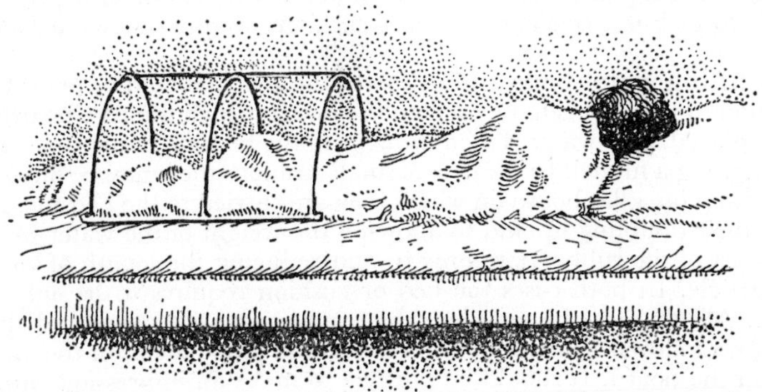

FIG. 24
When a cradle is put in the bed, place a blanket or sheet next to the patient, otherwise he may feel cold.

metal, for fear lest the heat, rapidly conducted, might burn the patient should he touch the bedcradle.

Bedrest. A bedrest or backrest is a light wooden or wicker frame, or canvas or cane covered frame placed obliquely behind the patient as he sits up in bed; pillows are arranged on this form of support against which the patient rests. It is probably provided for economy of pillows; some of the more modern hospital bedsteads have the back of the bed arranged on a hinge which permits it to be swung forward to form a similar type of support.

A patient supported on a bedrest may need an air ring cushion, as the lower part of his back is apt to become sore from continuous sitting. His head should be supported by a specially soft pillow placed at the nape of his neck—otherwise his neck muscles will grow tired of supporting the weight of his head. When the head of a patient nods backwards and forwards it is reasonable to suppose that he was placed in position by a nurse without the necessary imagination for visualizing this particular form of discomfort.

Bedtables. Small tables are provided which fit across the knees of a patient as he sits up in bed; they may be employed for meals, or for reading or other light work, but when one is used for him to lean forward on, in an effort to assist very difficult breathing, it is often described as a *heart table.* When a patient with dyspnoea has to sit in this position for a considerable time it is important to take care that, as he leans forward, the lower part of his back is supported by a pillow, and that his back, shoulders and arms are covered by a light warm wrap. When a bedtable is used as a heart table it must have feet or castors which can be fixed, so that it will not move when the patient leans on it.

Some tables have a head rest provided, and this should be padded; it is movable and can be raised and lowered so that the patient's forehead is properly supported as he sits.

FILLING AIR AND WATER BEDS AND PILLOWS

Full-size air and water beds are used in cases of helpless patients who are liable to bedsore. In some instances cushions or ring pillows are utilized.

In filling water beds and pillows, the article should be placed in the position in which it is to be used on the bed in which fracture boards have been placed. The water is then brought to the bedside in jugs and the bed filled, using a funnel. In the case of small cushions they may be filled in the bathroom on a flat board on which they are carried to the bedside, to prevent their doubling up and so allowing the weight of the water to fall on one part of the rubber, straining it, and reducing the length of service of the article. In both cases the bed or cushion requires to be only partly filled. All air must be expelled, the stopper screwed down and the bed tested as follows: Pronate both forearms and place them on the bed as it lies on the board. It should be possible to make an impression with both arms and, with one, the hard surface beneath should be distinguished. It is a very good plan for every probationer who is being taught to fill these articles, to practise filling a cushion and sitting or lying on it, letting the air or water out as the case may be until she considers it comfortable. She will be surprised at the little inflation that is necessary and would never have believed it without this experience.

In filling air beds, either a footpump or a handpump should be used. This is advisable also in filling cushions, but there may be occasions when a nurse will be faced with the difficulty of filling a cushion without this appliance, in which case she should blow it up by mouth, covering the nozzle with a piece of gauze in order to protect her lips. All air cushions and beds should be tested if there is any doubt about them by placing in water after inflation, when if a hole is present the air will bubble through into the water.

When large water beds are used, the temperature of the water should be about 105° F. The bed should be covered with a blanket as its surface is apt to get chilled and strike cold to the patient. Sometimes a water cushion or pillow filled with water at a temperature of 120° is used in the treatment of shock in infants, as it provides a large warm surface on which the infant can lie during treatment.

Water beds and cushions when in use require emptying and refilling every fortnight as the water tends to decompose. Some sisters aim at obviating this by putting a little formalin in the water.

Chapter 6

Positions Used in Nursing

The positions described are:—Supine—Prone—Semirecumbent—Fowler's—Left lateral—Sims's semiprone—Lithotomy—Trendelenburg's—Rose's—Genu-pectoral —Orthopnoeic—Hyperextension—Head suspension—Postural drainage

The positions used in nursing vary with the needs of the patient—as a rule patients are nursed in recumbent, semirecumbent or erect sitting positions. Nurses would have no difficulty in realizing the possible uses of the various positions and the best way of maintaining them in comfort, if they would devote half an hour to placing themselves in the different positions. The practice becomes very interesting when a group work together, putting one another in the various positions, and usually results in wholesome firsthand criticism of the manner of handling and moving the model.

The dorsal recumbent or supine position is lying flat on the back with one soft pillow, the knees being straight or very slightly flexed over a pillow. This position provides for full relaxation and is the one in which many acutely ill patients are nursed. It is contraindicated in elderly persons, or any who may be subject to bronchitis, or liable to contract hypostatic congestion of the lungs; also in all surgical abdominal cases where drainage is necessary, and after operations on the breast or thorax, and in a great many other conditions. It is also contraindicated in most long-standing illnesses and in neurological conditions, as it is apt to become depressing—partly because of the difficulty of carrying on any little occupation in this position, and partly because the patient is not able to see and take an interest in the life which is going on around him.

This position is also used for examination of the front of the trunk, but for examination of the abdomen the knee pillow should be removed. It is also used for examination of the rectum and vagina provided the thighs are flexed and outwardly rotated.

Prone recumbent position. In this position the patient lies on the front of the body. A pillow is placed beneath the chest, and usually one arm lies beneath the body in a hollow below this pillow. A second pillow is provided on which to rest the side of the face, the arm on the side to which the face is turned lying flexed beside this pillow.

This position is not very often employed; it is useful when there is danger that bedsores may form on the back, and it also prevents and relieves flatulent distension; it is occasionally used to facilitate drainage from the front of the body, as for example in the case of a peri-umbilical abscess.

Dorsal elevated or semirecumbent position. The patient lies on his back with his chest raised on several pillows. It can also be maintained by elevating the top of the bed on blocks so that the patient lies on an incline. This position is freely used, both in medical and surgical nursing. It is the one in which most gastric cases are nursed, most chronic and subacute and some acute chest conditions; many patients after a general anaesthetic and after abdominal or pelvic operations, except when the erect sitting position is indicated. Practically all convalescent patients favour this position.

A pillow is placed beneath the knees and secured to the sides of the bed, or it may be rolled in a drawsheet which can be firmly tucked under the mattress at the sides to keep it in position, or the ends of the drawsheet may be twirled round, tied with cord and fastened to the top of the bed. In some instances a footrest is employed. All these devices are designed to prevent the patient from slipping down and so assuming the recumbent in place of the semirecumbent position.

Fowler's position. This position was introduced by an American surgeon who elevated the top of the bed on 24-inch blocks, and so secured a semirecumbent position (q.v.); but for all practical purposes what is described as Fowler's position in England is a more erect one in which an effort is made to maintain the patient in a sitting posture as nearly upright as possible.

The position may be maintained by means of the *Lawson-Tait Fowler-position bed*, or by propping the patient up by means of backrest and pillows, or by using only pillows. The arms should be supported on pillows so that the patient sits with his forearms supported, as in an armchair. As he is sitting erect a ring air cushion is frequently employed to prevent soreness over the sacrum. When pillows are used, a knee pillow is employed to help maintain the position arranged as described in the semirecumbent position.

Uses. This position is used whenever drainage of the abdominal cavity is desired, and in most cases after operation on the upper part of the stomach and duodenum. It makes breathing easier in cases of dyspnoea, by facilitating the movement of the diaphragm and therefore aids expansion of the lungs, and for this reason is employed in many chronic and in some acute conditions of the chest.

Left lateral position (see fig. 37, p. 186). This must not be confused with Sims's position (see below). The left lateral position is used when a patient is turned on to his side for purposes of washing and rubbing his back as in the routine treatment for the prevention of bedsores. It is also frequently used for giving any form of enema, for the insertion of a suppository, the taking of the temperature by the rectum, or for any treatment to, or examination of, the perineal region.

Sims's semiprone position (see fig. 38, p. 186) is one in which the patient lies partly prone, and on her left side. Her right arm lies on the bed in front of her and the left is behind her. Both knees are drawn up, the right being rather more flexed than the left, and lying on the bed in front of it, thus rendering the position fairly steady. The left side of the face rests on a small pillow placed under the cheek.

This position is used for examination of the vagina; the effect of it is to cause ballooning of the vagina when a Sims's speculum is introduced, thus facilitating examination of the vaginal walls. It is also useful when a rectal treatment is to be undertaken, should it be considered necessary for the anus to be more clearly visible than is possible in the left lateral position. Alternatively a modified left lateral position, as shown in illustration, fig. 39, p. 187, may be used for examination of the vagina.

The lithotomy position is obtained by flexing the hips and knees as the patient lies supine; the pelvis is raised and brought down until the sacrum rests on the edge of the table upon which the patient lies. The position is maintained by special devices attached to many operating tables, or by means of Clover's crutch.

It is used for examination of the genito-urinary tract, and for operations on the lower part of this, the rectum and the perineum.

Trendelenburg's position. In this, the top and centre of the table is tilted so that the head is lower than the pelvis; the lower end of the table is hung down at right angles and against it the legs are fixed at the ankles. All modern operating tables are adaptable, and the best way to obtain this position is to fix the patient's *ankles only* on to the lower flap of the table as the legs lie, with the knee joints of the patient exactly over the hinge of the table, so that when the end is let down at right angles the legs are flexed, as when sitting on a chair. Unless the ankles are fixed the patient will slip down into the anaesthetist's lap when the table is tilted, and if this happens an attempt to fix the knees will result in pressure on the peroneal nerve; but if the ankles are firmly fixed the straps can only impinge on the soft parts of the calf of the leg and thus pressure on this nerve as it passes over the head of the fibula will be avoided.

Some tables have shoulder rests, and if these are used they require careful adjustment for each patient, otherwise the trunk may lie so heavily against these rests as to cause pressure on the brachial plexus of nerves, resulting perhaps in paralysis of the arms, which may seriously disable the patient long after he has recovered from the effects of the operation which he has undergone. Two important points have therefore to be considered in getting a patient into Trendelenburg's position, but if these are attended to the surgeon is relieved of anxiety and the patient of possible serious injury.

Trendelenburg's position is used during the performance of operations through the anterior abdominal wall, and on the organs of the pelvis and lower part of the abdomen. It is also used in the treatment of syncope during anaesthesia.

Placing the foot of the bed on high blocks obtains a similar position, and this is used in the treatment of shock and in the arrest of bleeding from the lower limbs.

A position the *reverse of Trendelenburg's* is employed for operations on the organs of the upper part of the abdominal cavity.

Rose's position is one in which the head of the operating table is let down so that the head hangs over it. It is used in operations on the mouth and throat, as in the removal of tonsils and adenoids, in order to prevent blood from entering the larynx.

Genu-pectoral position. In this position the patient rests on his knees, arms and chest. To obtain it, he is asked to kneel on the bed and, keeping his thighs upright, to bend forward until his chest rests on the bed; he then places his arms in yard-position on each side of his head. His head is turned to one side and his face rests on a small pillow. This position is used when the effect of gravity is employed as in the administration of high colonic lavage and also in visceroptosis, in which case the patient is asked to occupy this position for several intervals during the day in order to assist in replacing the dropped organs.

Orthopnoeic position. This is used in cases of dyspnoea, usually of heart disease, when the patient is unable to obtain any relief and finds it extremely difficult to breathe unless he is sitting up and leaning forward.

The erect sitting position is maintained by means of backrest and pillows. In addition the patient is given some form of support, such as a bedtable, on which to rest his arms in front. In some cases a headrest on which the forehead can be placed is also provided. Nurses will notice the nodding movements of the head which occur with every respiratory act when dyspnoea is marked, and the provision of a headrest in such cases adds considerably to the patient's comfort.

Hyperextension is used in the treatment of some forms of spinal disease, but as a rule some apparatus is utilized to maintain the position.

Head suspension may be used in diseases and injuries of the neck, but in this case also some form of fixation is employed, to obviate the difficulty of maintaining immobility during the performance of the various necessary nursing measures.

Postural drainage is the placing of a patient in such a position that secretion (sputum) drains out of the cavities of the lung in the case of tuberculosis, and out of the dilated alveoli in the case of bronchiectasis. The *lower lobes* are most often affected and the method of tipping shown in the Nelson bed (fig. 40, p. 187), is that adopted. The *upper lobe* drains best when the patient is sitting up. The *middle lobe* drains when the patient lies flat, and the *back parts of the lobes* when the patient lies on his face. The physician will inform the nurse which lobes are affected and in what position he wishes the patient to be placed for postural drainage purposes. The patient usually lies in the special position required for several long or short intervals during the day.

Chapter 7

Local Applications

Fomentations and stupes—Applications of cold: icebag, cold compress, evaporating dressing, Leiter's coils, ice poultice—Poultices and plasters: antiphlogistine, linseed, mustard, charcoal, starch, mustard plaster, belladonna and opium plasters—Liniments—Ointments and glycerines—Application of a leech—Counterirritants: rubefacients, vesicants and cupping

Local applications are applied for many purposes—they may be hot or cold; contain antiseptic, sedative, stimulating, soothing or antispasmodic substances. They may be applied in a number of different ways, including fomentations, plasters, poultices, evaporating dressing, wax dressing, liniment and paint.

HOT APPLICATIONS

Applications of heat may be applied dry, or moist; the latter are considered to be more penetrating than dry applications.

Fomentations are also called *stupes* in some instances; a fomentation may be a surgical dressing, either when applied in an aseptic manner or when of an antiseptic nature; it may be used as a medical treatment in order to provide moist heat and in this case a simple fomentation is employed.

A medical fomentation can be made by wringing out a piece of old flannel or blanket in very hot water. Any soft absorbent material may be used; when wrung out it must be shaken to allow the steam to escape so that the patient may not be scalded. When applied every few minutes there is no need to cover this dressing; but when applied at intervals of 2 hours or so, it is usual to cover it with either a piece of dry absorbent material or a piece of waterproof.

To prepare and apply a fomentation a wringer is used (see fig. 41, p. 188). The fomentation is then removed from the wringer and shaken to let steam escape. A fomentation must not be applied over broken or abraded skin. The fomentation may be covered by a piece of dry flannel or by cotton wool, or a sheet of jaconet may be placed over it, which may also be covered by cotton wool. In all cases the covering material should be larger than the fomentation as the purpose of the former is to retain the heat (see fig. 42, p. 188). The application is then bandaged on.

Medical fomentations may be changed every hour or every two, three or four hours. Before changing, the old one should be removed and the skin carefully inspected to see if it has been too freely reddened. In all cases in which the skin is tender it should be smeared with a little vaseline or olive oil before the moist application is made. If any interval of time should elapse between the removal of one hot dressing and the application of the next the area should not be left exposed, but should be covered with a layer of warmed cotton wool until a fresh application is made. The material used for this type of fomentation may be dried and used over again. It is usually convenient, when employing medical fomentations, to have two or three pieces of flannel or blanket in use alternately, but the material should always be quite dry before being used again—otherwise the cold wet material will cool the water and the fomentation will not be quite as hot as it might be.

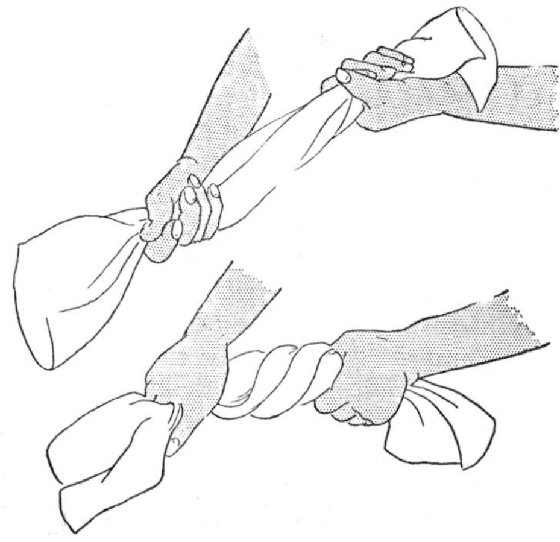

FIG. 25

Take hold of the wringer as shown in the upper drawing, then twist and stretch; this wrings out the water. Keeping the grip with the left hand, take again the first position with the right, and repeat wringing until all water is squeezed out.

Alkaline or *soda fomentations* are sometimes ordered in the treatment of painful arthritic or rheumatic conditions. A teaspoonful or two of sodium bicarbonate is sprinkled over the fomentation before the water is poured on. The amount depends upon the size of the fomentation and the nurse should try to manage so that one or two teaspoonfuls are used with each pint of water.

Hypertonic saline fomentations. These may be ordered for the relief of tension of the tissues when congestion and swelling are causing pain, as in cellulitis. Two drachms of salt or magnesium sulphate are added to the fomentation for each pint of water used. As the skin is tense it is advisable to smear it with liquid paraffin or olive oil before applying the hot moist application.

Sometimes a drug which may be of either a soothing or an irritating nature is added to a medical fomentation, and this form of application is often described as a *stupe*. The drugs most commonly employed are opium as a sedative, belladonna as an antispasmodic, and turpentine as an irritant.

Turpentine stupe. Preparation is made as for a medical fomentation, and from *two to four drachms of turpentine are sprinkled on to the flannel before the water is poured over it*. Although this method is almost universally used, it has one disadvantage in that the turpentine may not mix freely with the water, and therefore not be well diffused over the whole dressing. This disadvantage will be obviated if, instead of sprinkling the turpentine over the flannel, one or two drachms of turpentine mixed with a little olive oil are smeared on the skin over which an ordinary medical fomentation is then applied. As turpentine is a very powerful irritant the skin will be reddened fairly quickly—some skins being more sensitive than others—and the nurse should raise a corner of the dressing 10 or 15 minutes after its application, and at intervals following its application. When the skin is well reddened the dressing should be removed and the skin wiped over with oil or alternatively dried and powdered, and some warm cotton wool then lightly bandaged on.

A turpentine stupe may be used as a counterirritant in cases of bronchitis, pleurisy and pneumonia to relieve pain in the chest. It is also frequently ordered for the relief of abdominal distension.

Opium stupe. When preparing this application from 20 to 60 minims of tincture of opium are sprinkled evenly over the flannel *after* it has been wrung out. This method is used to conserve the drug which is readily soluble in water, and the opium is used as a sedative application.

Belladonna stupe. This may be prepared in exactly the same way as an opium stupe, using tincture of belladonna in place of opium, an alternative method being to paint the skin with glycerine of belladonna, and then to apply a medical fomentation over this. Belladonna is a sedative, but is also very valuable for its antispasmodic properties, being used for the relief of pain and particularly that of lumbago.

Surgical fomentation. This is a form of aseptic dressing which may be applied over a wound, either boracic or white lint being used. The articles required include sterile towels, wool and swabs, Cheatle's forceps in lotion, sterile instruments such as those suitable for the performance of a simple surgical dressing, dissecting forceps, sinus forceps, pointed scissors, probe and artery forceps. Some antiseptic lotion in a sterile bowl for cleansing the wound and receptacles for soiled dressings and used instruments should be provided. The fomentation should be prepared ready for boiling (see fig. 43, p. 189) and a bandage should be supplied.

To prepare the fomentation, a double fold of lint is placed in a wringer, which is then put into a sterilizer or saucepan, with the ends hanging out over the sides, and the dressing is boiled. After boiling for 10 minutes the fomentation is wrung dry and handed to the doctor or nurse who is to apply it. He or she lifts the fomentation out of the wringer—using two pairs of forceps—shakes it as before described in order to free the material of all steam and then applies it. This dressing may be covered by a piece of sterilized wool or jaconet and wool, and bandaged on.

An antiseptic fomentation may be made by using 1–80 carbolic, a weak solution of perchloride of mercury or lysol, instead of water, in which to wring the fomentation.

Hot dry applications may be made by means of a rubber hot-water bottle, but great care must be taken not to burn the patient, and it is inadvisable to have the water hotter than 120° F., as the patient is very likely to hug it closely to himself. The bag should be covered with a flannel cover.

The next most commonly used form of dry heat is an *electrically-heated compress* made of flexible material which can be adapted to the surface of the body. It is fitted with a heat regulating switch on the wall plug adjustment.

Another method of making an application of dry heat is by means of a *bran* or *salt bag*, which is just a small cushion lightly filled with bran or salt, heated in an oven between two enamel plates and applied reasonably hot. Care must be taken to avoid injury to the skin.

APPLICATIONS OF COLD

Cold applications are frequently used in order to limit inflammation, especially when of non-bacterial origin, and in the early stages of injury. Cold is useful in limiting the effusion, which rapidly follows on injury, especially injury to a joint; it is also effective in the diminution of bleeding when applied over the bleeding part, and will relieve congestion—as in cerebral congestion and cerebral haemorrhage—and it is sometimes used for the relief of pain. Most cold applications require the addition of ice.

Ice is fairly often used in nursing, either as an application of cold, or for patients to suck if they especially wish to have it, although this is not advisable as it tends to crack the lips.

It is possible that a probationer nurse will feel rather appalled when first she sees a block of ice with which she is expected to deal, and she may be quite at a loss how to tackle it. Ice is best kept in a piece of blanket unless an ice chest is available. A large block may be broken by striking it with a hammer whilst it is wrapped in a piece of blanket—the use of the blanket deadening the sound and preventing splinters from flying about. Small pieces are most easily broken off, either by using an ice pick, or a strong pin—a small hatpin, for instance, such as nurses frequently wear to keep their caps in position. In order to deaden the sound when breaking ice the block should stand on a double fold of old blanket, either on a plain deal table or on a block of wood.

Icebag. An icebag is the commonest form of cold application used, and it is frequently applied to the head in cases of cerebral haemorrhage, or to relieve headache when this is due to congestion. Nurses frequently forget the value of an icebag in this respect, yet they will not be backward in suggesting contemptuously that a contemporary who is studying hard might put a wet towel on her head! An icebag is also applied locally as an aid in the arrest of bleeding.

Icebags, or *icecaps* as they are most often called, are made of rubber, and are of different shapes and sizes though generally they are round or oval. Some are helmet-shaped for close application to the head, and long narrow ones are supplied for use round the neck.

To fill an icebag (see fig. 48, p. 191), first inspect it to see that it has no holes and that it will hold air when inflated—that it is not perished, and that the screw cap fits and has an adjustable rubber ring for greater security.

The ice is prepared by chopping it into convenient pieces about the size of a walnut, and if allowed to stand a moment or two any sharp corners which might injure the bag will disappear. Sprinkling salt over the pile of prepared ice will make a better freezing mixture. The ice is then put into the bag until the latter is half full, and the bag is grasped by one hand, the air expelled and the stopper screwed on. The surface of the bag should be wiped dry, and it is then put into a flannel bag which should fit well, or it may be wrapped in a piece of flannel, and applied to the part ordered.

An icebag should rest lightly on the skin, and except in the case of the head it should *always be suspended from a cradle* so that, although the covered bag touches the skin, the patient does not receive the weight of it. In cases of meningitis when an icebag is applied to the head it is advisable to take the precaution of tying the bag to the rail or head of the bed.

Icebags should be kept half filled with ice, the nurse watching to see how often it needs replenishment, which will depend on the temperature of the patient and the heat of the part to which application is made, and also upon the size of the bag that is used. The skin over which the application is made should be inspected for mottling, which would indicate that the application should be discontinued for a time. The neglect of this precaution might in certain cases result in gangrene and frostbite.

To store an icecap. Like other rubber articles it should be handled from time to time to preserve its elasticity, and when empty it should be drained until dry and then mopped out with a soft cloth to ensure this. It should afterwards be slightly inflated with air so that the interior surfaces of the rubber do not lie together, and it should be kept in its own cover or wrapped in a piece of material to protect it as it lies in the box in which it is kept.

Compress. Two types of compresses are commonly employed; one described here as a cold compress, and the other as a moist dressing, because it is not always kept cold.

Cold compress. A single layer of material which permits of evaporation is essential for the application of a *cold* compress. This is a means of keeping a part cool by evaporation of water from the material used, and when once a nurse realizes this point she will not attempt either to make use of a double fold of material or to cover the material up.

The linen used is wrung out of iced water, laid on the part affected, and then changed as soon as it is warm. This type of compress when used as an application to the forehead may relieve headache. When applied to a sprained joint it will limit effusion of fluid into the joint, and so relieve congestion and pain.

In all cases a compress should be changed frequently—when a very small dressing is used, as in the case of an eye, a dozen applications may be prepared at once and, having been wrung out of water or lotion, be placed lying ready on a block of ice at the bedside. This treatment is usually ordered to be given for say 15 minutes every hour, changing the compress every 30 to 60 seconds in order to ensure constant application of cold, and it therefore requires a nurse in constant attention at the bedside.

When the area treated is larger, and the congestion less severe, the compress may be changed once every 10 or 15 minutes, as when an application is made to a sprained ankle.

Moist dressing. This is applied by wringing out two or three layers of some soft absorbent material in cold water. Lint, flannelette or linen, with a layer of wool sandwiched between two layers, may be used, and this dressing can be retained in position by means of a gauze bandage. It is changed every half-hour or every hour, is soothing when applied over painful parts, and is particularly valuable for relieving pain and discomfort in catarrhal laryngitis.

Evaporating dressing. Evaporation and consequent chilling is more rapid when spirit is applied to the water—a mixture of one part of spirit to three parts of water being very usual. Methylated spirit is frequently used but as this has an unpleasant odour a little lavender water might be added.

Various evaporating lotions are used, a fairly common one being a mixture of lead and opium which is applied for the relief of very painfully bruised or congested parts.

Leiter's coils. By means of coils of flexible material such as lead or rubber, a continuous application of cold may be made to a part, iced water being constantly run through the coil.

To apply. The arrangement of coils is applied to the skin over a layer of lint or flannel, and secured in position either by straps or bands which are attached to the apparatus; or it may be lightly bandaged on, provided that when rubber is used the pressure is not sufficient to compress the tubing. A length of rubber tubing—a yard or two—passes from each end of the coil, and a sinker is attached to the distal end in each case. One end of tubing is placed in a receptacle above the level of the patient's head. It may be hung from the bedrail or from the top of the locker, or suspended by means of a bedside stand. This receptacle contains water in which large pieces of ice are placed, large pieces being used since these will not melt so rapidly. The water then flows, by siphonage, through the coil of tubing which is lying on the patient, and by means of a second length of tubing is carried from the lower end of the coil into a receptacle which stands on the floor by the bedside. It is important for the nurse to see that the receptacle from which the water is running does not become empty. A very easy way of managing this method of treatment is to alternate the upper and lower poles—for example, by elevating the bedside pail when it is full of water and placing the upper one, now almost empty, on the floor. Large pieces of ice are placed in the water in the pail which now becomes the receptacle from which the water is flowing.

Ice poultice. This form of cold application may be made to a small area as in the case of an eye, instead of applying cold compresses; or it may be made to a large area in cases in which a cold application is made to the chest, for example, in cases of pneumonia.

To prepare. Two pieces of guttapercha are chosen, of the size required for the application, with a thin layer of wool on one piece, which reaches within half an inch of the edge of the tissue all round. Ice is chopped into small pieces, sprinkled with a little salt as in filling an icebag, placed evenly on the layer of cotton wool and covered by a second similar layer, and over this is placed the second piece of guttapercha tissue. The edges of three sides of tissue are now moistened either with chloroform or turpentine, pressed together and so sealed, since either of these substances dissolves the tissue and makes it slightly tacky. The air is then carefully pressed out of the poultice, and the fourth margin is sealed in the same way.

To apply. As in all applications of cold, it is necessary to see that the patient's skin is free from abrasions and that there is a layer of lint or flannelette between the application and the patient's skin. The poultice should be renewed as soon as the ice melts.

As guttapercha tissue is rather expensive, the pieces used need not be discarded, but the sealed margins may be cut off and the good pieces used again. This will render the second application only slightly smaller.

POULTICES AND PLASTERS

A *poultice* or, as it is also called, a *cataplasm*, is a hot application of moist, soft consistency, made of some mealy substance which retains heat comparatively well. Linseed meal is commonly used for this purpose, with mustard in some cases added to it to render the application more stimulating to the circulation.

A *plaster*, or *emplastrum*—not necessarily a hot application—usually consists of a paste tacky in substance and containing drugs which may be either irritating or soothing in character. The best examples are *belladonna* and *opium plasters* applied as soothing applications, and a *mustard plaster* used as a counterirritant.

Antiphlogistine is a preparation of clay and is used in the method of applying heat most common today. The clay contains a number of volatile oils, including methylsalicylate, and is supplied ready prepared in tins. The length of time it retains heat as compared with other forms of poultice, and the volatile substances which it contains, render it a very favourite application. Alternatively, cataplasma kaolin co. is used.

The articles required for the *application of antiphlogistine* include the necessary amount of clay in an upright container which can be heated in a saucepan of water over a stove or gas ring, but it is important to see that the bubbling water does not run over into the clay. The contents of the tin should be stirred by a metal spatula so that it is heated evenly throughout, and the nurse will test the heat from time to time by lifting some antiphlogistine on the spatula and applying it to the skin of her forearm.

A *poultice board* is required and some *lint* or *flannelette*, on which to spread the mixture, together with a *pad of wool* to cover the poultice and a *bandage* or *binder* and *safety pins* with which to secure it in position.

To apply. The clay may be spread directly on to the patient's skin, which should be free from abrasions or cuts, and covered by a thin layer of wool, which is a very comfortable method provided the application is not too hot; but the more practical method is to spread the antiphlogistine with the heated spatula on to the smooth side of a piece of lint to about half an inch in thickness, leaving a margin of an inch or more all round the edge. The edges of the lint should not be turned over on to the clay as this would make a hard bulky edge which soon becomes uncomfortable when the application is worn. The poultice is then covered by a piece of warm fluffed-up cotton wool and lightly bandaged on.

When the poultice is removed the skin should be washed and gently dried, and any little bits of dried antiphlogistine adherent to the skin should be removed with olive oil swabs. The skin should then be powdered and covered with warm cotton wool, secured in position by means of a gauze bandage.

Linseed poultice. As this poultice must be applied hot, all the utensils used for the preparation of it should be placed in hot water to become thoroughly heated, and the linseed should be warm. Care should be taken, however, only to warm the amount of linseed meal that is required, since repeated warming tends to dry the meal by removing the volatile oils.

The *articles required* (see fig. 44, p. 189) are, *linseed meal*, ready warmed in a bowl, and *olive oil*. A small bottle of olive oil, holding about two ounces, should be at hand in the poultice cupboard. The oil should be heated before it is used, and this little bottle may be heated by standing it in hot water. The olive oil may be used to spread on the surface of the poultice as described below, or else it may be smeared over the patient's skin before the poultice is put on.

A metal *spatula* should be standing ready in a jug of hot water.

Some *teazled tow* or *linen* will be required, on which the poultice is to be prepared. Tow is best, as the air between the fluffed-out particles of it acts as a good non-conductor of heat and helps to retain heat in the poultice. Moreover, tow is lighter and warmer than linen.

A *poultice board* will be required on which to prepare the application, and either two *earthenware dinner plates* ready warmed, or a *warmed bowl* or *warm towel*—any one of these can be used for conveying the poultice to the bedside.

A *layer of wool*, larger than the poultice, should be supplied to cover it. Some sisters use jaconet, but this is not invariable as many of them think that the employment of jaconet over any hot moist applications is apt to make the skin sodden.

A bandage or *binder*, and *safety pins*, will be needed to retain the poultice in position.

To make and apply the poultice. The required quantity of boiling water should be poured into the *earthenware bowl* in which the poultice is to be mixed. Only experience will teach how much water will be required, but roughly half a pint of water will make a poultice for the throat while about a pint and a half will be needed for a poultice for the chest.

The warm linseed is then put into the water in handfuls until the water appears to be well soaked up. The mixture should now be stirred with the metal spatula and the nurse continues to sprinkle linseed meal into it until the mixture begins to leave the sides of the basin. She then stirs it thoroughly well, not taking too long about it, as steam is rising all the time and the mixture is rapidly becoming cool; she turns it out on to the prepared tow which is lying on the poultice board, and spreads the mixture evenly but quickly to the desired thickness, which varies, but for average purposes may be from about a quarter to half an inch in thickness. Finally, the nurse pours a little of the warmed olive oil over the entire length of the blade of the spatula and, with one clean sweeping stroke, smears this oil in a thin film across the surface of the poultice. The tow is then turned over the edge of the linseed all round with the same rapid twisting movements that a cook uses when she twists paper over the rim of a jar or jampot. The poultice is placed on the wool on which it is to be applied; it may be rolled or folded and then put into the article which has been provided for carrying it to the patient's bedside.

Having reached the bedside the nurse informs the patient that she has brought his poultice, exposes the part to which it is to be applied and inspects the skin to see that it is quite free from any abrasion or injury. If the poultice is to be applied to any part of the trunk, she first places the binder ready in position, and then unrolls the poultice and tests its heat on the skin of her own forearm, and applies it gently to the patient's skin, lifting it off and on, and not permitting the weight of the poultice to lie on him until he can bear the heat of it. She must encourage him in this and should judge more by the degree of redness the heat causes than by the patient's opinion, because some patients are afraid of being burned and will not bear anything; while others, overanxious to help, will willingly bear heat which would result in a blister.

Poultices may be ordered to be applied two-hourly, or four-hourly, but as a linseed poultice does not retain the heat longer than thirty minutes or an hour, according to its size, it should be removed when its heating power has ceased, especially if it makes the patient uncomfortable and restless.

When *removing a poultice* the nurse takes to the bedside some olive oil swabs, with which to remove any particles of linseed adherent to the skin, some dry wool to dry the skin and powder, and a layer of warmed cotton wool with which to cover the part—which is lightly bandaged on by means of a gauze bandage. The skin should be inspected to see if it has been unduly reddened, in which case it might be necessary to smear it with olive oil instead of drying it. Whenever a reddened area is to be dried, it should be blotted dry, not rubbed.

Mustard poultice. A linseed poultice with mustard added is described as a mustard poultice, but the amount of mustard to be used is generally ordered in a definite proportion to the linseed. When this is left to the nurse she may consider the proportions of 1 part of mustard to 15 of linseed sufficient for a child of three, 1 to 10 parts for an older child, and 1 to 5 for an adult. She should be careful to get her proportions accurately measured, but this may easily be done by ladling out say fifteen spoonfuls of linseed to one spoonful of mustard, as suggested in the first instance.

Another important point is to see that the mustard is well mixed with the linseed so that it is uniformly distributed over the whole application. This may be done by rubbing the mustard into the linseed meal as fat is rubbed into flour in making pastry; or the necessary amount of mustard may be mixed to a paste with tepid water beforehand, and added to the hot water with which the poultice is to be mixed before the linseed meal is sprinkled in.

In *applying a mustard poultice* the nurse must take care not to blister the skin. She will apply the poultice as described in the case of linseed, but she should not leave the bedside for long. After from 10 to 15 minutes she should raise the edge of the poultice and inspect the skin, where she may find a varying degree of erythema due to the action of the mustard. She should then inspect it at more frequent intervals and remove when the skin is well reddened—it should be a deep pink, but not angrily red. The same precautions should be taken as in removing a linseed poultice, but in this case it is always advisable to smear the skin well with olive oil, and then to cover it with a piece of lint.

Charcoal poultice. A charcoal poultice is very occasionally ordered for application to some offensive sore. Charcoal is deodorant and drying in character. It is too drying to be used undiluted, and is therefore mixed with linseed meal in the proportions of one part of charcoal to four or five parts of linseed. This poultice is meant to be an antiseptic application, and ome antiseptic lotion, such as 1–60 or 1–80 carbolic, is accordingly used nstead of water for mixing the poultice. As far as possible, asepsis is maintained, and the face of the poultice is covered by a single or double layer of sterile gauze.

To prepare and apply. The carbolic lotion is ready boiling in a saucepan on a stove or gas ring. The prepared mixture of charcoal and linseed is sprinkled in the boiling liquid and stirred with the spatula, great care being taken to see that it does not become too dry. The spatula may be considered sterile. The mixture is now poured out on to a piece of sterile int, smeared evenly across with the spatula and covered with the sterile gauze. The edges are turned over. The back of the poultice is placed on a piece of sterile wool and outside this lies a piece of jaconet. It is then applied to the sore.

Starch poultice. A starch poultice is used to remove dried crusts, mainly in scabby skin conditions such as impetigo. The starch is prepared in a state of soft consistency and sets in a jelly round the scabs, thus softening them. It is usual to add to the starch some very mild antiseptic, such as boracic acid or borax, which tends to soften the scabs. The thickness of the poultice must depend upon the depth of the scabs, and it may be any thickness from one to one and a half or two inches as required. It is essential for the scabs to be completely covered.

To prepare. Starch is made as for laundry purposes—that is, some powdered starch is mixed to a smooth paste with a little cold water, the borax is added, and boiling water is poured on until the desired consistency is obtained. As a guide to quantity, from 1 to 2 ounces of powdered starch and from 1 to 2 drachms of borax can be mixed to a smooth paste with from 2 to 3 ounces of cold water. This will require from 1 to 1½ pints of boiling water, and the size of the poultice will be sufficient to cover the patient's head.

The nurse will find that success will be attained if she attends to the following points: When pouring the boiling water from the kettle on to the paste of starch, she should pour the water on quickly and stir very slowly, until the starch begins to thicken, when she will notice that it is changing from a white clearness to a dirty opacity. At this point she should pour the water on very slowly and stir very rapidly; she will then notice that the starch appears to cook and thicken, and now very accurate judgement is necessary in order to obtain the exact consistency required. It is quite worth practising, and the nurse will realize that quantities given in textbooks are of very little value as starch varies very much.

The mixture is next poured on to a piece of old linen, and if this has been wrung out of water and is damp, the starch will adhere more closely and will not so readily fall off the surface of the linen when the poultice is lifted off the board. A good margin should be left, but it is not necessary to fold the linen over at the margins. This is a matter of choice. The mixture which has been poured on to the linen should be allowed to cool to a comfortable temperature before it is applied. The face of the poultice may be covered with gauze.

To apply. The part to which the poultice is to be applied should be cleaned with olive oil swabs as well as possible without causing pain. Olive oil or vaseline should be smeared round the edges, where the starch will cause discomfort by sticking to the skin when it begins to dry. The starch poultice may be covered either by jaconet or only by a layer of wool and then bandaged in position.

To remove a starch poultice. The nurse should take to the bedside som olive oil, boracic swabs, dissecting forceps, receivers, and a freshly pre pared poultice if the application is to be repeated—if not, some linen o lint which is soaked in olive oil for application to the affected area an some wool to cover it.

She removes the poultice with great care, very slowly and gently easing with the dissecting forceps any scabs that have become loose, i order to get as many as possible away on the poultice. She puts the poultic into the receiver prepared, inspects the skin and, using dissecting forcep and olive oil swabs, tries to detach loose particles of scab and to rende the skin as clean as possible, gently mopping any bleeding points with th boracic swabs provided.

Plasters. See also p. 106, in which the composition of a plaster i described.

Mustard plaster. This substance, which is frequently used as a counterirritant, may be applied in the form of a *mustard leaf* or a *mustar plaster*—the latter is also sometimes described as a *mustard poultice*, but a poultices usually consist of a soft mass, applied hot, the term is apt to b confusing.

A mustard plaster may be prepared by mixing mustard and flour together either in equal parts for a strong plaster; or using one part of mustar to four or six of flour when a weaker application is desired. The mustar and flour should be mixed together with a small quantity of water, and i should be free from lumps and quite smooth and of a consistency that ca be spread with a spatula or knife. The mixture is spread on to either paper gauze, linen or lint, to a thickness of about an eighth of an inch. Th application should be made to the size that has been ordered, and it may be four, six or eight inches square; the surface of it should be covered wit one or two layers of gauze—one layer is sufficient if the mesh is close— and, after inspection of the skin to see that it is in good condition, th plaster may be applied and covered with a piece of cotton wool slightly larger than the plaster, and lightly bandaged on.

Mustard is a very powerful irritant. The nurse should raise the corne of the plaster from five to ten minutes afterwards and note the degree o reddening, and remove it altogether when the skin is thoroughly pink, picking off any bits of mustard with olive oil swabs, smearing the skin with olive oil, dabbing it dry and powdering it. It should be covered with a piece of lint or a thin layer of cotton wool as a protection to the somewhat painfully red, irritated surface. Mustard is never used for blistering (see Blisters, pp. 117–19), as it is very irritating and causes a nasty slough which takes a long time to heal and results in a scar. It is very important, therefore, that all nurses should realize that in no circumstances whatever should a blister be allowed to form. The application should be removed before the skin becomes oedematous and dark red, as this state would result in blistering even when the plaster had been removed.

Mustard leaf. This is a preparation of mustard ready prepared on a piece of paper which very often has the instructions printed on the back or on the envelope in which the article is supplied by the chemist. The usual instructions indicate that the application should be moistened by soaking it in tepid water for a few minutes, shaken to free the paper of moisture and applied to a suitable area of the skin, gently covered, held or lightly bandaged in position for a few minutes—not more than 20—and subsequently treated as described in the case of mustard plaster.

Belladonna and opium plasters. These two plasters are commonly used for the relief of muscular rigidity, spasm and pain. It is usual for the doctor to state the size which is to be applied, from 4 to 6 inches square being a usual application. The plaster, after being slightly warmed by holding the back of it against a jug of hot water, should be pressed on to the skin with the hands until it adheres, care having been taken that the area of skin is whole and free from abrasions. It may be necessary to snip the edges in order to make it fit without creasing, as creases in plaster are apt to become uncomfortable and may lead to soreness. As a rule this type of plaster is left on until the edges curl up, though it may sometimes be ordered for a specified time.

A belladonna plaster is occasionally applied to the breast in order to limit the secretion of milk when a mother has lost her baby. It is important to watch her carefully for any signs of belladonna poisoning.

LINIMENTS

Liniments are soapy, oily preparations containing drugs which are rubbed into the skin, usually in order to produce a local effect by stimulating the circulation, and so effecting some degree of counterirritation or resulting in soothing of spasm and pain, according to the ingredients contained in it.

To apply a liniment. Having arranged the patient in a position in which he can be relaxed and comfortable throughout the application, the pillows and bedclothes should be rearranged so that the part to be treated is easily accessible. The articles required at the bedside are a tray on which is placed the liniment, a gallipot into which the amount of liniment to be used is to be poured, and a bowl of hot water in which the gallipot can be placed so that the liniment will be warm before it is applied. A towel or two are needed to protect the bedclothes, and on one of these the nurse wipes the back of the hand in which the liniment is transferred from the gallipot to the patient's skin. A pad of wool, bandage and safety pin should be provided for covering the area afterwards.

Liniments in common use include: *A.B.C. liniment*, containing aconite, belladonna and chloroform, used for the relief of pain in lumbago, neuritis and rheumatism; *camphorated oil*, containing camphor, which is used as a mild counterirritant for application to the front and back of the chest in cases of laryngitis, tracheitis and bronchitis; *oil of wintergreen*, or the equivalent chemical preparation, *methylsalicylate*, which is specifically used in the treatment of rheumatism. In these three instances, and in most other cases except where contraindicated, the liniment is warmed before use. A little is poured on to the palm of the hand, and rubbed well into the skin, the process being repeated for a duration of from 10 to 15 minutes until the skin is well reddened. It is important for all nurses to realize that this reddening of the skin is an indispensable part of the treatment.

The area which has been treated is then covered with warm wool, to protect the personal clothing from the liniment which may remain on, in order to keep the part as warm as possible so that more effective absorption occurs.

Iodine. Preparations of iodine are painted on to the skin either because of its antiseptic action, as in preparation for cutting operations, or in order to act as a counterirritant.

Before applying iodine it is very important that the skin should be dry. Iodine is a preparation in alcohol, which readily evaporates when exposed to the air. If evaporation does not take place, a blister will be caused when the part is covered up by personal or bed clothing, because of the retention of the iodine vapours. It is important, therefore, that a surface of skin painted with iodine should not be covered up until the nurse is sure that the skin is perfectly dry.

Application. The articles required at the bedside are a tray on which is placed a bottle of iodine, a gallipot into which a small quantity can be poured just before it is required for use, either a camelhair brush or a cotton wool swab in forceps, with which to apply the iodine, and a layer of lint or linen to cover the part so as to prevent soiling of the patient's personal clothing or bedclothes.

The patient should be prepared as for the application of liniment. The bedclothing needs particular attention as iodine stains linen very badly. The nurse should be quite sure as to which is the area to be treated and the exact size of this area. A layer of iodine should be painted very evenly over the skin, allowed to dry, and the process then repeated. It is a good plan to apply the first layer in vertical strokes, the second in horizontal strokes, and so on. Application will be made until the part is either a light brown or a dark brown as required. A nurse might overdo this application, not realizing how dark a colour she will obtain until the iodine has dried, but if this happens it is possible to wipe off some of the iodine with swabs wet with alcohol.

If the patient complains of burning after the application has been considered dry and covered up by the nurse, she should inspect the area to see what has happened. It may be that the patient has perspired and the skin become wet. In this case she should wipe the skin over with alcohol and allow it to dry before it is covered up again.

OINTMENTS

Ointments are preparations of fatty substances either of lanoline or lard, or of liquid paraffin or vaseline, containing in many cases a drug for application to the surface of the body.

Ointments may be used:

(*a*) To protect an abraded or raw surface, and in this case the base should be non-absorbent in character—liquid paraffin or vaseline. In addition to protecting the part, the ointment may contain some healing substance, such as zinc, eucalyptus or menthol, or some antiseptic substance such as creosote or carbolic, or something with antiparasitic properties, such as mercury. When the ointment is to be used for either of these purposes it is usually spread on lint or gauze. If the surface to which it is to be applied is raw or abraded, the articles used should be sterile.

To spread ointment on lint, the nurse should prepare an ointment slab and spatula or knife, and if the ointment is hard she will require a jug of hot water in which to heat the spatula. The ointment may be spread on the smooth side of lint or linen. It should be evenly and thickly spread, like evenly buttered bread. If the ointment is required to be applied in strips as in the case of Scott's dressing (see below), it is best to spread it over a sheet of material first and then to cut it into strips of the desired size as in this way time is economized and the edges of the material are more evenly covered with the ointment. When an application is to be made to the face, a piece of lint of the desired size is spread with ointment and a mask is made, by cutting holes for the eyes, nostrils and mouth.

(*b*) An ointment may be used for the purpose of counterirritation, and in this case it should be rubbed in vigorously.

(*c*) When an ointment is used in order to convey a drug into the circulation by absorption through the skin, the treatment is carried out by inunction, which is described on p. 322. In this case the base used is of an animal fat which will be readily absorbed, such as lanoline.

When ointment is used to protect the skin round an opening made of some part of the alimentary tract, as in a case of gastrostomy, duodenostomy or colostomy, the nurse has to consider whether the secretion from the wound is likely to effect alteration in the fat used. If, for example, the discharge contains pancreatic fluid, this will alter the character of animal fat, and in such a case, therefore, she must use some preparation which will not be affected, such as liquid paraffin or vaseline.

Scott's dressing. This is an application of mercury—unguentum hydrarg. co.—containing mercury, olive oil and camphor, but although it is prepared in the form of an ointment its mode of application requires special description.

The ointment is rather hard and should therefore be warmed before it is spread on the lint or linen, which should then be cut into strips of about 1½ to 2 inches wide. It is usually applied to a joint in order to reduce inflammation, such as may occur in chronic synovitis of the knee. The ointment application is covered up by strapping firmly applied, and by this means not only an application of mercury but at the same time an application of pressure is employed, which will facilitate the reduction of the swelling as the mercury produces its effect.

To apply. The joint should be washed, thoroughly dried, and shaved if necessary. The strips of linen spread with ointment are applied from 2 or 3 inches below the joint to 2 or 3 inches above it. The first strip is applied well below, and is crossed on the outer aspect of the joint; the second and subsequent strips overlap each preceding strip by half an inch and are carried up to above the knee. Strips of strapping slightly wider than the strips of linen are then applied in the same way, beginning on the skin half an inch below the first layer of linen and continuing over the joint to half an inch above the top layer. The strapping is applied firmly and each layer is crossed, over the outer aspect of the joint, so that the crossings lie directly one above the other and form an even pattern (see fig. 111, p. 238). This application will require to be removed every week. The indication for renewing it will be that it becomes loose as the inflammatory condition of the joint lessens, the swelling decreases and the joint becomes reduced in size. Before making a fresh application the nurse should wash the area thoroughly with hot water and soap to remove all stale ointment.

The strapping should be covered by a firm bandage as the mercurial ointment is black and may stain the patient's personal clothing. Moreover, there is less danger that the strapping may become curled up at the edges if it is kept in position by means of a bandage.

Scott's dressing contains 12 per cent of mercury, and the nurse should therefore know the symptoms of mercurial poisoning and be able to recognize any early symptoms that may show themselves. It is advisable when caring for such patients as are submitted to this treatment to make careful inquiries regarding their appetite, as one of the earliest symptoms of mercurial poisoning is nausea, loss of appetite and a nasty taste in the mouth.

APPLICATION OF WAX, UNNA'S PASTE AND GLYCERINE PREPARATIONS

Wax. Either *paraffin wax* or *ambrine wax*, which is a proprietary preparation, may be used as a dressing for inflamed and raw surfaces. In addition, ambrine wax is used for the relief of many painful conditions.

Method of application. In the case of paraffin wax, it should be heated to 130° F., while ambrine wax may be heated to 140° or 150° F. To apply ambrine wax to an inflamed area in which there are some raw surfaces, the wax should be heated and kept standing in a container of very hot water so that it does not lose heat. Forceps and wool swabs will be required with which to apply the wax, and flakes of cotton wool to cover it, and these will be secured in position by a bandage.

Saline solution and swabs should be supplied with which to wash the area, and sterile towels to dry it thoroughly. It is a very important part of the preparation that the skin should be thoroughly dry, as wax will not adhere to a moist surface, but instead, will be seen to rise from it in blisters.

The area having been cleansed and dried, the wax will be painted on to the skin, in an even layer, the nurse having first tested the temperature on the skin at the flexure of her elbow, with a swab of wool. Having applied the first layer smoothly on the skin, it is covered with wisps of wool, the edges of each layer of wool being fastened on to the wax beneath by use of a swab dipped in the hot melted wax. When the dressing is sufficiently firm, a layer of cotton wool is placed over it and this is bandaged on.

When properly applied the wax will be seen to be closely adherent to the skin so that, when the dressing is changed, it has to be detached. It peels off readily, since the wax is of a soft, pliant nature.

A wax dressing is valuable for all superficial inflammatory lesions, and also for burns of the first, second and third degrees. When used for either of these purposes it is usual to change the dressing after 24 hours—the second dressing can be left on for several days.

Unna's paste. This is a soothing preparation containing zinc oxide, glycerine, gelatine and water. It is used in the treatment of dry eczema and for many irritable skin conditions. It is also specially valuable in the treatment of chronic ulcers, including varicose ulcers.

Application. The paste is melted in a gluepot, or by placing it in a saucepan of hot water on a gas ring. The part to which it is applied must first be thoroughly cleansed, and as far as possible crusts and scabs should be picked off; if the skin is hairy it should be shaved. The melted paste is then applied, with a broad camelhair brush, to a thickness corresponding to that of a rubber glove, so that a pliable covering is made on the skin. This first layer is either covered by a layer of gauze, or wisps of wool may be used as described in the application of wax. Further layers of paste are painted over this, and the process is repeated until the dressing is of the desired thickness. This application does not need covering with an outer layer of wool, as it forms a firm and gelatinous casing—any superfluous wool on the surface can be picked off, and a bandage carried over the paste to protect it.

An Unna's paste dressing can be left on for a week or ten days, when it will require to be changed—if a second dressing is employed it may be left on for two or three weeks. *In the treatment of varicose veins* an application of Unna's paste is sometimes made in conjunction with the application of an elastoplast bandage. This is also a proprietary preparation, the bandages have a certain degree of elasticity and when applied fairly tightly give considerable pressure which tends to improve the circulation of the limb.

Glycerines. The preparations of glycerine most commonly used are *glycerine of borax*, used in cleaning the mouth; *glycerine of belladonna*, which is used to relieve pain in neuritis and rheumatism, phlebitis and thrombosis—it also lessens secretion and therefore assists in the termination of inflammation by resolution which is aimed at in the treatment of thrombosis; *glycerine of ichthyol* is an antiseptic substance which smells rather like tar and is prepared from fossilized fish—it is a very valuable local application for the relief of inflammation, and is particularly useful in the inflammation following severe sunburn, mosquito and bug bites. It is used for the treatment of the inflammation which occurs in erysipelas, and also as a local vaginal application in cases of chronic discharge.

Both belladonna and ichthyol are dark in colour, and being glycerine preparations become absorbed by lint, wool and bandage used as coverings, so that care must also be taken to avoid staining of the patient's personal or bed clothing.

APPLICATION OF LEECHES

Leeches are bloodsucking parasites which are used to relieve congestion and pain, particularly in eye surgery. They are also used to relieve cyanosis, when applied to the chest in cases of cardiac congestion, and in the same situation for the relief of pain in pneumonia.

The articles required, in addition to the number of leeches, will be several test tubes threequarters filled with cotton wool—each leech will be collected in a tube, tail end in, and by this means will be applied to the patient's skin. Some warm water is needed in order to prepare the skin. Soap and antiseptics may not be used. The object is to render the skin slightly red and moist to attract the leech, and for this reason also the skin should not be dried. A leech likes a moist surface, and is used to attacking its prey under water.

A piece of lint or linen with a tiny hole cut in the centre will be required, through which the leech will be allowed to bite the patient. The body of the leech may be allowed to remain in the test tube, or the tube may be withdrawn and then the leech will be on the piece of lint—the slimy parasites should never be allowed in contact with the patient's skin.

A bowl of 1–20 carbolic is provided in which to place the leech when it falls off, and this solution will destroy the leech which can then be put down the sluice.

Pads are needed to form a pressure dressing in case the leech bite bleeds more than is desired, and these may be made of rounds of lint, increasing in size from small to large ones. Strips of lint can be arranged starwise over the bite and, as all the strips will cross over the point of the bite, the greatest pressure will be applied here (this method is illustrated in fig. 45, p. 190); or two rolls of lint may be used, one across the other. Whatever form of pressure dressing is employed, it must be either strapped or bandaged in position.

A fomentation may be employed if it is considered necessary to encourage the bleeding to continue.

To apply. If possible explain to the patient what is going to be done, but do not let him see the leeches. Having prepared the skin and left it damp, place the piece of lint with the hole in the centre over the part to be treated; collect the leech in a test tube and render the lint taut upon the skin, so that the leech does not get away beneath the lint, but bites exactly where the hole lies. When the leech is holding well, the test tube may be gently withdrawn and the leech then rests lightly on the lint.

If a leech refuses to bite, the skin may be pricked with a sterilized needle to withdraw a tiny drop of blood. This method is better than applying milk, as the latter may not be sterile.

A leech should never be pulled off or its teeth will be left in the wound and may give rise to sepsis. If there is any reason for removing it before it has had its fill and is ready to fall off, a sprinkle of dry salt on its head will render it thoroughly uncomfortable, and it will loose its hold.

A leech draws a very small quantity of blood, and the amount withdrawn is useful enough when taken, say, from near the eye; but when leeches are applied to the chest it is usual to follow their removal by fomentations in order to extract more blood, and thus as much as half a pint of blood may be removed.

If the leech bite continues to bleed, it may be necessary to use a pressure dressing which has been previously described. As the leech feeds, it secretes a substance called *hirudin* from glands in the region of its head which prevents clotting of the blood it sucks into its stomach. Some of this substance gets into the patient's tissues and prevents clotting there. It is because of this that bleeding may continue.

A leech bite always leaves a tiny white triangular scar like a bird's footmark, which persists for a long time, and such scars are sometimes observed on patients admitted to hospital.

COUNTERIRRITANTS

A counterirritant is a means of producing superficial irritation or inflammation with the object of relieving a symptom arising in the deeper tissues—such as pain—or with the object, by bringing blood to the surface, of relieving a more deeply seated congestion. Counterirritants act thus by producing a condition of hyperaemia, and by this means they alter the blood supply of the part to which they are applied; alternatively, their effect may be produced by reflex stimulation of an organ which may be associated with the area of skin to which the application is made.

Counterirritants are classified according to the effects they produce.

Rubefacients are those which cause reddening of the skin. Many of the applications already described, all applications of heat—including those to which some irritating substance has been added—turpentine and mustard act as counterirritants. Any means which produces hyperaemia can be included, such as the brisk rubbing of a part, as for example when a liniment is rubbed in, and if the liniment should contain a substance stimulating to the circulation, such as camphor or turpentine, the effect is enhanced.

Painting the skin with different chemicals, such as the iodine painting already described, and the application of various irritating substances such as a mustard plaster are other means of reddening the skin and so producing a form of counterirritation.

Vesicants. The degree of counterirritation, next in severity to reddening, is the production of a blister. An agent is chosen which produces a fairly clean blister, only raising the epidermis and leaving a comparatively well-stimulated raw area beneath, which will heal fairly rapidly without sloughing or scarring. *Cantharides* is the substance mainly used for this purpose, and it is prepared from a blistering fly prevalent in South America and Spain. It is supplied in the form of plaster, ointment and fluid—*liquor epispasticus*—and as collodion—*collodion vesicans*. Probably the most convenient form for ready application is the prepared plaster, made up on strong linen which has a green back, and is marked out in inch squares very conveniently for cutting up, since the majority of blisters are ordered to be either half an inch or an inch square. The active side of the plaster is blackish grey colour and slightly tacky in consistence.

In all cases, the area of skin which is to be blistered must be aseptically prepared; therefore, in whatever form the blistering agent is used, the nurse must also take to the bedside the articles needed for cleaning the skin and for covering the blister. The articles required include materials for cleansing the skin, a blistering agent which may be fluid, ointment, or specially prepared plaster. If blistering fluid or ointment is employed a sterilized glass rod should be supplied with which to rub the blistering agent into the skin.

To apply blistering plaster. Having prepared the skin, and cut the plaster to the size ordered, if cut square the corners should be snipped off as this will provide a round blister rather than a square one, and the blistered area will heal the more readily from not having angular corners into which fluid might collect and so delay the process of healing. The blistering plaster is applied to the prepared skin and pressed firmly on to it. It is a slight advantage to warm the blistering plaster beforehand, by holding its back against a jug containing hot water.

When applied, the plaster may be covered by a layer of gauze or wool which should be very lightly bandaged on, in order not to cause pressure on the blister as it rises. A rather more scientific method of covering is arranged as follows: Take a piece of guttapercha tissue 4 inches larger than the blistering plaster used. Fold a pleat into it vertically up the middle, and horizontally across the piece of tissue (as shown in illustration, fig. 46, letter D, p. 190). This is placed over the plaster and retained in contact with the skin by the application of small strips of strapping, as shown in the illustration.

As the blister rises, the pleat which lies over the plaster gradually unfolds, and this has two advantages—(1) the progress of the rising blister can be observed, and (2) there is no pressure upon it which would give rise to pain.

The application of blistering ointment. Having cleaned the skin, the area to be blistered should be outlined with an oily substance—either olive oil or vaseline—evenly applied in the form of a circle by means of a dressed glass rod or tiny camelhair brush. A probe or glass rod is then dressed with cotton wool, covered with the blistering ointment and rubbed vigorously over the part to be treated. The rubbing should be continued for a few minutes until the area is well reddened.

Blistering fluid. The application is made in much the same way as described above for the application of ointment. A point to be remembered in this case is that one layer of fluid will not blister a fairly tough skin, and it will certainly not produce a blister on a part that has been previously treated. Blistering fluid requires to be thoroughly well rubbed into the area treated.

Collodion vesicans. This is a special form of collodion which contains a blistering agent. To apply it, the skin is prepared, and the area may or may not be marked out with oil as described above—this depends upon the proficiency of the nurse who is to make the application. The collodion is painted on to the prepared area. This application need not be covered, unless the patient is restless, in which case it will be advisable lest the collodion be rubbed off. When this blister rises the layer of collodion will be seen adherent to the risen skin.

To help a blister to rise. A cantharides application should result in blistering within 6 to 8 hours, and in some cases the blister may rise much earlier than this. If the application does not produce a blister within this time, it may be that the material used was stale and had lost its potency; or it may be that the patient has a particularly tough skin—in either case it would be advisable to apply heat over the blister. An application of dry heat such as a hot-water bag may be sufficient, or fomentations or poultices may be needed. If this is not effective, it would be advisable to get some fresh material for the blister, and to pay very great attention to reddening the skin when applying it, in order to create a good hyperaemia before the blistering agent is applied.

To dress a blister. When a blister has risen the nurse should take to the bedside the following articles: Sterile dissecting forceps and scissors, with which to snip the blister and so evacuate the fluid and, if desirable, remove the dead epidermis. Some dry absorbent wool swabs, with which to catch the fluid as it runs out of the blister. If this fluid is allowed to run over the adjacent skin, seeing that it contains blistering agent, it may cause irritation.

A dressing suitable for the raw area is also supplied, and this may be zinc or any other healing ointment, spread on lint, or alternatively gauze soaked in liquid paraffin and flavine may be used. The dressing applied should be the exact size of the blistered area, and should be kept in position by some means which will not retain fluid, but will permit of evaporation. Any serum exuding from this raw area will contain blistering agent and, if it is confined, may continue to injure the tissues beyond the effect which was intended by the original application.

To retain the dressing in position. Strips of strapping may be used to retain the dressing in position, and these may be applied all round the margins of it, or in the form of a 'gate' (see fig. 46, letter E, p. 190).

To cut a gate of strapping, take a piece at least double or treble the size of the blistered area, fold it and cut strips out, so that the strapping is similar to a three, four or five-barred gate in appearance. By this means the dressing is kept adherent all round its edges and has one or two strips of strapping across it, and yet it permits air to reach the dressing, so that evaporation readily takes place.

The dressing will require changing twice a day at first and then once a day. Healing takes place fairly rapidly.

A flying blister. By this is meant that a blistering agent is applied for a short time, long enough only to redden the skin, and a number of these applications are made round a given area.

Cantharides is one of the drugs which are irritants to the kidneys. It is therefore important to test the urine for albumin for a day or two after its application, for fear lest any untoward effects have been caused. The administration of liberal bland fluids will, by stimulating urinary secretion, tend to prevent any irritation.

CUPPING

Cupping is a form of counterirritation by which the dilation of the subcutaneous blood vessels is effected. Heated glass cups are used and a partial vacuum created; the prepared cup or glass is applied to the area to be treated, and consequently the superficial tissues are attracted into it to fill the partial vacuum, thus bringing a good deal of blood to the surface. Some special cupping glasses, described as *Bier's* or *Klapp's suction cups*, have rubber bulbs attached, by means of which the vacuum can be created after the glass object has been inverted on to the skin, thus obviating the trouble of heating the glasses.

Conditions in which cupping may be ordered are inflammatory conditions of the chest such as bronchitis and pleurisy in which case one to two dozen cups will be applied over the chest wall. An application is made over the loins for the relief of renal congestion in acute nephritis. Cupping is one of the most comfortable forms of treatment used in lumbago, since it results in the relief of rigidity and pain more rapidly than does any other form of treatment.

Application of dry cupping. It does not matter very much in what way the vacuum is created. A nurse who is experienced can manage this by using a flaming torch with which to heat the glasses. The following is quite a useful way for nurses to practise using this application, and it is also quite effective and has the additional advantage that it is unlikely that the patient will be burnt by this method.

The articles required (see fig. 47, p. 191) are cupping glasses, a little methylated spirit in a bowl, a pair of dissecting forceps, some small squares of blotting paper, and either a box of matches or a lighted taper. Vaseline and swabs, with which to smear the edges of the glass in order to make it adhere more closely to the skin, should also be provided.

Method. Holding the cup upright in her hand, the nurse drops part of the blotting paper into the methylated spirit, lifts it out by means of the dissecting forceps, and lights it in the flame; she then drops the morsel of lighted paper into the cup she is holding and, before the blotting paper has burnt out, inverts the cup on to the area of skin she wished to treat. She will notice that the cup adheres closely, and that the tissues rise into the partial vacuum created. The process is repeated until sufficient cups have been applied. They should not be placed too closely together. The nurse should watch the skin under the cups very carefully; it will soon become pink, and eventually be a deep bluish red. The cups should be removed before any mottling occurs, and before petechial points of haemorrhage appear on the skin.

To remove a cup. The cups are usually allowed to remain on for some 10 to 20 minutes. To remove, steady with one hand placed on the cup ready to lift it off as air is allowed to enter beneath it. The nurse inserts her thumbnail under the edge of the cup, and will hear the noise made by the rapid entry of air, and as the cup is loosened it is lifted carefully off. The cupped area will be very sore and tender and should, therefore, be covered by warm wool which may be lightly bandaged on, pressure being avoided.

When a second application is made it is advisable to avoid putting the cups in exactly the same position—the rim should not rest on the same spot as before.

Wet cupping. This treatment consists in the withdrawal of blood by incisions made in the skin before the cupping glasses are applied. The vacuum thus created results in drawing blood into the cups, but it is a means of bloodletting which is rarely employed today. If the nurse is ordered to prepare the articles she will require materials to render the skin surgically clean, and sharp knives for making the small incisions. The cupping glasses should be sterile.

The forms of bloodletting used today are venesection, and for small quantities the application of leeches.

Chapter 8

General Applications

General treatments for the reduction of temperature—Tepid and cold sponging, exposed sponging—cold packing—Brandt's bath—Ice cradling—Affusion—Applications of heat—Hot baths and hot sponging—Radiant heat baths and electric blankets—Hot wet pack—Hot dry pack—Vapour bath—Hot air bath—Warm baths and medicated baths—Aerated and foam baths

GENERAL TREATMENTS FOR THE REDUCTION OF TEMPERATURE

General applications of cold are chiefly employed for the reduction of temperature. The water used is considerably below the temperature of the body. When immersion in a bath is employed, the water quickly absorbs heat and in this way the temperature of the body is fairly rapidly lowered; when packs and spongings are used, cooling is produced mainly by evaporation of the water applied to the surface of the body. Evaporation is more rapid and more effective when the surfaces which are being treated are being exposed to the air. When this method of sponging is adopted the treatment is described as 'exposed sponging'.

In some cases a liquid which evaporates more rapidly than water is employed—such as some form of alcohol, or a mixture of alcohol and water. The more rapid the evaporation produced, the more effective will the cooling process be.

In addition to its effect in lowering the temperature of the body, the result of an application of cold improves the patient's general condition. This is brought about owing to an increased circulation of blood in the subcutaneous tissue, which is one of the reactions expected to follow an application of cold, and partly also because of the reduction of toxaemia which results from stimulation of tissue activity and is followed by an increased elimination of the excretory waste products, particularly those from the skin and kidneys.

The reduction of toxaemia, accompanied by relief of general discomfort, will in many cases render restless patients more comfortable and more peaceful, and so conduce to sleep.

At the commencement of a general application of cold, the patient may shiver violently, but this should not continue. In the first place it is due to contraction of the involuntary muscles in the skin in an endeavour to produce heat, and this is accompanied by contraction of the involuntary muscles in the blood vessels of the skin which should soon be followed by an improvement in the circulation generally, when the shivering will cease. Prolonged shivering would be an indication that the treatment should cease and would suggest that the patient's general condition is too low to respond to the treatment by the expected reaction. Nurses will rarely, if ever, meet with this emergency, as the physician will have considered the patient's condition before a general application of cold is ordered.

As the result of improvement of the circulation the action of the heart is improved, and this is manifested by a fuller and stronger pulse; but when a fairly drastic application of cold is made the pulse may become weak and rapid and barely perceptible at the outset, and if such untoward symptoms are very marked a dose of brandy is often given, to facilitate promptness of reaction, and a few minutes later the expected improvement will be noticed. Tepid and cold spongings are the applications of cold generally made. Cold packs, Brandt's bath, ice cradling and affusion are more rarely employed.

SPONGING

Either tepid water (*tepid sponging*) between 75° and 80° F., or cold water (*cold sponging*) below 70° F., may be used for the reduction of temperature, and this form of treatment is frequently employed when it reaches 103° F. or over. In some cases of delayed toxaemia, sponging is employed whenever the temperature reaches 102° F.

The **articles required** (see fig. 51, p. 194) are, *tepid* or *cold water*, and either a jug of cooler water or some pieces of ice, in order to keep the temperature of the water even, as the heat of the patient's body is transferred to it by the sponges used. A *lotion thermometer* should be kept in the water so that any rise of temperature can be observed. It is usual to begin the sponging with water at the maximum degree of temperature mentioned, namely 80° F., gradually cooling it to 75° F.

Several sponges will be required; some sisters use four, others use six or eight. Two sponges should be used alternately, for the actual sponging treatment, and the spare sponges may be placed in contact with different parts of the skin of the patient's body, such as the nape of his neck, the axillae and groins. He may be given a sponge to hold in his hands, the object of these extra sponges being to cool parts of the body where heat proves very uncomfortable, and in parts where the skin is thin, and a liberal blood supply present—as in the axillae and groins—where rapid cooling may take place.

A *face towel* is supplied for drying the face—the only part of the patient's body which is dried. The water is allowed to evaporate from the remainder of the skin, as it is by this evaporation that cooling takes place.

A tray should be ready prepared for the ordinary routine treatment of the back, and this will be performed at the termination of the sponging.

Two thin bath blankets or bathsheets are placed—one beneath and one above the patient—unless a sheet—which is cooler—is preferred for covering him. Some sisters put a mackintosh beneath the under blanket, but this should not be necessary if the sponging is carefully performed and the water not allowed to run on to the bed.

A pail should be ready at the bedside in case it becomes necessary to change the water, as might happen when tepid sponging is being carried out, because the heat of the water rises rapidly, and the addition of cold water to the basin may not be sufficient to keep the temperature of the water even. It is a good plan to have two basins at the bedside, one of very cold water in which to wring the sponges out after taking them off the hot body, before transferring them to the second basin which contains the tepid water that is being used for sponging.

Method. The patient having been prepared ready stripped beneath a sheet or blanket as described, his face is sponged and dried. This makes him feel more comfortable, and if extra sponges are used these are then placed against the parts of the body chosen. The nurse now proceeds to work with two sponges alternately—first the upper extremity is sponged, working on the arm on the opposite side of the bed to that on which the nurse is standing. She grasps the hand of the arm undergoing treatment and, holding the sponge as full of water as possible, passes it slowly over the skin from the top of the shoulder to the fingertips, taking care to see that small beads of water are left on the skin. The hand with which the nurse holds the sponge must be relaxed, otherwise she will squeeze water out of it, and little rivulets will run on to the bed.

Having made the first stroke she places the used sponge in the cold water to cool it and proceeds with the next stroke; eight or ten strokes should conclude the treatment of an upper limb, and this should occupy from two to three minutes. The limb is then placed by the side of the patient's body either beneath the covering sheet or allowed to lie above it. The other arm is then sponged in the same way. It gives the patient pleasure if he is allowed to dabble his hand in the bowl of water at the conclusion of the treatment of each arm, and the basin may be held over the bed for this purpose or allowed to rest on the bed, and whilst the hand is in the water the nurse swills the tepid water up over the forearms as far as she can.

The stationary sponges are changed from time to time as considered convenient, but they should, if possible, be changed from at least four to six times during the treatment.

The front of the body is next treated, and the strokes of the cool wet sponge over the front of the chest should be made in circles, not just backwards and forwards, as vertical strokes with a cold wet sponge might cause the patient to flinch or gasp. At the sides of the body, the strokes may be vertical, but the subcutaneous tissue is thick in this area and the sponging hereabouts should occupy from three to four minutes.

The lower extremities come next, one limb being sponged at a time. It may be flexed at the hip and knee, with the foot placed flat on the bed, but it must be supported by the nurse; or the limb may be sponged lying flat on the bed and lifted whilst the under part is treated. The treatment of the lower limbs should occupy from eight to ten minutes, and roughly from twelve to fourteen strokes of the sponge from top to bottom will be sufficient. If it can be managed, a basin should be placed on the bed and each foot in turn held in the basin, the nurse swilling the water up over the lower leg as she did in the case of the forearm. After removing the foot from the water and placing the bowl on the locker, she should separate the toes and remove any excess water from the hollows between them.

Special attention should be paid to the groin, the inner aspect of the thigh and the popliteal space. The skin is comparatively thin in these areas, and hot spots are very frequent here, and treatment of these materially assist in cooling the body by a reflex effect.

Finally the patient is turned, if permissible, and his back is sponged. The tissues of the back are very thick. Long sweeping strokes should be made with the wet sponges, and special attention paid to the thick muscles on either side of the spine. At least five minutes should be taken in sponging a back—and more, if as so often happens the patient finds it very comforting and soothing. In order to save turning the patient again, the toilet of the lower part of the back is carried out for the prevention of pressure sores. The bath blanket or sheet beneath the patient is taken out, the patient's personal clothing put on, and the bed made up as usual.

Throughout the treatment, whenever possible a cold compress should be kept on the patient's forehead, and changed as often as necessary in order to keep it cool. He may also have a hot-water bottle at his feet, although this is not invariably used.

Recording the temperature. The temperature is taken ten minutes after the sponging and the result charted—a fall of between two and three degrees being considered satisfactory. The temperature obtained by

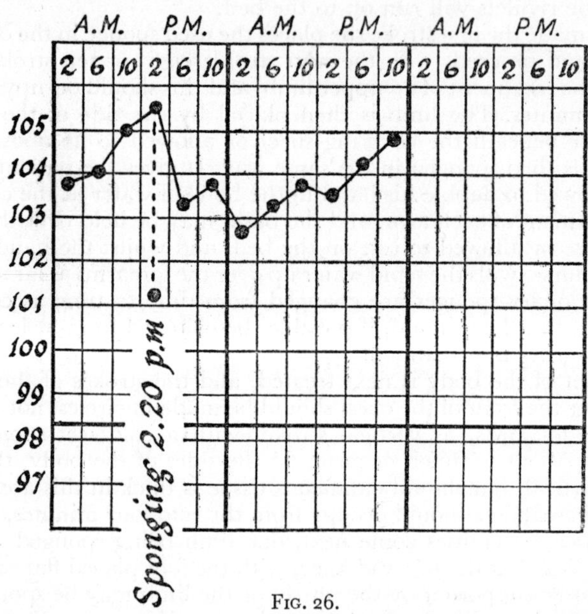

Fig. 26.

Tepid sponging for reduction of temperature in high fever. Note that the effect of sponging is maintained for 24 hours, when the temperature is very high again. At this point sponging would, very likely, be repeated.

sponging a patient or reducing fever by any similar method is charted as described on the accompanying illustration.

Observation of patient's condition. The general condition of the patient should be very carefully watched for any signs (already indicated on p. 121) which would suggest that the reaction expected would be retarded or absent. Untoward signs include weakness and irregularity of the pulse; pallor or cyanosis; anxiety of facial expression, the appearance of perspiration on the face; complaints of palpitation and sighing or irregularity of respiration. Such signs are comparatively rare, and they are more likely to be caused by injudicious movement and undue exposure of the patient during this treatment than by the cold applications themselves. Should they occur, however, treatment might be suspended for a time and the patient given a warm drink; a stimulant may be necessary in some cases, and he should be covered up and kept warm for a few minutes before the treatment can safely be continued.

Exposed sponging. This more drastic form of treatment is carried out in exactly the same way as described above, but the patient, instead of being covered by a sheet, lies naked and exposed on the surface of his bed, wearing only a loincloth, or a towel to cover his loins. The exposure of the surface of the body to the air causes rapid evaporation and cooling, and the treatment must be quickly performed if chilling is to be avoided.

COLD PACKING

Either cold or iced water may be employed in the application of a cold wet pack.

The **articles required** and the method are shown in illustration fig. 52, p. 195.

BRANDT'S BATH

Brandt's bath is the most drastic form of cold application that is ever practised; it is both cumbersome in use and severe in its effects. It is rarely employed.

Method. A bath is wheeled to the bedside and the patient is lowered into the water. The shock of immersion may be serious. The pulse and colour should be watched and a stimulant given if necessary.

The *duration of the bath* may be three minutes, or from five to ten minutes. For a first treatment the temperature of the bath is not usually lower than 85° F., but for subsequent treatments, and even in the first instance if the patient can stand it, the temperature of the bath may be lowered 10° or 20° by gently pouring in iced water at the corners and stirring it up to reach the surface of the body whilst the patient is undergoing treatment. In this way the temperature of the water may be lowered to 65° F.

At the termination of the treatment the patient is covered by a light blanket or bathsheet and allowed to remain undisturbed for half an hour. At the end of this time his temperature is taken in order to record the effect of the bath, his clothes are put on and his bed made up as usual.

ICE CRADLING

Ice cradling is a form of cold application which is gentle compared with those already described and, although it may be used for the reduction of fever, it is more generally used *to cause a gradual reduction of the temperature of a patient's bed during very hot weather, or in very hot climates.*

The **articles required** and the method of application are shown in fig. 54, p. 197.

AFFUSION

Affusion is a method of reducing temperature by pouring cool or cold water over the body of a patient who lies on a mackintosh and sheet, the mackintosh being so arranged that water can be directed from it into a pail or pails at the bedside. The patient may wear a cotton garment, or he may be stripped and covered only by a single layer of cotton sheet. By means of small watering cans water is sprinkled over his body and allowed to run into the pails at the bedside. The height from which the water is poured increases or decreases the tonic effect of this treatment and of the consequent reaction.

APPLICATIONS OF HEAT

By a general application of heat the heat of the body is increased, loss of heat is prevented and perspiration is induced. As a result of increased activity of the sweat glands, the rate of the elimination of fluid is promoted. In this way the work of the kidneys is relieved, and this form of treatment is therefore especially useful in cases of renal failure in which symptoms of suppression occur.

The immediate result of a hot application is to stimulate the nerve endings in the skin and, as this increases the activity of the central nervous system, the pulse rate also is increased. In certain cases some degree of congestion of the internal organs, particularly of the brain, occurs, and it is to prevent the discomforts associated with this—such as headache and throbbing of the veins of the head—that a cold compress is applied to the head during the administration of any general application of heat.

A little later on in the treatment the stimulating effect is followed by relaxation; and during this time the patient feels drowsy and comfortable; but the vital organs, previously stimulated, share in this depression, and it is for this reason that careful watch is kept on the pulse throughout the administration, so that any untoward degree of depression can be anticipated, the treatment discontinued and first aid measures—including rest and stimulants—applied before any serious symptoms can arise.

Generally speaking it may be said that the hot applications requiring the least disturbance of the patient are to be preferred—that vapour and hot air baths are rarely employed and that the tendency is to use radiant heat and not bathing.

HOT BATHS AND HOT SPONGING

Apart from cleansing baths, hot baths and hot spongings may be employed:

(*a*) As a prophylactic to possible infection, and for the relief of shivering in persons who have been exposed to severe wetting and chilling.

(*b*) As a prophylactic treatment at the outset of a severe cold in order to assist the skin to act, thus promoting diaphoresis and stimulating the subcutaneous circulation.

(*c*) For the relief of fatigue following physical strain in conditions of exhaustion.

(*d*) As an application of warmth in the treatment of shock and collapse, particularly in cases where dehydration is a marked feature, as in infants suffering from diarrhoea and vomiting.

(*e*) In spastic conditions, as when employed for the relief of muscular rigidity in convulsions, and for the relief of restlessness in cases of chorea.

The **articles required** for bathing in a bath include under these special conditions a bath half full of water at a temperature of 100° F. The temperature will be raised gradually when the patient is in the bath to 105° or 110° F. Bath blankets—one is used to cover the patient's shoulders as he sits in the bath, and this blanket might be spread over the back part of the bath; a second blanket being used to cover the top of the bath so that the patient is sitting with his shoulders protected and the bath covered, and his body, thus in contact with the steam rising from the water, is in no danger of becoming chilled. A cold compress might be needed for his head during the treatment, and he should be given hot drinks if possible. A chair with warm blankets or bathsheets should be placed in readiness beside the bath on which he can sit and be dabbed dry before he is carried back to bed.

Throughout the treatment the nurse should stand by, taking the patient's pulse at the temple, watching his colour, the expression of his face for anxiety and distress, and the signs of perspiration which may be expected upon it. Any softness, irregularity, compressibility of pulse, or general signs of distress would indicate the necessity for removing the patient from the bath at once and laying him flat between warm blankets until he had recovered. A stimulant might be required.

The duration of the bath should be from 10 to 15 minutes. At the end of this time the patient should be placed on the chair beside the bath, wrapped in warm bathsheets, gently dabbed dry and put back to bed to rest. His bed clothing should be warm woollen and he should have a blanket next to him as he will probably go on perspiring. The effect of the bath as regards the perspiration produced should be particularly noted. He should be given fluids throughout as these will make up for the amount of water lost by the skin, and prevent exhaustion or prostration.

RADIANT HEAT BATHS AND ELECTRIC BLANKETS

A form of heat sometimes employed as a general application is administered by placing cradles fitted with electric light bulbs, anything from 12 to 30, arranged in rows on the apparatus, over the patient as he lies on the bed. The patient may be stripped and lying between blankets, the cradles being placed over him covered by blankets and quilt which should be tucked in at the bottom and sides of the bed, and carried closely up to the patient's neck. A thermometer is hung at a convenient point on one of the cradles where it can be conveniently inspected. Opinions differ as to whether the patient's body should be unshielded from the radiant heat or protected by a blanket of non-inflammable flannelette.

The patient having been placed in position the current should be turned on and the rising temperature of the bed carefully watched. Radiant heat cannot be borne at a greater temperature than 120° F. or a little over. The patient's skin should be kept under constant observation, as if he perspires it is possible that he will be badly burnt. During the administration of this form of treatment, the patient will probably feel uncomfortable, complaining that the heat in various isolated spots is almost impossible to bear. This is due to the fact that wherever moisture collects on the skin the heat rays seem to be absorbed, resulting in this uncomfortable degree of burning, which will not be relieved until the moisture has evaporated and the skin become quite dry again—and in the meantime, unless sweat is wiped off, the patient may be badly scalded.

The electric blanket is principally used in the treatment of mild degrees of shock. It is a large heating pad in which heat is generated by a current, run off the mains supply; the temperature is thermostatically controlled.

The electric blanket is placed on the bed and covered by an ordinary woollen blanket. It is heated, when possible, for two hours before it is required for a patient. The patient is placed on top of the woollen blanket and covered by another blanket. By this method the increase in body heat averages half a degree Fahrenheit per hour. If the patient is wrapped in the electric blanket the rate of rise increases but this method is not advocated.

The principle underlying the use of the electric blanket is the conduction of heat to the patient which prevents the loss of metabolic heat. This causes the patient no discomfort. Burns are less likely to occur than with an unshielded cradle but one disadvantage is that whereas with the cradle the temperature of the air around the patient's body can quickly be raised to a given degree and maintained at that level, in the case of the electric blanket the heat is invariable and the blanket only raises the body temperature half as quickly as the cradle.

HOT WET PACK

The articles required for a hot wet pack (see fig. 49, p. 192) are a long bed mackintosh which, covered by a dry blanket, is placed beneath the patient to protect the mattress.

A second dry blanket is placed over him, and he lies stripped of his personal clothing between these blankets.

Two thin old blankets are required for the wet pack, and a large wringer, if possible with sticks at each end for wringing. The blankets folded in the wringer may be placed in a sink or small bath. It has been found by experience that if water of 180° to 200° F. is poured over the pack in the bath, by the time the blankets are soaked through and wrung out the application is a little less than 120° F., which is about the required temperature.

The hot wet blankets are shaken until free of steam and the patient is gently and carefully wrapped in them.

A cold application—either a compress or icebag—should be provided for the head. Hot drinks will be administered to the patient during the treatment. A urinal should be ready at hand as patients, even those suffering from nephritis, are often stimulated to pass urine during this treatment, and this is possibly the result of some reflex stimulation of the kidneys occurring as the result of the general application of heat to the skin.

Several dry blankets may be placed round the patient after he is enclosed in the pack.

The *duration of the treatment* is from 20 to 30 minutes. The patient must be carefully observed for changes in colour, any signs of apparent distress, and for the presence of perspiration on his face, which would indicate that the treatment was being effective. The nurse standing by should wipe the perspiration from his face as it is apt to be very distressing to him, but she must be able to report to what extent he has perspired. Observation is made of the pulse at the temple—any weakness or irregularity might indicate the necessity for stopping the treatment. The patient should be given hot drinks throughout. If he complains of discomfort as the result of these, cool drinks may be given.

At the termination of the treatment the wet blankets should be gently taken away and the patient left lying undisturbed under hot dry blankets, lightly packed round him, and with several hot-water bottles in the bed, so that he may go on perspiring for an hour or so. He may then be sponged to remove sweat and make him feel fresh, and his bed is made in the usual way.

HOT DRY PACK

The patient is wrapped in hot dry blankets, surrounded by hot-water bottles, and is given mild diaphoretics such as spirit of nitrous ether, or hot lemon drinks. In some cases pilocarpine is ordered.

A hot dry pack is probably most often used as a simple nursing measure in the treatment of the early stages of a common cold, at the onset of influenza, or after a very severe wetting in order to prevent chilling. In this case it is usually preceded by a hot bath. In hospital practice a hot dry pack is used in certain cases of suppression of urine, when pilocarpine, which is a very powerful diaphoretic drug, is ordered. The patient is put into the pack before the drug, which is administered by hypodermic injection, is given, as it acts very quickly. Note should be made of the quantity of urine passed.

VAPOUR BATH

A vapour bath is an application of water vapour to the body which is made in order to increase the activity of the skin. It is rarely used. Some means by which steam can be passed into the bed in contact with the patient's body is employed. The temperature of the bath should not generally be raised above 120° F. The general condition of the patient should be carefully noted throughout the treatment. One form of apparatus used is shown in fig. 50, p. 193.

HOT AIR BATH

The same apparatus (see fig. 50) may be used but hot air, not vapour, is passed into the bed so that dry, hot, moving air is constantly supplied over the patient's skin. He feels no discomfort from this as, owing to convection, evaporation of moisture from the surface of the body is materially assisted.

The following points are of considerable importance, and must be carefully attended to:

(1) The heat of the bed must be very gradually raised, and it should take at least twenty minutes for the temperature to reach 140° F.—the average degree of heat employed when hot air is introduced. The mean range is from 120° to 180° F. For a first treatment it may be found impossible to proceed above 120° F.—much depends on the extent to which the skin is active. The treatment should be terminated if the skin does not act, as in this event, the patient is merely being made uncomfortable, his temperature is rising and the treatment is being harmful rather than beneficial to him. Nurses must realize the importance of this point and make accurate and careful observation of the state of the patient's skin.

(2) As the body is losing heat by evaporation of moisture induced by convection, another point of importance is that no two skin surfaces should be permitted to lie together, as this would prevent evaporation; the lower limbs should therefore be slightly separated and the arms should lie on each side of, but away from, the sides of the body.

WARM BATHS AND MEDICATED BATHS

Warm baths at a temperature of 95° to 100° F. are used for a variety of conditions. Possibly their most important use is in the treatment of insomnia, when lying in warm water soothes the circulation generally and results in relaxation of muscle and a reduction of the activity of the brain, so probably inducing sleep. When a warm bath is continued for longer than an hour and a half to two hours at a time, it is described as a continuous bath.

For the administration of *a continuous warm bath*, some means must be secured to keep the water at a constant temperature, and there must therefore be an outlet for cool and an inlet for warm water. The patient should be made comfortable or he will suffer from cramp and fatigue. He should be suspended in a hammock as he lies in the water, with his buttocks resting on a ring air cushion; air pillows might be arranged to support his back, and his head and neck should rest on a specially devised horseshoe-shaped air cushion. It is always advisable to provide a footrest, or otherwise he is liable to slip down the bath. The bath should be covered and only his head exposed above the covering. The room should be quiet and gently lighted so that irritating stimuli are absent. It is inadvisable to leave a patient lying in a bath, and a nurse should therefore be in attendance.

Warm baths are also used in the treatment of many cases of skin disease, particularly at the outset of the treatment when it is necessary to remove crusts and scabs. For this purpose some antiseptic may be added to the water.

Emollient baths are used in cases of skin irritation, the substances frequently employed including *powdered borax*, ½ pound to 30 gallons; *bran*, 2 to 3 pounds; *linseed* or *oatmeal*, 1 to 2 pounds. Bran, linseed and oatmeal should be added to the water by being tied up in a strong bag and boiled in a large saucepan containing half a gallon of water—the mucilage so obtained is then added to the bath. *Starch*: 1 pound of starch mixed to a paste with cold water, made into a mucilage by pouring on boiling water, is added to the bath. *Glycerine*, 10 ounces to a bath.

Antiseptic baths, used for the relief of parasitic skin conditions, include *sulphur*, 2 to 3 ounces to a bath; *creosote*, 1 to 2 drachms; *carbolic* of the strength of 1–300 may be used. This requires a little calculation, but if the bath is of the capacity of 30 gallons, 16 ounces of pure carbolic thoroughly mixed in 5 pints of boiling water and added to the bath will be found to give the correct quantities. *Iodine:* 1 ounce of tincture of iodine is added. *Mercury*, a dilution of 1–8,000 is the usual strength ordered. This can be attained by dissolving 30 tablets of perchloride of mercury in 30 gallons of water.

Astringent baths. These are used in cases of irritable skin conditions. Examples are *alum*, ½ pound to 30 gallons; *boracic acid*, sufficient to make a 2½ per cent solution, or alternatively 2 to 3 pounds of boracic acid may be added to 30 gallons of water; *tannic acid* is sometimes ordered, but the amount is always specially prescribed in each case.

Acid and alkaline baths. *Alkaline baths* are frequently ordered in cases of chronic rheumatism, 1 pound of *sodium bicarbonate* being added to 30 gallons of water.

An *acid bath* is obtained by adding a *gallon of vinegar* to the water, or 5 *ounces of hydrochloric acid* may be added, but this should be specially ordered.

Stimulating baths are used to increase the circulation in the subcutaneous tissues and are believed to have a tonic effect on the general system. Examples of these are the ordinary *cold bath*, followed by a brisk rubbing; *sea water bath*, obtained by adding 7 pounds of sea salt to 30 gallons of water; *mustard bath*, obtained by adding a pound of mustard to a bath of water, and it is advisible either to have the mustard in a muslin bag, or to mix it to a smooth paste before it is added to the water.

AERATED AND FOAM BATHS

In the administration of an aerated bath air under pressure is passed into the water by means of a special apparatus. Bubbles of air, rising through the water to escape on the surface, cause movement by displacing the water through which they pass. This results in stimulation of the circulation in the skin which causes the heart to beat faster at first, but after a few minutes acts as gently graduated exercise would do, and increases the tone of the cardiac muscle. This improves the force and volume of the pulse, and thus the circulation of the blood in all organs is improved and the functions of the body are increased and metabolism is consequently carried on at a slightly higher rate, cellular activity is stimulated and a general feeling of wellbeing is brought about.

In the use of foam baths in medicine a foam-producing herb extract is employed. From 1 to 2 ounces is usually put into a small quantity of water at the bottom of a bath, and an air-distributing apparatus is placed at the bottom of the bath, covered by the water. Gas, carbon-dioxide or oxygen, or air under pressure, is then passed in by means of this apparatus and escapes into the water which contains the foam-making extract, as fine bubbles of air, until the bath is half or three-quarters filled with foam.

A foam bath may be given for a variety of purposes. When it is used in order to increase the activity of the skin, as in chronic rheumatism and neuritis, the temperature of the water used to produce the foam is about 115° F.; the bath is filled with foam and when the temperature of the small quantity of water at the bottom of the bath—some 3 or 4 inches—has cooled to 98° F., the patient is allowed to get in.

As he becomes used to the heat of the foam bath the temperature of the water at the bottom of the bath may be increased; and he sits in the bath for about half an hour perspiring freely. The sweat is constantly wiped from his face and brow by the nurse in attendance, who should watch his colour for any signs of distress and take his pulse at the temple. A foam bath is comfortable, since foam does not exert pressure as does water, and it may be prolonged without causing fatigue.

In addition to the promotion of sweating the effect of this bath is to cause relaxation and dilatation of the superficial blood vessels, and the blood pressure is consequently slightly lowered.

After a foam bath, the patient should be wrapped in warm blankets and allowed to lie still and rest for from an hour and a half to two hours; he may be given any warm drinks of his choice and will probably go on perspiring for some time. When the action of the skin becomes less and the patient has rested, he is sponged with warm water and allowed to have his own clothing on and, if he is in bed, his bed is made as usual.

Chapter 9

The use of Enemata and Suppositories

The administration of an enema—The use of a flatus tube—Varieties of enemata—Giving enemata to babies and infants—Suppositories

An **enema** is an injection into the lower bowel. The word is usually employed when the injection is given with the object of washing out and evacuating the contents of the bowel. In a few instances it is given for purposes of treatment of the bowel, or the introduction of fluid and drugs which are meant to be retained and absorbed. These include astringent, sedative, stimulating and anaesthetic substances.

An enema which is to be returned may be given by means of a rubber catheter and tubing and funnel, or by an irrigation can (see fig. 55, p. 198), or by Higginson's syringe to which a short rubber tube is attached as the use of an unguarded bone nozzle is inadvisable, because the mucous lining of the rectum can be so easily injured or even perforated by it.

Requisites. The apparatus shown in fig. 55 consists of an irrigation can, tubing and rectal catheters, short flatus tube, soap solution, swabs, lubricant and a thermometer. A mackintosh and drawsheet to protect the bed may, but should not usually, be necessary.

The solution to be injected should be prepared in the reservoir at the desired temperature. It is sufficient to say that unless otherwise ordered the fluid should not be hotter than 90° to 100° F.

Preparation of patient. If the patient is in a fit condition the proposed treatment and the result expected should be explained to him; for example, if a cleansing enema is to be given, he should be told that this enema will be injected very slowly and carefully and that he will retain it for probably a quarter of an hour, when it will be returned with an evacuation of the bowel. Tell him also that the necessary bedpan will be at hand should he desire to use it earlier, but that the best results will be obtained by his co-operation, in retaining the enema for a short time.

The bed should be screened and the articles placed ready on the right-hand side. The bedclothes are then turned down to the foot of the bed leaving the patient covered with a blanket. If it is possible to move him it is best to give the enema with the patient in the left lateral position; he is brought to the right side of the bed, his personal clothing moved out of the way, his knees drawn up and the uppermost leg is flexed across the other, resting on the bed in front of it, in order to steady his position. The pillows should be comfortably arranged. It is important to ensure that the patient is quite comfortable, and then he will be be relaxed during the performance of the treatment.

The rectal catheter is lubricated and passed four or five inches into the rectum. A pint or a pint and a half of fluid is ordinarily used for a cleansing enema; it should be slowly administered, taking about 5–7 minutes. If the patient complains of any discomfort the nurse should stop the treatment for a few moments, encourage him by telling him that all is going well, see that he is breathing evenly, getting him to breathe through his mouth if necessary in order that his muscles, particularly those of the abdomen, should be fully relaxed.

When all the fluid has been injected the nurse watches the patient carefully and, when a suitable moment comes and he appears relaxed and comfortable, gently withdraws the rectal catheter. If she notes that this seems to act as a slight source of irritation, which might stimulate peristalsis, she might separate the catheter from the apparatus and secure the end of it with a rubber tubing clip or spigot instead of withdrawing it.

She covers the patient with all his bedclothes but does not necessarily alter his position; it is better if he can continue to lie quite still for a short time, but she should stay near him, and if he expresses a desire to return the injection she should attempt to avoid this happening by explaining the necessity of retaining it. A folded towel pressed against the anus or holding the buttocks pressed together in order to restrain that bearing down feeling which makes the patient think that the return of the injection is imminent may help.

Observation. The contents of the bedpan should be inspected and a report on the character of the result of the enema made, as to whether it is merely coloured fluid, contains only particles of faeces or is a good action. The character of the stool should be stated, and whether it is constipated or not; the presence of any abnormal constituents or abnormalities of shape, colour, etc., and the passage of flatus should be noted.

When an enema is given to relieve retention of urine it is important to discover whether urine is passed and for this purpose the returned enema must be measured and compared with the quantity given, unless evidence from some other source is obtainable.

When an enema is given in order to be retained similar preparation is made, but the injection should be administered *very slowly* and always be preceded by passing a flatus tube. For example, if from 4 to 6 ounces of starch is given in order to allay bowel irritation, about 10–15 minutes would be occupied in administering it. When saline is administered, 8–10 ounces may be given in 20 minutes, see fig. 58, p. 199 (unless the drip method is utilized when a special apparatus is employed). The rate of flow then varies from 40 to 60 drops per minute.

The enema should be given with the patient in a position in which he can remain, so that he need not be disturbed for some time after the injection, and he should not be subject to any irritation or anxiety about the matter.

To *pass a flatus tube* the anal region should be swabbed clean, the tube lubricated and passed into the rectum, sufficiently far to tap the flatus beyond the internal sphincter. The distal end of this tube is attached by means of a glass connexion (see fig. 57, p. 199) to a piece of rubber tubing with a sinker or funnel attached to its free end. This enables the end of the tubing to be retained in a bowl of water or lotion, and by this means the flatus from the bowel can be made to bubble through the fluid and the amount of flatus expelled can be roughly estimated.

Varieties of enemata. These are divided up into groups, named according to the result to be obtained or the substance which is to be used.

An evacuant enema is given for the purpose of emptying the lower bowel. Plain warm water is the simplest form, and this is sometimes described as a simple enema—*enema simplex*—though this term is also generally used to describe a soap-and-water enema, more correctly designated—*enema saponis.*

Soap-and-water enema. A good common yellow soap, a quarter of an ounce to a pint of water may be used. The soap should be finely shredded before mixing. Soap jelly is made by dissolving soap in water in such proportion as to form a jelly. To prepare an enema, an ounce of this jelly is added to a pint of water.

In hospital practice a prescription containing pure soap may be available or some pure soap jelly.

From 1 to 2 pints is usually ordered—the soap must be thoroughly dissolved and mixed with the water and, if ordinary soap is used, the mixture should be strained through a fine sieve or gauze to remove any particles. The injection should be given warm, at about the temperature of 80° to 90° F., and not above 100° F., and all soap bubbles should be removed from the top of the fluid as these hold air.

In some hospitals it is the routine practice to add half to one ounce of olive oil to a simple enema in order to make it less irritating and more lubricating.

Olive-oil enema. From 6 to 20 ounces of warmed olive oil constitutes an olive-oil enema, although many authorities advocate the mixing of from 4 to 8 ounces of olive oil with equal quantities of warm water or soap and water; the nurse should therefore inquire as to the practice of the hospital, or the wishes of the physician before she gives this enema. In some cases a soap-and-water enema will be ordered to follow an olive-oil enema an hour or so later.

An olive-oil enema is given with a large catheter, or a rectal tube and glass funnel, and the apparatus should be prepared in hot water to keep the rubber as pliable as possible and so facilitate the passage of the warmed oil. The apparatus should be immersed in soap and water after use in order to cleanse it of oil.

Olive-oil-and-glycerine enema. Equal parts of olive oil and glycerine may be administered in the same way as the enema described above.

Glycerine enema. A small quantity of glycerine—from 2 to 8 drachms—is injected into the lower bowel in order to extract water from the walls of the rectum and so facilitate the breaking up and passage of hard, impacted faeces which may be lying there. A special vulcanite glycerine syringe is often provided for this purpose, but its use is to be deplored as the hard nozzle may injure the rectum. It is better to use a short rectal tube and glass syringe for this injection (see fig. 59, p. 200).

A mixture of glycerine and warm water is frequently used to obtain evacuation of the bowel when a slightly lubricant effect is desired. Two to four ounces of glycerine with equal quantities of water is the usual proportion given, and it is given by means of a catheter and funnel.

Purgative enema. Although a cleansing enema produces an evacuation of the bowel it is not definitely purgative. A purgative enema contains some purgative substance.

Castor-oil enema. Two to four ounces of castor oil is mixed with double this quantity of olive oil and given by means of a large rubber catheter, tubing and funnel.

Ox-bile enema. Two to four drachms of ox bile is mixed with 4–8 ounces of starch mucilage or warm water.

Magnesium-sulphate enema. One to two ounces of magnesium sulphate is mixed with 4–8 ounces of starch mucilage or warm water.

Aloes. Twenty to thirty grains may be given slowly in mucilage or warm water.

It will be noticed that only small quantities are injected in these instances. The object is that the enema shall be retained for an hour, two hours or more, and so effect a better action. Should a purgative enema not be returned within four hours, it may be followed by a small soap-and-water injection. A magnesium-sulphate enema is also employed as a special treatment for the relief of oedema in cardiac and renal cases by assisting in the elimination of water.

Carminative enema. A carminative enema assists in the expulsion of flatus.

Turpentine. One ounce of turpentine is usually mixed with two ounces of olive oil, unless a special prescription is ordered. The mixture is shaken up in order to emulsify it and then added to a pint of soap-and-water enema solution. An alternative mixture is 1 ounce of turpentine added to 4 ounces of olive oil or to 4 ounces of starch mucilage.

Asafoetida. Thirty grains of asafoetida are administered in a small quantity—about 4–6 ounces—of starch mucilage.

Alum. Two ounces of powdered alum are dissolved in from 1 to 2 pints of tepid water.

Molasses. Three ounces of molasses well mixed with 3 ounces of warm milk may be given. Black treacle may alternatively be employed. Some physicians order the treacle to be given in 15 ounces of warm water or mucilage, instead of in milk.

Anthelmintic enema. This enema is used in the treatment of threadworms which migrate to the lower part of the bowel.

Infusion of quassia.

Cold salt and water. A hypertonic solution is made by adding two drachms of salt to a pint of water.

Astringent substances decrease the secretion of mucus by causing constriction of the blood vessels in the bowel wall. An astringent enema is ordered in the treatment of dysentery characterised by diarrhoea; the stools containing blood and mucus. The substances employed are specially ordered in each case, and include *nitrate of silver solution,* 0·2 per cent, and *tannic acid,* 2 per cent.

Sedative enema. A sedative substance added to an enema diminishes the number of stools, and is therefore used in the treatment of some forms of diarrhoea, particularly in typhoid fever.

Starch and opium is the commonest sedative mixture administered by the rectum, from 20 to 60 minims of tincture of opium is mixed in a small quantity—usually 2–4 ounces—of starch mucilage; the mixture is given cool and injected very slowly.

Starch mucilage, barley mucilage, gum tragacanth, or any other mucilaginous substance may be administered to allay irritation and diminish the frequency of stools. A small quantity (not more than 5 ounces) is given, the object being to form a coating on the inner surface of the mucous membrane. This tends to relieve tenesmus.

Starch mucilage is made by mixing 2 drachms of powdered starch to a smooth paste with a little cold water, and then pouring boiling water up to a pint on to it as in making starch for laundry purposes. The preparation should be sufficiently tacky to coat a spoon lightly.

Stimulating enema. A stimulating enema is given to allay shock as in the treatment of dehydration following loss of body fluid or collapse. It also increases body heat and for this reason is administered in the state of coma and collapse which follows opium poisoning.

Normal saline, which is practically a teaspoonful or a drachm of salt to a pint of water, can be obtained in almost any circumstances and is the fluid ordinarily used. In hospital it is usual to have special tablets containing 40 or 80 grains, and either one 80-grain tablet or two 40-grain are used to the pint. Some authorities advocate that saline should be given at a slightly higher temperature than the average enema, but generally speaking it is better for all rectal injections to be not hotter than 100° F. A saline may be ordered as one single treatment such as is given when a patient is brought back from the operating theatre and it is desired to increase his body heat at once. Or salines may be administered at regular intervals, over a period of time, to patients who are in a state of collapse, or to those who are dehydrated by the continual loss of body fluid, as in cases of profuse bleeding, or vomiting, and also to those who for some reason are unable to receive an adequate amount of fluid by the usual means. The apparatus shown in fig. 55, p. 198, may be employed or a tube and funnel may be used as in fig. 56, p. 198. A flatus tube should first be passed.

Continuous administration of rectal saline is often better treatment than the giving of small quantities at intervals—for the description of methods see pp. 153–4.

Coffee. Five ounces of strong black coffee to which a pinch of salt has been added is sometimes administered as a stimulant in the treatment of the coma and collapse following opium poisoning.

Nutrient enema. At the present time pre-digested foods are not given by rectum but the capacity for absorption of fluid by the bowel is made use of in many instances. For purposes of feeding, a solution of glucose is used; in order to allay thirst, plain water may be administered; and, in order to prevent or combat any possible acidosis following an operation, water containing a teaspoonful of sodium bicarbonate to the pint may be given. The value of normal saline has already been mentioned.

Medicinal enema. Medicines may be given per rectum under certain conditions, particularly in the case of unconscious patients, in disorders of the stomach and when vomiting is persistent.

When this method of drug administration is used it is customary for the physician to order double the dose that would ordinarily be given by mouth.

Anaesthetic enema. Rectal administration of certain drugs is sometimes employed for the purpose of induction of general anaesthesia.

Avertin is employed in a 2½ per cent solution as a basal narcotic to produce anaesthesia. The amount of avertin used is 1 to 2 grains per pound of body weight, and the dose is carefully worked out for each patient. The average total quantity administered varies from 4 to 8 ounces as required.

In preparation, the patient is given an aperient or an enema the previous evening, and in some cases a sedative such as sulphonal is given overnight. A light breakfast may be taken on the morning of the operation. Before avertin is administered the patient is prepared for the operating theatre. In some cases an injection of morphia and atropine is given, in all cases the patient is permitted to pass urine, any special clothing employed for theatre use is put on, and dentures are removed. Everything should be done as quietly as possible, all fussiness or anything that will irritate the patient being avoided, particularly if the case happens to be one of thyrotoxicosis. He may then either be put on the trolley on which he is to be conveyed to the theatre, or the canvas of the stetcher on which he is to be lifted may be placed under him as he lies on his bed, the latter method being preferable as it ensures that the patient will lie comfortably in his bed during induction. The injection is made by means of a catheter, tubing and funnel—there is no necessity to move the patient into the left lateral position as the injection can be given while he lies on his back. A flatus tube is passed, the injection is slowly made, the nurse watches the patient carefully and as soon as he falls asleep or becomes unconscious she ceases the administration even though the full amount ordered may not have been given. The injection is made as slowly as it can conveniently be given; some authorities prefer that only half the amount ordered should be administered at first, and then a short pause made—and the administration is continued until the patient becomes unconscious.

Ether. Ether may occasionally be given by rectum in order to produce general anaesthesia, but as colitis may result it is now rarely employed. The mode of administration is as follows: the lower bowel is washed out, usually the evening before; a hypodermic injection of morphia and atropine is administered half an hour before the rectal injection of ether is to be made, and the patient is prepared for a general anaesthetic as described in the case of avertin. A 5 per cent solution of ether and oil, well shaken up in order to ensure emulsification, is slowly passed into the rectum by means of a catheter and funnel. The amount of ether to be given is always specially ordered.

The nurse watches the patient carefully throughout the administration. His legs will first become numb, then his arms, and finally he will become unconscious.

In order to prevent colitis, immediately the operation is over, colonic lavage is administered until all odour of ether has disappeared.

Giving enemata to babies and infants. Although the term enema is used, when this treatment is given to a tiny baby the rectum is merely irrigated with from 2 to 4 ounces of plain water or weak boracic lotion, at a temperature not exceeding 80° F. As a rule the infant is placed on the nurse's lap, her knees are protected by a mackintosh, the infant's buttocks are slightly raised on a folded towel as he lies on his back, the fluid is allowed to run in very gently, and is then siphoned back into a receptacle placed on the floor or on a stool in front of the nurse.

With children over two years of age a small quantity—from 4 to 6 ounces—of water, containing very little soap, making a weak solution, ıay be administered gently with a catheter and funnel. The child should e placed upon a chamber to evacuate his bowel.

The nurse may attempt to frustrate any urgent desire the child may have) return the fluid immediately, by pressing his buttocks together for a few ıinutes. If there is any tendency to prolapse of the rectum the child ıould not be placed on a chamber but should be allowed to return the nema while lying on his side on the bed, the nurse catching fluid and ıeces into a receiver as they are ejected.

Enema rash. In some—comparatively rare—instances a rectal in- :ction, particularly one of soap and water, is followed by an enema ash. This is very similar to a serum rash and usually combines the char- cters of an erythematous, urticarial, and papular rash.

SUPPOSITORIES

Suppositories are usually cone-shaped, solidified preparations contain- ıg lubricants or drugs. A *glycerine suppository* is made of glycerine, solidified vith gelatine. It is used when it is desirable to empty the rectum of faecal ontents which for some reason may have become arrested there.

A glycerine suppository may be dipped in warm water, which renders t lubricated; other types of suppository need vaseline. With the patient n the left lateral position, as for giving an enema, the suppository should e passed beyond the anal canal into the rectum by means of a gloved inger. When a suppository is given to children it is necessary to hold the uttocks pressed together for a few moments, otherwise it will immediately e ejected. Great care must be taken to insert the suppository slowly and arefully in order to prevent injury to the mucous membrane of the owel.

Suppositories containing belladonna, and morphia or opium, are made ıp with a base of oil of theobroma, except in hot countries, where this vould melt, when purified beeswax is used instead. When the suppository :ontains any substance which is to be retained, its administration hould be preceded by the passage of a flatus tube (see fig. 60, p. 200) in rder to leave the rectum quite free of air; or by the administration of an :nema if the rectum is loaded with faeces.

After the insertion of a suppository which contains a sedative it is important to lace the patient in a position in which he will be quite comfortable and ıble to rest.

Chapter 10

Irrigation, Lavage, Douching and Catheterization

Gastric lavage—High colonic irrigation—Catheterization and bladder irrigation and drainage—Vaginal douching

GASTRIC LAVAGE

The washing out of the stomach is performed for the removal of poison which has been swallowed, and in some cases in order to cleanse the stomach before an operation is performed upon it, as for example when a patient with an acute abdominal condition is vomiting large quantities of fluid. Gastric lavage is also sometimes employed in the treatment of post-operative vomiting when this symptom is troublesome and persistent.

The **apparatus required** includes (see fig. 61, p. 201) a *Jaques's rubber stomach tube* with a *funnel* attached.

A *mouth gag* and *tongue forceps*, a *lubricant* for the tube, plenty of lotion and a lotion thermometer, a mackintosh and towel may be needed to protect the bed, a pail for the returned fluid and either articles for cleansing the patient's mouth after the treatment, or a mouth-wash, if he is in a condition to use one, should also be provided.

Method. There are instances in which a stomach is cleansed by passing a Ryle's tube (as described in the administration of a test meal on p. 173). This method is undertaken when a surgeon wishes the resting juice to be withdrawn and the stomach cleansed by passing in a small quantity of fluid by means of a large syringe and withdrawing or aspirating this fluid back by the same means.

But for gastric lavage employed for washing poison out of the stomach large quantities of fluid should be used, as described by H. K. Marriott in 'The Treatment of Acute Poisoning' and employed by him at the Middlesex Hospital. Dr. Marriott also advocates either the use of Trendelenburg's position on an operating table, or having the patient lying prone on a couch, with his head supported over the end. In these positions there is no danger that the regurgitation of fluid around the tube in the pharynx will fall into the trachea, which happens in unconscious cases when the cough reflex is absent.

When the patient is in position his false teeth are taken out and, if he is unconscious, a mouth gag is inserted. The tube is lubricated and passed into the mouth, slight pressure on the tube as it reaches the posterior wall of the pharynx will direct it into the oesophagus; it is then passed quickly on, until the mark on the tube (20 inches from the end in the case of an adult and 10 inches for a child) is at the level of the lips—the tube is now in the stomach.

Half a pint of lotion is now poured in, and siphoned back into a receiver

—in a case of poisoning plain water is used—this specimen is kept for examination. Washing out of the stomach is then continued, using a pint at a time until the fluid begins to return clear and odourless. Anything up to two gallons may be required.

When the treatment is over, the tube is withdrawn and either the mouth is cleansed or the patient given a mouth-wash. The soiled tube should be washed in tepid water, and boiled after use. If a nurse has performed this treatment, she would be expected to make a report on the amount of lotion used, the state in which it was returned and the presence of any blood, mucus and bile, and the odour. It may be necessary to save all the fluid for the inspection of the doctor.

HIGH COLONIC IRRIGATION

In this treatment fluid is injected in fairly large quantities into the bowel. It is used in the treatment of colitis and diverticulitis, and in other cases in which toxaemia is marked and thought to be aggravated by absorption from the bowel as, for example, in eclampsia. The fluids used include normal saline, plain warm water, a solution of potassium permanganate 1 grain to the gallon, and many other slightly antiseptic, and sometimes slightly mucilaginous, liquids may be ordered. At least 8 pints should be prepared and in many cases up to 20 may be used. The temperature of the fluid should never be above 100° F., and the nurse should work from the right side of the bed.

The condition of the patient has to be taken into consideration, and this must be observed throughout the treatment, the pulse being taken before the treatment begins and again afterwards, and a comparison carefully noted.

Almost any apparatus suitable for rectal injection may be utilized. Some sisters use a tubing and funnel, others like a graduated 2-quart irrigation can. A soft rectal tube should be attached, for passage into the rectum. The container or pail for the returned fluid should also be graduated so that the nurse can always know how much fluid is for the moment lost—that is, how much is at any given moment in the patient's bowel.

The treatment of colonic irrigation is divided into two parts, one described as irrigation and the second as lavage.

Irrigation. The patient lies on his back in the dorsal position with his shoulders flat on the bed and a soft pillow under his head. Fluid is run through the apparatus first in order to expel air, and the rectal tube is then inserted carefully into the rectum, allowing a little fluid to precede it, in order to facilitate its passage. Up to 2 pints of fluid are allowed to run in, the nurse watching the patient carefully for any signs of discomfort, pausing if she sees these, and then continuing. Not more than 2 pints should be lost with the patient in this position. The fluid should be very gently injected, having the can or funnel just above the level of the bed to ensure that the rate of flow is slow. The can is then lowered to the level of the floor, and the fluid allowed to run back into it. The can may be raised or lowered alternately to perform the process of irrigation; or, larger quantities of fluid having been prepared, continuous irrigation, in and out, may be made into the bedside pail. When the irrigation process is complete the first fluid used is siphoned back.

Lavage. For this, the patient lies first on his side, in the left lateral position, and one pint is slowly injected. He turns on to his right side, and this is repeated. He then slowly assumes the knee-chest position and a third pint is injected. He rests for a minute or two if he can—that is, if the discomfort is not too great—and is then allowed to evacuate his bowel of the 3 pints of fluid on a special bedpan capable of containing this quantity.

If the patient is not capable of getting into the knee-chest position an alternative plan is to employ the left lateral, the dorsal and the right lateral positions in this order.

The nurse carefully observes the general condition of the patient immediately after the treatment, inspects the returned fluid, and reports the presence of undigested food, bile, blood, mucus, casts, worms or other foreign bodies, the colour and the odour of the fluid, and the occurrence of any pain, difficulty, or spasm during the procedure. Careful comparison should be made between the initial amount prepared and used, and the amount returned. If at any time during the procedure there should be any difficulty in returning the lost fluid, the nurse should elevate the irrigation can, run rapidly in about 4 or 5 ounces, equally rapidly lower the receptacle, when she will find that the fluid will begin to siphon back.

CATHETERIZATION

The act of catheterization taps the urinary bladder, and is carried out by means of a urethral catheter.

Types of Catheters. *Urethral catheters* vary in length and shape for male and female patients. The *female catheter* is short and fairly straight, and is made of glass or metal. *Male catheters* are longer and curved, and they are usually made of metal or hard rubber. Metal ones are curved; some having a specially large curve are prostatic catheters, designed for use when the prostate gland is obstructing the passage of an ordinary catheter into the male bladder. The hard rubber catheters just mentioned are made of rubber composition or gum elastic. Examples of hard rubber catheters for tapping the male bladder include the ordinary straight *gum elastic* catheter, the *coudé* catheter which has a short curve at the tip, the *bicoudé* which has a double curve and the *olive-headed catheter* which has a bulbous portion immediately behind the tip.

Soft rubber catheters have many uses, as for catheterizing the bladder, for the administration of rectal injections, and for nasal feeding.

Self-retaining catheters may be employed for keeping the bladder empty; these have bulbous ends which prevent the catheter from slipping out; in order to insert the catheter a special director is employed which temporarily straightens out the end. A self-retaining suprapubic catheter is passed into the bladder through a wound in the lower part of the anterior abdominal wall, above the pubes.

Ureteric catheters are fine instruments, long enough to be passed along the ureter into the pelvis of the kidney, in order to collect a specimen of urine from one side only, or for the injection of fluid into the renal pelvis. The method of application is described on p. 145.

A *uterine catheter* is made of soft rubber and has graduated markings upon it to indicate the distance the catheter is passed into the uterus. For the introduction of a uterine catheter, the anterior vaginal wall is retracted and a special pair of introducing forceps is employed; the rubber catheter is clamped between the blades of this instrument and guided into the uterus. This catheter is used for the introduction of glycerine in the method of treatment described by the late Dr. Remington Hobbs for uterine drainage in cases of puerperal sepsis.

An *intratracheal catheter* is employed for the introduction of anaesthetics by this route.

A *eustachian catheter* is used to test the patency of the eustachian tubes; or to enable inflation of the tube to be carried out when obstruction is complained of. (For types of catheters see also figs. 62 and 64, pp. 202–4).

Female Catheterization. The articles required for this procedure (see fig. 63, p. 203) include *two sterile catheters*—two being supplied in case one should be soiled in a first attempt at passing the catheter.

Some mild *antiseptic lotion* and *sterile swabs* will be required for cleansing the vulva and some stronger lotion for cleansing the hands of the nurses.

Three receivers will be required, and one of these should be sterile as it is needed to collect the urine and a sterile specimen may be wanted. The other two are required for the soiled swabs and the used catheter.

A sterile measure should be provided for the urine and a sterile specimen glass and test tubes.

Position of the patient. If possible the patient should lie on her back, with one or two pillows supporting her head and shoulders; her thighs should be flexed and abducted. She can be made very comfortable in this position if her feet are placed flat on the bed. The bed should be screened; a good light must be provided and it is advisable to place a hot-water bottle in the bed.

Procedure. The patient is lying in the position described and the bedclothes are divided so that some are used to cover the upper part of her body and others cover the legs and thighs. So arranged it is easy for the nurse to separate these by manipulating the movement of them with her elbows (after she has scrubbed up) should she have to work alone, without an assistant.

The nurse should work from the righthand side of the bed—unless she is lefthanded. She should place sterile towels above and below the pubes and then separate the external labial folds with the fingers of her left hand, holding them apart until the catheterization is over. The vulva should be carefully cleansed, paying special attention to cleansing the vestibule and urethral orifice. The latter should be inspected to see that it is normal in size and character.

The sterile receiver should then be placed on a mackintosh or towel on the bed, between the patient's legs and ready to receive the urine. The nurse should pick a catheter out of the lotion in which it is lying, shake it gently to free it of moisture, hold it about an inch from the open end, and if it is a glass catheter, inspect it carefully to see that it is not cracked or broken. It should be gently inserted into the opening of the urethra, without having touched any other part. The nurse should notice whether the patient is relaxed or rigid; if she is holding herself stiffly, this may be overcome by asking her to open her mouth slightly and breathe through it; concentrating on this, she may relax. If there is any difficulty in passing the catheter, it is important that force should not be used; any real difficulty experienced would necessitate the use of a rubber, not a glass, catheter. In a normal case the catheter can be passed with ease, and the urine will begin to flow into the receiver provided for this purpose; it should be held steadily and, when urine ceases to flow, if the catheter is withdrawn slightly it may tap urine which is at a lower level in the bladder.

Finally, when urine has ceased to flow, the catheter is gently withdrawn; if the nurse places a finger over the open end, she will find she can withdraw the catheter without spilling any drops of urine; when she removes this finger and inverts the catheter, it will empty itself as its contents will fall by force of gravity.

The catheter should be carefully inspected again, to see that it is still intact. It would be a serious complication if a catheter were to be broken in the urethra, as retention of small pieces of glass might cause serious injury. A nurse should never attempt to remove this, should it happen; she ought to send for a doctor and get ready some lotion and swabs and long narrow forceps which he may require to use.

After catheterization the patient is dried, the bed remade and the patient left comfortable; she should be given a hot-water bottle and a warm drink and be tucked up in bed.

Report of the time of catheterization, the amount of urine obtained; any difficulty experienced or pain caused and the character of the urine with notes on the presence of any abnormality should be made immediately, before these points are forgotten, and the urine should either be tested by the nurse or sent to the laboratory for examination.

Precautions. The strictest asepsis should be maintained and carried out for the purpose of catheterization, in order to prevent the entry of micro-organisms into the bladder which would give rise to cystitis.

A nurse should realize that patients who need regular catheterization do get cystitis when there can be no possible reflection on the surgical technique practised, and that this probably occurs because the tone of the bladder is lowered either owing to frequent retention or, in some cases, as when the prostate gland is enlarged in men, or after the operation of radical hysterectomy in women, because the bladder is never properly emptied and because the residual urine, however small the quantity may be, acts as an irritant.

The use of a glass or metal catheter is contraindicated in midwifery practice, in the case of very nervous patients and children, and after operations on the perineum. A soft rubber catheter should be employed in these cases.

Whenever the bladder is very seriously distended and the condition has persisted for some time, it is inadvisable to empty it rapidly, by catheterization. It is better to draw off the urine very slowly, and even to close the end of the catheter by a spigot and allow two intervals of from 10 to 30 minutes to elapse before completely emptying the bladder.

When a rigor occurs soon after a catheter has been passed—this is described as a *catheter reaction*—the patient should be put to bed, warmly wrapped up and given hot lemon drinks. A doctor may consider it necessary to order some quinine. The patient's temperature should be taken at frequent intervals of 15–30 minutes as long as it continues to rise.

URETERIC CATHETERIZATION

The collection of a specimen of urine from each kidney separately is arried out by means of ureteric catheterization when it is necessary to ıvestigate the function of each kidney. If, for example, one kidney is to e removed (nephrectomy), it is necessary that the function of the other 'hich remains should be as perfect as possible.

A ureteric catheter is also employed for the injection of fluid into the elvis of a kidney as in the performance of pyelography by the retrograde ıethod (see p. 169).

The *articles required* include a cystoscope, together with the articles for atheterizing the bladder and for the provision of fluid in the bladder hich is necessary before a cystoscope can safely be passed. The cystoscope mployed in this instance has special canals at each side of the telescopic ody, for the passage of the fine, long ureteric catheters. This instrument passed into the bladder; the surgeon looks along the telescope and sees ıe opening of each ureter and guides the ureteric catheters into these; assing each one some distance along the ureter, if possible as far as the elvis of the kidney. A general anaesthetic is sometimes used as the passing f a ureteric catheter is uncomfortable; but, if the patient is willing to have carried out without an anaesthetic, he can be of use to the surgeon; as ıe patient can usually feel when the catheter is in the pelvis of the kidney.

The urine drips down the ureters and is collected in two small sterile lass tubes, which are fitted into a small frame attached to the handle-like nd of the cystoscope; the distal end of each catheter is placed in this eceptacle and the urine is collected in it.

IRRIGATION OF THE BLADDER

The bladder is irrigated in order to cleanse it before operation, and as art of the treatment necessary to assist its healing. It is also irrigated in pecial cases to arrest bleeding from the bladder, and in the treatment of ny inflammatory condition.

The frequency with which this treatment may be made and the nature f the solution used for the purpose vary enormously. In inflammatory onditions irrigation is carried out every 4 hours, some bland fluid which not likely to irritate, such as normal saline or an alkaline solution, being mployed.

The character of the solution to be used, and the effect expected, the ate of flow in and out of the bladder, the temperature of the solution, he amount of pressure, and whether a high or low pressure flow is to be sed, are all points of the greatest importance.

The *articles required* for washing out a bladder include those necessary or catheterization (see fig. 63, p. 203). The following items will be eeded in addition: A Y-shaped glass connecting tube which has three rms, will be required, one limb being attached to the catheter which vill be in the bladder, a second to the tubing which is passing to the ınnel or irrigation can from which fluid is being served to the bladder, vhile the third limb will carry a piece of rubber tubing in the direction f a pail which is placed on the floor in order to receive the flow of fluid eturning from the bladder. A clamp or tap is inserted into the rubber tubing just below its attachment to the funnel or irrigation can used as service tank, and this is adjusted as required to regulate the rate of flo of the fluid (see fig. 65, p. 204).

An adequate amount of the solution which is to be used should be avai able, and a lotion thermometer to ascertain that it is prepared at the co rect temperature. The bed should be protected by mackintoshes an

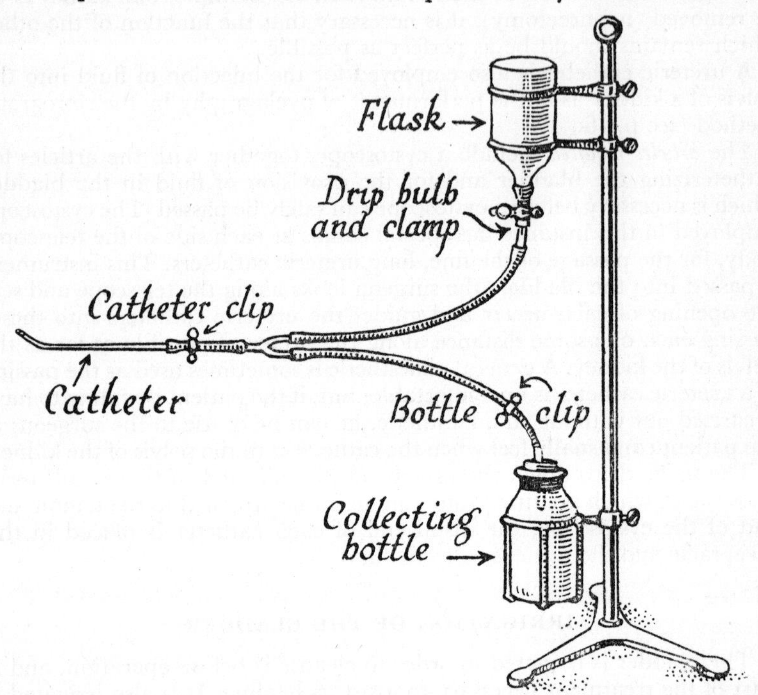

FIG. 27. DUKE'S APPARATUS FOR INTERMITTENT BLADDER IRRIGATION AND DRAINAG

towels, and articles for the washing and rubbing of the back should be a hand for use after the treatment in order to leave the patient comfortabl fixed up in bed.

Procedure. The patient and bed should be prepared as for catheteri zation (see p. 143); the patient lying on his back with thighs flexed an abducted. He must be warmly covered as it will probably take 20 minute to irrigate a bladder with several pints of fluid. The irrigation can may b suspended above the level of the bed—a foot above gives a moderat amount of pressure—and this is made possible either by the use of a specia bedside stand or by some apparatus fixed to the bedhead.

The catheter is passed and the bladder emptied. The catheter is nc withdrawn, but is connected to a glass connexion which communicate with the Y connecting tube mentioned above. Before it is connected up the clamp on the tubing below the irrigation can is released and some flui run into the tube, so that air is expelled, otherwise air would be passe into the bladder possibly causing discomfort or pain.

The clamp is then adjusted to permit of the flow of lotion into th bladder at the rate required; but when from 6 to 10 ounces have been passed in the flow is arrested, and the bladder allowed to empty, by releasing the clamp on the rubber tubing which hangs over the pail, below the Y glass connexion. The irrigation is continued, either until a given amount of fluid has been used or until the returned fluid is quite clear and free from any odour. If treatment is continuous the catheter is allowed to remain in the bladder; when treatment is intermittent the catheter may be removed. The patient should have a hot drink and be warmly wrapped up after bladder irrigation.

Tidal Drainage of the Bladder. Dr. Munro of Boston, U.S.A., introduced tidal bladder drainage. The Laurie-Nathan apparatus shown in fig. 28 is a recent modification of Munro's method. The apparatus is first assembled and then boiled. The flask filled with warm lotion is placed on the stand at the bedside, the screw clip being closed; the siphon tube (C) is fixed at the level shown. A catheter is passed and a spigot inserted. The screw clip (A) is then loosened and the tubing (B) and (D) filled with fluid to expel all air, the spigot is removed from the catheter and the tube (D) is connected to the catheter. Great care must be taken to exclude air or the apparatus will not function.

The bladder is distended to a certain level which is determined by the height to which the siphon is fixed above the level of the symphysis pubis—in the illustration given this is shown as about 7 inches. The lotion is

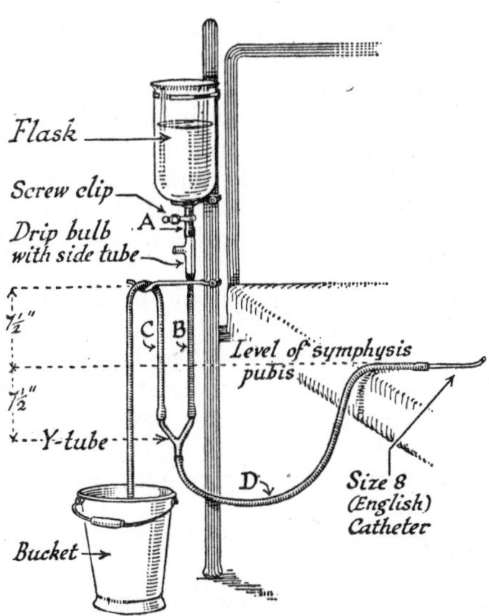

FIG. 28.—LAURIE-NATHAN'S APPARATUS FOR AUTOMATIC TIDAL DRAINAGE OF BLADDER.

(It is important to assemble the apparatus with the tubing of the sizes and lengths given below.)

A. Four inches of rubber tubing, ¼ inch diameter.
B. Sixteen inches of tubing of the same bore.
C. Two yards of pressure tubing, ⅙ inch diameter.
D. One yard of pressure tubing of the same bore.

The dotted line represents the level of the symphysis pubis which is taken as approximately the level of the catheter in the bladder.

graduated to drip at 60 drops per minute so that the bladder fills slowly, and when pressure within the bladder reaches the level of the siphon tube the bladder automatically empties. It is the nurse's duty to see that the flask is not allowed to run dry, that the free end of the siphon tube is always above the fluid in the collecting bucket, the level at which the surgeon arranges the siphon tube is not altered, and that the glass Y connexion hangs free and is not tucked in with the bedclothes, and that the tubing does not get kinked. The amount of fluid added to the reservoir and emptied from the bucket must be recorded. The catheter is changed every few days. Great care must be taken not to permit air to enter the apparatus when changing the catheter.

Duke's apparatus (see fig. 27) is sometimes alternatively employed. By this means the bladder is kept empty and can be irrigated at intervals. The catheter constantly drains the bladder. To flush the bladder—close the clamp below the Y connexion and release the clamp above the drip bulb, then allow half to one pint of fluid to pass into the bladder. Now close the clamp above the drip bulb and release the clamp below the Y connexion and the bladder will empty. By this means intermittent flushing of the bladder can be carried out at intervals.

VAGINAL DOUCHING

Irrigation of the vaginal canal is usually described as douching. It is performed in order to cleanse the vagina when a woman is wearing a pessary and as treatment in some cases of discharge and before an operation on the lower part of the female genital tract. Vaginal douching is also employed in the treatment of inflammatory conditions of the vagina, cervix, ovaries and tubes and in the emergency treatment of severe uterine bleeding.

The *solution* used varies—many mild antiseptics are employed, including boracic lotion, Condy's fluid, lysol and iodine in the strength of half a drachm to the pint of water, perchloride of mercury 1–5,000 and flavine 1–4,000.

For cleansing purposes the lotion should be warm; in the treatment of inflammatory conditions it should be hot—about 100° F.; and for the treatment of bleeding it is used very hot, up to 110° F.

The condition of the external genitalia should be inspected carefully before a hot douche is given; it may be necessary to smear the parts with a lubricant in order to protect them from injury by the hot solution.

The **articles required** (see fig. 67, p. 206) include a mackintosh and towel to protect the bed.

Sterile towels to place over the bedclothing, which is divided in the middle.

Two glass douche nozzles, an irrigation apparatus or douche can with tubing and clamp, sufficient lotion and a lotion thermometer.

Lotion and swabs to cleanse the vulval region and a bowl for soiled swabs and a receiver in which the douche nozzle will be placed after use. A douche pan and cover.

Method of giving a douche. As a rule the patient lies on her back with the legs drawn up and knees separated (but a douche can be given with equal convenience to a woman lying on her side). The bedclothes are divided and separated so that the patient and her legs are covered and only the vulval region is exposed. This region is covered by a sterile towel. The patient is placed on the pan. The nurse washes her arms and hands, removes the towel over the vulva with forceps to avoid soiling her hands—as the patient may have touched this towel—she then separates the labia and cleanses the vulva with swabs and lotion, inspects the glass nozzle to see that it is intact, allows some lotion to flow through from the irrigation can and inserts the nozzle into the vaginal canal. She should move the nozzle about in order to irrigate the walls and vault of the vagina.

When the treatment is over, the glass nozzle is removed and inspected carefully to see that it has not been broken during the treatment. If the patient can sit up, she may do so for a few minutes, as the erect position favours more complete drainage of the vagina. The toilet of the vulva is completed by drying both the lower part of the vagina and the external parts. The bed is rearranged and the patient made comfortable.

The lotion used should be inspected and any abnormalities noted and reported.

Chapter 11

Artificial Feeding, the Administration of Fluid and Blood Transfusion

Methods of artificial feeding—Channels for the administration of fluid—Blood transfusion: direct and continuous—The grouping of blood—Rhesus factor.

ARTIFICIAL FEEDING

Food may be introduced into the body in the following ways—by means of an oesophageal tube passed through the mouth, by the nose in nasal feeding, and by the rectum in rectal feeding. It may also be administered by means of openings artificially made as when food is introduced into the oesophagus by oesophagotomy, into the stomach by gastrostomy, and into the small intestine by duodenostomy or jejunostomy.

General rules for consideration which will be found applicable in most cases. Only liquid food can be used. The temperature of the food should be between 95° and 100° F. The amount given must be measured and recorded, and in most cases the liquid should be strained, otherwise the tube through which it is passed may be blocked.

When the patient is conscious and capable of knowing what is being carried out, the treatment should be explained to him and the character of the feeding described. If the patient is delirious or difficult to manage help may be required to steady him during the administration of the feeding. In the case of a very young child it is wise to wrap him in a blanket so that his arms cannot be unexpectedly used to pull the tube away, should he suddenly become frightened.

Any medicines or stimulants the patient may be having should be administered either before or after the feeding, to save passing the tube a great number of times.

The apparatus should always be clean, moist and warm; the patient must be comfortably arranged, the nurse being very gentle and no force ever being used.

NASAL FEEDING

For nasal feeding a fine catheter is passed through the nose and on into the oesophagus for about 4–6 inches. The **articles needed** (see fig. 68, p. 207) are:

A *mackintosh* or *towel* to protect the bed.

A *fine rubber catheter*, No. 3 or No. 4, should be attached by a fine glass connexion to a short length of rubber tubing, which has a glass funnel attached at its other end. This should be boiled and placed in warm water, ready at the bedside. A rubber tubing clamp may be useful, but most nurses learn to control the rate of flow by pressure of their fingers on the rubber tubing.

A non-irritating *lubricant*, such as liquid paraffin, is usually supplied, either to apply to the end of the catheter or to cleanse the interior of the nostril. As the catheter is moist it will be slippery enough, provided the cavity through which it is to pass is lubricated.

Saline swabs are better for cleansing the nose than boracic, as the latter is astringent and slightly irritating. *Dry swabs* should be supplied in order to dry the edges of the nostril when the tube is removed after the feeding has been given.

The quantity of food to be given should be warmed and standing ready in the measure in a bowl of water; a *lotion thermometer* should be provided in order to ascertain the temperature of the feeding.

Method. When possible have the patient propped up, but the feed can be given in any ordinary position. Having placed the mackintosh and towel in position to protect the bed in case of accident, cleanse the nostril that is to be used, choosing the one seen to provide the clearest passage, lubricate it and insert the tube gently but quickly, some 6 or 8 inches, passing it in a backward, *not* an upward direction.

See that it has not come forward and curled up in the mouth, listen with the ear against the funnel as the movement of air may be heard if the tube is in the trachea. Look at the patient and see if he is at all cyanosed, whether he is coughing, and whether he appears to be quite comfortable. If in doubt withdraw the tube and try again.

When satisfied that the tube is in the oesophagus, pour a little sterile water into it and allow this to trickle down, checking the flow by constricting the tubing—the absence of distress will confirm the fact that the tube is not in the trachea. Give the feeding, then pour a little water down to clear the tube, pinch the tube close up to the nostril and withdraw it rapidly. Inspect the nostril and dry it or lubricate it if necessary.

Some sisters recommend that a nurse should ask the doctor in charge of the case to be present when giving the first nasal feeding to any patient, but this only applies to the inexperienced. Sometimes the tube is left in, and it should then be clamped at the end of the feeding, and fastened up on to the side of the temple by means of a piece of strapping.

OESOPHAGEAL FEEDING

The articles (see also fig. 68, p. 207) which will be required are similar to those for nasal feeding. It is necessary to protect the bed, strain and warm the feeding; the mouth should be cleaned and a lubricant which is pleasant to taste should be provided for applying to the end of the tube; glycerine and lemon is excellent for this purpose.

The **apparatus** consists of a Jaques's oesophageal feeding tube, with a funnel attached. A mouth gag will be needed if the patient is obstreperous, and since he may feel sick, or be sick, a vomit bowl and towel should be provided. Articles for cleansing the mouth when the tube is withdrawn should be at hand.

Method. The patient should be sitting up if possible, supported by pillows. The mackintosh and towel are arranged around his neck and under his chin, and he may be permitted to hold a receiver or vomit bowl if he is convinced he will feel sick. The tube is lubricated and passed gently over the tongue, and, putting it in at the corner of the mouth, it is passed to the pharynx; slight pressure on the tube will deflect it and cause it to pass into the pharynx without impinging on the posterior wall of the fauces, and, the patient being asked to swallow, the tube is easily guided into the oesophagus. There is a mark on the tube and, when this is near the lips, the tube should be in the stomach.

The feeding is gently poured into the funnel and runs along the tube into the stomach. When all has been passed, a small quantity of water may be given, in order to leave the tube clear of fluid food. The nurse should then compress the tube and quickly withdraw it. The patient may rinse out his mouth for himself or else the nurse may clean it for him.

As a rule from a half to one pint is given at a time and a patient on oesophageal feeding is usually fed every 4 hours.

RECTAL FEEDING

The apparatus required for rectal feeding is the same as that used when salines are administered by this route (see p. 153 and fig. 58, p. 199).

OESOPHAGOTOMY, GASTROSTOMY AND DUODENOSTOMY FEEDING

Artificial feedings by means of openings made into the oesophagus, stomach or duodenum have certain points in common and the general principles of feeding by these methods can therefore be considered collectively.

If the tube has been left in the wound, or an opening made, the apparatus required consists of a glass connexion which can be attached to this and a short length of rubber tubing with a funnel through which fluid food can be poured into the stomach. The apparatus should be boiled and placed ready in warm water. The food must be strained; a little sterile or plain water should be supplied to pour in first, in order to test the patency of the tube; a little water is also used to clear the tube after the feeding. The bed should be protected.

Method. As a rule there is a surgical dressing around the tube in order to protect the skin sutures which have been inserted to approximate the edges of the wound. It is advisable to arrange for the tube to pass through this dressing so that it need not be changed every time the patient is fed. The distal end of the tube should be closed by means of a clamp or spigot, and the tube may be attached to the exterior of the dressing, by means of a safety pin binding it down to the bandage. It should be covered with a towel.

On arrival at the bedsid ethe bedclothes should be protected, the tubing liberated and the spigot removed; the glass connexion is then attached to the tube and a little water poured in through the funnel and tubing. If the passage is clear, the prepared feeding may be given. The tube is then cleared by passing some plain water through, the spigot reinserted and the tube fastened down and covered.

When the tube is not left in the wound, the lining of the organ—in the case of gastrostomy, the stomach wall—is brought up to and fastened to the skin of the anterior abdominal wall. A catheter must therefore be provided, and it is passed through this opening into the stomach and the feeding given by means of catheter, tubing and funnel.

In this case the wound requires to be treated as an ordinary surgical dressing, and aseptic precautions should as far as possible be taken.

Any oozing of the contents of the organ on to the surface of the skin will cause soreness around the opening. To prevent this, it may be necessary to use an ointment dressing, the base of which should be liquid paraffin or vaseline, as lanoline or lard would be affected by the digestive juices.

THE ADMINISTRATION OF FLUID AND BLOOD TRANSFUSION

The administration of fluid by a variety of channels is very important in the treatment of dehydration. By *dehydration* is meant the deprivation of the tissues of water, which occurs whenever large quantities of fluid are lost to the body by vomiting, diarrhoea or bleeding; and also whenever fluids are not circulating in the body as occurs in conditions of toxaemia and collapse.

The *symptoms of this condition* include a rapid, thready, running, low tension pulse; marked thirst, furring of the tongue and dryness of the mouth; the face is pinched and drawn and the eyes, deeply sunken in the sockets, appear dull and listless. The abdomen is retracted, and in severe cases the skin has the appearance of being shrivelled, as is a leaf when the sap is down.

Babies and infants very rapidly become dehydrated, and when this happens the temperature rises rapidly, as the heat-regulating mechanism is easily disturbed in infants.

The *channel by which fluid may be administered* is primarily the mouth but, if for any reason this is contraindicated, fluid may be given per rectum, by subcutaneous or intramuscular injection—though the latter method is comparatively rare—and by intravenous and intraperitoneal infusion.

The fluids employed include plain water, normal or isotonic saline 0·85 sodium chloride, isotonic dextrose (glucose) 5 per cent, gum saline, water containing sodium bicarbonate 1 drachm to the pint, a 25 per cent haemoglobin-Ringer solution, and transfusion of fresh blood, stored blood of different ages, blood plasma and blood serum (see p. 157). The amount given depends on certain factors: (*a*) whether any fluid is capable of being taken by mouth; (*b*) the need of the patient as demonstrated by his present condition (see symptoms of dehydration, above); (*c*) the efficiency of the circulation which becomes devitalized and lowered when prostration and collapse are marked. In such serious cases, apart from the use of the intravenous method, only small quantities of fluid can be given at first. The administration may be made at frequent intervals, more considerable intervals, or continuously. The latter is resorted to when the means chosen is either the rectum or the subcutaneous or intravenous route. In the latter case, as much as 6 to 10 pints may be administered during 24 hours.

Proctoclysis—or the administration of fluids per rectum. The *apparatus required* is a rubber catheter, attached to a tubing and funnel when small quantities are administered at intervals (see fig. 58, p. 199). For continuous administration some form of vacuum flask is supplied, together with rubber tubing and catheter, into which a drip connexion, either Ryall's or Laurie's, is inserted (see fig. 29, p. 156). Above the connexion is placed a rubber tubing clamp in order to regulate the flow,

Rectal feeding

and this regulation is then inspected by means of the drip connexion, the average rate of flow being from 40 to 60 drops per minute.

Before a rectal administration can be made the lower bowel must be emptied, by an enema if necessary, and the expulsion of gas obtained by passing a flatus tube (see fig. 58, p. 199). Should the administration be continued over a number of days the bowel should be rested by discontinuing the flow at regular intervals, every other hour, one hour every three hours, according to need.

Hypodermoclysis—or subcutaneous injection. By means of this method fluid is absorbed principally by the lymphatics. All the apparatus used must be sterile and the skin into which the needles are to be inserted should be cleansed. The injection is made into some part where the tissue is loose such as the abdomen, axillae or thighs. The *apparatus* consists of one or two special needles attached to rubber tubing. If two needles are used, a Y-shaped connexion is employed, and the upper end of that is attached to a single piece of tubing and a funnel when only small quantities are to be given; or to an irrigation can or vacuum flask if the administration is to be continuous, necessitating the preparation of larger quantities (see fig. 69, p. 207).

A similar drip connexion and tubing clips as before mentioned are used. The skin is purified, the saline is allowed to run through the apparatus to expel air, the tubing is clamped, the needles inserted as in the administration of hypodermic injection and the flow regulated. Some means should be taken to prevent the needles from either slipping out or being pulled out by any tension on the tubing. As a rule a small piece of elastoplast placed across the blunt end of the needle is sufficient support.

During the administration, the nurse stands by the bedside and keeps the apparatus in working order, watching carefully for any tension of the skin under which the fluid is running. This must be avoided, and the rate should be so managed that the fluid is actually absorbed as rapidly as it flows in—otherwise, if it runs in too quickly, the resultant pressure may cause a sloughing of the tissues. The formation of an abscess is another, rather more remote, danger, but as this is solely due to bad surgical technique it should be negligible, and hardly calls for mention here.

The amount that can be administered depends entirely on the absorptive powers of the tissues and no dogmatic statements can be made with regard to this. Occasionally when a subcutaneous infusion is to be made to infants, very small quantities only may be permissible, and in this case it may be administered by means of a 10-c.c. or 20-c.c. syringe.

INTRAVENOUS INFUSION AND BLOOD TRANSFUSION

Venesection may be performed whenever large quantities of fluid, either saline or 5 per cent glucose, are to be administered or blood transfusion is to be made. The instruments required are shown in fig. 70, p. 208. Alternatively a needle may be employed.

Estimation of the haemoglobin content of the blood made at the outset and again at intervals during the transfusion in cases who are bleeding, acts as a guide to the rate of administration needed to compensate for loss of blood. *Continuous blood drip transfusion* has proved of considerable value in haematemesis, in marked anaemia and in post-operative bleeding. It can e given before, during and after operation and in this way reduces the sk in operating on patients who are seriously ill, dehydrated and anae- ıic. A vein in the forearm is opened and the cannula inserted. In Dr. Iarriott's method a reservoir which contains the blood is suspended about feet above the level of the bed and fitted with a nickel gauze filter to rain clots. The blood is delivered to the patient from an opening at the ottom of the reservoir, the rate of flow being observed by a Laurie drip ıbe and controlled by a screw clip. The blood in the reservoir is kept ıixed by allowing a gentle stream of oxygen to flow into it; this is filtered y the insertion of three cotton wool filters at intervals in the tubing pass- ıg from cylinder to reservoir. The reservoir is also fitted with an outlet for xygen. Very gentle bubbling is necessary and the fact that the mixing is dequate can be seen by the layer of from 2 to 3 inches of froth on the ırface of the blood. In addition to mixing the blood so that the red cells o not collect at the bottom of the reservoir, oxygen also oxygenates it.

EMERGENCY TRANSFUSION APPARATUS FOR INTRAVENOUS INFUSION

The Emergency Transfusion bottle contains 180 c.c. of anti-coagulant nd is fitted with a screw cap.

For taking blood the metal cap, having been removed, is stood on a sterile owel and a rubber bung containing two holes is inserted; two short glass ıbes pass through this bung. One is connected by a piece of rubber ıbing, containing a window, to the needle for withdrawing blood, and ıe other to a piece of rubber tubing which contains two cotton wool lters. The free end of this tubing is attached by means of a glass con- exion to a Higginson's syringe (see fig. 71, p. 209) which the patient olds in his hand and squeezes gently, thus maintaining the circulation in is arm and the flow of blood from the vein to the bottle. Three hundred nd sixty cubic centimetres of blood are withdrawn, the rubber bung is emoved, the metal cap replaced and the bottle labelled. The blood is ored at 4° C. and can be kept at least for a fortnight and sometimes for a ıonth depending on the rate of haemolysis.

For giving blood the bottle is taken from the cold chamber, inverted once r twice and warmed by standing in a bowl of water at blood heat for at ast half an hour. The metal cap is removed and a rubber bung contain- ıg one long glass tube plugged with cotton wool to act as an air-inlet and lter and one short glass tube guarded by a 'gas mantle filter' is inserted. 'o the short tube a length of rubber tubing is attached containing a aurie drip bulb and screw clamp for regulating the flow of blood when ıe bottle is inverted and hung over the patient's bed. The lower end of ıe tubing is attached to a needle by means of a record fitting adaptor; lternatively Kaufmann's syringe (see fig. 73, p. 209) or cannula may be sed. (The same method is also convenient for the administration of plas- ıa, glucose, saline, etc.)

In the *nursing care* of a patient who is having a blood drip transfusion it important to see that the rate of flow ordered—usually 30 to 60 drops a ıinute—is maintained. If the flow ceases clotting will take place in the annula and provide an obstruction to subsequent flow and necessitate hanging the vein. If the patient complains of pain in the arm this ıould be reported as it may be due to phlebitis. In the administration of continuous infusion of blood it has been found advisable to change the vein after 24 hours, as there is a tendency to phlebitis when a vein has been used for some time.

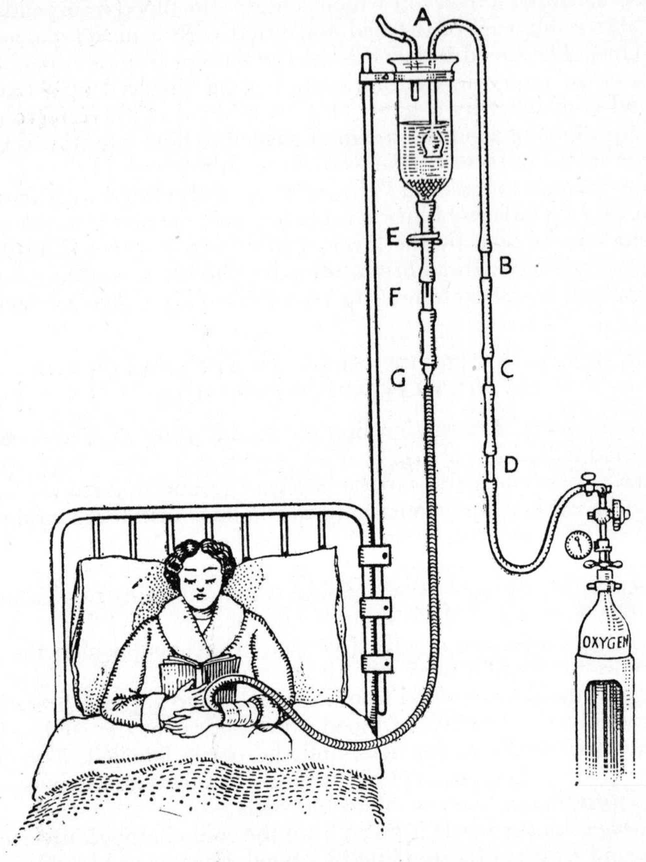

FIG. 29. ADMINISTRATION OF BLOOD TRANSFUSION.

(A) Reservoir with perforated rubber bung through which two glass tubes pass—th tube conveying the oxygen ends in an inverted thistle funnel—the oxygen bubble through the blood and escapes by means of the second shorter tube. At the bottom c the reservoir is a gauze filter. (B), (C) and (D) three cotton wool filters inserted in th tubing conveying oxygen to the reservoir. (E) rubber tubing clip. (F) Laurie's drip bulb (G) graduated glass connexion—from the lower end of which pressure tubing convey the blood to the cannula inserted in a vein of the forearm.

COMPLICATIONS IN INTRAVENOUS INFUSION

A *rigor* is the complication most often heard of. It is now considered to b due to dead organisms in the solution used, owing to being prepare with imperfectly distilled water, and it is a very rare occurrence indee when this point is attended to.

Pain in the chest accompanied by some distress of breathing or general restles ness may occur. This is thought to be due to too rapid administratio resulting in dilatation of the right side of the heart. Decreasing the rate of infusion will usually give relief; if it does not do so, the treatment is usually stopped.

In blood transfusion *some degree of haemolysis* may result from rapid breakdown of the red blood cells. This will be followed by jaundice, symptoms of which may be accompanied by a rise in temperature and rigors. Rapid haemolysis might prove fatal, but as the *grouping of blood* (see note below) is undertaken in order to avoid such a catastrophe, it is unlikely to occur.

Sepsis will only occur if there has been faulty surgical technique.

Thrombosis and *phlebitis* may occur locally.

GROUPING OF BLOOD

In order to prevent a blood transfusion being complicated by haemolysis of the red blood cells due to non-compatibility of the bloods of donor and recipient, the blood of humans has been classified into four groups. In this country the nomenclature O, A, B, AB, which is based on the agglutinogenic content of the blood, is employed.

New Terminology.	Old Terminology. (Moss system)	Number of people in each group.
AB (Universal Recipient) . .	I	Under 5%
A	II	About 40%
B	III	About 10%
O (Universal Donor) . . .	IV	About 40%

To facilitate recognition of the different blood groups when these are stored, a definite colour-scheme is used in labelling the blood.

Group	AB	White	Group	A	Yellow
,,	B	Pink	,,	O	Blue

The rule for transfusion is that the donor's cells should not be agglutinated when in contact with the recipient's serum. It will be seen that a patient of AB (or I) group is a *universal recipient* and may receive cells from any group.

An A (or II) group patient may receive blood from groups A (II) and O (IV).

A B (or III) group patient may receive blood from groups B (III) and O (IV).

An O (or IV) group patient may receive blood from group O (IV) only.

Thus it will be seen that group O (IV) is a *universal donor* and may give to any of the four groups.

PLASMA AND SERUM

Plasma and serum are superseding blood for transfusion purposes as these substances are more easily stored. *Agglutinin-free plasma* is the ideal one. It is made by mixing fresh blood from the various groups, particularly A and B, and can be used for every individual of whatever blood group he may be. *Dried Plasma* is also prepared which can be redissolved in sterile water and made up to the ordinary concentration of blood proteins, or a higher concentration can be prepared. By this means a higher percentage of blood proteins can be administered in a given quantity of fluid.

Serum is also employed, and it possesses certain advantages. It is easily prepared and is more stable than plasma and does not clot. It is useful when prolonged storage is necessary; it can be transported long distances and into warm climates.

MERITS OF FLUIDS AVAILABLE

Transfusion is performed with two main objects (*a*) *restoring the oxygen-carrying capacity of the blood*, as in the treatment of the anaemias when fresh blood is needed because the red cells are essential, and (*b*) in order *to restore the blood volume and blood pressure* when any innocuous fluid which can be retained in the circulation may be employed. For this purpose the blood derivatives are best—stored blood, prepared plasma and serum as these contain blood proteins.

Other available fluids include gum saline, isotonic saline (normal saline) and isotonic glucose. Of these gum saline is the most efficacious, but all these fluids are evanescent, and the transfused fluid rapidly leaves the circulation and is excreted by the kidneys.

RH OR RHESUS FACTOR IN BLOOD

Blood grouping as described above has been made in order to avoid putting non-compatible bloods, which would cause haemolysis of the red cells, together in giving blood transfusion. Another, more recently investigated factor which causes red blood cell destruction, particularly in the foetus and newly born, has been described as the rhesus factor because it is found in the Rh cells of rhesus monkeys. About 85 per cent of humans are rhesus-positive, the remaining 15 per cent being rhesus-negative.

Haemolytic disease in infants has been traced to the fact that the mother being Rh-negative, the father Rh-positive, the infant may be Rh-positive but, owing to the mixture in the foetal blood the mother's blood develops antibodies to the rhesus factor which will destroy the red blood cells of the foetus or the newly born. This is not the only cause of haemolytic disease in infants, but it is a cause which in the past has, in some cases, proved fatal. With the knowledge that is now available it is possible to transfuse blood into the infant containing the Rh factor and in this way the infant is kept alive until all the antibodies to the Rh factor present in his blood at birth have been eliminated and the new red blood cells being formed are no longer destroyed.

Chapter 12

Aspiration and Drainage of Body Cavities

Aspiration of the pleural cavity and the pericardial sac—Tapping the abdomen—Drainage of the subcutaneous tissue—Lumbar puncture and cisternal puncture

ASPIRATION AND TAPPING

The nurse will be expected to prepare both patient and apparatus for the performance of different forms of aspiration and paracentesis, or tapping, in order to remove fluid from the various cavities of the body. The *operation of paracentesis* consists of passing a hollow needle into the cavity from which the fluid is to be taken; the fluid, being under pressure in the cavity, will then run out as when a beer barrel is tapped. The term '*aspiration*' is used to describe the evacuation of a cavity when the fluid will not run out in the same way, and where some form of suction has to be employed in order to procure its evacuation, as in the case of the pleural cavity.

The chief reasons why any form of evacuation of a cavity is undertaken are: (1) for examination of the fluid contained in it; (2) for the relief of pressure caused by the fluid; and (3) to remove fluid in order to replace it by some other substance, such as saline, or serum.

With regard to the preparation of the apparatus and of the patient a few general rules may be laid down. In preparing apparatus *strict asepsis* is essential in order to prevent infection. The *inspection of the apparatus* is very necessary in order to see that it is in good working order; otherwise time will be lost and the patient will be inconvenienced by the delay. Great care should be taken to see that *any sharp instruments are really sharp* and that the *stilettes fit the needles* for which they are intended, and that in the same way trocars fit the cannulae. In the latter case it is very important that the trocar should only extend to the edge of the cannula. When a bevelled trocar is used, as in the case of Barker's needle for lumbar puncture, it must exactly fit the bevelled edge of the needle.

With regard to *preparation of the patient*, the nature of the exploration should if possible be explained to him. He should be told that as little discomfort as possible will be caused, and that a local anaesthetic will be used so that he does not feel the injection or puncture. The skin should be prepared as for a surgical operation. The patient must be made exceedingly comfortable in the position he is to adopt, as he may be required to maintain it for several minutes. If he moves, it may interfere with the operation, particularly in exploration of the pleura.

In addition, the nurse ought to know the effects that are expected from the investigation made, and she should be familiar beforehand with any untoward symptoms which may possibly arise during the performance of it. She should watch both the patient and the physician or surgeon, and be able to anticipate the wants of both without their having to give expression to them. She should supply the necessary specimen bottles with bungs or corks to fit, and have the appropriate pathological labels ready at hand.

She should have inquired beforehand whether the specimen is to be sent at once, as may be required in cases where it is essential that it should be delivered warm to the laboratory; in this case she should have ready some fluid at body temperature in which the test tube or other receptacle can be placed.

ASPIRATION OF THE PLEURAL CAVITY, OR THORACENTESIS

This operation is performed for the relief of symptoms in cases of pleural effusion, and also in some instances in order to collect a specimen of fluid for examination. The articles required include: *Potain's aspirator* (see figs. 74 and 75, p. 210), or an aspirating syringe may be employed.

Hypodermic syringe and needle, charged if necessary with a local anaesthetic. *Ethyl chloride* may be necessary.

Articles for cleansing the skin, including alcohol or some antiseptic, together with swabs for its application, and a receiver for soiled swabs.

Sterile test tubes for the reception of specimens of the fluid and some form of bowl or large receiver for the collection of further fluid should be provided.

Sterile towels and dressings—gauze and collodion, and either adhesive strapping, elastoplast, bandage or binder for securing the dressing in position, may be required.

A *sputum cup* should be at hand in case the patient wishes to use it, and a dose of *stimulant* should be provided such as brandy and water, in case he feels weak and faint.

The aspirator should be tested as follows—Insert the rubber bung with its connecting tubes into the glass bottle. Attach the pump to the proximal side and place the tubing on the distal side in a bowl of sterile water. Then adjust the taps, having the proximal tap opened and the distal one closed. The tap is open when it lies horizontally or in a line with the tubing, and closed when it lies at right angles, across the tubing. Having made certain that the rubber bung fits well into the neck of the bottle, to prevent the entrance of air, and seeing that all other connexions are similarly secure, the nurse then pumps rapidly and rhythmically for two or three minutes.

To test the vacuum, she then turns off the tap on the proximal end, and turns on the distal tap, when, if a vacuum has been formed, water will rush into the flask from the porringer of water in which the distal tube is lying.

Preparation of the patient. Having told the patient the nature of the operation, and allowed him, if it seems at all reasonable, to see the apparatus that is to be used, including the small size of the needle with which the puncture is to be made, and the local anaesthetic which is to be used to prevent his feeling even the tiny prick of this, he is placed in position. As a rule he is arranged either leaning forwards over a bedtable or pillow, on his knees, with his arm on the side to be treated carried well forward across his body in front of his chest in order to separate the intercostal spaces and keep the scapula well up out of the way. Or he may be arranged lying on the unaffected side with a firm pillow under his chest, so that he lies with his trunk flexed laterally over the pillow. The arm on the affected side is arried up over his head and the patient may grasp the rail at the bedhead, r clutch the mattress, or have his hand held in this position by a nurse.

The skin is then prepared, the bedclothes rearranged and towels are laced around the area of injection. The physician applies the local naesthetic and passes the needle into the chest. The needle is then at-ached to the tubing on the distal side of the aspirator bottle in which a artial vacuum has been created, and if the needle has tapped the fluid in he cavity this will flow into the bottle.

The nurse assures the patient that all is going well, and tells him that if e wishes to cough or move he must first inform her. She watches his colour nd pulse very carefully and reports any change.

When the operation is completed the needle is withdrawn and the punc-ure sealed by collodion or covered by the dressing provided. The appara-us is removed to a convenient place, the patient is made comfortable in is usual position in bed, given a stimulant if necessary—if not, he is given drink, and the nurse then clears the apparatus away. She has already nquired what is to be done with the fluid, and collected a specimen if ecessary; the remainder of the fluid should be measured and inspected or colour, odour and any abnormal appearance, and then thrown way.

She may now proceed to clean the apparatus. Fluid from the body prob-ly contains albumin, which is a coagulable substance. To cleanse the ubing and apparatus it may be reassembled as described when testing it, nd clean, cold water drawn through it several times; when quite clear of ll albuminous fluid an antiseptic may be drawn through—preferably one f a non-soapy nature such as 1–20 carbolic. The bottle, and the stopper vith its connecting tubing, may then either be sterilized by boiling or dis-nfected by soaking in carbolic 1–20 for one hour. At the end of this time he apparatus should be dried. Spirit may be drawn through it in the same vay as the water, or spirit may be syringed through the tubing. The tubing nd connexions should then be well shaken to free them of excess spirit, nd hung up to dry before being replaced in the box in which the appara-us may be kept. The glass bottle should be thoroughly polished with a dry luster. The aspirating needle and hypodermic syringe and needle used nay be cleaned as described on p. 623.

ASPIRATION OF THE PERICARDIAL SAC

The same apparatus as previously described may be employed, but, as he amount of fluid withdrawn from the pericardial cavity is small com-pared with that from the thoracic cavity, a 10 or 20 c.c. syringe and needle re usually found to be adequate. The front of the patient's chest is ex-posed, and he may either lie on his back, or be propped up with pillows. As considerable shock may attend this operation the nurse should watch he patient very carefully for changes of colour and irregularities of pulse.

TAPPING THE ABDOMEN, OR PARACENTESIS ABDOMINIS

Tapping the peritoneal cavity for the removal of fluid is usually under-aken for the relief of troublesome symptoms produced by ascites. It is im-portant for the nurse to realize that the removal of a large quantity of fluid will decrease the intra-abdominal pressure, and may give rise to cor siderable shock to the patient.

The **articles required** (see figs. 76 and 77, p. 211) include a *scalpel* fc making the initial incision in cases in which a large trocar and cannula employed.

A *trocar* and *cannula* of the size required, which may be an ordinary larg abdominal instrument, or Southey's tubes, may be employed. Rubbe tubing should be supplied of a suitable size to fit the trocar and cannul and it should be long enough to convey the fluid from the abdomen to th receptacle provided for it. When a large quantity of fluid is expected, as usually the case, a pail is placed at the bedside for its reception.

A *sterile specimen bottle* may be required if a specimen of the fluid wanted. *Sterile towels* and *sterile dressings* will be needed and an *abdomin binder* either of the usual many-tailed type, or of a special type designe for the application of pressure during the escape of the fluid from th abdominal cavity, in order to overcome the rapidly decreasing intra abdominal pressure, and so combat the ill effects which might result.

A *stimulant* should always be at hand and water or some other drink fc the patient who may need it during the operation.

Instruments provided should include dissecting forceps, scissors an needles; also sutures for suturing the edges of the small incision, togethe with *suitable dressings*, binder and safety pins.

Preparation of the patient. The patient will be propped up in sitting posture, as required by the degree of ascites present. As the pun ture is made in the midline it is essential for the bladder to be empty, an when collecting the apparatus the nurse must provide a suitable bedpa or urinal, and also have ready at hand the articles for catheterizing th patient.

The binder should be placed ready behind the patient in case it necessary to use it as described above during the escape of fluid.

The skin is prepared, anaesthetized, the incision made and the troca inserted. The rubber tubing provided is attached to the distal end of thi and the end of the tubing is placed in a receiver into which the fluid is t pass. The tubing should be long enough to reach to the bottom of th article provided for the reception of the fluid.

It is very important to watch the patient's pulse carefully, and the nurs should stand at the patient's bedside with her hand on the pulse, and if loses volume and tone she should at once give the patient a dose of th stimulant which lies ready at hand, and at the same time adjust the binde in order to help maintain intra-abdominal pressure.

At the termination of the treatment the cannula is removed. If an initi incision was made, a local anaesthetic is used and the wound sutured; suitable sterile dressing is applied, the binder firmly adjusted and secure in position by safety pins. The patient should be made comfortable in h bed, but should be moved as little as possible, since the movement of patient who has just undergone an operation is liable to induce shock. Th patient must be very carefully watched for some hours, and the binde which must not be allowed to get slack, should be readjusted from time t time.

Drainage of the subcutaneous tissue may be carried out by mea of *acupuncture*—when minute punctures are made in the skin by means of sharp sterile scalpel, the fluid which runs out being collected in large pads of sterile gauze and wool; or *Southey's tubes* may be employed. These tiny tubes are shown in illustration, fig. 77, p. 211, each one consisting of a silver cannula; in the illustration under figure A one silver cannula is depicted with the trocar inserted ready for use, and a second is shown with tubing attached after the trocar has been withdrawn.

A number of these cannulae may be employed; they are introduced into the oedematous tissue of the legs and thighs and the fluid drains either into bowls or receivers placed in the bed, or into a large pad of gauze and wool, which is changed as soon as it is saturated. It may be necessary to use a small strip of elastoplast to prevent the cannula from slipping out if the patient is restless.

The limbs that are being drained should be kept warm by being wrapped in cotton wool and the weight of the bedclothes should be removed from them by means of a low bedcradle.

LUMBAR PUNCTURE

Lumbar puncture is performed to tap the fluid in the *subarachnoid space* or, as it is sometimes called, the *theca.* It may be performed for several reasons: (*a*) to remove cerebrospinal fluid for examination purposes, (*b*) to remove fluid preliminary to the introduction of drugs, saline or serum, etc., (*c*) to ascertain the pressure of the cerebrospinal fluid, in which case a glass manometer is fitted to the apparatus used (Greenfield's apparatus), and (*d*) to remove fluid for the relief of intracranial pressure in a variety of cases including meningitis and conditions of oedema of the brain.

The apparatus generally used (see fig. 78, p. 212) **is a Barker's lumbar puncture needle.** It is a long needle with a finely bevelled point, and is fitted with a stilette, which is also bevelled, so that when placed in the correct position it completely fills the point of the needle, and the two together present a smooth bevelled cutting edge. Barker's needle is so adapted that the stilette has a little metal projection on the hilt which fits into a corresponding groove on the hilt of the cannula so that when these two are adapted the stilette is in the correct position. This special needle is made so that it will fit on to a record syringe, which should also be ready sterilized in case it may be required for withdrawing fluid should the pressure in the theca be exceedingly low.

One or two *sterile test tubes* should be in readiness for the collection of specimens of the fluid. In handling these test tubes two points are of importance—the fluid collected may be infectious, as in cases of cerebrospinal meningitis, and it is therefore important that the outside of the tube should not be contaminated. If it becomes contaminated the surface should be washed with alcohol, and the nurse who handles it should wash her hands. The second point is that in some cases the fluid should be conveyed warm to the laboratory where it is to be examined.

A *local anaesthetic* should be supplied, either novocain 2 per cent and a hypodermic syringe, or an ethyl chloride spray.

Antiseptic lotions and swabs will be required for cleansing the skin; any antiseptic may be employed, but iodine should be avoided if an ethyl chloride spray is to be used, as the effect of freezing skin painted with iodine is to render it tough. A *collodion dressing* is usually applied to the puncture.

A *drink* should be supplied in case the patient feels faint or weak as the result of the treatment, and in some cases a stimulant may be used.

Preparation of the patient. This operation is usually performed with the patient lying in the left lateral position with his thighs flexed on the abdomen, the knees flexed on the thighs and the head and shoulders drawn forward on to the front of the chest, so that the spine is as thoroughly flexed as possible and, therefore, the vertebral spines will be comparatively well separated, thus facilitating the passage of the needle between them.

The skin is cleansed over the area to be treated. As a rule the interval between the second and third or third and fourth lumbar vertebrae is punctured. If the nurse is in doubt as to the position of these bones, she can determine the level of the second or third lumbar vertebra by drawing her finger in a straight line from the top of the crest of the ilium to the middle of the patient's back. She should hold the patient in the curled up, flexed position whilst the puncture is made.

Another position in which this operation is sometimes carried out is to have the patient seated on a stool and leaning forward on some support placed in front of him, or, if he can manage it, with his hands clasped round his knees. The nurse stands in front of him and places her hands on the posterior aspect of his shoulders and keeps his trunk flexed, allowing him to rest his head against her side.

After lumbar puncture has been performed, the foot of the patient's bed should be elevated for some hours. If serum or any other fluid has been injected, this will facilitate its circulation more rapidly round the brain and cord. If fluid has been removed, it prevents the headache which might result from suddenly draining the fluid away from the ventricles of the brain.

Cisternal puncture is performed when it is desirable to obtain cerebrospinal fluid, or to inject serum or some other fluid, when this cannot be performed by lumbar puncture. A needle, similar to Barker's needle but shorter and finer, is passed beneath the skull, between it and the first cervical vertebra, into the *cisterna magna*, which is the portion of the subarachnoid space lying between the cerebellum and the medulla oblongata.

The back of the head is shaved as far up as the external occipital protuberance, the skin cleansed and a local anaesthetic applied; when the needle is inserted the head should be held forward on to the chest.

Cisternal puncture may be performed in conjunction with lumbar puncture in the investigation of spinal canal obstruction. Differences in the composition and in the pressure of the spinal fluid above and below the point of obstruction may be a guide in diagnosis (see also lipiodol injection p. 167).

Chapter 13

Some Investigations and Tests

X-ray examination of the alimentary tract—The use of lipiodol in X-ray examination—Encephalography and ventriculography—Examination of the function of the gallbladder—Examination of the function of the kidneys—Examination of the urinary bladder—Examination of the sigmoid colon—Gastric analysis—Glucose tolerance test. (See also pp. 509, 420, 471, 473, 532, *and* 558 *for the tuberculin tests, the Widal test, tests used in the diagnosis of some of the infectious diseases, the Wassermann reaction and tests of pregnancy)*

In order that a nurse may the more intelligently understand and appreciate the treatment which is being carried out, she ought to have some idea of the nature of the commoner investigations and tests which she will, from time to time, see undertaken and for which she may have to prepare her patient as well as, in some cases, the apparatus.

DIAGNOSTIC X-RAY EXAMINATION

General notes on considerations to be made on taking any patient to the X-ray room for examination. The patient should be suitably clothed; all articles used should be such as can be easily removed and rearranged without exposure of the patient. Some easily manipulated garment, such as a shawl or small blanket or shoulder wrap, should be at hand to cover the patient's shoulders if he has to wait for any reason—such as the recharging of a plate carrier or whilst a film is developed.

The clothing should be quite free from all articles known to be impervious to X-rays, such as metal buttons, and such things as keys or a watch should be taken out of the patient's pockets. Silk garments should not be worn. If the head is to be X-rayed all hairpins, slides, combs and ribbon should be removed. Dentures should be taken out, at the last moment, and kept safely. If splints are used, wooden ones are preferable, metal should not be used; bandages should not contain safety pins and strapping ought not to be employed.

The patient should be informed, as clearly as possible, what is to be done and the help expected from him. He will have to lie very still, and great pains should be taken to see that he is comfortably placed on the table or other piece of apparatus on which he is to lie, or rest.

X-rays were first employed in the diagnosis of conditions in tissues which, because of their calcium content, are opaque to X-rays, such as the bones, and in cases of urinary stone. Later, X-rays began to be employed in the examination and diagnosis of conditions of the alimentary tract. At first, bismuth was administered for examination of the upper part of the tract, and barium for enemata. At the present day, the use of barium has superseded that of bismuth almost entirely; a *barium meal* consists of about 4 ounces of barium in a pint of Horlick's malted milk, or cocoa. In a *barium enema*, 1 to 2 pounds of barium are mixed in 4 pints of mucilage of tragacanth.

Examination of the alimentary tract is undertaken for a number of reasons and to diagnose a great number of conditions and diseases, including:

(*a*) *stricture of the oesophagus*. In this condition the barium will be observed above the obstruction when complete.

(*b*) *cardio-spasm*. The barium will lie curled up at the cardiac orifice, owing to closure of the latter by spasm.

(*c*) *examination of the stomach*. Normally the contour of the organ will be regular in outline and the waves of peristalsis will be seen passing along it at regular intervals. In the event of disease or abnormality, the stomach may be seen to be dilated; in carcinoma there is often irregularity of filling, with deformity of the contour of the stomach; in peptic ulcer, the crater of the ulcer can be seen, accompanied by spasm of the corresponding segment of the organ. The rate of emptying of the stomach is usually investigated; it may empty quickly when the organ is hypertonic; alternatively, a residue will be seen, after 4 hours, in cases of pyloric obstruction.

(*d*) *visceroptosis*. The stomach or any part of the intestine—particularly the caecum—may be seen to be displaced.

(*e*) *examination of the large intestine* The appendix should be seen to fill and empty normally; any narrowing of the lumen of the gut would be noticed; arrest of the passage of the barium would be caused by obstruction, spasm or stricture; in diverticulitis small pouches would be seen.

Preparation of a patient for X-ray investigation of the alimentary tract. A light diet should be given for a few days before the examination is to be made; any medicine containing bismuth must be omitted during this period. For examination of the stomach and small intestine the patient should be fasting from the previous evening; for examination of the colon a light breakfast is allowed.

In order to empty the alimentary tract, an aperient such as castor oil, from half to one ounce, should be given 48 hours before the time of examination, and in some cases this is repeated again, 24 hours before. It should be followed by a simple enema, 6 hours beforehand, if necessary. In many cases a dose of any aperient the patient is familiar with may be substituted for castor oil; but aperients that are known to cause flatulent distension—such as magnesium sulphate—should be avoided. Some flatulence is invariably present after the use of any aperient, and to overcome this many physicians order a dose of pituitrin, or arrange to have a flatus tube passed a short time before the examination is to take place. When the stomach is the site of examination an opiate mixture may be ordered 4-hourly, or 6-hourly, for 12 hours before the examination.

X-ray examination of the stomach is usually carried out early in the morning. The prepared barium meal is given in the X-ray room, and the first examination made about 9 o'clock (see fig. 79, p. 213), subsequent ones being carried out at intervals of three hours, in order to note the rate at which the barium passes along the tract. It is very important that a patient undergoing this examination should be kept warm, and permitted to rest comfortably, either in his own bed, or in a rest room adjoining the X-ray department. It is essential that everyone, including the patient himself, should clearly understand that, until the final examination has been made, he may not have anything by mouth—neither food, drink nor medicine. He will be feeling very weak and tired after his long and difficult fast and, as soon as the last examination has been made, he should be given a light meal.

When the colon is the site of examination, a barium enema will be given to the patient in the X-ray room (see fig. 80, p. 214). It is important to remember that mackintoshes should not be used as this material is impervious to X-rays.

Lipiodol examination. Lipiodol is a fatty substance which contains a certain amount of iodine and is opaque to X-rays. It is used for several examinations:

(*a*) for *inspection of the character of the bronchial tree*, in cases of bronchiectasis. About 4 c.c. of the substance is passed into the trachea, by introduction through the crico-thyroid membrane. The patient lies on the side which is to be examined and the lipiodol trickles down into the branches of the bronchi, which can then be seen on X-ray examination (see fig. 81, p. 215).

(*b*) in the *diagnosis of the position of tumours of the spinal cord*. It is injected into the subarachnoid space, usually at the base of the skull, and will trickle down and become arrested at the site of the tumour.

(*c*) to determine the presence of *stricture of the fallopian tubes*, the preparation of lipiodol being injected into the uterus under pressure, in cases suspected of sterility and, if this is due to stricture of the tubes, the lipiodol will be seen held up, and unable to pass the stricture, on subsequent X-ray examination (see fig. 82, p. 216).

(*d*) injected into *sinuses* to facilitate investigation of their extent by X-ray examination.

Encephalography and **ventriculography.** In both these investigations radiograms are taken after the withdrawal of fluid from the ventricles of the brain and its replacement with air. The examination is undertaken as an aid to diagnosis of the presence of a tumour of the brain which would cause displacement of the fluid injected into the ventricles.

Ventriculography is only undertaken as a last measure, as it requires a surgical operation. Holes are drilled in both parietal bones and air is injected directly into the ventricles.

In *encephalography* lumbar puncture is performed, and air injected into the theca rises and fills the ventricles. The patient is given morphia gr. $\frac{1}{4}$ and hyoscine gr. $\frac{1}{150}$, or gr. $\frac{2}{3}$ of omnopon before the investigation is made. The articles required for the performance of encephalography are shown in fig. 83, p. 217. The patient sits on a stool, the lower part of his back is uncovered and a sterile towel is draped over his clothing; it is kept in position by means of 2 towel clips. Lumbar puncture is performed, and 5 c.c. of fluid are withdrawn. Then 5 c.c. of air are drawn through sterile cotton wool into an easily moving glass syringe and injected into the theca.

The withdrawal of fluid and its replacement by air is repeated until from 50 to 60 c.c. of fluid have been withdrawn and the same quantity of air has been injected. During the treatment the patient's head is slowly raised and lowered in order to get better diffusion of air in the ventricular spaces. He is X-rayed in different positions as air being light will tend to rise, so that when for example he is placed on his right side air may be expected to show in the left ventricle.

As the result of this investigation the patient will have very severe headache; he is taken back to the ward and put to bed and is generally given a dose of morphia for the relief of pain. His bed should be elevated at tl foot on blocks 12 inches high in order to encourage the circulation of cer brospinal fluid in the ventricles which have been drained. The headacl usually subsides in 24 hours; in the meantime the patient should be e couraged to take plenty of fluid to drink. His pulse should be recorded ar in some cases the physician will wish the blood pressure to be taken als

For *diagnostic examination of the kidneys* see p. 169; and of the *gallbladd* see below.

EXAMINATION OF THE FUNCTIONAL ACTIVITY OF THE GALLBLADDER

The gallbladder normally empties its contents into the duodenum. I its function of storing bile, it also concentrates this substance and, whe diseased or disordered, this function may be impaired. Direct examinatic of the gallbladder has been proved unsatisfactory and the examinatic described below as *cholecystography* has entirely superseded this method.

Examination of the character of the bile can be made by means Lyon's system of gallbladder drainage.

Cholecystography. *Graham's test.* Dr. Graham discovered th opaque salts were removed from the blood by the liver and concentrate in the gallbladder. This rendered it possible to investigate the outline the gallbladder by X-ray examination.

Preparation. The routine general preparation is carried out as describe on p. 165. The very light evening meal given the day before should b entirely devoid of butter, milk and all other fats. The examination is to b made fasting, and the patient should not be given any medicine or pe mitted to see or smell food, for fear of stimulating the activity of the gal bladder.

A special dye (opacol) is used. It may either be taken by mouth or i jected intravenously. If given by mouth 6 grammes, or even 8 gramm for a fat person, are given with citric acid and sugar at 6 p.m. the evenin before the examination is to take place, and photographs are taken nine and twelve the following day. When the dye is administered by th intravenous route, it is important that none of the dye should be permitte to escape into the tissues during the administration, as this would result ulceration and sloughing; moreover, the administration of the dye shoul be followed by passing a small quantity of sterile saline through the needl into the vein so that it is completely washed out before it is withdraw

If the gallbladder is concentrating normally a shadow of the organ wi be seen on X-ray examination (see fig. 85, p. 219). When gallstones ar present there will be lack of uniformity of shadow, and if there is n shadow it indicates that the gallbladder is not concentrating and is there fore not functioning normally. It is of interest for the nurse to know th a good outline should show in a normal gallbladder at the first examin tion; at the second examination it should show a mere shadow, and at th third examination it should be empty.

The first examination is made at 9 a.m. and the second at about 1 noon. If shadow is still visible at noon a third examination is made, bu before this a meal rich in fat is given. A cup of cocoa, with bread and bu ter, and egg, is frequently employed. This causes the gallbladder to empt

Lyon's gallbladder drainage. This is also described as *non-surgical drainage of the gallbladder*, and is carried out by the administration of a small dose of concentrated magnesium sulphate poured into the duodenum by means of a Ryle's tube.

Preparation. The patient is given a comparatively non-fatty supper the previous evening. Lean meat, brown bread and stewed prunes are frequently given. He is then told not to swallow his saliva when he wakens the next morning, but instead to rinse his mouth out with a mild antiseptic wash.

Method. A Ryle's tube is passed, and the resting juice drawn off the stomach, as in the preparation for a test meal (see p. 172). The patient is then turned on to his right side and the tube is passed a little farther, in the hope that it may enter and lie in the duodenum. Twenty c.c. of 25 per cent magnesium sulphate solution is introduced by means of a record syringe attached to the end of the tube, at the lips. Fifteen minutes later fluid is drawn off at short intervals by means of the record syringe until a bright yellow specimen is obtained. This is labelled '*Specimen* 1'. It is tested with litmus, and if found to be acid the tube is considered to be in the stomach. A funnel is then attached to the duodenal tube and sterile water poured down into the stomach; this may stimulate peristalsis and cause the end of the tube to be carried through the pylorus into the duodenum.

Specimens are collected at intervals until a dark coloured alkaline specimen is obtained, and this is labelled '*Specimen* 2'. When no more fluid can be obtained, 50 c.c. of the magnesium sulphate solution is poured in. This causes the gallbladder to act, and when a golden brown specimen is obtained it is put up in a glass labelled '*Specimen* 3'.

EXAMINATION OF THE FUNCTIONAL ACTIVITY OF THE KIDNEYS

The examination of the functional activity of the kidneys is an important part of the preparation of a patient for an operation on any part of the genito-urinary tract. This examination includes *chemical examination of the urine* (see p. 69), *microscopic* and *bacteriological examinations of the urine*, *examination by means of direct X-ray*, by *pyelography*, by *estimation of the percentage of urea in the blood* and the *function of the kidney in concentrating the urine and eliminating urea.*

For obtaining a direct **X-ray examination of the kidneys,** the routine general preparation is carried out. The patient is kept on low diet for several days beforehand and an aperient is given, as described in the case of examination of the alimentary tract, followed by an enema if necessary. Means are taken to see that the colon is free from gas. A light breakfast may be given.

Pyelography means the making of a photograph of the pelvis of the kidney. The history of the investigation of the urinary tract is very interesting. At first, ureteric catheters were used. These were rendered opaque by the insertion of rings of gold so that the position of the catheters was visible on X-ray examination. The next step was the use of collargol, a substance opaque to X-rays, injected by means of the ureteric catheters in order to show the outline of the kidney pelvis. The next step was the discovery that substances with a large iodine content were opaque to X-rays, and could be administered in a form which was rapidly secreted by tl kidney. Two methods of pyelography are described—(1) cystoscopic, ar (2) intravenous.

Cystoscopic examination is carried out in the X-ray department a ureteric catheters are passed into the ureters. (For apparatus used s fig. 86, p. 220.) These are left in but the cystoscope is withdrawn. A war solution of the opaque iodine compound is then injected by means of syringe—the pelvis of the kidney will hold about 5 c.c. of fluid. As a ru the patient is not given a general anaesthetic, and the passing of tl cystoscope and the ureteric catheters, and the injection of the fluid, m therefore cause some discomfort. The patient should be watched very car fully, and asked to let the doctor know what sensations he experiences; patient can usually tell when the ureteric catheter has reached the pelv of the kidney. The injection of fluid may give rise to fairly considerab discomfort, due to the fact that the pelvis does not hold as much as normal one might be expected to hold, and in this case the physician w cease injecting the fluid. The administration of a mild analgesic, such aspirin, will tend to minimize the fears and painful impressions the patie receives.

The *disadvantage of the cystoscopic method* is the discomfort caused by i and for this reason it is considered unsuitable for children or for nervo restless patients.

The *intravenous method* is most useful, especially in the examination persons who will not readily submit to the passage of a cystoscop Patients suffering from inflammation of the lower part of the urinar tract would suffer considerable pain from the passage of a cystoscope.

Intravenous pyelography is performed by the injection into the circulatio of a substance called *uroselectan*. It was first prepared by Professor vo Lichtenberg, and is a non-irritating compound, containing a little ove 50 per cent iodine. It is secreted very quickly and does not produce an toxic symptoms, and the urine in which it is contained is rendered opaqu to X-rays. As a rule about 20 c.c. are injected and an X-ray examinatio is made at intervals of 5, 15 and 30 minutes, when shadows of the kidney and ureters will be seen (see fig. 87, p. 221). If the patient refrains fro passing urine, the outline of the bladder can be seen later; but, in order t investigate thoroughly the lower part of the ureter, the bladder should b emptied as opacity here obscures examination of the pelvic ureters.

Urea concentration test. (MacLean's test.) Investigation of the func tion of the kidney is carried out during the treatment of medical an surgical conditions. In the former it is largely used as an aid to diagnosis In the latter it enables the surgeon to determine any disability of the rena function and forms a preliminary investigation to any operation, par ticularly those on the genito-urinary tract. After all operations, the bloo urea rises, and the kidneys therefore require to be in specially good con dition in order to perform the extra work put upon them, for, should the fail, the patient may die of uraemia.

Preparation of the patient. A light evening meal is given, and after this th patient is not allowed any fluid, medicine or food. At a given hour th next morning, say 7 a.m., the patient passes urine, and this is saved in glass labelled '*No.* 1'. He is then given 15 grammes of urea in 100 c.c. o water. He passes urine at 8 a.m., 9 a.m., and 11 a.m.—that is, 1, 2 and hours after the administration of urea. These specimens are collected and placed in glasses labelled '*No.* 2', '*No.* 3', and '*No.* 4'.

The urine collected is examined—the normal amount of urea in urine is 2 per cent; but, as urea acts as a diuretic, the urine obtained immediately after its administration will be more dilute and the first specimen may therefore be expected to contain only 1·5 per cent, which is accepted as normal. The amount of urea will rise in the second specimen, and the last one will contain the highest quantity, which should be 2 per cent. If the kidney is disabled, the percentage of urea found in the urine will be lower than normal, and will not rise in the later specimens as it should.

Blood urea test. As a general rule analysis of the blood for its urea content is made at the same time as the urea concentration test. A specimen of blood is taken before urea is administered, and at one or two intervals after its administration.

The normal percentage of blood urea is 20 to 40 milligrammes per 100 cubic centimetres. In uraemia, arteriosclerosis, acute nephritis, chronic interstitial nephritis and other conditions in which the kidney is disabled, it may be as high as from 200 to 300 milligrammes per 100 c.c. A blood urea of over 200 is very serious. In chronic parenchymatous nephritis the blood urea content is abnormally low.

Indigo-carmine dye test. An intravenous injection of indigo-carmine is found to render the urine of a normal subject a deep blue colour in from 7 to 10 minutes or perhaps a little longer. This test is sometimes performed in the investigation of the renal function; if the time is delayed, or the colour only pale blue, the kidney is considered to be disabled.

Renal efficiency test. (Van Slyke's test.) In order to determine with comparative accuracy the function of the kidney with regard to the normal constituents contained in urine and the presence of any possible abnormal constituents, particularly albumin, the following investigation is made. No preparation is necessary.

First thing in the morning, whilst the patient is still fasting, his bladder is emptied by means of a catheter. The catheter is left in position, with a spigot placed in the free end. Exactly one and two hours later the bladder is evacuated and the specimens obtained are sent to the laboratory for examination.

EXAMINATION OF THE URINARY BLADDER

Cystoscopy. Examination of the urinary bladder by means of an instrument called a cystoscope is carried out in order to inspect the cavity of the bladder and the condition of the openings of the ureters which enter it.

A cystoscope consists of a telescope, fitted with lenses. An electric bulb is passed into the telescope. It is rather a large instrument, like a metal catheter, and is passed into the bladder through the urethra; as a rule a general anaesthetic is not employed; in the case of men an injection of percaine or novocaine is made into the urethra (see fig. 88, p. 222).

Preparation for examination. The instrument is sterilized—preferably in formalin vapour, since this does not necessitate wetting. It may, alternatively, be prepared by separating the different parts and standing them in a tall vessel in lysol or spirit; the distal end, which contains the lenses, should not be covered by solution, as these will be fogged if fluid get between them. The electric bulb should be tested to see that it is workin before the apparatus is handed to the surgeon for insertion into th urethra and bladder. A spare bulb should always be supplied.

Method. The patient should be informed of the nature of the procedur and he should be placed in the lithotomy position. He must be covere so that there is the least possible exposure and his legs should be encased i long woollen stockings. A catheter is passed and the bladder is emptied; tubing and funnel are then attached to the catheter which is in the bladde and sterile lotion is run in—5 to 10 ounces being used, in order to disten the bladder and enable the surgeon to see all parts of it. The lotion use should be warm.

Sigmoidoscopy. For this investigation the instruments shown i fig. 89, p. 223, are required. The colon must be empty, therefore the patien is given an aperient two days before the investigation, and 12 hour beforehand the colon is irrigated.

In some cases a general anaesthetic is given, but in the majority of case the patient is given morphia gr. $\frac{1}{4}$ half an hour beforehand. The examina-tion may be made with the patient in the left lateral position or kneeling resting on the elbows. The instrument is supplied with an introducer; thi is lubricated and it is then passed through the anal canal. The introduce is then withdrawn and the surgeon puts his eye to the lens, the electri power which illuminates the lamp is turned on, and the passage of th instrument along the rectum is carefully directed.

GASTRIC ANALYSIS

Analysis of the gastric secretion is carried out as an aid to diagnosis b helping to discern the behaviour of the stomach, its absorptive power and the condition of its secretions. The commonest method in use is by th administration of a test meal which aims at discovering the activities of th stomach during the process of gastric digestion.

A **fractional test meal**, the method of Rehfuss, is most commonl employed today, and the articles used for this (see fig. 90, p. 224) includ a Ryle's stomach tube, a mild lubricant and a record syringe of 20 c.c capacity.

A pint of oatmeal gruel which has been prepared by putting 2 oz. o oatmeal into a quart of water and boiling it gently until it has been re-duced to a pint, and a feeder or drinking cup from which the patient take this fluid.

A sterile flask for the reception of the *resting juice* with a capacity of abou half a pint; and a flask of similar capacity for the reception of the *residua fluid*.

Eight to ten sterile test tubes numbered in order, into which 10–15 c.c of fluid from the stomach will be put every 15 minutes. Some physician like a piece of filtering paper placed at the open end of each test tube, s that the fluid received is filtered at once.

A towel is provided for the patient to place under his chin, and receiver in case he feels that he is going to be sick.

The patient should be told the nature of the examination. He will no suffer any inconvenience from it and may be given something interestin to read so that his attention will be occupied; a woman might knit or sew as she pleases.

Method of administration. The test meal is given on an empty stomach, usually at an early hour in the morning, say at 8 or 9 a.m. The patient will have had a light supper, early in the evening, of a carbohydrate nature. Two or three hours after this he will be given one or two charcoal biscuits and should not take any other food or drink until after the test is carried out the following morning.

At the time of the test the patient swallows the tube. It should be moist, but as it is usually brought to the bedside in a bowl of warm water no other treatment will be required. Some sisters use a small quantity of liquid paraffin to lubricate the tube, though this is not necessary. The tube is put in at the corner of the patient's mouth and he is encouraged to swallow it—put in in this way there is less likelihood that the tube will impinge on the posterior pharyngeal wall which would make the patient retch. The end of the tube will reach the stomach when the first mark on it is at the level of the lips. The 20 c.c. syringe is then attached to the distal end of the tube and the contents of the fasting stomach, that is the *resting juice*, is withdrawn; the quantity is noted, and it is put into the sterile flask labelled ready to receive it.

The patient now takes the gruel; if he finds it difficult to drink a pint the nurse can pass some of it into the stomach through the Ryle's tube. Specimens of about 10 c.c. are now, by means of the metal syringe, withdrawn every 15 minutes for two to two and a half hours, until eight to ten specimens have been obtained. These are placed in the test tubes ready numbered. At the end of this time, if the stomach is not empty, the remainder of the contents are withdrawn and put into the flask labelled '*Residue*'. The tube can then be removed, and the patient may be given a mouth-wash and a suitable feeding or light meal.

Investigations which will be made as a result of this test will prove:

(1) *The amount of resting juice.* In the normal this is from 60–120 c.c. In abnormal conditions it may be very much increased and in carcinoma it may rise to 400 c.c.

(2) *The amount of hydrochloric acid present.*

(3) *Any charcoal present.* Charcoal should have been passed off during the night, and its presence will show delay in the activity of the stomach.

(4) *Excess or absence of hydrochloric acid.* In the absence of HCl, lactic acid may be present.

(5) *The odour of the specimen*—particularly any foul odour, which would suggest dilatation of the stomach.

(6) *The amount of residue.* A large amount would indicate that the stomach is very slow in emptying.

The colour should be noted—whether clear or not, and whether it contains bile, showing that there is regurgitation from the duodenum, or blood, which indicates oozing from the stomach, or any excess of mucus.

The method of gastric analysis described above—a fractional test meal—also gives information regarding the degrees of acidity at different intervals; the time when bile, blood or excess mucus may appear, and the time the stomach takes to empty.

Alcohol injected by means of Ryle's tube, is occasionally substituted for gruel in a fractional test meal. Only 100 c.c. of seven per cent alcohol is employed as compared with 500 c.c. of gruel. Samples of stomac contents are taken every half-hour for one and a half hours.

Ewald's test meal. Other less often used tests for gastric analys include Ewald's. In this test the patient is given a slice of dry toast and cup of tea without sugar or milk on a fasting stomach. A stomach tube passed and the meal removed after an hour or so.

Boas's meal consists of half a pint of gruel passed into the stomach an removed in thirty minutes. (The method of passing a stomach tube h been described in the administration of gastric lavage, on p. 140.)

Histamine is used in examination of the contents of the stomach i order to make a differential diagnosis between a true and a false achlo hydria; it is a most powerful stimulant to the secretion of HCl. Th

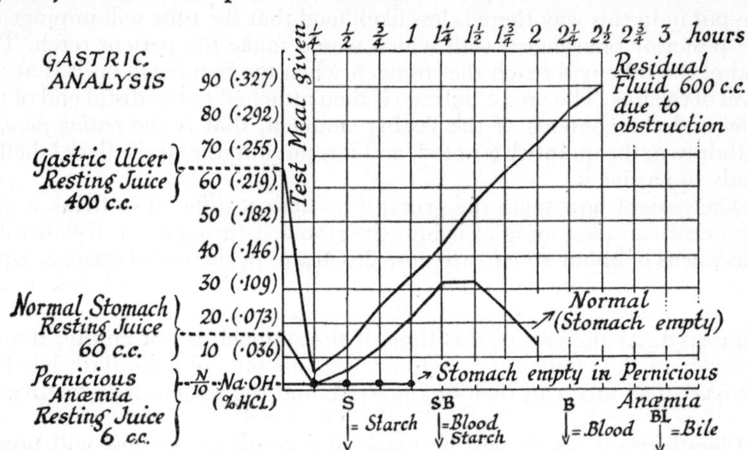

FIG. 30. CHART SHOWING GASTRIC ACID CURVE—IN A CASE OF GASTRIC ULCER COMP CATED BY PYLORIC OBSTRUCTION—IN A NORMAL STOMACH—AND IN A CASE OF PERNICIC ANAEMIA.

stomach is prepared as for a fractional test meal, the fasting juice wit drawn, and the stomach washed out with plain water. A hypoderm injection of histamine, 0·5 milligramme, is given and half an hour lat from 10 to 15 c.c. of gastric fluid is withdrawn and tested. The absence acid, determined by using Günzberg's reagent, confirms the diagnosis of true achlorhydria such as exists in pernicious anaemia.

Histamine is a poison which causes a sudden fall in blood pressure; it therefore used with caution in pernicious anaemia, a disease in which th blood pressure is usually low.

GLUCOSE TOLERANCE TEST

Since the blood always contains some sugar, it can reasonably b expected that its sugar content will be highest immediately after a me rich in carbohydrates, and lower several hours after a meal, and lowe when fasting.

In a normal person the fasting blood sugar is about 0·08 to 0·12 per cen the resting blood sugar being about 0·12 to 0·15 per cent. After rapi bsorption of glucose there is a quick rise in blood sugar up to just below he *renal threshold*—this on the average is 0·18 per cent. At this level the nsulin factor, or the mechanism which controls the storage of sugar in the ody, comes into play and prevents the percentage of blood sugar from ising above the renal threshold limit. Instead, it begins to fall steadily and radually until the resting level is again reached.

The *renal threshold* is the term used to describe the maximum percentage f blood sugar possible without its being secreted in the urine. It is also ometimes described as the *leak point of the kidney*, meaning the point, or ercentage of blood sugar, at which sugar would begin to leak out of ne body by way of the kidney. The accompanying chart shows what

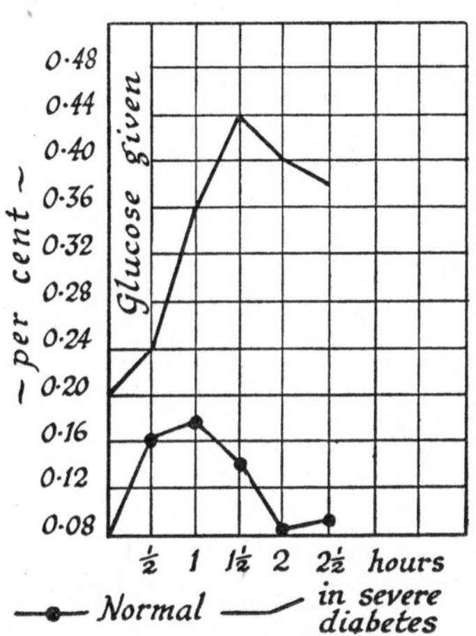

IG. 31.—SHOWING THE BLOOD SUGAR CURVE CONSEQUENT ON A GLUCOSE TOLERANCE TEST IN A NORMAL PERSON AND IN A CASE OF SEVERE DIABETES.

ctually happens in a normal subject when a dose of glucose is given order to test the function of the sugar-controlling mechanism of the lood.

In diabetes there is deficiency of insulin with the result that the storage nechanism is disordered. There is, therefore, no control, and varying egrees of hyperglycaemia occur after the administration of glucose. The ccompanying chart shows a blood sugar curve in a very serious case of iabetes, as compared with the normal. The fasting blood sugar is 0·2 per ent; in half an hour it rises to 0·36 and after one hour reaches a naximum of 0·44 per cent. It then begins slowly to fall.

Comparison with the chart demonstrating the behaviour to be expected the normal subject shows that the resting blood sugar is 0·08 per cent— rose to 0·17 per cent, which is below the renal threshold margin, and fell uickly. At the end of two hours it is seen to be almost as low as at the tarting point, which demonstrates perfect functioning of the sugar-controlling mechanism.

The test is carried out as follows—A sample of the patient's blood taken before breakfast when he has fasted all night. He is then given 50 rammes of glucose in 100 c.c. of water and specimens of his blood are taken at half-hourly intervals for the next 2 hours; three specimens c urine are taken at hourly intervals. In the normal subject the fasting bloo sugar may for example be 0·12 per cent—within half an hour it will ris to just below the renal threshold. It may rise to 0·17 per cent, but will the begin to drop quite rapidly and in two hours will have fallen to the restin level again.

Chapter 14

The Application of Splints, Plaster of Paris, Extensions and Strapping

Types of splints—Plaster of paris—The use and application of extension—Skeletal traction—Splint and plaster sores—Closed plaster method—Application of strapping

Splints are rigid structures employed to give support and protect the parts of the body to which these are applied. In an emergency a splint may be made of any fairly stiff material. Cardboard, wood, walking sticks and umbrellas are commonly used as emergency splinting.

The splints used in hospital may be of light metal, aluminium, or malleable iron, of poroplastic felt or of wood, leather or steel. Plaster of paris is a very favourite splint as it can more easily be modified and adapted to the body, and can also be prepared in a variety of thicknesses and degrees of strength.

The side of the splint which is to be placed next to the body is usually padded, either with felt or wool in the case of metal splints or by a specially prepared padding stitched on. The articles required and the mode of procedure in padding a wooden splint are illustrated in fig. 92, p. 225.

The padding of a splint is designed to prevent pressure of the hard framework of the apparatus, which is bandaged to the affected part, from injuring it and the padding must be adequate for this purpose; the sides, ends and edges of the splint must be covered and when the splint is applied the nurse should examine it to see that these parts are covered and not pressing into the skin.

A nurse should be familiar with the splints in use in the hospital in which she is working and know how to apply them. Many splints are named after the surgeon who designed them: such are the Thomas's leg splint and Hodgen's splint which are shown in fig. 33, p. 179. Other well-known ones are Carr's, Neville's and McIntyre's splints. Splints are also described according to their shape as straight, angular, gutter splints, etc.; others are designated according to their use as a cock-up splint for the hand, a talipes splint, an angular foot and leg splint and so on.

Plaster of paris splints are made by using muslin bandages into which fine dental plaster has been rubbed, the bandages are then rolled loosely and after being soaked in tepid water are applied wet to the part; the plaster sets fairly quickly, in a few minutes, and the splint dries and hardens. (See figs. 94–102, pp. 227–30.)

The articles needed to apply plaster of paris are shown in fig. 93, p. 226. The part for which the splint is intended should be shaved if the plaster is directly applied to the skin; but when the skin is first protected with a layer of wool, a domette or lint bandage, shaving is not necessary. When preparing the patient the nurse should protect the floor around the bed and the patient's bedclothing and personal clothing with dust sheets for fear lest splashes of wet plaster should fall on these.

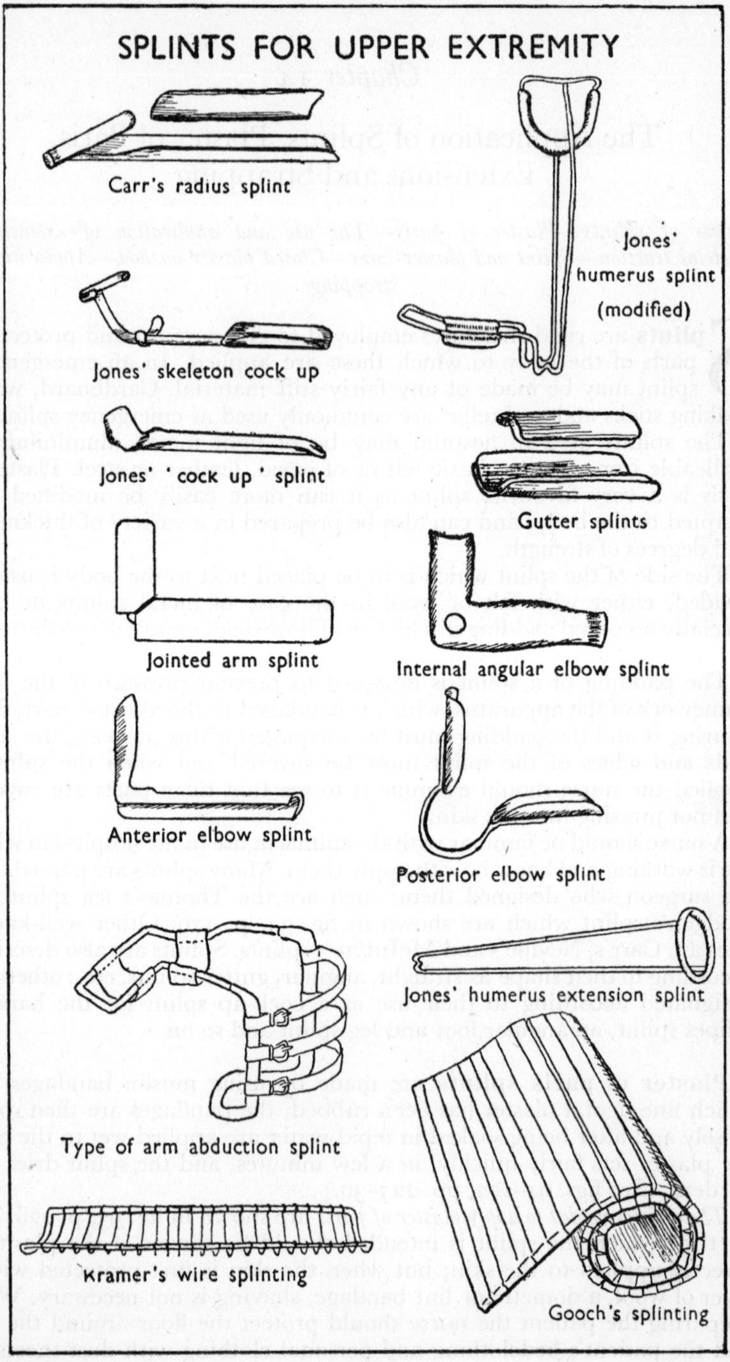

SPLINTS FOR UPPER EXTREMITY

Carr's radius splint

Jones' humerus splint (modified)

Jones' skeleton cock up

Jones' 'cock up' splint

Gutter splints

Jointed arm splint

Internal angular elbow splint

Anterior elbow splint

Posterior elbow splint

Jones' humerus extension splint

Type of arm abduction splint

Kramer's wire splinting

Gooch's splinting

FIG. 32.

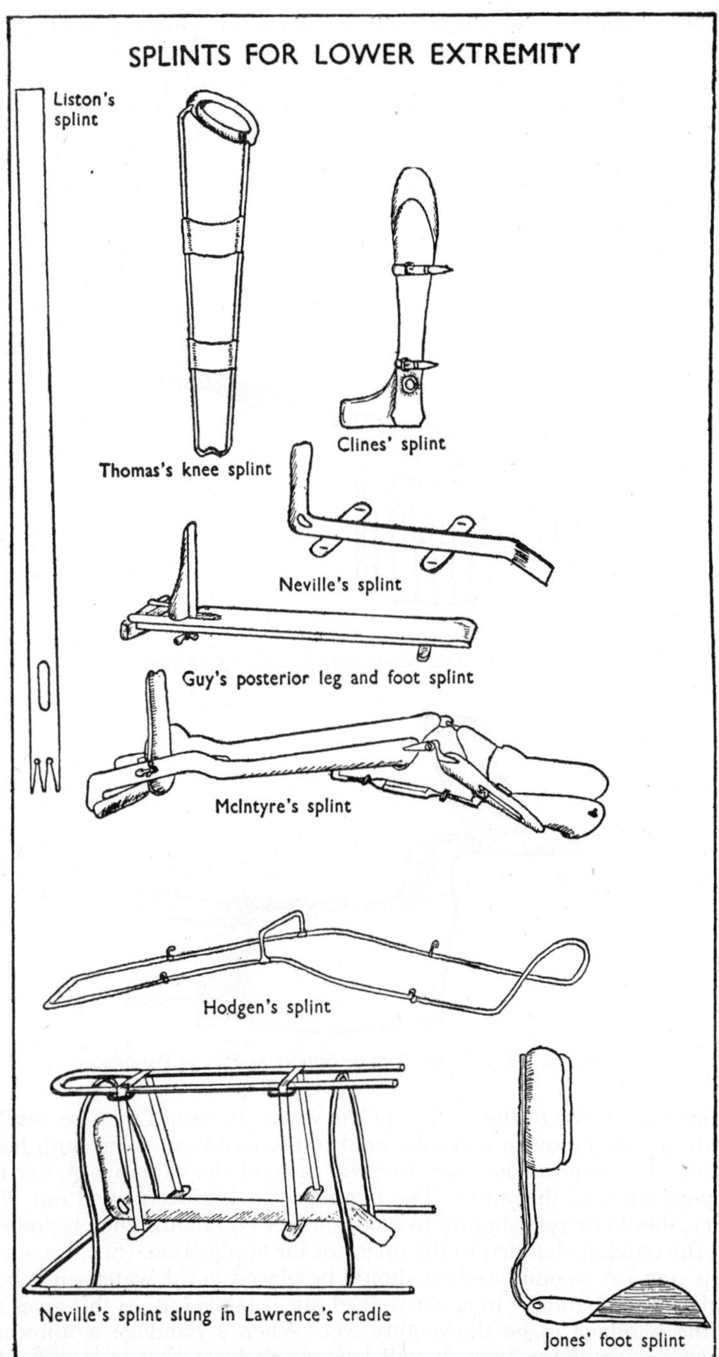
SPLINTS FOR LOWER EXTREMITY
Liston's splint
Thomas's knee splint
Clines' splint
Neville's splint
Guy's posterior leg and foot splint
McIntyre's splint
Hodgen's splint
Neville's splint slung in Lawrence's cradle
Jones' foot splint

FIG. 33.

Those handling the plaster will usually wear gowns to protect thei clothing and gloves to protect the nails and skin of the hands (sinc plaster of paris makes the skin dry and uncomfortable).

Tepid water should be supplied for soaking the bandages; hot wate delays setting and cold water makes the plaster set too quickly. Whe soaking a plaster bandage it should be placed carefully into the wat (which must completely cover it); it will be soaked through when bubbl

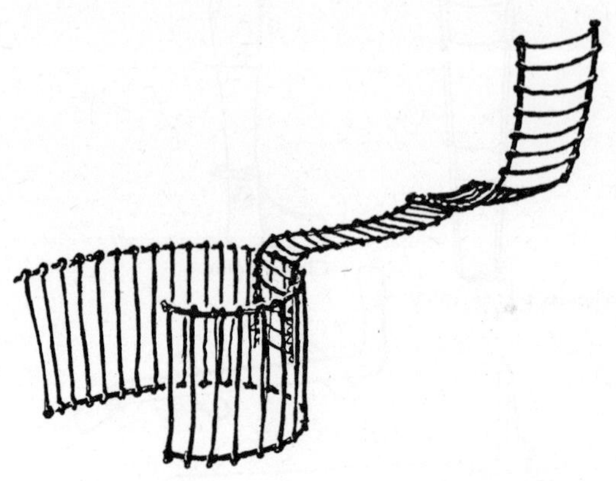

FIG. 34. AEROPLANE (ARM ABDUCTION SPLINT) IN KRAMER'S WIRE.

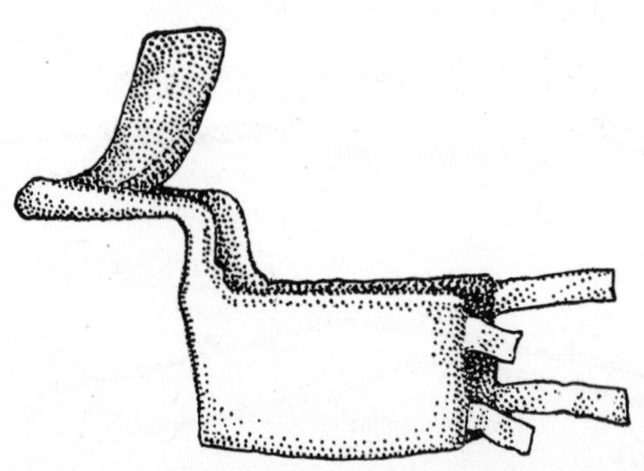

FIG. 35.—THE SAME TYPE OF SPLINT AS FIG. 34 PADDED.

of air cease to rise to the surface of the water. It should then be carefull lifted out—if the nurse will take hold of the bandage, using both hand and gently compress the ends, this will prevent the valuable plaster fro slipping out into the water. The bandage, having been lifted out of th water, should be very slightly twisted; the free end should then be loosene and the bandage handed to the operator for application. (See figs. 95 an 96, p. 227.) A second bandage should be placed in the water—it is bette to place each bandage in as the soaked one is taken out, as this gives tim for the bandage to be thoroughly wet. When a bandage is allowed t remain in water too long, it will become so loose that it is difficult t handle, and the plaster will set and stick to the bottom of the bow

Plaster of paris bandages cost several pence each and wastage should, as far as possible, be avoided.

In the application of plaster of paris strengthening bands and pads can be incorporated as needed, over the flexures of joints for example, where strain may be experienced. These are prepared as shown in figs. 97 and 98, p. 228. Another method of strengthening the plaster splint is by the incorporation of malleable iron splints, and strips of metal.

When finished the surface can be made smooth by moulding the wet plaster with the hands, by the addition of plaster of paris paste made by mixing some loose plaster with water. When quite dry the surface may be polished with talcum or varnished with some rapidly drying varnish. The provision of a smooth surface renders the plaster less liable to injury and wet. The edges should be trimmed with the plaster knife provided. The date of operation and/or application of the plaster and the length of time it is to be worn may be written on the plaster (see fig. 102, p. 230). At the same time the plaster is marked where it is to be cut for removal. Fig. 103, p. 230, shows the method of handling plaster shears.

THE USE AND APPLICATION OF EXTENSION

Extension by one means or another may be applied to almost any part of the body, more usually to the limbs and the head. The object of this form of treatment is to effect greater immobilization than can be attained by the application of splints or plaster of paris.

Immobilization by means of extension is employed:

(*a*) to correct deformity by overcoming the spasm of large muscles recently subjected to injury as in the case of a fracture of a limb, or muscles irritated by the existence of disease as occurs in tuberculous affections at joints;

(*b*) to maintain the correction of deformity produced by reduction of a fracture or dislocation;

(*c*) to prevent pain, such as may occur when the diseased parts of a joint rub together as occurs for example in tuberculous joint disease.

The commonest methods of applying extension to a limb are: by *traction on the skin* as when adhesive plaster or Sinclair's glue is used, and by *skeletal traction* when some form of apparatus is applied to part of the skeleton below the affected part.

Strapping extension. The articles required for this application are shown in figs. 104 and 105, pp. 231–2. The skin of the leg should be shaved, the strapping extension prepared to fit the patient for whom it is intended, either of the two varieties of extension shown in fig. 105, p. 232, being employed. When a Thomas's splint is used the separate strips of strapping placed one on each side of the leg are used—the strapping is notched as shown, lampwick is used to obtain the pull from the lower end—note the two different ways in which this may be fixed to the strapping; in one instance a loop of strong holland tape is sewn on to the end of the strapping and the lampwick fastened by means of a nautical knot; in the other the lampwick is stitched to the end of the strapping. The strapping extension is then applied as shown in figs. 106, 107, pp. 233–4. Note that the malleoli are not covered by strapping, but that a layer of bandage is first placed round the ankle to prevent the edge of strapping from impinging on th skin. The extension is placed fairly well back on the leg so that the foot not plantar-flexed by it—having the strapping forward produces th deformity and it is an error commonly made. In order to render th strapping sticky the back of the plaster should be placed against a jug hot water, laid over a radiator or held in front of a fire. Turpentine shoul not be used as it irritates the skin.

When the form of strapping extension with a spreader and cord employed, weights are used. Fig. 109, p. 236, showing a patient in bed wit this extension applied, indicates the use of weights, and fig. 110, p. 23 gives some idea of the extent a patient with a fractured femur (fo example) may help himself.

Skeletal traction is very commonly used today. The extension appara tus shown in illustration, fig. 108, p. 235, is employed. Either a transfixio pin, or more rarely ice-tong calipers, are used.

For application of transfixion pin the skin should be prepared, and a the sterilized pin is bored through the bone by a drill, a local or genera anaesthetic will be needed. A sterile dressing is placed round the poin of insertion of the pin on the skin and traction is made by fixation of th ends of the pin to a specially devised stirrup-shaped apparatus, from th base of which cord is passed over pulleys on the special apparatus attache to the type of bed employed and, by means of weights, extension is mad on the limb. Either a Thomas's knee splint or a Hodgen's splint employed with slings attached by means of clips (see illustration, fig. 109 p. 236) in which the limb rests as in a hammock.

Special points in nursing patients wearing splints, plaster or extensions. Th general attitude of the patient should be watched and discomfort relieve whenever possible. A small pillow under an arm or leg, in the nape of th neck or the small of the back may help. Cradles should be employed when ever possible so that the weight of bedclothes does not rest on a splinte limb.

The extremities should be watched for indication of interference wit the circulation to a limb particularly. The toes and fingers should b warm and not blue and cold after a splint or plaster has been applied It is important to avoid footdrop; the heel should not rest on a splint, no the foot hang over so that the tendon of Achilles is made sore.

The nurse should be very familiar with the effect the surgeon desires t obtain by any application the patient is wearing and see that this is no interfered with, the slightest alteration of the position of a splint or an movement of an extension appliance being reported without delay. Whe weights are employed these must hang free of the bedstead; the treatmen will be interrupted for example if the weight rests on the bedstead or eve touches it, or rests on the floor.

SPLINT AND PLASTER SORES

When any fixed apparatus is badly put on, sores may be caused, eithe because the apparatus is inadequately or badly padded, or it may be to loose or too tight, the pressure being unevenly or too tightly applied.

Sometimes a patient will imagine he is called upon to bear any discom fort which comes his way; the application of a splint or plaster of paris one of the occasions when he should be warned about this, and asked to report any discomfort, so that it may be investigated. Children are the worst offenders, as they so quickly get used to discomfort that sores may arise without the making of any complaint; and the first indication the nurse has of the condition is an offensive smell or discharge. But children who are uncomfortable are often restless at night, and such an occurrence should never go unreported in surgical nursing. Once noticed it should be investigated.

In some cases discomfort or pain due to pressure soon results in tingling and burning sensations, and swelling of the distal parts will occur if the pressure is uniform over the circumference of a limb.

Treatment. Many splint appliances have, by the nature of the treatment required, to be tightly applied, as for example when correction of any deformity has to be made. But if one spot becomes painful, attempts should be made to relieve pressure at that point for a time—the use of a small ring pad of wool may be tried though, as the putting of wool between a painful spot and a splint usually increases the pressure, such relief is often only temporary. The nurse had better try to distribute the pressure more evenly and, if she cannot alter the bandages for this purpose, she should have everything in readiness for the surgeon to do so when he next visits the ward, or even request him to come for this purpose.

CLOSED PLASTER METHOD

Mr. Winnett Orr during the war of 1914–18 taught the value of rest in the treatment of wounds by enclosing the wounded limb in plaster of paris. After the war he continued to work and experiment and write, and to him is ascribed the *principles* of the 'closed plaster method'. During the war in Spain Dr. Trueta demonstrated to the world the advantages of this method.

Principles. *Cases must be treated early*, within six hours, before serious infection has become established.

Debridement, which includes removal of all contused tissue, blood clot, injured muscle that seems to be inelastic when touched, is absolutely essential. (See note below.)

Given these conditions any wound may be encased in plaster of paris. Blood and discharge soaks through the plaster which may become very offensive.

Nursing Points. Keep the limb *well elevated*. Watch the colour of the toes or finger ends which are always left exposed. Note whether the patient complains of pain, or numbness and tingling. Observe how quickly the plaster becomes soaked, and the odour. The temperature will usually rise and should be watched, but unless accompanied by signs of toxaemia it is not considered important. Upon these points being accurately observed and reported, the surgeon will determine how the case is progressing and whether interference with the plaster is necessary or not.

The 'closed plaster method' is *not* considered satisfactory when cases are not treated early; when infection has undoubtedly invaded the fascia covering muscles and local debridement is impossible. In such cases dead muscle tissue is present and there is danger of gas gangrene and with the 'closed plaster method' this danger would be greater.

APPLICATION OF STRAPPING

It may be necessary to shave the skin before applying strapping This point should be considered. Holland-backed adhesive strappin should be warmed to make it adhere better. Zinc oxide strapping i adhesive. No creases or wrinkles should be allowed as these caus soreness. When strapping is applied round the circumference of a lim it must be firm and even but not tight. After application the extremitie of the limb should be examined to see that the circulation has not bee impaired.

Elastoplast is frequently used as a support and to retain dressings i position as an alternative to strapping. It is pliant and slightly elastic When applying elastoplast it is important to maintain a slight, eve stretch on the material. When taken round a limb the tension must b very even.

H

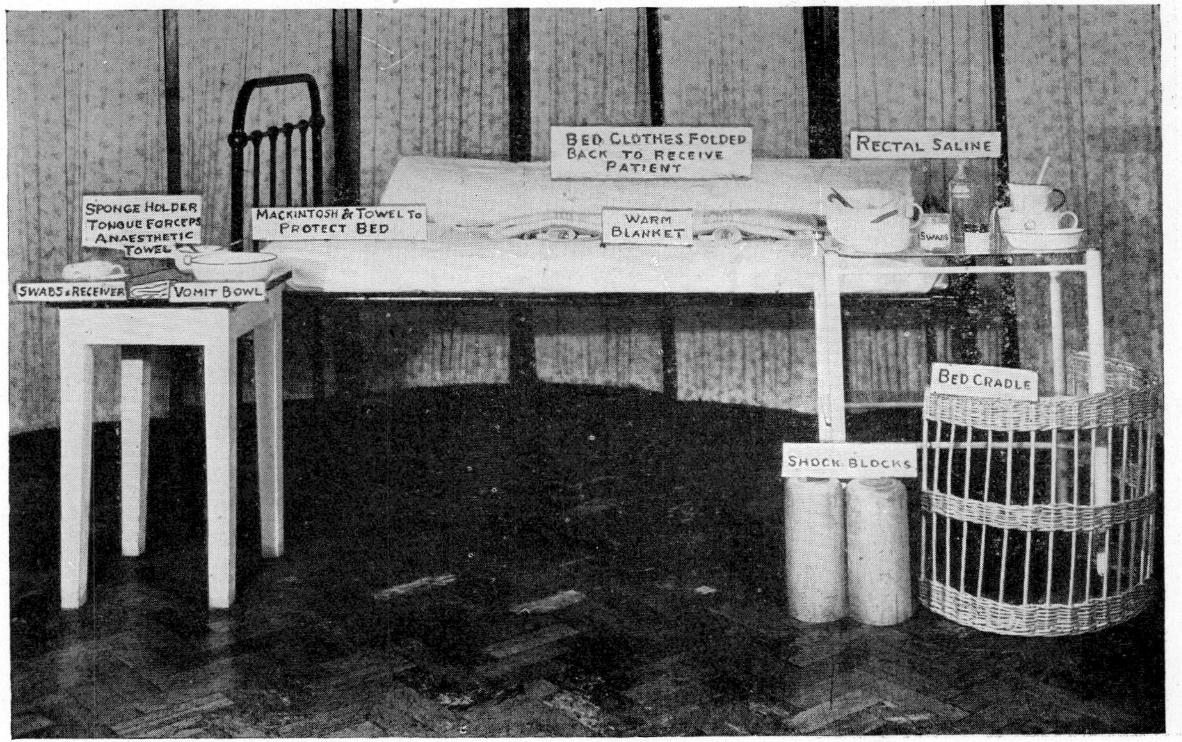

FIG. 36.

see page 88.

OPERATION BED PREPARED FOR A PATIENT RECOVERING FROM A GENERAL ANAESTHETIC.

The articles on the table at the head of the bed are required in all cases. At the foot of the bed various appliances are shown which would be required in special circumstances.

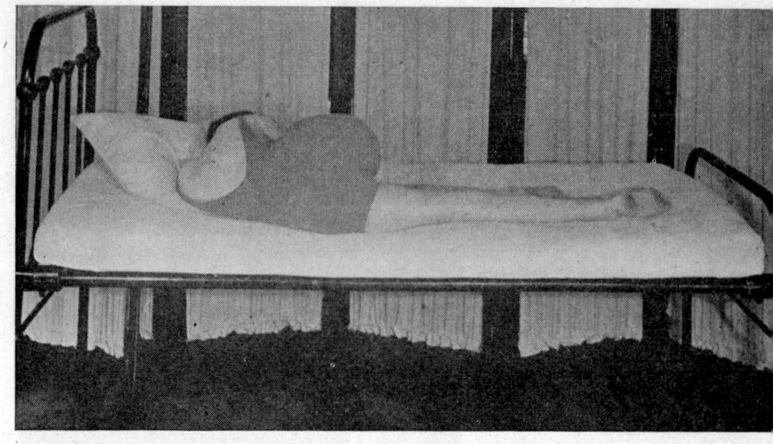

FIG. 37.—*see page* 97. THE LEFT LATERAL POSITION.
The left lateral position, as would be used for examination or treatment of the rectum.

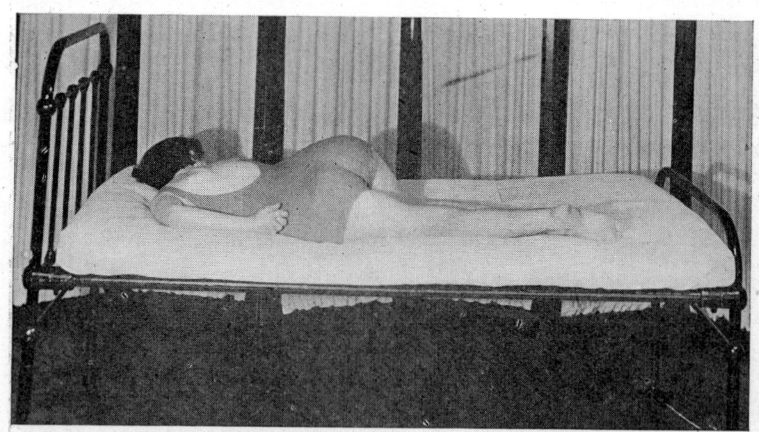

FIG. 38.—*see page* 97. SIMS'S SEMI-PRONE POSITION.
Sims's semi-prone position, as used for vaginal examination.

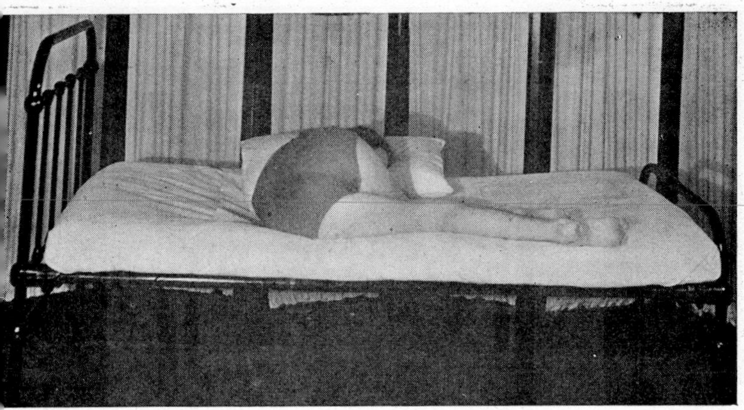

FIG. 39.—*see page* 98. MODIFICATION OF THE LEFT LATERAL POSITION. Modification of the left lateral position, as used for vaginal examination.

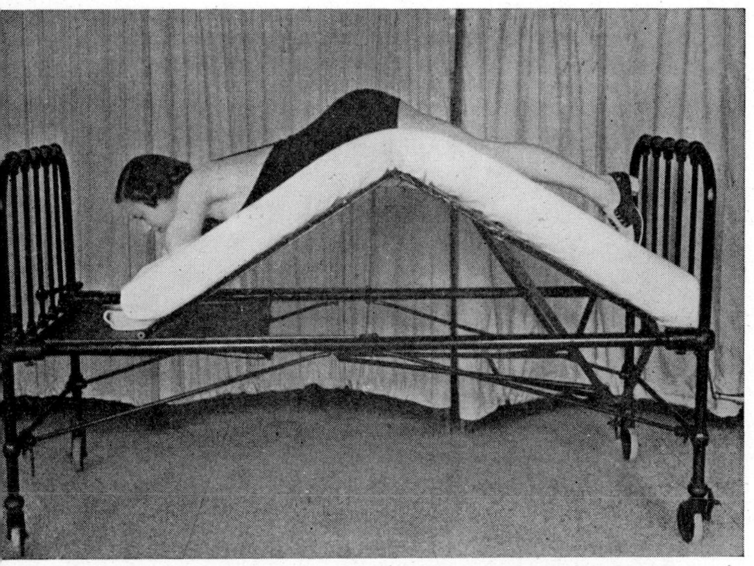

FIG. 40.—*see page* 99. POSITION USED FOR POSTURAL DRAINAGE OF LUNGS. Nelson's bed is shown in the illustration.

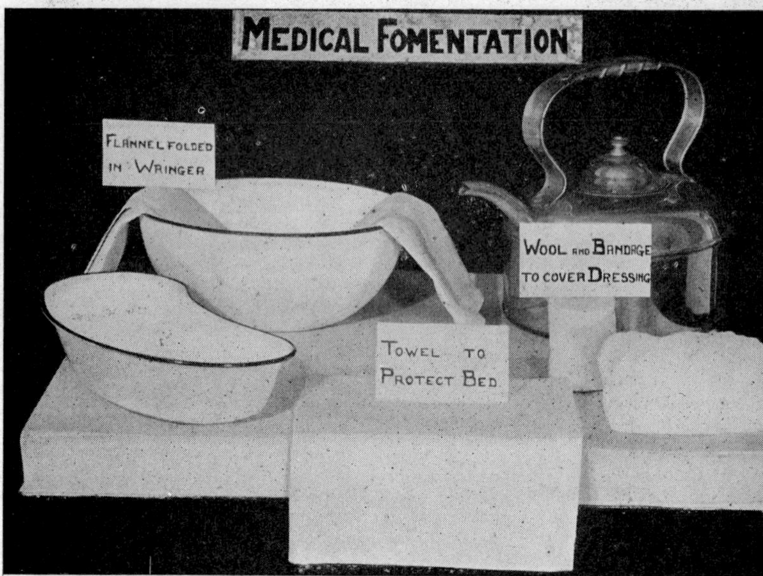

FIG. 41.—*see page* 100. Pieces of flannel, blanket, lint or any other absorbent material may be used as a medical fomentation.

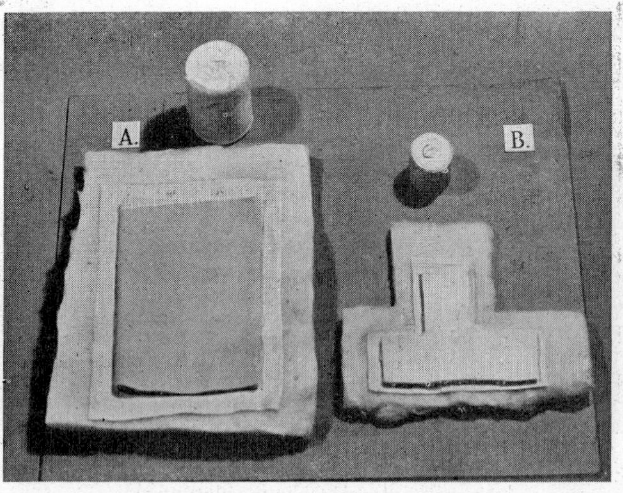

FIG. 42.—*see page* 100.

METHOD OF CUTTING MATERIALS FOR FOMENTATION.

(A) Note that the lint is double; the jaconet is one inch larger and the wool larger again than the jaconet. (B) Method of cutting a finger fomentation.

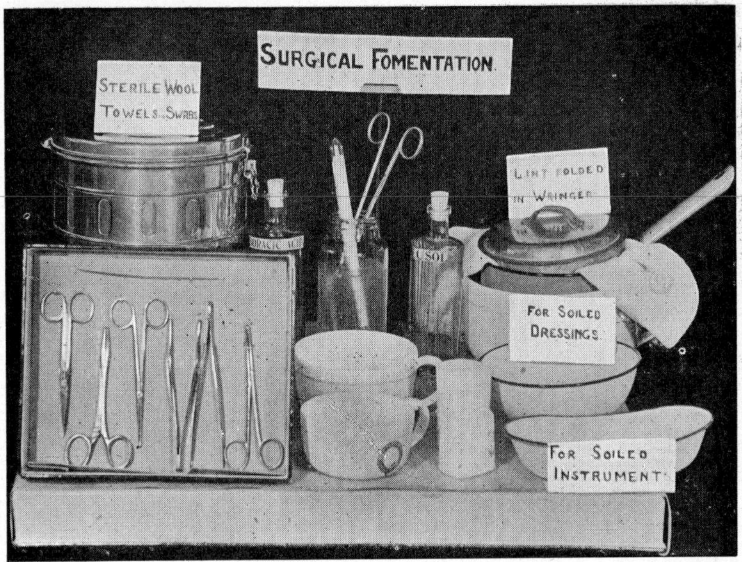

FIG. 43.—*see page* 102. Instruments: Scissors; sinus, dissecting, dressing and artery forceps, probe, sterile towels and dressings; lotion and thermometer. The fomentation may be boiled in a saucepan or a sterile wringer and lint may be used.

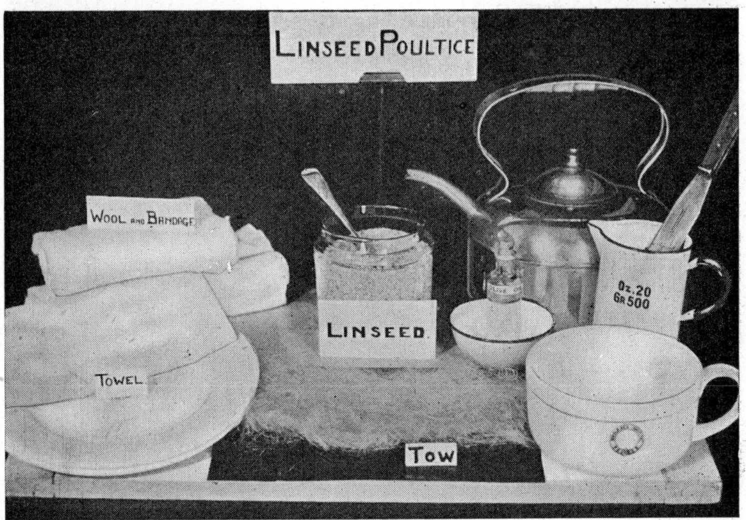

FIG. 44.—*see page* 106. All articles are warm, a small bottle of olive oil is standing ready in hot water, the spatula is in hot water, plates and towel, wool and binder are warm and the delf porringer supplied for mixing the poultice contains hot water so that it may be as warm as possible.

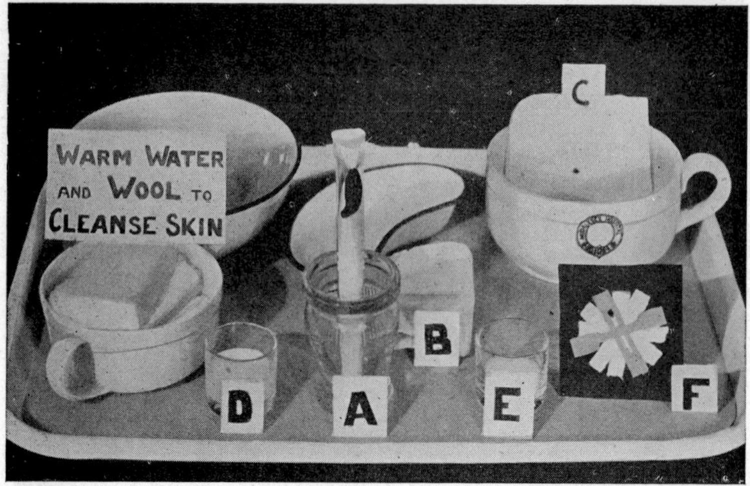

FIG. 45.—*see page* 115. APPLICATION OF LEECH. (A) Leech in upper $\frac{1}{3}$ of test tube, the lower $\frac{2}{3}$ being filled with cotton wool. (B) a square of linen for handling leech if necessary. (C) a piece of lint having a hole cut in it, through which the leech is applied (see above). (D) warm milk. (E) salt. (F) method of applying a pressure dressing in order to arrest bleeding, after removal of leech, if necessary.

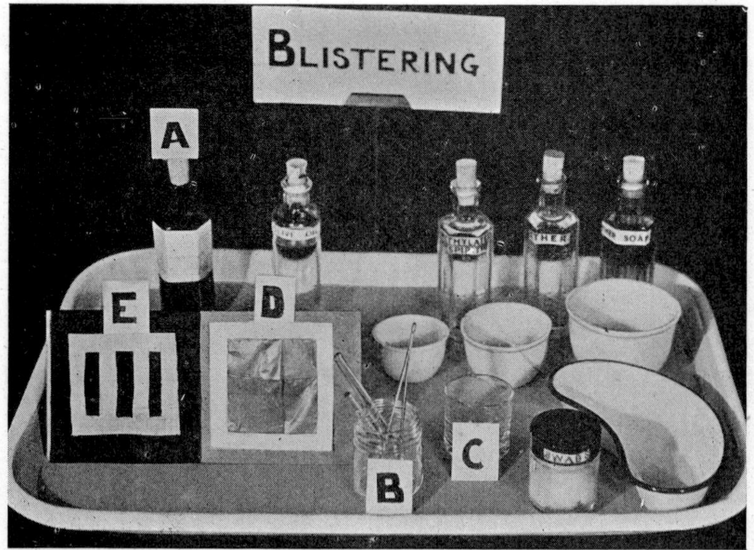

FIG. 46.—*see page* 117. APPLICATION OF BLISTERING AGENT. (A) Blistering fluid. (B) glass rods. (C) olive oil. (D) method of covering blistered area with gutta-percha tissue and (E) method of preparing a 'gate of strapping' with which to cover a dressing after removal of the raised epidermis when the blister has risen. In addition articles for cleansing the skin, before blistering, are provided.

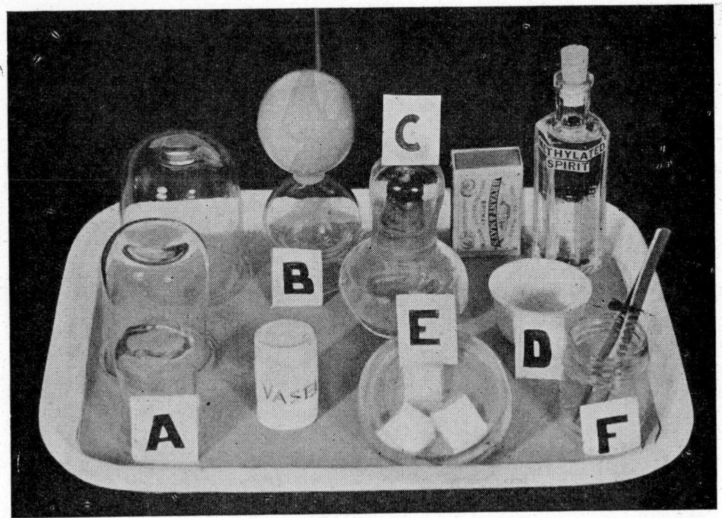

FIG. 47.—*see page* 119. CUPPING.
(A) Cupping glasses. (B) one example of Bier's suction cups. (C) spirit lamp. (D) a small quantity of methylated spirit in a gallipot. (E) squares of blotting paper. (F) forceps for handling the lighted blotting paper. Vaseline is provided to smear the edges of the cups.

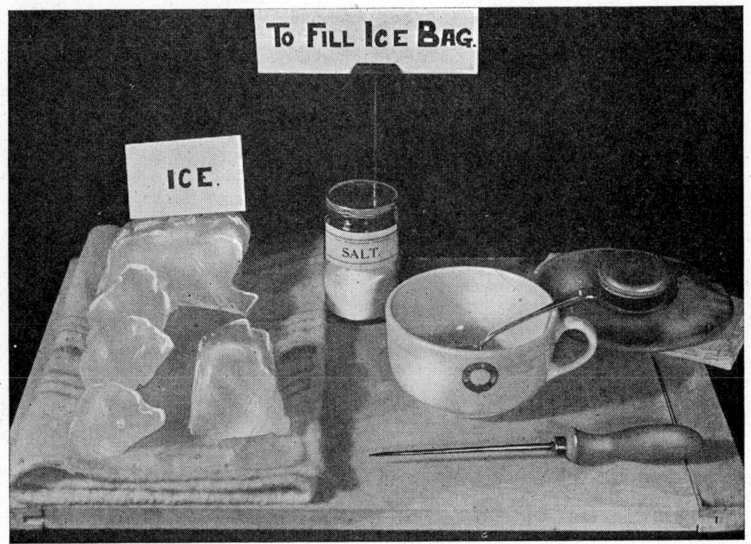

FIG. 48.—*see page* 103. The bowl and spoon are supplied to mix chopped ice and salt together in order to make a better freezing mixture.

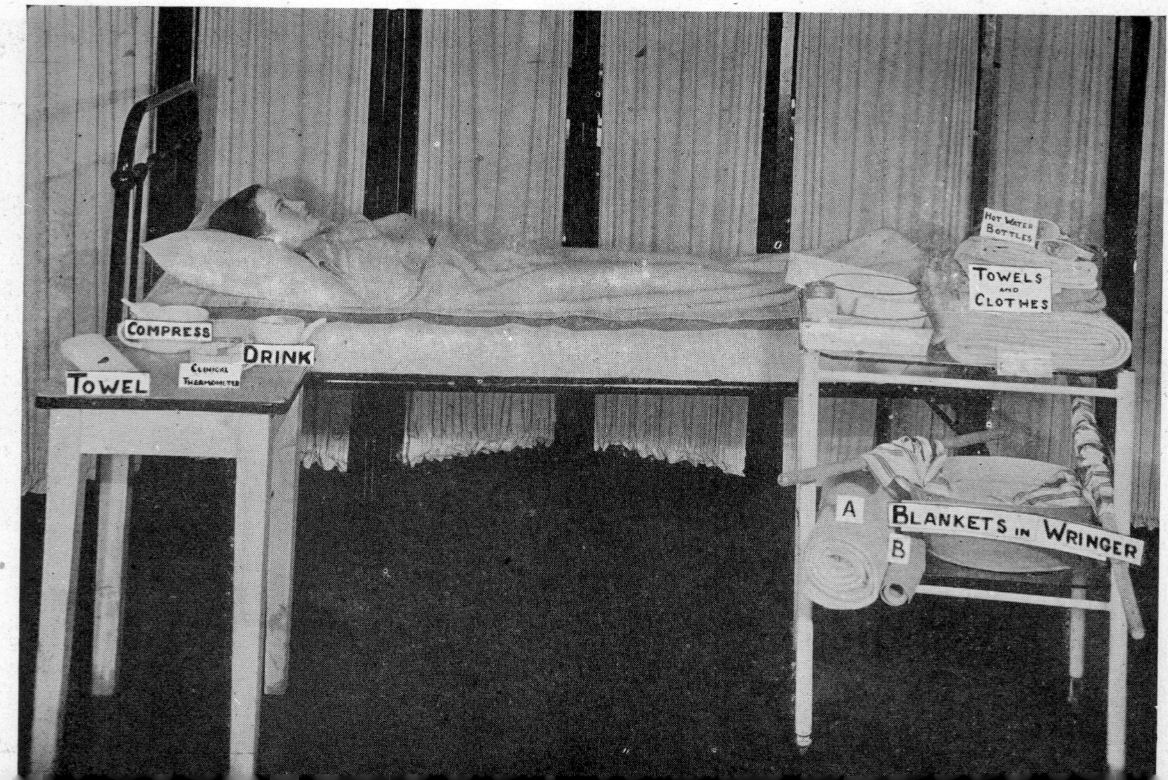

Fig. 49.—*see page* 128. The Application of a Hot Wet Pack.

The patient is lying on a blanket and long mackintosh and is covered by a dry blanket. The hot wet blankets are ready in the bath on the lower shelf of the wagon which is of metal. (A) dry blanket and (B) long mackintosh ready to cover the patient when he is wrapped in the hot wet blankets.

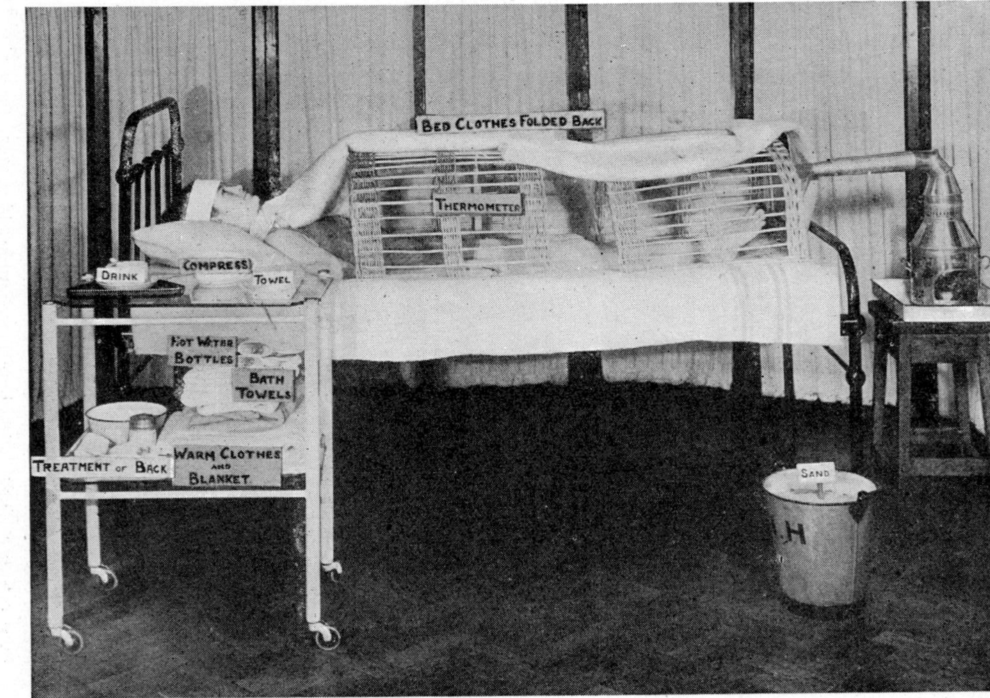

Fig. 50.—*see page* 129.

The Administration of a Vapour or Hot Air Bath.

In the example shown Allen's apparatus is employed, the bed-clothes are folded back to show the position of the patient lying stripped so that the hot air or vapour can freely circulate around him. The position of the bath thermometer hanging from the upper cradle can also be seen.

When in operation the bed clothing is tucked in on both sides of the bed. It is tucked snugly round the patient's neck, and fitted closely over the apparatus at the foot of the bed. It is important to so arrange the bed that the hot air or vapour is retained in the bed and cannot escape through cracks or openings.

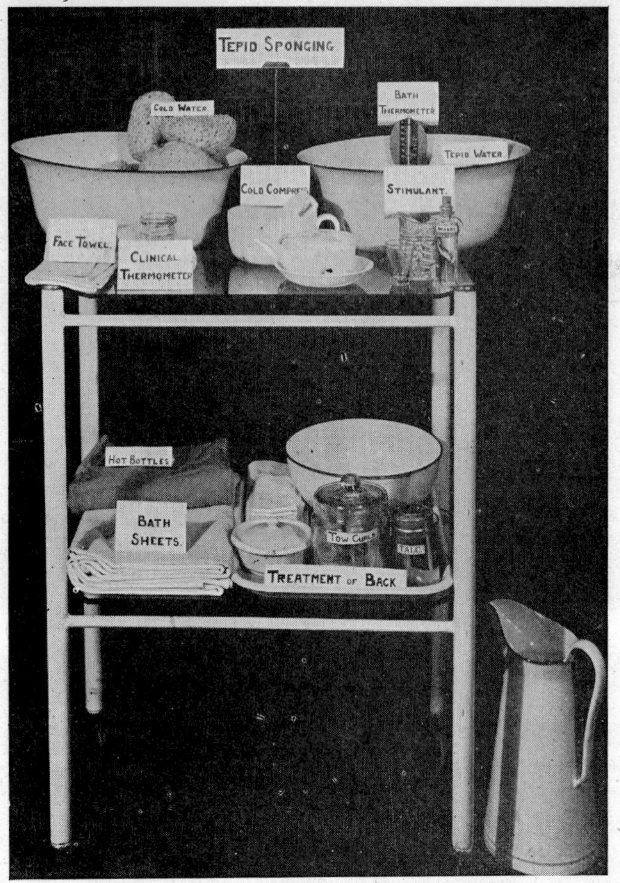

Fig. 51.—*see page* 122. Tepid Sponging.

Upper Shelf. Clinical thermometer. Bowls for water, bath thermometer and sponges. Cold compress for patient's forehead. Feeder containing drink. Stimulant.

Lower Shelf. Bath sheets, hot-water bottles and articles for the treatment of back and other pressure points.

A jug of cold water.

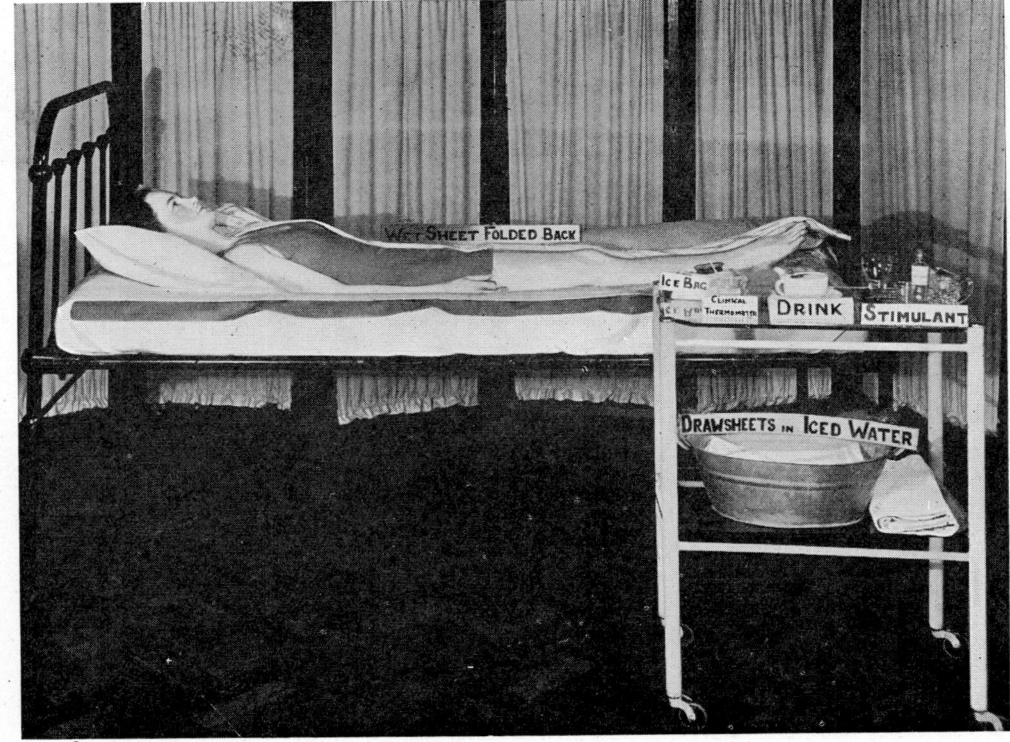

FIG. 52.—*see page* 125.
THE APPLICATION OF A COLD PACK.

The patient lies on the bed on a wet sheet and long mackintosh and is covered by a second wet sheet. The sheets are wrung out in iced water (see lower shelf of waggon). On the top shelf are a clinical thermometer, an ice bag for patient's head, a drink ready prepared and a stimulant in case of need. In the illustration the top wet sheet is folded back to show the position of the patient.

The wet sheet over the patient is tucked in closely to his body. Steam rises from the wet sheet as evaporation, which reduces the patient's temperature, takes place. The wet sheet is changed every few minutes. Duration of treatment is 10 to 20 minutes. The patient's pulse and general condition must be noted throughout. The patient should rest after the treatment. As a rule the temperature will be reduced from 2 to 2½ degrees Fahrenheit.

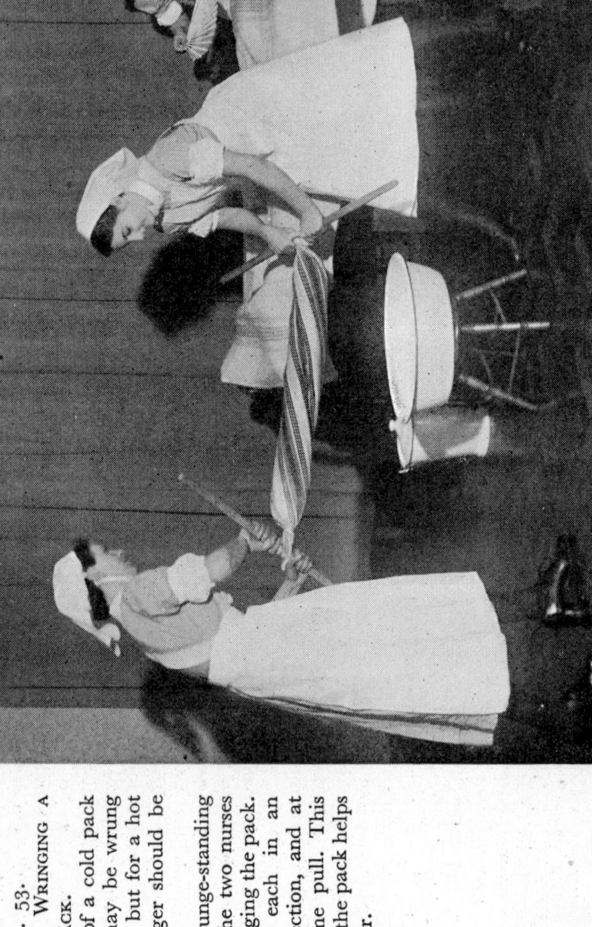

Fig. 53.
Method of Wringing a Pack.

In the case of a cold pack the sheets may be wrung out by hand but for a hot pack a wringer should be used.

Note the lunge-standing position of the two nurses who are wringing the pack. They twist, each in an opposite direction, and at the same time pull. This stretching of the pack helps to expel water.

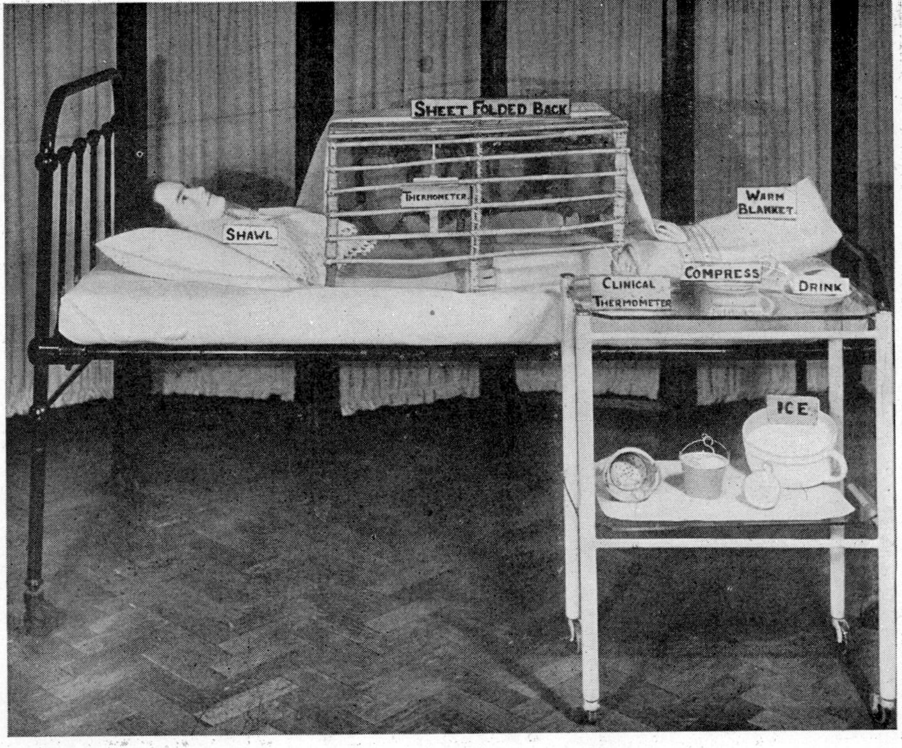

Fig. 54.—*see page* 125.—Ice Cradling. For ice cradling the patient lies between sheets, the shoulders are protected by a covering and the feet must be kept warm. The ice cradle is placed over the patient's body. A shawl covers the shoulders and the feet are wrapped in a warm blanket. A thermometer is suspended from the cradle. The cradle is covered by a sheet which is raised a little to allow air to pass over the patient. This aids evaporation and cooling. On the upper shelf of the waggon are a clinical thermometer, cold compress and prepared drink in a feeder.

In the accompanying illustration the sheet is folded back so that the general arrangement of bed clothing and the position of the thermometer can be seen.

The sheet covering the ice cradle (and patient) is looped up at each side so that cool air circulates freely over the patient's body. A cold compress on the forehead or an ice bag to the head will add to the patient's comfort. The treatment may last several hours or it may be continuous.

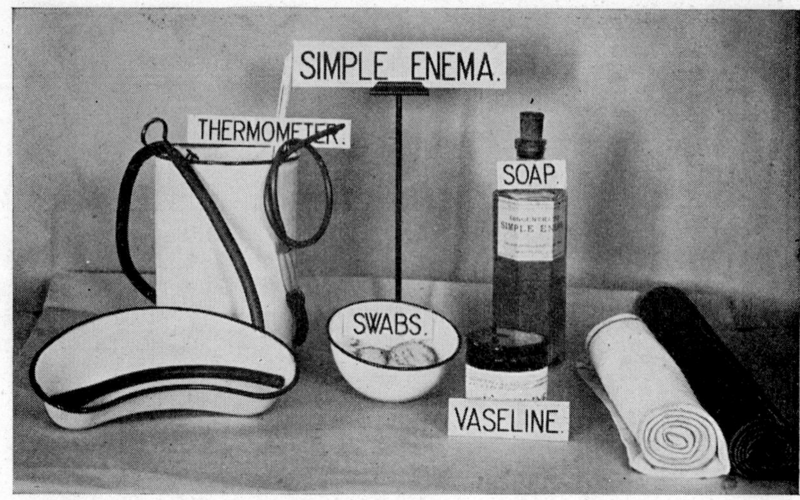

FIG. 55.—*see page* 133. ARTICLES FOR GIVING AN ENEMA. Irrigation can, tubing and rubber catheter. Flatus tube. Swabs. Lubricant, Soap solution. Thermometer.

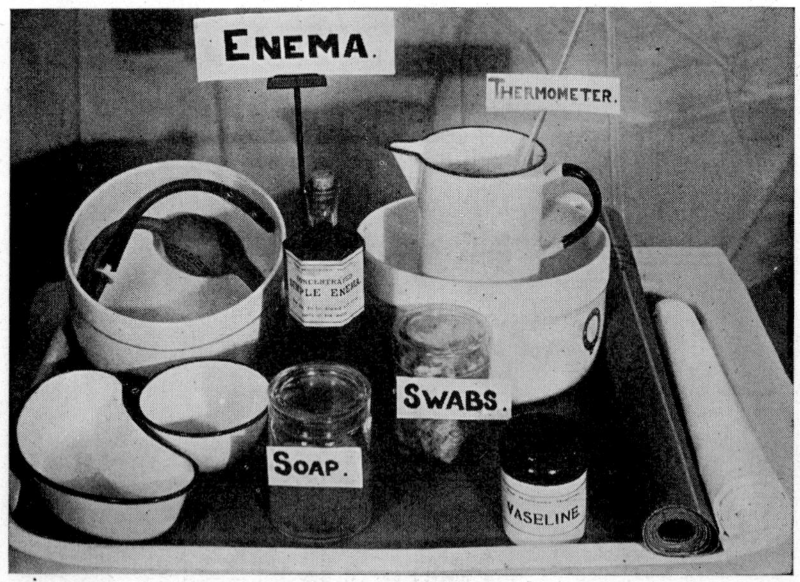

FIG. 56.—*see page* 133. In some cases Higginson's syringe is used for giving an enema but when this is employed a soft rectal tube *must* be attached to the hard bone nozzle.

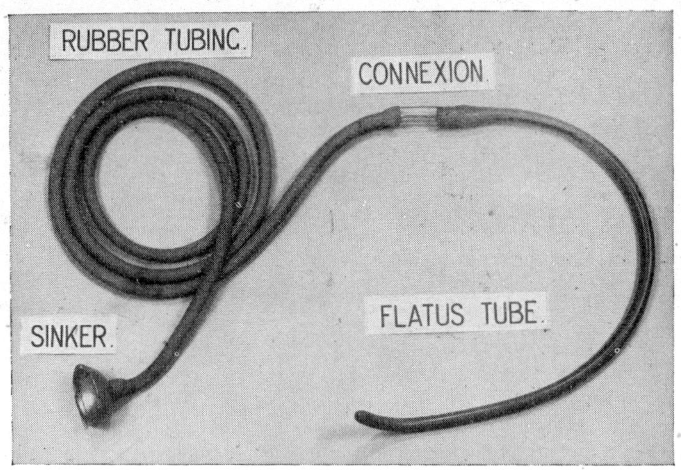

FIG. 57.—*see page* 134. FLATUS TUBE.
A length of rubber tubing which carries a metal sinker is attached. The sinker (alternatively a small funnel may be employed) serves to keep the free end of the tubing immersed in a basin of lotion so that the passage of flatus bubbling through the lotion can be noted.

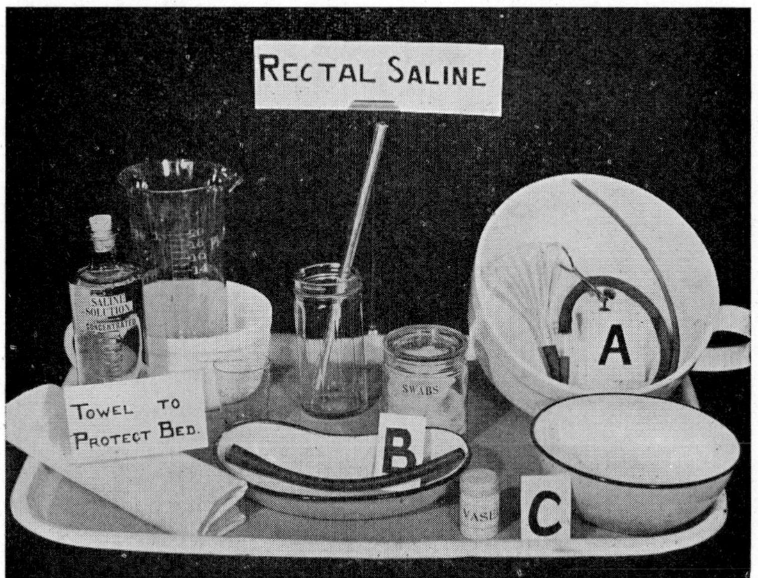

FIG. 58.—*see page* 153. (A) Catheter, tubing and funnel. (B) short rectal tube which is passed before the saline is given, so that flatus may be expelled. Brown wool swabs are provided to cleanse the anus and a receiver (C) for the used swabs. A lubricant may be needed for the rectal tube and rectal catheter. The prepared saline is standing in warm water. A lotion thermometer is provided.

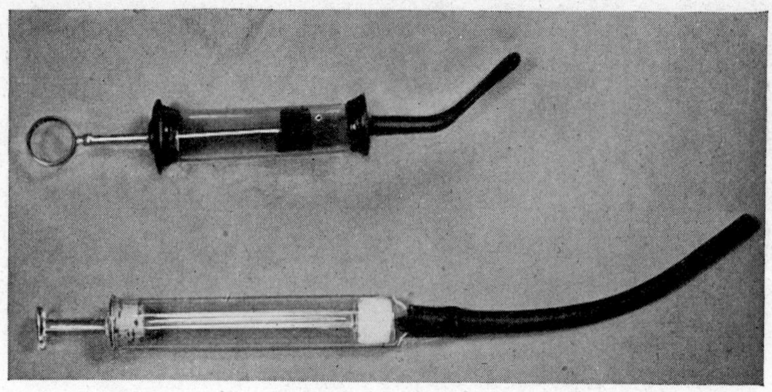

Fig. 59.—*see page* 135.

Syringes for Administration of a Glycerine Enema.

When a mixture of glycerine and warm water is employed a rectal catheter is used as in illustration Fig. 58, p. 199.

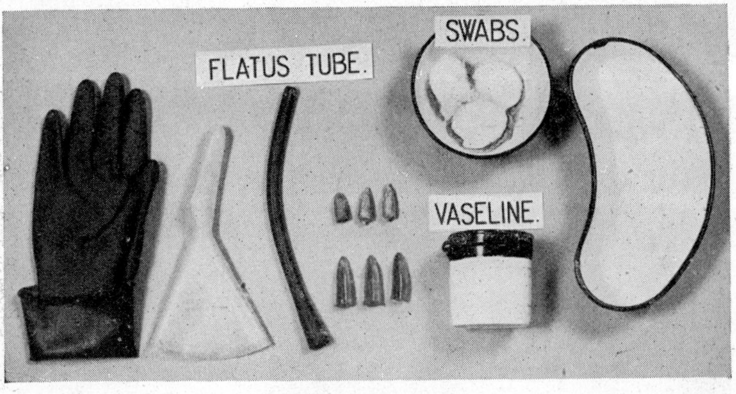

Fig. 60.—*see page* 139.

Articles for the Administration of a Suppository.

A flatus tube should be passed before inserting a suppository which is to be retained.

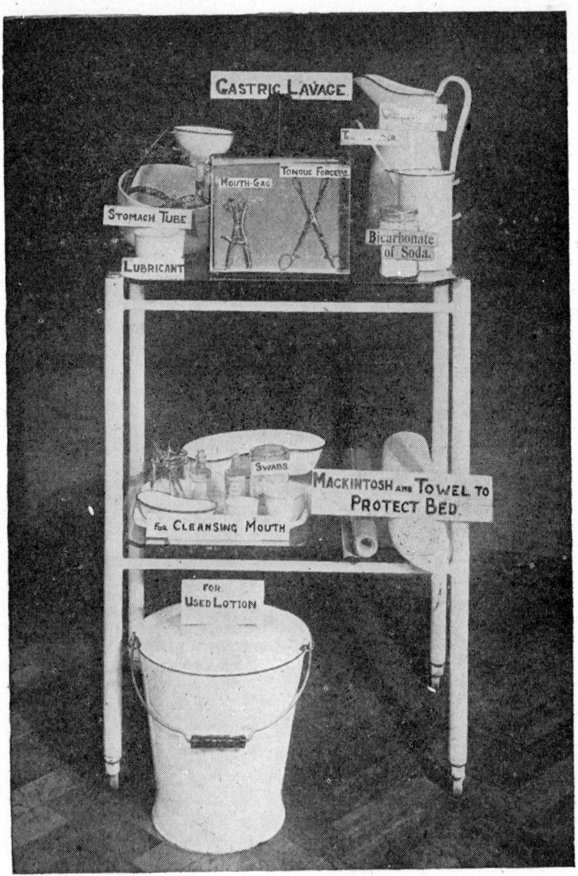

FIG. 61.—*see page* 140.

ARTICLES FOR GASTRIC LAVAGE.

UPPER SHELF. Stomach tube (Jaques's pattern), lubricant, mouth gag and tongue forceps, lotion and thermometer.

LOWER SHELF. Mackintosh and towel, receiver in case of vomit and for used tube, articles for cleaning the mouth. Pail for used lotion.

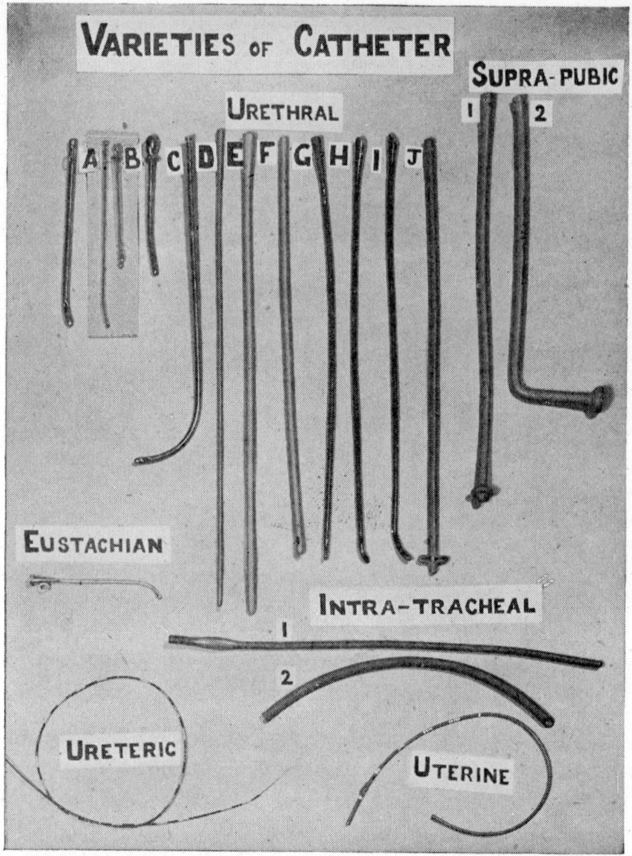

FIG. 62.—*see page* 142. Urethral catheters shown are (A) and (B) for female, metal and glass. The short ones are Kidd's pattern. (C) prostatic catheter. (D) rubber, (E) Harris's, and (F) whistletip patterns. (G) composition, olive-headed, (H) coudé, and (I) bicoudé patterns. (J) Malécot's two-winged pattern (this type is also used for suprapubic drainage). Suprapubic catheters shown (1) De Pezzer's and (2) Joll's patterns.

Intratracheal (1) silk web and (2) rubber Magill's pattern are employed for the introduction of anaesthetics by this route.

A uterine catheter is a soft rubber catheter with a terminal eye used for injection of substances into the uterus.

Ureteric catheters are passed along the ureters to the pelvis of the kidney, *see p.* 145.

Eustachian catheters are passed into the eustachian tube to test its patency in an extensive examination of the ear.

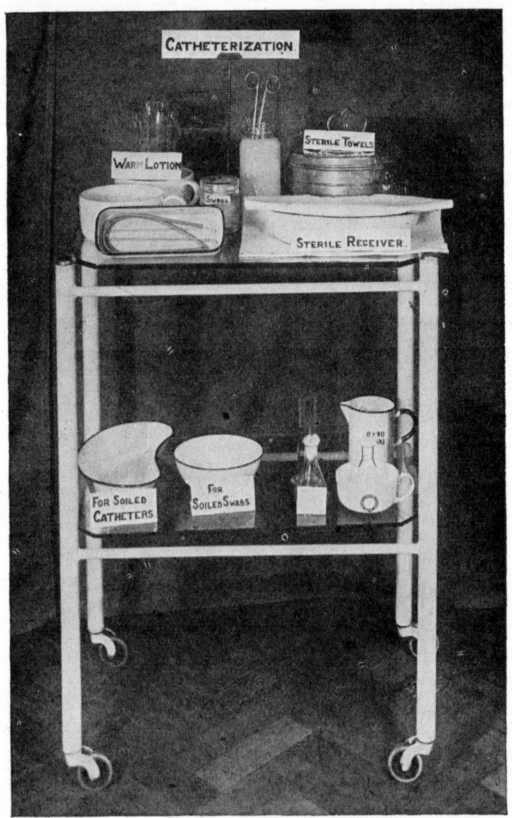

FIG. 63.—*see page* 143. On the UPPER SHELF of the wagon two rubber and two glass (female) catheters are in a small tray. The sterile receiver (on the right) is for collection of the urine. Swabs and lotion are needed for cleansing the vulva and urethral orifice. On the LOWER SHELF a variety of specimen flasks and pathological department labels are provided.

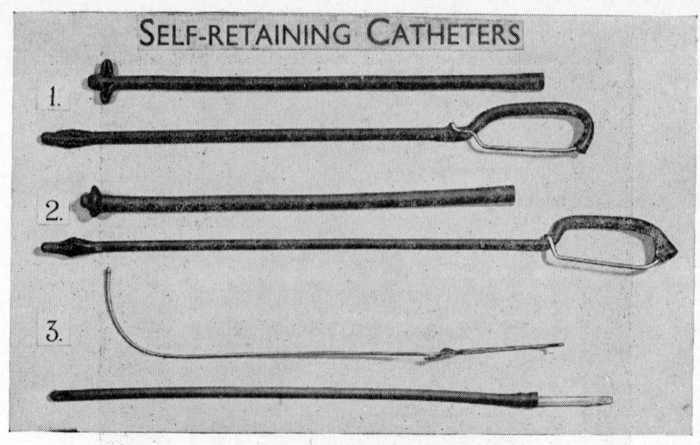

FIG. 64.—*see page* 142.
1. Malécot's catheter, without and with introducer.
2. De Pezzer's catheter, also with introducer.
3. Harris's rubber catheter and metal introducer.

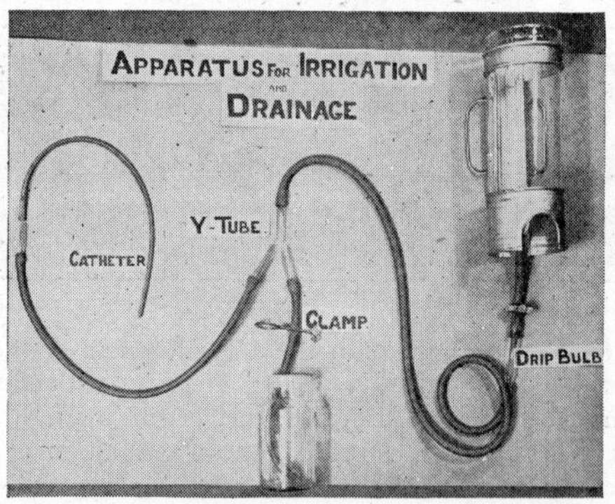

FIG. 65.—*see page* 145. Duke's apparatus consists of irrigation can, tubing, Y-shaped glass connexion, catheter and collecting bottle. Note the position of the clamps.

To fill the bladder release the clamp below the reservoir of fluid and close the outlet by closing the clamp below the Y-connection.

To empty the bladder close the clamp below the reservoir and release the clamp below the Y-connection. (*See also* pp. 146–7.)

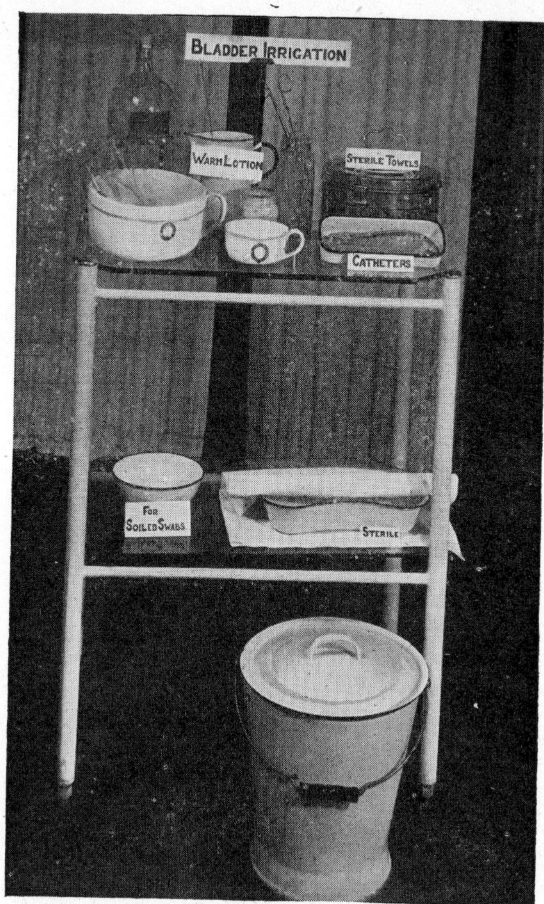

FIG. 66.—*see page* 145.
ARTICLES FOR BLADDER IRRIGATION.
(*see also Fig.* 27, *p.* 146)

The glass funnel and rubber tubing and connexion for catheter are ready in the porringer to the left of the top of the wagon. Catheters and sterile towels are on the right. Swabs and small porringer of lotion are provided for cleansing urethral orifice. A thermometer is provided for testing the heat of the lotion used.
The sterile receiver on the bottom of the wagon is for the reception of the urine which is first drawn off, in case a specimen is required.

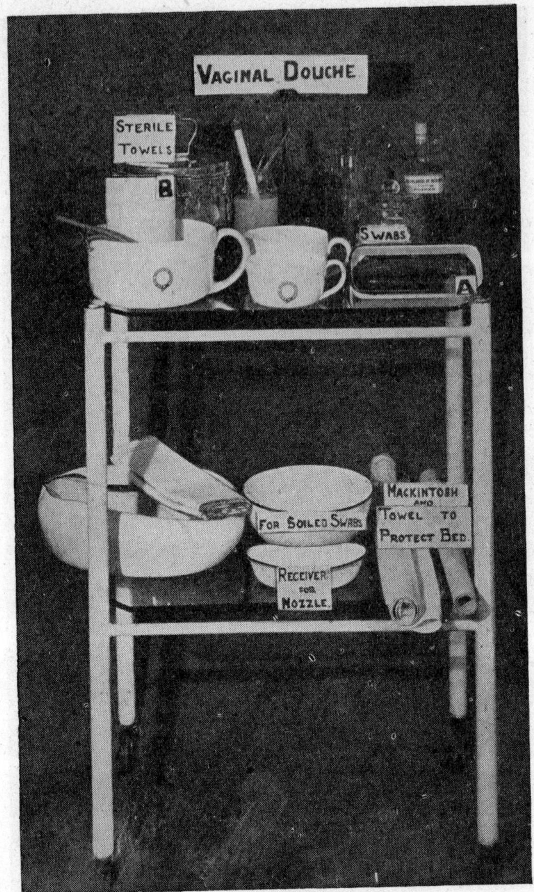

FIG. 67.—*see page* 148.

ARTICLES FOR VAGINAL DOUCHING.

UPPER SHELF. (A) Glass douche nozzles. (B) Douche can, tubing and clamp. Lotion, thermometer, measure and swabs.

LOWER SHELF. Mackintosh and towel, douche pan and cover, bowl and receiver for soiled swabs and used douche nozzle.

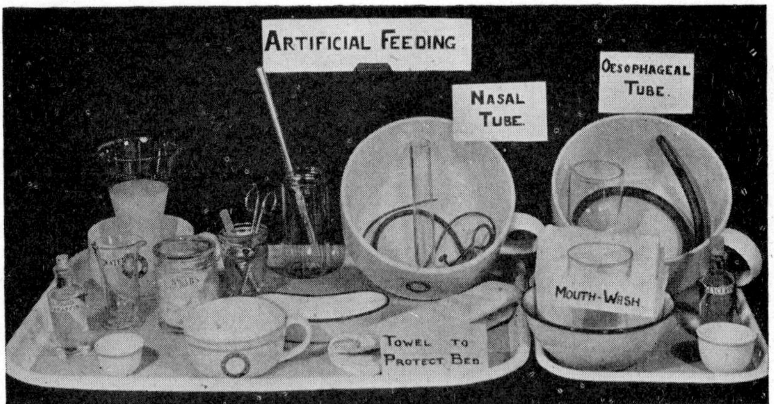

FIG. 68.—*see page* 150. ARTICLES FOR ARTIFICIAL FEEDING.
In nasal feeding articles to cleanse and lubricate the nostrils are required—swabs, lubricant and forceps. Note the small size of a nasal catheter as compared with an oesophageal tube. In both nasal and oesophageal feeding the fluid given should be warm. After oesophageal feeding the patient should either be given a mouth-wash or have his mouth cleaned.

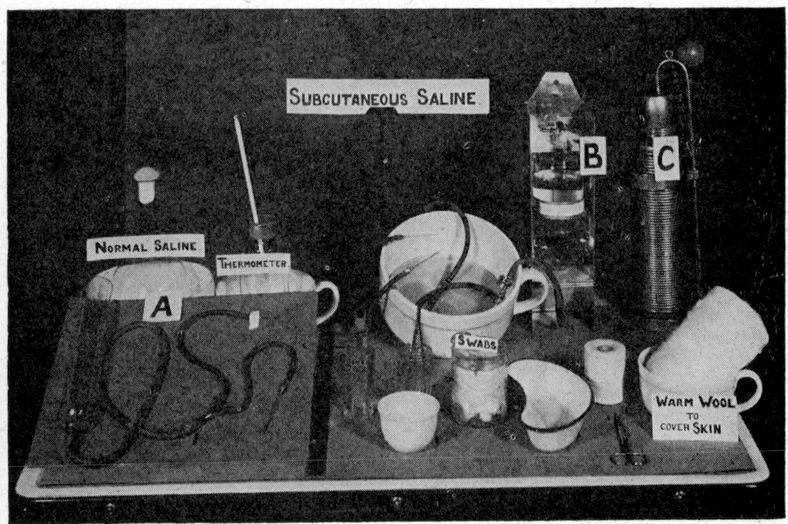

FIG. 69.—*see page* 154. ARTICLES FOR SUBCUTANEOUS INFUSION OF FLUID.
Three types of apparatus are shown for the administration of subcutaneous saline. (A) graduated funnel, tubing, Y connexion and two needles—the upper of the two needles is fixed in position by means of a strip of elastoplast to prevent its slipping out of the skin. (B) apparatus for continuous infusion fitted with rubber tubing clamp, drip bulb, tubing and two needles. (C) Souttar's vacuum flask.
In addition articles are needed for cleansing the skin, warm wool to cover the part undergoing infusion, and scissors to cut the strips of elastoplast.

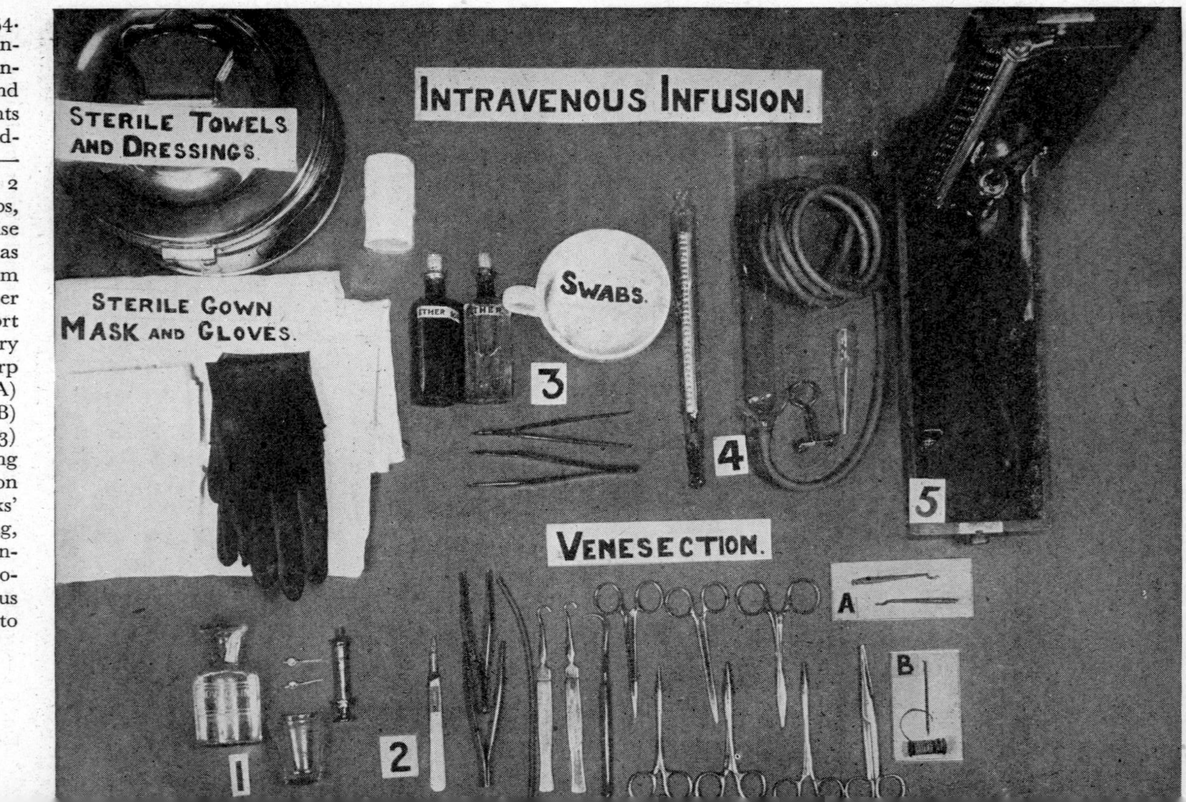

FIG. 70.—*see page* 154. Articles shown include:—(1) Local anaesthetic, syringe and needles. (2) Instruments for venesection—reading from left to right—Bard Parker's knife, 2 pairs dissecting forceps, rubber tubing to raise vein, 2 blunt hooks as retractors, 1 aneurysm needle, 3 pairs spider forceps, 3 pairs short Spencer Wells' artery forceps, 1 pair sharp pointed scissors. (A) glass cannulae. (B) needles and silk. (3) Articles for cleansing the skin. (4) Lotion thermometer, Horrocks' flash, rubber tubing, clamp, and glass connexion. (5) Sphygmomanometer apparatus with pressure bag to act as tourniquet.

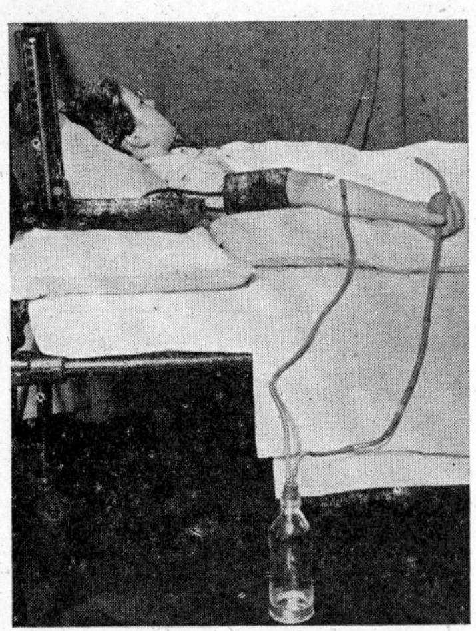

FIG. 71.—*see page* 155.
APPARATUS FOR TAKING BLOOD.

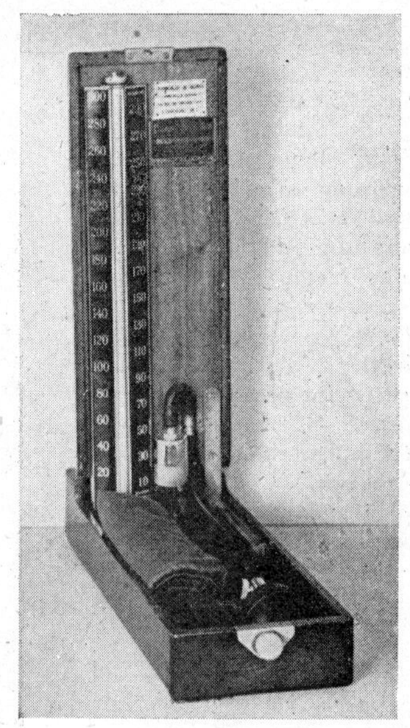

FIG. 72.
SPHYGMOMANOMETER.

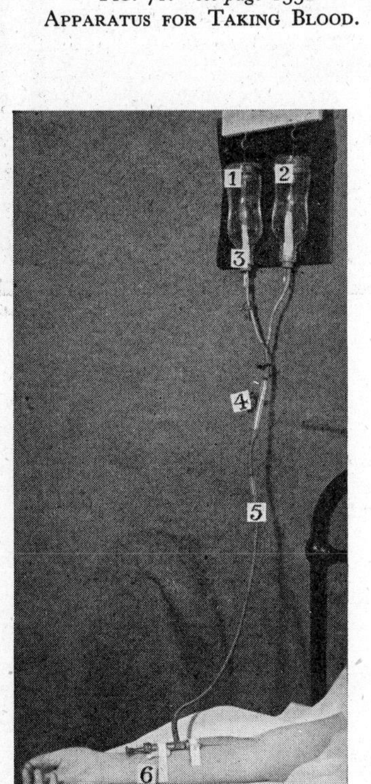

FIG. 73. —*see page* 155.
APPARATUS FOR GIVING BLOOD.
(1) and (2) bottles for blood. (3) Rubber bung through which glass tubes pass. (4) tubing tap attached to Laurie's drip bulb; by means of a syringe air collecting in the tubing can be removed. (5) glass window for noting level of air in tube. (6) Kauffman's syringe for giving blood.

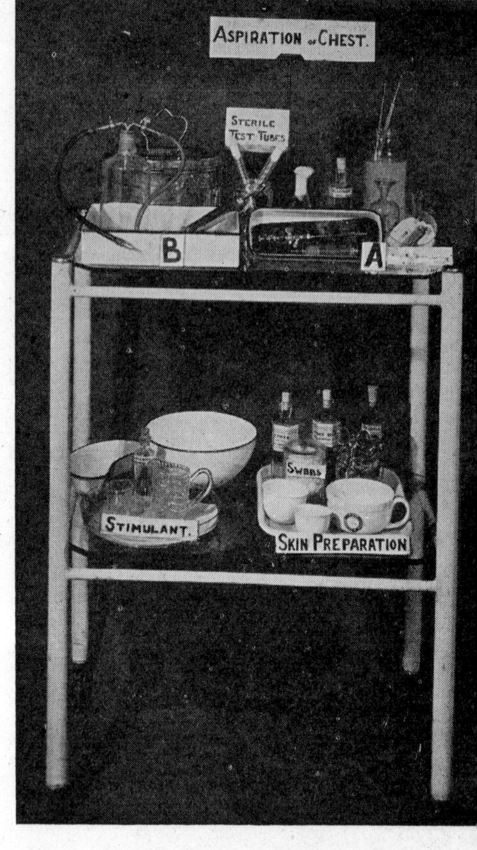

FIG. 74.—*see page* 160.
UPPER SHELF. Local anaesthetic, hypodermic syringe, exploring syringe, aspirator, sterile towels and swabs. Specimen tubes and flask.
(The method of testing the aspirator is described on page 160.)
On the LOWER SHELF is found articles for preparation of the skin.
A stimulant in case the patient needs one.
Basin and receiver for soiled swabs and used instruments.

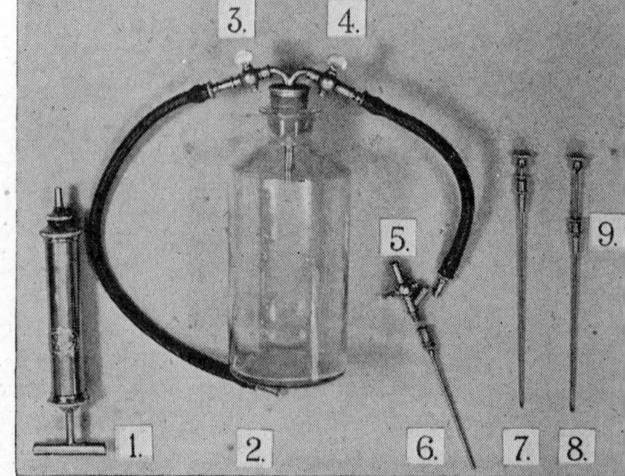

FIG. 75.—*see page* 160.
POTAIN'S ASPIRATOR.
(1) Pump. (2) Aspirating bottle. (3 & 4) Taps controlling inlets. (5) Connexion between tube and needle. (6) Needle or cannula. (7 & 8) Trocars to fit hollow cannula. (9) Collar or trocar to fit cannula.

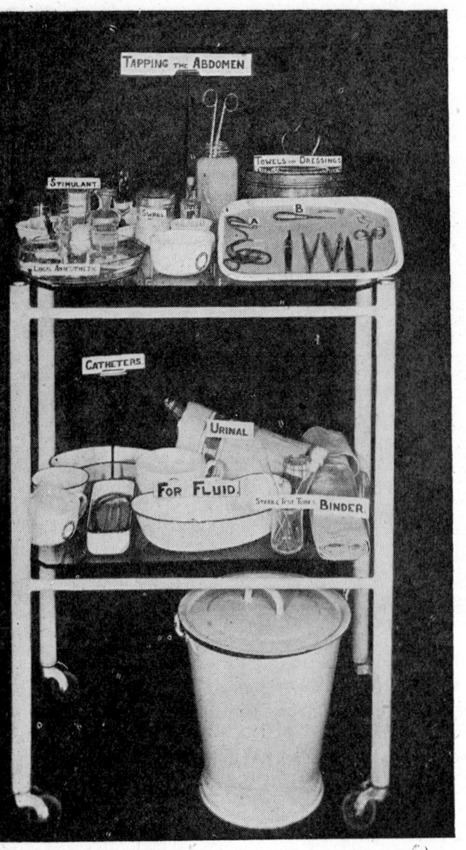

FIG. 76.—*see page* 162.
ARTICLES FOR
ABDOMINAL PARACENTESIS.

UPPER SHELF. Instruments (Fig. 69). Local anaesthetic, articles for cleansing skin, stimulant.

LOWER SHELF. Urinal. Catheters in case required. Sterile flasks for specimens. Receiver. Abdominal binder for use when required.

When a large trocar is employed a pail should be provided as the fluid will flow quickly. But when tiny trocars are used, the fluid will drain away more slowly, and may be collected in a receiver placed in the bed, or be permitted to drain into cotton wool which will be changed as it becomes saturated with fluid.

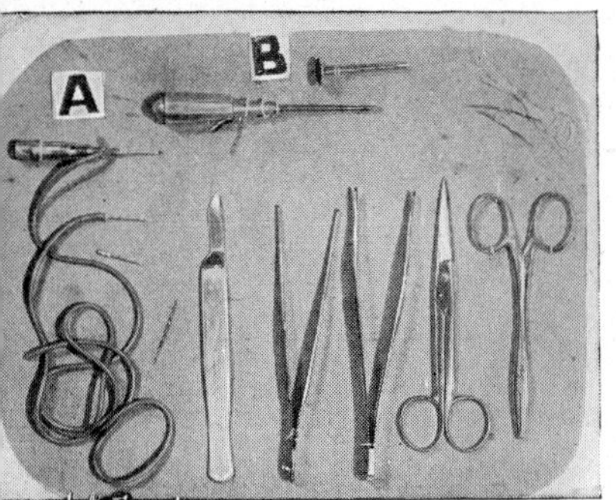

FIG. 77.—*see page* 162.
INSTRUMENTS FOR TAPPING.

(A) Southey's trocar and cannula. When this is used a tiny incision may have to be made for which scalpel, dissecting forceps and a stitch may be required.

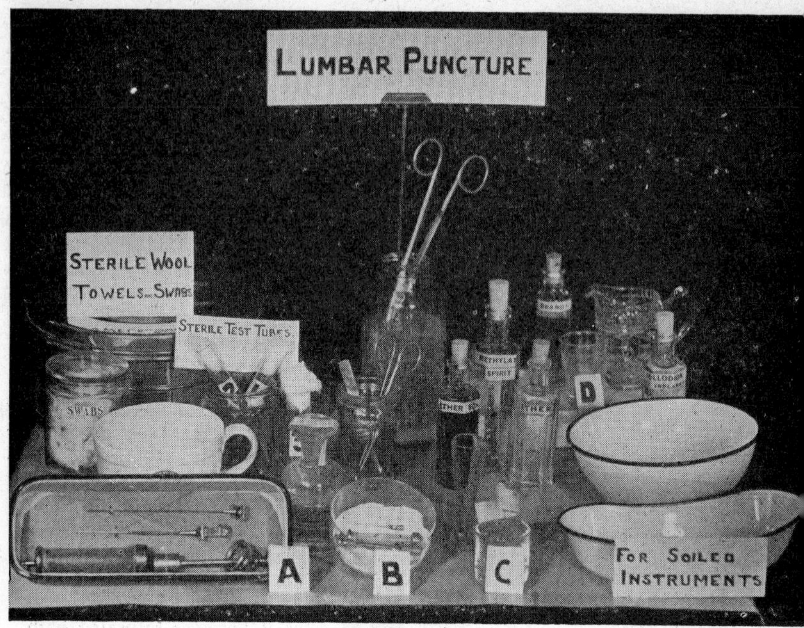

FIG. 78.—*see page* 163.

ARTICLES FOR LUMBAR PUNCTURE AND INTRATHECAL INJECTION OF SERUM. (A) Exploring syringe and Barker's needle. (B) Hypodermic syringe and local anaesthetic. (C) Phial of serum in water at 99 deg. F. (D) A stimulant in case of need. Sterile towels and dressings, collodion and strapping. Articles for cleansing the skin. Sterile specimen tubes and flasks (*see also Fig.* 75, where Greenfield's manometer for measuring the pressure of the cerebro-spinal fluid is shown).

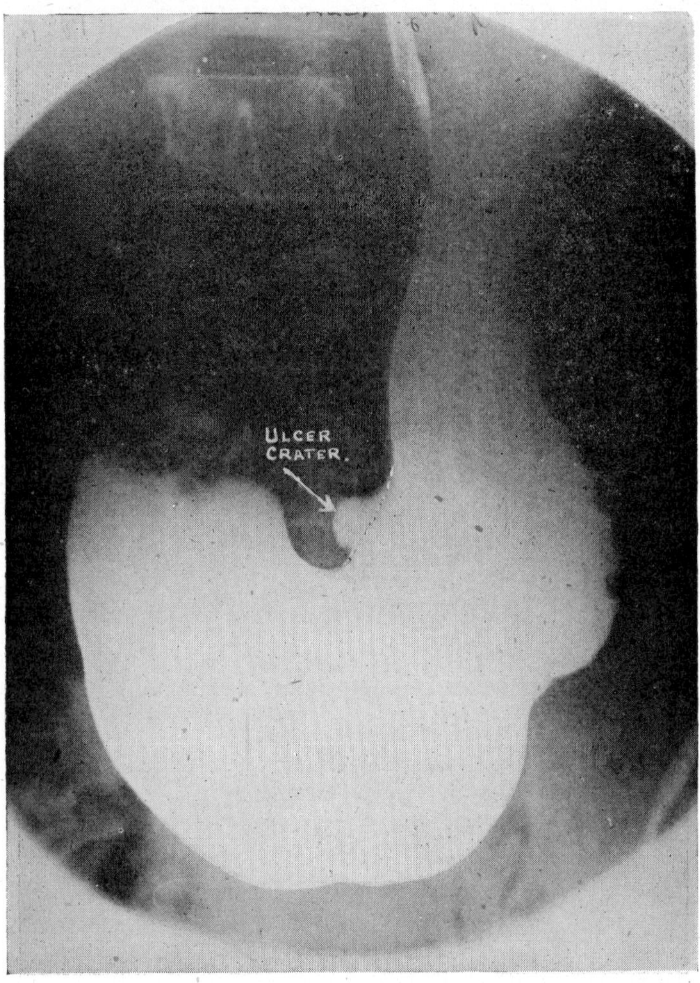

Fig. 79.—*see page* 166.

Barium Meal Examination of Stomach Showing Ulcer Crater. The dotted line represents the normal outline of the lesser curvature. Note also the constriction of the stomach, opposite the ulcer.

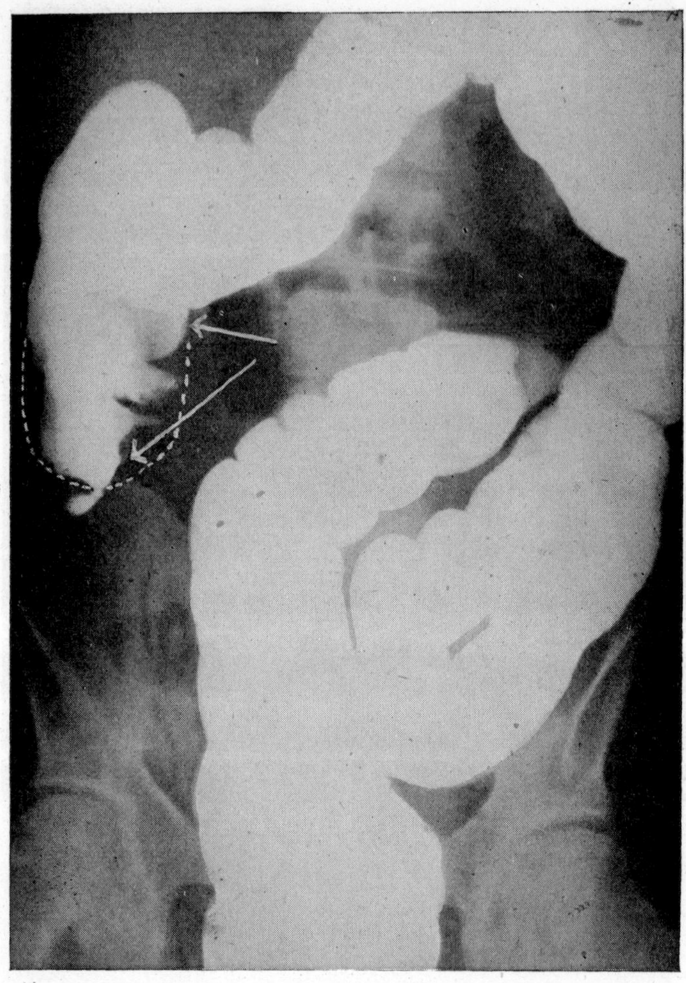

FIG. 80.—*see page* 167.

BARIUM MEAL EXAMINATION OF COLON SHOWING FILLING DEFECT IN CAECUM. The dotted line represents the normal outline of the caecum. The alteration in the contour of the caecum is due, in this case, to carcinoma.

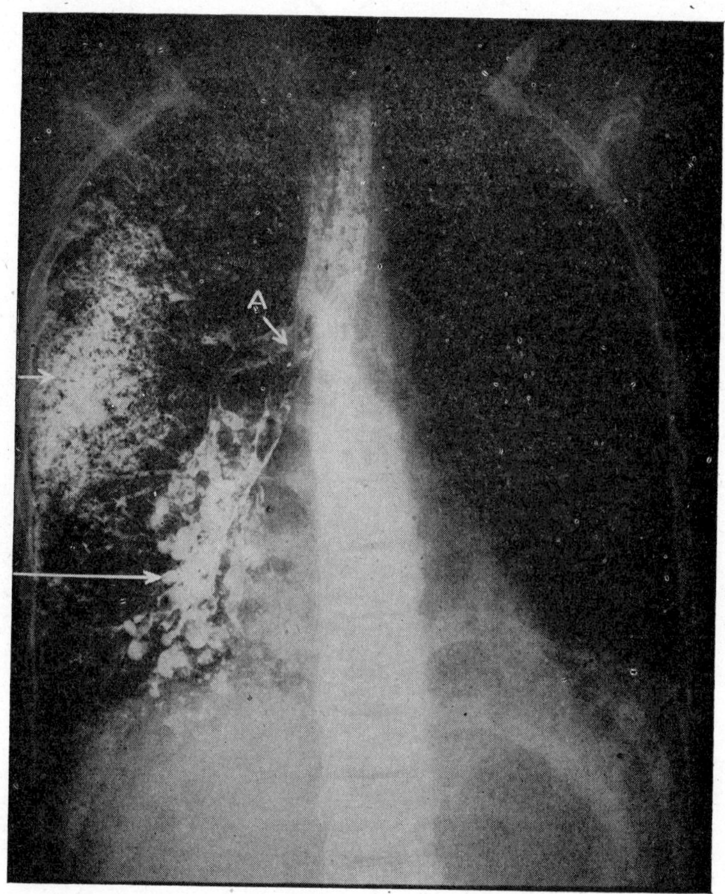

FIG. 81.—*see page* 167.

LIPIODOL EXAMINATION OF BRONCHIAL TREE.

(A) indicates position of right bronchus dividing into eparterial and hyparterial bronchi. (B) shows distribution of lipiodol in normal alveoli and (C) bronchiectasis in lower lobe due to dilatation.

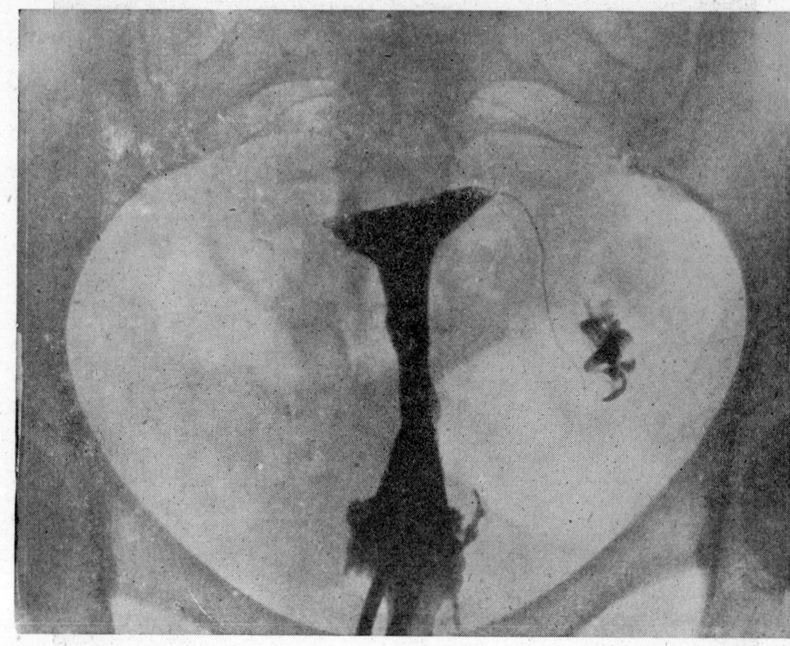

FIG. 82.—*see page* 167. HYSTERO-SALPINGOGRAPHY.

Examination of the patency of the uterine tubes. The opaque medium used is lipiodol. The shape of the uterus can be seen and the fine uterine tube on the left. The opaque medium shows the outline of the tube and the shape of its fimbriated end. Subsequent examination would show that the lipiodol had dripped from the tube into the pelvic cavity. In this patient the right tube is not patent, it may be absent. The examination proves that only one tube functions.

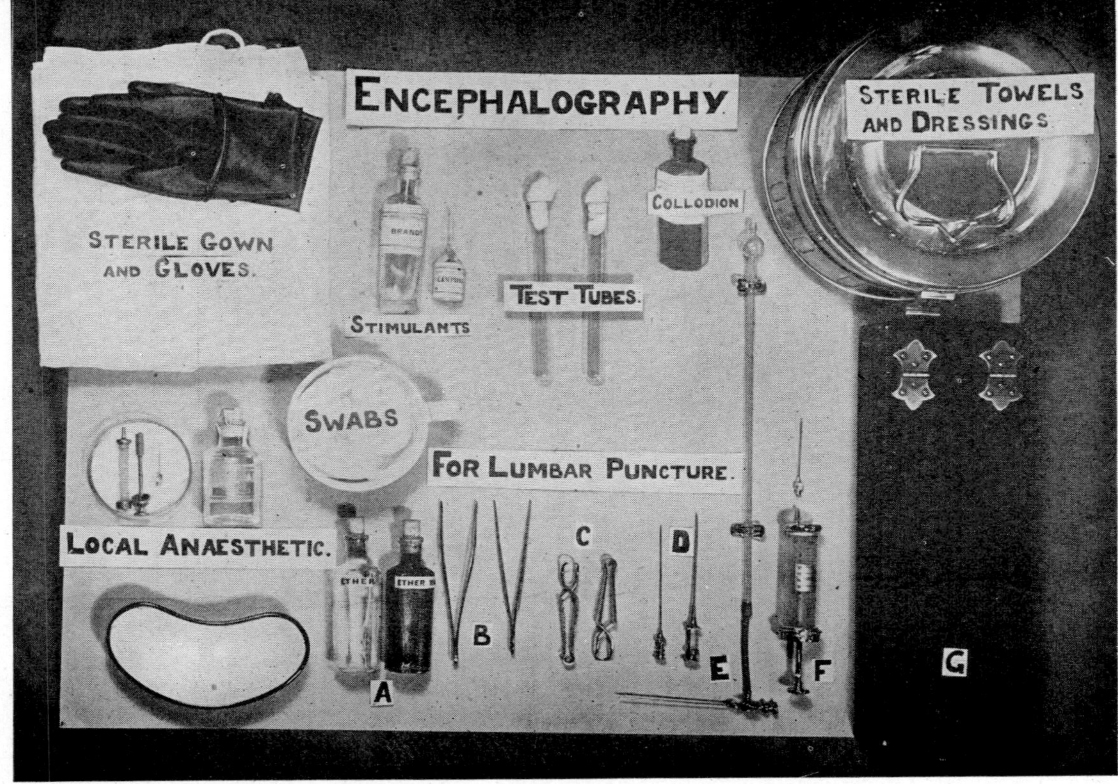

FIG. 83.—*see page* 167. The articles shown include sterile towels, dressings and swabs, gloves, local anaesthetic. (A) Articles for cleansing the skin. (B) Dissecting forceps. (C) Towel clips. (D) Barker's needle. (E) Greenfield's manometer. (F) Twenty c.c. syringe and needle. (G) Sphygmomanometer. Collodion for sealing the puncture. Sterile test tubes for specimens of fluid.

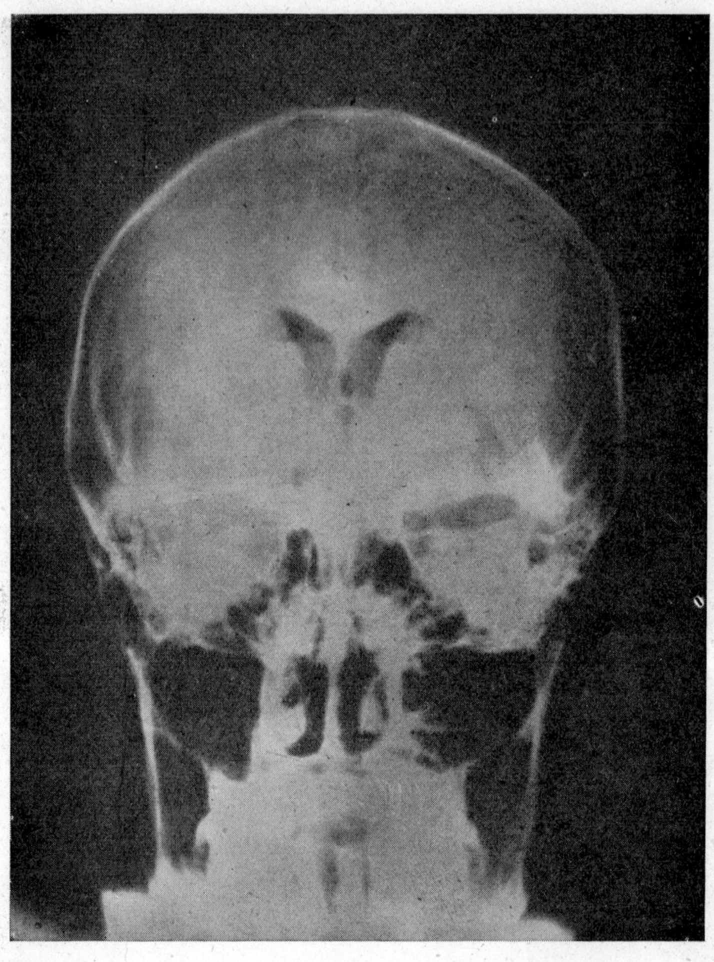

FIG. 84.—*see page* 167. ENCEPHALOGRAM.
Showing the anterior and posterior horns of the lateral ventricles filled with air.

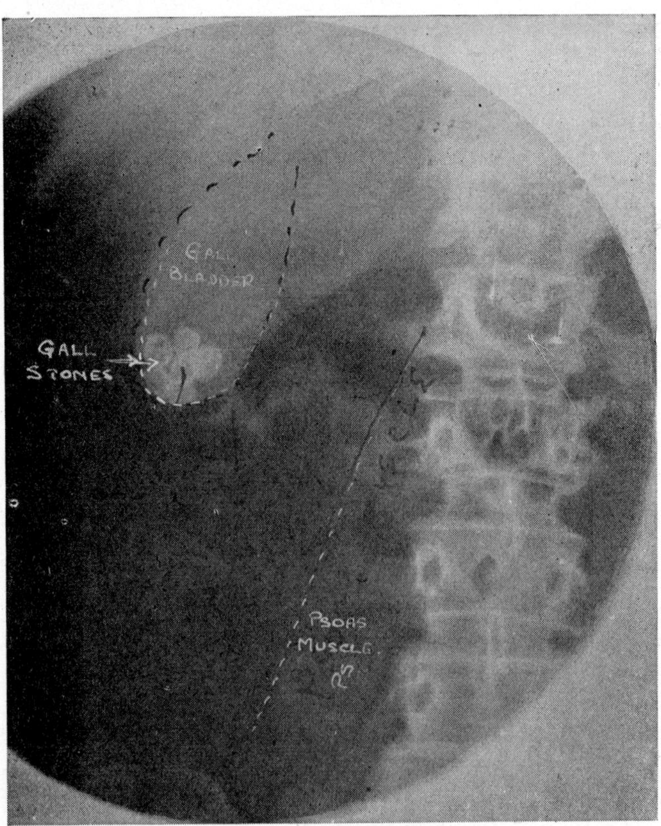

FIG. 85.—*see page* 168.

CHOLECYSTOGRAM SHOWING GALLSTONES IN A DYE-FILLED GALL BLADDER.

The gall bladder is outlined, the positions of the gallstones indicated and the psoas muscle is outlined.

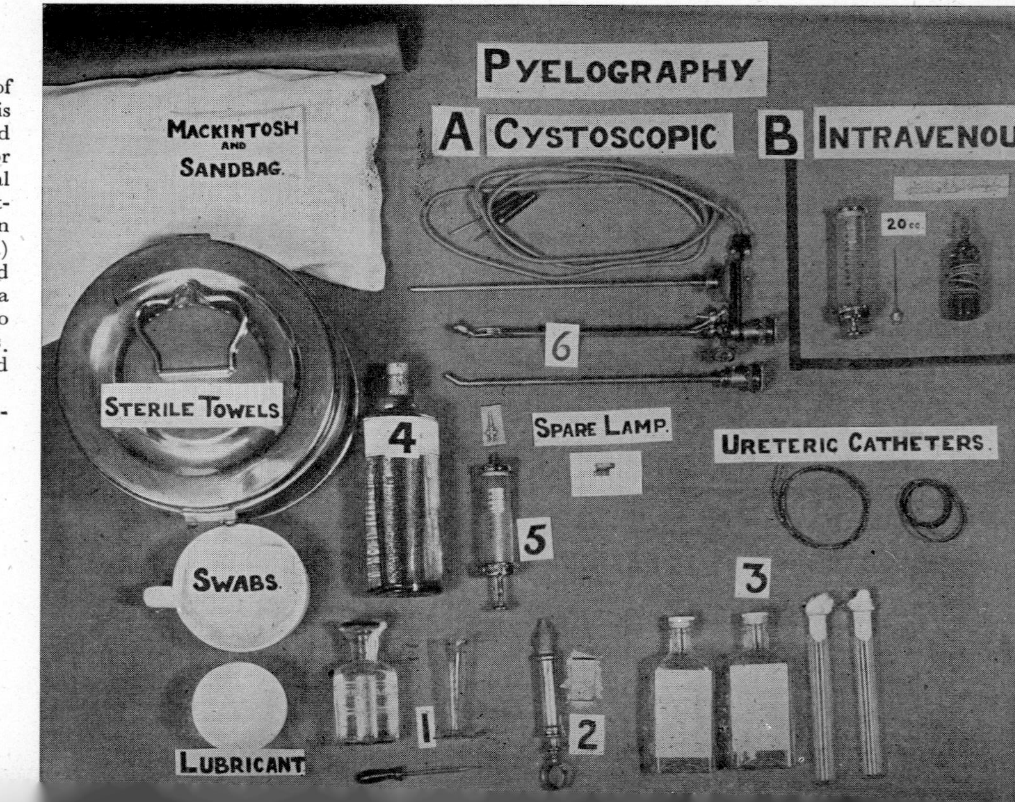

FIG. 86.—*see page* 170.
For the retrograde method of pyelography (A) cystoscopy is necessary. The articles required are (1) local anaesthetic for urethra in males. (2) urethral syringe. (3) sterile specimen bottles or test tubes for the collection of urine from each ureter. (4) sodium iodide solution. (5) record syringe of 20 c.c. capacity with a special connexion for fitting on to the end of the ureteric catheters. (6) cystoscope with telescope and outer sheath.
For *intravenous pyelography* (B) uroselectan is provided.

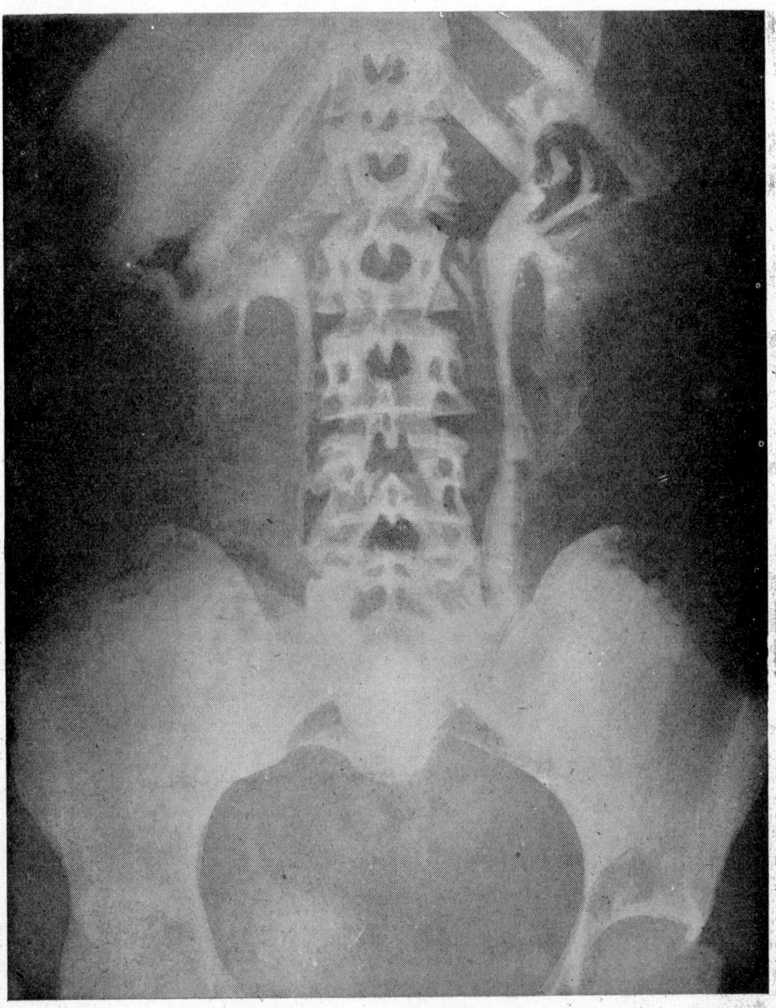

FIG. 87.—*see page* 170. UROSELECTAN EXAMINATION.
The outline of pelves, calices and ureters is shown by the dye. Upper, middle and lower calices can be distinctly seen.

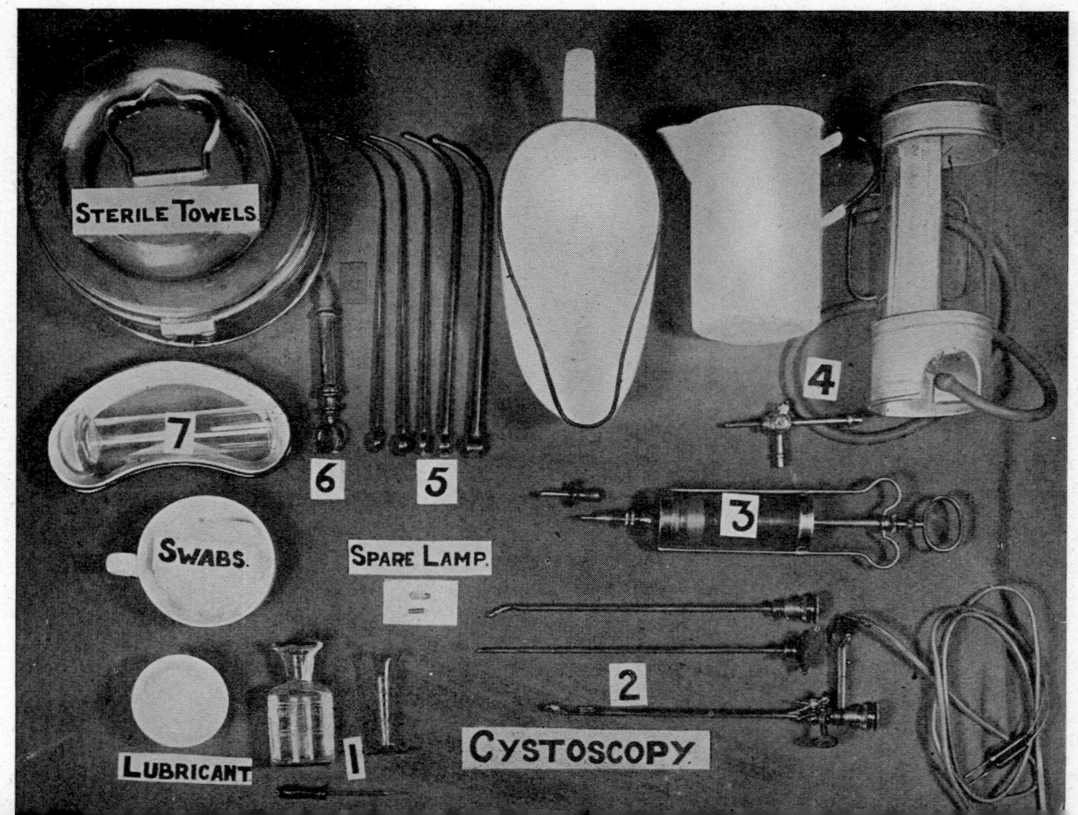

FIG. 88.—*see page* 171.
The articles required for cystoscopy include (1) local anaesthetic and pipette for female urethra — a male urethral syringe is numbered six. (2) cystoscope with telescope, outer sheath and lead for attachment to transformer. (3) bladder syringe with extra nozzle for attachment to cystoscope. (4) irrigation can with tubing and special metal attachment for cystoscope. (5) and (6) urethral dilators and syringe for male patient. (7) sterile glass for specimen of urine. A special boat-shaped receiver is supplied.

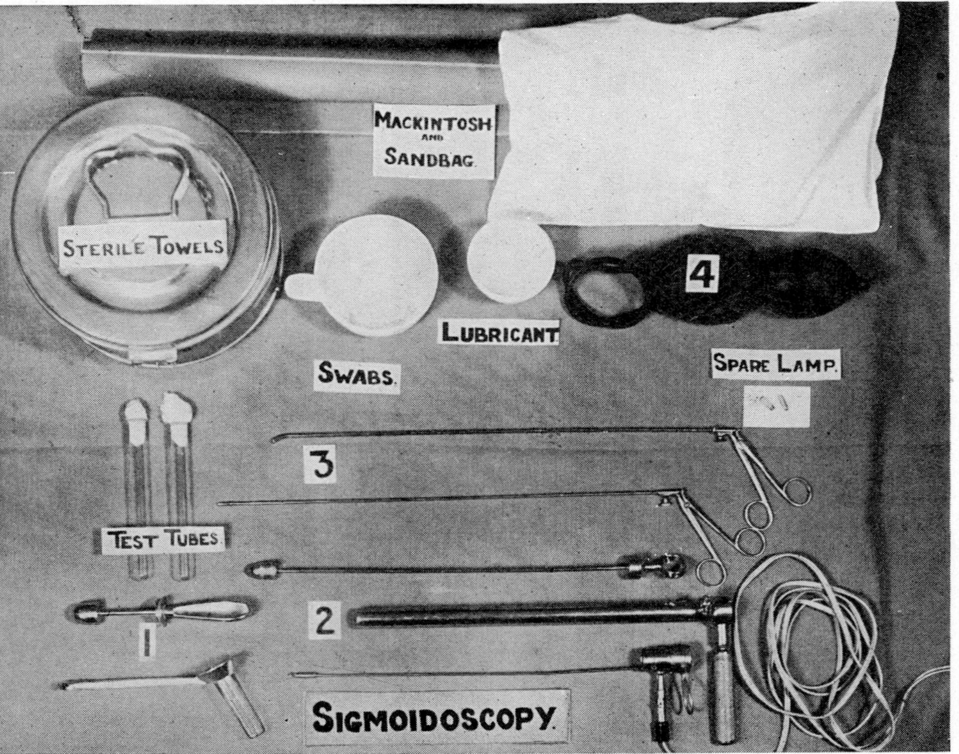

Fig. 89.—*see page* 172.
The articles for sigmoidoscopy include (1) Proctoscope. (2) Sigmoidoscope. (3) Two pairs Patterson's forceps. (4) Bellows for inflating sigmoid flexure. Sterile towels, swabs and lubricant, mackintosh and sandbag and sterile test tubes for the collection of specimens are also required.

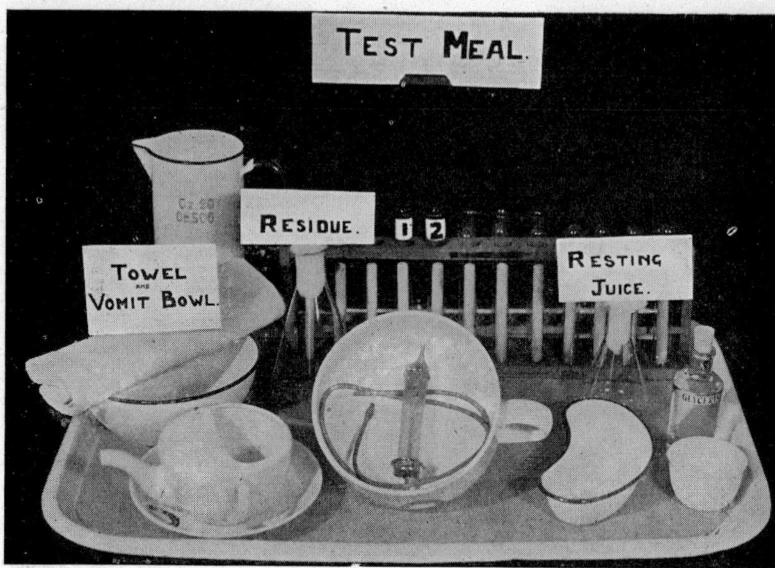

FIG. 90.—*see pages* 172.
A Ryle's tube and 20 c.c. syringe are in the porringer on the front of the tray. Glycerine is provided to lubricate the tube. Specially large flasks are provided for the resting juice and residual fluid and a number of test tubes labelled 1, 2, etc., for the specimens of stomach content withdrawn every 10 to 15 minutes (see above).

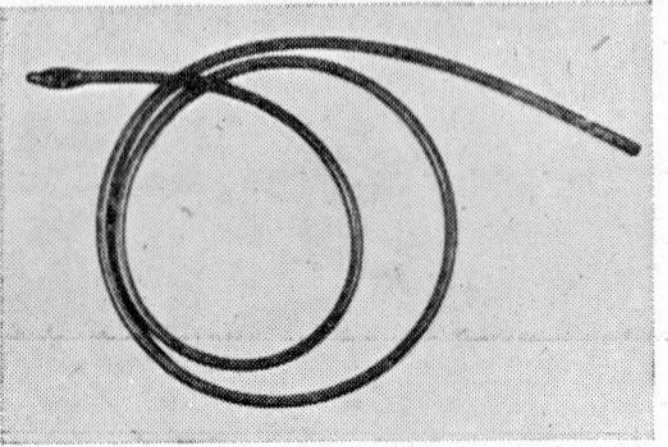

FIG. 91.—RYLE'S TUBE.
Note the bulbous, slightly weighted, end of the tube.

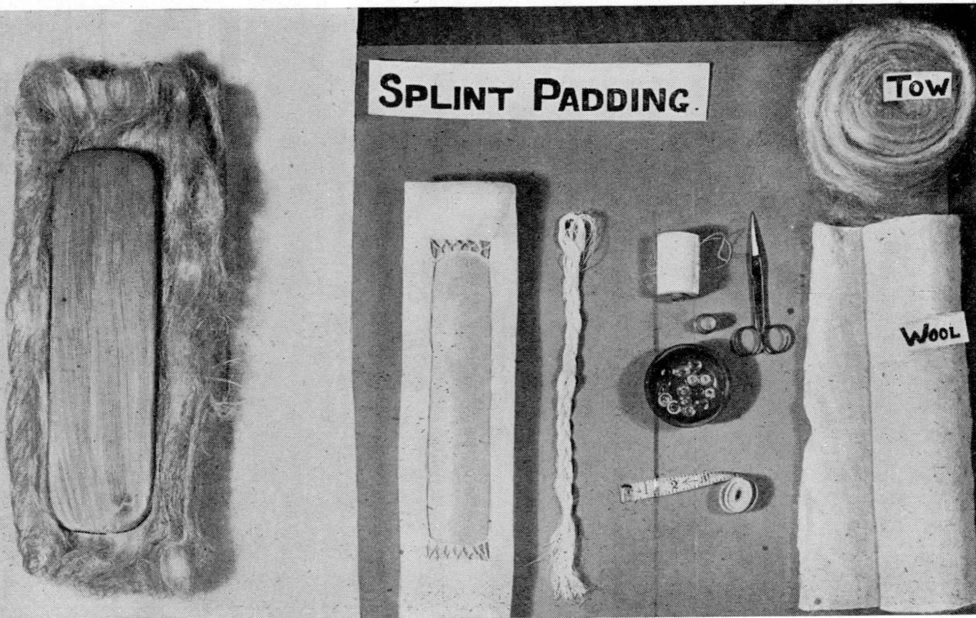

FIG. 92.—*see page* 177.

On the *left* a wooden splint is shown on a prepared pad of tow and wool. On the *right* the articles required for splint padding are shown and a padded splint completed.

These articles are:

A piece of linen large enough to cover padding and splint.

Needle, strong thread, thimble and scissors.

Brown wool and tow. The tow is teazled to make it soft and free from lumps. The brown wool is cut large enough to cover the front and the edges of the splint.

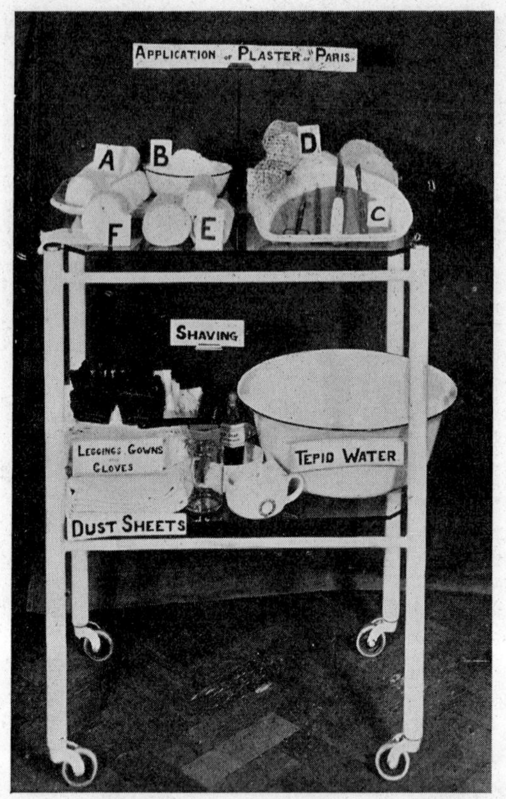

FIG. 93.—*see page* 177.

UPPER SHELF. (A) Plaster of paris bandages. (B) Powdered plaster of paris. (C) Plaster knives and scissors. (D) Cotton wool bandages. (E) Lint bandages. (F) Roll of stockinette.

LOWER SHELF. Dust sheets and protective clothing for the operator. Articles for shaving the skin. Large bowl (or pail) for tepid water.

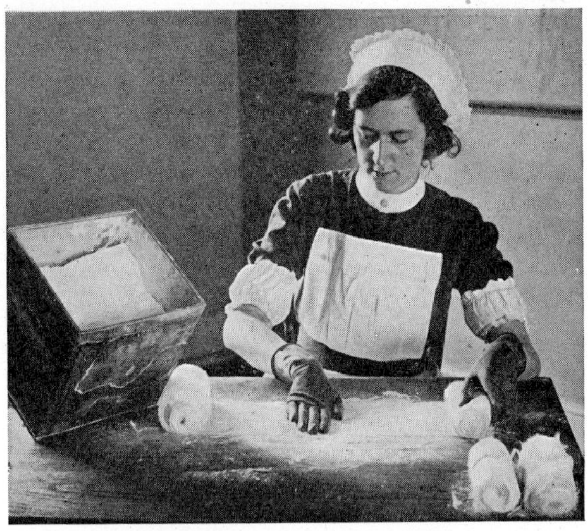

FIG. 94.—*see pages* 177–80. MAKING PLASTER BANDAGES. Fine dental plaster of paris is rubbed into the meshes; the bandages are lightly rolled and stored in tins.

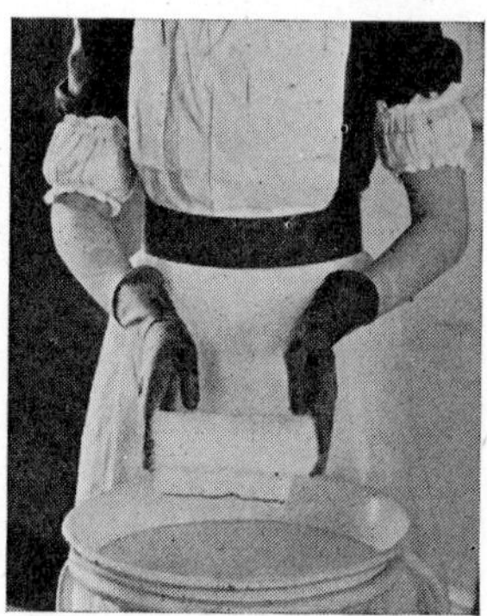

FIG. 95.
PUTTING A PLASTER BANDAGE IN TO SOAK.
A dark thread is run through the free end of the bandage in order that the end may be more easily distinguished.

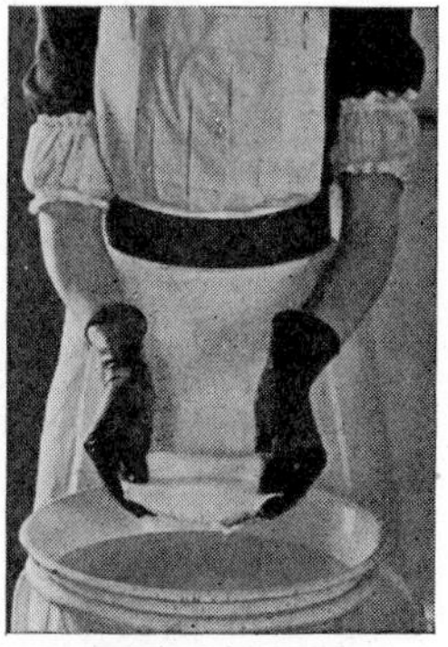

FIG. 96.
When the bandage is soaked it is lifted out, the ends are slightly compressed before the bandage is handed to the operator. The nurse, in handing a plaster bandage, slightly loosens the free end.

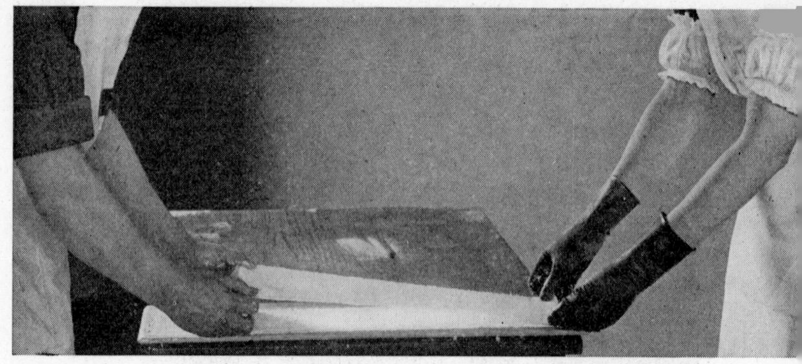

FIG. 97.—*see pages* 181.
A pad or slab is made by soaking a bandage and carrying it backwards and forwards as shown.

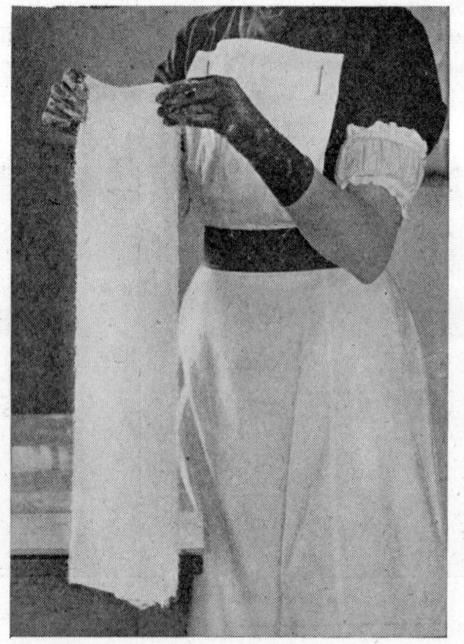

FIG. 98.
The completed slab ready to be handed to the operator.

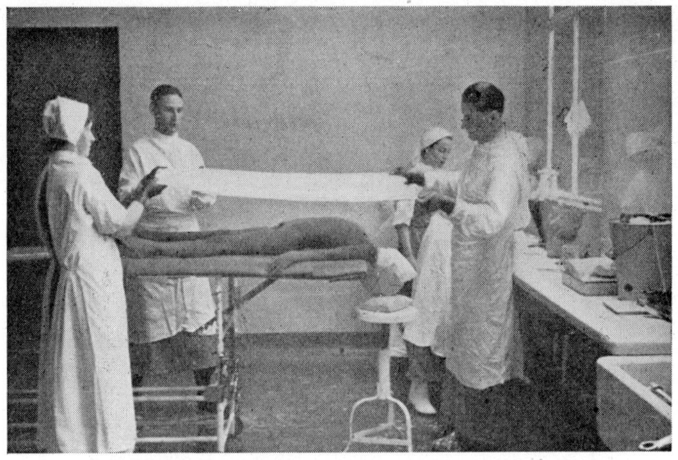

FIG. 99.—*see page* 181.
Using a plaster of paris slab to make an anterior plaster case.

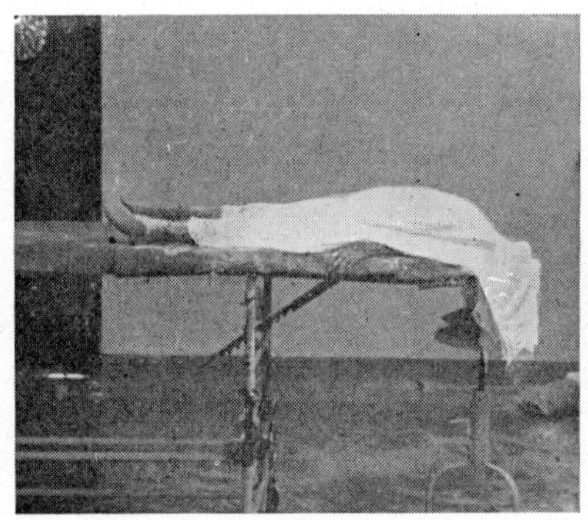

FIG. 100.
The plaster slab (in Fig. 98) in position on the patient.

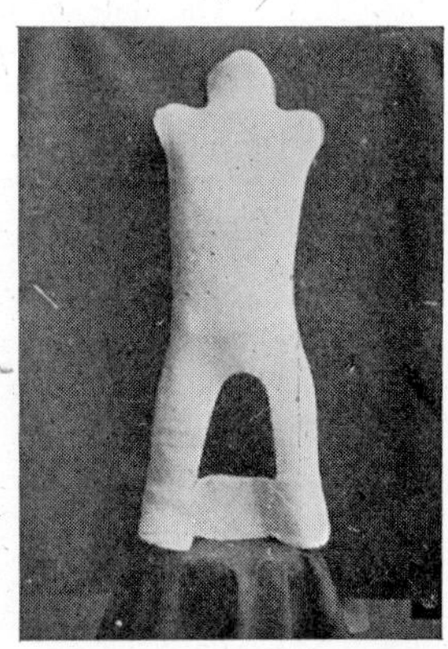

FIG. 101.
The completed anterior plaster case.

(*Photographs are kindly lent by Mr. F. P. Fitzgerald*)

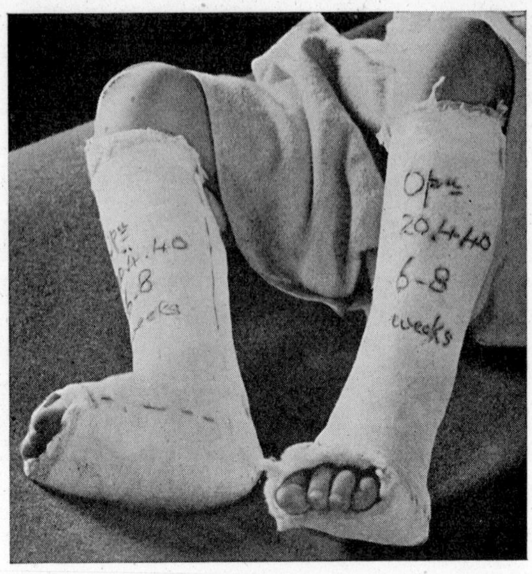

FIG. 102.—*see pages* 177–80.
The date of operations, and the time the plaster is to be worn is written on it with indelible pencil. The plaster is marked where it is to be cut.

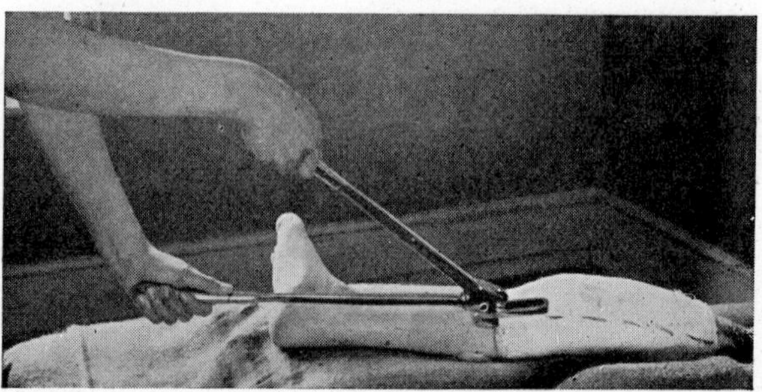

FIG. 103.
Cutting along the line on a marked plaster with plaster shears.

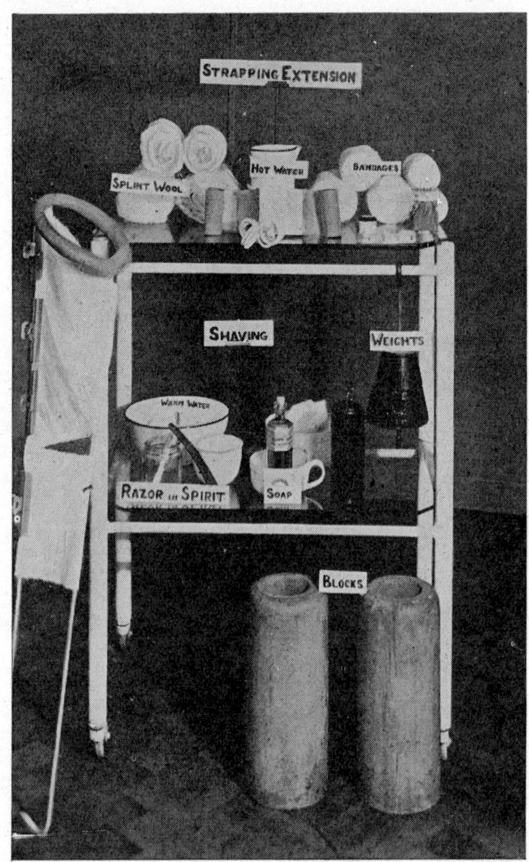

FIG. 104.—*see page* 181.

UPPER SHELF. Strapping extension as in Fig. 105. Hot water to warm the strapping. Splint wool, bandages, needle and cotton.

LOWER SHELF. Articles for shaving the skin, weights, bed blocks.

A Thomas's leg splint is shown ready prepared with bandage slings, for the leg, held in position by clips.

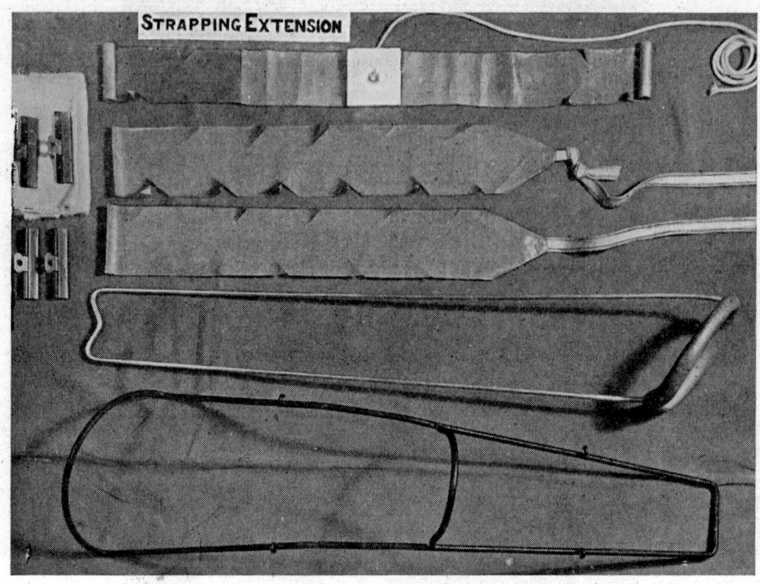

FIG. 105.—*see pages* 181–2. STRAPPING EXTENSIONS.

The prepared strapping extension at the top of the picture has a strapping spreader inserted. This is made of wood, with a hole in the middle through which cord is passed for the suspension of weights. This method of strapping extension may be employed in conjunction with a Liston splint or with Hodgen's or Thomas's splint as shown in Fig. 109.

The other examples given above are those employed when fixed skin traction is used. The ends of the strapping are then tied to the lower end of either the Hodgen's or the Thomas's leg splint.

In the lower of the two examples a piece of lamp wick is firmly stitched to the end of the strapping; in the other a firm loop is stitched on and the lamp wick is knotted through this loop. Lamp wick is used because it is strong, firm, and does not slip. (*See also Figs.* 106–7.)

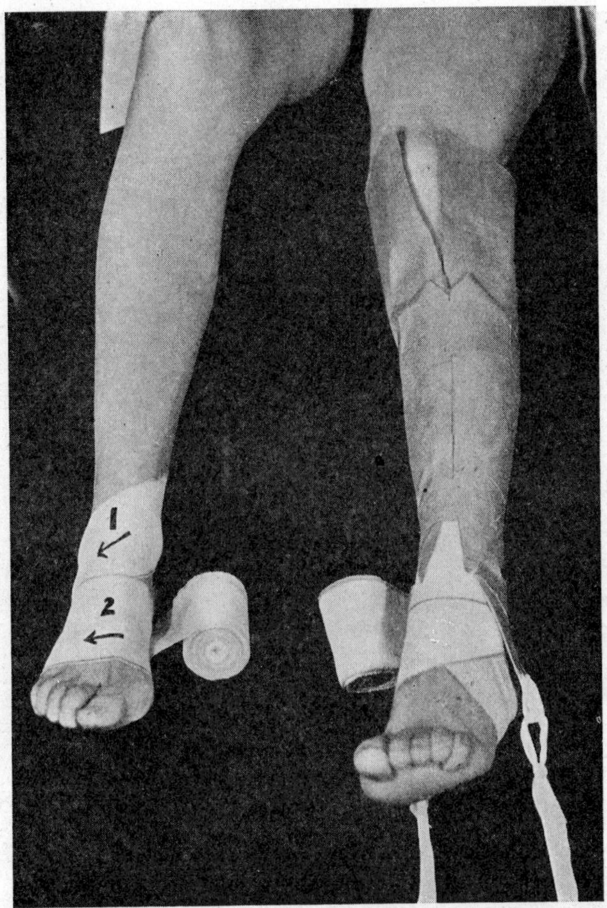

FIG. 106.—*see pages* 181–2.

APPLICATION OF STRAPPING EXTENSION TO LEG.

RIGHT LEG. A bandage is applied over the foot and malleoli to protect the bony prominences.

LEFT LEG. The strapping extension is in position and adherent to the skin of the leg. The bandage, as shown on the right leg, is now carried up, over the strapping (see next figure).

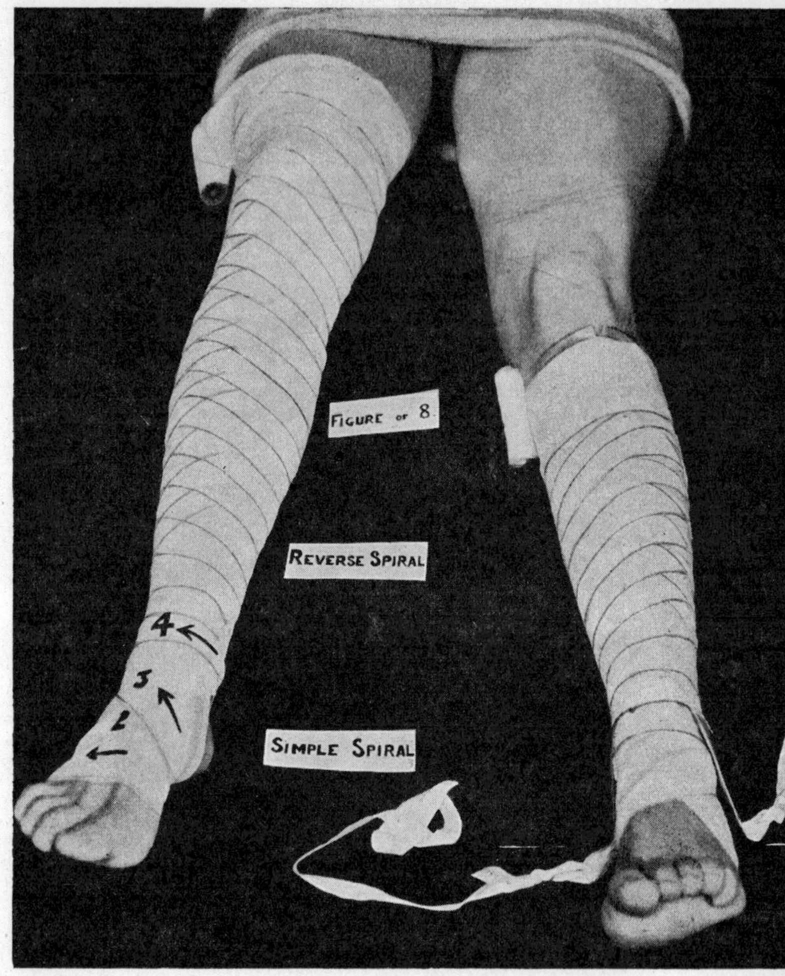

FIG. 107.

APPLICATION OF STRAPPING EXTENSION TO LEG.

LEFT LEG. This shows the strapping extension illustrated in Fig. 106. It is nov covered by bandage. Note that the strapping has been turned down at top, belov the knee, sticky side outwards. The bandage is carried round over the sticky strap ping which prevents the bandage slipping.

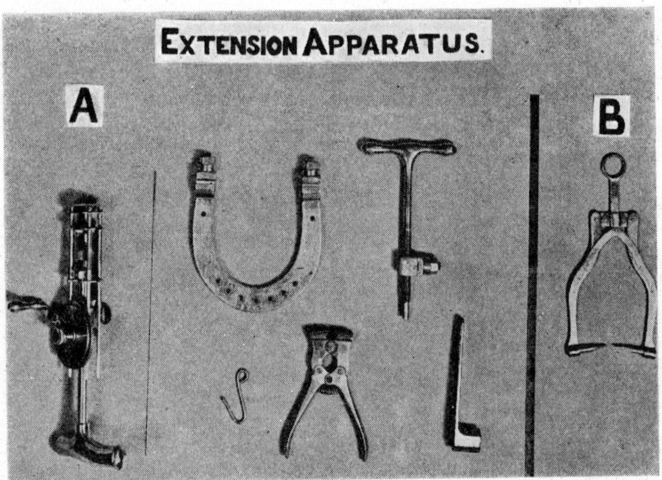

FIG. 108.—*see page* 182. (A) Kirschner's drill and wire, stirrup and hook, wire cutters and instruments for tightening nuts. (B) Icetong calipers.

When skeletal traction was first employed almost invariably icetong calipers (*see* B *above*) were used. The points of the calipers are inserted into the cancellous tissue of the bone, but there is a tendency for these to slip and in time experience showed that the use of a pin or wire passed through the end of the bone was preferable. It is more comfortable and there is no chance of the pin slipping.

The pin is sterilized and bored through the bone by a drill. The ends of the pin or wire are then fixed to a specially made stirrup and from this, cord is carried to pulleys placed on the special bed apparatus. Weights are suspended from the cord.

The pin or wire is firmly attached to the stirrup and made secure by having the nuts tightened up. When properly applied the pin does not slip and there is little discomfort even at the beginning of the treatment.

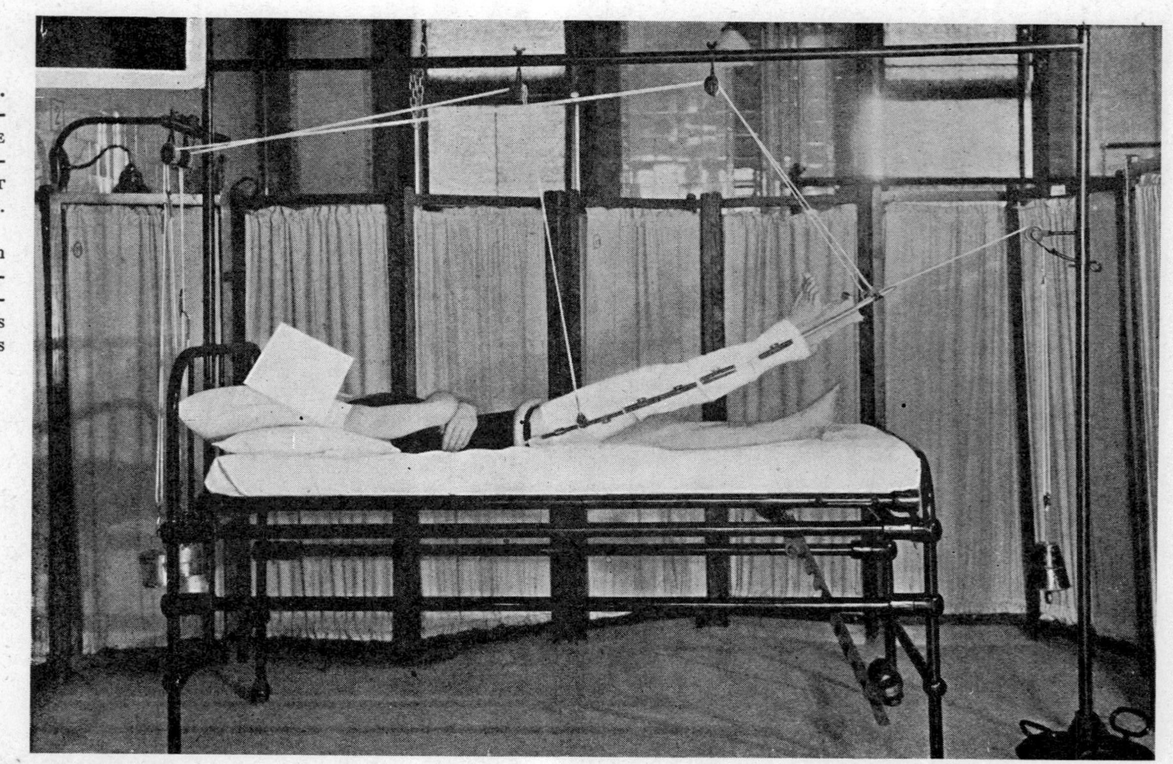

FIG. 109.—*see page* 182. APPLICATION OF STRAPPING EXTENSION IN THE TREATMENT OF FRACTURE OF THE RIGHT FEMUR (*see also Figs.* 105 *and* 110).

In the example shown Thomas's splint is employed and the extension is made by means of strapping, pulleys and weights.

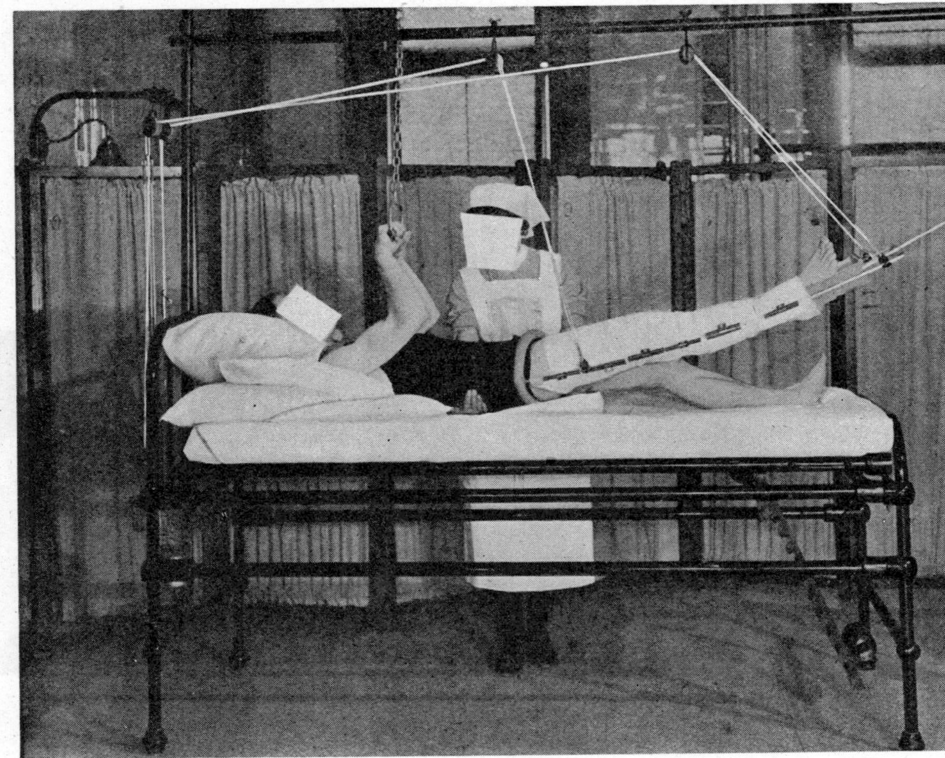

Fig. 110.

The same patient as in Fig. 109. Note the physical effort the patient is making to raise himself from the bed. Provided the broken bone is adequately splinted, the patient may move about freely in bed. Movement is exercise, and by this means the patient can keep fit, but the exercise he is allowed depends on his general state of health.

A man with a broken leg, for example, who is otherwise quite fit, should be made to realise that the more he moves about in bed and the more he does things for himself, so much the better will he be, and if he keeps fit he will find that when he begins to get up he will have less difficulty in taking up his usual mode of life and occupation.

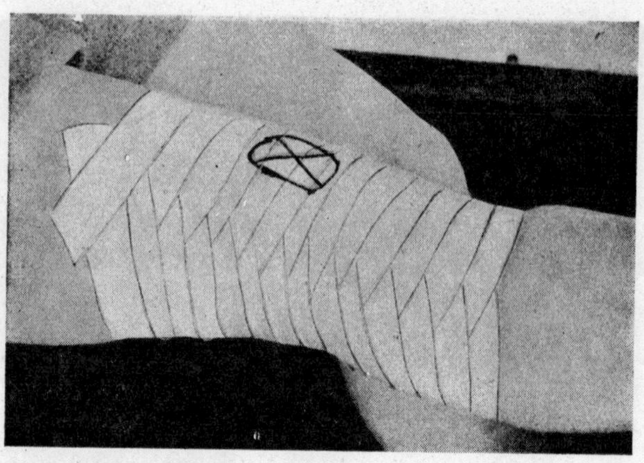

FIG. 111.—*see page* 113.
Strapping applied to knee, as in applying Scott's dressing. The position of the patella is shown.

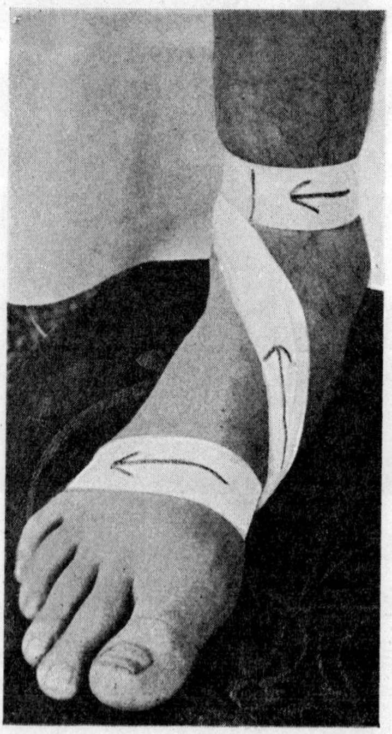

FIG. 112.
Strapping applied to the foot after Goldthwaite's method. The first turn is round the metatarsals, the second up over the internal arch and the third round the ankle. The arrows indicate the direction of the strapping. The effect of the strapping in supporting the arch can be seen.

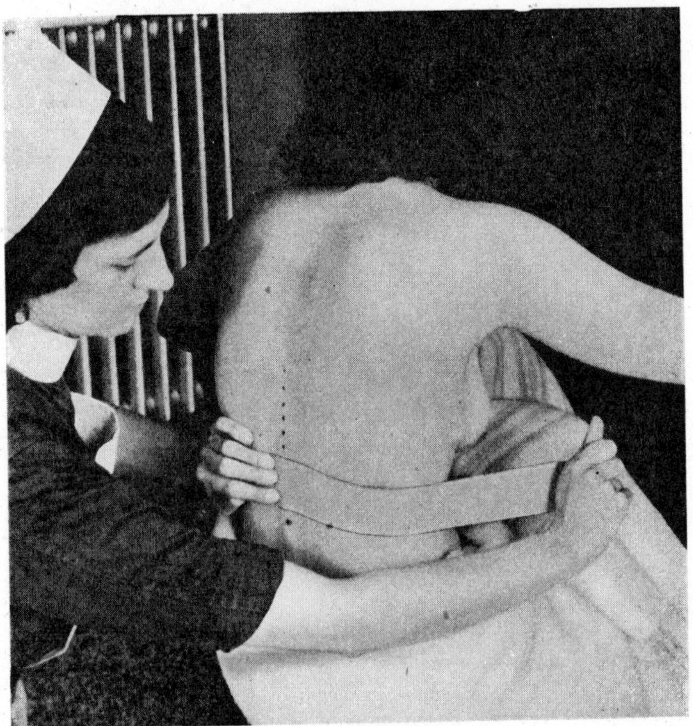

FIG. 113.—STRAPPING OF CHEST.

Note that, for the purpose of demonstration, the vertebral spines are marked. The strips of strapping are all prepared. Application is made from below upwards, over the lower ribs first, with *the chest in full expiration*. Each strip must extend from beyond the spine (as shown) at the back, round the chest, and to the opposite side of (that is beyond) the sternum in front.

The operator fixes one end of the strip of strapping over the spine by placing her fingers on it (as shown). She then gets the patient to breathe *in* and then *out*. The patient must empty the chest as much as possible and is instructed to *blow* the air out of his chest. The operator says "continue blowing, go on, right out" until she is assured the chest is as empty as possible. She then, with her other hand, carries the free end of the strapping round the side and front of the chest where it is firmly fixed. The subsequent layers of strapping are then applied. (*See Fig.* 114.)

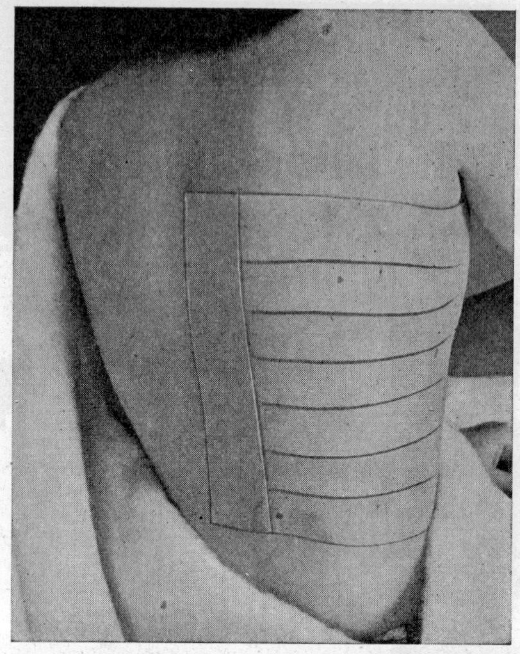

FIG. 114.—STRAPPING OF CHEST.

When the chest is strapped, a strip of strapping is placed, vertically, over the ends of the strips, back and front, in order to prevent the ends of the strips being disturbed.

The patient is not allowed to raise his arm when his chest is being strapped, because raising the arm would interfere with full expiration. The object of strapping the chest is to prevent the full range of respiratory movement.

In Fig. 113 the arm of the patient is being held out of the way by an assistant. But notice that the arm is merely held away from the chest wall; it is not elevated because raising the arm would partly fix the ribs and full expiration would then be difficult.

Chapter 15

Bandages and Bandaging

Types of bandages—Materials used in bandaging—Rules for the application of a roller bandage—Examples of bandaging—Triangular bandaging

There are varieties of bandage, examples including the *roller bandage* made from strips of material of convenient lengths and from half an inch to eight inches wide. These bandages should be prepared without selvedge; in many cases raw edges are used; in the woven bandages the edges are firm but not hard. A roller bandage should be closely and firmly rolled, with all the edges even.

The *triangular bandage* or *sling* is made by taking a square of material; for a large sling a piece 40 inches square is chosen. If this is folded over once triangle-wise and then cut across, it will make two bandages. A triangular bandage is described as consisting of a long side—the base—opposite to which is the point or apex, and two short sides and two ends (see p. 253).

Special bandages include the T-shaped bandage, plain and many-tailed binders and the four-tailed binders. A *T bandage* is made by taking two strips of material, from 4 to 5 inches wide, and stitching them together in the form of the letter T. It is used to retain dressings on the perineum. In the case of a male patient the strip of material carried up in front of the pubes is divided into two, one being placed on each side of the scrotum, in order to avoid discomfort.

A *plain binder* is made by stitching two strips of material together, so forming a double layer. It should be sufficiently long and wide to retain a dressing, or to give support to any part of the trunk to which it may be applied.

A *many-tailed binder* or bandage, the bandage of Scultetus, is made by stitching strips of material together in the middle third of their length, leaving the ends on either side free, in tail formation.

A many-tailed bandage can be made in an emergency by tearing a piece of material into shape, and it is useful for example, when a limb is to be bandaged which may not be raised or lifted from the bed; the bandage, with the tails at one side rolled or folded up, can be slipped under the limb by pressing down on the pillow or mattress on which it lies; then, by taking the tails across in front of the limb, a dressing may be retained in position and changed without movement of the limb.

The *four-tailed bandage* is made by taking a piece of material of the desired length and width and tearing it towards the centre to form four tails (see p. 248).

Materials used for bandages. *Cotton*, *linen*, *muslin*, *gauze* and *calico* are fairly cheap materials. *Flannel*, *flannelette* and *domette* are warmer than cotton, a little firmer and more expensive. *Crêpe* material is used where slight elasticity is required and *elastic* and *rubber* bandages where firm support is needed. For warmth and protection, *lint* or *cotton wool* bandages are used. *Starch* and *plaster of paris* bandages are employed where a very firm surface is required to act as a splint.

Some of the **uses of a bandage** have been outlined as the materials employed were named, but, in addition, the uses of a bandage may be classified as follows:

The provision of support and protection.

Retention of splints, dressings and other apparatus in position.

Retention of a limb in some definitely fixed position.

Prevention of swelling by firmness of the application.

To arrest bleeding as when an Esmarch's rubber tourniquet is employed.

To lessen external sources of irritation and so to relieve spasm.

The application of firmness in bandaging may also lessen muscle spasm.

Rules for roller bandaging. A neatly rolled bandage of correct length and width should be chosen, and held firmly in the hand. The operator should stand facing the patient at one side of the bed and, unrolling several inches of the bandage, place the unrolled material against the skin of the patient in an oblique direction, from within outwards and from below upwards in the case of the limbs and chest, and from above downwards in bandaging the abdomen, unless an ascending spica of the hip is incorporated, in which case the direction will be from below upwards. The reason for the direction given above is that the bandage fits better and is more easily retained in position by covering first the slimmest parts. The bandage should be held in the right hand when bandaging the right side, and in the left hand when bandaging the left side, and a nurse should be able to bandage equally well with either hand. Pressure should be applied very evenly, and to effect this the bandage is unrolled in contact with the skin of the patient or with the dressing which is to be covered—a bandage should not be unrolled first and then dragged round the part to which it is applied, as this would result in creases or wrinkles and would thus provide a very uneven pressure.

As a general rule two-thirds of the preceding turn are covered by the oncoming turn when bandaging a limb, and half the preceding turn is covered when bandaging the head. A pattern, such as is made when a reverse ascending spiral or figure of eight is employed, should be arranged to lie on the outer side of the limb unless contraindicated, for example, by a wound in this situation. A pattern should never lie over a wound or over a bony prominence because the greatest pressure falls where the bandage crosses as in the formation of a pattern. Any pattern should be evenly spaced, one above the other.

In bandaging a limb for the purpose of retaining a splint in position, it is inadvisable to cover the fingers or toes; if these are left free they can easily be inspected for changes in colour and temperature when the bandage is complete.

Modes of application of a roller bandage. A bandage may be applied in *circular turns* as when one turn covers the other completely; this may be used on the neck or trunk, but circular turns round the limbs tend to cause constriction and, with the exception of an occasion when a bandage is used as a tourniquet, should not be employed for fear of interfering with the circulation in the limb below the bandage.

A *simple spiral bandage* is commenced by placing the tail of the bandage against the limb in a direction from above downwards; the bandage is then carried round the limb and upwards and outwards—so fixing the bandage which is then carried up the limb in a series of spiral turns.

A *reverse spiral* is begun in the same way to fix the bandage but, as it is carried round the limb from within outwards, the bandage is turned down on itself as it passes over the middle and outer third of the anterior aspect of the limb, which results in the formation of an inverted V pattern on the outer aspect (see figs. 115 and 116). The thumb of the free hand is used to steady the bandage as the reverse turns are made.

A *figure of eight* is commonly employed when bandaging over a straight joint, or one which is not required to be moved. A *figure of eight bandage* for the knee joint when extended is shown in figs. 117 and 118—the mode of application being indicated by arrows.

(Bandaging is so essentially a subject which can only be taught by practical demonstration, that no attempt is made to describe the movements in detail. A number of illustrations are appended which may help the student nurse in her practical work.)

Bandage for hand and forearm. A and B. In the first illustration (fig. 115) the bandage is carried obliquely, from the radial to the ulnar border as indicated by 1, around the fingers—2, and up over dorsum of the hand—3; the head of roller, indicated as 4, is carried down over

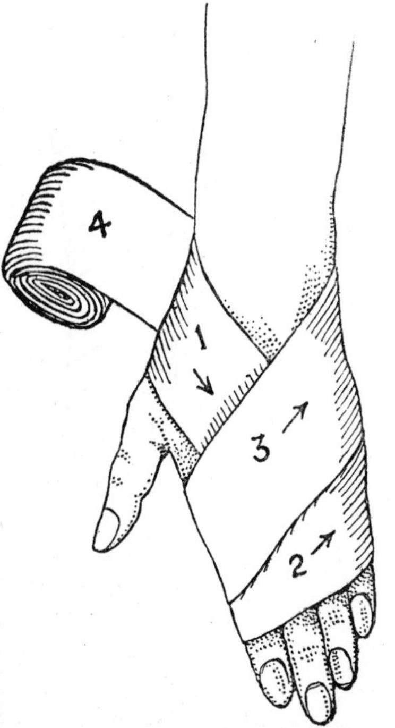

FIG. 115.—" A " BANDAGE FOR HAND AND FOREARM.

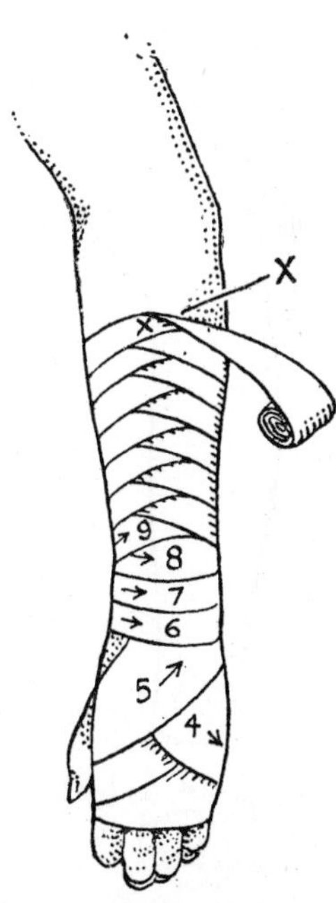

FIG. 116.—" B " BANDAGE FOR HAND AND FOREARM.

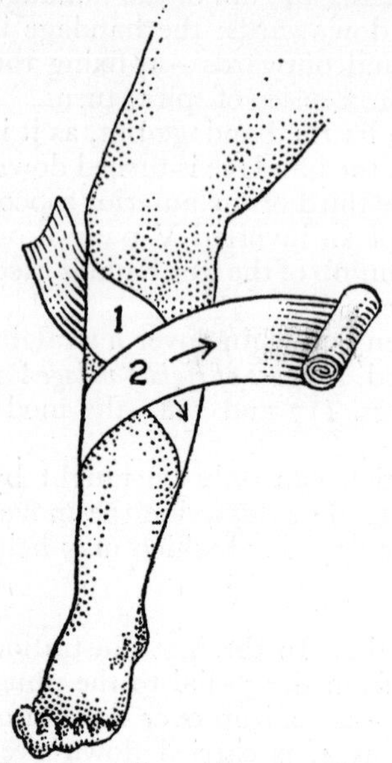

FIG. 117.—FIXING TURN TO COMMENCE FIGURE OF EIGHT BANDAGE.

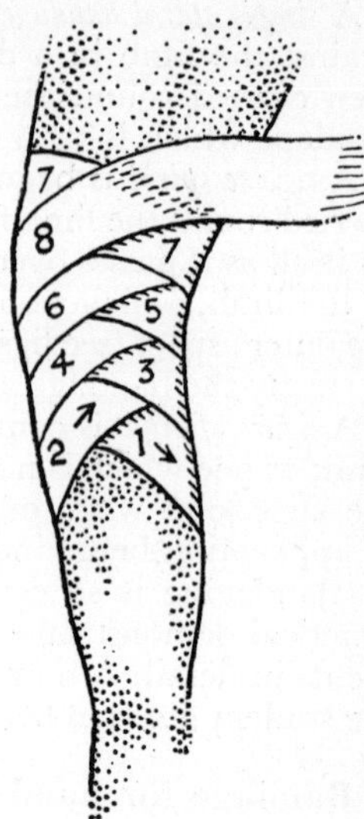

FIG. 118.—FIGURE OF EIGH BANDAGE APPLIED TO KNE JOINT.

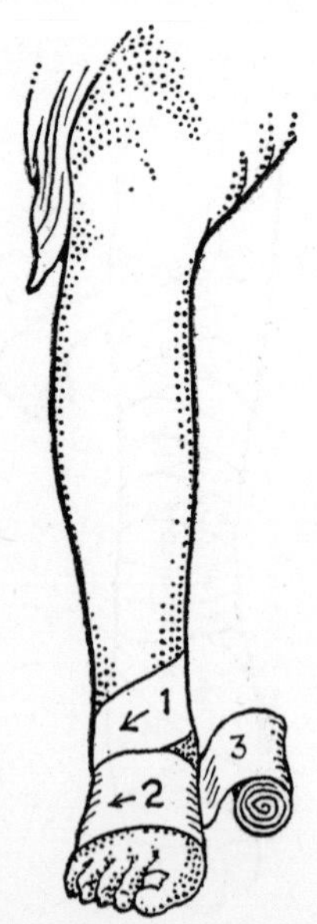

FIG. 119.—"A" BANDAGE FOR FOOT AND LEG.

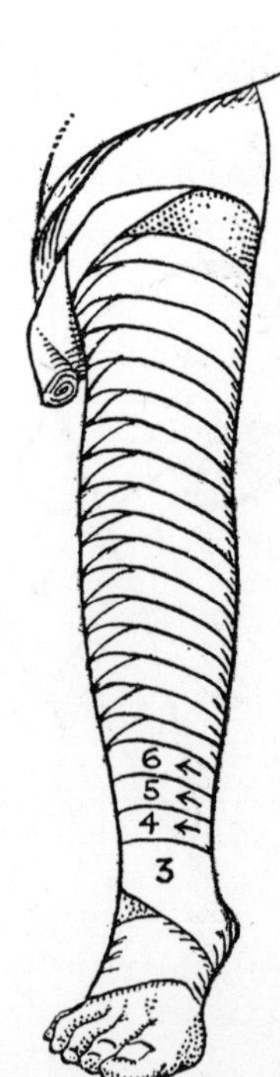

FIG. 120.—"B" BANDAG FOR FOOT AND LEG.

ɔrsum of hand (fig. 115); it is then taken round palmar aspect and ɔwards to the ulnar side of wrist, as 5. Three circular turns of an cending spiral are made round wrist as indicated by arrows. The first cending reverse spiral turn is indicated as 9. The mode of reversing e bandage is shown at the last turn, the point at which the bandage is versed on itself is indicated as X.

Bandage for foot and leg. A and B. This is similarly arranged and e direction of the turns is indicated by figures and arrows. In bandaging limb, a figure of eight is employed over a joint which is extended and a vergent spica over one which is flexed (see next figures).

In a *divergent spica*, application is made as shown in figs. 121 and 122, of ıe elbow and ankle. In both instances the tail of the bandage is first laid

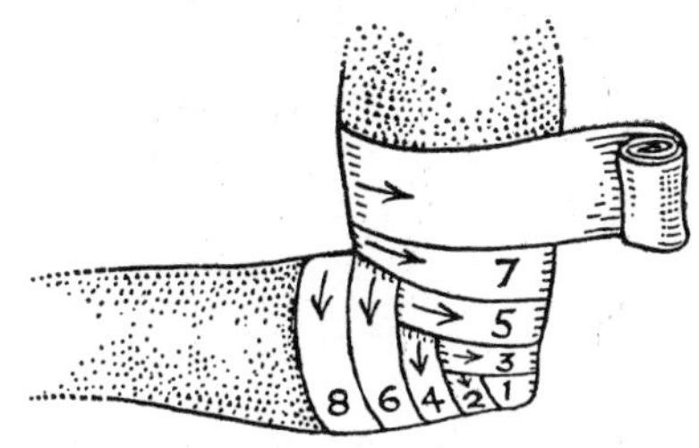

FIG. 121.—DIVERGENT SPICA APPLIED TO ELBOW.

bliquely across the joint from within outwards, and then carried over the pex as indicated by 1. It is then carried alternately below and above the ɔint leaving only half the preceding turn uncovered at first, and in the ırns made later one third is uncovered. The direction of the bandage is ıdicated by arrows.

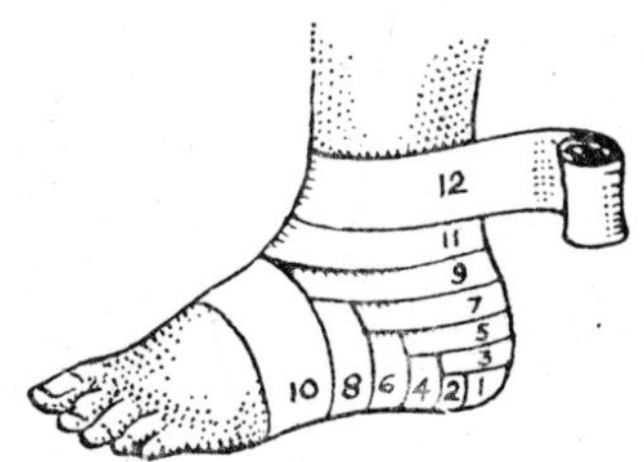

FIG. 122.—DIVERGENT SPICA APPLIED TO ANKLE.

An ascending spica of the shoulder (see fig. 123). The tail of the andage is placed obliquely on the shoulder in a direction from before ackwards and downwards as 1, it is then taken round the arm and rought up on the inner side. The bandage is then carried across the houlder, over the upper part of the scapula and across the back to the xilla of the opposite side, across the front of the chest (see turn 2) and is ontinued over the shoulder; and the turns are repeated as often as necesary in order to cover the dressing. The bandage is finished as shown overeaf.

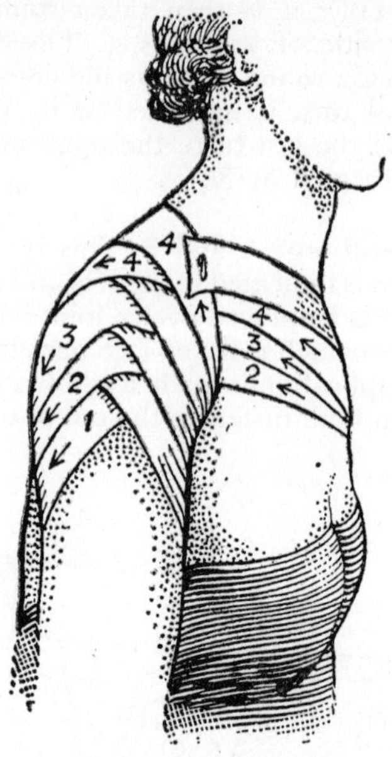

FIG. 123.—ASCENDING SPICA APPLIED TO RIGHT SHOULDER.

A descending spica of the groin. The tail of the bandage is lai obliquely in a direction from below upwards, as shown in fig. 124. Th roller is then carried round the back of the trunk to the opposite side an brought forward again as 2 in fig. 125. It is then taken over the oute

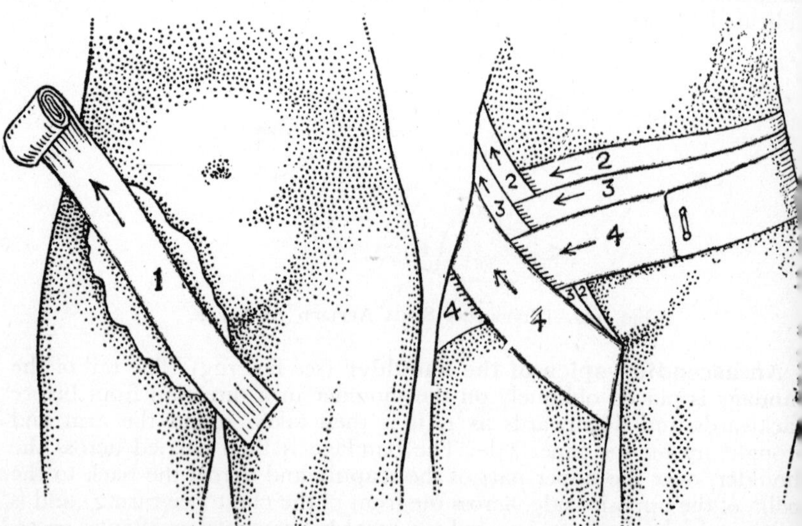

FIG. 124.—COMMENCEMENT OF DESCENDING SPICA OF RIGHT HIP.

FIG. 125.—DESCENDING SPICA OF RIGH HIP SHOWN COMPLETED.

spect of the thigh and round to the groin where it exactly covers the tail f the bandage shown in fig. 125. The first complete turn is indicated by 2 1 fig. 125, subsequent turns by 3 and 4.

Bandage to cover an eye. In both illustrations the right eye is overed. A pad is placed over the closed eye; the first turn of the bandage carried round the head in the direction indicated; the second turn is arried over the occiput at the back of the head and brought under the

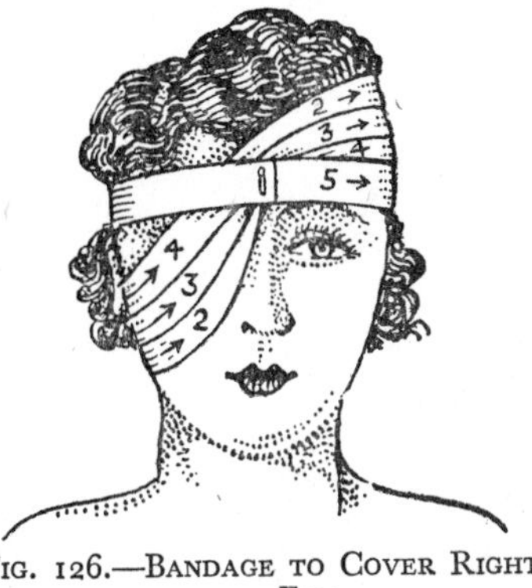

'IG. 126.—BANDAGE TO COVER RIGHT EYE.

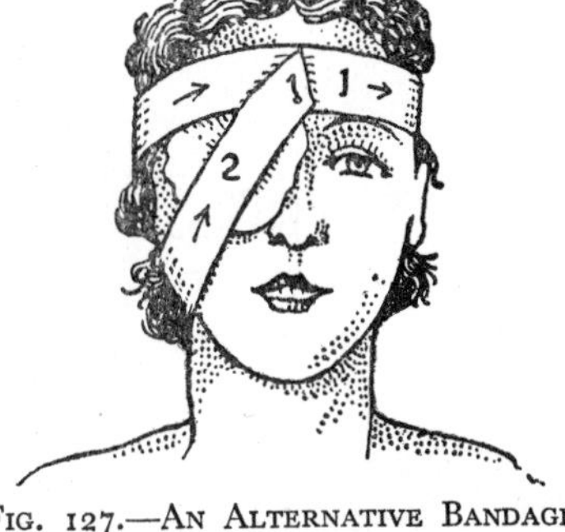

FIG. 127.—AN ALTERNATIVE BANDAGE FOR THE EYE.

ar and up over the cheek as shown—this turn is then carried up on to the ide of the head as indicated by 2. Subsequently, turns 3 and 4 are applied s indicated, and the bandage is completed by another circular turn, over he first one, around the head.

When it is considered undesirable to cover the pad over the eye com- pletely, as, for example, in patients who are undergoing frequent treatment o the eye, a bandage may be applied as shown in fig. 127.

A bandage to cover an ear may be required after an operation such s radical mastoidectomy. In fig. 128, the left ear is shown covered; in

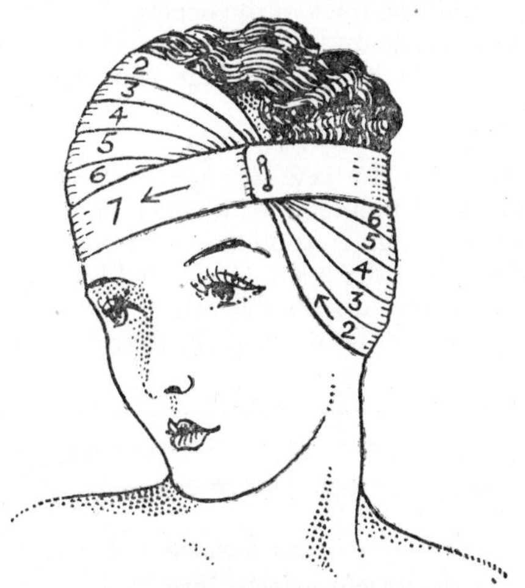

FIG. 128.—BANDAGE TO COVER LEFT EAR (SINGLE MASTOID BANDAGE).

fig. 129 both ears are treated. In the first illustration a fixing turn of the bandage is first applied round the head, it is then carried beneath the occiput at the back and brought round below the dressing over the ear, fairly low on the neck, as indicated by 2. This turn is carried up over the opposite side of the head. Subsequent turns are taken in the same direction as in 3, 4, 5 and 6; and finally a circular turn (7) is taken round the head. If the safety pin is carefully placed it can be used to secure all turns of the bandage where these cross at the side of the head (see fig. 129).

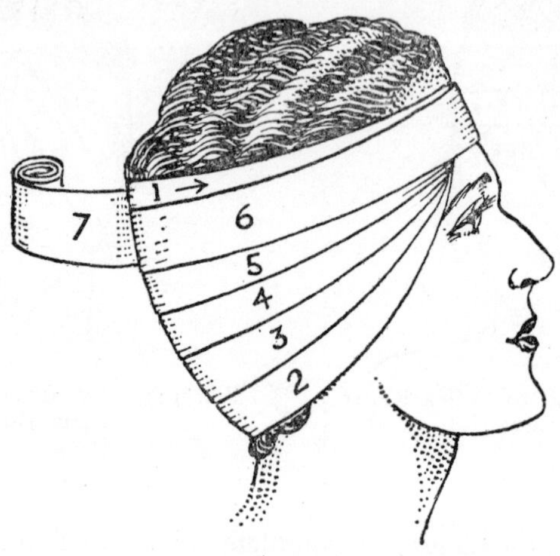

FIG. 129.—DOUBLE MASTOID BANDAGE (BOTH EARS COVERED).

In fig. 129, where both ears are covered as in the application of a double mastoid bandage the bandage may be commenced from either side. In the illustration given the bandage is carried from right to left. A circular turn round the head fixes the tail of the bandage; it is then carried down on one side, round the back of the occiput and up on the other side, being turned up on one side and down on the other to get the neat effect shown where the margins of the bandage converge towards the outer angle of the eye.

A bandage to support the jaw (see figs. 131 and 132) may be applied by means of a four-tailed bandage, or a roller may be employed. In the latter case a looped bandage is applied—three turns are made—the *first turn*, standing on the top of the head—indicated by an arrow—is brought down one side of the face, up on the other, and then taken obliquely across the head (2), below the occiput, in front of the chin (3), round

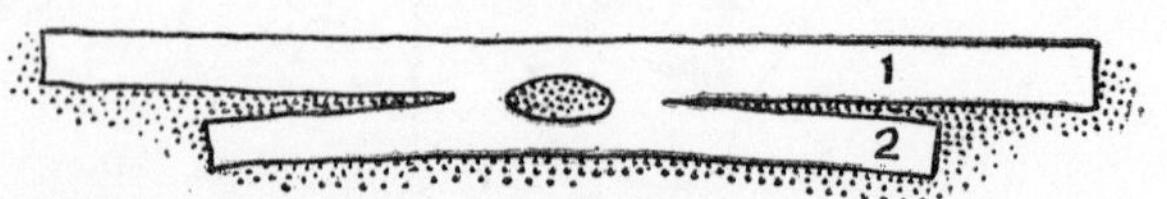

FIG. 130.—FOUR-TAILED BANDAGE FOR THE JAW.
(1) upper tails 40 inches long,
(2) lower tails 30 inches long.

elow the occiput and obliquely across the opposite side of the head to e pinned or stitched; the bandage finishes where it started at the point ndicated by an arrow (see fig. 132).

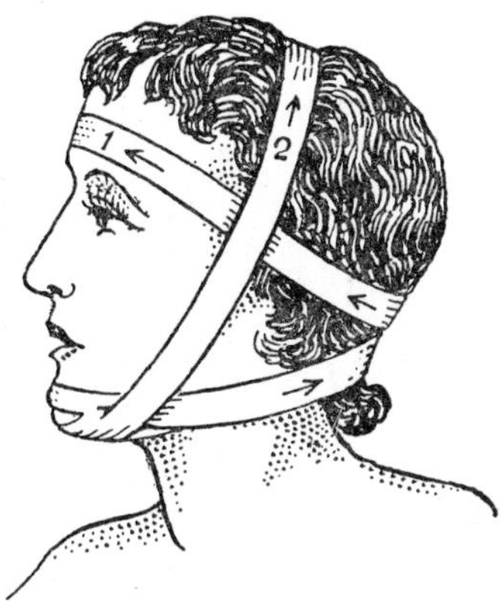

FIG. 131.—FOUR-TAILED JAW BANDAGE APPLIED.

When a *four-tailed bandage* is used to support the jaw, a piece of material ½ inches wide is chosen, cut as shown in fig. 130. The wide part is placed over the chin, the upper tails which are 40 inches long are taken round, below the ear, to the occiput where the ends are crossed and carried obliquely across the side of the head, to be fastened over the forehead in ront. The lower tails are carried up the side of the head and fastened on op, as indicated by arrow 2.

A bandage applied to support the arm in the case of an injured shoulder (fig. 133). The forearm lies across the front of the chest, a layer of wool being placed between the skin surfaces and a pad in the axilla of the injured side. The bandage is applied round the trunk and over the elbow ixing the arm to the side of the body.

The first turns are round the body and over the elbow in the direction indicated by arrow 1; having fixed the arm, the bandage is carried across the back of the chest, beneath axilla and over the shoulder of the opposite side as in 2, then across back of chest again, down to below elbow and up over the anterior aspect of the chest, and over the injured shoulder as arrow 3. As many turns as required to support the elbow, forearm and hand are employed and the bandage is finished in front as shown.

To **retain a dressing in one axilla and over the front of one breast** an application as in fig. 134 may be employed. The first turns are carried round the trunk in the direction shown by arrows 1 and 2, the third turn is taken slightly obliquely over the front of the chest, and on to the outer aspect of the arm; from here it is carried downwards round the arm and up as indicated by 3; this turn over breast and shoulder is repeated as often as necessary to cover any dressing on the upper part of the breast.

To **retain dressings on the side of the neck** a bandage as shown in fig. 135 may be used. The tail of the bandage (which would ordinarily

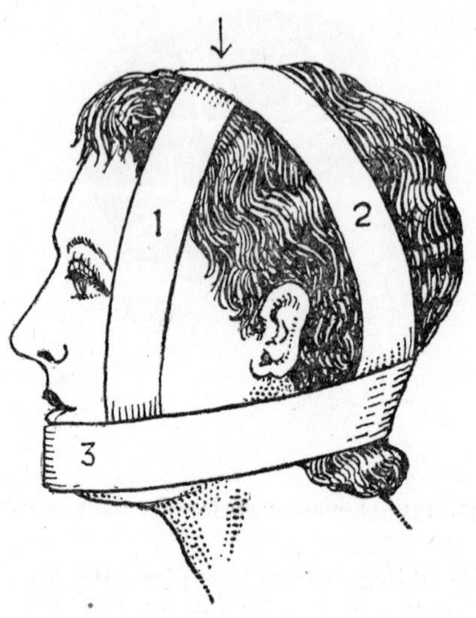

FIG. 132.—ROLLER BANDAGE TO SUPPORT JAW (LOOPED BANDAGE).

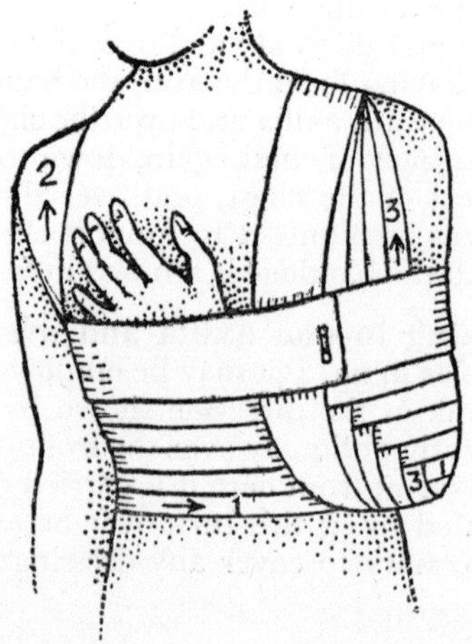

FIG. 133.—BANDAGE TO SUPPORT ARM IN A CASE OF INJURY TO THE SHOULDER.

be covered but has been left exposed to indicate its position) is indicated as letter A. From here the bandage is carried round the arm, in order to fix the end, as 1. It is next taken round the opposite side of the neck and under axilla as 2. The next three turns are taken round the neck in the form of a simple ascending spiral. The fifth turn, after passing beneath the

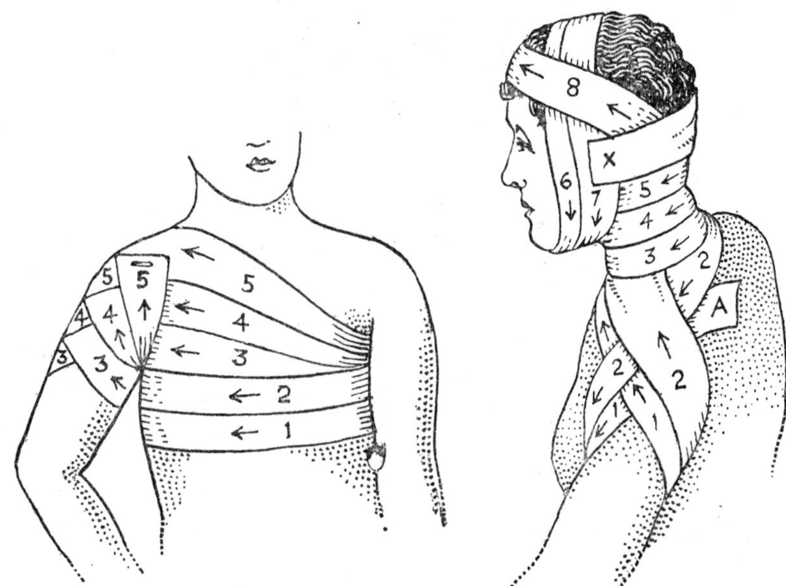

FIG. 134.—BANDAGE TO COVER DRESSING FOR BREAST AND AXILLA.

FIG. 135.—BANDAGE TO COVER A DRESSING ON THE SIDE OF THE NECK.

chin, is carried up on the opposite side of the face (in front of the ear), and down on the near side as 6—the seventh turn is a repetition of this except that it lies behind the ear on the opposite side so that the ear of the unaffected side is not covered by bandage. The seventh turn after passing beneath the chin is carried across the side of the head as shown in turn 8, and then round the head to be finished as X.

To **cover a dressing at the back of the neck** (see fig. 136), the bandage may be commenced from either side—in the illustration it is carried from right to left. Arrow 1 indicates a circular turn round the head, the next turn (2) is brought obliquely across the back of the head, carried beneath the chin, high on the neck, and round the opposite side to the front of the head again. Subsequent turns are made as indicated by figures and arrows.

A **bandage to retain a dressing on a stump** is arranged similarly to the well-known capeline used for the head. In fig. 137, the first turn is taken over the end of the stump as indicated by 1; subsequently the bandage is carried backwards and forwards as indicated by 2 and 3, and 4 and 5, until the stump is covered; circular turns are then carried up the limb for as far as necessary in order to prevent the bandage from slipping down. In a very restless patient it would be advisable to continue the bandage over the hip joint as an ascending spica for one or two turns.

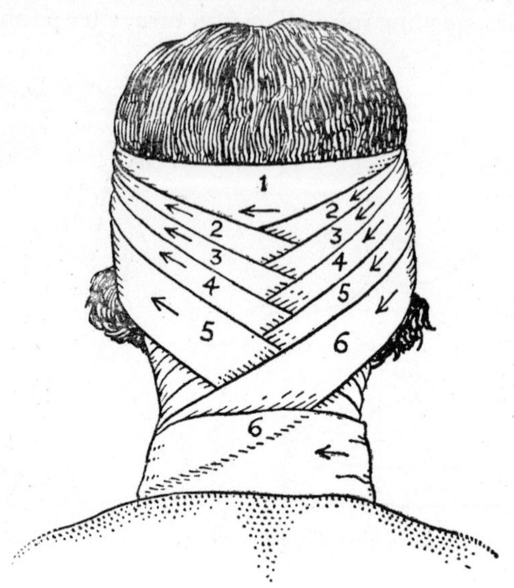

Fig. 136.—Bandage to Cover Dressing on Back of Neck.

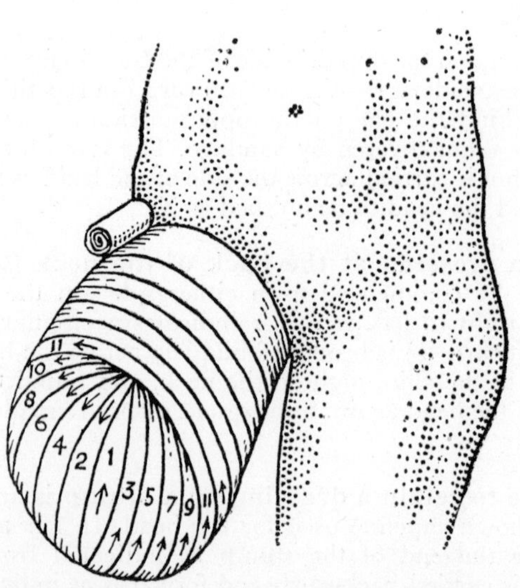

Fig. 137.—Bandage to Retain a Dressing on a Stump.

THE TRIANGULAR BANDAGE

The triangular bandage was first used by Professor Esmarch. It is readily improvised from a triangular scarf or piece of material. Unbleached calico is frequently used as it is cheap and strong. The bandage may be used whole as the *large arm sling*, or it may be folded broad to form the *small arm sling*, and folded narrow to form the *cravat bandage*. In one form or another the triangular bandage can be applied to practically every

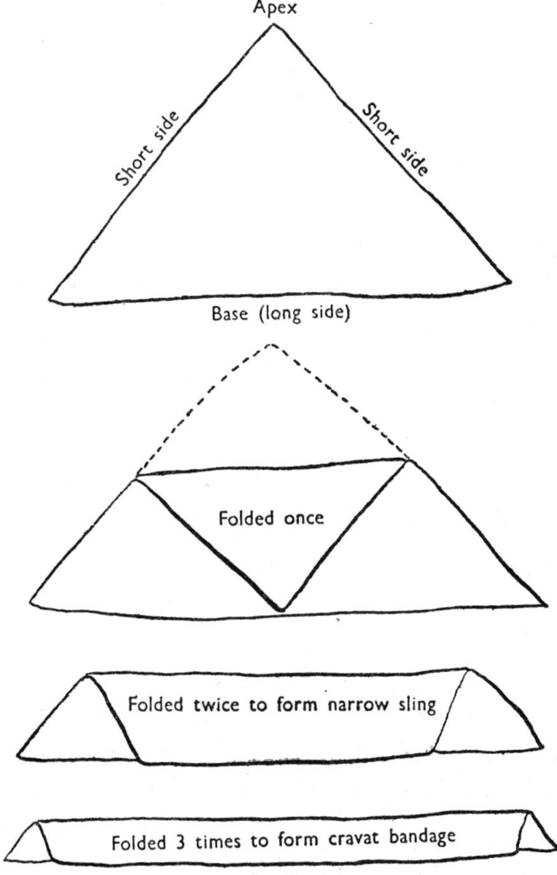

part of the body. The unfolded bandage is employed where it is desired to cover a fairly large area. The bandage folded broad is used to retain dressing in position and apply splints to different parts, and the narrow bandage or cravat sling is employed principally to tie splints together, to act as a fixing point for a wider bandage and as the cravat sling shown in fig. 140. Some examples of the use of the triangular bandage are appended.

Large arm sling (to support elbow). The unfolded bandage is placed over the front of the chest as in fig. 138; A, with the apex towards the injured side. The forearm is flexed and placed in front of the bandage which is then taken up over it. The two ends are tied in a reef knot and the apex is brought round and pinned to the bandage in front of the arm as in B.

The forearm must be supported and the hand as far as the knuckles. The hand must always be placed at a level slightly higher than the elbow.

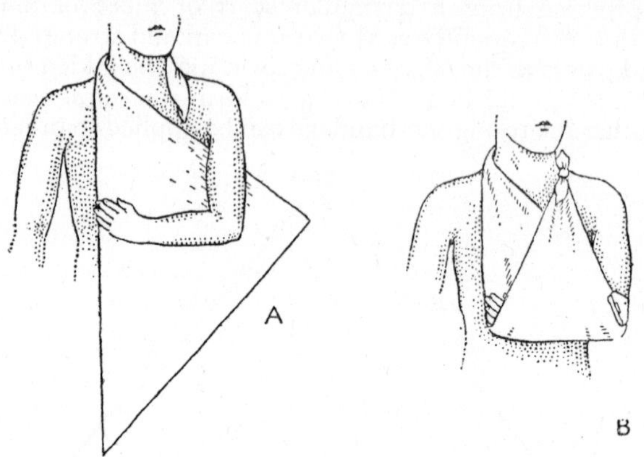

Fig. 138.—Large Arm Sling Applied to Support Elbow.

Small arm sling. The triangular bandage folded broad is used for this, it is applied as shown in fig. 139. It may be tied at either side of the neck, but the support obtained is firmer when tied on the unaffected side as shown.

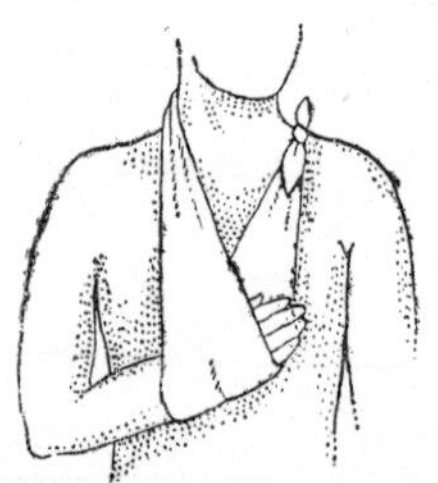

Fig. 139.—Small Arm Sling to Support Forearm.

Cravat sling. For this, the triangular bandage folded narrow is used. The bandage is placed round the neck with one long end crossed over

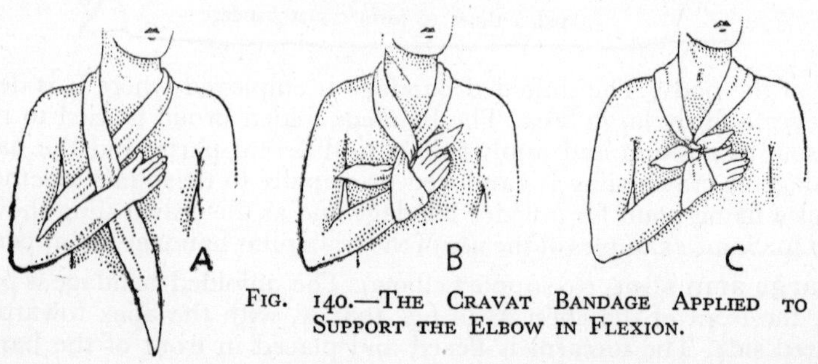

Fig. 140.—The Cravat Bandage Applied to Support the Elbow in Flexion.

ne short end as shown in A. The elbow is flexed. The long end of the andage is taken up in front of the wrist and passed behind the two olds as they lie crossed on the chest, this brings the two ends opposite ach other as in B. The two ends are then tied in a reef knot well down n to the wrist so that the patient is unable to withdraw his hand from he cuff. The completed bandage as shown in C is similar to the collar nd cuff retention brace; it is used to support the elbow in flexion.

Sling for support of elbow. The unfolded triangular bandage is placed n front of the chest (fig. 141), one end being taken up over the injured side nd the apex lying towards the unaffected side. The end that is hanging lown is then taken up over the forearm which lies across the chest with he fingers directed towards the opposite clavicle. The ends are tied at the ide of the neck as in B. The apex of the bandage is then carried up to the houlder of the injured side and when pinned to the bandage in front of the lavicle of this side as in C, it will be found that the whole forearm is upported from the elbow to the ulnar border of the hand and fingers.

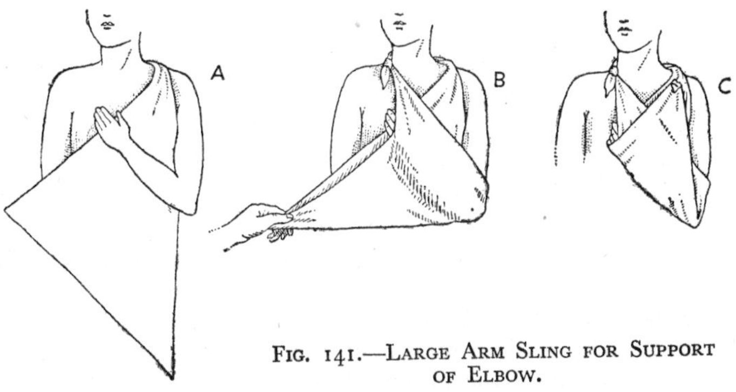

FIG. 141.—LARGE ARM SLING FOR SUPPORT OF ELBOW.

The St. John's sling (to support shoulder). This is used when the shoulder is injured and painful, properly applied it gives good support.

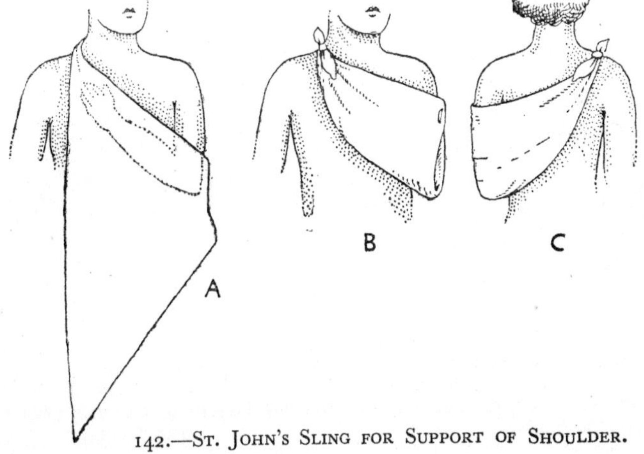

142.—ST. JOHN'S SLING FOR SUPPORT OF SHOULDER.

The arm of the injured side is flexed and an unfolded triangular bandage placed in front of it as in A (fig. 142). The elbow is supported and the base c the bandage is tucked beneath the forearm (between it and the front of th body), the free end of the bandage being carried across the back to mee the other end on the opposite shoulder. These ends are tied. The ape which lies beside the injured elbow may be placed and pinned in front c or behind the elbow, or turned in and pinned as shown in the illustratior

Triangular bandage for breast. By cutting an armhole as shown i fig. 142, and making small gussets as indicated by inverted arrows alon the base of the bandage, a triangular bandage can be used to retain :

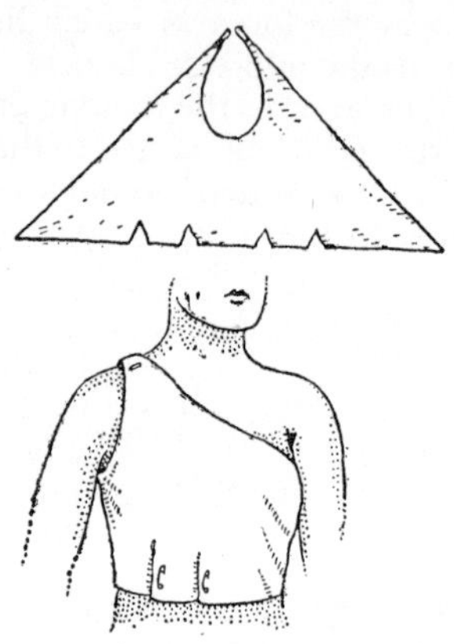

FIG. 143.—MODIFIED TRIANGULAR BANDAGE APPLIED TO RETAIN DRESSING ON THE BREAST

dressing on the breast in such cases as those who after radical mastectom may be undergoing radium treatment and require dressings to be com fortably retained during the period of reaction. The bandage is pinnec on the shoulder.

Barrel jaw bandage.

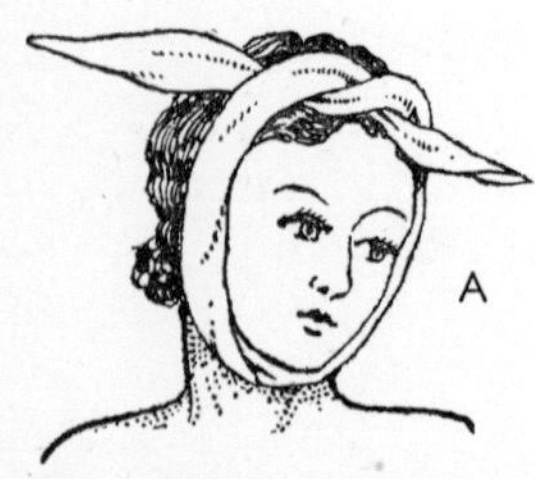

FIG. 144.—THE FOLDED BANDAGE IS TAKEN FROM BENEATH THE CHIN AND THE ENDS ARE CROSSED ON THE TOP OF THE HEAD AS SHOWN.

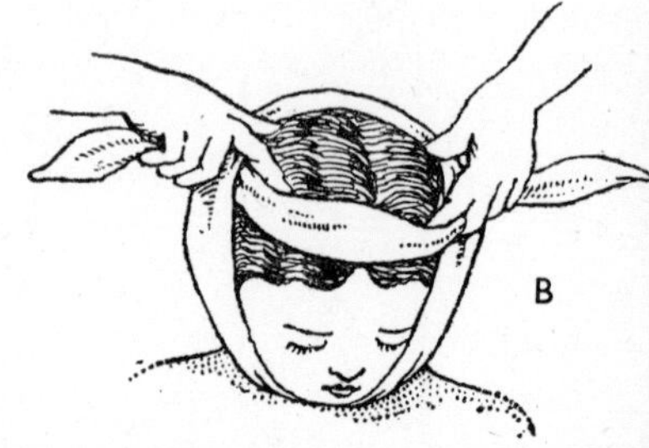

FIG. 145. THE ENDS ARE OPENED BY THE FINGERS AS SHOWN. ONE PASSES IN FRONT OF THE FOREHEAD AND THE OTHER BEHIND THE OCCIPUT.

Barrel jaw bandage. The barrel bandage may be applied by means of a strip of bandage material or by using a triangular bandage folded narrow, see below. See also figs. 144–145.

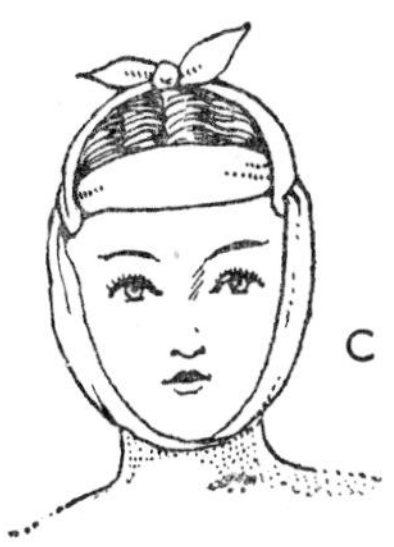

Fig. 146.—Traction is Made on the Ends until the Jaw is Firmly and comfortably Held by the bandage, the Ends are then Tied on Top of the Head.

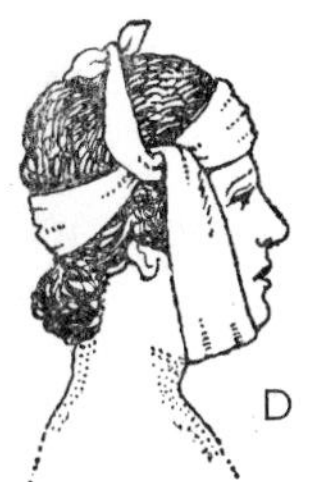

Fig. 147.—Side View of the Completed Barrel Bandage which is Easy to Apply and Comfortable to Wear.

Section 2

The Feeding of Adult Patients and Infants, Elementary Dietetics

Chapter 16

Food and Feeding of Adult Patients

Classification of foods—The use of proteins, carbohydrates and fats—The value of water to the body—The use of salts, vegetables and fruits, milk and eggs—The preparation of milk for invalid feeding—Serving food to patients—The administration of fluid diet—The balance of fluid in the body

That she may help in the proper feeding of a patient, it is necessary for a nurse to have some knowledge of the different classes of food and of their value to the body. The combustion of food in the body provides heat and energy and makes possible the growth of new tissue and repair of waste, and provides, moreover, the material which enables the various systems of the body to perform their different functions.

For a diet to be adequate it must contain proteins, fats and carbohydrates, water, salts and vitamins; and for it to be well balanced it must contain the first three in moderately definite proportions. The amount of protein and fat is small compared with the quantity of carbohydrate provided as suggested by most physiologists. The following table is an average one:

Proteins	80–100	grammes	320 C.
Fats	80–100	,,	720 C.
Carbohydrates	500	,,	2000 C.

The Calorie is the unit of heat, each Calorie represents the amount of heat required to increase the temperature of 1 litre of water 1° C.

Foods may be classified as *organic*, such as those obtained from animal and vegetable sources—proteins, fats and carbohydrates, each one containing different proportions of carbon, hydrogen and oxygen; and *inorganic* foods such as water and salts.

Protein is also described as nitrogenous food, as in addition to containing carbon, hydrogen and oxygen it contains nitrogen and also phosphorus and sulphur. The nitrogen in protein is composed of a series of amino-acids; some proteins contain all the important ones, and are described as *first class* or *complete*—examples are milk and meat; others contain fewer and are *second class* or *incomplete* proteins—examples of these include vegetable proteins, particularly those contained in peas, beans and lentils. This protein is called *legumin* and these substances are described as legumes, or pulses.

Reference to the table, given below, will show that protein food contains 4·1 Calories per gramme, but protein is not generally used for the production of heat and energy, and the amount contained in a well-balanced diet, is sufficient to repair the waste of the body tissue only. In certain diets, where carbohydrate and fat have to be restricted, protein is used in larger quantities in order to provide a source of heat and energy but, generally speaking, the loss of energy which is caused through the excretion of the waste products of protein is so considerable that it is commonly considered inadvisable to use protein for the production of heat. Protein moreover is more expensive than carbohydrate. It is estimated that:

1 gramme of protein	contains . .	4·1 C.
1 ,, ,, fat	,, . .	9·3 C.
1 ,, ,, carbohydrate	,, . .	4·1 C.

The amount of protein contained in various diets will be seen in those described as *high* and *low protein diets* in the table given on p. 276. A high protein diet contains about 120 grammes and a low protein diet 50 grammes.

Lean beef and mutton contain about 10 per cent protein. Fish is one of the most easily digested protein foods, and poultry comes next in regard to ease of digestion and assimilation, chicken being best because it is tender; duck or goose is not suitable for invalid diet as the flesh contains a good deal of fat.

Internals. The value of the internal organs of animals varies in usefulness, but *sweetbread* (the pancreas) and thymus are easily digested foods. *Tripe* is very easily digested provided it is boiled for a long time. *Tongue* is usually tender and can be used instead of lean meat as it has the same food value. *Heart*, *kidney* and *liver* are very dense in structure, and this renders them tough and difficult to digest; liver contains glycogen and cannot be used as meat when carbohydrate foods are restricted, but it is a particularly valuable article of diet in the treatment of severe anaemia.

The chief end-product of the internals of animals is uric acid, which is excreted in the urine—internals are, therefore, contraindicated in the treatment of gout and chronic rheumatism, as well as in fibrositis and other conditions where excess uric acid is excreted.

Carbohydrates. These include starches and sugars, which contain carbon, hydrogen and oxygen, and are mainly of vegetable origin and classified into three groups according to their complexity or simplicity:

Polysaccharides—animal starch, e.g. dextrose and glycogen.

Disaccharides—cane sugar, beet and milk sugar.

Monosaccharides—These are the simplest ones into which all others must be reduced before they can be made use of in the body—examples of these are glucose or dextrose, and fructose.

Carbohydrate foods provide heat and energy, and are reduced to glucose in the tissues and stored in the muscles and liver as glycogen; a great increase in the intake of carbohydrate would lead to storage of fat in the tissues. Starchy foods are also described as *farinaceous*. The main ones are true cereals, others are starch. Cereals are obtained from the grain of plants and the seeds of grasses, and include wheat grain, such as flour from which we make bread; semolina and macaroni are preparations of wheat. Oat grain is supplied from oatmeal, and barley is used as pea barley in thickening soups and broths, as barley water for invalid feedin and is a source from which malt is obtained in brewing beer. Rice con tains large quantities of starch and is a favourite milk pudding. Tapioc and arrowroot are preparations of starch obtained from the roots of plant

Fats. Fats, composed of fatty acid and glycerine, are mainly derive from animal sources, although some are vegetable. Fat is a fuel food but i is very difficult for the body to digest and assimilate it. Excess is stored a fat in the subcutaneous tissue around the kidneys and heart, and othe internal organs, and in the interstices of muscle tissue. The amount of fa varies in an average diet from 80 to 100 grammes, and if, for example, diet contains 100 grammes of fat and protein, 500 to 600 grammes of car bohydrate will be added to this; the proportion of fat to carbohydrate i therefore 1 to 5 or 6, but fat is sometimes added in considerable quantitie in the administration of special diets and the treatment of diseased con ditions.

For example—whenever a high Calorie diet is required, fat is the articl of diet added, in which case the choice of fats should be the more easil assimilated ones, such as milk fat, which is administered in wastin diseases such as pulmonary tuberculosis where as much fat as the patien can comfortably be persuaded to take is added to the diet.

Fat is added in very considerable quantities when a ketogenic diet i given; this diet is so named because the fat content is pushed far enough t produce a condition of ketosis. It was first utilized in America in th palliative treatment of cases of epilepsy, as it had been observed that per sons suffering from epilepsy who had accidentally developed ketosis wer free from fits during this period. It has more recently been adopted in thi country in order to produce a highly acid urine in the treatment of bacil luria due to the presence of *Bacillus coli*. In the condition of ketosis th alkalinity of the blood is slightly decreased and the urine becomes highl acid.

Water. Water is essential to the tissues of the body, about three to fou pints being supplied daily with an average diet—probably half thi quantity is taken in as drinks, water, lemonade, tea, etc., and the othe half is contained in the food eaten. For example, large quantities of wate are contained in all food, and some fruits and vegetables contain over 9 per cent of water. The bodily excretions eliminate 4 to 5 pints a day— from 40 to 50 ounces as urine, perhaps 1½ to 2 pints as sweat, in addition t moisture present in the expired air which is saturated with water vapour and the water present in faeces. It is an interesting fact that water doe not undergo any change in its passage through the body.

Water is required for the functional activity of all the organs, and fo the carrying out of all chemical processes in the body upon which lif depends. It is not possible to live many days without water. It helps in th regulation of the body temperature, particularly as the loss of heat, which forms part of this mechanism, is made possible by the evaporation o moisture from the surface of the body. By means of water the chemica agents are conveyed to and from the different parts of the body.

Water serves to dilute the substances taken in as food. These cannot be swallowed until they are comfortably moist; they cannot be acted upon by the different enzymes, responsible for changing them chemically, until they have been dissolved. Water is also essential for diluting the waste products of the body, and any poisonous products which may get into the body, and by so diluting them to render it possible for such waste products to be eliminated by the kidneys. It is in order further to dilute these products that water is liberally provided in the treatment of most febrile conditions when metabolism is rapid and the breakdown of tissue greater than normal.

The administration of increased fluid volume is indicated in all conditions of toxaemia; in most febrile conditions and when the rate of metabolism is increased; and where the administration of fluid acting as a diuretic will increase the urinary output; many cases of constipation may be relieved simply by the addition of water to the diet. In nursing sick patients many symptoms of discomfort may be obviated and others relieved, particularly those associated with a dirty mouth, thirst, constipation, insomnia, restlessness and delirium, by the administration of copious drinks of water and other watery drinks at regular frequent intervals.

Restriction of fluid. Fluid is restricted in conditions of oedema such as occurs in advanced cardiac and renal disease; in cases of high blood pressure accompanied by arteriosclerosis in which rupture of an artery may occur, and give rise perhaps to the condition of cerebral haemorrhage. In these instances fluid is restricted to 1–1½ pints a day. In the administration of a ketogenic diet, mentioned on p. 286, fluid is very carefully restricted, as little as from 8 to 15 ounces per day being allowed.

In the administration of diets in which fluid is restricted to a given amount, it is necessary to take into consideration the actual fluid value of certain foods, particularly fruits, as for example plums, apples and oranges, which contain almost their total weight in water, so that a large plum may be providing an ounce or two of fluid, and an apple three ounces.

In dilatation of the stomach, when the fluid accumulates in the distended organ, the amount given is carefully considered; it may be restricted, or a normal amount of fluid may be given, though this must be administered in small quantities at a time. In the dietetic treatment of obesity, the fluid intake is also graduated. In some persons a considerable amount of their excess in weight is due to fluid, and with these it is sometimes advisable to restrict fluids at meals, allowing them to be taken only between meals.

Salts and condiments. Salt is used to flavour food, but in addition it is essential if osmosis is to take place, since its presence regulates the concentration of fluid in the tissues. The presence of salt is necessary in the stomach for the secretion of hydrochloric acid. *Salt is restricted* in cases of oedema, as when fluid is retained in the tissues the administration of salt would result in a greater collection. It is also restricted in nephrosis and in all conditions where the function of the kidneys is disabled, because salt is eliminated by the kidneys, and its restriction therefore lessens the necessary work of these organs. Other common condiments include pepper, mustard, vinegar and spices, which are chiefly used for flavouring.

Vitamins are essential food factors which have definite physiological and also therapeutic value. A balanced diet must contain sufficient vitamins. These substances are classified into:

Water-soluble vitamins	B and C.
Fat-soluble vitamins	A, D, E and K.

Information as to the sources and special values of the different vitamins is contained in a chart in Appendix II, on p. 822, and some information on this subject is also included in the note on deficiency diseases on p. 433.

Vitamin therapy is possible today because of the many potent preparations of vitamins available such as halibut- and cod-liver oil, rose-hip syrup and black-currant purée. Synthetic preparations of some of the vitamins are also available, notably that of vitamin C or ascorbic acid.

The protective foods. The foods described as protective contain the essential vitamins, fats, first class protein, and salts including iron, phosphorus and calcium. In order to maintain good health definite amounts of these substances must be provided, daily, in the meals taken. The amounts vary according to the age of the individual and the type of work done. Children, women during pregnancy and whilst feeding their infants require more than other individuals. Protective foods are needed in larger quantities in the treatment of deficiency diseases (see p. 433).

Vegetables and fruits have very definite value as articles of diet. *Green vegetables*, such as cabbage and spinach, contain some valuable mineral salts, such as phosphorus and potash, and in spinach iron is present in considerable quantities. When cooked, most of the salts contained in green vegetables pass into the water and it is for this reason that good cooks use vegetable water for soup stock, etc., and whenever possible cook vegetables in very small quantities of liquid.

In addition, vegetables provide considerable bulk in the intestine, and are therefore valuable in the treatment of that form of constipation which is due to sluggish peristalsis, the bulk helping to stimulate the activity of the intestine. Vegetables would, however, be contraindicated in constipation due to spasm, as in these cases peristalsis is irritated and occurs irregularly, so that for this type of constipation a bland non-irritating diet is desirable. When eaten uncooked, green vegetables are valuable for their vitamin C content.

Root vegetables such as potatoes, carrots, parsnips, turnips, Jerusalem artichokes and beetroot contain starch in varying quantities. Potatoes provide the most prolific source of starch, and because of their starch content these vegetables have to be specially limited in the administration of a diet of low carbohydrate value, as in the treatment of diabetes and in obesity.

A potato is a good source of vitamin C which is contained immediately beneath the skin of it. It is for this reason that potato cream is advocated in the treatment of scurvy; this is made by carefully collecting the potato beneath the skin of one boiled in its jacket and mixing it to a creamy consistence with a little cool milk.

Fruits contain large quantities of water, very small quantities of carbohydrate and some cellulose, their natural sweetness being due to fruit sugar. Banana contains more carbohydrate than most other fruits and, in addition, a little protein. Some fruits contain more cellulose than others, examples of these are apples and lemons which are particularly useful as laxatives in the treatment of constipation. Lemons, oranges, grapefruit and tomatoes contain citric acid. Grapes contain tartaric acid. It is because of their acids that these foods are frequently made into drinks and used as mild diuretics.

Milk and eggs are so largely employed in the feeding of invalids that a note on their value may be useful to nurses. The value of milk as invalid food lies in the fact that in addition to the presence in it of all the foods mentioned in a well-balanced diet, these are present in the forms most easily assimilated by the body, and quite naturally so, since milk is intended for the young of man and animals. Each milk is specially suited to the young of the animal for which it is intended, and it is for this reason that cow's milk requires special treatment before it can be rendered suitable for the young baby.

The protein of cow's milk consists largely of caseinogen, which forms a heavy curd. For this reason it is citrated or diluted, and in some cases peptonized, when used for invalid feeding; and humanized when employed for baby feeding. The carbohydrate of milk being lactose is readily used by the body. Milk fat is almost an emulsion—it is separated in tiny globules, which being lighter than the fluid rise to the surface as cream. The mineral salts needed by the body are contained in milk, with the exception that cow's milk contains insufficient iron for baby body building. The vitamin content in milk depends upon the feeding of the cows; pasture-fed cattle yield milk rich in vitamins A and D, and some B and C are present but the two latter are rapidly destroyed when the milk is heated.

The uses of milk. Milk as a food makes the least demand on the digestive and excretory organs, and there are many ways of modifying it to increase its usefulness in invalid feeding. Most febrile cases can be given diluted milk, as a rule 5 ounces of fluid are given to such cases every 2 hours. The protein of milk is one most easily dealt with, and it provides the least possible amount of waste matter for elimination by the kidneys. Milk and water can therefore be given in most cases of acute nephritis and acute rheumatic fever.

Because of its nourishing properties milk is an excellent addition to the diet where the Calorie value is required to be high. An ounce of milk provides 20 Calories, so that the addition of one or two pints of milk to the diet is an excellent means of adding some 400–800 Calories in the treatment, for example, of patients who are convalescent after certain wasting diseases and acute illnesses.

THE PREPARATION OF MILK FOR INVALID FEEDING

Most of the methods used aim at reducing the density of the curd. The rennin present in the normal stomach curdles milk, but by *diluting* the milk with barley water or soda water, half and half, or in the proportion two-thirds of milk to one-third of water, or *citrating* the milk by the addition of 2–4 grains of potassium citrate to the ounce, the amount of this curd can be reduced.

Peptonizing is carried out whenever further action upon the curd is advisable, and is a process by means of which the protein in the milk is predigested. A Fairchild's peptonizing powder is added to 5 ounces of water and 1 pint of milk, and the mixture is then heated to 105° F., and kept at that temperature for 10–15 minutes. It is then either rapidly cooled by placing it on ice, or heated to 150° F. in order to stop the action of the peptonizing agent.

Separation of the curd of milk results in the preparation of *whey*. Whey contains fats, sugar, salts and the vitamins, in fact everything except the protein which is contained in the curd which has been separated. Whey is prepared by heating milk to 100° F. and adding one drachm of rennet (a preparation of rennin) to each pint, letting it stand in a cool place until set, and then stirring it with a fork to break up and separate the curd and draining the whey off through muslin. *Lemon whey* can be made by adding half an ounce of strained lemon juice to a pint of milk; *white wine whey* is made by adding a gill (4 ounces) of white sherry to a pint of milk. In both cases the curd is separated and the whey drained off through muslin.

Skimmed milk is used when the greater part of the fat is required to be removed, as in the treatment of some cases of jaundice where extreme nausea is a feature of the symptoms.

Lactic acid milk is made by adding 45 minims of lactic acid to a pint of milk and stirring it in very slowly drop by drop, in order to avoid curdling the milk. It is used in the treatment of marasmus babies, particularly when this condition is due to diarrhoea and vomiting.

Junket can be made by adding a drachm of rennet to a pint of milk as described in the preparation of whey, but it is served only when the milk is set. It may be coloured and flavoured. *Milk jelly* is prepared by adding a quarter of an ounce of leaf gelatine to each half-pint of milk. The gelatine is dissolved in a small quantity of milk and the mixture allowed to set in a cool place. Milk can be varied by the making of milk tea, coffee and Bovril, milk being used instead of water in the preparation of these beverages.

Eggs. The Calorie value of a hen's egg weighing 2 ounces is 80. Eggs are very valuable as an article of diet because they contain a quantity of useful protein—albumin—in the white of the egg. This is coagulated by heating, and is therefore most easily digested uncooked and may be given as *albumin water*. This is made by cutting the white of an egg in order to break up the membrane and mixing it with 5 to 10 ounces of cold water. It may be mixed with the same quantity of lemonade instead. Albuminized drinks should be strained through muslin, before they are served.

Egg drinks. Egg flip may be made with the whole egg, or only the white used. In both cases the white should be whipped until it is a stiff froth, and either milk, a mixture of milk and cream, cream and sherry, or milk and brandy may be added. The drink should be flavoured to taste.

The yolk of an egg contains a fairly large amount of fat which provides vitamins A and D, but the presence of lecithin and cholestrin renders it indigestible, and egg yolk as an article of diet is contraindicated in the treatment of conditions of the liver and gallbladder, in many cases of obesity and in all persons subject to biliousness.

POINTS TO BE CONSIDERED IN SERVING FOOD TO PATIENTS

Having considered the types of food available and the need of these, the conditions in which special types of food are indicated in some cases and contraindicated in others, the nurse should next realize that food must be properly cooked in order to render it digestible, and, although this may not be her duty, it is nevertheless within her province to see that the food is invitingly served. It is usually considered inadvisable to discuss food with patients except in so far as to consult their wishes and likes and dislikes with regard to it, in a purely general way, as soon as they have settled down in hospital.

The value of any one meal to a given person, whether healthy or ill, ay be assisted or retarded by the state of mind in which it is approached. 'o have to face a meal after fatigue, after hurry, anxiety and worry will il to give the maximum result. On the other hand, this will be best btained by a peaceful, contented, happy state of mind contributed to by heerful surroundings and if possible by congenial company. Care should e taken to avoid monotony in diet and, although this may not be alto- ether within the scope of a probationer in hospital, it is possible in many nstances to make little alterations. The night nurse, for example, might ary the arrangements for breakfast, so that a patient on full diet is not iven the same meal each day. Again, with regard to the evening meal, n many hospitals it is possible for the nurse to plan small dishes of jelly, ruit salad, etc., and so to do much to add to the variety of the diet and ive pleasure to her patients. If mince or shepherd's pie is served for upper it can be made more inviting, appetizing and palatable by the imple addition of small crisp pieces of toast. In the case of a patient on nilk diet, small variations can be made—a little fruit juice and sugar vill serve to make milk pudding more appetizing to some.

Punctuality in serving meals is important, and absolute regularity must e observed in the administration of fluid feedings and special diets. Most f these are given two-hourly or four-hourly, and unless one has been a atient on a special diet it is impossible to visualize the (possible) pleasure he thought of the next meal, however small, will give. The patient care- ully observes the time it is due, he watches his nurse leave the ward for the itchen and thinks he will get his diet next: if it does not come, he is disappointed, and perhaps by the time it arrives the pleasurable anticipa- tion has given place to painful, irritable anxiety—especially in the case of men—in which case the digestion of the meal may be seriously impaired. Patients with poor appetites and a distaste for food have to be gently persuaded to take it, yet they should never be forced. A little change of dish, an alternative diet if possible, or a simple measure such as taking the patient's plate away and rearranging the food upon it, may secure the eating of the food.

Preparation of the patient. The ward should be quiet and orderly, all unpleasant sights should be removed, any very seriously ill patients should have screens placed round their beds, no visitors should be per- mitted, in order that the patients may eat undisturbed and unobserved. However busy nurses may have been during the morning or evening, they should now concentrate on being happily engaged in the work of the moment—which is serving the patient's meal.

The preparation of the patient for his food is of the utmost importance, and he should be comfortably supported by pillows, his shoulders being protected from chill; if necessary a knee pillow should be inserted in order to prevent painful stretching of the hamstring muscles as the patient sits up or leans forward. The bedtable should be placed where it will be comfortable; if only a tray is used some provision must be made for adequate support in a place the patient can conveniently reach (see preparation of trays, below). The table napkin or diet cloth should be placed within reach of the patient, or if he is helpless it should be arranged for him. As far as possible a meal should not be given after a distressing treatment or painful dressing.

Preparation of tray and delivery at bedside. Trays must be daintily prepared and have clean traycloths, if these are used. The tray should be complete with all necessary articles placed in the most convenient position for the patient to reach, such as a drink, condiments, etc. The glass or cup containing the drink should never be so full that it can be spilled or is capable of splashing over as the patient makes a slight movement in bed. Small helpings should always be given and all food placed very neatly on the plate; the patient's wishes ought to be consulted as to whether he likes gravy with meat, sauce with fish and so on. Cold food should be served on a cold plate, and hot food on a really hot plate. Only one course is served at a time, and the soiled articles from the previous course should be removed before it is delivered. Hot water plates ought to be provided whenever there is a long distance to cover between kitchen and bedside and in cold weather and whenever patients are being nursed in the open air. The tray should be removed the moment the patient has finished, so that he can be made comfortable in bed and rest, and so fulfil the requirements necessary for perfect digestion of the meal.

Whenever a patient requires help with his food this must be generously given, without his feeling that he is being hurried in the slightest. If hot food requires to be cut up this should be done in the kitchen on a hot plate if possible, and not at the bedside where it will be getting cold during the process. When a helpless patient requires to be entirely fed with food and drink a diet cloth or table napkin should be tucked underneath his chin, over his personal clothing and bedclothes in case of accident. In giving a drink to a very helpless patient the head should be raised by the nurse placing her arm underneath the patient's pillow and elevating his head and shoulders; the drink is then put to the patient's lips and small mouthfuls given at a time. A patient can stem the flow from a feeder with a spout by putting his tongue against the opening in it; but this should not be necessary as if the nurse watches her patient carefully she will note when he has enough fluid in his mouth to be comfortable, and she will accordingly lower the utensil whilst he swallows. A patient should be allowed time to breathe between mouthfuls, as he cannot both breathe and swallow at the same time. Longer rest should be given at intervals in all cases, and most particularly when swallowing is difficult or painful and whenever dyspnoea is present.

Food chart. When a food chart is kept it is used to indicate the amount of food taken. A nurse should always report on the amount of food a patient has eaten. Whenever a tray is taken away from a patient's bedside the amount of food left should be observed and reported to the head nurse or ward sister.

Waste food. In large institutions any waste food is sold as pigwash, but pig owners object to the presence of eggshells, tea-leaves or fruit skins or stones, and other odd articles which sometimes find their way into this receptacle, including screwed-up bits of paper, empty tins, etc. It is part of the economy of the hospital to sell waste food as pigwash and it is, therefore, most definitely the duty of every nurse and probationer to see that the quality offered for sale is of a good order. In cases of infection all waste food has to be burnt. In some large hospitals for the treatment of pulmonary tuberculosis, waste food is sterilized and then given to pigs.

THE ADMINISTRATION OF FLUIDS

Patients are sometimes ordered fluids *ad libitum*. This does not mean the amount the patient wants but the greatest amount he can be persuaded to take by a good nurse who has an intelligent interest in the patient's welfare and knows what he ought to have. As in the administration of all special diets, regularity and promptness are most important. In such cases it is usual for the patients to be given a drink every two hours, in many cases five ounces will be given at a time, water being given in between each nourishing drink. In addition the nurse should be on the look-out for opportunities to give an extra drink at any time, as for example when a patient wakens from a short sleep or doze, after a little talking or after making his bed or performing some other treatment for him. The nurse must not consider her duty done when she has placed a feeder of drink on the patient's locker—she has also to see that he drinks it within a reasonable time.

A patient on fluid diet should have his mouth cleaned regularly, at intervals of either two or four hours, and usually before a nourishing drink is to be given. Whenever possible after a milky feeding has been administered a small drink of water should be given in order to prevent the milk from clinging to the patient's mouth as milk is a food which quickly decomposes, and becomes a very ready medium for the growth of organisms and so results in the formation of sordes and crusts on the teeth. Milk should always be given very slowly, as it is sometimes quite difficult for patients to digest even diluted milk.

For a patient on a nourishing fluid diet, a definite plan ought to be followed and, taking a case of lobar pneumonia on such a diet, the following table is useful, and the plan adopted is to give the patient 2 pints of milk and 1 pint of meat broth, in addition to 3 pints of water or other simple drink. In the following arrangement care should be taken to space the more nourishing articles of diet evenly throughout the day, and yet at the same time to avoid monotony:

6 a.m.	Milk 5 ounces, water 2 ounces, flavoured with tea. (The patient looks upon this as an early morning cup of tea.)
8 a.m.	Milk 5 ounces, water 2 ounces, flavoured with Horlick's or Ovaltine.
10 a.m.	Chicken broth or other light nourishing soup, 7 ounces.
12 noon.	Milk 5 ounces, and water 2 ounces, and if eggs are permitted a beaten egg is added to this, and it might be looked upon as lunch.
2 p.m.	Beef tea or light soup, 7 ounces.
4 p.m.	Milk 5 ounces, water 2 ounces, flavoured with tea or coffee (the afternoon drink).
6 p.m.	Chicken broth or other light nourishing soup, 7 ounces.
8 p.m.	Milk 5 ounces, and water 2 ounces, and if an egg is permitted the second egg might be given here; if not, the feeding might be flavoured with Ovaltine or Horlick's or, if Benger's food is permitted, this could be given and regarded as the evening meal.
10 p.m.	If the patient is not asleep, milk 5 ounces and water 2 ounces can be given.

By this arrangement, the patient has received 35 ounces of milk, and a pint of broth. The night nurse will give the patient probably five to ten ounces of milk during the night.

Water, lemonade or barley water should be near at hand and the nurse should make a rule of giving the patient three to four ounces of one or other of these drinks at the intervals between the feedings—say at 7, 9 and 11 a.m., and 1, 3 and 5 p.m., and so on. This will give eight drinks, totalling about 30 ounces, which is the minimum the patient should receive. By judicious management double this quantity can easily be given. Some care ought to be taken in order to avoid following a drink of milk by lemonade. Barley water or water should be employed after milk, and lemonade given after soup.

It is sometimes difficult for patients to swallow fluids and easier for them to take soft solids; in these cases some of the foods can be made into a cream or jellied. Any fluid may be jellied by adding a quarter of an ounce of leaf gelatine to every half-pint of liquid, and in this way lemonade, tea, Bovril, milk, beef tea, etc., can be given in the form of jelly. This method is particularly useful in cases of palatal paralysis which may complicate diphtheria, when the soft palate does not rise to close the posterior nares during the act of swallowing, and fluid is regurgitated down the nose. Most fluids can be frozen, and then when almost solid briskly whipped to the consistency of thick cream—given in this way they are comforting and soothing to patients with very sore throats and are particularly useful for children after tonsillectomy has been performed.

BALANCE OF FLUID IN THE BODY

Water accounts for about 65% of body weight. It is contained in the blood vessels as plasma (5%), in the tissue spaces as interstitial fluid (20%), and in the body cells, including the red blood cells as intracellular fluid (40%). The endothelium of the capillary walls and the cell walls permit fluid to permeate or pass from one part to another, the direction and the amount of fluid being determined by the amount of protein and salts contained in the various parts.

The intake and output of fluid. Water is derived from drinks and from water contained in all foods; even dry foods contain some water; it is also derived from the oxidation of proteins, fats and carbohydrates. The *average daily intake* is 2·5 litres. The *average daily loss* is estimated at from 250 to 500 c.c. in the expired air, about 500 c.c. from the skin apart from sweating which causes greater loss, and about 100 c.c. in the faeces which is increased in diarrhoea. The amount eliminated as urine depends on the fluid intake, on the amount lost in expired air and by the skin, but on an average the fluid lost in urine is about 1 to 1·25 litres. The amount of water in the body is kept fairly constant by increase in intake indicated by thirst, and by variations in the urinary output to balance changes in the water lost by the skin and lungs required to maintain a normal body temperature. The water intake and output is increased in the tropics and during physical exercise.

Dehydration. Pathological decrease in the body fluid causes disturbance of metabolism, circulation and renal function. Dehydration may be due to a primary loss of water as in vomiting, diarrhoea and excessive bleeding, or it may be due to a reduction in the salt content of the body but in many cases of dehydration water loss and salt loss are combined.

Dehydration also occurs when the vital reflex centres are depressed or disorganized as in grave states of septicaemia and toxaemia, in conditions of shock, collapse and prostration, and in some conditions of chemical toxaemia. In these circumstances the need of increased fluid intake is manifest, but at the same time the condition of the patient may be so low and so lacking in vitality that any fluid given by mouth will remain in the stomach, or if given by rectum will lie in the colon and not be absorbed, and therefore cannot reach the circulating fluids and so will not relieve the grave condition from which the patient is suffering. It is in such cases as these that the administration of fluid by the more direct routes such as the intravenous, subcutaneous and intraperitoneal methods is so important.

When a grave state of dehydration exists the patient looks like a shrivelled leaf, his skin is crinkled, his eyes are deeply sunken and his abdomen is boat-shaped.

Retention of fluid is the other extreme. It occurs in certain types of nephritis owing to the fall in the blood-plasma protein due to massive albuminuria. When the protein content of plasma falls below 4 per cent, the fluid cannot be attracted back again into the blood stream and oedema occurs. It is in order to relieve this condition that the high protein diet introduced by Epstein is employed in the treatment of chronic parenchymatous nephritis.

Congestive heart failure is another condition where fluid is retained in the tissues. In this case it is due to venous back pressure. Owing to increase of pressure in the veins, stagnation and retention occur. Fluid is retained in the tissues in considerable quantities before its presence can be detected by oedema. It increases the weight of the patient and could be discovered in this way. It could also be detected by decrease in the urinary output which is the first sign of decompensation in congestive heart disease. It is important therefore that a careful record of the intake of fluid and the urinary output should be kept.

Retention of salt in the tissues is another cause of fluid retention. The theory put forward is that salt retention attracts fluid in order to maintain the isotonic concentration. The cause of salt retention is not understood but it is a well-known fact that the condition is relieved by giving a salt-free diet.

Chapter 17

The Feeding of Infants

Composition of milk—The preparation of milk for infant feeding—Precautions in feeding—Weaning an infant

It is very unfortunate for an infant to be deprived of its own mother's milk. During the first month of a baby's life any artificial food must be much diluted, the best substitute being cow's milk suitably modified. Four to five weeks should be taken in which to reach the ideal dilution of equal parts of milk and water; but if the infant is very tiny, say one or two weeks old, it may take a little longer to reach this.

A baby needs 50 Calories per pound of body weight per day at first; after seven months it may be reduced to 45 Calories, and after 12 months to 40. He also needs 2½ ounces of fluid per day per pound of body weight. If therefore a tiny baby weighs 8 lb. and requires to be artificially fed, 20 ounces of fluid should be given and the food value of the feedings ought to be 400 Calories.

Composition of milk.

	Human milk		Cow's milk	
Protein	2%	(caseinogen 0·6% lactalbumin 1·4%)	4%	(caseinogen 3·4% lactalbumin 0·6%)
Fat	2·5%		3·5%	
Sugar	7%		4%	
Mineral Salts	·25%		·75%	
Vitamins				

The protein in cow's milk is largely casein, which makes great demands upon the infant's stomach as curd is formed by the action of rennin and hydrochloric acid on it. Lactalbumin, which forms the bulk of the protein of human milk, is not affected by rennin. Human milk is sterile. Cow's milk, when it is obtained from a reliable dairy, can be considered safe if it is "tuberculin tested", or "accredited"; but other cow's milk may contain dirt and a large percentage of organisms, particularly coliform and tubercle bacilli, and must be boiled for five minutes before use as by no other means can it be rendered safe for infant feeding. Some of the vitamin content is destroyed by boiling, but vitamin C can easily be added to the diet in the form of orange juice. The sugar in human milk is greater in quantity than in cow's milk; the form in both milks is lactose, but in adding sugar when cow's milk is humanized dextri-maltose or cane sugar is used—glucose is not advisable and lactose is thought to produce fermentation and cause sore buttocks. The fat present as cream is in fine globules in human milk, that of cow's milk being coarse and large by comparison.

To modify fresh cow's milk. As the average percentage of protein is 4%, fat 3·5% and sugar 4%, a simple method of modifying cow's milk

) approximate the composition of human milk would be as follows. Take ne pint cow's milk, add one ounce of sugar which increases the sugar y 5% raising the total content to 7%; add one ounce of dairy cream hich contains 33% fat and therefore adds 1·5% to the mixture, giving total of 3·5% so that the percentage now more nearly resembles that f human milk (see above).

The addition of one or two grains of sodium citrate to each ounce of he mixture will make the curds smaller and more digestible.

As the child grows older the strength of the mixture should be increased, o that after the fourth month the mixture will contain two parts of milk o one part of water, and when they reach the age of 18 months infants an take undiluted cow's milk.

Proprietary brands of dried and condensed milk are sometimes used for infant feed-ng. Dried milks represent the 12 per cent solids present in cow's milk— per cent each of fats, carbohydrates and proteins. To make a humanized nixture take 10 drachms of dried milk, 20 ounces of water, 1 ounce of ugar and 1 ounce of dairyman's cream.

Condensed milk is a preparation in which the water is partly evaporated. good example is Ideal milk which is fresh cow's milk superheated and wo-thirds of the water evaporated, nothing being added. This can be ised with advantage in dealing with very sick infants. To prepare a nodified unsweetened milk for a healthy infant take 4 ounces of the milk, 16 ounces of water and add 1 ounce of sugar and 1 of cream.

Calorific value. The Calorie value which should be allocated to a baby as already been mentioned. In order to determine whether food of the orrect calorific value is being administered, it is useful to know the Calorie alue of the substances used. Cow's milk contains 20 Calories per ounce, nd Ideal milk 49 Calories. Lactose and cane sugar are of equal value— 114 Calories per ounce; thick cream contains 112 Calories to the ounce; New Zealand cream is richer, containing 180 Calories.

Example: a baby weighing 8 pounds requires 50 Calories per pound— 400 Calories. He requires 2½ ounces of fluid per pound of body weight— 20 ounces. The milk mixture described as humanized milk contains 20 Calories to the ounce, 20 × 20 = 400. This is supplied as follows:

Cow's milk	10 ounces	= 200	Calories.
Water	10 ,,		
Dextri-maltose	1 ounce	= 108	,,
Cream	1 ,,	= 100	,,
		408	,,

Precautions in feeding. Warm the milk mixture before feeding to 100° F. by standing it in warm water for ten minutes; too hot feedings destroy the mucosa of the mouth and gullet, too cool feedings give rise to colic and diarrhoea. A cover should be used to retain the heat during feeding time. It is important to see that the hole in the teat is the right size—neither too large, which would deliver the feed too rapidly, nor too small, which would render the work of the infant too difficult. The ideal position for feeding a baby is on the nurse's lap with his head resting on her arm, adopting, as far as possible, the position of an infant feeding at the breast. In holding the bottle it should be tilted so that the feed is agai the neck of the bottle all the time, otherwise the baby may suck in ai After feeding the infant should be raised to bring up wind, and the placed warm and dry in his cot. Tiny babies require three-hourly feeding and larger ones who can take more at a time may be fed four-hourl Babies should be comfortable during their feeding and therefore wet an soiled napkins should be changed beforehand.

Feeding bottles should be rinsed in cold water, washed and boiled afte use, and they should be cleansed with a bottle brush and boiled and store in sterile water until they are needed. Teats should be cleaned with sal washed and boiled.

A *nurse ought to know whether a baby is thriving on the diet he is having, or no and the chief indications of this are:*

(1) *Weight*, whether stationary or decreasing—both are unsatisfactory too rapid increase in weight is also unsatisfactory—what is required is regular gradual increase. An infant should double his birth weight in or 6 months, and then gain at the rate of 1 lb. per month during the nex 6, and weigh 28 pounds at the end of 2 years. (See accompanying weigh chart, fig. 148.)

If the weight appears unsatisfactory, a test feed is useful in breast-fe infants and, in order to determine the amount taken, the infant is weighe before and after the feed in exactly the same clothing.

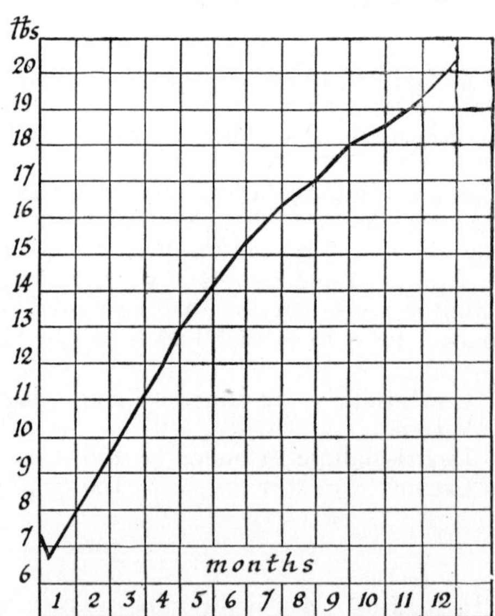

FIG. 148. WEIGHT CHART OF A NORMAL INFANT.

(2) *Vomiting* may indicate inability to digest the feeding, in which cas it should be further diluted and then gradually increased again. Or vomit-ing may be merely regurgitation or posseting, which may be due to a too rapid taking of the feed, to too large feedings, or to injudicious handling of the infant after feeding.

(3) *Condition of stools*. An infant may have diarrhoea or constipation, and the latter usually indicates underfeeding, particularly when combined with failure to gain weight. Overfeeding usually gives rise to colicky pain, the child screaming and drawing up its legs immediately after feeding; stools may be unduly large, or peristalsis may be rapid giving rise to green frequent stools. The stools should always be observed for the presence of undigested food—curds, fat, and any other abnormalities.

(4) *Crying* usually indicates abdominal discomfort. It may be due to hunger caused by underfeeding, to abdominal distension resulting from overfeeding, to constipation, or to discomfort caused by being cold and wet or overheated by too many clothes.

Wasting, or *marasmus* (athrepsia), is often brought about by injudicious feeding over a long period; the infant becomes wasted and dehydrated, with sunken eyes, dried skin, and flattened abdomen (the shape of a soup plate)—all symptoms which markedly demonstrate loss of body fluid. By the time the infant is in this condition he has lost all ability to take or to digest any food except the most dilute, and what he is able to take is quite insufficient for growth at a normal rate. This most serious condition accompanied by severe toxaemia and fever renders the infant acutely ill. In this state he is unable to resist even the mildest infection he may meet.

In the treatment of such a marked degree of wasting the food of this infant must be increased as rapidly as possible in order to supply the necessary protein for body building, and it is in such cases as these that lactic acid is so often used, seeing that it is of value in compensating for the low hydrochloric content present in the gastric juice of weakly babies. (For the mode of preparation of lactic acid milk, see p. 264.)

WEANING AN INFANT

The developing child requires some hard object to bite on at six months; a month or two later he may be given a crust or a piece of hard apple so that he can learn to masticate, but care must be taken to see that he does not bite off and swallow large pieces—these should be taken out of his mouth. At 8–9 months of age one feeding at about midday can be substituted by a small meal of some cooked cereal and milk, or bread and milk. A few days later a second meal may be added, the cereal meal being given at a time corresponding to breakfast and the midday meal to consist of mashed potato or breadcrumbs and the red gravy of meat, followed by a very small quantity of steamed custard and a little fruit juice. Still later, a cereal evening meal may be added.

In all baby feeding regularity is most essential, and by the time the infant is 12 months old he should be having three meals a day—breakfast 8 a.m., dinner 12.30 and tea 4.30. One to one and a half pints of milk a day should be given in addition, and this should be taken as a drink at breakfast and tea, and a cupful should be given before going to bed at 6.30. No food is to be permitted between meals.

The foods most suitable at this age may be taken from the following list. It will be noticed that very sweet foods such as jams, jellies and cakes are not included, and these should be avoided until the child is about 2 years; cooked meat other than mince should not be given until the child is over 18 months. Pastries, condiments and cheese must be avoided.

Cereals. Toast, bread (a little), toast fried in bacon fat, rusks an porridge.

Fats. Butter and dripping in fairly liberal quantities.

Meat foods. Eggs, lightly boiled, poached or scrambled (not fried). Vege table soups and chicken broth, Irish stew, minced freshly cooke beef and mutton, steamed fish and boiled chicken.

Vegetables. Boiled mashed potatoes, carrots and turnips. Cabbage an cauliflower, vegetable marrow and spinach.

Puddings. Milk puddings, steamed custard and boiled suet pudding Cooked apple, the pulp of cooked plums and prunes.

Fruits. Raw apple, minced unless the child will masticate thoroughly. Orange juice, and skinned and stoned grapes.

It is very important to teach the child to eat deliberately and not hurriedly to masticate thoroughly and not to swallow until quite ready. Drink shoul be taken between mouthfuls only.

Between the age of 18 months and 2 years the child ought to be taugh to speak correctly, to walk, to control and regulate micturition, to hav regular habits of bowel evacuation, to wash his hands before eating an to clean his teeth.

He requires regular meals and regular sleep. A child of this age usuall wakens about 6 a.m.; he should immediately empty his bladder, and ma have a drink of water or milk and water; he must remain in bed withou disturbing other people until 7.15, but he may have a toy to play with or book to turn over the pages. At 7.15 he will be washed and dressed ready fo breakfast at 8 o'clock. After breakfast he should immediately have an actio of the bowels before play or other interest can be entertained. He may pla and be amused until 10.30 when he should be put to rest in his perambulato in the open air. He will sleep for an hour or more, but he may not get u until 12 noon, when he should empty his bladder, be washed and prepare for dinner at 12.30.

Dinner should take nearly an hour, and he must sit quietly until 2 o'cloc when he may be taken out in his perambulator until 4 o'clock. Tea is at 4.3 and after tea he may play or be amused until 6 o'clock, but this play shoul not consist of excited romping or he will be kept awake. At 6 o'clock he bathed and prepared for bed; he may have a cup of milk, cocoa or brot and a finger or two of toast or a biscuit with it. He should be lifted t pass urine about 9.30—this ought to prevent his being disturbed durin the night, and he should sleep all night.

After 18 months, tea may be made a little more interesting by th addition of jam, but pips should not be allowed, and one piece of plai cake may be given. Sweets should not be eaten between meals, but on or two sweets may be added to the midday meal.

Chapter 18

Elementary Dietetics

Diet in diabetes, nephritis, cardiac conditions, gout and rheumatism, malnutrition, obesity, peptic ulcer, hypochlorhydria and hyperchlorhydria, jaundice, anaemia, constipation and colitis—High and low Calorie diets—Calcium and iron diets—Ketogenic diet—Diet in deficiency diseases (see also Vitamin Chart, Appendix II) —Diet in coeliac disease

DIABETES MELLITUS

Diabetes mellitus is a constitutional disease in which carbohydrate metabolism is defective. The islets of Langerhans are disordered so that the internal secretion of the pancreas is diminished, the glycogenic function of the liver is disorganized so that sugar cannot be stored, and the percentage of blood sugar is higher than normal. In order to remove this sugar from the blood large quantities of sugar-laden urine are excreted and the tissues of the body are thus deprived of fat, owing to the very rapid combustion that takes place.

The *chief symptoms* are wasting and hunger, thirst, glycosuria, polyuria, and the presence of acetone and ketone bodies in the urine. The danger of diabetes is coma, which is brought about by the retention of acetone and ketone bodies in the tissues.

The dietetic treatment of diabetes is divided into three parts:

(1) A period of preliminary starvation; during this time the pancreas is at rest, glycosuria is relieved and the blood sugar decreased to normal.

(2) A period lasting about 2 weeks follows in which the amount of diet is slightly increased, the effect on the blood sugar content noted, and the urine tested for sugar.

(3) A final period, during which the amount of diet is increased to supply the needs of the body, and insulin is added if necessary.

Formerly the limited amount of diet a diabetic patient could take was the difficulty experienced in treating this condition. Then followed the discovery of insulin and its effect on the treatment, which enabled more sugar and starch to be taken so that a patient could have the amount of food he required in order to carry out his work and live a comparatively normal life, but at first the difficulty of giving a sufficiently varied diet was experienced, and it was partly to meet this difficulty and also to help patients plan their own diets that the Line Ration Scheme was introduced by Dr. Lawrence. This scheme is largely used by patients who are treated in their own homes, and it is also in use in many hospital and nursing home units.

At the present time, when the services of specially trained dietitians are available in hospitals and elsewhere, it is becoming increasingly the practice for the physician to prescribe the diet in grammes of carbohydrate, protein and fat. He may, for example, prescribe 105 grammes of carbohydrate, and 70 each of protein and fat. The dietitian prepares the meals, if the patient is not having insulin the nurse will give the amount of carbohydrate prescribed, evenly, at each of the four meals of the day. When the patient is having insulin, she will concentrate the amount of carbohydrate pre scribed into the two main meals before which insulin is given.

The object of treatment is to provide a diet of sufficient Calorie valu to supply the needs and maintain the weight of the body and permit th patient to carry on his usual mode of life without increase of the bloo sugar beyond the normal limits of 0·09–0·12, or the reappearance of suga in the urine.

NEPHRITIS

Acute nephritis due to bacterial infection necessitates complete res for the kidney. In these cases the urine will be found to contain blood and will probably be very much diminished in quantity.

In the dietetic treatment the minimum of protein will be given and fluid will be limited to 2 pints in 24 hours until the urine contains less blood an albumin, showing that the disease is abating and the degree of inflam mation of the kidney becoming less severe. Some physicians eliminate al protein, including milk protein, for the first 10 days, giving only glucos up to half a pound a day, in lemonade or barley water. Other physician give a pint of milk and a pint of water during the 24 hours so that th patient is receiving a little protein.

The amount of fluid is increased as the condition becomes less acute and after 2 or 3 weeks 2 pints of milk and 1 pint of water may be taken Later, such things as Benger's food and arrowroot, milk pudding an bread and butter, may be added to the diet; but protein, particularly mea protein, and salt and condiments should be omitted until convalescence i thoroughly well-established.

Chronic nephritis is divided into two main types, in one of which known as *chronic parenchymatous nephritis*, the main substance, that is th tubules of the kidney, is involved. The kidney is large and pale and th patient also is swollen and pale because he is anaemic and his muscles ar flabby and oedema is present. His urine contains large quantities of albu min which represent heavy loss of protein to the body.

Treatment. In the dietetic treatment of this form, the loss of protein ha to be made good, so that a high protein diet is administered—an exampl of this diet is given below. The protein used should include eggs and fish and meat. Fat should be limited as the body tissues deprived of protein find it difficult to use fat, and ketosis may develop. Because of the oedema fluids should be restricted to 35–40 ounces a day. In some cases of oedema salt is omitted or limited.

A high protein diet contains from 100 to 120 grammes of first-class protein; some second-class protein may also be given, though this is not invariably included.

The following is an example of the type of meals a patient may have when on this diet:

Breakfast. One or two eggs or 4 ounces of fish with bread (unlimited) and butter. Tea with milk and sugar.

Dinner. Lentil soup or soup made with milk. Meat 4 ounces or fish 6 ounces. Vegetables (peas, beans and lentils contain protein but it may not be possible to give this type of vegetable every day as it renders the diet monotonous). Milk pudding or egg custard.

Tea. One egg, or some cheese or meat sandwiches may be given (it is usual to give 1 ounce of minced meat or chicken in sandwich form). Tea with milk and sugar, bread (unlimited) and butter.

Supper. Meat or fish as at dinner, bread (unlimited) and butter, milk pudding or a drink of milk.

Chronic interstitial nephritis. In this condition the interstitial tissue rather than the tubules of the kidney is affected. The kidneys are small and red in character. This disease is associated with arteriosclerosis and hypertension and high blood pressure. The patient may be passing large quantities of pale urine because the kidneys fail to concentrate, and it may contain only a trace of albumin. On examination of the blood the urea content is markedly high, as the urinary waste products are being retained to a very injurious extent. Uraemia frequently complicates this type of chronic nephritis.

The *treatment* consists of a low protein diet, in order to lessen the retention of urinary waste products in the blood. Apart from this the patient should lead an easy uneventful life as described in the treatment of high blood pressure.

A low protein diet contains less than 60 grammes of protein. The meals a patient may have when on this diet are indicated in the following example:

Breakfast. Fruit and one or two slices of bread and butter. Tea with milk and sugar.

Dinner. A little chicken or fish soup. A moderate amount of protein—2 or 3 ounces of fish, two vegetables, such as potatoes and green cabbage. Stewed fruit or fruit salad, or cornflour mould made with fruit juice, or a cereal such as tapioca cooked in fruit juice (not in milk).

Tea. A little bread and butter, salad or jam. Tea, with milk and sugar.

Supper. Salad and fruit and bread and butter with lemonade and glucose to drink.

Bread is limited in a low protein diet as it contains considerable protein. Preparations of fat-soluble vitamins A and D may be required as the patient is having little fat because he is deprived of red meat and eggs.

DIET IN CARDIAC CONDITIONS

In all cases of *acute heart disease* a low diet, usually milk only, is adopted. In *chronic heart disease* a comparatively low and easily digested diet is given. The meals chosen should be small in quantity and given at frequent intervals of 2 or 3 hours. Such articles of diet as milk, easily digested proteins such as fish, and very well cooked farinaceous foods are employed. It is advisable for the diet to be fairly dry, fluids being given between rather than with meals, as one of the main principles of treatment is to avoid distension of the stomach, because its proximity to the heart would give rise to indigestion, palpitation and cardiac embarrassment.

Stimulating fluids such as tea, coffee and alcohol should as far as possible be avoided, but a small cup of weak tea may be given on awakening in the morning as it relieves nausea and the same may be taken after th early afternoon nap.

When oedema is present in heart disease fluids are restricted and salt i restricted or eliminated from the diet.

Hyperpiesis. By this term high blood pressure is understood, and i the middle-aged this is most commonly associated with arteriosclerosi

Treatment. In hyperpiesis the nutrition must be maintained, and there fore drastic lowering of the diet is not indicated. As a rule red meat pro teins are limited to once a week, fish and chicken being taken on othe days. In middle age there is a tendency to obesity, and as cases of hig blood pressure will be taught to lead a quiet moderately uneventful lif they may tend to become fat; this is to be avoided, and therefore carbo hydrates should be moderately restricted to this end. Stimulants whic may increase the rate of the circulation are inadvisable; alcohol shoul not be taken and tea and coffee only in strict moderation; if the patien can be persuaded to accept the restriction, and the deprivation is not to seriously felt, such beverages should be limited to a cup of weak chin tea twice a day.

The patient should be advised to lead a very even life and go to be early and rise as late as possible; a day in bed a week is very advisable and if the patient has a tendency to obesity the day in bed a week may b a day spent on orange juice only. Life should be as free as possible fron worry and anxiety.

The dietetic treatment and the general mode of life, advised above fo cases of hyperpiesis, can be applied to cases of *arteriosclerosis* and *aneurysr of the large vessels.*

DIET IN GOUT AND RHEUMATISM

The diet which is described as *purin-free*, is frequently advised in cases o gout and chronic rheumatism. The internals of animals contain comple purin substances known as nucleo-proteins. The vegetables classed togethe as legumes—peas, beans and lentils—and other vegetables, including asparagus and onions, contain vegetable purins and are included in th foods contraindicated in gout and rheumatism. Foods which can be freel used and considered purin-free include eggs, milk, milk products, cerea foods, cabbage, lettuce and cauliflower; potatoes can be used in moderatior as these contain only very small quantities of vegetable purin.

In **acute rheumatism** diluted milk is the main diet, especially while the temperature is high. Lemonade and barley water can be given freely as the fluid intake ought to be increased because perspiration is very marked in these cases, and the loss of fluid requires to be made good. When the acute febrile stage is over chicken broth and milk foods may be added to the diet.

In **chronic rheumatism, myositis and fibrositis,** the diet should be purin-free, and only those foods mentioned above should be used. Rich fat food should be avoided, particularly pastry, fat fish such as herring, salmon and sardine, highly spiced foods and prepared sauces and stimulants.

MALNUTRITION

Generally speaking malnutrition is associated with loss of weight, and ith this factor digestive disorders are a very primary cause. *Absence of ppetite* will cause loss of weight and a nurse may help a physician in nding out whether there is definite disinclination and lack of desire for od, or whether the small amount the patient is taking is due to his avoidg food for fear of painful or unpleasant consequences. The former is true ck of appetite, in the latter case appetite may be normal.

Disease of the stomach and intestine (see peptic ulcer diet) and disease of e colon are very usual causes of loss of weight. The possession of *too few eth* would make digestion unsatisfactory and so give rise to loss of weight. *septic focus* somewhere in the body may, by absorption of toxins from this cus give cause to toxaemia and result in loss of weight. The *fear of getting t* may become an obsession, even in quite young people, while in others eir profession may demand the acquisition of a slim figure. Such sychological factors in regard to wasting and malnutrition cannot be easonably overlooked today.

In taking the history of a patient suffering from malnutrition, habits of fe should be investigated, particularly with regard to the amount of od taken and the amount of fluid, the regularity as to times of meals and e time allowed for meals, the times for retiring and rising, the amount f physical exercise taken during work and play, the amount of rest vailable and of sleep obtained, and whether sleep is continuous or terrupted. The regularity of bowel action and the action of the skin nd kidneys should also be carefully considered.

An acute febrile condition is associated with loss of weight, but this veight will usually be replaced during convalescence. The so-called wastng diseases, including tuberculosis, demand a diet of high Calorie value. n exophthalmic goitre the patient may have a normal appetite and eat vell, and yet lose weight owing to the increased rate at which metabolism s being carried out.

The *treatment of malnutrition* depends entirely on the cause. A nurse may e able to assist by tempting the appetite, and the rules for feeding a atient (on p. 264) may suggest how she can make his food appetizing nd the diet varied. Whenever a diet of high Calorie value is to be given, nilk, cream and butter should be added as far as the appetite and good vill of the patient will permit. Mealtimes should be free from worry and nxiety. A rest period of thirty minutes during which the patient lies on is bed totally unoccupied and relaxed should precede each meal, and a est of an hour and a half or two hours should follow the two main meals f the day.

OBESITY (see also p. 441).

Many persons who consider themselves overweight take to injudicious limming, with consequent harm to the body, and it is therefore advisable or every woman who is in the nursing profession, even in the capacity of nurse student, to realize the fundamental factors upon which the diet f obesity may be undertaken with comparative safety and without harm o the subject; and to realize further that in the majority of cases it is nadvisable to limit the diet to any extent except under the direct observation of a medical practitioner—and particularly is this so in th case of women over forty.

The *principles governing the dietetic treatment of obesity are:*

(1) The provision of a diet of low Calorie value in order to reduce th weight—carbohydrates therefore should be restricted.

(2) To incorporate into that diet sufficient food to satisfy the appetit prevent hunger and supply roughage sufficiently for the avoidance o constipation.

(3) The provision of the necessary *minimum but adequate amount of prote* (at least 3 ounces), and the administration of *sufficient fat* to act as a lubr cant and provide enough of the vitamins A and D, and the provision o *sufficient carbohydrate* to avoid the production of ketosis.

(4) Sufficient fluid should be taken to avoid thirst, but it should b given between and not with meals.

(5) Adequate exercise ought to be undertaken.

The *rate of loss of weight* will depend on the intake in food and the ou put in work and energy. If, for example, a working woman, considerabl overweight, desires to reduce, she might safely do this on an intake o 1,500 to 1,700 Calories instead of the normal one of over 2,000 and i such a case might expect to lose about 2 pounds per week. This rate of lo would be considered safe; more rapid loss, say at the rate of 3 pounds week, could be maintained by a patient on less diet, spending most of he time resting, but for the former a rate of loss of 2 pounds per week woul be all that should be attempted.

A patient being allowed about 1,500 Calories might have a diet simila to the following examples of meals:

Breakfast. Tea, with milk but no sugar. Two Vita Wheat biscuits. On boiled egg or a little grilled fish and a little butter (about ounce).

At 11 *a.m.* In order to give something to satisfy the patient and preven his desiring to eat too large a meal at midday an apple may b given.

Dinner. Two ounces of meat, or 4 ounces of fish. A large helping o green vegetables and a second vegetable, either parsnips, harico beans, peas or lentils. Salad, fresh fruit, stewed fruit (sweetene with saccharine).

Tea. Tea with milk but no sugar. Two Vita Wheat biscuits and ounce of butter and some salad.

Supper. Two ounces of lean ham, or 3 ounces of fish or som cheese. Two Vita Wheat biscuits. Salad, fresh fruit and lemonad sweetened with saccharine.

As a rule 3 pints of fluid should be taken in the 24 hours including glass of hot water on rising and going to bed.

Limitation of fluid intake and of salt is advocated when there is retentio of water in the tissues.

PEPTIC ULCER (see also p. 380).

Both gastric and duodenal ulcers are included under this heading a an ulcer usually occurs on the parts exposed to the irritation of gastri juice.

The **symptoms of peptic ulcer** vary slightly according to its position, and as a general rule the patient will complain of indigestion, which may be continuous or recurrent, while the pain varies with the site of the ulcer. In the *duodenal type* it comes on at a fairly long interval after a meal and is relieved by taking food or alkalis. In *gastric ulcer* the pain is more in the middle line, comes on a short time after a meal, and is relieved by vomiting and also by the administration of an alkali and bismuth.

The **dietetic treatment** of gastric and duodenal ulcer is very similar, and in practically no other condition does dietetic treatment occupy such an important position. It is essential therefore that nurses in charge of these cases should have a clear knowledge of the principles governing this mode of treatment.

(1) The diet should be *bland* and *non-irritating*, and it should not stimulate the flow of gastric juice, because, as already mentioned, this acid fluid acts as an irritant to the ulcerated area and so prevents healing. The principles applied, therefore, must be those of rest in all its phases, particularly as regards the physiological chemical activity and the mechanical movements of the organ in order to reduce the work and so rest the diseased part.

(2) The *amount of food given must be small* in quantity and the intervals between feedings should be very short so that there is no intervening time for the accumulation of gastric juice.

(3) The *protein used* should be one that is easily combined with the hydrochloric acid, so that the acid content of the stomach is readily fixed by it. For this purpose milk protein is advised by Dr. Lenhartz.

(4) The *fat content* of the diet should be high, because fat acts as a deterrent to gastric movement, and so helps to allay spasm.

(5) Whenever the dietetic treatment has to be sustained over a considerable time, it is important to ensure a *good calcium content* and an *adequate vitamin supply* and the Calorie value of the diet should be reasonably high. To supply vitamin C, which is invariably lacking in this diet, strained orange juice may be given.

Lastly, many of the peptic ulcer dietaries employed to-day are modifications of two very well-known ones briefly described below—Lenhartz and Sippy. (For Meulengracht's diet, see p. 384.)

The Lenhartz Diet. This was first introduced in 1904 and has been modified since. The principles already given in the preceding pages are employed in the administration of this method. Dr. Lenhartz used *egg protein.* The regime began by giving one egg per day, increasing by half an egg per day until at the end of a week four eggs are being given. Later, the eggs are reduced as fish is added to the diet.

At the outset 3 ounces of *milk* are given on the first day, to be increased by 1½ ounces per day until the patient is having about 12 ounces by the end of the first week. On the eighth day 5 ounces are added and subsequent increases of an ounce per day are added until the patient is receiving 23 ounces.

Sugar and starch. Six drachms of sugar are given on the third day, gradually increased until the patient is having 14 drachms at the end of 3 weeks. Two drachms of arrowroot are given on the sixth day and continued throughout the second week. Three ounces of blancmange are given on the eighth day, and slightly increased during that week. Rusks may be given on the ninth day, about threequarters of an ounce, and increased until the patient may be having 4 ounces of rusks at the end of a fortnight.

Fat. Three-quarters of an ounce of butter is given on the tenth day, 1 ounce on the eleventh day, and 1½ ounces on the twelfth and subsequent days.

Thirst is relieved by salines, until the patient is having sufficient fluid for this purpose.

Calorie value. During the first week the Calorie value of the food given is a little below 1,000. This results in loss of weight; during the second week it reaches 2,000. Many modifications may be made by the end of the second week and the diet could quite easily be arranged as a series of regular meals—for example:

Breakfast—8 *a.m.* Poached egg, two or three rusks with butter, ¼ pint of milk.
Light lunch—10.30 *a.m.* Two buttered rusks and ¼ pint of milk.
Dinner—1 *p.m.* Steamed fish with butter and rusks, steamed custard with sugar, and water to drink.
Tea—4 *p.m.* A meal similar to breakfast.
Supper—7 *p.m.* Blancmange or milk pudding, rusks and butter, ¼ pint of milk.
Light nourishment—10 *p.m.* Five to six ounces Benger's food.
During night—One or two drinks, 4 or 5 ounces of milk may be given.

Sippy's diet was introduced in 1915. This treatment aims specially at keeping the stomach free of hydrochloric acid and is carried out by the administration of fat such as cream and olive oil, and by the giving of atropine before feeding followed by large doses of alkalis after feeding.

Three ounces of a *milk cream mixture* are given every hour from 7 a.m. to 7 p.m. *Lightly cooked eggs* are added after a few days, and *well-cooked starchy foods* at the end of a week.

The *alkalis* generally used are sodium bicarbonate 10 grains, magnesium carbonate 10 grains, alternately with bismuth carbonate 10 grains —the administration of magnesium and bismuth being so regulated that the bowels are kept acting regularly and diarrhoea and constipation avoided. Half an ounce of olive oil is given before alternate feeds and $\frac{1}{50}$ gr. atropine hypodermically before the other feeds.

Diet in *Haematemesis* including Meulengracht's and Dr. Witts' diets are mentioned on page 384.

Advice to convalescent patients. (1) The regular habits formed in hospital should be carefully observed and continued and meals should be small, regularly taken, and the intervals between them short. (2) All food should be taken very slowly and well masticated before swallowing. (3) As far as possible fluids should be taken between meals rather than with meals. (4) All foods cooked in fat should be most rigorously avoided. (5) The hygiene of the mouth should be carefully carried out at least twice a day and regular visits paid to the dentist. (6) A regular action of the bowels is essential every day, and the patient should realize that the action must be adequate, and that a small constipated stool is not sufficient. (7) If possible the patient should not smoke, but if this is a very great deprivation he may be permitted one or two cigarettes a day.

HYPOCHLORHYDRIA

Deficiency of hydrochloric acid in the gastric secretion is met with in pernicious anaemia and in other secondary anaemias; it is marked in advanced cases of cancer and occasionally occurs in normal persons.

Dietetic treatment. Easily digested foods should be chosen, and any foods which are known to inhibit gastric digestion should be avoided as far as possible. Small meals should be taken and the food should be finely broken up by chopping and mincing whenever possible. Toast should be taken in preference to bread, as it is easier to masticate. Condiments and extractives which help to stimulate the gastric juice may reasonably be used. The administration of hydrochloric acid before and during meals is advised.

HYPERCHLORHYDRIA

An excess of hydrochloric acid in the gastric juice occurs in most forms of dyspepsia and in cases of peptic ulcer.

In the **dietetic treatment** everything which will help to fix the hydrochloric acid is used, and therefore milk, egg and fish proteins are valuable. All articles likely to stimulate the secretion, such as condiments and spices, extractives and alcohol, should be carefully avoided.

JAUNDICE (see also p. 393).

This is more often a symptom of a disease than a disease in itself. It is generally divided into obstructive jaundice and non-obstructive; apart from infective catarrhal jaundice, and haemolytic types, most forms are due to obstruction. In these cases the bile does not enter the duodenum as it should and is being absorbed by the blood stream, giving rise to the symptoms which are present.

The **dietetic treatment** aims at the relief of symptoms. A light easily digested diet should be given with liberal supplies of fresh fruit and vegetables; fats should be avoided and in some cases even milk fat cannot be taken; milk puddings should be made with skimmed milk; meat extracts, condiments and stimulants should not be taken. Bland fluids should be given freely in order to aid the excretion of bile, which is present in excess in the blood, by means of the kidneys and the skin. The bowels should be kept acting regularly, since constipation is apt to occur owing to the absence of bile, which is normally a stimulant to peristalsis.

ANAEMIA (see also p. 359).

There are a number of varieties of anaemia, but in all cases, whether it be primary—a disease of the blood—or secondary, following haemorrhage or accompanying some cachexial condition, there is either diminution in the quantity or in the quality of the blood. All cases of anaemia, therefore, require a good nourishing diet, but it is in the treatment of pernicious anaemia that dietetic treatment has proved so particularly valuable.

Pernicious anaemia. In the treatment of this condition liver diet is now universally employed. This was first instituted by Drs. Minot and

Murphy, who found that on a diet of liver cases of anaemia improved; a much as half a pound of raw liver a day was administered, preference bein given to calf's liver, though pig, lamb and ox liver may be used.

At the present time valuable preparations of liver extract are availabl and these are substituted for raw liver, and alternatively desiccated hog' stomach is used.

In addition *hydrochloric acid* is given. The diet should also contain larg *quantities of fresh fruit and green vegetables* including tomatoes. By 'a larg quantity' at least half a pound of fruit and threequarters of a pound o vegetables should be understood.

Fats and carbohydrates should be limited because of the tendency to develo lardaceous degeneration of some of the hard organs, including the live and kidneys. Fat should be limited to about 2 ounces per day—therefor bacon, cheese and cream should be avoided as far as possible and mil should be used only sparingly.

DIET IN CONSTIPATION

The causes and symptoms of this condition are dealt with on p. 389 The dietetic treatment depends on whether the subject is suffering fron tonic or atonic constipation.

For *atonic constipation* a **high residue diet** will be given, and thi means that the patient is to be given as much fruit and green vegetable as possible with plenty of carbohydrate foods.

A **low residue diet** is employed in the treatment of *tonic* or *spasti constipation*. In this diet all fruits and green vegetables are omitted and als foods such as brown bread. Care has to be taken in the preparation of th diet to see that no harsh particles are included. Milk and cream may b given.

When the patient is convalescent and is first allowed a little fruit i should be passed through a sieve so that it is as finely broken up as possible A raw apple grated and pressed through a sieve is an example of what i first given.

As patients who are on a non-residue diet for some time may not ge enough vitamins B and C, small quantities of strained orange juice should therefore be given, and some preparation containing vitamin B, such a Marmite or yeast.

COLITIS (see also p. 386).

Colitis may be acute or chronic; in ulcerative colitis the stools contai blood and mucus and are frequently passed.

The diet in these cases varies with the treatment adopted by the physician; in some instances a low residue bland diet is employed and care is taken to eliminate all irritating particles by creaming and straining the foods used. Another method adopted is the restriction of fats giving a little Bovril and Marmite and dry toast first; then, as improvement is manifested, gradually building up a moderate, light, fat-free diet; but milk as an article of diet and eggs are not given until fat is added in the final stages of treatment.

More recently cases of acute colitis with frequency of stool as a sympton have been treated by Moro's apple purée diet; raw apple is grated and pressed into a mould and allowed to stand, and the patient is given as much as he will eat of this, and nothing else, for every meal for from 2 to 4 days. It appears to be successful as the stools decrease from 8 or 10 to 1, 2 or 3 a day, the character of the stool improves and the patient begins to make progress.

HIGH AND LOW CALORIE DIETS

A *low calorie diet* is found in the example given on page 280 in a diet for obesity. This may contain as little as 1,000 Calories and the patient will lose weight on this diet.

A *high calorie diet* is employed in order to produce an increase in body weight; it is given during convalescence from disease and in the treatment of certain wasting diseases, as in tuberculosis.

When providing a high calorie diet, sugars, starches and fats are increased. Sugar may be given as glucose and brown sugar used in preparing fruit drinks, as well as in sweetening foods; all foods rich in starch, such as bread, cakes, puddings and sweets are employed, and fat is provided in the form of fat meats and as milk, cream, butter and cheese.

In the provision of a high calorie diet in the treatment of pulmonary tuberculosis, fat is given in large quantities, as the object is not only to increase the weight of the patient, but to provide a diet rich in vitamins A and D as well. Many patients do not tolerate fat well and some are disinclined to take sweet foods, so that in every instance the wishes of the patient and his likes and dislikes have to be considered; for this reason it is impossible to lay down a diet table suitable for every occasion, but the following dietary for one day is suggested as an example:

Breakfast. Two or three ounces of cereal with cream and sugar. Two rashers of bacon and two eggs (fried). Toast, butter and marmalade. Coffee or tea, with milk or cream and sugar.

Midmorning. A milk drink of 6 ounces with 1 ounce of cream. Biscuits and butter with Marmite (the latter being employed to give the necessary amount of vitamin B in a diet of high calorie value).

Lunch—1 *p.m.* Meat or fish, about 6 ounces. Potatoes, fried or baked; or boiled potatoes mashed with butter and milk may be given. Vegetable, with butter or sauce containing cream or butter. A steamed pudding, apple charlotte, baked custard or milk pudding, or bread and butter pudding are all excellent. (A steamed pudding with jam sauce or white sauce is of very high calorie value.) A sweetened fruit drink.

Tea—4.30 *p.m.* Tea with milk and sugar, bread and butter, and jam sandwiches and cake.

Supper—7.15 *p.m.* Soup, thickened and containing cream. Savoury such as cheese soufflé, macaroni cheese, or potato pie with thickened gravy. A pudding (such as one of those suggested for lunch). Cheese, butter and biscuits. (Three courses may be given, but the alternative course had better be soup or cheese.) A sweetened fruit drink.

At night. A milk drink of 6 ounces with 1 ounce of cream, biscuits and butter.

DIETS RICH OR LOW IN CALCIUM AND IRON

Diet rich in calcium (*high calcium diet*) and diet in which the calcium content is low (*low calcium diet*) may be ordered. In certain abnormal conditions of the body the utilization of calcium may be disordered and special dietetic care may be required to estimate the intake and output of calcium by means of a diet described as—*a calcium balance diet*.

The foods rich in calcium are milk, eggs and cheese; these will be given liberally in a high calcium diet and omitted from a diet of low calcium value.

In the nursing care of patients who are on a *low calcium diet*, *low iron intake diet* or a *calcium balance diet* all the water taken into the body has to be distilled. The utensils used by the patient for feeding purposes are washed in distilled water, all food is cooked and prepared with it, the patient's teeth should be cleaned with it, and if he has to have an enema or a saline injection this also must be prepared with distilled water.

KETOGENIC DIET

A ketogenic diet is rich in fat. It renders the urine highly acid and causes acidosis. It was used in the treatment of chronic infections of the urinary tract due to *B. coli*, but is rarely employed today, having been superseded by mandelic acid treatment (see p. 404).

The diet prescribed may contain 50 grammes of protein, 250 grammes of fat and 20 grammes of carbohydrate. The fat is given in the form of butter, cream and bacon fat.

DEFICIENCY DISEASES

The group of diseases described as deficiency diseases indicate that the cause is due to the absence of certain vitamins present in food essential in diet to health and wellbeing. These diseases are frequently caused by dietetic errors, and the history of the diet should be very carefully investigated and suitable foods administered. (See Vitamin Chart, Appendix II.)

Rickets produces constitutional changes. There is deficiency of calcium in the bones, and dentition is delayed. The infant is pale and flabby. He may be irritable and restless, and may have convulsions, diarrhoea and night sweatings. Rickets does not usually develop until after the age of six months, and it responds to the administration of cod-liver oil and irradiated ergosterol in which vitamins A and D are freely contained. The dose of vitamin D required to cure rickets is 2,000 to 3,000 I.U. daily.

The *diet* includes fresh cow's milk and cream, orange juice, fresh fruit, fruit pulp and green vegetables. Bacon and butter should be given liberally. Lightly cooked eggs and protein—fish protein and red beef gravy from underdone beef, and freshly cooked red beef minced may be used. Carbohydrates should be limited, especially sweets and cakes. The following is a *sample day's dietary* for an infant aged eighteen months with rickets:

Breakfast—8 *a.m.* Two ounces of porridge and ½ ounce of cream. Quarter of a slice of bread fried in bacon fat with a small piece of fat bacon. Five ounces of milk.

Light lunch—10.30 *a.m.* Four ounces of milk and a buttered rusk.

Dinner—1 *p.m.* Three ounces of freshly cooked minced beef—plenty of red beef gravy, ½ ounce of breadcrumbs and 1 ounce of potato. An ounce of well-cooked minced cabbage. A little custard and fruit pulp. Water to drink.

Tea—4.30 *p.m.* A lightly boiled egg, 2 well-buttered rusks, or half a slice of well-buttered bread cut into fingers. Milk to drink, 5 ounces.

On going to bed—6 *p.m.* A small drink of milk.

Xerophthalmia is a condition in which hardening or keratinization the cornea occurs. This is due to deficiency of vitamin A, and responds treatment by administration of sufficiently large doses of this vitamin.

Night blindness is due to inability of the retina to adapt itself to arkness. Vitamin A is of importance in maintaining this function.

Scurvy. This disease is due to deficiency of the antiscorbutic vitamin nd, when it appears, it occurs most commonly between the ages of 6 nd 18 months.

The infant responds rapidly to *dietetic treatment.* He is usually being arti-cially fed on some proprietary milk preparation devoid of antiscorbutic itamins without having these added to the diet. Fresh cow's milk should e given and orange and lemon juice, tomato juice and potato cream. 'he infant may be in a very bad state with sore tender gums, his limbs nay be very tender to touch and he is easily hurt when handled. The nouth should be kept very clean and, if it is difficult to get the food taken he child may be fed by the nasal tube. He requires very gentle handling. mprovement will occur quickly as the response to treatment is always apid.

Beri-beri is due to deficiency of thiamin (vitamin B1). It is a disease haracterized by polyneuritis. Two types are described (*a*) *dry beri-beri* in vhich muscular wasting and weakness is marked and (*b*) *wet beri-beri* haracterized by oedema; there is also anasarca and ascites.

Treatment consists in the administration of a well-balanced diet. Yeast nd Marmite are given as these two substances contain large quantities f vitamin B1.

Pellagra is a disease which occurs when the diet is deficient in milk and neat, which contain the necessary *nicotinic acid* and riboflavin or one of he vitamin B2 entities. This disease is characterized by symmetrical areas f dermatitis on the exposed parts of the body such as the hands and fore-rms, forehead and face. There is loss of appetite, soreness of the mouth nd loss of weight.

Treatment. The patient is put to bed and the symptoms are treated. He is given a diet rich in milk and eggs, butter, meat, fruit and vegetables, nd liberal doses of yeast. The areas of skin affected should be covered in rder to protect them from the light which is irritating in this condition.

DIET IN COELIAC DISEASE

Coeliac disease is considered to be due to the inability of the infant to bsorb fats, a large amount of fat appearing in the stools which are large, pale and greasy. There is great wasting.

The *dietetic treatment* should be of a minimum calorie value, entire devoid of fat and with carbohydrates limited. Protein forms the base the diet and dried milk, white of egg, orange juice, green vegetables ar bananas, as many as 6 or more a day, are given. As improvement begi carbohydrates are gradually added and then fats given in small quantitie

Vitamins A and D are given to prevent rickets and substances whic help in the assimilation of fats, such as bile salts, are prescribed in sma doses.

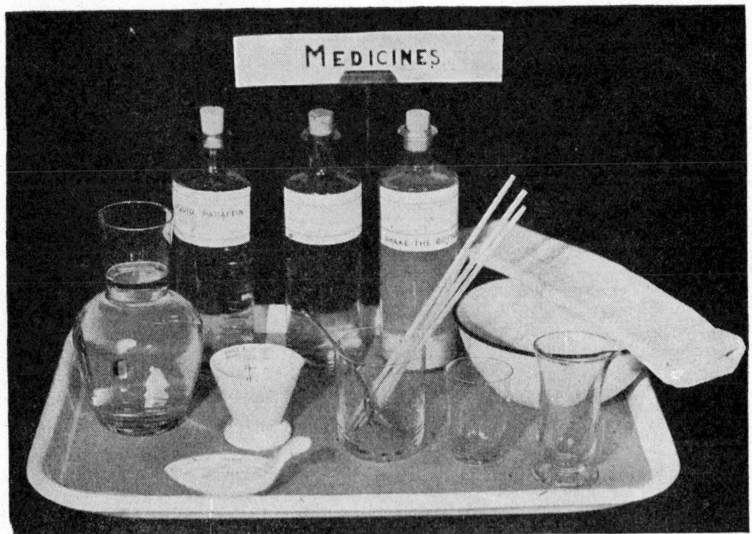

FIG. 149.—*see page* 311. On a tray for giving medicines provide water to dilute the medicines, bowl of water and glass cloth for washing and drying medicine measures. A delf oil cup or spoon is used for giving oil and emulsion. Straws are required for medicines containing iron.

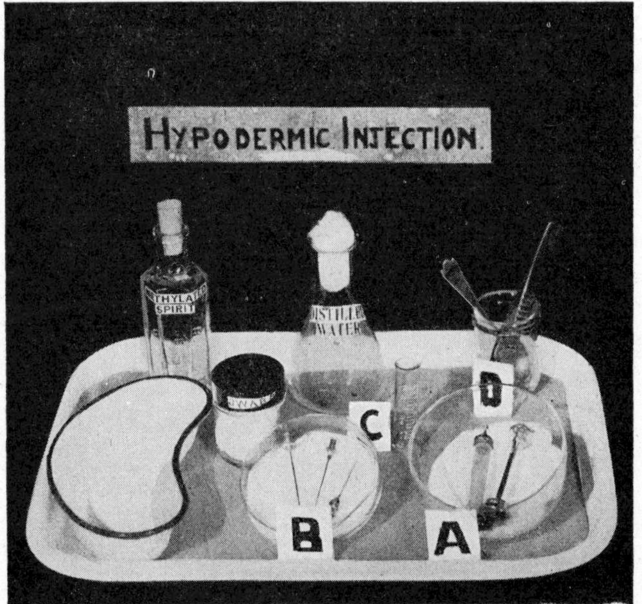

FIG. 150.—*see page* 313. (A) Hypodermic syringe. (B) needles to fit syringe. (C) a small minim measure. (D) small dissecting forceps, spoon. In addition swabs and spirit are needed for cleansing the skin and some distilled water in which to dissolve the drug when it is put up in tablet form.

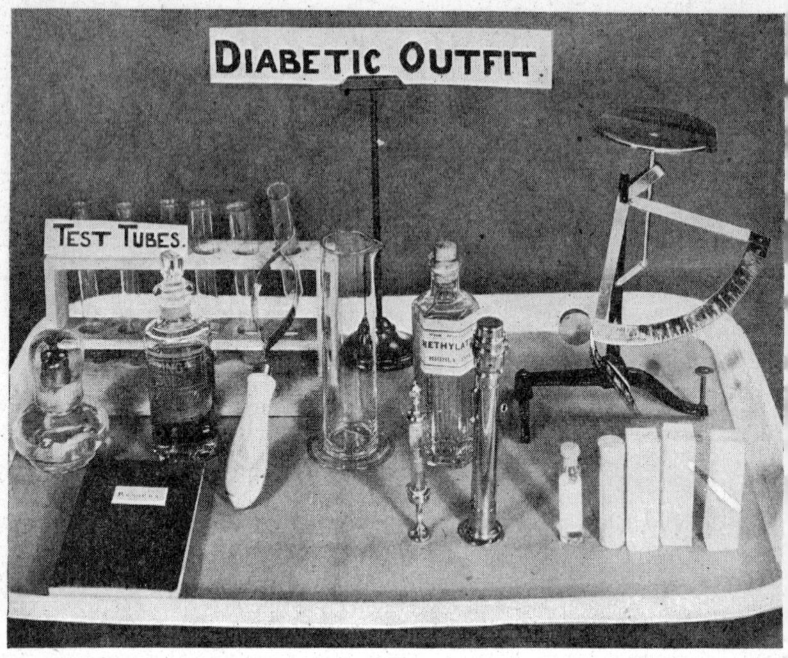

FIG. 151.—*see page* 439. The outfit includes a spring balance; in front of this is shown a supply of insulin with insulin syringe and special pocket case, and spirit for cleansing the skin. Urine testing apparatus and record book are shown on the left of the picture.

A patient with diabetes should be trained in the management of his own diet, in the testing of his urine and the administration of his insulin. He should be familiar with the different types of insulin (*see page* 437) and be able to mix doses of soluble insulin with protamine zinc insulin if these are ordered together. He should also know the symptoms which suggest the onset of hypoglycaemia and be able to deal with this. Fuller instructions on this subject will be found on page 438.

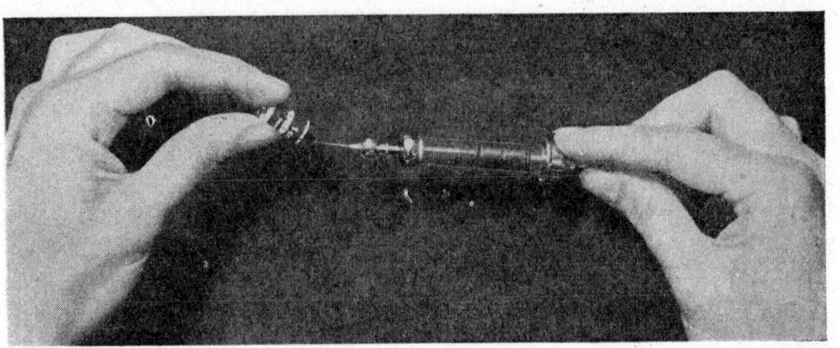

FIG. 152.—*see page* 313.
CHARGING A HYPODERMIC SYRINGE FROM A PHIAL.

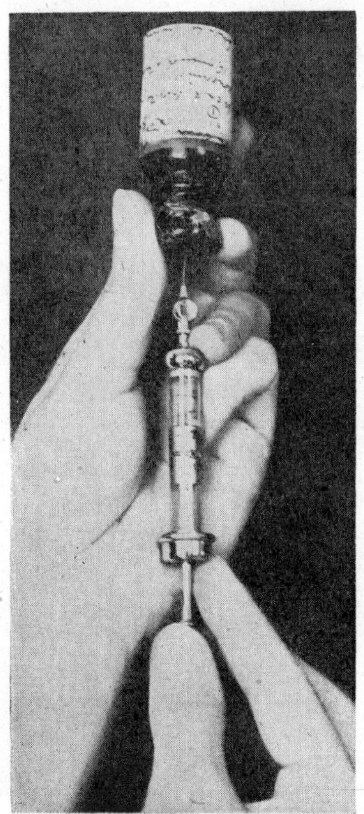

FIG. 153.—*see page* 314.
CHARGING A HYPODERMIC SYRINGE FROM A RUBBER-CAPPED BOTTLE.

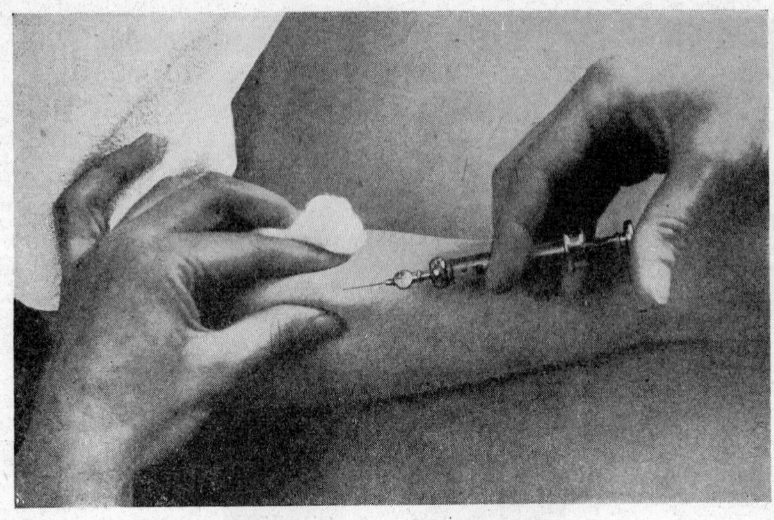

FIG. 154.—*see page* 314. GIVING A HYPODERMIC INJECTION.

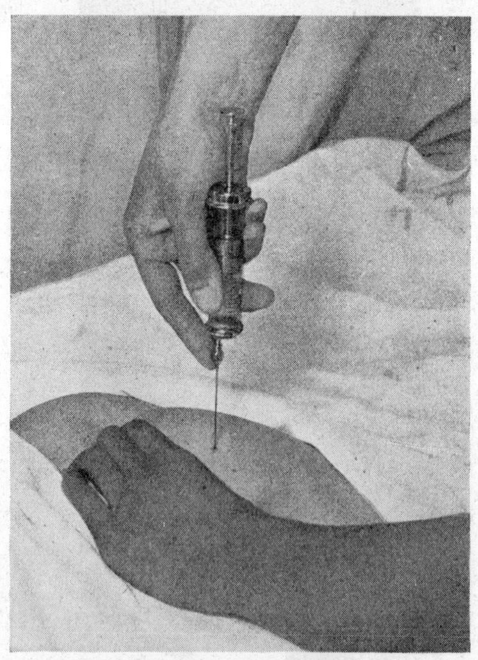

FIG. 155.—*see page* 315. GIVING AN INTRAMUSCULAR INJECTION INTO THE BUTTOCK. The needle, held at right angles to the skin. is plunged up to the hilt into the muscle, at the upper and outer quadrant.

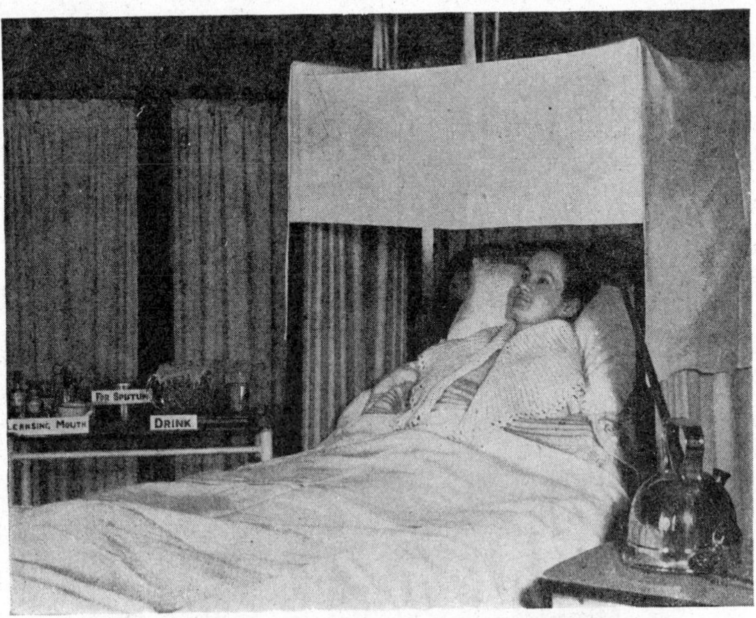

FIG. 156.—*see page* 318. CANOPY FOR USE WITH STEAM KETTLE.

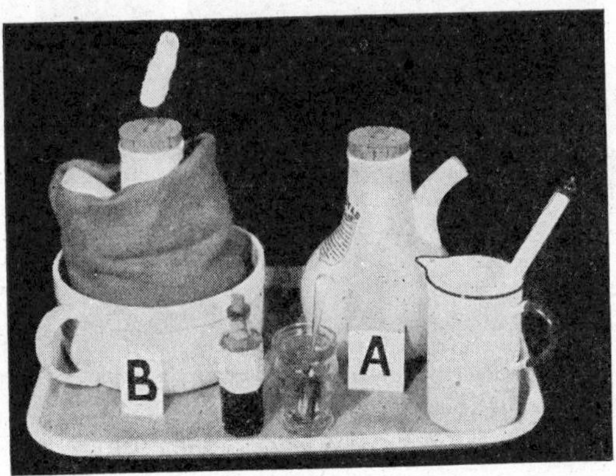

FIG. 157.—*see page* 317. ARTICLES FOR STEAM INHALATION. (A) Nelson's inhaler showing the correct position of glass mouthpiece. (B) Inhaler prepared for use, in flannel cover and standing in a delf porringer. The mouthpiece is covered with gauze as it may be too hot for the patient's lips to rest on it.

The bottle on the tray contains friar's balsam—a spoon is provided for measuring the one or two drachms required. In some cases a thermometer will be needed.

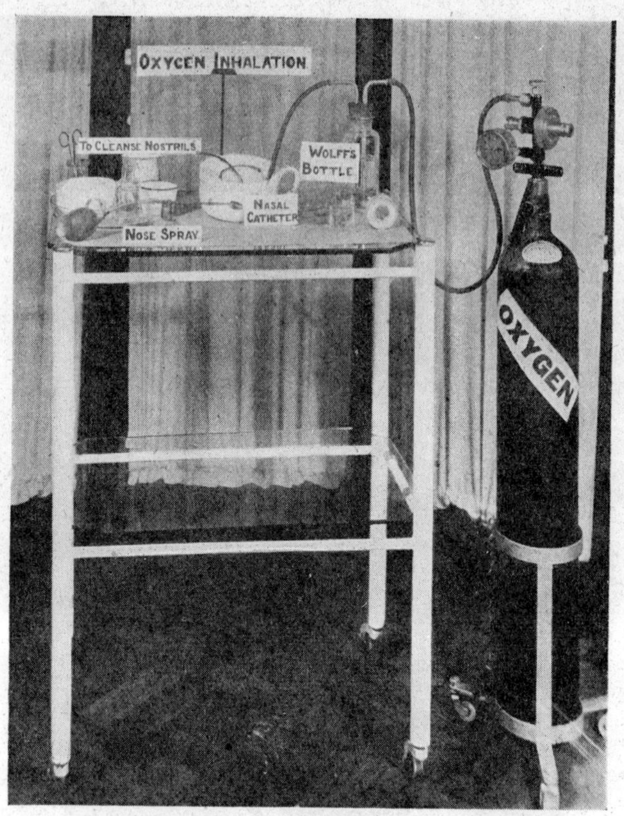

FIG. 158.—*see page* 319.

FOR INTRANASAL ADMINISTRATION OF OXYGEN.

The nostrils should be clear, the catheter is lubricated and passed backwards into the pharynx. (*See also Figs.* 164 *and* 165 *on pages* 318–19.)

Oxygen requires to pass through water in order to moisten it; for this purpose a flowmeter and humidifier may be employed (*see Fig.* 159), or Wolff's bottle may be used.

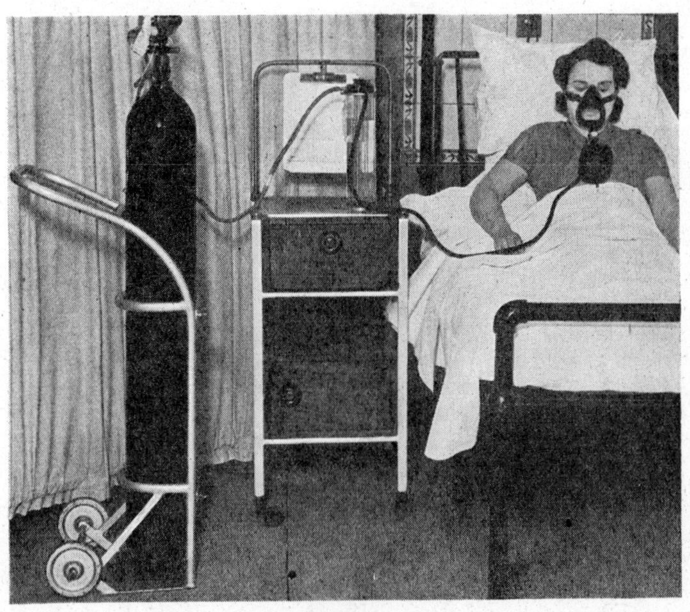

FIG. 159.—*see page* 319.

B.L.B. (BOOTHY, LOVELACE AND BULBULIAN) OXYGEN INHALATION APPARATUS IN USE. *The mask can be seen in detail on page* 320. In the illustration the oxygen is passed through a flowmeter and humidifier. The use of a humidifier can be dispensed with, as the reservoir breathing bag, being closed by a small glass stopper at the distal extremity, collects moisture as the patient breathes in and out of the bag.

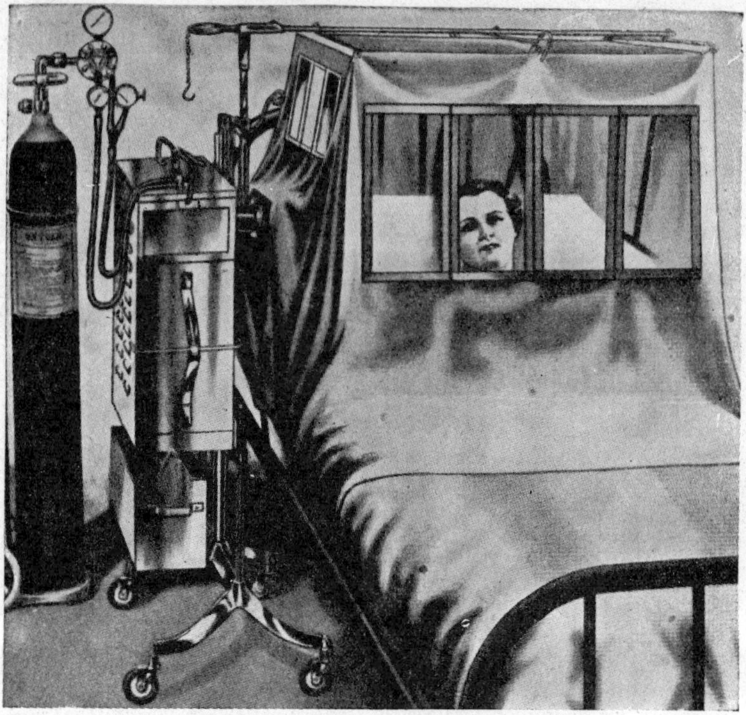

FIG. 160.—*see page* 320. PATIENT IN HEIDBRINK'S OXYGEN TENT.

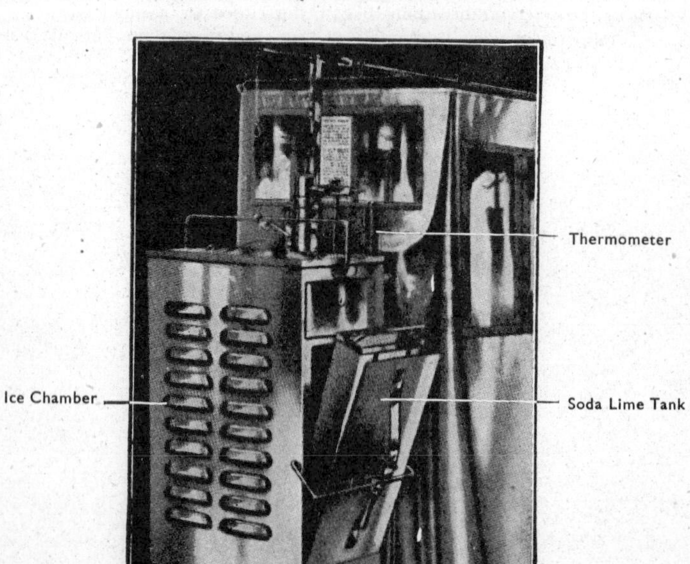

FIG. 161.—SHOWING ICE CHAMBER AND SODA-LIME TANK APPARATUS.

Section 3

The Administration of Drugs and Medicines. Elementary Materia Medica. Poisons and Poisoning

Chapter 19

Administration of Medicines and Drugs

'he origin and dosage of drugs—Idiosyncrasy and intolerance—Weights and ıeasures—Modes of preparation of drugs—Classification of drugs—The pre- ·ription—The safe custody of medicines and drugs—Rules for giving medicine— 1odes of administration of drugs—Inhalations, including administration of oxygen—The use of sera and vaccines—Chemotherapy

Medicines and drugs used in the treatment of disease are derived from three main sources. The majority are of *vegetable origin*, being obtained from the leaves, roots, stems and seeds of plants—as, for xample, digitalis from the leaf of the foxglove, and colchicum from the eeds of meadow saffron. A fair number of drugs are derived from *mineral ources*, principally salts of iron, mercury, arsenic, lead and phosphorus, nd a few from *animal sources*—usually the extracts of endocrine organs uch as the pituitary body, and the thyroid gland, adrenalin from the uprarenals and insulin from the pancreas.

Before a drug can be ordered its dose must be standardized. The majority are tandardized by *chemical means*, and they are then supplied as a solution ontaining a certain percentage of the active principle of the drug. In a ew instances, however, where the drug is obtainable in a pure crystalline orm a certain weight of it—e.g. so many grammes or grains or fractions f a grain—will be given.

The other method of standardization is *biological*, by which the effect f a drug on an animal is determined.

Having arrived at the standardization of any given drug, its dose for he adult is then laid down by the compilers of the British Pharmacopoeia, nd this is determined by the *strength* of the drug. A certain dose for the dult man is given, but in practice this has to be modified according to he age of the person, and to some extent according to his size—for example large fat man weighing 18 stone will require considerably more than a ittle lean man of 8 or 9 stone. A woman is considered to require slightly ess than a man, but here again size and weight have to be taken into onsideration.

A child requires a correspondingly smaller dose than an adult, and in ractice this is determined in several ways, one of the more common ways of calculating the dose required for a child being by means Young's rule—Take the age of the child over the age plus 12, e.g.

$$\frac{\text{Age } 2}{2 + 12} = \frac{2}{14} = 1/7\text{th of the adult dose.}$$

Idiosyncrasy or undue sensitiveness to the action of a drug sometim exists in a person, and is a factor which will materially alter the size the dose to be given. Some people are sensitive to, and can only tolera small doses of such drugs as aspirin, sodium salicylate, quinine ar potassium iodide. A dose of ordinary size in these cases produces manifest tions of what are described as *untoward symptoms*—in reality symptoms poisoning though a poisonous dose has not actually been given. *Potassiu iodide* results in *iodism*, manifested by coryza, laryngitis and an eryth matous rash. *Quinine* gives rise to deafness, headache, nausea, subnorm temperature and shivering. *Sodium salicylate* causes hissing and ringi noises in the ears, headache, deafness, nausea and malaise, and an eryth matous rash.

The **cumulative effect** of a drug has also to be considered, and th means that drugs can and should only be given at the rate at which the will be absorbed, produce their effect, and then be excreted. It is impor ant to remember that some drugs take longer to be excreted by the kidne than others, and this is why some medicines are ordered every 3 or 4 hour some every 6 hours or four times a day, and others three times day.

Some drugs are known to tend to accumulate in the body and therefo more definite precautions are taken to prevent this. Digitalis, for exampl is given only every 6 hours, and arsenic is another drug which will accum late. If this fact is ignored, untoward symptoms may develop. *In the case digitalis* probably a powerful action of the drug would occur at first, th pulse becoming slow and the urine more plentiful; later, if these sym toms are not reported and means taken to prevent further accumulatio the pulse would become irregular in character, the urine suppressed an as the patient gradually became poisoned by digitalis, nausea and vomitin would develop. The *cumulative action of arsenic* would give rise to sympton of disorder of the alimentary tract, including nausea, vomiting and dia rhoea; and later, as the symptoms became intensified, the patient would b markedly dehydrated as the result of a continual loss of fluid, and if th administration of the drug is not omitted neuritis will develop, followe by paralysis of the muscles that control the wrist and ankle.

Increased tolerance. Some persons develop an increased toleranc for a drug, when repeated doses—even quite small doses—are taken over fairly considerable time. They then need an increasingly large quantit of the drug before it will produce any effect. This is a very dangerous facto especially as this tolerance to the drug invariably develops in the case hypnotics and narcotics—such for example as morphia, leading to th desire for it, and resulting in an addiction to its use. For example, a mo phia addict may require to take up to 5 grains of morphia early mornin before he can even face the beginning of his day's work, following this b similar doses once or twice throughout the day until by night time he ha had from 15 to 18 grains of the drug.

WEIGHTS AND MEASURES

Imperial System.

Weights (Avoirdupois)

Unit of weight—1 grain (gr.)

1 grain	(gr.)	the unit of weight
1 ounce	(oz.)	contains 437½ grains
1 pound	(lb.)	contains 16 ounces

Capacity (Imperial fluid measure)

Unit of measure—1 minim (min. or m.)

1 minim	(min.)	the unit of measure
1 drachm	(fl. dr.)	contains 60 minims
1 ounce	(fl. oz.)	contains 8 drachms
1 pint	(pt.)	contains 20 fluid ounces

Relation of capacity to mass in the Imperial measures. The measures of mass nd capacity are not quite the same. One minim weighs less than one ain—it takes 109 and a fraction minims to equal in weight 100 grains; nd therefore it is taken that 110 minims equal in weight 100 grains, nd whereas one part in 100 parts ordinarily make a 1 per cent solution, has to be taken that in the Imperial system 1 grain in 110 minims of ater equals a 1 per cent solution. For example the British Pharmacopoeia reparation of morphia for hypodermic use is a 2½ per cent solution; eaning that 2½ grains of morphia are contained in 110 minims of water. therefore a nurse is asked to prepare ¼ of a grain of morphia for inction into a patient she must remember this—as 2½ contains 10 fourths the whole, if she divides 110 by 10, this equals 11 minims, and ¼ of a ain will be contained in that quantity.

Metric System.

Weights

Unit of weight—1 gramme (gm.)

1 milligramme	(mg.)	0·001 gramme
1 centigramme	(cg.)	0·01 ,,
1 decigramme	(dg.)	0·1 ,,
1 gramme	(gm.)	the unit of weight
1 dekagramme	(Dg.)	10·0 grammes
1 hectogramme	(Hg.)	100·0 ,,
1 kilogramme	(Kg.)	1,000·0 ,,

Measures

Unit of measure—1 millilitre (ml.) or
1 cubic centimetre (c.c.)

1 centilitre	(cl.)	10 c.c.
1 decilitre	(dl.)	100 c.c.
1 litre	(l.)	1,000 c.c.

The unit of weight—the gramme—equals the weight of 1 millilitre olume of water. Because of the relationship between the units of weight nd measure in the metric system, dispensing is made easier.

Some equivalents of British to Metrical System.

17 minims	=	1 cubic centimetre
1 drachm	=	4·0 grammes
1 ounce	=	30·0 ,,
1 pint	=	568 cubic centimetres
35 fluid ounces	=	1 litre
2 pounds 3 ounces	=	1 kilogramme

MODES OF PREPARATION OF DRUGS

Aceta. Solutions in acetic acid. Examples are: aceta scillae, which is us as a stimulant expectorant.

Aquae. Solutions in water, which are usually preparations of volati substances, such as chloroform and peppermint. The dose is fro 1 to 4 drachms, and these solutions are used as flavouring.

Bougies. Small rods of oily substance, prepared with glycerine ar gelatine, containing drugs used for insertion into the ear, nose ar urethra. The bougie is slightly heated in a little oil or warm wate and then inserted into the canal where it dissolves, so that the dru contained in it comes into contact with the walls of the orifice.

Confectiones. Pastes of the consistency of thick jam, made of suga preparations containing a drug. Amongst the best examples ar confection of senna and confection of sulphur, both of which ar used as laxatives, the dose being from 1 to 2 drachms.

Collodia (Collodions). These are solutions of pyroxin dissolved in eth or alcohol, and should be kept in closely sealed bottles. Sever varieties of collodion are described. *Simple collodion* is used to se small punctures. *Flexile collodion* is a form containing some oily su stance such as castor oil, it is used to paint over irregular surfac because by reason of its oily nature it works its way into crevic and cracks and it is used in such situations to retain dressings i position. *Collodion vesicans* is a preparation of collodion containir cantharides, which is a blistering agent.

Cataplasmata. Soft moist plasters of various kinds commonly calle poultices, which are applied locally as applications of heat, and i some cases contain a drug.

Cachets. Little wafer paper boxes used for the administration of insolub or nauseating drugs. Examples are quinine, aspirin and guiac carbonate.

Capsules. Flexible gelatine containers, which hold from 5 to 30 minim The tiny ones are round and the larger ones egg shaped. They ar filled through a minute hole at one end which is afterwards seale by collodion, and are used for the administration of unpleasar tasting drugs of a liquid character, including fish-liver oil, castor oi creosote, cascara sagrada and paraldehyde.

Cigarettes. A cigarette in which a drug replaces tobacco, the commone example being the stramonium cigarettes which patients smok inhaling the fumes for the relief of asthma.

Collunarium. A nosewash.

Collyrium. An eyewash.

Decocta. Liquid preparations made by boiling solid substances in water for from 10 to 20 minutes, with the result that the active principle of the substance used passes into the water. Example—decoctum aloes, dose ½ to 1 drachm.

Emplastra. Substances used as plasters by smearing on holland or silk with a heated spatula. Examples are lead (plumbi) plaster and belladonna plaster. When ordered the size of the plaster is specified and also the length of time it is to be kept on.

Emulsiones. Mixtures of oil or fat and water, which are usually rendered more permanent by the addition of a gum or alkali. Examples include paraffin, and cod-liver oil emulsion.

Enemata. Fluid preparations for injection into the lower bowel.

Essentiae. Essences are solutions of volatile oils in alcohol. An example is essence of peppermint. The dose of an essence is small, usually a few drops, on sugar.

Extracta. Extracts may be solid or fluid, the former are prepared by evaporating the expressed juice of plants. Examples—extract. cascarae segradae, 2 to 8 grains, and extract. colchicum, grains ¼ to 1.

Fluid extracts are prepared by extracting a substance in a liquid. The liquid is then partially evaporated to make a stronger solution of the drug. Examples are liquorice extract (ext. glycyrrhizae. liq.) prepared in water, and extract of nux vomica prepared in alcohol.

Fomenta. Fomentations are wrung out of hot water to which drugs may or may not have been added.

Gargarisma. Gargles are liquid preparations for application to the mouth, fauces and throat.

Glycerines. These are substances in which glycerine is used as a solvent. Examples are glycerine of borax, used in cleaning the mouth; glycerine of ichthyol, used as a local preparation for the relief of inflammation; and glycerine of belladonna, used for the relief of pain.

Granules. Little pills. Example—Nativelle's granules of digitalin, dose 1/400th to 1/60th of a grain.

Guttae. Drops for instillation into the eye.

Haustus. A haustus is a single draught, the dose usually being large, as much as from 1 to 2 ounces. Example—haustus sennae co., which contains, in addition to senna, magnesium sulphate and liquorice.

Infusa. Infusions are made by pouring either hot or cold water on a dry substance in a vessel, and allowing it to stand for a variable time. The tea we drink is an example of infusion.

Infusion of senna, which is made by soaking a number of senna pods in cold water for several hours, is a well-known laxative.

Other infusions include infusion of digitalis and infusion of gentian (infusio gentianae co.). The dose of each of these is ½ to 1 drachm.

Injectiones. These are concentrated preparations of solutions of specia drugs used for hypodermic injection. Examples are injectio mor phinae hypodermica, and injectio apomorphinae hypodermica.

Inhalationes. Inhalations are administrations of volatile substances i water in which the vapour of the water is inhaled.

Insufflationes. Spraying with powders, usually on to the walls of cavitie such as the pharynx and nose.

Lamellae. Small thin disks made with gelatine or glycerine used to dro into the eye. Examples are atropine and eserine disks.

Linctus. Substances of a sticky nature used as a sedative when a coug is irritable and ineffective. They contain a basis of syrup and gly cerine, and in some cases sedative drugs are added, a linctu accordingly being described as a simple or an opiate linctus.

Linimenta. External applications of soapy and oily preparations used a counterirritants or as sedatives or antispasmodics for the relief c pain according to the ingredients contained in them. Many of thes contain alcohol, chloroform, belladonna, turpentine or menthol. I applying a liniment it is important to rub it in warm, and to con tinue rubbing until the skin is well reddened.

Liquores. Solutions of special drugs, in many cases of very potent ones in water. In the following instance the solution contains 1 grain c the drug in 110 minims of water, making a 1 per cent solution Liquor morphinae hydrochloridi; dose 5–30 minims.

Lotiones. Watery mixtures for external use. Examples are lotio rubr which contains zinc, lavender water and a colouring preparation and lotio nigra, or blackwash, which is a mercurial preparation.

Mella (Honey). Example—mella boracis, which is used for cleaning th mouth when glycerine of borax is found to be too astringent.

Misturae. Mixtures are solutions of substances suspended in water o mucilage. Most of the medicines commonly prescribed are mixtures

Nebulae. Oily or aqueous preparations sprayed on to areas by means c an atomizer.

Olea. Oils. Examples include oil of cloves, oil of turpentine and oil c cajuput.

Pastes. A preparation similar to ointment but containing powder (e.g Lassar's paste).

Perles. Little gelatine capsules (see also Capsules).

Pessaria. Solid conical substances, similar in shape to suppositories, mad up with cocoa butter, and used for insertion into the vagina in orde to bring a drug into contact with the vaginal wall.

Pigmentum. A preparation in the form of a tacky paint for local applica tion. Example—pigmentum Mandl, used as a throat paint.

Pillulae. Pills containing a drug, and usually coated with sugar or silver

Pulveres. Powders. Examples—Gregory's, Dover's, pulv. jalapae co.

olutiones. Watery preparations containing a dissolved solid substance, such as for example a saline solution, and solutions of glucose and sodium bicarbonate.

Those containing a more powerful drug are frequently made up in a uniform strength of 1, 2 or 4 per cent. Examples include preparations of cocaine.

uppositoria. Cone-shaped substances for rectal administration, usually prepared with a basis of gelatine, or oil of theobroma. One example is the glycerine suppository, with is used to evacuate the rectum. Other examples include belladonna and opium suppositories.

The pessaries used for vaginal administration are sometimes described as suppositories.

yrupi. Sugary liquid preparations used for flavouring medicines. A example is syrupus lemonis.

'abellae. Tablets. Nitroglycerine prepared with chocolate—trinitrin.

'incturae. Tinctures. Solutions of the active principle of the drug in alcohol. Examples are tincture of digitalis, tincture of opium, the dose of either being from 5 to 15 minims; tincture of strophanthus, dose 2 to 8 minims; tincture of belladonna, dose 15 to 20 minims. Tinctures are prepared in alcohol which is scarce at present and in many cases an alternative, authorized under the 'Shortage of Drugs' order, must now be employed. Most of the authorized alternatives are liquid preparations in water which have the same therapeutic value as the tinctures formerly used.

'rochisci. Lozenges. These are usually made with a fruit basis, and may contain a sedative, astringent or antiseptic agent.

Jnguenta. Ointments are semi-solid preparations of a fatty substance containing an active drug, and intended for external use.

'ina. Liquid preparations in which sherry is used as a solvent. Examples —vinum antimoniale, dose 10 to 30 minims; vinum ipecacuanha. (The 1932 edition of the British Pharmacopoeia altered the name of this latter preparation to tincture of ipecacuanha.)

'apores. Preparations by which the inhalation of volatile drugs is rendered possible, when exposed to the air.

CLASSIFICATION OF DRUGS WITH EXAMPLES

Anaesthetics are drugs which produce loss of sensation when applied ocally, and loss of consciousness when a general administration is made.

Anthelmintics are drugs used in the treatment of worms or intestinal arasites. There are three kinds of worms which chiefly infest the alimenary tract in man—tapeworm, roundworm and threadworm and, less requently, the hookworm (for symptoms and treatment see p. 389).

Male fern (filix mas) is used in the treatment of tapeworm in the form f extract of male fern. It is nauseating and is therefore frequently given n capsule form, the dose being from 45 to 90 minims.

Santonin is the drug which is specifically used in the treatment of rounc worm and in some cases in the treatment of threadworm. The dose is fror 1 to 3 grains. Santonin may render the urine yellow in colour and ma also cause the patient to 'see yellow' (yellow vision).

Thymol, from 15 to 30 grains, is used in the treatment of hookworm.

Infusion of quassia 1 per cent is given as an enema in an attempt to clea the lower bowel of threadworm.

Antidotes are drugs used to produce an opposite effect in order to com bat symptoms of poisoning, as for example where atropine is administere in cases of morphia or opium poisoning.

Antipyretics are drugs which lower the temperature of the body. Thes are rarely used for this purpose today, though they are employed when, i addition to lowering the temperature, they have a specific effect in th treatment of certain diseases.

Examples are quinine sulphate or quinine hydrochloride, used in dos of from 1 to 10 grains in the treatment of malaria; salicylic acid, dose to 10 grains which is specific in rheumatism; aspirin, antipyrin and ant febrin—dosage 5 to 10 grains—are used as analgesics for the relief c neuralgia and myalgia, and also as diaphoretics to reduce temperature.

Antiseptics are substances used to prevent the growth of organism when applied externally. Therapeutically, antiseptic substances are use to produce some effect on one or other of the systems of the body, but the must of necessity be given in very weak solutions, otherwise their actio would be injurious to the tissues.

Examples include—*respiratory antiseptics*—creosote, minims 1–3; *saliva antiseptic*—such as potassium chlorate; *intestinal antiseptic*—such as guiac carbonate, dose 5–10 grains. Hexamin, dose 15–30 grains, acts as *urinary antiseptic* and also as a *biliary antiseptic*.

Antitoxins. These are substances opposed to the action of toxins in th blood, and are administered in the form of antitoxin serum. The dos varies according to the disease for which it is used. Scarlet fever ant toxin is administered in doses of 10–20 c.c. Diphtheria antitoxin an tetanus antitoxin are prepared in units—the dose varying from 3,00 units upwards.

Astringents are substances which lessen secretion by causing contrac tion of the lumen of the blood vessels in the walls of the tissue to whic they are applied.

Examples of these include tannic acid, which is contained in many c the throat paints, and also given in the form of an enema in the treatmen of some forms of diarrhoea. An example of an astringent, given hypc dermically to produce its effect on an organ for which it is specific i action, is ergot, the dose of extract of ergot being from 30 to 60 minim It acts by stimulating contraction of the blood vessels in the uterus an arresting haemorrhage.

Cardiac Drugs. See Stimulants, also p. 308.

Carminatives. These are substances which result in expulsion of flatu or gas, from some part of the alimentary tract, either upper or lowe They act by stimulating contraction of the involuntary muscle containe n the walls of the canal. They are usually ordered to be given occasionally r as required. *Examples* of those administered by mouth include oil of ajuput and oil of peppermint, dose 1–3 minims. These may be ad-ninistered on a lump of sugar. Other examples include cloves, ginger, lill water and sal volatile.

Carminatives which may be administered by the rectum include tur-pentine, and asafoetida (see also Enemata).

Cholagogues (see Purgatives).

Diaphoretics are substances which increase the action of the skin and re therefore used in the treatment of febrile conditions when the skin is ot and dry, and also in the treatment of chronic nephritis, with oedema, n order to assist the elimination of water from the body by causing the kin to act. A similar effect can be produced by a local application of eat to the skin. *Examples of diaphoretics* are pilocarpine nitrate—dose rom $\frac{1}{120}$–$\frac{1}{5}$ grain—which acts very quickly, so that the patient should e prepared for sweating by wrapping him in blankets, surrounded by ot-water bottles before the drug, which is given hypodermically, is dministered; sweet spirits of nitre (spirit of nitrous ether), 15 to 60 ninims; and liquor ammonium acetate, 2 to 8 drachms.

Diuretics. These drugs increase urinary output, by stimulating the unction of the kidney. Only very mild alkaline substances such as potas-ium citrate can ever be used as diuretics in the treatment of acute ephritis. All drinks are diuretic, including tea. Other articles of diet, which are diuretic in action, include theobromin in chocolate, and caffeine n coffee.

Examples are potassium citrate, potassium acetate and potassium artrate, dosage 15–60 grains; liquor ammonium acetate, 2–8 drachms; iquor ammonium citrate, 2–6 drachms; infusion of buchu, 1–2 drachms. *Urea*, dose from 15 to 240 grains, is also used as a diuretic.

Mercury is a powerful diuretic. It is used in the form of Mersalyl in loses of 8 to 30 minims. One dose may result in the output of 7 to 8 pints of urine. The use of mercurial diuretics in the relief of cardiac edema is described on p. 353.

Guy's pill which contains three important diuretic drugs, mercury, squills and digitalis is another method of giving mercury.

Emetics. These substances produce vomiting, either by irritating the mucous membrane of the stomach or by stimulating the vomiting centre in the medulla. *Examples* of the former type include mustard, 1 table-spoonful to a tumbler of water; or salt, 2 tablespoonfuls; and tartar emetic, 2–4 drachms. *Examples* of the latter type include tincture of ipecacuanha, which is given in fairly large doses of 10 to 30 minims; and apomorphine hydrochloride, dose from $\frac{1}{20}$–$\frac{1}{6}$ grain, given hypodermically. This is used to induce vomiting in unconscious patients.

Expectorants. As a rule expectorants increase the amount of secretion from the lungs, and in this case they are described as stimulating ex-pectorants. These are used when cough and sputum are present as in the later stages of bronchitis. *Examples of stimulating expectorants* are am-monium carbonate, 5–10 grains; ammonium chloride, 5–60 grains; infusio senegae co., ½–1 drachm; syrup of Tolu, ½–1 drachm; tincture of scillae, 5–30 minims.

Potassium iodide, dose from 10 to 30 grains, and sodium bicarbonate dose from 10 to 60 grains, are frequently included in stimulating expectorant mixtures, as they dissolve mucus and render expectoration easier.

Another group of drugs which increases the amount of expectoration by its stimulating action on the respiratory centre, is nux vomica, and its active principle, strychnine.

Depressant expectorants are used when a cough is ineffectual and painful and serves no useful purpose, and therefore is better inhibited. *Examples* include any soothing syrupy preparation in the form of a simple linctus which may contain glycerine, and one or two fruit syrups, such as syrup of prunes and lemons. More powerful ones contain an opiate, either heroin, opium or morphine.

A linctus is usually given in doses of from 1 to 2 drachms, and it should be sipped slowly from a warmed teaspoon.

Hypnotics and Narcotics. *Narcotics* are substances which produce abnormally deep sleep. General anaesthetics are narcotics. Barbiturates specially prepared for 'basal narcosis' have a similar action. Other drugs including morphia, grain $\frac{1}{8}$–$\frac{1}{3}$; heroin, grain $\frac{1}{25}$–$\frac{1}{8}$; hyoscine or scopolamine, grain $\frac{1}{200}$–$\frac{1}{100}$; and more recently pethidine hydrochloride, 100 milligrammes and physeptone, 5 to 10 milligrammes, are, because of their pain relieving properties, sometimes used and classed as narcotics.

Hypnotics or *soporifics* are drugs which produce sleep and have no effect on pain. These drugs are used in the treatment of insomnia but there is a tendency to become habituated to taking them. *Examples* include the *bromides* which are depressants of the nervous system. Potassium bromide, ammonium bromide and sodium bromide are given in doses of 15 to 30 grains. Sedobrol is a proprietary preparation of bromide containing 1[illegible] grains of the drug in each tablet; the tablets are brown, and when dissolved taste like meat juice. One or two tablets are given at bedtime. The *synthetic preparations* form a large group of hypnotics including:

(*a*) *Halogen derivatives*. Chloral hydrate, dose 10 to 20 grains; this drug is often combined with potassium bromide. Chloralamide and chlorbutol (Chloretone) are other examples given in doses of 5 to 20 grains.

(*b*) *Paraldehyde*, dose 30 to 120 minims, is a powerful hypnotic.

(*c*) *Sulphones*. Sulphonal, dose 5 to 20 grains, is a good hypnotic but slow in action.

Urea derivatives. Barbitone (veronal) dose 5 to 10 grains and sodium barbitone (medinal) 5 to 10 grains are examples. Then come the large class of *barbituric hypnotics* which include luminal, dose ½ to 2 grains, used in the treatment of epilepsy and chorea beginning with ½ a grain twice a day; dial, dose 1½ to 3 grains, sodium amytal, dose 3 to 9 grains, and nembutal, 3 to 9 grains. Sodium seconyl is a rapidly acting preparation which is capable of producing hypnosis in from 15 to 30 minutes.

Two drugs which contain a little morphia and opium respectively are di-dial (containing morphia) dose ½ to 1½ grains; and Dover's powder or pulv. ipecacuanha and opium, dose 5 to 10 grains, which is often given at the onset of influenza because it is a diaphoretic also.

Laxatives (see Purgatives).

Mydriatics are drugs used to dilate the pupil of the eye.

Examples are atropine and homatropine, in ½ to 2 per cent solutions instilled as necessary to produce, and maintain the desired effect.

Myotics are substances which cause contraction of the pupil of the eye and include eserine and pilocarpine, instilled as above. (Opium causes contraction of the pupil of the eye, which is one of the earliest signs of the overdose of this drug, but it is not used as a myotic.)

Purgatives. Aperient drugs are usually given by mouth. In a few instances rectal administration is made (see Enemata). The hypodermic administration of pituitrin—dose from 5 to 10 units—which acts as a stimulant to peristalsis, is used in the treatment of paralytic ileus.

Purgatives are classified, according to the severity of their action, into *laxatives*, *simple purgatives*, and *drastic purgatives* or *cathartics*. They are further classified according to the manner in which their effect is produced, as *lubricants*, such as liquid paraffin, dose 1–8 drachms; *hydragogues*, which extract water from the blood, such as concentrated doses of magnesium sulphate; and *cholagogues*, which stimulate the gall-bladder to empty itself and also stimulate the liver in its production of bile. Examples include salines, mercury and aloes. Other substances act as aperients because they increase the food residue and therefore add to the bulk of the contents of the intestine—among food substances producing this effect are fruits, green vegetables and wholemeal bread.

The action of the bowel may also be affected by drugs acting on the neuromuscular mechanism. In spastic constipation belladonna is administered, and by its antispasmodic action effects relaxation of the contracted gut and so relieves the constipation resulting from this.

Conversely, when the walls of the bowel are relaxed and lacking in tone, or dilated, the administration of small doses of strychnine or nux vomica will increase the tone and stimulate contraction of the muscle in the walls of the gut.

Examples of laxatives. Syrup of figs, 1–4 drachms; confection of senna, 1–2 drachms; liquid magnesia, 1–2 ounces; pulv. glycyrrhizae co., which contains sulphur, senna and liquorice root, is given in doses of 1–2 drachms.

Simple purgatives include aloes, in the form of pil. aloes, 4–8 grains, extract of aloes, 2–8 grains. Cascara is given as extract of cascara sagrada, 2–8 grains. In tablet form, and liquid extract of cascara, dose ½–1 drachm. This form is bitter and very often objected to by patients, and is therefore usually given in capsules. A proprietary drug, which is quite pleasant to take, is cascara evacuant, dose ½–1 drachm. Gregory's powder contains rhubarb and magnesia. Phenolphthalein, 1 to 5 grains, is usually combined with liquid paraffin.

Salines remove a good deal of water from the bowel. Magnesium sulphate and sodium sulphate are given in doses of ½ to 2 drachms dissolved in water.

Seidlitz powders are an example of a saline aperient. These are prepared in two packets. A blue packet which contains sodium bicarbonate and sodium potassium tartrate and a white packet containing tartaric acid. The contents of the blue packet are dissolved in half a tumbler of water, the contents of the white packet are added, the mixture is briskly stirred and the fluid is drunk whilst in effervescence.

Drastic purgatives. Calomel ½ to 3 grains. Calomel may be given as a single dose of one, two, or three grains. Or it may be given in ¼ grain or ½ grain doses, until a maximum of 1 to 3 grains has been given. Calomel should always be freshly obtained as it becomes altered and converted into perchloride of mercury when kept. As a general rule calomel is either combined with another purgative or followed by a saline aperient in order to prevent the drug accumulating in the system.

Pulv. scammony co., 10 to 20 grains, and pulv. jalapae co., 10 to 60 grains, are used when it is desirable to obtain a watery action of the bowel, as, for example, when oedema is present. Pulv. jalapae co. contains jalap, ginger and cream of tartar.

Pil. colocynth, 2 to 4 grains, is a very strong aperient. It is frequently combined with hyoscyamus which is an antispasmodic and prevents pain being produced by the griping action of the colocynth. Hyoscyamus belongs to the belladonna group of drugs and therefore this substance should not be used as an aperient for patients suffering from glaucoma.

Castor oil when given in large doses, of from ½ to 1 ounce, is a strong purgative. Croton oil, in doses of from ½ to 1 minim, is prescribed in apoplexy and cerebral compression when a very rapid action of the bowel is desired.

Styptics. Any drugs used to arrest bleeding by local application are described as styptics. An example may be found in the use of adrenalin 1-1,000 for packing the nasal cavity before an operation. Tincture of ferri perchloride is another example. Most astringent substances are styptic in action.

Stimulants. Stimulants usually act either by means of the circulation or through the central nervous system, by stimulating the different special centres and so producing an effect on the function of some particular organ. *For example*, apomorphine stimulates the vomiting centre in the medulla and makes the patient sick. Some of the expectorant drugs produce their effect by stimulating the respiratory centre. Strychnine is a stimulant to the general circulation. Caffeine, coramine and camphor are cardiac stimulants.

Speaking more generally the term stimulant is used to imply the administration of some form of *alcohol*. In hospital practice, brandy is most commonly used. The dose for infants is from a few minims up to ½ drachm. The adult dose is from ½ to 1 ounce at a time, not more as a rule than 2–3 ounces being given in the 24 hours. Brandy should never be given at the same time as other medicines, and it should always be diluted—one part of brandy to two parts of water. Port wine is a stimulant sometimes given to convalescent patients as an aid to improving their appetite. As a rule 2 to 3 ounces are given each day with meals. Champagne is an expensive form of alcohol. It is given in small doses frequently to patients who are very ill and who for some reason are incapable of taking or retaining other forms of liquid.

Alcohol acts as a general stimulant to the circulation and so increases for the moment the sense of wellbeing. Because of its rapid effect it is, therefore, a very valuable cardiac stimulant in emergencies such as fainting and syncope. The exhilarating effect of alcohol, however, is followed by depression of the central nervous system.

Stomachics are drugs used to stimulate the activity of the stomach one group being described as *bitters*, which stimulate the flow of saliva and gastric juice. They are bitter to taste as the name implies and include infusion of calumba co., infusio gentianae co., and infusio tincturae aurantii. The dose of each is from 30 to 60 minims. They are used in many tonic preparations and are gastric tonics.

Stomachic substances may also act by increasing the movements of the stomach. Tincture of nux vomica, dose from 10 to 30 minims, is an example of this type.

The function of the stomach is improved in cases of achlorhydria by the addition of dilute hydrochloric acid, dose from 5 to 60 minims. This drug is given with orange juice and taken during, and about 10 minutes after, food.

Tonic drugs are used to improve the tone of the general health. *For example* (see Stomachics), gastric tonics such as gentian may be used to stimulate the appetite, thus resulting in increase in weight and general physical improvement.

Other tonic substances such as iron act by improving the quality of the blood, which may be given in the form of Blaud's pill, from 1 to 5 grains; or it may be combined with another drug, as in ferri et ammonii citrate, dose from 5 to 15 grains, or in a mixture, such as Parrish's chemical food, which contains iron, phosphates and calcium among other ingredients. The dose is from 30 to 120 minims. Sometimes iron is administered with arsenic, which is a nerve stimulant, thus combining two forms of tonic substances in one mixture.

Preparations of iron should always be carefully dealt with, as iron stains the teeth. When liquid preparations are used, they should be given through a straw, and the teeth should be well brushed afterwards.

Strychnine is a general tonic to the circulatory system as well as a respiratory stimulant, and it is contained in many tonic mixtures and preparations. Easton's syrup is one example, containing $\frac{1}{60}$ grain of strychnine in each drachm. In addition it contains iron, which is a blood tonic, and quinine which acts as a nerve and gastric tonic.

UNDERSTANDING A PRESCRIPTION

The word prescription is derived from *prae* meaning 'before', and, *scribo*, I write. It is the usual manner in which drugs are ordered and contains instructions from the doctor to the dispenser as to the ingredients to be used, and the manner in which the medicine is to be administered.

It is usually written in Latin, partly because this is a universal language and therefore the prescription written in it can be dispensed in most civilized countries, and partly because the majority of patients cannot read Latin and some physicians think that it would not be good for a patient to know exactly what drug he is having.

A prescription is divided in to five parts:

(1) The *heading*, which indicates the name of the patient. Beneath this in the left-hand corner is written R meaning *recipe* or 'take thou'.

(2) *Names of the substances prescribed* come next. Each occupies a separate line, and is followed by the symbol of the weight and measure to be used and the amount to be included in the mixture.

(3) The *instructions to the dispenser* as to how the medicine is to be prepared, as to whether it is to be a liquid, pill, powder, etc.

(4) *Directions as to mode of administration.* This also may be in Latin for the instruction of the dispenser, but it is also written clearly in English on the label for the use of the nurse and patient.

(5) Lastly, at the bottom right-hand corner, the doctor writes his initials or signature, and in most cases adds the date.

For special precautions taken in the writing of prescriptions containing dangerous drugs, see note on p. 331.

THE SAFE CUSTODY OF MEDICINES AND DRUGS

In hospital practice all drugs are checked as they are received from the dispensary.

The *medicine cupboard* is usually kept or placed in a room adjoining but not in the ward.

All poisons are kept in a separate cupboard, in which different compartments or shelves may be allocated to different types of poisons—for example, lotions, liniments etc., may be in one part, and the very potent drugs used for hypodermic injection in another part of the cupboard. As far as possible all poisons should always be in the same place, so that a nurse going to a cupboard in a hurry will automatically put her hand in the direction in which she expects to find that for which she is looking, though this must not be relied on. In addition, the poison cupboard should be lit from inside, and failing this precaution the nurse should use a torch when the light is poor. Poisons are kept in bottles distinguishable to the touch by being ridged or grooved, and to sight by being coloured blue or green. A nurse should never be permitted to change the label on any bottle containing poison—this should only be done by the dispenser who is responsible for issuing the poison in any particular bottle.

The *poison cupboard must always be kept locked*—in some instances a double locked cupboard is used, but the important point is that the key should never be kept in a so-called 'safe place', but should always be on the person of the sister or head nurse in charge of the ward, who as far as possible should herself always handle the contents of this cupboard. A junior nurse should never be permitted to administer drugs to a patient.

Certain special substances including vaccines, antitoxin sera and insulin, together with other drugs of animal derivation, require to be kept in a *cool place*. A trained nurse should be familiar with the customary dose of the drugs in constant use that may be ordered; if in doubt, she should verify the dose, and she may even query a dose if she considers it excessive in amount, though such a query should of course be made with tact—a nurse should never be afraid to ask questions about the dosage and action of drugs—the number of dangerous drugs on the market is so various and they are so often made up in different strengths that she need never be ashamed to show her ignorance on this matter and should always be ready to learn.

As far as possible trained nurses should make themselves familiar with new drugs introduced from time to time. The action of any drug given to a patient should be ascertained, so that its effects can be noted, and any untoward symptoms quickly observed.

A nurse should be very strict with regard to the checking of drugs. During her hospital training she will be impressed by the ritual with which the checking of a dangerous drug is carried out, and the meticulous precision observed by everyone concerned, so that if she remains faithful to the training she has received she will not be likely to err.

(See also the note on the administration of the Dangerous Drugs Act, on p. 331).

RULES FOR GIVING MEDICINES BY MOUTH

Medicines must be given punctually and, as they are most readily absorbed on a comparatively empty stomach, they are usually given between meals and feedings. They are given at stated hours, such as 10, 2, and 6; or 11, 3, and 7, unless the medicine is specially required to be given in relation to food.

A gastric irritant, such as arsenic or iron, is given after food. Medicines employed to produce a general beneficial effect on the wellbeing of the body, to produce increase of weight and improve the changes which make up metabolism are also given after food. Examples of such medicines are malt and cod-liver oil.

Medicines given to allay spasm, such as chalk and bismuth, to inhibit secretion, such as belladonna, atropine and olive oil, to affect the reaction of the gastric juice, such as hydrochloric acid or alkalis, and bitters, which are given to stimulate the gastric secretion, are all given before food; though when alkalis are used in the treatment of peptic ulcer, with the object of reducing the acidity of the gastric juice fairly constantly, they are given after meals.

Aperients are usually given on an empty stomach, last thing at night, especially when the drug employed is laxative in its effect and acts slowly, taking from 10 to 12 hours to produce its effect. Aperients which have a rapid action, such as the saline aperients, are given on a fasting stomach first thing in the morning, half an hour before the first drink of tea is taken.

A nurse should have a good working knowledge of the time an aperient she may be asked to give will take to act, and she should administer the medicine at a time which will allow the patient to be as little disturbed as possible by its action later. Strong purgatives like large doses of castor oil and colocynth act in from 4 to 6 hours; hydragogue purgatives, like salines and jalap, may act within 2 hours. Drugs such as these should not be given at the patient's bedtime or the result will be that he will be disturbed in the early morning hours.

The *articles required for giving a dose of medicine* are shown in fig. 149, p. 289. In some cases the patient's bedcard will be required to verify the prescription, although in most wards the sister or head nurse checks the prescription written on the bottle of medicine with the original on the prescription card as soon as the medicine is received by her; a distinguishing mark is made by the ward sister on the bottle to show that the prescription has been checked. But whenever the medicine contains a dangerous drug the bedcard should be produced and the dose checked by a second person with the prescription on the card at each administration.

The **administration of medicines** requires the greatest possible care and thoughtfulness, as well as undivided attention. Whilst pouring out and delivering medicines, a nurse should not attend to any other matter; there should be no general conversation or chatter; the nurse engaged in giving medicines should not be spoken to, or otherwise interrupted, except in a case of emergency. The directions on the medicine bottle label should be read carefully, before and after pouring out the dose of medicine.

Bottles containing medicine should always be shaken but not by an up and down movement which causes froth to form on top of the fluid; the nurse should place one finger on the cork to prevent its flying out, and then shake the bottle, using a side to side, swinging pendulum-like movement, inverting the bottle completely once or twice during the process.

In *pouring out a dose of medicine*, the bottle should be held with the label uppermost, and the fluid be poured out away from the label, any drips being caught with a swab of cotton wool before replacing the cork.

The marked medicine glass or measure should be held with the marks against the light, just above the level of the eye, so that the person pouring out the medicine has to raise her head slightly to look at the level of the fluid in the glass. The surface of fluid in a small measure is not flat, it has a curve—called the *meniscus*—which is lowest at the centre so that, if the measure is held just above the level of the eye, the lowest point of the curve of the meniscus may be considered to be on a level with the marking on the medicine glass.

As far as possible medicines should be poured out at the bedside of the patient for whom they are intended, but in all cases the medicine should be delivered to the patient before any sediment can settle. The nurse should stand by the patient until the medicine has been swallowed, and if permissible a little water may be given afterwards or the mouth may be rinsed. In administering medicines which have an unpleasant flavour the mouth should always be rinsed afterwards, and peppermint water is a very pleasant preparation to use for this purpose. Medicines that stain the teeth are usually administered through a straw and the teeth brushed immediately afterwards.

Oily preparations may require special preparation, and in all cases if permissible they may be followed by a section of orange given to suck. In administering castor oil, for example, it should be disguised in some such way as the following. Take an oil measure, which is made of delf or earthenware, and warm it. Pour in some orange or lemon juice and float the dose of castor oil on to this, cover with more fruit juice, taking care not to shake or move the measure about, so that the oil is kept floating inside a covering of fruit juice. In taking it to the patient advise him to open his mouth and pour it quickly to the back of it and swallow at once in order to avoid movement of the fluid which would result in his tasting the castor oil. Giving a little bread to chew, or bread and salt, after the administration of any unpleasant form of oil, tends to relieve the mouth of the nauseating sliminess. If the patient is not allowed solid food he may spit out the bread, or alternatively he might rinse out his mouth with peppermint water.

In giving *tablets*, *pills*, *cachets* and *capsules*, they should be delivered in a spoon and accompanied by a large glass of water. *Cachets* may be softened by placing them in a spoonful of water before swallowing. *Powders* should be unfolded, collected to the middle of the packet and poured on to the centre of the protruded tongue. The patient should be given water sufficient to swallow the powder. If he objects to this mode of administration, the powder may be buried in a spoonful of jelly or jam, provided these form part of the patient's diet.

Effervescing powders should be dissolved in half a tumbler of water and drunk whilst effervescing.

Pills. Some patients find it extremely difficult to swallow pills, and the nurse should, in such cases, be very patient and try various means—the pill may be buried in jelly or jam, or in a piece of bread, if the patient is allowed these. It may, however, have to be crushed and given as a powder.

Giving medicine to children. As far as possible the medicine should be made pleasant to taste. The nurse may have to be firm, but force should never be used. A child can usually be persuaded to swallow his dose of medicine by having a sweet, a nice drink or a little fruit or other similar treat after it. In some children's wards it is usual practice to give the daily ration of fruit in small pieces at medicine times. A tiny child should have his cheeks gently held together by the nurse, and the medicine administered by means of a spoon; if the child cries he will only breathe through the medicine, thus gargling with it for a few seconds and, when he stops to breathe in, he will swallow the dose.

MODES OF ADMINISTERING DRUGS

By *way of the alimentary canal*, either by mouth, which is by far the commonest route used, or by means of the rectum. All drugs taken by mouth are passed to the liver in the portal circulation and excreted in large quantities by the kidneys without remaining long in the circulation.

By *hypodermic* or *subcutaneous injection.* By this route drugs enter the circulation through absorption by means of the lymphatics, and many drugs, that would be injuriously affected by the digestive juices if given by mouth, are administered in this way, including adrenalin, insulin and some forms of liver extract.

By *intramuscular injection.* By this route more rapid action is made possible, and many of the preparations of drugs suspended in oil and preparations of quinine are administered thus.

Intrathecally, or by means of the cerebrospinal fluid route, and this method is chosen in the treatment of some forms of meningitis (for mode of administration, see lumbar puncture, p. 163).

Intraperitoneal route. This method is most commonly adopted for the administration of saline and, more recently, sera have been given in this way with excellent results and with less danger of complications than when given by the intravenous method.

Intravenous method (for mode of administration, see p. 315.

By the skin by inunction and ionization (see p. 322).

By inhalation (see also p. 316).

By **subcutaneous or hypodermic administration or injection.** By this means drugs reach the blood stream more rapidly than when given by mouth. It is also employed in many instances where the drug does not remain potent when it is administered by the mouth, owing to the affecting of its action by the digestive juices.

The *apparatus required* is a hypodermic needle, which should be sharp, and a syringe capable of holding 15–20 minims. Some swabs and possibly some mild antiseptic, or alcohol, should be provided to cleanse the skin. See figs. 150 and 152–4, pp. 289–92.

Method of administration. There seems to be a considerable amour of uncertainty amongst nurses as to whether the drugs which are put u in solid form, in tablets or tabloids, may or may not be boiled in a te spoon over a spirit lamp in preparation for administration.

The following solutions may be sterilized by boiling without bein injuriously affected: Morphine hydrochloride, pilocarpine nitrate an strychnine sulphate; but in the case of such drugs as the following, th distilled water should be boiled first to render it sterile and then allowe to cool to about 100° F. before adding the hypodermic tablet: Apo morphine hydrochloride—atropine sulphate—digitalin—eserin—emetin hydrochloride—heroin hydrochloride (diamorphine)—hyoscine hydro bromide—morphine and atropine—morphine, atropine, and strychnine— morphine and hyoscine—strophanthin.

Charging a syringe. There are different methods of handling the tablet but it should not be touched by fingers since inflammation may occur a the site of injection if aseptic technique is not observed. Some sisters kee a small sterile spoon in the dish with the hypodermic syringe and needle while others prefer to use a tiny minim glass. The tablet should be shake out of the tube into the spoon or glass, which should be dry so that, if mor than one tablet is shaken out, the unwanted ones can be replaced in th tube. Ten to fifteen minims of distilled water may be added to the table in the spoon or glass and when the tablet is dissolved the whole of th fluid should be drawn up into the syringe.

Another method is to shake the tablet from the spoon into the barrel o the syringe, replace the piston, and then draw up into the syringe th 10–15 minims of distilled water as desired. A sterile swab may be hel firmly over the lower end of the syringe whilst it is gently shaken up and down in order to help mix the drug contained in the dissolving table with the water.

Methods of charging a syringe from a phial and from a bottle are show in figs. 152 and 153, p. 291.

Having charged the syringe the air should be expelled by holding the syringe, needle pointing upwards, and slowly pressing the piston into the barrel, until all air bubbles have been expressed from the needle and a drop of the solution is seen at the end of it.

In giving a hypodermic injection the nurse should first explain to the patient that he is going to have a slight prick, but, as the needle is sharp, it will not hurt very much. Then, choosing a portion of tissue fairly well covered with fat, such as lies over the supinator longus muscle on the extensor aspect of the forearm, cleanse the skin with ether or alcohol on a cotton wool swab, and then either grasp the tissue between the thumb and forefinger of the left hand, or, if preferred, stretch the skin by pressure of the forefinger and thumb, but in this case care should be taken to avoid bruising; the needle is then inserted beneath the skin parallel with the surface, grasp of the tissue is relaxed and the solution is gently, but not too slowly, pressed out of the barrel of the syringe by gentle pressure on the end of the piston, either with the thumb or the palm of the hand. The needle is then withdrawn and as it leaves the skin a swab is placed over the puncture and held there for a few moments. If a tumour of fluid is visible, gentle massage in an upward direction away from the puncture should be used to disperse it. All hypodermic injections should be given in an upward direction as this corresponds with the flow of the lymphatic stream by means of which the drug is about to be carried into the blood. It seems needless to say that in no circumstances should such an injection be made over a joint or over any part in which the fascia is taut. An injection made into such a locality gives unnecessary pain as the fluid, penetrating the dense tissue, causes local pressure.

The intracutaneous route. For this method, which is employed with comparative rarity, an especially fine needle is necessary as *the drug is injected into the substance of the skin and not beneath it.* It is sometimes used in the administration of local anaesthesia, and also in the administration of toxin and antitoxin in the Schick and Dick tests, and also in the Schultz-Charlton and Mantoux tests.

Intramuscular route. This is used when more rapid absorption is required than that obtained by the subcutaneous route, as for example in the administration of serum. It is also used when the substances injected, such as oily preparations, and preparations of quinine, might prove irritating if given more superficially.

The *apparatus required* is similar to that for subcutaneous injection, but a larger syringe is used, since from 5 to 10 cubic centimetres are usually given. As in this method the needle is larger, and therefore makes a larger puncture, it is usual to provide a small collodion dressing to cover or seal this. The fluid to be injected should be warmed to the heat of the body by standing the phial in water for 10 minutes before administration, so that less pain may be caused and the fluid more quickly absorbed.

Method. Having charged the syringe and prepared the skin, a large muscle is chosen, such as that of the buttock, the outer aspect of the thigh or the scapula region for the administration of large quantities, the deltoid and supinator longus being the sites commonly used for smaller quantities. The needle is plunged deep into the muscle at right angles to the skin—in the case of the buttock the needle is plunged right up to the hilt, the nurse steadying its passage through the skin by a forefinger placed on the hilt of the needle. The injection should then be slowly but steadily made.

Intraperitoneal route. Drugs are rarely administered by this route, but it is one which is quite commonly used for the administration of saline to dehydrated babies; and more recently it is being used for the administration of serum, which by this route is found to be almost as rapidly effective as by the intravenous method, with less possibility of the occurrence of dangerous complications.

Intravenous route. This is used when the most rapid action of the drug possible is necessary, as in diabetic or insulin coma, when insulin or glucose is necessary, but cannot be administered by any other route. To administer a small quantity of fluid by this route *the following articles will be required*—a 5 or 10 c.c. syringe and needle, ready sterilized, and if these have been placed in water they must be rinsed in saline or distilled water before an intravenous injection is made. For a larger quantity a Horrocks's flask should be provided (see fig. 70, p. 208). It is becoming an increasing practice, however, to sterilize the articles used for this purpose either by boiling them in liquid paraffin or by dry heat in an oven. An exceedingly sharp, finely graded needle is necessary, otherwise it may only pass over the surface of the vein as the physician attempts to insert it.

Ether and swabs will be required, with which to cleanse the skin, and dry sterile swab to place over the puncture for a few minutes when th needle is withdrawn. Some physicians order a small collodion dressin to be applied.

A light rubber tourniquet is applied to the arm in order to compre the veins so that the one chosen for injection stands well out, and whil the tourniquet is being adjusted, if the patient is conscious and capab of movement, he should be asked to close his fist and flex and extend hi forearm, or to open and close his fist.

Method. A doctor usually gives this injection. He will charge the syring and expel all air, whilst the nurse steadies the patient's arm and is read to loosen the tourniquet when the doctor gives the word. He passes th needle into the distended vein, taking care to keep in the lumen of it, an not to pass through the vein—it is for this reason that the nurse keeps th patient's arm very still—and when once in the vein he will require th tourniquet to be very gently loosened. He then withdraws the piston s that a little blood enters the syringe, showing the needle is in the vein makes the injection slowly and evenly and, when this is completed, with draws it. At the same time the nurse places the dry sterile swab over th puncture, flexes the arm on to this and holds it steady for a few moments If the slight oozing of blood which may occur does not cease, she applie a collodion dressing.

INHALATIONS

The gases, vapours and fumes of drugs are inhaled either in order t produce a local effect on the upper respiratory passages through whic the vapour passes, or to influence the circulation in the lungs and s either increase or decrease the bronchial secretions, or to allay spasm o the tubes by effecting alteration in the vasomotor control of the blood vessels, or bronchial vessels. Inhalations are also used as a means of producing the absorption of a drug through the lungs when a general effect is required as in the case of the induction of a general anaesthetic by this route, or when rapid absorption is known to occur and produce an effect on one of the other systems of the body, as in the administration of amyl nitrite in the treatment of angina.

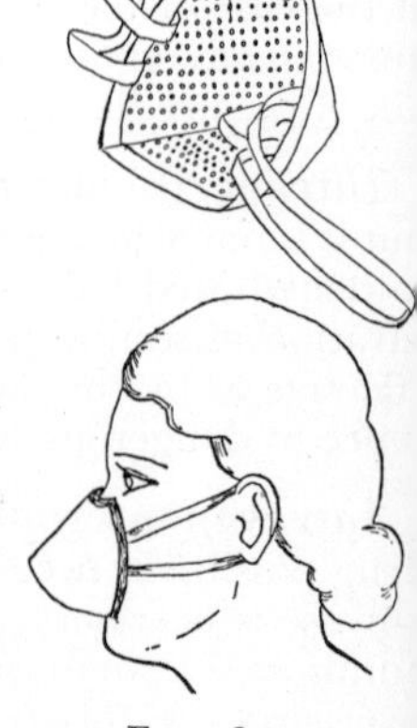

FIG. 162.

Burney-Yeo's inhaler—above, the interior is shown; below, the inhaler.

The drugs most commonly used to relieve congestion in the upper respiratory passages are menthol and eucalyptus, administered either on gauze or in water. *Those used as a respiratory disinfectant* in purulent bronchitis and lung abscess include creosote, carbolic, iodine, oil of pine and friar's balsam.

Any of these disinfecting substances may be given by means of a *Burney-Yeo inhaler*, which consists of a frame of perforated zinc the edges of which are bound, the inhaler being worn over the nose and mouth. A few drops of the drug—as ordered—are placed in the pad in the inhaler, which is then retained in position by elastic over the ears. Another method of administering this type of drug is by means of a 'creosote bath'. One ounce of creosote is rapidly vaporized over a lamp placed in a closed room in which the patient sits or lies. His eyes are protected by goggles and his nose is lightly plugged with cotton wool. He remains in this 'bath' for a definite period, or periods, each day, as ordered by the physician.

Ammonia, which is inhaled in cases of fainting and syncope, irritates the mucous membrane and also reflexly stimulates the respiratory, cardiac and vasomotor centres, thus improving the circulation. It must be applied to the nostrils with caution, and the eyes should be kept closed, as otherwise the conjunctiva will be very seriously irritated by it.

Amyl nitrite is used in the treatment of some forms of angina pectoris. Tiny capsules containing two or three minims of the drug are crushed in gauze and held to the nose for the patient to inhale, and, as the immediate effect produced is flushing of the face head and neck, as the drug causes dilation of the arterioles and capillaries, its effect on the spasmodically contracted coronary blood vessels is thereby demonstrated. Amyl nitrite is also sometimes used to relieve spasm of the bronchial tubes in *cases of asthma.*

Stramonium. The dried leaves of this plant are burned and the smoke inhaled, or stramonium cigarettes may be smoked provided the patient can inhale the smoke into his lungs. Stramonium relaxes the spasm of the bronchial tubes and is *used in the relief of asthma.*

The leaves may be ignited in a small bowl and held under the patient's nose. He should be instructed to close his eyes in order to avoid irritation by the smoke. If the leaves are not obtainable a little powdered stramonium may be ignited in the same way. Some sisters use a shallow dish, and make a stiff paper cone, placing the large wide open end in the dish and causing the patient to inhale the smoke out of the other, narrow end. Leaves of *belladonna* may be used in the same way and for the same purpose.

Steam inhalations. Some of the drugs—such as menthol and eucalyptus—employed for the relief of nasal congestion, and the antiseptic drugs used in purulent bronchitis, may be combined with hot water and the vapour inhaled, but the volatility of the drug has to be considered when this method is used. Those which vaporize easily should be put into water not exceeding 120° F.; those which vaporize less readily may be placed in the receptacle first and have the water poured over them. It is impossible to inhale the steam from water hotter than 160° F. This is a point that all nurses should know and remember, as the patient may otherwise be caused considerable inconvenience and may even have his upper respiratory passages injured.

Nelson's inhaler (see fig. 157, p. 293). This inhaler is supplied in various sizes, the average being that in which two pints of water will fill the inhaler to a point below the air inlet. This should never be covered, as if air cannot reach the fluid in the vessel the vapour cannot rise. The mouthpiece, which should always be boiled, is made of glass, and passes through a cork which fits the neck of the inhaler. It should be placed in the direction shown in fig. 163, p. 318, or in the direction opposite to the air inlet, because, if it lay in the same plane as the inlet, when the patient breathed into the inhaler he would force steam out of the air inlet on to the region of his chest, and the moisture penetrating his clothing might scald him.

The inhaler having been filled, it should be delivered to the bedside covered by a flannel bag which fits it, and standing in a wooden bowl or porringer as indicated (fig. 157, letter B). The patient sits up or leans over on one side, while the nurse arranges the apparatus and instructs the patient to place his lips to the mouthpiece—which may be protected by a piece of gauze—and to breathe in so that he receives the steam. He may breathe out into the inhaler, but this will cause steam to rise through the outlet, and it is better if he will remove his lips for a moment from the mouthpiece whilst breathing out. In many instances the nurse will have to stand by the patient's side steadying the inhaler for him. To inhale the steam which will rise from two pints of water will occupy from 15 to 20 minutes.

In some cases, particularly that of one with chronic bronchitis or winter cough, the patient is likely to be familiar with this treatment and so to be able to hold the inhaler for himself. It may be placed on a bedtable in front of the patient as he sits up in bed and, as it is adequately protected with a flannel cover and by the bowl or porringer in which it stands, the patient is not likely to be burnt.

After a warm inhalation the patient must not move about or go into places where the temperature varies but should remain in the same room.

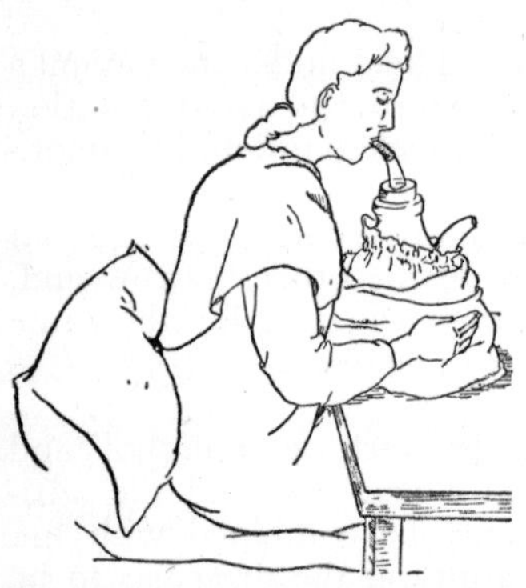

FIG. 163.—THE USE OF NELSON'S INHALER.

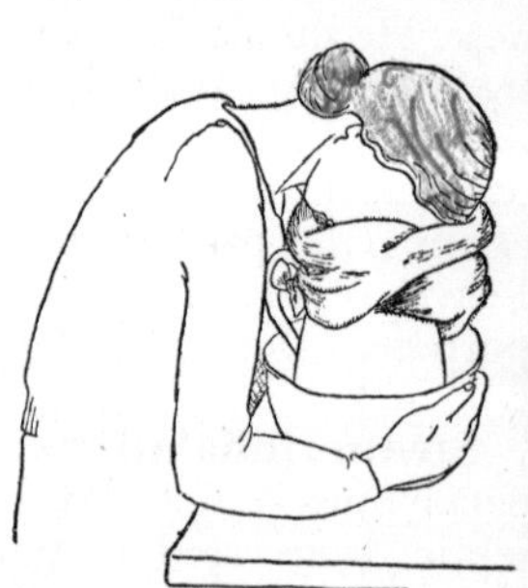

FIG. 164.—METHOD OF INHALING FROM A JUG DRAPED WITH A TOWEL.

Jug inhalation. Any ordinary jug or a two-pint delf jam jar may be used for the purpose of an inhalation; but in this case, as there is no mouthpiece, the patient may wear a towel over his head in order to form a canopy under which to collect steam, or the mouth of the jug may be draped with a towel turban fashion to render the opening small enough for the patient to apply his nose and mouth to it, as shown in fig. 164.

A *steam kettle* is used when required to maintain a constantly moist atmosphere; when the *steam tent* method is employed a kettle of boiling water is arranged to admit steam into the tent, the latter contrived by use of a light covered-in framework attached to the bed. The tent should not be hotter than 75° F.; it is necessary for the tent to be well ventilated, and for this purpose air inlets and outlets should be provided. A steam tent is rather cumbersome and has been largely superseded by the modification of placing only a *canopy* over the head of the bed and providing a steam kettle as shown in fig. 156, p. 293. By this method the difficulties of nursing a patient in a tent and of properly ventilating the tent are obviated.

Administration of oxygen. Deficiency of oxygen in the blood, which s described as *anoxaemia*, is always serious, because the production of nergy and heat by oxidation of food materials in the tissues depends upon he presence of an adequate supply of oxygen in the blood. Deficiency of xygen may arise in a number of conditions including cardiac failure —when the pulmonary circulation is poor—in disease of the lungs, as neumonia, in chronic conditions of the lungs including emphysema, and n phosgene and chlorine gas poisoning. Anoxaemia also follows severe aemorrhage when the haemoglobin content of the blood becomes low. It occurs in cases of shock and collapse when the circulation of the blood s depressed, and as a result of carbon monoxide poisoning because the haemoglobin combines with this gas rather than with oxygen. It also occurs when the absorption of oxygen is reduced owing to a very high altitude—as when flying or mountain climbing.

When *carbon dioxide* is administered either it is combined with oxygen in a 5 or 10 per cent mixture, or dual cylinders—one of carbon dioxide and the other containing oxygen—are coupled together on one stand, the tube leading from each cylinder being connected by a Y-shaped connexion piece to a single tubing which passes from the stem of the Y and conveys the mixture which is then regulated by the different valves on each of the cylinders and so administered to the patient.

A variety of apparatus is employed for the administration of oxygen. It is ideal to have a fine adjustment valve attached to the oxygen cylinder and a combined flowmeter and humidifier. A Wolff's bottle may alternatively be used.

Nasal catheter. Extra holes are cut in the end which is lubricated and passed 4 inches into one nostril and fixed to the patient's face with strapping. By giving oxygen at 4 litres per minute a concentration of 30 per cent can be delivered.

Nasal tubes. Tudor Edwards's spectacle frame catheter carrier or Marriott's catheter carrier may be employed. Both carry cycle valve tubing

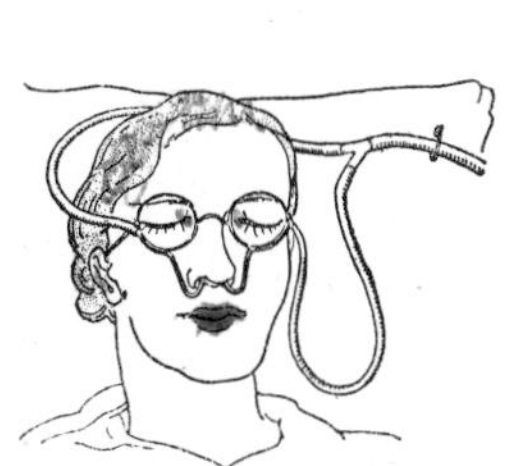

FIG. 165.—TUDOR EDWARDS'S SPECTACLE FRAME CATHETER CARRIER.

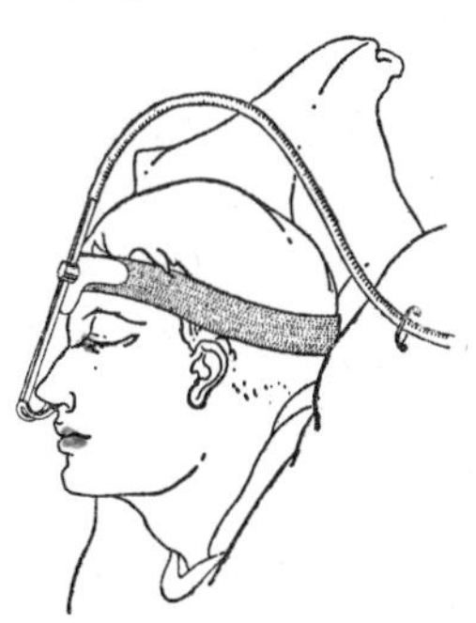

FIG. 166.—MARRIOTT'S HEAD-PIECE AND CATHETER CARRIER.

which is lubricated with liquid paraffin and percaine, or cocaine ointment, and passed into the nostrils. This form of tubing is more comfortable than the nasal catheter.

B.L.B. inhalation apparatus (Boothy, Lovelace, Bulbulian). This consists of three parts, the mask which fits the nose, hollow tubes pass from this into one single tube, through a connecting regulator device to the reservoir-breathing bag. The mask is adjusted by straps. The concentration of oxygen depends on having the airports on the connecting device open or closed. With all holes closed the patient receives over 90 per cent oxygen when delivered at 6 to 7 litres per minute. He receives about 75 per cent, with two airports open when delivered at 5 litres per minute, and 50 per cent, when delivered at the rate of 3 litres per minute. This apparatus will probably replace the use of the oxygen tent, except for cases with facial injuries and those who will not tolerate wearing any apparatus—children, for example.

There are two types of mask, the nasal one shown below, and an oronasal mask, covering nose and mouth, for use when nasal breathing is obstructed.

Oxygen Tent. When a patient, owing to facial injuries or because he will not tolerate it, cannot wear the B.L.B. mask, or if a high concentration of oxygen is necessary, a tent is used (see figs. 160 and 161, p. 296).

The Heidbrink tent is one of the latest, it is made of oiled cloth and is tucked under the mattress at the head and sides and under a blanket in

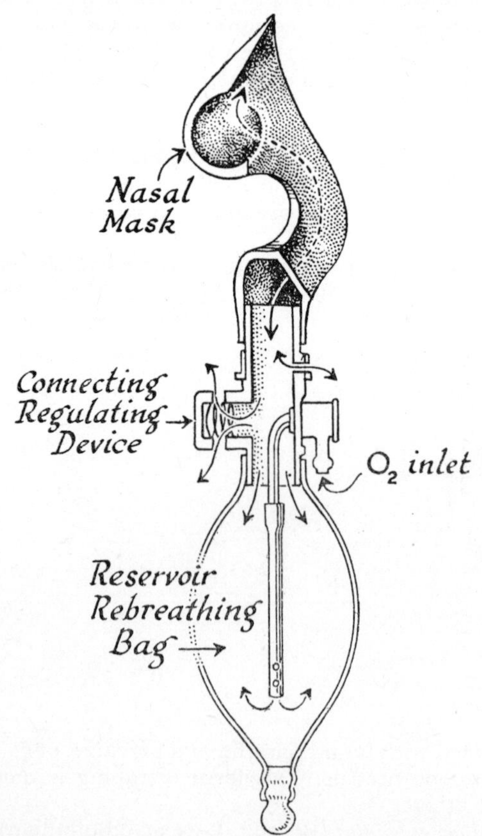

FIG. 167.—B.L.B. OXYGEN DELIVERING MASK IN SECTION (SEE ALSO FIG. 159, p. 295).

ont. The tent is first flooded with oxygen, then a flow of 4 to 5 litres er minute will maintain a service of 40 to 50 per cent oxygen in the ent.

Oxygen is passed into the tent by means of an injector. The pressure f the flow of oxygen causes the tent air to be syphoned out and drawn, with the oxygen, through the soda-lime tank and ice-chamber. The soda-ime removes carbon dioxide from the circulating tent air and the ice ontainer serves several purposes; it causes condensation of the exhaled moisture and maintains relative humidity, and it maintains the temperature of the circulating tent air within a reasonable limit. A thermometer which for purposes of reading is outside the tent is attached to the chamber. The bulb of the thermometer lies in the tent-circulating air-outlet stream, and so records the temperature of the tent air. The temperature should be maintained at 60 or 65° F. and may be regulated by running less of he oxygen through the ice-chamber.

The tent air should be analysed in order to ensure that the percentage of oxygen decided upon by the physician is maintained. The *absorber* illustrated (see fig. 168) contains an ammonium chloride solution which absorbs oxygen. The bell tube with a fine capillary tube attached is inserted in the solution. The syringe is graduated (backwards) and the figures from 1 to 100 represent percentage.

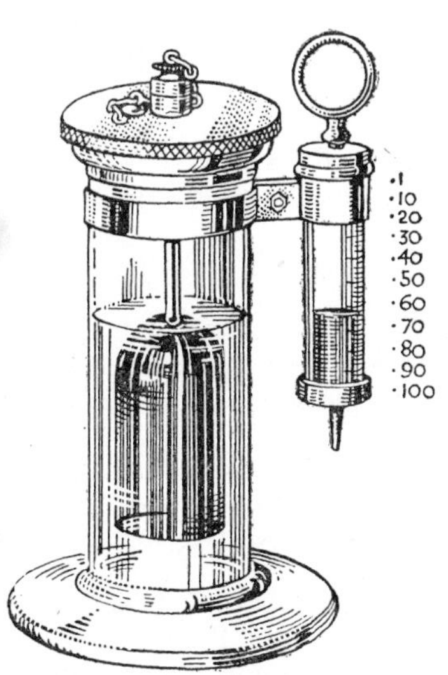

Fig. 168.—Oxygen Absorbing Apparatus with Syringe Graduated Backwards from 100 per cent to 1 per cent.

To take a test of the tent air. Note the level of the absorbing fluid in the capillary tube, then open one of the zipp fasteners of the hood and plunge the syringe in and draw up the piston —the syringe is filled with tent air. Then gently squirt the air into the absorber when it will displace the absorbing solution in the bell tube; allow 20 to 30 seconds. Now gently withdraw the piston until the solution in the capillary tube rises to its previous level. Lift the syringe and read—the reading, 40 or 50 or whatever it may be, is the percentage of oxygen in the tent, because the oxygen has been absorbed by the ammonium chloride.

Precautions regarding fire. The inflammable nature of oxygen must never be forgotten and any articles likely to cause fire, or even any manipulations likely to result in sparks must be most studiously avoided. For example, smoking, the use of matches, lighters, night-lights, gas, electric light switches, wireless, an electric bell push (a hand bell can be provided) and in the case of children all sparking toys, toys provided with flints, toys which can be wound up and will run quickly down so causing friction, must not be used in the tent. It is important also to avoid causing sparks in combing the hair, or moving artificial silk or woollen clothing briskly. All such movements likely to cause sparking must be slowly and carefully carried out. Serious accidents have been caused by lack of sufficient precaution in these respects.

By means of the skin. Inunction is the mode most commonly employed when drugs are applied to the skin in order that they may be absorbed and so produce their effect elsewhere in the body.

The best examples are the use of belladonna in the form of a plaster and mercurial inunction by means of an ointment.

For mercurial inunction the skin should be prepared by washing with hot water and soap, and then drying it well, in order to soften the skin and bring blood well up to the surface. A soft part of the skin is chosen, such as the skin on the inner aspect of the arms or thighs, or of the axillae or groins, or the skin at the sides of the abdomen. When the axilla is chosen or whenever the part chosen is hairy, it should be shaved, because the friction employed while rubbing in the ointment will drag on the hairs and cause pain and discomfort or even produce soreness.

The amount of mercurial ointment and the strength in which it is to be used will always be specially mentioned on the order. The amount should then be carefully weighed, and warmed, and well rubbed in, a little at a time until the whole amount has been used. A note should be made of the area of skin treated. Mercurial inunction may be ordered daily or every other day, and different areas of skin should be used in turn as mercury is an irritant and may give rise to dermatitis. Mercury is a poisonous drug, and the nurse who is using it should therefore protect her hands either by using a solid glass applicator or by wearing rubber gloves.

Ionization. By this means the drug is driven into the tissues locally by electricity, ions being used of some of the salts of the drug that has been specified. (This treatment is carried out by those specially qualified in medical electricity.)

THE USE OF SERA AND VACCINES

Serum is the liquid part of blood which has been separated from the solid part. When quantities of serum are needed blood is usually taken from an animal, although this is not invariable.

An *antitoxin serum* is that obtained by collecting serum from an animal that has been immunized to some such disease as diphtheria or tetanus, by having been inoculated with the toxin. This serum is given in doses varying from 1,000 to 100,000 units or more.

An *antibacterial serum* is obtained from an animal that has been immunized by inoculation with the bacteria of the disease. Examples of this type are antistreptococcal, antipneumococcal, and antimeningococcal sera which are usually given in doses of 10, 20 or 50 c.c.

In both instances, the blood serum taken from the animal contains the antitoxin, or antibacterial substance, which will neutralize the action of the toxin or organism and so raise the resistance to that particular disease of the person to whom it is administered. If a sufficiently large dose is given, the effect may be to confer immunity, lasting for a certain time, and in this case the serum will be used as a *prophylactic measure*.

When serum is administered during the course of a disease as part of the treatment it is described as a *curative measure*. In this case it acts by supplying the ready prepared neutralizing substances and so helps the atient's body to combat the disease from which he is suffering. Sera are sually given in the early stages of acute infections when the toxins are irculating in the tissues and the production of antibodies is relatively slow. At this time the administration of the ready prepared antibodies contained n the serum is an invaluable treatment.

In the preparation of serum the horse is frequently used as, being a large nimal, it is possible to take a considerable quantity of blood from it without inconvenience. In the case of diphtheria and tetanus, the horse s injected with toxin, and after a time is bled from the jugular vein, he serum is separated, some antiseptic added, and the serum is then oncentrated so that a small dose of antitoxin serum will contain a large amount of the antibody. The process of concentration at the same time emoves a great deal of the protein material, and therefore the possibility of any serum reaction becomes less likely. On an average, antidiphtheria erum contains 1,000–2,000 units in each cubic centimetre.

Human convalescent serum is employed for the administration of antitoxin n measles and mumps.

Administration of serum. Serum may be administered in a variety of ways, including intravenously, intrathecally, by the intraperitoneal oute, intramuscularly, and subcutaneously. It is important that serum hould be warmed to body heat before it is administered, and this can be done by standing the phial in a bowl of water at this temperature and not any hotter, for ten minutes until the serum is of the same heat as the water. If the serum is placed in very hot water the antibodies contained n it might be destroyed by the heat. Whatever mode of administration s chosen very strict asepsis is essential.

Anaphylactic shock. After the administration of an initial dose of serum in some cases, but more often when the patient has had serum before, and also in cases which are asthmatical, or have any tendency to allergic conditions, there is danger lest immediate and serious shock should follow rapidly on serum administration.

The symptoms come on rapidly and may even begin to appear during the administration of the serum, in which case it should be stopped. Symptoms commonly met with are restlessness, pallor, dyspnoea; a rapid, feeble, irregular pulse, muscular twitchings, rigor and convulsions; and in serious cases the patient lapses into coma, and death may occur. Treatment is by the administration of adrenalin and atropine hypodermically.

If danger of anaphylaxis is suspected the patient is desensitized to serum protein before administering the whole dose. This is carried out by the administration of a tiny dose—say, 0·01 c.c.—given intracutaneously; if the patient is sensitive this will be followed by a reaction which will be demonstrated by the appearance of an urticarial wheal at the site of injection. The first test is usually followed in from half to one hour by giving 1 c.c. of serum subcutaneously, and if no local reaction arises it is then considered safe to give the whole dose within an hour or two.

Serum Sickness. A milder degree of anaphylaxis, designated serum sickness, may arise eight days after administration. These symptoms include a *serum rash*, which is multiform in character and very irritable, *joint pains*, and a rise of temperature and malaise. Skin irritation may be relieved by calamine lotion.

A vaccine is a preparation rather different from a serum. It consists o dead germs, or the toxins which have been obtained from them, suspende in saline solution; a vaccine therefore contains the same irritating sub stances as does a germ, but in a much weaker form, since in most instance the germs are dead before the vaccine is made. A vaccine acts an an *antigen* a substance which stimulates the patient's tissues to produce antibodies

Vaccines are used in the treatment of subacute and chronic conditions in order to raise the patient's degree of resistance to the disease. They are also use to confer an active immunity, as for example, in scarlet fever and diph theria, and in some cases they are used as an aid to diagnosis and in othe cases to test an individual's susceptibility to a certain disease.

Vaccines are usually administered hypodermically in doses of a con venient size, i.e. in doses of ½–1 c.c. They may be supplied in phials of thi size or in small rubber-capped bottles, sealed with paraffin wax. The labe states the strength in millions per c.c.

After the administration of a vaccine, certain reactions occur. The nurse shoul anticipate and be able to recognize the severity of these.

Local reaction. This occurs at the site of inoculation and is demonstrate by the ordinary changes of inflammation, with the usual signs of redness swelling and heat.

General reaction. As the result of the inoculation the general constitutio is disturbed and the patient suffers from malaise, headache and a rise ir temperature.

Focal reaction. In any case where there is a focus of disease, as the resul of the administration of a vaccine, the symptoms will be temporarily increased. For example, should the vaccine have been administered during the course of pulmonary tuberculosis, as is tuberculin, a focal reaction wil be demonstrated by an increase in cough and sputum.

CHEMOTHERAPY

History. The use of chemicals as therapeutic drugs which act directly on the causal organisms of disease dates from the use of quinine in the treat- ment of malaria. In 1907 Ehrlich produced a synthetic preparation of arsenic specific in the treatment of syphilis, the world-famous '606'. Since then synthetic drugs have been produced which are useful in the treat- ment of tropical diseases most of which are due to tiny parasites called protozoa but it is comparatively recently, since 1935, that chemothera- peutic drugs have been produced capable of acting on the germs of many of the acute bacterial infections.

In 1935 Domagk demonstrated the use of *prontosil* in haemolytic strep- tococcal infections in animals. Prontosil is broken down in the body into a more simple compound known as *sulphanilamide*. The group of drugs described as *sulphonamides* dates from and includes sulphanilamide. *Sulphanilamide* was first tried out in the treatment of puerperal sepsis by Drs. Colebrook and Kenny in 1936 who found that taking a fairly large series of cases over a period of almost two years the mortality in puerperal sepsis was, by the use of sulphanilamide, reduced from over 20 per cent to below 5 per cent. Thus the value of sulphanilamide in the treatment of haemolytic streptococcal infection was proved and other infections due to the same class of organism such as other forms of septicaemia, erysipelas, tonsillitis, osteomyelitis, and scarlet fever were successfully treated. But its alue in dealing with other infections was less satisfactory and considerable esearch led to the production of other drugs all based on sulphonamide out being modified compounds of it and these drugs are now classed as he sulphonamide group of which only a few are mentioned in these pages.

Sulphapyridine (M & B 693) was first tried out by Whitby at the Middlesex Hospital in the treatment of *pneumonia*. It is also valuable in a ariety of infections including cerebrospinal fever and other forms of neningitis, gonorrhoea, and gas gangrene.

Sulphathiazole or thiazamide (M & B 760) is particularly valuable in taphylococcal infections and infections of the urinary tract.

Sulphaguanidine is valuable in the treatment of infections of the intestine, and has proved of particular value in the treatment of bacillary dysentery.

Sulphadiazine is a preparation claimed to be less toxic than sulphathiazole which is used for the same purposes.

Many other new compounds include *sulphapyrazine*, *sulphamethazine*, *ulphamerazine* and *succinyl sulphathiazole*, an alternative to *sulphaguanidine*.

As each new compound is produced an attempt is made to find a drug less toxic or more valuable in one or other sphere.

Action of the Drugs. All these compounds are bacteriostatic rather than bacterocidal. They prevent the action of the organisms and inhibit their growth. Some drugs act better on one group of organisms than others and become the drugs of choice for use in a certain disease. The best effect of the drugs is produced by maintaining an adequate concentration in the blood stream.

Mode of Administration. The sulphonamide compounds are usually given by mouth. They are rapidly absorbed in the small intestine and in order to maintain an adequate concentration of the drug in the blood it is necessary to give it at regular intervals, day and night. If a patient vomits after taking his dose the physician must be informed as he may wish the dose to be repeated. This is one of the instances when a patient *should* be wakened from sleep in order to be given his medicine.

Sulphonamides may only be given on prescription and, except in very small doses their use in patients who are up and going about is inadvisable.

Dosage. The compound is prepared in tablets containing 0·5 gm. (half a gramme or 7½ grains), they may be swallowed with a drink of water or crushed and mixed with water or milk. The dose usually recommended is 4 tablets *statim* and then 2 tablets four-hourly for 4 to 5 days: the dose is then reduced to 1 tablet four-hourly for the following 2 to 3 days. Larger doses are occasionally ordered. In the case of infants the dose is a quarter of a tablet for those under 3 months, half a tablet between 3 and 12 months, and one tablet for older infants. Children tolerate the drug well.

Observations and precautions. Certain toxic effects may occur; nurses should watch for cyanosis, pallor, jaundice, skin-rashes, headache, giddiness, haematuria and uraemia. In a few instances haemolytic anaemia or agranulocytosis (see p. 361) may arise; in order that the onset of this grave complication may be recognized immediately regular routine blood counts are made. Agranulocytosis may be successfully treated by penicillin. Alteration of the haemoglobin pigments may result in methaemoglobin or sulphaemoglobin giving rise to dusky cyanosis, this is not serious as it does not interfere with the oxygen-carrying capacity of the blood.

During the administration of sulphonamides by mouth, nausea and vomiting may be a troublesome accompaniment. This may be avoided (1) by powdering the tablets and giving them in milk or in sodium bicarbonate solution; (2) by giving the drug in smaller doses and more frequently, instead of two tablets every four hours, one may be given every two hours.

A soluble form of M & B 693 'dagenan sodium' is available for intramuscular injection when vomiting with the oral compound is persistent, and in cases in which it is essential to get a high concentration of the drug in the blood without delay.

Plenty of fluid should be given, at least six pints a day is the amount recommended, as barley water, water and weak tea, in order to prevent the formation of crystals in the pelvis of the kidney.

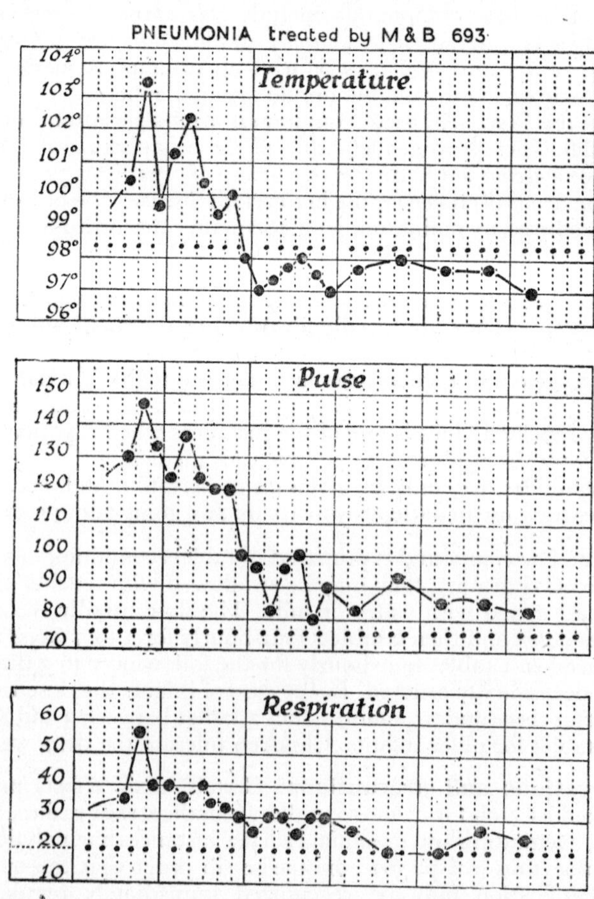

FIG. 169.—CHART OF A CHILD OF FIVE

On admission M & B 693, 2 grammes, followed by 0.5 gm. four-hourly for two days and a half. Then, as the temperature was normal and the general condition good, the dose was reduced to 0.5 gm. twice daily, and 36 hours later the drug was discontinued.

The bowels should be kept acting by the use of liquid paraffin and of emata when necessary. The amount of urine passed should be noted, nd it should be tested for albumin.

The accompanying chart illustrates the result obtained from giving I & B 693 to a little girl of five years. She was admitted in the early days f pneumonia, seriously ill, very cyanosed, and suffering from marked yspnoea with a typical expiratory grunt and movement of the alae nasi. Ier temperature declined within 36 hours after the initial dose and she nade an uneventful recovery.

Local Application of Sulphonamide powder either alone or combined with enicillin is made in the case of wounds likely to be infected or which re infected, in severe burns and in the treatment of certain skin infections uch as impetigo; and recently it has been employed within the peritoneal avity in cases of acute abdominal infection. When nursing any of these ases it is essential to be on the watch for the symptoms of toxaemia lescribed above.

PENICILLIN

Penicillin is a new substance. It is not a sulphonamide. It is an antibiotic vhich means that it is produced from a living substance, in this case a nould, and that it is destructive in action to pathogenic organisms. It was liscovered by Fleming in 1929 quite accidentally, who, whilst making xperiments, noticed that a mould had grown on some of his culture lates and that when this was incubated the bacteria, in the parts overed by mould, did not grow. This mould is *Penicillium notatum*, imilar to the mould which forms on jam. In 1940 Professor Florey and iis fellow workers at Oxford produced an extract from the mould capable of being used for therapeutic purposes.

Uses and characteristics. Penicillin acts on a great many pus-producing organisms including staphylococci and streptococci. There is no danger n giving an overdose of penicillin. It is claimed to be virtually non-oxic when given systemically and not injurious to the tissues when pplied locally. Untoward symptoms are rare, they include headache, nalaise and an urticarial rash which can usually be controlled by a small lose of ephedrine or benzedine. The action of penicillin is not affected by he presence of pus. It is rapidly excreted by the kidneys and therefore dministration must allow for this and be prescribed in such a way as to nsure the continuous presence of the drug in the blood stream. Penicillin s affected by exposure to the air and should be treated with care and only uncovered when in use.

Preparation. There are several varieties of penicillin typed as 1, 2, 3, and all preparations contain a proportion of each type. *White penicillin* (as distinct from yellow) in this country contains over 90 per cent of pencillin 2; it is purer and more stable than the others but more xpensive.

Methods of administration. *Systemic application.* Penicillin may be given by *intravenous*, *intramuscular* or *subcutaneous* injection. An injection is given every three hours. For continuous injections the Indrip, electric clockwork or other special drip apparatus is used which will deliver the required amount evenly over the 24 hours. Some physicians prefer a simple apparatus for delivering the required amount every one or two hours. Some use a needle kept *in situ* which must be properly protecte from sepsis and to which a hypodermic syringe can be attached.

Subcutaneous injection is rarely employed as it is painful. Some worke use ½ to 1 per cent procaine with the penicillin solution in order to avoi pain both for subcutaneous and intramuscular injection.

Intravenous injection is used in some very severe infections and in th treatment of syphilis.

As it is essential to maintain penicillin in a steady concentration i the blood, the necessity of three-hourly injections renders the treatmen very tiresome for the patient and various devices have been though out in order to reduce the frequency of the injections such as the use c some apparatus for continuous injection mentioned above. Probably th most effective method is the more recent use of an oily solution such a the British Pharmacopoeia preparation of penicillin in beeswax and peanu oil. By this means absorption is slower and injections can be more widel spaced.

The preparation of the syringes used for the injection of penicilli is important. These may be sterilized in oil, or in a paraffin bath a 130° C. To sterilize the syringe it is filled with oil and emptied. This i repeated six times, the needle is then attached and the procedure is agai repeated six times.

Alternatively the syringe and needle may be prepared by boiling fo 15 minutes, or it may be prepared by storage in spirit. In the latter cas it is essential that all trace of spirit should be removed by washing th apparatus carefully and drawing saline or sterile water through th syringe and needle before use.

To inject penicillin. Choose the sites carefully. Then map out th areas to be used each in turn so as to avoid having both sides of the bod painful and difficult to lie upon at the same time. If a local anaestheti is being used, draw 2 per cent procaine into the syringe after it has bee charged with penicillin. Use about half the quantity of anaesthetic as c penicillin, this means that one-third (the lower part) of the syringe wil be charged with procaine. Expel the air, attach the syringe to the needl already in position and inject slowly and evenly.

Local application of penicillin is made by means of powder, cream ointment, spray or by soaking gauze in a given concentration and applyin it to the surface of a wound. Penicillin may also be combined wit sulphathiazole, one form of which is flavazol, or with plasma powde When combined in a powder each gramme contains 1,000 units o penicillin. The cream contains 200–400 units per gramme. Ointmen is more stable than cream as it is prepared in a fatty base instead of a oil-water emulsion. Penicillin lozenges contain 500 units per lozenge These are used in the treatment of infections of the mouth and throat Penicillin may be applied to the nasal cavities in the form of drops o as snuff and it is also applied to the rectum in the form of suppositories.

Inhalation. The use of penicillin as an aerosol in the treatment o pulmonary infections has been investigated. It is atomized and inhale in the form of a fine mist. By this means penicillin has a two-fold effect (*a*) it acts as a local application to the respiratory tract and (*b*) it i absorbed into the blood stream. It has been demonstrated that a highe

oncentration of penicillin is found in the sputum than when administra-
.on is made by the systemic methods. One of the methods employed is he use of Rybar's inhaler. The inhaler is loaded with ½ a c.c. of penicillin approximately 45,000 units), the patient breathes out and then, whilst ıhaling, the bulb is squeezed sharply several times, he then holds his reath for a short time and finally breathes out. This method is useful or patients who are able to co-operate with their treatment. Penicillin nay be combined with oxygen and carbon dioxide in a penicillin vapour :nt. This last method is used for patients who are dangerously ill.

Oral administration of penicillin has not so far been considered a success s it is affected by the acid gastric juices but experiments are being nade of giving penicillin to children by mouth.

DISEASES OF WHICH THE ORGANISMS ARE PENICILLIN SENSITIVE OR INSENSITIVE

Sensitive

Adenitis
Anthrax
Blepharitis
Boils
Bronchitis (acute)
Broncho-pneumonia
Cancrum oris
Carbuncles
Erysipelas
Gonorrhoea
mpetigo
nfantile dermatitis
aryngitis
Mastoiditis
Meningitis
Ophthalmia neonatorum
Otitis media
Osteomyelitis
Pemphigus
Puerperal infections
Quinsy
Relapsing fever
Septic skin infections
Stys
Syphilis
Sycocis barbae
Tetanus
Tonsillitis
Weil's disease

Insensitive

Bacillus coli infections
Dysentery group
Cholera
Chickenpox
Enteric group
Herpes zoster
Infantile paralysis
Influenza
Measles
Mumps
German measles
Scabies
Smallpox
Tuberculosis
Typhus
Whooping cough and most of the diseases and conditions due to viruses.
Infections of the newly born. Infections of the urinary tract and septicaemia depend for treatment on the causal organism. In some cases the organism may be penicillin sensitive and in others it may not be so.

It should however be remembered that any of the diseases listed above nay be complicated by some other disease or condition which will espond to penicillin. For example, scabies may be complicated by mpetigo, influenza or measles by broncho-pneumonia, chickenpox by ome septic skin infection and so on.

In addition there are a number of diseases ordinarily responding sulphonamides such as erysipelas and types of pneumonia which certain instances may not respond to this group of drugs but may b successfully treated by penicillin.

Other antibiotics include *streptomycin* which is used in the treatme of tuberculous meningitis and miliary tuberculosis. *Aureomycin* an *chloromycetin* are effecting revolutionary improvement in the treatme of enteric and typhus fevers.

Nursing observations. The general condition of the patient will b seen to be improving, he becomes less toxic and more cheerful. H appetite improves and he begins to sleep well. At first these symptoms ar not always accompanied by a decline of fever and a patient may continu to run a high or swinging temperature for some days after general improve ment has been noticed. When penicillin is locally applied the signs of in flammation will disappear and pus will be replaced by a serous exudat

Hormone therapy is the term applied to indicate the therapeutic use c the group of drugs of endocrine origin. These are different from othe drugs in that they are normally present in the body. Their functions ar studied by the effects produced when these substances are present in exces and they are employed to relieve the symptoms which result from de ficiency of these substances and also in order to produce the known effects as for example when *adrenalin* or *epinephrine* is employed to stimulate th sympathetic nervous control of involuntary muscle and when *pituitar extract* is given to stimulate the uterus, the intestinal muscle or th involuntary muscle in the walls of the blood vessels.

The endocrine preparations most commonly used are those of th following:

Gland	*Extract and dose*
Pancreas	Insulin 10 to 15 units.
Thyroid	Thyroideum ½ to 5 grains.
Parathyroid	Parathormone 20 to 40 units.
Adrenal	Adrenaline $\frac{1}{600}$–$\frac{1}{120}$ grain. Liquor adrenalina hydrochloride 2 to 8 minims.
	Extract of adrenal cortex 5 to 40 units.
Pituitary (posterior lobe)	Liquor pituitary 2 to 5 units. Oxytocin 2 to 10 units. Vasopressin 5 to 10 units.
Pituitary (anterior lobe)	Extracts of the growth hormone, the gonado tropic, thyrotropic, and adrenotropic are thos principally used.
Ovary	Oestrone preparations such as oestradiol an stilboestrol (a synthetic preparation) and cor pus luteum hormone progestin are employed
Testis	Androsterone and testosterone are examples o testicular gland extracts.
Liver and Stomach	Extracts of the liver and stomach are know also to contain some hormonic preparation.

Vitamin therapy (see p. 262 and Appendix II).

Chapter 20

Poisons, and the Treatment of Poisoning

Dangerous Drugs and Poisons Acts—Poisoning and its treatment—Examples of poisoning, including gas poisoning (for Food poisoning, *see p.* 495)

DANGEROUS DRUGS AND POISONS ACTS

The **Dangerous Drugs Acts** were passed to control the sale and use of habit-forming drugs. The drugs which come under the Act are *morphine*, *cocaine*, *ecgonine*, *diamorphine* (heroin) and all preparations containing heroin—no matter how little.

Pethidine hydrochloride and *physeptone* are chemical compounds with an action similar to that of morphia which have recently been added to the habit-forming drugs.

The parts of the Acts which specially concern nurses include the following:

(1) Any amount of the drug, or medicine containing the drug, can only be used for the individual patient for whom it is ordered. These drugs can only be obtained on a doctor's prescription; and, in hospital, when this prescription is ordered on the patient's bedcard. The prescription must contain the patient's name and date, the exact amount of the drug to be given, the number of doses, and the signature or initials of the doctor. The prescription cannot be repeated, unless specifically ordered at the time of writing.

(2) The stock of all such drugs should be kept in the poison cupboard in the ward and can only be supplied on the written requisition of the sister to the dispenser. The cupboard must be kept locked. The drugs contained in this cupboard can only be issued and used on the written instructions on the medical card of a patient by the physician who is responsible. When the sister issues these drugs for use from this cupboard, they must be checked by a second person, and a note made of the amount issued.

The **Pharmacy and Poisons Act, 1933,** was brought into being to restrict the sale and use of poisons. This is accomplished by including them in a number of schedules to which restrictions and exemptions apply. Schedules 1 and 4 are of interest to nurses, the former listing a very large number of drugs including arsenic, belladonna, digitalis, insulin, pituitary extract, nux vomica, etc. These must be kept under lock and key and the amount given checked before administration.

To be able to purchase these drugs the purchaser must be known to the chemist, submit a signed statement of the purpose for which they are required and give name and address. Liniments and other poisonous substances for external use must be in poison bottles. Substances in schedule 4 can only be supplied upon a prescription, whch is valid for one occasion only, unless directed by the doctor to be repeated. The drugs in this schedule include the barbiturates, veronal, etc., atophan, amidopyrin, nitrocreosols and sulphonal.

POISONING AND ITS TREATMENT

Poisons may be taken by mouth, by hypodermic injection, or they may be absorbed through the skin or reach the blood stream by being inhaled. They may be taken accidentally or intentionally, and certain general principles are laid down for use in case of poisoning.

Remove the poison from the stomach by giving an emetic or washing out the stomach, except when the poison taken is a strong corrosive, acid or alkali, in which case a demulcent is given.

Give an antidote when possible, that is, if the character of the poison is known.

Treat the patient for shock by application of heat, by raising the foot of the bed or couch on which he lies and by giving him strong black coffee to drink or by rectal injection. Give rectal salines.

If the patient is drowsy, try to keep him awake and, particularly if his pupils are pinpoint, which may indicate opium or morphia poisoning, do not allow him to relax for a moment.

If the patient is in pain, and not writhing about excessively, apply heat to the abdomen and prepare the hypodermic of morphia which the doctor will probably order.

If breathing is very shallow and slow, or has ceased, perform artificial respiration, provided that the respiratory passages are first clear of any obstruction, and, if oxygen and carbon dioxide are available, give inhalations of these.

Antidotes include morphia for atropine and belladonna poisoning, atropine for morphia and opium poisoning.

An acid, such as 4 ounces of vinegar, is used to neutralize poisoning by alkalis.

An alkali, such as Epsom salts $\frac{1}{2}$ ounce in 4 ounces of water, is used to neutralize acid poisons.

Emetics include mustard, 1 tablespoonful, or salt 2 tablespoonfuls, in 8 ounces of water; tincture of ipecacuanha, 30–60 minims given in water; and apomorphine hydrochloride, grains $\frac{1}{20}$–$\frac{1}{6}$ administered by hypodermic injection.

Demulcents. Milk, butter, olive oil, white of egg, gruel and barley water are the commonest demulcents employed when a corrosive acid or alkali has been swallowed.

Stimulants. Brandy and whisky in water may be given by mouth; ether, 30–60 minims, or strychnine hydrochloride, $\frac{1}{64}$–$\frac{1}{32}$ of a grain may be given hypodermically; aromatic spirit of ammonia, $\frac{1}{2}$–1 drachm in water, or strong black coffee containing a little sugar may be given by mouth. Inhalation of smelling salts, and electrical current (faradism) applied locally, are other means of stimulating a drowsy patient.

SOME EXAMPLES OF POISONING

When corrosive acids and alkalis have been taken, the surfaces of the lips and mouth will be destroyed, and there will be considerable pain in the mouth, throat and stomach, accompanied by collapse. In such instances the treatment indicated is to avoid emetics or lavage, to give one or more demulcents and to treat the patient for shock pending the arrival of a physician.

Carbolic acid makes the lips and mouth white and hard, pain and collapse are very marked, and the urine is suppressed and green in colour (carboluria). When pure carbolic has been taken the treatment is as above, but if the patient has swallowed a solution of 1–20 or 1–10 the stomach may be washed out with permanganate of potash solution, white of egg may be given as a demulcent, and magnesium sulphate in water as an alkali. Shock should be treated and stimulants administered freely.

Oxalic acid (salts of lemon). This is not as destructive as pure carbolic so that stomach lavage can be administered with care. Lime and chalk should be given and the shock treated.

Prussic acid (hydrocyanic acid). In this case the breath smells of bitter almonds, the respirations are sighing and gasping in character, the patient soon becomes unconscious with fixed staring eyes and dilated pupils.

Treatment. An emetic may be given, as this acid is not powerfully corrosive—that is, if the patient is not severely collapsed. Inhalations of ammonia should be given and stimulants administered freely. Shock and collapse should be treated.

Lysol. This is one of the exceptions in which the stomach is washed out when a corrosive has been taken. Brandy and water 1–4 is used for this purpose, and 4 ounces of magnesium sulphate solution are left in the stomach. Shock and restlessness should be treated.

Arsenic (weed killer). Acute arsenical poisoning is accompanied by nausea, vomiting, diarrhoea and severe dehydration. The *treatment* consists in washing out the stomach and giving demulcents.

Belladonna, and its active principle atropine, results in dryness of mouth and dilatation of pupils; the skin becomes hot and dry, the patient is flushed, the temperature is raised, the pulse is rapid, and there is restlessness and delirium.

Treatment includes the giving of emetics—in addition pilocarpine nitrate, gr. $\frac{1}{4}$ is given hypodermically—and the administration of sedatives to relieve the restlessness.

Cocaine. Acute cocaine poisoning results in respiratory and cardiac failure with marked syncope. The *treatment* includes the administration of inhalations of ammonia and amyl nitrite, the giving of aromatic spirit of ammonia by mouth, and the use of strychnine hypodermically.

Chloroform. The result of poisoning by chloroform is depression of the cardiac, respiratory and vasomotor centres followed by failure of respiration and failure of the heart's action. The *treatment* is artificial respiration, the provision of fresh air, inhalations of ammonia and amyl nitrite, and the administration of powerful cardiac restoratives, such as coramine and ether, hypodermically.

Lead. In acute lead poisoning the mouth is dry and there is a metallic taste in the mouth, a blue line about the gums, sensations of nausea, cramplike pain in the muscles and intestinal colic.

The *immediate treatment* consists of rest in bed and applications of heat to the abdomen, with the administration of stimulants; attempts will afterwards be made to eliminate the lead from the system by the administration of small doses of Epsom salts. The patient should be removed from the possible source of lead contamination to which he is evidently susceptible.

Mercury. Symptoms include soreness and swelling of the gums, loosening of the teeth, a metallic taste in the mouth, nausea, diarrhoea and vomiting, followed by collapse. The *treatment* is to wash out the stomach and give demulcents, particularly albumin water; shock is treated by stimulants and heat.

Narcotics, including all hypnotics. As the patient will be drowsy and difficult to arouse, if he is not already in a coma, *the treatment aims at keeping him awake; emetics* are given, potassium permanganate being generally used for this purpose, and *stomach lavage* is employed for patients who are unconscious. *Stimulants* such as coffee, administered either by mouth or rectally, and such stimulants as atropine, coramine and strychnine are given hypodermically. *Artificial respiration* is performed when necessary.

Phosphorus. Taking phosphorus results in pain in the throat and abdomen, with vomiting, and the vomit may be luminous in character.

Treatment. An emetic of copper sulphate, 1 grain to the pint, is administered, followed by Epsom salts. Demulcents such as white of egg may be given, but oils should be avoided as these render phosphorus more soluble, and therefore result in further absorption of the poison.

Strychnine (vermin killer). Symptoms of strychnine poisoning are muscular twitchings, cramp and convulsions. The *treatment* is to wash out the stomach, administer sedatives, give plenty of fluids and eliminate as far as possible all external stimuli, which would excite twitchings or convulsions—the patient is usually nursed in a darkened and quiet room.

GAS POISONING

Gas poisoning, whether deliberate or accidental, may be a very rapid cause of death. The places in which poisonous gases are likely to be met are in the shafts of mines, the battened-down holds of ships, in garages where motor-car or aeroplane exhaust gases are not diffused freely and rapidly enough and in places where high explosives are employed. Leaks from gas mains occurring in an ill-ventilated confined space may also give rise to gas poisoning.

The **symptoms of carbon monoxide poisoning** begin as dizziness, pass on to faintness and result in collapse which is followed by failure of respiration. If the subject remains exposed to the gas and untreated, death from deficiency of oxygen, anoxaemia, will occur. The lips and fingernails take on a characteristic cherry-red colour, but this is not invariable.

Carbon monoxide is not a poison. It is lack of oxygen which gives rise to the symptoms which are so severe and may terminate fatally. It so happens hat the haemoglobin in the red blood cells has a much greater affinity for arbon monoxide than for oxygen, so that whenever the former gas is vailable the haemoglobin will combine with it, rather than with oxygen.

Treatment. The patient should lie down, no exertion being permitted. 'resh air and artificial respiration are valuable; inhalation of carbon lioxide 7 per cent in oxygen should be given if available. A patient with noxaemia is grey and cold, and as soon as he is breathing satisfactorily he shock from which he is suffering should be treated.

Section 4

Medical Conditions and Diseases and Their Treatment and Nursing

Chapter 21

Introductory

The observation of symptoms—Insomnia, the importance of rest and sleep in the treatment of disease—Varieties of pain, including types of colic—The manifestation of indigestion as a symptom of disease—Delirium

The practice of medicine is an ancient tradition, of Greek origin. Hippocrates is designated 'the Father of Medicine', and the oath which Hippocrates expected his students and followers to take before a degree was conferred upon them contains the sentiments of generosity and duty which have characterized the members of the medical profession throughout the ages.

In this oath the young physician promises to use his knowledge for the benefit of his patients—'to give no deadly drug to any, though it be asked of me, nor will I counsel such, and especially I will not aid a woman to procure abortion'. He further promises that whatever house he enters he will go there 'for the benefit of the sick'. 'Whatsoever things I see or hear concerning the life of men, in my attendance on the sick, or even apart therefrom, which ought not to be noised abroad, I will keep silence thereon, counting such things to be as sacred secrets. Pure and holy will I keep my Life and Art.'

A nurse may learn a good deal from studying the Hippocratic oath. Patients and their relatives often speak freely to a nurse, and what she learns about the patient and his family in this, or any other way, she must learn to look upon as sacred professional secrets.

In the progress of the science and practice of medicine many other sciences have derived from it, as anatomy, physiology and psychology. Others have been adopted as essential to it including botany, chemistry, physics, pharmacology and bacteriology. As the study of medicine extends a tendency has developed to separate this vast science into various fields by specialization. In the wards of a general hospital, for example, will be found units devoted to the care of nervous diseases—in psychological medicine; skin diseases—in dermatology; the care of sick children—in pediatrics; as well as special units for the care of cases of infectious disease and pulmonary tuberculosis.

In the following pages an introductory chapter deals with the observations of some fairly common symptoms met with in disease. Then follow an outline of the care of diseases of the organs of the circulation and respiration, of digestion, of the urinary tract, the nervous system, of metabolism, the endocrine organs, diseases of the skin and communicable diseases.

Symptoms may be described as evidence of disease. They are classified as *subjective symptoms*, which can be and often are complained of by the patient because they distress and worry him; other symptoms, which are not so evident to him but which are more often discovered by the doctor on examination, are described as *objective*.

Symptoms are also classified as *local* or *focal* when they occur in a definite part, and *general* or *constitutional* when they affect the various systems of the body. In inflammation, for example, the local symptoms present are heat, redness and swelling, and the general are those associated with any rise of temperature which may accompany the condition, or which may be due to a general disturbance of the body associated with the local discomfort. For example, a patient suffering pain will be unable to sleep, and this results in sensations of fatigue and weariness, headache and general aching pains, loss of appetite, and in time it will be the cause of loss of weight.

A great deal of the work of a nurse lies in her constant observation of symptoms, and her ability—which should be fostered and trained—to report on her observations with accuracy, not minimizing any one point, or ever exaggerating even in the slightest degree. Her work will probably be most valuable in connexion with the subjective group of symptoms the discovery of which does not require special examination.

The observations made regarding the condition of a patient on admission (described on p. 20) will suggest a number of points which may help a nurse to give a doctor some assistance in his initial examination. The nurse will be more useful to him in this way if she has an idea of the various symptoms which may arise in association with disease of the different systems of the body, as outlined below.

The digestive system. *Subjective symptoms* include thirst and dryness of the mouth, heartburn, loss of appetite and difficulty in swallowing food or drink, flatulence, indigestion, abdominal pain, vomiting, constipation or diarrhoea. *Objective symptoms* include the condition of the mouth when examined, such as the state of the tongue, whether dry or moist, pale or red, clean or dirty, furred or fissured; the lips, whether dry and cracked, and the presence or otherwise of any sordes on them; the condition of the abdomen, whether distended and whether any irregularities are present such as visible peristalsis or a very obviously enlarged liver or spleen.

The circulatory system. The presence of dyspnoea, palpitation or pain, feelings of faintness, the character of the pulse (which is described in detail on p. 48); any pulsation of the veins of the neck, the presence of a malar flush or of cyanosis or pallor, coldness of the hands and feet, blueness of the tips of the fingers and toes and of the ears and nose; the presence of any oedema, and whether the skin pits on pressure.

The respiratory system. (For types of dyspnoea, see details on p. 53. The character of the sputum is described on p. 74.) Pain in the chest should be considered and also the character of the pain, and whether it is dull and aching or sharp and shooting; the presence of dilatation of the alae nasi combined with the marked distress which accompanies laboured breathing should also be noted.

Urinary system. The quantity and character of the urine should be investigated and compared with the normal as described on p. 68. Any difficulty or frequency of micturition should be observed and the urine tested for abnormalities.

Nervous system. The observation of fits, convulsions and coma are described on pp. 427–33. The condition of the eyes should be noted, particularly as regards the colour of the sclera, irregularity of pupils, the presence of squint and ptosis, and protrusion of the eyeball (exophthalmos).

Any sensory symptoms present should be considered, such as pain, numbness, tingling, sensitiveness to touch (hyperaesthesia) and loss of sensation (analgesia). The condition of the skin, whether dry or harsh, shiny or moist, and any evidence of the presence of a rash. The presence of any paralysis, and whether this is of the spastic or flaccid type, and the position in which the limbs lie when resting. Any difficulty the patient has in speaking or hearing should also be noted.

A number of symptoms in which the accurate observations of the nurse are invaluable have already been described in dealing with observation of the temperature, pulse and respiration, and excreta and discharges, including observations of urine, stool, vaginal discharges, vomit and sputum. Three other symptoms—insomnia, pain and indigestion—in which the observations of the nurse will be particularly valuable are appended here, including notes on some of the measures which might be taken to procure their alleviation, and also the observations necessary when a definite form of treatment is ordered—such, for example, as absolute rest.

INSOMNIA

It is becoming increasingly common for patients to approach their doctors or attend at the consulting rooms of highly specialized neurologists, complaining of insomnia. Possibly the treatment of this, which may be a difficult neurological problem, can hardly be considered to be within the province of the nurse, although she will often be expected to help (see note on neurological nursing, p. 426).

Nursing measures in insomnia. A nurse in a general hospital ward will often be faced by the problem of a patient who for some reason or another is unable to go to sleep. It is her duty to attempt to discover the cause, and she should investigate the different possibilities. For example, the patient may be hungry or thirsty, too cold or too hot, or his feet may be cold, his position uncomfortable—he may be lying on creases, on a moist sheet, or on crumbs. If he is wearing any surgical apparatus this may be uncomfortable, a bandage may be too tight, or a splint may be hurting at some particular point. He may be conscious of lack of movement of air around him, or he may wish to empty his bladder, or to use the bedpan.

Some of the symptoms of the complaint from which he is suffering may be very irritating and troublesome—he may be in pain or have a headache, his skin may be hot and dry, or he may be perspiring heavily; or again he may have marked restlessness, or be suffering from dyspnoea, palpitation, flatulence or indigestion, or be exceedingly uncomfortable because he has a very high temperature.

Various little nursing attentions may be carried out in an attempt to relieve discomfort and to obtain the relaxation that is so necessary if the patient is to lie quiet and still, breathing regularly and with his eyes closed —all of which are so important if he is to get to sleep. These measures include giving the patient a warm, light nourishing drink, allowing him to empty his bladder, altering his position, rearranging his pillows, so that he is supported and his head is not nodding, straightening his sheets, tightening the undersheet, rearranging the drawsheet so that he lies on a cool part of it. Sponging his hands, and in some cases warm sponging the entire body, combing and brushing the hair, smoothly stroking the forehead may be effective, or carrying the hands down over the side of the face and neck over the jugular veins may soothe. A cold compress or the application of an icecap may sometimes be effective in the relief of headache.

It is equally important to see that the patient is not facing or in any way irritated by a light; on the other hand, the patient may be distressed because he is in the dark and the provision of a suitably shaded nightlight may give the confidence which will render it possible for the patient so worried to relax.

It is inadvisable to allow patients who are sleepless to read, and it is a great mistake to allow a patient to think that counting sheep going over a stile will help—this is an effort of concentration which will certainly keep him awake—but it is very important to get him to understand that muscular relaxation is necessary, and help him to practise this; and if, at the same time, he will think 'What a marvellous thing it is to go to sleep', or 'What a wonderful thing sleep is', he will find his body becoming gradually more relaxed.

A nurse should be very careful to avoid making a noise. She must move quietly, close doors gently, and make up fires without fuss or undue haste. There must not be any whispering, or clattering of utensils, and she should see that beds do not creak. It is a great pity that so many of the hospitals in which our sick are nursed are placed in the centre of some of our largest cities, often in the midst of traffic which is continuous until long past midnight and begins again at four or five in the morning.

During sleep certain quite definite changes occur: the cerebral circulation is diminished and the blood pressure falls slightly; metabolism is maintained at a lower level than during waking hours, and possibly the reason why people who are overtired are unable to sleep is that the fatigue products, produced in their muscles, result in the stimulation of certain metabolic activities which temporarily hinder the attainment of sleep.

The *causes of insomnia* are too numerous to detail, but they may be divided into nervous fears and physical conditions, the latter being manifested by the painful symptoms which are preventing relaxation.

The use of sedatives. In certain diseases the prognosis is rendered very grave unless reasonable sleep can be obtained, and to this end sedatives may be ordered, but the nurse should clearly understand that these are a last measure, and that they are drugs which by their action depress certain faculties and centres, and so may possibly give rise to an accumulation of toxins which would not occur during natural sleep.

When a patient is ordered a sedative the nurse must take pains to prepare him beforehand for sleep, so that, for example, he will not be likely to ask for a drink or a bedpan fifteen minutes after the sedative has been administered —all these matters should have been previously attended to. Any treatment the patient is having should have been performed; if the temperature is being recorded four-hourly and the sedative is ordered half an hour before this falls due, it should be given then, and a note made of the alteration in time—not that the patient would be wakened should he have fallen asleep, but, by the application of common sense, to get as perfect a record of the temperature as possible.

Report on sleep. With a patient for whom the nurse knows that sleep is of vital importance, she must make a very careful record of the amount obtained, and this should also be done whenever a sedative has been given. It is a good plan to include in the report:

(*a*) The amount of sleep obtained altogether in hours and minutes.

(*b*) The duration and the actual time of the longest sleep the patient had; e.g., he might have slept from 1 a.m. to 2.15 a.m.=1¼ hours.

(*c*) The character of the sleep should also be noted, whether it was quiet sleep, or restless and disturbed, or whether the patient slept only in short, fitful periods.

REST AND SLEEP

Rest might be considered to be the principle of practically all treatment of abnormal conditions, both of body and mind. In many diseases, particularly those associated with the febrile state and states of toxaemia, there is excessive wasting and destruction of the tissues of the body and deleterious effects are produced on the muscular system; this is productive of strain on the circulatory system and, by the state of rapid breakdown of tissue, extra work is thrown on the urinary system. All these, and many other systems thus undergoing overwork and suffering from fatigue, cry out for rest.

Rest of the body is obtained by keeping the patient in bed; but he should lie quietly in bed, not restlessly fidgeting, jerking and turning.

Rest of mind is of even greater importance, and to ensure this there must be absence of all worry, irritation, excitement and anxiety and all mental effort should be avoided.

Further, in addition to the physiological rest, generally indicated above, *mechanical rest* of one or more of the organs may be obtained. For example, rest of the eye may be secured by covering it; or the instillation of some mydriatic, which paralyses the ciliary muscle, produces a similar effect. A limb may be rested by binding it securely on to a splint.

Absolute rest indicates that the patient does not do anything for himself. He lies flat in bed with one pillow. He is washed and fed by the nurse. Two nurses are employed to move him whenever this is necessary. He is not allowed to read, talk, sew or perform any other kind of work.

The term 'absolute rest', however, is used with a variety of meanings. Some doctors say the patient is having absolute rest when he is at rest in bed, but performing the ordinary sanitary and toilet offices for himself. The nurse must therefore clearly understand what any individual physician means and requires when he orders a patient absolute rest, and until she gets this interpretation from him she should proceed as previously indicated.

The application of rest in the treatment of disease will be mentioned in each instance. It is sufficient to state here that in certain conditions it is the only possible available treatment as, for example, it is instanced in the frightened, rigidly still attitude of a patient suffering from an attack of angina; and again, in the importance attached by every ward sister in the nursing of pneumonia to the degree of rest which the nurse is able to provide for her patient, since this may be the sole means of preventing ultimate and fatal heart failure—when every pulse beat has to be economized and every irritating stimulus, however slight, eliminated in order to obtain the maximum degree of rest.

Healthy sleep is practically the most perfect condition of rest for mind and body and is looked upon as one of the most important factors in the treatment of disease. A patient should never be wakened from sleep—unless specially ordered, as in most cases sleep is more important than either food or treatment. Therefore, it is better to miss giving the patient a feeding, or recording a four-hourly temperature, for example, than to risk wakening him. On the other hand a patient who is apparently asleep may be in a condition of stupor, and it is very important that a nurse should be able to recognize the difference.

There is another aspect that must be considered with regard to sleep—speaking for a moment of the normal person, it may truly be said that lack of sleep never killed anyone, and the layman's idea that a person who does not sleep will eventually become mad is grossly inaccurate. But it must be recognized that a patient who during his normal life begins to sleep badly will most certainly be worried about it, and so worrying may contract the habit of sleeplessness—thus introducing one of the possible causes of insomnia.

PAIN

Pain is a very common symptom in disease and it often provides the physician with valuable information. It varies much in extent and degree, and is apt to be a very distressing symptom, producing not only physical but also mental distress. Although pain may accompany some normal physical processes, as instanced in the pains of labour, it is usually an indication of an abnormal condition of disease.

Another point to be taken into consideration is the *reaction of the individual to pain*, certain persons tolerating pain more readily than others. In some instances the degree of concentration may intensify the suffering; yet on the other hand, if the mind can be distracted, the pain is less severely experienced. The *memory of pain* is another very important factor, including the memory of any painful experience which may not necessarily have been physical, such as the induction of anaesthesia by the inhalation methods which the use of the barbiturate preparations has done so much to obviate.

Varieties of pain. It is very important when dealing with patients to be able to follow carefully their description of the pain they have experienced and to apply it in a way that may help to determine the cause of the suffering. The presence of pus in the tissues is usually indicated by a throbbing pain; disease of bone gives rise to a gnawing, aching pain; pressure on nerves may result in tingling sensations, numbness, hyperaesthesia or analgesia; chronic inflammatory conditions of a nerve such as occur in chronic neuritis and rheumatism give rise to a dull aching pain particularly when the part is at rest and when it gets warm; acute nerv lesions such as neuralgia are characterized by shooting pains.

Pressure caused by a too tightly applied splint or by plaster of paris i usually indicated by a hot burning pain, and the pain of a serous mem brane is always sharp and shooting in character as is the pain of pleurisy.

Most adults can give some lucid description of pain, but in dealing wit infants and tiny children it may be necessary for the nurse to differentiat between a cry of pain and one that is due to temper or hunger. Generall speaking any restlessness, particularly at night, indicates pain in a child— a tiny child may be seen to put his hands frequently to his face, whic might indicate earache, or the pain of cutting teeth; or the child might ro its head about on the pillow or bang its head, although head banging i usually due to some nervous condition.

Observation on pain in special regions. A nurse may be called upon to hel determine the cause of pain in some special region, particularly in head ache and in colic.

Headache is a very common complaint and the causes appear to b endless. It is important to decide the situation of the pain—whether it b frontal, or occipital, or whether half the head or the whole is involved Again, the character of a headache varies very much—it may be an acut unbearable pain which will only respond to the administration of drugs such as morphia, or a constant dull aching pain, or a pain as if pressur is being brought to bear upon the head, a penetrating pain of a borin character, or throbbing in character, or a very intense pain only occurrin at intervals. In most of these the patient is not utterly disabled, but is abl to carry on with his ordinary routine duties, though he may be definitel suffering very grave, and perhaps unnecessary discomfort, and therefor the cause should always be investigated.

Causes. In investigating the cause of headache the physician will usuall go through the different systems and try and find out first whether th headache is associated with disorders of digestion or with constipation Defective sight is another fairly common cause, and in this case the pain may occur over the eyes or at the occiput when the visual area is fatigued, so that a frontal headache at the end of the day and an occipital headach on waking in the morning might be considered an indication of eyestrain Abnormalities of blood pressure cause headache—which in low blood pressure is due to anaemia of the brain, and in high blood pressure is probably due to pressure and congestion. Mental strain or any worry and anxiety frequently cause headache, and this includes the case of a child over-working at school or being unduly anxious about his lessons, or that of an older student who is being pressed to reach a standard of which he is not really capable. Many diseases of the central nervous system have headache as a symptom, and any injury which gives rise to concussion of the brain or spinal cord will give rise to headache.

Another very constant cause of headache, particularly in diseased con-ditions, is toxaemia, and this is met with in nephritis particularly and in jaundice and toxaemia due to sepsis or constipation. A persistent headache may be traced to the presence of septic teeth or tonsils, a septic appendix or gallbladder, or infected cranial sinuses. Headache is a frequent symptom at the onset of many febrile diseases, particularly an acute attack of influenza, pneumonia and typhoid fever, scarlet fever or smallpox, and the headaches associated with erysipelas and tetanus are severe beyond description.

Another very potent cause of headache in women is interference with or disturbance of the functions of the reproductive organs; ovaritis and uterine displacements (for example) are associated with headache. Many women suffer severe headaches at the onset of menstruation and again at the menopause.

Treatment. As far as the nursing is concerned the aim will be to relieve the headache—it is the physician's business to discover the cause, although the nurse will be able to help by her observations and also by the fact that a woman patient will very often confide in her concerning matters which she might not so willingly discuss with the physician.

An application of cold to the head will give some relief in most headaches, and this may take the form of an icebag, cold compress, Leiter's coils, or evaporating lotion. A hot bath, by stimulating the circulation and bringing blood to the lower extremities and skin, may also give relief; the application of heat or of some form of counterirritant, such as a mustard leaf at the back of the neck, may relieve the pain by a reflex effect. In headaches associated with low blood pressure or fatigue, a stimulant such as tea or coffee, a little caffeine or sal volatile may give relief; those due to a high blood pressure or to cerebral congestion may be relieved by the administration of a small dose of concentrated magnesium sulphate solution which produces some degree of dehydration.

Drugs should be very carefully used and should never be advised by a nurse, because a person afflicted by persistent and continuous headache may become addicted to the use of drugs. Different preparations of aspirin, phenacetin and antipyrin are sometimes ordered by physicians, particularly when a headache is producing marked insomnia, which is quite definitely lowering the vitality of the patient.

The usual considerations to be taken regarding further measures for the relief of headache include care in advising the patient regarding his diet and mode of life, particularly with regard to avoiding repeated fatigue and to obtaining sufficient sleep and rest; the condition of the bowels should be considered, as even if the patient has a daily bowel action he may still be constipated, as the stool may be insufficient in amount, and the amount of urine passed should be very carefully considered and the urine itself tested.

Colic. Colic is an intermittent, usually acute pain, produced by the contraction of the involuntary muscles contained in the walls of some of the hollow viscera and tubelike structures passing from one organ to another, particularly in the case of the ureters in renal colic and the bile ducts in biliary colic.

Gastro-intestinal colic. This is the commonest type of colic, and is due to a variety of causes. It may be the result of taking indigestible food, or of food poisoning. The ingestion of lead gives rise to lead colic or painter's colic. The colic met with in prussic acid poisoning is very acute. In some persons colic appears to be of nervous origin, as anxiety and worry give rise to an attack. During an attack of gastro-intestinal colic the patient is seized with pain in the abdomen, and may describe his intestines as 'all tied up in knots'; he grasps his abdomen with both hands, curls himself into a ball and draws his knees up on to his abdomen. In a few moments the attack subsides and he falls back more or less exhausted. This type of colic may be accompanied by diarrhoea or vomiting, or constipation may be present, particularly in the form due to lead colic. The severity of the pain results in a considerable degree of shock, which is probably contributed to by fear of the impending and almost certain attacks of pain; the patient is extremely restless, his face is pinched, his expression anxious and his pupils often dilated with pain, his temperature is usually subnormal, his pulse weak, his respirations shallow and rapid and his skin cold and clammy.

Treatment. The treatment is aimed at the cause; but apart from this, when a nurse is in charge of a patient with intestinal colic she must try to relieve it, and applications of heat to the abdomen during the attack may cause it to abate. As a general rule an aperient should *not* be administered, but in the case of children, who may be suspected of eating indigestible food, a dose of castor oil *may* be administered. If a doctor is available he may order the addition of a little laudanum to this. For severe intestinal colic morphia will probably be ordered. The nurse should always see that the patient is kept very warm, his cold wet skin should be wiped dry between the attacks and, if the patient can take fluid, small drinks should be given.

Renal colic is due to the passage of some abnormality down one or both ureters—this may be crystals, stones or a bloodclot. The pain begins in the loin and passes down the affected side to the groin and then to the inner side of the thigh; it is markedly severe, and strong men have been known to twist the brass rail of a bedstead in the agony they suffer during an attack of renal colic. This pain is accompanied by great restlessness and anxiety, and frequently also by vomiting, and is followed by a considerable degree of shock. It is also accompanied by a constant desire to pass urine, though micturition may be painful. There is usually some degree of haematuria.

Treatment. Morphia is usually ordered for the relief of pain in renal colic. During the attack the nurse should do her best to alleviate the pain by hot applications over the loins or by the use of counterirritants and by encouraging the patient to take hot baths. The cause must be investigated, and medical treatment aims at keeping the urine diluted. It is therefore good nursing treatment to administer large quantities of fluid during an attack of renal colic.

Biliary colic. The pain in biliary colic is similar to that in renal colic and is due to a similar cause. In this case probably a gallstone or some thickened bile is blocking a bile-duct and the increased peristalsis giving rise to pain is nature's effort to expel the foreign body along the duct. The patient will describe this pain as knifelike in character, passing from the right side over the epigastrium and up to the right shoulder. It is severe, the patient is restless and rolls about in bed writhing with pain, and although vomiting accompanies the attack it brings no relief. The attack is followed by collapse. Jaundice may follow an attack of biliary colic if a stone blocks the common duct, though not otherwise, so that jaundice is not considered a symptom of biliary colic, but a symptom of blockage of the duct. (See also cholecystitis, p. 395.)

INDIGESTION

Indigestion or dyspepsia is a very common symptom which may be due to an enormous variety of causes, including the partaking of badly cooked meals and unsuitable foods; eating too rapidly, too frequently or too infrequently; the injudicious use of tea, coffee, alcohol or tobacco; neglected dental hygiene, constipation, disorders and diseases of the stomach, and a number of other causes which include worry and bad temper and other emotional excesses.

When a nurse is asked to make observations on the condition of a patient who complains of indigestion, she must first bear in mind the large number of contributory causes which may be involved; she should next note which foods disagree with her patient and which he can take without discomfort; whether the indigestion complained of occurs after every meal or only at certain times of the day. In the case of peptic ulcer (for example) the pain will be experienced at a varying time after meals; in disorders of the gall-bladder the discomfort may accumulate towards the end of the afternoon and the beginning of the night. A nurse should also notice whether it is a full or an empty stomach which produces discomfort. In some cases of duodenal ulcer the pain is relieved by taking a small quantity of food; in others, as in gastric ulcer, pain can only be relieved on emptying the stomach by vomiting.

It is essential for nurses to remember that indigestion is not only associated with disorders or diseases of the stomach. There is a vast field of reflex causes of indigestion, and it is not an exaggeration to state that indigestion may be the only troublesome symptom complained of in the early stages of many serious conditions such as cardiovascular disease. It may for example be the first symptom of a slight degree of hypertension of the heart associated with arteriosclerosis and high blood pressure; or again, it may be a very distressing symptom in coronary thrombosis; whilst the part which indigestion plays in any functional derangement of the heart is more common than either palpitation or tachycardia.

Reflex indigestion may also occur whenever any part of the alimentary tract is displaced, disordered or diseased. It is well known that constipation and visceroptosis give rise to indigestion, but it is less well known that even slight displacement of the lower part of the large intestine which may for example arise as a result of enlargement of the uterus by a fibroid tumour, or simply as the result of retroversion of that organ, very slightly altering the position of the pelvic colon, may be the cause of the symptom. Appendicitis and cholecystitis may be disguised for months under the cloak of indigestion, and—to mention one or two other organs—disease of the lungs and kidneys may be manifested for a considerable time by indigestion. Many nurses are familiar with indigestion as one of the recognized modes of onset of pulmonary tuberculosis which, accompanied by nausea and vomiting, render the victims so difficult to care for, as the food needed in the treatment of this wasting disease becomes so difficult to administer. Few perhaps realize the discomfort that indigestion produces in many cases of pneumonia—the patient, desperately inconvenienced by his many distressing symptoms, does not differentiate between pain in his chest and pain due to indigestion, and it is for this reason that in such cases small doses of easily digested fluids should be given, distension of the stomach being carefully avoided because of its close proximity to the heart, which is bearing the strain of the grave toxaemia from which the patie is suffering.

Before the treatment of indigestion can reasonably be undertaken investigation the cause and diagnosis of the condition should be made. The nurse's part will to contribute an accurate report of any observations she may have mad or any history she may have been able to elicit.

A diseased stomach will be treated by rest but, apart from the treatme of severe haematemesis, when two to three days' complete starvation m be considered as a preliminary, rest to the stomach does not mean keepi it empty. The principles of treatment undertaken in these cases includ

(1) A choice of food which is bland and non-irritating, such as dilute or citrated milk or white of egg.

(2) The administration of small quantities, 1½–3 ounces at first, i creasing to not more than 5–6 ounces at intervals of 1½–2 hours. diseased stomach functions most easily when it contains a small quanti of non-irritating food.

(3) Fluid is essential for the wellbeing of the body and, in cases disordered digestion, it ought to be given half to three-quarters of an ho before food, rather than with it.

(4) As one part of the alimentary tract is so dependent upon other part the teeth should be carefully examined and the hygiene of the mout maintained in as perfect a state as possible; the hygiene of the colo should be similarly considered and constipation carefully avoided.

DELIRIUM

Delirium is a confusion of the mind which may vary from slight dis turbance to severe mania. It occurs easily in children as the result of slight rise of temperature or gastro-intestinal disorder. In adults it accom panies more grave states of fever and toxaemia. The mind is confuse and the patient does not recognize his surroundings, he may lie quietl chattering to himself or become noisy and violent. *Acute delirium* when th patient shouts and struggles is very exhausting and he quickly become prostrated. In *coma-vigil* he lies with wide-open eyes, staring at the ceilin and quietly muttering. This form accompanies grave toxaemia, as i typhoid fever. In *delirium tremens* the patient is terrified, he imagines h sees unpleasant moving objects such as snakes and vermin; he is restles and covered with perspiration. Unless the condition can be relieved h will become gravely exhausted (for treatment of D.T.s, see p. 658).

In the nursing of delirious patients, a patient who is attempting to get out of bed should be given a bedpan or urinal in case the desire to pass urine or stool is making him restless. He should also be given a drink or offered some form of nourishment as he may be hungry. A delirious patient should generally be humoured rather than restrained. The nurse must discover the best treatment for each; some resent being touched, others will relax if gently handled. Some can be reassured, others will be more excited if spoken to. A nurse must never show that she is afraid; she must act kindly but firmly and without any hesitation.

Chapter 22

Diseases and Disorders of the Heart, and Organs of Circulation

Pericarditis, endocarditis, myocarditis—Congenital heart disease, functional heart disease—The symptoms, treatment and nursing of cases of heart disease—Cardiac syncope—Angina pectoris—Cardiac asthma—Coronary thrombosis and embolism—Diseases of the blood vessels: aneurysm, arteriosclerosis, arteritis, atheroma, thrombo-angiitis obliterans, Raynaud's disease, phlebitis, varicose veins—High and low blood pressure—Diseases of the blood: anaemia, haemophilia, purpura, polycythaemia, agranulocytosis, splenic anaemia, lenkaemia—Diseases of the lymphatic system: adenitis, lymphangitis, and lymphadenoma

VARIETIES OF HEART DISEASE

Heart disease may be congenital or acquired. Practically any form of microbic disease can affect the heart, acute rheumatism, influenza, diphtheria, pneumonia, acute nephritis, and streptococcal infections of the ear, nose and throat, such as tonsillitis, may all be causes of heart disease.

Acquired heart disease may affect the pericardium, myocardium or endocardium, producing *pericarditis*, *myocarditis* and *endocarditis* respectively, and one, two or all three of the layers of the heart may be involved in the infection. *Organic heart disease* may be acute or chronic. *Functional disorder of the heart* may exist apart from organic changes.

PERICARDITIS

Pericarditis is commonly associated with acute rheumatism. It is very disabling and is the source of much of the cardiac disease met with in children and young people. The *changes* which take place in the pericardium vary according to the stage of the disease. In the early stage a layer of fibrin is formed between the pericardial layers, rendering the surfaces slightly roughened and causing pain on movements. A little later on in the disease the serous membrane secretes fluid in excess and this, poured out between the layers, separates them and causes the pain to be less, but the pressure of the fluid in the pericardial sac further embarrasses the action of the heart. Much later in the disease, the fluid is absorbed and the roughened layers of membrane adhere together, adhesions form between them and the condition known as an *adherent pericardium* arises. In addition adhesions form on the outer surface of the pericardium and cause it to become fixed to the adjacent structures, such as the diaphragm.

Symptoms. In addition to the symptoms mentioned later (on p. 350), which are found in all forms of heart disease as the result of cardiac failure, *certain symptoms arise which are characteristic of pericarditis*. *Pain*, due to rubbing together of the inflamed serous membrane, is felt over the sternum in the precordial area.

The *rate of the pulse is increased* owing to embarrassment of the action c the heart.

Dyspnoea occurs, breathing is thoracic in character and very rapid, an abdominal movement is absent. The patient has to be propped up o pillows in order to lessen the discomfort.

In a severe case of pericarditis the patient is very ill indeed and may di from cardiac failure. If he recovers, some of the fluid may be removed (se aspiration of the pericardial sac on p. 161). If adhesions form the ape beat is seen to produce a wide ripple of movement instead of the usua small impulse, and in children the intercostal muscles may be indrawn b the tug exerted with each contraction of the heart which is bound dowr by adhesions to the wall of the chest.

Treatment. When pericarditis is rheumatic in origin *salicylates* ar administered. Gaultherium ointment spread on lint is applied daily ove the precordium both to reduce the inflammation and to relieve the pain. Alternatively some form of hot application such as antiphlogistine, or a mustard leaf may be used.

The *nursing care* of pericarditis includes observation of the chart for variations in temperature and careful watching of the pulse and respiration as collapse may occur. This would be met by omitting the salicylates and giving heart stimulants. The patient must be kept in bed for three months at least after the temperature and pulse are normal. Getting up should be very gradual and walking very limited for nine months; games requiring physical effort should not be allowed for two years.

ENDOCARDITIS

Endocarditis, or disease of the endocardium, affects the valves of the heart and produces *valvulitis* or *valvular disease*. As the result of inflammation of the valves *deposits of lymphoid tissue* form on them; later on, tiny growths described as *warty vegetations* are formed; and, still later, *fibrous tissue* is deposited and, when this contracts, it results in scarring which may produce narrowing of the valvular orifice.

As the result of the changes described above the affected valve or valves —as a rule the aortic and mitral valves are affected in endocarditis for valvular disease—undergo one of two changes:

(*a*) *Incompetent closure of the valve* results in *regurgitation of blood*, or *leakage* into the chamber behind the valve because, owing to the presence of adhesions, it is unable to close properly.

(*b*) *Obstruction* or *narrowing of the valvular orifice* may be present, and in this condition, described as *stenosis*, part of the lumen of the valve is permanently closed by the contracted fibrous tissue—which results in scarring—and the passage of blood through the opening is partially obstructed.

Symptoms of valvular disease. The symptoms present vary according as the mitral or the aortic valve is affected. In *mitral disease* the pulmonary circulation is first affected and the symptoms are—*palpitation* and *dyspnoea* on exertion, with a characteristic *malar flush* and, in severe cases, marked *cyanosis*. *Pain* over the heart is complained of, and this is associated with palpitation. As heart failure occurs the feet and ankles swell towards the end of the day.

In *aortic disease* the systemic circulation is primarily impaired and *the* *tient is pale*, complains of *dizziness and faintness* on the least exertion and as *pain behind the sternum* due to the insufficient supply of nourishment to e cardiac muscle. The pain is anginal in character (see also angina, n p. 354).

Acute infective endocarditis (malignant or ulcerative endocarditis) a very severe form of an acutely infective character which results in lceration of the valves; small particles of the friable ulcerated tissue reak away and, travelling in the circulation, give rise to the formation f *embolic abscesses* in various parts of the body. The patient is seriously l; the temperature is high, and rigors occur; there is marked wasting and rave prostration. Acute infective endocarditis may occur during the ourse of pneumonia, otitis media, scarlet fever and other infective conitions when the organism causing either of these diseases attacks the eart. The condition may end fatally in a few weeks unless the patient esponds to penicillin.

Treatment. The patient should be kept at rest in bed. Adequate doses of enicillin are given regularly, day and night over a period of six to eight veeks.

MYOCARDITIS

Myocarditis is inflammation of the myocardium; it may be due to any nicrobic infection and is found associated with acute rheumatism, inluenza, typhoid fever and diphtheria. The condition may be acute or ubacute and an acute myocarditis may become chronic.

Symptoms. The function of the heart is seriously affected in myocarlitis, the sounds are feeble, the rate increased, the rhythm irregular and he heart is dilated and flabby. *Palpitation* and *dyspnoea* occur on slight exertion, and the danger of fatal heart failure is always present.

CONGENITAL HEART DISEASE

Congenital heart disease is due to defective development of the heart. It may be present in a serious or in a minor degree. Serious disease may be due to the absence of a septum—a *bilocular heart*. There may be absence of either a ventricular or auricular septum, giving a heart with three chambers—a *trilocular heart*. Both these conditions are incompatible with any length of life.

Less serious disease is seen when there is incomplete development of a septum and the blood on both sides is mixed. Another form is described as a *patent ductus arteriosus*, meaning that the opening which exists in the foetal heart, between the pulmonary artery and the aorta, does not close at birth, as it should do, and that consequently arterial and venous blood mix and the baby is cyanosed and is called a *blue baby*. *Dextrocardia* is the transposition of the heart to the right side of the chest.

The **symptoms of congenital heart disease** are cyanosis and *dyspnoea*, which may be serious and alarming and is constant or paroxysmal, according to the severity of the condition. If the baby survives he will be subject to bronchitis and broncho-pneumonia and to infective conditions. If he grows up, clubbing of the fingers may be seen, and th conditions of cyanosis and dyspnoea usually persist.

FUNCTIONAL HEART DISEASE

Functional heart disease is also described as D.A.H., or *disorderly actio of the heart*, or the *effort syndrome*, because the action is deranged althoug there is no organic disease present.

The *cause* may be of nervous origin resulting from a disturbed emo tional state, or it may be due to the excessive use of alcohol, tobacco o. drugs.

The *symptoms* of functional heart disease are very numerous an may be much more distressing to the patient than the symptoms of seriou organic disease. Symptoms such as indigestion, constipation, palpitation breathlessness, insomnia, sweating, fainting and tremor are frequent.

The *treatment* includes the investigation for the presence of toxaemia which might be a contributory factor, and the general standard of healt should be improved.

SYMPTOMS OF FAILING CIRCULATION

Symptoms of failing circulation arise from the failure of the heart to pump blood into the organs, or to pump it with sufficient force to return the blood in the venous system back to the heart. This disability of function is described as 'back pressure' because, instead of the return of the blood to the heart for proper maintenance of the circulation, stagnation tends to occur in the various organs, resulting in impairment of their function because their blood supply is poor and ineffective.

At first the **circulatory system** will be affected and *the symptoms of pulse changes*, including irregularity of rhythm, rapidity and weakness will appear. *Pallor or cyanosis* may be present, depending on whether the systemic or pulmonary system is first affected; *coldness of the extremities* occurs as the result of a diminished blood supply to the limbs; *oedema* will arise as the result of inability of the venous system to convey its load of fluid back to the heart, and there is danger of bedsores, owing to diminished blood supply to the skin. *Anasarca* is generalized oedema.

Symptoms which arise as a result of *interference with the functioning of the respiratory system* include *dyspnoea*, *cyanosis*, *orthopnoea*, *cough* and *expectoration*. There may be *slight haemoptysis* and some degree of *bronchitis* may be present. In advanced disease *oedema of the lungs* occurs.

The symptoms associated with *disorder of the alimentary tract* include *loss of appetite*, *nausea*, *indigestion*, *constipation*, *flatulence* and *vomiting*. Disorder of digestion is also a cause of palpitation.

As regards the **excretory system**, the *amount of urine is usually diminished* and it may contain a small quantity of albumin. As the skin does not act freely, owing to defective circulation and the consequent insufficient supply of blood, it becomes dry and parched and is liable to be injured by friction and pressure. *The bowels are usually constipated;* ineffective return of the venous blood from the lower part of the intestine and rectum, owing to congestion of the liver, may give rise to congestion of the veins of these parts and result in haemorrhoids.

Symptoms affecting the *nervous system* are *headache*, complaints of *altera-n of vision* and *noises in the ears*, *irritability of temper*, *sleeplessness*, *night fears* ıd, in serious cases, *delirium*. A rise of temperature will usually only occur hen the cause of the heart disease is specific or infective in character, as rheumatism and infective endocarditis.

TREATMENT AND NURSING

The treatment of heart disease is usually divided under three eadings—**rest, diet** and **drugs.** With the first two nurses will be rimarily concerned, and in the application of all nursing measures it is ıerefore essential to bear in mind the need for absolute rest, and it ıould be remembered moreover that rest for the whole person, physical nd mental, automatically provides rest also for the disordered heart.

Type of bed. The bed should be comfortable, the patient should be kept dequately warm and may have a hot-water bottle to his feet and a light lanket next to him; if the weight of the bedclothes is sufficient to cause iscomfort they should be elevated by means of a low bedcradle. Some sters advocate the use of a blanket bed.

Position of patient. The position adopted must depend on the symptoms resent; in acute heart disease it will be possible to nurse the patient ecumbent; in chronic heart disease in which dyspnoea is present the atient will have to be supported in an erect sitting position. It is im-ortant that support should be adequate, and that there should be no ollows or spaces permitted between pillows. The head should be sup-orted on a small head cushion, and the arms should be placed on pillows t the sides of the patient so that he sits armchair fashion.

Rest must be adequate, and a patient with severe heart disease should ıot be permitted to make any effort—he should be washed and fed, very ently moved, and carefully lifted when necessary, so that his muscles do ıot contract during the strain of movement. His locker should be out of each, and he should be warned against raising his arms.

Later, when improvement occurs and he is allowed to do things for him-elf, his activities should be very carefully graduated; at first he might lean his teeth, and help to hold his feeding cup; next, he might wash his ace and hands, and so on. It is important to count the patient's pulse be-ore any active movement is made, and it should be counted again after-wards; if the effort has been too severe the pulse will not return to its original rate. This should be used as a guide throughout.

Sleep is necessary as it is the best form of rest, and yet no one sleeps as lightly or as badly as does a patient with heart disease. Nurses require to exercise great ingenuity in obtaining the best possible conditions to secure sleep for their patients, particularly with regard to maintaining their physical comfort; the correct degree of warmth, the provision of a low, non-irritating light, the reassurance that someone is within call and will hear the slightest sound—all of these things need careful attention.

Other factors which may induce rest for the heart include the perfect functioning, as far as it can be obtained, of the excretory organs; *the skin should be cared for* and bedsores prevented; *the bowels should be regulated* to act once or twice a day, producing a soft solid stool, or even watery stools, in order to remove fluid from the body and also to ensure that any possi-bility of constipation is avoided, as the passing of a constipated stool is a very great physical strain. The *amount of urine passed should be measured* ar compared with the intake of fluid, and the urine should be tested daily f albumin. Diuretics such as novurit may be employed (see below).

Chart. It is usual to keep a four-hourly chart in cases of heart disease, n only as a record of the temperature but also to obtain a regular record the pulse; and, besides the rate, the volume, tension, regularity and rhyth should be very carefully noted and any changes reported to the physicia without delay. When taking the pulse very definite observations should b made of the expression of the patient's face, for any manifestation anxiety; of his eyes, for signs of fatigue; his lips, for pallor and cyanos —and his general colour should also be noted—thus ensuring prop observation of many important points.

Diet. *The main factors* in the administration of diet in heart disease ar that it should be light, and easily digested, and that the feedings should b regularly and frequently administered, giving only small quantities at time because the stomach lies in close relation to the heart, and if th stomach is filled to capacity, or even only moderately filled, the weakene heart may be embarrassed.

In *acute heart disease* when the heart is failing, as in acute rheumatic car ditis or endocarditis, only diluted milk feedings will be given. As improve ment takes place, a light diet may be ordered. As a rule, protein and sal are limited, though a little protein such as white fish may be given, bu the diet should consist mainly of well-cooked farinaceous foods. It shoul not be too fluid, particularly if oedema is present, and fluid is in all suc cases best taken between rather than with meals.

Drugs. Digitalis, strophanthus and quinidine are the drugs mos commonly employed in the treatment of heart disease.

Digitalis acts as a heart tonic, slowing and strengthening the ven tricular contractions and prolonging the period of rest or diastole. It i given six-hourly because it is absorbed slowly.

Dosage: Digitalis folia, ½ to 1½ grains
Tincture of digitalis, 5 to 15 minims
Nativelle's granules of digitalin, $\frac{1}{600}$ or $\frac{1}{240}$ of a grain
Cat unit tablets, one tablet is given for every 10 lb. of body weight
Digoxin prepared from *digitalis lanata*, dose, 0.75 to 1.5 milligrammes.

Larger doses are employed to effect *digitalization* at the commencement o treatment, and it is in these cases particularly that careful watch should be kept.

In *nursing* certain precautions should be taken and the following observa- tions made. A patient having digitalis should be in bed, he should be warned against making any sudden or violent movements. When having large doses he should be kept on absolute rest. The *pulse* should be noted for irregularities, coupling of the beats, and decrease in rate. A pulse below 60 should be reported at once. *The rate of the heart beat should be counted at the apex.*

The *urine* should be measured and the increase noted; digitalis is a diuretic, *failure to produce diuresis* may mean that the drug does not suit the patient. Decrease in the quantity of urine indicates digitalis poisoning.

Nausea and *vomiting* may occur.

Strophanthus is usually employed when digitalis is not well tolerated. Tincture of strophanthus 2–5 minims may be given or *strophanthin* dose $\frac{1}{[illegible]00}$ to $\frac{1}{100}$ of a grain by the intramuscular or intravenous route.

Quinidine, one of the alkaloids of cinchona, is used principally in cases of auricular fibrillation. The dose is 3 to 10 grains; a test dose of 3 grains is given in case the patient has an idiosyncrasy; if no symptoms of toxaemia arise an average dose of 5 to 6 grains is then given every three hours for several days. The drug will only be continued if it suits the patient.

In the *nursing care* it is important to keep the patient quite quiet in bed, on absolute rest if possible. The bowels should be made to act regularly and effectively every day. He will usually complain of headache. Nausea, vomiting, abdominal discomfort and pain, and diarrhoea indicate toxaemia, and in some cases the patient becomes very ill. An erythematous rash may develop.

Drugs used in cardiac oedema. *Mersalyl* is an official and *Esidorne, Neptal, Novasural, Novurit* and *Salyrgan* are trade preparations of mercury employed as diuretics for the relief of oedema in cardiac failure. The urinary output may be increased, up to ten pints during the 24 hours following the administration of one of these preparations. The degree of dehydration produced by passing large quantities of urine may be accompanied by fatigue and malaise, but these symptoms usually disappear after a day or two.

Administration. The patient, if up and about, should go back to bed. He is given thirty grains of ammonium chloride every six hours for two days in order to make the urine acid. He is then given one of the mercurial preparations either by the intravenous or intramuscular route (Novurit is sometimes given in the form of suppositories). The dose is repeated at weekly or fortnightly intervals as found necessary to keep the patient free from a serious degree of oedema.

SUDDEN CARDIAC FAILURE OR SYNCOPE

This is a complication which may arise in any case of acute or advanced chronic heart disease. The patient will feel faint and may collapse, his breathing will become difficult and shallow, his pulse rapid and irregular, his face pale, his lips pale and blue, and beads of perspiration will collect over the brow and face.

This condition requires *immediate treatment* by the administration of cardiac stimulants including coramine and alcohol. In addition, hot fomentations may be applied over the region of the heart, and external heat applied by means of hot blankets, hot-water bottles and an electric cradle. A hot rectal saline should also be administered. Oxygen should be given.

CARDIAC ASTHMA

Cardiac asthma is a form of paroxysmal dyspnoea, similar in character to asthma, which occurs in heart disease. The patient is acutely distressed and unable to rest or sleep, as he is so frequently disturbed by painfully distressed breathing.

Nursing. The nurse will do everything she can to secure the patient's comfort in bed, and seeing, for instance, that he is adequately supported and well propped up with pillows, she will constantly administer oxyge which will be found to give slight relief. Stimulants will be given con paratively freely, and the nurse will be on the look-out for the signs c fatigue which indicate the necessity for administering these. In most case relief is only obtained after the administration of morphia. The prognos is grave.

ANGINA PECTORIS

Angina pectoris may be due to interference with the nutrition of th cardiac muscle, owing either to degenerative changes in the vessels supply ing the heart, or to impairment of the heart muscle.

The *symptoms* include pain, which characteristically commences over th region of the heart and radiates down the left arm. The patient has a sens of tightness about the chest, and he becomes rigid as he feels that he is i danger of immediate death. His face becomes ashen grey and his skin col and clammy. The pulse may vary, and in many cases the blood pressure i raised during an attack. Each attack begins suddenly, and it is usuall brought on by exertion. (See also coronary thrombosis, below.)

Nursing treatment during an attack. Nurses must be familiar with the drug which may be ordered in the treatment of angina, and be able to appl them without delay. In some cases amyl nitrite is inhaled from minut glass capsules, the capsule being broken in a piece of gauze or a handker chief and held under the nostrils. In other cases chloroform is inhaled fron a piece of absorbent material; in others again, some form of nitroglycerin is administered in tablet form.

The patient should rest whenever the attack occurs; if he is standing in the street he should keep still and be supported as well as possible, but i he is at home he should sit down and be comfortably supported. It is in advisable for him to lie flat as, owing to the constriction of the chest, h feels he cannot breathe.

Between attacks great attention should be paid to the maintenance o a good tone of general health, constipation must be avoided, and a nourishing, easily digested, diet taken. A reasonable amount of sleep i necessary, and all strain and worry should be avoided.

CORONARY THROMBOSIS AND CORONARY EMBOLISM

Cardiac infarction may be brought about by coronary thrombosis or em bolism. The former is commonly due to atheroma of the coronary vessel and the latter occurs as a complication in infective endocarditis.

Symptoms. In some cases there will be a *history of previous attacks of angina* (see above) but unlike angina this attack usually occurs during rest. In a very acute case the patient complains of severe pain over the heart, radiating to the neck and arms and also over the abdomen; he may have nausea and vomiting. In appearance he may be grey or cyanosed, his skin will be covered with sweat and his breathing distressed. He is restless and anxious.

The treatment of this form of cardiac attack is rest, morphia is administered and the patient is kept as quiet as possible; he should be confined to bed.

DISEASES OF THE BLOOD VESSELS

Aneurysm. An aneurysm is a dilatation of the walls of an artery. It is frequently associated with degenerative changes in the walls of the vessels and the aorta is the vessel most commonly affected.

In aneurysm of the aorta, the *symptoms* produced are those due to pressure on the neighbouring organs—dyspnoea, cough and sputum will result from pressure on the trachea—dysphagia will be due to pressure on the oesophagus—congestion in the veins of the head and neck will be due to pressure on the large veins returning the blood to the heart—a brassy cough is produced by pressure on the laryngeal nerves. In cases of aneurysm of the innominate or either of the subclavian arteries there may be inequality of the two radial pulses, as the blood takes a little longer to flow past the dilatation, and the pulse on the affected side may be slightly delayed.

Nursing and treatment. If admitted to hospital a patient with an aortic aneurysm is kept in bed in order to give him the necessary rest, and it will be important to see that he is not permitted to make any exertion. For a time he may be ordered absolute rest; later, he will be allowed to get up, and at this stage he should be warned against making vigorous movements.

As in the nursing of all cases of heart disease, the bowels should be kept acting regularly, the skin should be cared for, the diet should be light and easily digested, the patient should be free from worry and anxiety and should get a reasonable amount of sleep. In some cases there is considerable pain, and morphia may be ordered for the relief of this; in other cases the pain is intermittent and angina is a feature of the condition. Other drugs ordered include potassium iodide, arsenic and mercury, and nurses should be familiar with any untoward symptoms that might develop after the prolonged administration of these. Necessary details will be found in the section on drugs, p. 297.

Post-operative nursing care. In some cases of aneurysm *surgical measures* are taken. The aneurysm is separated from the vessel by proximal and distal ligature, which means that the circulation of the part, normally supplied by the vessel which has now been obliterated, has to be carried on by what is known as a collateral circulation—the vessels coming off above the area ligatured, anastomose with the capillaries of the vessels which arise from the artery below it; and, as when traffic is diverted in the city when a street is put temporarily out of use for the purpose of repairs, so in this case the traffic of the blood is permanently diverted into various side channels.

The most important points on the post-operative nursing care of such a case include observation of the circulation of the limb or affected part together with the maintenance of all possible nursing measures for keeping the limb warm. This may be accomplished by means of an electric pad, an electric blanket, well protected rubber hot-water bottles or the wrapping of the limb in warm wool. As sensation will be considerably impaired, owing to the lowered functional activity of the circulation to the part, heat can only be applied with great care, and the affected parts should be inspected every fifteen minutes or so. The position of the affected limb should be adjusted in order to help the circulation of the blood in the limb and the movement of the venous blood in the vessels.

Arteriosclerosis is a hardening of the walls of the arteries, whic causes a loss of elasticity and is frequently associated with a raised bloo pressure. Predisposition to this condition can be caused by a life of extrem tension and anxiety and it is also brought on by chronic toxaemia, and associated with such poisoning as that due to lead or the toxins of gou syphilis and chronic interstitial nephritis.

The *symptoms* are those of high blood pressure described in the no below.

Arteritis is inflammation of the walls of an artery.

Atheroma is degeneration of the large arteries, such as the aorta, an is a common cause of aneurysm.

Thrombo-angiitis obliterans (Buerger's Disease). This disease characterised by thrombosis of the arteries and veins in the extremitie usually in the legs. The cause is unknown. It affects men more tha women. The condition begins with numbness and pain which is increase by walking. The affected leg is red and shiny, the skin cold and the puls in the arteries of the foot are generally obliterated. The disease is progressive one; it may last for years. Gangrene of the limb may set in

Treatment. Rest in bed is recommended and massage and passive move ments of the leg. Protein shock therapy is useful in some cases.

Raynaud's disease is a vaso-motor disturbance of the blood vesse causing changes in the extremities. The fingers and toes become dea and pale, tingling and pain may be complained of. In more severe case the extremities go quite black, are extremely painful, and there is a tendenc to gangrene.

Treatment consists in protection from cold, and massage and electrica treatment. In severe cases sympathectomy may be necessary.

Affections of the Veins. Phlebitis is inflammation of the vei wall; it may be associated with varicose veins, thrombosis (thrombo phlebitis, see p. 567, is one type) or with gout and rheumatism. Th affected vein becomes swollen and painful; in the case of a superficial vei the skin becomes congested, oedema frequently occurs in the regio drained by the inflamed vein.

Treatment is rest and the application of belladonna. The patient shoul stay in bed and have a non-stimulating though adequately nourishin diet; the bowels should be kept acting regularly. After six weeks, massag may be given to help restore the circulation; when the patient gets up a elastic bandage should at first be worn.

Varicose veins are common in many people. The condition tends t run in families. Predisposing causes include occupations which necessitat standing, injury to superficial veins and phlebitis and thrombosis. Th veins most commonly affected are the internal and external saphenous, their tributaries, and the gluteal veins draining the back of the thigh.

Treatment is by injection and ligation. The patient has a bath on the day o operation, the limb is shaved from ankle to groin. A local anaesthetic is injected and a small incision made over the vein under treatment, it is dissected out, double tied, divided, and some sclerosing agent, 10 c.c. o quinine and urethrane, for example, is injected into the distal end and the nb is strapped from the ankle upwards. After one week the strapping is moved, and the stitches are taken out, the vein is examined and if necesry further injection of the lower parts of the vein made. In a few cases e patient is retained in hospital for a day or two, but he is not kept in d as rest is thought to predispose to the formation of pulmonary nbolism.

Contraindications to injection treatment are pregnancy, extreme age, raised ood pressure, severe constitutional disease, and a history of phlebitis or rombosis.

Complications include fainting, urticaria which would suggest an allergy the substance employed, allergic shock and collapse, and excessive action characterized by ascending phlebitis.

(Venous thrombosis is described on p. 658, and embolism on p. 377.)

HIGH BLOOD PRESSURE
(*Hyperpiesis*)

The walls of the arteries are normally elastic, contracting and relaxing cording to the pressure of blood contained in them, and the amount of essure exerted by the blood is described as the blood pressure. This is timated by means of a sphygmomanometer. Normally, the pressure gistered is described as being 100 plus the age of the subject; this is the stolic pressure, a systolic pressure above 140 being considered excessive persons under 50. The diastolic pressure is that found during the period diastole, or cardiac rest phase. The normal diastolic pressure is fairly nstant at from 70 to 80. In some cases of high blood pressure of the ypertensive type, it may be constant at 100, but this is a 20 per cent isability.

Symptoms of hyperpiesis. The blood pressure is high, in arterio-lerosis the artery is felt to be thick and tortuous under the examining nger, arterial tension is high and the pulse volume also is fairly full. With is type there is a tendency to cramplike pains in the muscles, and in the ecordial area which is suggestive of angina.

Other symptoms of hyperpiesis include headache, particularly frontal eadache made worse on stooping and on exertion.

Fullness and throbbing of the veins of the neck, with palpitation and me dyspnoea, on exertion.

Giddiness, nausea and vomiting.

Flatulence, indigestion and constipation.

Nervous depression, and in some cases there are complaints of visual ymptoms such as seeing spots of different colours, or blackness before he eyes.

There is a tendency to bleedings including epistaxis, haematemesis nd cerebral haemorrhage; and also to retinal haemorrhage and profuse nenstrual loss.

Danger. The danger of high blood pressure, particularly when associated vith arteriosclerosis, is that the disease is likely to be progressive and that he heart being overworked in order to maintain the circulation will evenually, sooner or later, suffer strain and become disabled in consequence. This condition is described as a hypertensive heart; the heart is enlarged, nd the apex beat can usually be felt 1 or 1½ inches outside the normal line.

As decompensation is now present, which means that the heart is failing

to compensate for the general circulatory disability, the diastolic pressu
will be raised in addition to the systolic pressure. All hypertensive cardi
cases are liable to the further danger of cerebral haemorrhage. The gr
matter is soft, and the hardened arteries passing through it receive ve
little support and, being degenerated, they may rupture, and any exerti
may increase the likelihood of this. Another danger is that of cerebı
thrombosis, since blood may clot in the narrow degenerated vessels throu
which it can only pass slowly.

Treatment. Before treatment is undertaken various clinical tests w
be carried out in order to determine as far as possible the cause of the co
dition. In addition to the physical examination of the chest the urina
function will be investigated, the urine will be tested for the presence
albumin, the quantity passed will be carefully noted and the blood ur
content determined. A cardiograph will be taken in order to determine t
regularity of the heart's action and, if any hyperthryoidism is suspecte
a basal metabolic test will be carried out.

The principal points in treatment are rest, and diet. At the outset t
patient may be kept in bed until the blood pressure becomes stabilize
In all cases the patient should be encouraged to lead a quiet uneventf
life, avoid fatigue, retire early and rise late, rest at very definite interva
during the day and have one day's complete rest in bed each week.

The *diet* should be reasonably reduced; it is inadvisable for patien
with high blood pressure to maintain their weight at a normal level an
it should be reasonably below this. Articles of diet which tend to produ
obesity should therefore be as far as possible eliminated. Red meat shoul
only be allowed once a week; fish, eggs and chicken may be taken, b
the patient may have large quantities of fresh fruit and vegetables; cond
ments should be taken sparingly, alcohol as far as possible omitted, an
stimulating drinks such as coffee and tea used only in very limited quant
ties. Smoking is generally considered inadvisable.

Another aim in treatment is to maintain the body fluids at a reasonab
low level. For this purpose fluid may be restricted to two or three pints

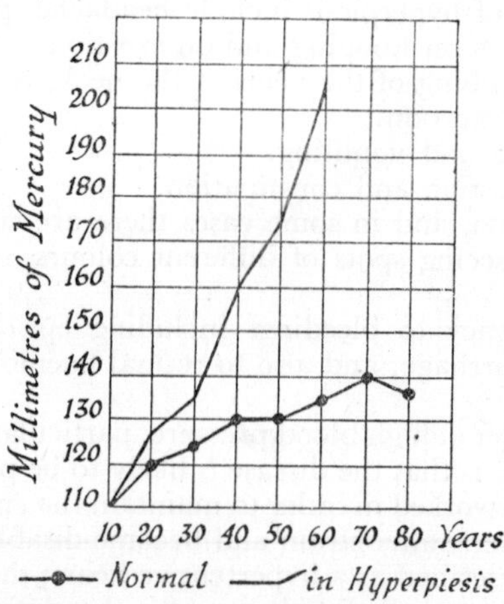

FIG. 170.—SYSTOLIC BLOOD PRESSURE GRAPH IN THE NORMAL PERSON AND IN A CAS
OF HYPERPIESIS.

ay. The bowels should be kept acting regularly and, as it is often con-
dered ideal for the patient to have at least two fluid stools a day, this
ıay be effected by means of a dose of calomel taken every week and a
nall dose of magnesium sulphate daily.

LOW BLOOD PRESSURE
(*Hypopiesis*)

A systolic pressure below 110 is considered abnormally low. Low blood ressure is met with in Addison's disease of the suprarenal glands, in con-itions of chronic wasting and in myxoedema. It also occurs in conditions f shock and bleeding when it is treated by applications of warmth and the dministration of fluid.

Patients with low blood pressure are usually anaemic and feel the cold ery much, the pulse is soft and of low volume, they are weak and avoid xerting themselves and often feel faint and dizzy.

Treatment. If immediate treatment is necessary, to relieve an attack f faintness or dizziness, adrenalin is usually ordered. The *general treatment* ıcludes rest, a liberal easily digested nourishing diet, plenty of fluids, and reatment for the relief of anaemia.

DISEASES OF THE BLOOD

Abnormal variation in the quality or in the quantity of the blood con-titutes a disease of the blood. The term *anaemia* indicates alteration in the ize of the red cells and their haemoglobin content. Formerly the anaemias vere described as *primary* when little, if anything, was known of the cause; ınd *secondary* when the anaemia followed some known condition, such as continued bleeding for example. More recently anaemia has been classi-ied according to the size and haemoglobin content of the red blood cells. The following is after Wintrobe's classification:

(1) **Macrocytic anaemia,** in which the red cells are larger than nor-nal. This type occurs in pernicious anaemia, and in anaemia associated vith disorder of the liver.

(2) **Normocytic anaemia,** in which the red cells retain their normal ize, as in anaemia after severe haemorrhage and in aplastic anaemia.

(3) **Simple microcytic anaemia,** in which the red cells are small and he haemoglobin content little, if at all decreased, is seen in chronic nfections and carcinoma.

(4) **Microcytic hypochromic anaemia.** The cells are small and the ıaemoglobin content is decreased. This type is seen in chlorosis (see below) ınd in cases where bleeding is constant and chronic.

The advantage of Wintrobe's classification is that it emphasises that in he macrocytic anaemias, when the red cells have their normal haemoglobin content, the cases are benefited by liver; but in the microcytic hypo-chromic anaemias, where the haemoglobin content is diminished, iron s indicated.

Primary anaemia or chlorosis, which is rarely seen today, was ormerly fairly common amongst girls in their teens, and is characterized by a greenish-yellow complexion, indigestion, loss of appetite, constipation, palpitation, difficulty of breathing—especially on effort—headache, swelling of the feet and ankles towards evening and some degree of insomnia. On examination of the blood the number of red cells is found to be very low and the percentage of haemoglobin, instead of being from 90 to 100 may be as low as from 25 to 30 per cent. The blood is watery in appearance and the colour index low.

This type of anaemia responds rapidly to treatment. Reasonable rest is advisable, with good nourishing diet; fresh air is beneficial, and tonics containing iron and arsenic produce rapid improvement; aperients may be necessary for the treatment of constipation at the outset, but the bowel should be regulated by the use of fresh fruit, vegetables and an adequate amount of water, as soon as possible.

PERNICIOUS ANAEMIA

Pernicious anaemia or Addisonian anaemia affects persons of middle age. It is considered to be due to lack of *haemopoitin*, which is an anti-anaemic factor produced by an 'extrinsic factor' in protein foods and an 'intrinsic factor' present in normal gastric juice.

Symptoms. The symptoms common to all types of anaemia are present—difficulty of breathing, palpitation, headache and general feelings of fatigue and weariness, loss of appetite and nausea, and swelling of feet and ankles occurs, particularly towards evening.

Certain symptoms are, in addition, characteristic of pernicious anaemia. The colour of the skin is lemon yellow, but the whites of the eyes are bluish white and stand out in contrast to the skin; the symptoms of indigestion are marked; the tongue is red and sore, and there is often marked nausea, vomiting and diarrhoea. In many cases some degree of paralysis of the limbs may be present, due to subacute combined degeneration of the spinal cord which occurs in many advanced cases and is an early feature in a few instances. The disease is characterized by marked achlorhydria, which may be responsible for the disordered digestion.

Examination of the blood reveals a diminished number of red cells; those present may be deformed and may be larger than normal while some are nucleated. The haemoglobin content of the blood is low, perhaps as low as from 40 to 50 per cent, this condition arising from the fact that there are so few red cells, though actually the amount of haemoglobin present in each cell is higher than normal.

Treatment. Originally, after the introduction of the *Minot Murphy liver treatment*, half a pound of raw liver was given daily. This has been replaced by liver extract which may be administered by mouth, by intramuscular injection or in very severe cases by means of the intravenous route, and has brought the prognosis of pernicious anaemia to such a standard that there is hope of permanent cure. A preparation of hog's stomach called *ventriculin* is employed as an alternative; some authorities consider that this is as valuable as liver, and that a hormone or similar substance is prepared in the stomach and stored in the liver, and that it is this material or hormone which controls the formation of blood cells in the bone marrow.

Hydrochloric acid is given in large doses in a dilute preparation in lemon or orange flavoured water, both before and during meals, in order to ttempt to make up for the deficiency in the gastric secretions. It is very isagreeable and it is therefore sometimes difficult to get the patient) continue taking this, but he should be encouraged to persevere with it.

In the nursing care of severe cases of pernicious anaemia the patient, being stless and anaemic, feels the cold severely and it is therefore necessary to eep him warmly clad and covered with light warm bedclothes. The ossibility of bedsores must be carefully guarded against. The mouth equires to be cleaned, as it is often sore, and the tongue, which is red and ainy, must be kept moist. The loss of appetite is a difficult feature to vercome. The symptoms of vomiting and of diarrhoea or constipation all for relief, and the former increases the difficulty of feeding the patient.

The many other troublesome symptoms that are present will require ursing attention as they arise, such as headache, general depression, aintness, marked malaise, sleeplessness and swelling of the feet and ankles. . severe case of anaemia therefore requires very similar nursing care to ne of cardiac failure.

Secondary anaemia, which presents the symptoms common to all orms of anaemia, as detailed above, may be due to one or more of , great many causes and, when severe, demands emergency treatment in he form of blood transfusion in order to give immediate relief. Subsequently the treatment is by the administration of iron.

Aplastic anaemia is due to an abnormal and probably degenerative ondition of the marrow, which interferes with its function in producing ed blood cells. These cases are desperately serious; the anaemia is exreme and often complicated by jaundice, and in many cases there is a ise of temperature.

Haemophilia is a disease of the blood in which there is inability to clot erfectly, so that subjects may bleed to death after a slight injury. It occurs nore markedly in males than females, and although there is little information to hand regarding treatment, it is necessary to try and prevent the ccurrence of injuries which will bleed.

Purpura is a disease characterized by the occurrence of bleeding into he tissues, and it is thought to be induced by toxic conditions, so that one of the first considerations is the investigation of this possibility. It is also net in scurvy, in serious cases of scarlet fever and in smallpox.

The grave anaemia which accompanies a serious state of purpura necessitates great care, carefully applied rest and the administration of blood transfusion.

Polycythaemia, also known as *erythraemia*, *Osler's disease* and *Vaquez's disease*, is an increase in the number of red blood cells. There is overactivity of the bone marrow, which manufactures red cells at a highly abnormal rate, and the spleen is enlarged.

In this disease deep X-ray treatment, applied in this case to the long bones, is carried out.

DISEASES AND CONDITIONS IN WHICH THE WHITE BLOOD CELLS ARE PRINCIPALLY AFFECTED

Agranulocytic angina or **Agranulocytosis** is a rapidly progressive disease characterized by marked diminution or loss of the granulocytes (polymorphonuclear leucocytes) in the blood. This condition is called *neutropaenia.*

The disease may be idiopathic, that is of no known origin, or it may follow the use of certain drugs, notably amidopyrine, compounds of arsenic and the sulphonamides. The condition of the patient is serious. Necrotic ulceration of the mucous membranes occurs, particularly of the mouth and throat. With the disappearance of the protective leucocytes the micro-organisms act unhindered, and the result is ulceration and destruction of the mucous surfaces which spreads with alarming rapidity. The patient becomes rapidly prostrate and in many cases fatal agranulocytosis occurs, but this condition can now be treated by penicillin.

Splenic anaemia or **Banti's disease** is characterized by marked enlargement of the spleen, and by diminution in the number of white cells—*leucopaenia*—the red cells and haemoglobin being also diminished. The *treatment* of this condition is splenectomy.

The condition of *leucopaenia* also occurs in pernicious anaemia and in influenza and typhoid fever.

Leucocytosis or **leukaemia,** on the other hand, is a condition of increase in the number of white blood cells. There are different types of this disease, and *some degree of leucocytosis* occurs in most conditions of prolonged suppuration or sepsis.

Lymphatic leukaemia is a condition in which there is a very large increase in the number of white cells, especially of the *lymphocytes*, and enlargement of the lymphatic glands all over the body. Normally the lymphocytes number from 25 to 30 per cent as compared with the white cells, but in this condition the number may be increased until they form 90 per cent of the total. This condition is very serious and the prognosis is grave; the disease may end fatally. *Treatment* by means of deep X-ray therapy has been employed, often with considerable success.

Spleno-medullary or **myeloid leukaemia** is characterized by marked enlargement of the spleen which may half fill the abdominal cavity; the bone marrow which is contained in the medullary cavity of the long bones is overactive, with the result that a large number of polymorphonuclear white cells are formed. The leucocytosis is marked, and this condition is also serious and the prognosis grave.

The *treatment* adopted is X-ray therapy, and in some cases good remissions of the disease occurs, though cure is unlikely.

DISEASES OF THE LYMPHATIC SYSTEM

The lymphatic system is part of the circulatory system, behaving, as it were, as the middleman, working between the tissues and the blood, and acting as a purifying agent which tries to prevent disease organisms or other poisonous products from reaching the blood from the tissues; but it is very likely, in conditions of disease, to become laden with dangerous waste matter, and this is demonstrated in conditions of lymphangitis and adenitis, when the lymphatic vessels and glands become inflamed, owing to the load of septic matter with which they have to deal in conditions of local sepsis, when the invading organisms are of a very virulent character.

Other conditions in which this function is demonstrated, when the glands in particular suffer and themselves become the site of disease, are surgical tuberculosis and secondary carcinoma.

Lymphangitis or inflammation of the lymphatic vessels is characterized by the presence of red lines under the skin; these are the inflamed vessels and can be traced to the nearest gland which may also be affected (see also adenitis, below). The area around the inflamed lymphatics is tender and swollen, and signs of general constitutional disorder will accompany the conditions when severe.

Lymphangitis is due to septic infection within a certain area—it may be that the focus of infection is in a septic finger or toe, and the lymphatics which drain this area will then be affected.

The *treatment* of the condition is to determine and then to treat the underlying cause; sulphonamides and penicillin are valuable; applications of heat, either fomentations or immersion in hot baths, will help. When the condition is complicated by cellulitis it may be necessary to incise and drain the infected area. The general care of the patient consists of the ordinary nursing attentions required in the treatment of a febrile and painful state.

Adenitis is inflammation of the lymphatic glands, one gland or more being affected. As in lymphangitis, when due to the presence of a septic focus, the glands which drain the area will be infected. In the upper limb the first lymphatic gland is at the front of the elbow; very important large groups of glands lie in the axilla and below the clavicle. In the lower limb the first groups are the popliteal glands, then come large groups of inguinal glands at the region of the groin. Several groups of glands lie in the neck, and these drain the region of the mouth, nose and throat which are so frequently affected by septic inflammatory conditions.

Adenitis may be *simple* when the gland is inflamed, enlarged, tender, red and hot, but does not suppurate; *suppurative adenitis* occurs when the inflammatory lesion progresses to the formation of pus. Adenitis may also be *tuberculous*, or *carcinomatous*, and a form of adenitis occurs in *actinomycosis*.

The *treatment of simple adenitis* is by the administration of sulphonamides and penicillin; *suppurative adenitis* necessitates incision and drainage of the infected gland; in *tuberculous adenitis* it is usual to aspirate the fluid and in some cases applications of X-rays and radium are employed.

When adenitis is severe it will be accompanied by a rise of temperature and the symptoms which are associated with this, and it will demand the ordinary nursing care applicable to such a condition.

Lymphadenoma, which is also called *Hodgkin's disease*, is characterized by a general enlargement of the lymphatic glands, affecting many or all of the glands; the spleen is enlarged and considerable anaemia is present.

It is a progressive disease, the enlarged glands exerting pressure on the nerves adjacent to them and giving rise to pain; all the symptoms of anaemia are present and the patient becomes gradually worse.

Treatment is directed to relieving the anaemia and improving the general health of the patient; in many instances the application of deep X-rays and radium to certain groups of the enlarged glands gives good results and by this means remissions in the course of the disease are possible.

Chapter 23

Diseases and Disorders of the Organs of Respiration

Catarrhal conditions of the respiratory tract: pharyngitis, laryngitis, tracheitis and bronchitis—Emphysema—Bronchiectasis—Asthma—The pneumonias: lobar, virus and broncho-pneumonia—Pleurisy—Empyema—Haemoptysis—Pulmonary embolism

For Influenza and Vincent's Angina, see chapter 34.
Pulmonary Tuberculosis is dealt with in chapter 35.

Diseased conditions of the respiratory tract are commonly classified according to whether the upper part is affected, as in the case of a cold in the head, or the lower parts as in capillary bronchitis.

In catarrhal conditions the discomfort experienced is due to interference with the function of the air passages in breathing. In most cases of catarrh the early symptoms of pain and obstructed breathing are due to dryness and congestion of the mucous membrane lining the passages. In the early stages of bronchitis the cough present will be painful, dry and suppressed.

In the later stages of catarrhal conditions the congested membrane secretes an excessive amount of mucus, the presence of which adds considerably to the discomfort in the case of a cold in the head, the running at the nose causing much inconvenience and soreness. In bronchitis, the increased secretion causes constant coughing in order to effect expulsion of the mucus filling the passages, and although this may be less painful than the dry suppressed cough of the early stage, the constant effort of coughing prevents rest and sleep and results in weariness and fatigue.

Disease of the lungs is another matter. In pneumonia, for example, large areas of both lungs may be incapacitated, and this will result in dyspnoea, which may be attributed to two factors:

(1) The *loss of an area of normally functioning lung tissue* owing to congestion and consolidation of a large portion of the organ (the lesser factor), and

(2) the greater factor, *strain on the heart* due to the inefficient oxygenation of the blood owing to the diminished respiratory area. This gives rise to dyspnoea and cyanosis and in severe cases will be followed by serious cardiac failure.

A description of the varieties of dyspnoea and cyanosis will be found in the observations upon respiration on pp. 51–4.

CATARRHAL CONDITIONS OF THE RESPIRATORY TRACT

Catarrh is a general term used to describe inflammation of a mucous membrane; in a common cold, the upper respiratory passages are affected, giving rise to *rhinitis*, spread of inflammation from the nasal mucous membrane to the pharynx causes *pharyngitis*, or *rhino-pharyngitis*, and in some cases *laryngitis* occurs.

A common cold is characterized by two stages. In the first instance the parts feel uncomfortably dry and hot, the membrane is congested and the nasal passages obstructed. In the *second stage*, *coryza*—a watery discharge from the nose—is present, because by this time the inflammation has progressed and the membrane is now secreting mucus very freely. At first this secretion is thin and watery, but after a day or two it becomes thicker and muco-purulent in character, and as the days pass it becomes offensive and thick like pus; later, as the catarrhal condition abates, the secretion diminishes.

The *treatment of a common cold* may be considered to be local and general. The *local treatment* consists in giving astringent inhalations in the early stages in order to diminish the congestion and relieve the obstruction; the use of steam inhalations will make breathing easier; the interior of the nasal cavities should be gently lubricated to keep them soft and free from cracks. Later, during the stage of severe coryza, the inhalations may be continued as congestion remains, and many proprietary articles are obtainable for use as nose sniffs and inhalations. The margins of the nostrils should be kept dry and free from soreness. The discharge is infectious and it should therefore be received on paper handkerchiefs or old soft rags which can be burnt; when the patient insists on using ordinary handkerchiefs these should be disinfected before they are washed, or washed and boiled separately from those of the remainder of the household.

General treatment consists in helping the skin to act and so improve the circulation; a hot bath, packing a patient up between hot blankets and hot-water bottles; the giving of a warm drink, such as lemon or hot whisky and the administration of a diaphoretic and sedative drug—either aspirin, or Dover's powder which contains opium and ipecacuanha—will help to ensure a good night's sleep and will also help the skin to act.

Whenever possible—and it is a pity this plan is so rarely considered possible—a patient during the first 3 or 4 days of having a cold in the head should stay in bed, partly for his own sake, in order to avoid the possibility of complications, but also for the sake of others, in order to avoid spreading the infection. If he can stay in bed, he may take an aperient on the second night, but otherwise the use of an aperient may only make him feel cold and uncomfortable and still further lower his resistance.

The pain experienced in the bones of the face when suffering from a cold in the head is due to infection of the sinuses; some degree of infection occurs in every instance, and the use of inhalations will help to relieve this and may possibly prevent serious infection.

When a person suffers from chronic colds, one following another in rapid succession, the cause should be investigated; it may be that the resistance of the patient to infection is lowered and that the use of a suitable vaccine will improve this.

PHARYNGITIS

Pharyngitis may be acute or chronic. **Acute pharyngitis** is usually associated with a common cold; it may, however, be present as a symptom of the onset of one of the infectious diseases, particularly measles and whooping cough.

The catarrh follows the same course as that described in the case of a cold in the head; at first the throat feels dry, swallowing is frequent in an endeavour to moisten it, and relieve the desire to cough; the cough is dry and irritating. The membrane of the pharynx will appear swollen, red and congested.

The *treatment* is very similar to that of a cold in the head, by the use c steam inhalations, and hot gargles will also help to relieve discomfort; th application of cold compresses to the front of the throat will sometimes b found to give relief. Penicillin is given as lozenges or in the form of a throa spray and when required it is also given by injection.

Chronic pharyngitis may follow repeated attacks of acute inflamma tion but it is more often brought on by the inhalation of irritating dus and fumes, and this may be associated with various trades; it may be du to the excessive use of tobacco, particularly cigarettes, or to excessive us of the voice. It may be associated with rheumatism or with the presence o a septic focus, locally, either septic tonsils or infected teeth.

The *symptoms* present are similar to those of acute pharyngitis; in man instances the throat is found to be relaxed and the uvula long and flabby the latter touching the walls of the pharynx and causing constant coughing

The *treatment of chronic pharyngitis* is primarily to investigate and treat an existing cause and to improve the general health. In the meantime th symptoms and discomfort must be relieved by the use of paints an gargles, which may be either antiseptic and astringent, or stimulating i character. The use of potassium chlorate, which may be employed locall as lozenges or given as a medicine, will help to keep the parts clean as thi drug is excreted through the salivary glands and therefore forms a con stant local application in the saliva which is being swallowed.

LARYNGITIS

Laryngitis may be catarrhal or it may be specific, as are the tuber culous and diphtheritic varieties.

Acute catarrhal laryngitis is usually due to spread of infectio from a cold in the head; it may, however, be due to inhaling irritatin particles, to overstraining the voice, or to excessive smoking; it is als associated with influenza, measles and whooping cough.

The structures of the larynx are inflamed, there is loss of voice, an irri tating cough and restrosternal soreness. These symptoms are accompanie by malaise and the patient may have a slight rise of temperature; he find it difficult to sleep as the cough is particularly troublesome at night.

The *treatment* is rest of the voice, which is the only way of resting th larynx; if the temperature is raised the patient should stay in bed, and i all cases it is advisable for him to avoid changes of atmosphere as changin from a warmer to a cooler one, or vice versa, will cause an attack of cough ing. Movement will also set up coughing, so that the patient should res quietly, if he will. It is important for the reason given above that the tem perature of the room in which the patient is nursed should be kept even day and night.

Local treatment by penicillin is often effective. Steam inhalations which moisten the air inhaled, will give relief; external applications of heat o moist warm compresses may help, and in some cases counterirritation i found to be of value.

TRACHEITIS

Inflammation of the trachea may be acute or chronic, and is usually associated with either laryngitis or bronchitis.

Acute tracheitis often begins as a cold in the head, but the symptoms soon show that the trachea is affected; there is a hard, dry, painful and irritating cough, accompanied by marked retrosternal soreness and pain; when the condition spreads to the larynx there is loss of voice. The cough is stimulated by movement and change of temperature, and is particularly irritating and troublesome at night when the patient is unable to sleep very much.

Treatment. It is necessary to keep a patient with tracheitis in bed. The trachea is a large respiratory vessel, very near the bronchi, and the condition may spread and give rise to a serious attack of bronchitis or bronchopneumonia if this precaution is not taken; subjects with tracheitis are moreover usually middle-aged or elderly persons in whom constant coughing and loss of sleep may soon give rise to cardiac strain.

The patient should be carefully watched for signs of more serious inflammation in the chest, a careful record of his temperature, pulse and respiration being kept; he may be given an aperient at the outset, and the physician will usually order a sedative to induce sleep. As the cough is dry and irritating sedative linctus will be required to relieve this; the diet should be light but nourishing, and the patient should have a jug of lemonade or any other drink he fancies at his side, as taking small drinks constantly will help to relieve the irritation which is making him cough.

The front of the chest may be rubbed with camphorated oil and covered with warm wool; poultices, if applied frequently, will give relief, and antiphlogistine is an alternative, though not as comfortable as the former. Penicillin may be of value and sulphonamides will help to prevent pneumonia.

BRONCHITIS

Inflammation of the bronchial tubes is described as *primary* when it occurs as the first symptom, and *secondary* when it is the result of spread of inflammation from the larynx or other part of the upper portion of the respiratory tract. It also frequently arises as a complication of influenza, measles and whooping cough.

Bronchitis may be *mild*, *severe* or *very severe*, and it may be *acute* or *chronic* When it affects the small tubes it is called *capillary bronchitis* (see bronchopneumonia, p. 374), this type being most commonly met with in infants. When affecting the large tubes it is described as *tracheo-bronchitis*, which is the type most commonly met with in elderly persons.

Bronchitis in elderly persons usually begins as a cold in the head and spreads to the large tubes giving rise to a troublesome cough which is dry at first. At this stage the sputum is scanty and mucoid, but later it becomes more abundant and muco-purulent in character and the cough becomes looser. Slight pyrexia usually accompanies malaise and the respirations are increased. The patient complains of soreness and pain behind the sternum and of slight dyspnoea. In extreme cases the dyspnoea is marked and it is then accompanied by cyanosis.

Treatment and nursing. The patient is kept in bed in a warm room (about 65° F.). The diet should be light and nourishing, and the bowels should be kept acting regularly. Sedatives may be necessary in order that the patient may sleep, as elderly people who do not sleep become very exhausted. Expectorants will be ordered. *Local treatment*, either rubbing the chest with liniment or applications of poultices or antiphlogistine may be ordered, and in some cases dry cupping is employed.

The *use of steam inhalations* will do much to relieve the dry harsh cough which is so distressing to the patient in the early stages of the disease. Inhalations of penicillin will reduce the amount of sputum and tend to prevent complications.

Chronic bronchitis. A form of bronchitis which occurs in some elderly persons winter after winter, and improves during the summer months, is described as *winter cough*. Such patients will be found in the chronic wards of hospitals year after year. The condition is commonly associated with other constitutional diseases, including diseases of the heart and kidneys.

The *symptoms* include cough, which is very troublesome at night, a large amount of muco-purulent expectoration is brought up and there is a varying degree of dyspnoea and cyanosis. There is usually slight fever. The pulse rate is slightly increased and the respirations are also increased; constipation is present, while the urine is scanty, highly coloured, and deposits urates on standing.

In the *nursing care and treatment*, the patient is transferred whenever possible to a warm, dry climate. When nursed in hospital wards a warm room is necessary. The diet should be very nourishing with the addition of cod-liver oil. Inhalations of penicillin are given. In some cases vaccine treatment is employed. Respiratory antiseptics are utilized and expectorants are usually ordered. The local applications mentioned above are also employed here.

It is in the *complications of bronchitis* that the seriousness of the condition is met. *Empyema* may occur, and the condition may also give rise to *emphysema* and *bronchiectasis*, but penicillin and/or sulphonamides will do much to prevent the development of complications.

EMPHYSEMA

In emphysema the air sacs have become dilated because the elasticity of the tissue in their walls has degenerated. Expiration cannot therefore be completed and as air is retained in the dilated sacs they are never completely empty. As the result of this the chest is always in a position of half expiration, and the epigastric angle is widened. Although this condition frequently follows chronic bronchitis it may also be brought on by whooping cough or by any very strenuous occupation in which forcible expiratory efforts are made.

The patient suffers from dyspnoea; he has intercurrent attacks of bronchitis and eventually his heart becomes disabled, and when this happens he is dyspnoeic even when at rest. The treatment aims at maintaining the general health.

BRONCHIECTASIS

Bronchiectasis is a dilated condition of the bronchi, with the formation of cavities which become filled with sputum. It occurs in patients in whom chronic coughing has weakened and dilated the walls of the air sacs, and is a complication of chronic pulmonary tuberculosis and chronic bronchitis. (For X-ray examination see fig. 81, p. 215.)

The *symptoms* include cough, which is paroxysmal in occurrence. Quite equently attacks of coughing occur in the morning, and also during the ay after intervals of rest. The sputum is offensive in odour, copious in uantity, dark in colour and deposits in three layers—a layer of pus at the ottom of the glass, then some brownish fluid surmounted by froth. As the esult of absorption of toxins, the patient's general condition becomes poor, ne temperature is intermittent in character and he looks toxic and, as ne years progress, he becomes very wasted.

The *nursing treatment* aims at maintaining the resistance of the patient by neans of a good diet. It is important that he should be placed in a suitable osition, i.e. head downwards for the purpose of drainage of sputum during nd after the attacks of coughing (see postural drainage, p. 99). Disnfectant inhalations are employed. Penicillin is given by intra-tracheal njection after postural drainage or by inhalation.

A *treatment* which has been found of value in these cases is collapse of the ung, which has been carried out by means of avulsion of the phrenic erve and by artificial pneumothorax.

ASTHMA

In asthma the patient suffers from attacks of expiratory dyspnoea which re brought on as the result of spasm of the muscle in the walls of the small ronchial vessels. There are various *causes of asthma*—in many cases an ttack is provoked by inhaling some foreign protein, in others it is provoked y the taking of some vegetable protein as food, but in many instances the ause cannot be determined.

In a typical case the patient may have some discomfort which indiates that an attack is coming on. In other cases he wakens out of a comortable night's sleep and immediately enters upon an attack. He sits up uffocating, almost unable to breathe, and his breath comes in wheezy aboured gasps, his face expresses fear, he is pale and anxious, his extremiies become cold and cyanosed, although his pulse and temperature may ot change. After a varying time he begins to cough in short severe aroxysms, which increase and eventually culminate in one which leaves he patient shaken to pieces and almost prostrated with fear and physical iscomfort. He then expectorates a little very sticky mucus and falls back xhausted—but usually relieved.

In some instances the attacks occur with little remission, and the patient ecomes the subject of *chronic asthma*.

Treatment. During an attack such as that described above, the treatnent aimed at is immediate relief, which in many cases can be obtained y the administration of 1 to 8 minims of *adrenalin*; but, as this has to be dministered hypodermically it becomes inconvenient for general use by he patient himself, and a Chinese drug, *ephedrin*, which in many cases is qually effective, is given as an alternative in half-grain doses by mouth. n very severe attacks some physicians consider a dose of morphia useful, ut there is a danger in this as the patient may become dependent upon he drug.

The *general health* of any patient who suffers from asthma should be naintained at as high a level as possible. He should particularly avoid neavy meals at night and any food which he finds it difficult to digest. It is advisable for him to sleep supported on several pillows. The bowe should never be constipated, and the hygiene of the nose and mouth shoul be very carefully attended to. Some patients find certain climates or atm spheres induce attacks whereas they can be quite comfortable in oth conditions, even in the immediate neighbourhood. This is a point f their own consideration as regards the choice of their mode of life.

THE PNEUMONIAS

Pneumonia is inflammation of the tissue of the lung. It may be acu or chronic. There are three types of *primary pneumonia*. These are all not fiable but secondary pneumonia is only notifiable in the case of influenz broncho-pneumonia.

Acute Primary pneumonia may be either *lobar pneumonia*, due t the pneumococcus, *atypical* or *virus pneumonia*, or *broncho-* or *lobula pneumonia* which occurs in infancy, childhood and old age.

Secondary pneumonia may occur as an acute pneumonia secondar to some other inflammatory condition in the lung, such as a pulmonar infarct, a growth, or to a lesion set up by the occlusion of a bronchi vessel, and to these cases the descriptive term 'pneumonitis' is sometim given.

Traumatic pneumonia, *post-operative pneumonia*, *inhalation pneumonia* and *hyp static pneumonia* are terms used to designate pneumonia secondary to som definite state or condition.

LOBAR PNEUMONIA

Lobar pneumonia is a disease of adults which follows a characterist course. It is due to the pneumococcus of which there are many type Types 1 and 2 are responsible for most cases of lobar pneumonia.

The *onset* is sudden, with headache and a rise in temperature an increased pulse and respiration, the temperature being 103° F. or over and the respirations as many as from 40 to 50. The patient is flushe with bright eyes, anxious facial expression, a dry dirty tongue, a hot skin he finds breathing very difficult, and is troubled by a short dry coug which he tries to suppress as every movement causes pain, and each act respiration terminates in a typical expiratory grunt.

The *disease is characterized by a very marked toxaemia*; it is a short sharp il ness, causing great strain on the heart, and it is this danger of heart failur that has to be ever borne in mind by the nurse who must be always on th look-out for symptoms similar to those described in an attack of syncop on p. 353.

Treatment and nursing. The *aim of treatment* is to maintain th patient's strength so that the work of the heart is supported, and to reliev toxaemia and prevent complications. On *admission* the patient will be pu into a comfortable bed, and whether he is given one, two or three pillow will depend upon the degree of dyspnoea present.

The sulphonamide drugs have revolutionized the treatment of pneu monia. Sulphapyridine (M. & B. 693) was first used but others of th group are also employed. Penicillin is of value in preventing empyema.

Chart. The temperature, pulse and respirations should be taken and charted four-hourly. Particular observation should be made of the pulse and respirations—the latter will be laboured and difficult throughout, but the pulse, if the heart is compensating, will maintain a fairly good volume, and be regular and not too rapid. Decrease in the volume and any rapidity say above 110 in the first few days, and over 120 after the third day, would be considered untoward. At the time of taking the pulse the nurse should make careful observation of the patient's general condition, noting his colour—pallor, greyness or cyanosis—the expression of his face for fatigue, his skin for the presence of cold sweat, his nose for any signs of dilation of the alae nasi, and his mental faculties for any tendency to wandering or delirium. She must also observe his sputum, note when it becomes tenacious, rusty or mucoid, and whether it is copious or scanty.

During the *course of the illness* the principal nursing duties include the maintenance of rest for the patient. It is important that he be saved all effort—he must not do anything for himself, he must be fed and washed and the sputum cup must be held for him. His mouth should be kept very carefully cleaned, all sordes being removed, and cracks and fissures treated in order to heal them. His lips should be kept constantly moist and lubricated with an oily preparation such as liquid paraffin. His nose requires similar attention as the nasal cavities tend to dry and become filled with crusts, which should first be lubricated and then removed.

The *position of the patient* in bed should be carefully considered, and whatever position is adopted should be adequately maintained so that he is entirely supported. He should be moved at intervals to avoid discomfort. He will frequently be found to lie on the affected side, and the nurse must be careful when she turns him on to the sound side as this will embarrass the movements of the chest and therefore diminish the work of the sound lung and so cause further strain on the already overtaxed heart.

The *personal clothing* should be of light woollen material which can be easily removed, and it should accordingly be made to open either at the back or front. Patients who are sitting up should have a gamgee jacket and a warm flannel bedjacket in addition. Patients who perspire a great deal might have a light blanket next to them. It is important, however, that the bedclothing should in all cases be light. Whenever there is any tendency to coldness of the extremities—indicating the onset of cardiac failure—external warmth should be applied and hot-water bottles given or a small electric cradle applied over the feet.

The *skin and excretory organs* should be attended to; the skin may be hot and dry or there may be free perspiration; in the latter case the patient will require frequent change of garments as he must not be left lying in damp clothing. The pressure points should be treated in order to prevent sores. The urinary output should be measured and the urine tested for the presence of albumin; albuminuria may accompany the onset of the febrile state without being considered serious but, when it occurs later in the illness, it may mean that the heart is failing. The bowels should be kept acting regularly, one or two soft solid stools a day being considered adequate. As the patient tends to be a dry, thirsty individual there is a natural tendency to constipation, and although the provision of adequate fluid may help to avoid this, in many instance aperients may have to be resorted to. It is usual, for example, to give the patient an aperient at the outset of the illness. Care should be taken in the choice of aperients, avoiding those inclined to the production of flatus, such as salines, and others apt to pro duce stimulation of the involuntary muscle and so give rise to griping an pain, such as colocynth, should also be avoided. As far as possible onl laxatives such as liquid paraffin and phenolphthalein should be employed

Sleep is all important in the treatment of pneumonia. The importance c rest has already been pointed out, and sleep is the ideal form of rest sinc during sleep not only are the muscles relaxed but the central nervou system is at rest, external stimuli being temporarily cut off. The nurse mus do everything she possibly can to obtain sleep for her patient, and the not on insomnia on p. 338 suggests measures which might be carried ou with this object in view. In many instances the physical discomfort is s great, despite all the nurse can do, that sedative drugs will have to b ordered, those most commonly employed being pulv. ipecac. co. et opi dose 10 grains (Dover's powder), and paraldehyde, dose 2–4 drachms, th latter being commonly given per rectum.

The suitable *diet* in pneumonia is rather a controversial subject, som physicians considering that, as the illness is so short, the provision c adequate fluids such as water and lemonade, up to 6 or 8 pints, provide that 6 to 8 ounces of glucose are administered each day, is sufficient Others like the patient to have nourishing fluids—in this case three pint of nourishing fluid, including milk, Benger's food and chicken broth ar employed, and 3 to 4 pints of watery fluids are given in addition. Th management of a fluid diet in a case of pneumonia might take the form o that described in the section on administration of a fluid diet under die section (p. 267).

Some degree of *delirium* occurs in a great many cases; it is to be expecte in chronic alcoholics, and in these cases the doctor will usually order stimulant from the beginning, in order to avoid the shock to the syster which occurs when alcohol is suddenly discontinued. It is important i attending these cases with delirium that movements should not be re strained more than is absolutely necessary, as such restraint increases th effort made by the patient and the principal aim in nursing all cases c pneumonia is to maintain rest. The note on p. 346, in which deliriur is discussed, is a guide to the nurse in her management of such cases.

Crisis. Reference to the chart shown on p. 45 will be an indication c the course and mode of termination—by crisis—which may be expecte between the fifth and tenth days in untreated cases. In some ir stances a *false crisis* occurs twenty-four hours or so before the true crisis A false crisis is unaccompanied by any abatement of symptoms or an decrease in the rate of pulse and respirations. When the *true crisis* com mences, the patient will be observed to be more comfortable, his coug easier, his sputum brought up with less effort, he will be inclined to sleep and the temperature will be found to be declining fairly rapidly, droppin from 104° F. to normal in 6 or 8 hours. This rapid decline can only tak place by loss of heat to the body, and the skin will be found to be actin freely. The nurse must watch for this, wipe the increasing perspiratio from the skin and change the patient's damp clothing, and apply extern heat in the form of hot-water bottles, or a hot bedcradle and warr blankets. She should persuade the patient to take warm stimulating fluic and nourishing drinks at this stage of his illness. He may sleep whilst th temperature is falling, but during this period he requires constantly watch ing and, since it is important for the nurse to know the rate at which it declining, his temperature should be taken without disturbing him. The danger at this point is of collapse. Any sign of greyness and pallor, or cyanosis, weakness of pulse, or shallowness of breathing must be treated by cardiac stimulation—the physician will order the stimulants which may be given in this emergency. The nurse should have ready, for the moment when the patient wakens, warm towels to rub him down, a warm bedgown to put on, and hot blankets to cover him. At the same time she should give him an opportunity to pass urine, which is more rapidly secreted at the time of the crisis, take his temperature and give him a warm stimulating drink and tuck him up when he will go to sleep again, and probably waken several hours later, thoroughly refreshed. The treatment which has just been described should then be repeated.

After the crisis the patient remains in a very serious condition for some time, being now very weak after an extremely short sharp illness, and is still in considerable danger from cardiac failure and collapse. He should not be permitted any exertion for a further week, and any signs of cardiac failure such as cyanosis, pallor or pulse weakness should be observed and treated.

At this time the amount of food may be suitably increased, the patient being gradually given a nourishing diet of high calorie value. After a week or ten days he may be permitted to wash his face and hands, and effort should be gradually increased until he is allowed to perform his own toilet. He may then be propped up and allowed to read in bed. When he is permitted to get up, half an hour is considered quite long enough on the first day, and this may be increased to an hour on the second. Convalescence is fairly rapid and is not usually complicated, but a fairly long convalescence, with rest from work and change of air, and a good liberal nourishing diet should be recommended.

Infection and isolation. Primary lobar pneumonia is a notifiable fever under conditions of epidemic. The sputum is infectious and teeming with organisms, and requires disinfection before disposal. In nursing cases of pneumonia in private houses, all feeding utensils should be kept separate, the sputum should be disinfected before disposal, the patient's handkerchiefs should be washed separately from those of the household, and the hands of attendants and visitors should be carefully washed after any contact with the patient.

Complications. *Pleurisy* may be regarded as a complication although it occurs in all cases of pneumonia when the inflammation spreads to the surface of the lung. *Empyema* may complicate convalescence. Other complications include *heart disease*, *otitis media*, *nephritis*, *meningitis*, *mal-resolution* of the lung and the formation of *lung abscess*.

VIRUS PNEUMONIA

This variety is called *pneumonitis*, *virus pneumonia* or *atypical pneumonia*. It is the type of pneumonia usually occurring in epidemics of influenza and it attacks young adults. It is due to a virus. There is an incubation period of 7–21 days.

The onset is insidious, the temperature rises to about 102° F. and the pulse increases to about 120 but the respiratory function is only slightly disturbed. There is a short dry cough. Mental confusion sometimes occurs.

After a week the temperature declines and the symptoms disappear. Complications are rare but the patient is left weak and tired after this illness and needs a long carefully supervised convalescence.

BRONCHO-PNEUMONIA

Broncho-pneumonia is also described as capillary bronchitis and as catarrhal pneumonia; it is met as a primary disease due to infection of micro-organisms and as a secondary condition as a complication of measles, whooping cough, influenza, and it may also arise as the result of the inhalation or aspiration of vomit, blood or saliva.

Primary broncho-pneumonia is most often met with in infants. The infant is very ill, he is flushed and cyanosed, his temperature is high and continues for from 8 to 10 days with slight daily remissions to terminate by crisis or lysis. The respirations are rapid, from 50 to 60 per minute, there is marked and distressing dyspnoea, with movement of the alae nasi, retraction of the sternum and recession of the intercostal muscles. The pulse is rapid, over 120, and becomes weak and running in character as the disease progresses. There is a short dry cough, but no expectoration, as tiny infants do not expectorate, usually swallowing any secretion brought up. At first the infant is restless, but as the days pass and toxaemia increases he becomes drowsy.

Treatment and Nursing. The infant should be in bed, propped up so that his head and shoulders are raised; he should be lifted for changing and feeding in order to get frequent changes of position. If secretion is brought up to the mouth, the nurse should endeavour to get it away so that it is not swallowed. Expectorants are not usually given to tiny infants, but if the heart is in a good condition tincture of ipecacuanha is administered in doses which will cause vomiting in order to assist in the bringing up of sputum. Sulphonamides for the treatment of pneumonia and penicillin for the prevention of empyema are the drugs employed.

The temperature of the room should be 65° F. and some physicians like a moist atmosphere—either a steam kettle boiling in the room, or a steam canopy may be provided. The chest should be rubbed with warm camphorated oil morning and evening and covered with wool or a gamgee jacket. The personal clothing should be light flannel and the infant protected from chilling.

The diet given is fluid, about 8 ounces of diluted milk containing 2 drachms of lactose every 3 hours being adequate. If curds appear in the stools or vomiting occurs the milk should be citrated (see p. 263). The temperature, pulse and respiration should be recorded every four hours; if the fever reached 105° F., the infant should be sponged, and inhalations of oxygen may cause improvement in colour and help to relieve the dyspnoea. The bowels should be kept acting regularly.

A tiny child or infant who is very ill—as is this one—requires constant company and his cotside should not be left; the nurse should touch him gently, take hold of his little hand, stroke his brow, and in this way let him see he is loved and cared for, and this will help the contentment which s an aid to the rest that is so essential if this short sharp serious illness is o be brought to a successful termination.

PLEURISY

Inflammation of the pleura may be acute or chronic. Acute pleurisy accompanies most cases of pneumonia. It is also common in pulmonary uberculosis and may be one of the modes of onset of this disease.

Two main varieties are described, **dry pleurisy** in which the membrane is inflamed but there is no exudate, and the roughened fibrous membrane rubbing together gives rise to considerable pain.

The *symptoms* in this variety are a short sharp shooting pain, increased on movement of the chest, as on taking a deep breath or when the patient coughs. The cough is short, dry and suppressed, and the patient is unable to rest, unable to sleep because of his pain, his temperature is usually raised, his respirations rapid and shallow, and his pulse slightly quickened. He tends to lie on the affected side in order to limit the movements which are giving him pain.

The second variety is described as **pleurisy with effusion** and in this type considerable fluid has been secreted and the two pleural membranes are separated. By means of this they are kept from rubbing together and the pain due to friction is not present. The presence of a quantity of fluid in the pleural cavity considerably embarrasses the breathing, however, and gives rise to dyspnoea. When respiratory distress is present cyanosis occurs and, when there is a large quantity of fluid, the heart may be displaced. The other symptoms mentioned in dry pleurisy, which are those associated with a rise in temperature, are also present.

Treatment. A case of pleurisy is treated as a febrile case, the patient is kept in bed, given an aperient at the outset, and a four-hourly record of the temperature, pulse and respiration rate is kept.

In *dry pleurisy* some means may be taken to help immobilize the affected side such as the application of a tight binder, or strapping the chest; counterirritants may be ordered to relieve pain, and either a form of heat such as antiphlogistine, or a mustard plaster may be used. Sedatives will usually be necessary to relieve pain in order that the patient may sleep.

In *pleurisy with effusion*, if the fluid is embarrassing the action of the heart some of it will be removed. In many cases this condition persists for weeks and the fluid is gradually absorbed. Penicillin is of value in preventing complications.

In all cases of pleurisy the *ordinary nursing measures* employed in the nursing of any febrile case are required, with, in addition, special care in each case. In dry pleurisy everything should be done to prevent pain, and in pleurisy with effusion the chief point to be considered will be relief of the embarrassed breathing by maintaining a suitable and comfortable sitting position in bed.

EMPYEMA

Empyema is a collection of pus in one or both pleural cavities. It may follow pleurisy, pneumonia or pulmonary tuberculosis. It is the complication which would be suggested in any of these cases by a secondary rise in temperature following the subsidence of the initial attack of the disease.

Symptoms. The chief symptom is irregular and intermittent pyrexia, accompanied by an increase in the rate of pulse and respirations. As the fluid in the pleural cavity is pus, unless it is removed the patient will rapidly assume the appearance of one suffering from septicaemia. His skin will be grey and unhealthy looking, his cheeks flushed; he will become wasted and considerable sweating will occur. The appetite will be lost and malaise will be marked. As a rule there is some pain in the side and a cough is present. When the fluid becomes large in quantity the action of the heart and lung will be embarrassed.

Treatment. In all cases the chest will be explored and a specimen of pus examined, to discover the organism that is producing the condition. In cases in which pus-producing organisms are found, penicillin solution, 1,000 units per c.c., is injected into the cavity after operation. Resection of rib may be necessary to remove pus and blood clot.

The *post-operative nursing care* is described in Chapter 46.

HAEMOPTYSIS

The spitting of blood occurs in a number of conditions but most particularly in disease of the heart (mitral disease), and as a complication in pulmonary tuberculosis.

A *severe attack of haemoptysis* is a very alarming condition, the patient sometimes coughing up a large quantity of blood. It is usually frothy, mixed with sputum and bright red in colour, and if the reaction is tested it will be found to be alkaline.

The **first aid treatment** is of primary importance in such a case, and the patient should be put to rest in a sitting position wherever the attack has occurred; his respiratory passages should be cleared of bloodclot by putting a finger at the back of the throat and clearing it out; he should then be given sips of cold water—he may wash his mouth out first, in order to avoid the nasty taste of blood, and then have a drink. His clothing should be loosened about the neck and chest and he should be allowed to breathe fresh air; he should at the same time be reassured as he will be very terrified, and he must be warned to avoid any effort and even to suppress coughing as far as possible.

As soon as possible he should be very carefully lifted into bed, but the effort of undressing him should not immediately be undertaken—he should rest for a time first. In the meantime, his pulse and colour should be very carefully noted, the degree of shock observed and treated as necessary. He may be given iced water by mouth, and the nurse should prepare a hypodermic injection of morphia as the physician will probably order this on arrival. He may also order various substances for the arrest of bleeding, such as preparations of calcium and coagulin ciba.

Once the patient is comfortably in bed and undressed, he may be placed in a sitting position or, if the bleeding has been very severe and shock is present, it may be found necessary for him to lie down. Suspending an cebag over the affected side, if this is known, does much to reassure the patient, and it also helps to keep him lying quietly, in order to preserve contact with the cold application.

The **nursing treatment** during the days following a severe attack of haemoptysis is very similar to the nursing care of any patient who has bled seriously. Rest is essential, the diet should be low, cool and non-stimulating, the bowels should be kept active by the use of saline aperients, and all movements and excitement, worry or anxiety should be prevented. The admission of visitors should be very carefully controlled and only those that will help to keep the patient calm, and not excite him, should be admitted.

PULMONARY EMBOLISM

An embolism is a foreign particle moving in the circulation, usually a small portion of bloodclot, and when it is circulating in the lungs it is described as a pulmonary embolism. It reaches the pulmonary circulation from the right side of the heart where it enters the pulmonary artery; the particle may have been brought to the heart by way of the venae cavae from some distant part, as when a pulmonary embolism occurs as a complication of some pelvic or abdominal operation; it may also be due to marked slowing of the circulation which happens in some forms of heart disease when bloodclot forms in the right auricle and is carried thence to the lungs. If the clot, or other particle, is big enough to obstruct a large artery in the lung, instant death occurs; the patient may be found to have died without any apparent distress, or he may sit up, look grey, gasp for breath and fall back on his pillows dead.

Symptoms. When the embolism blocks a smaller artery, only a portion of the lung will be deprived of blood, and the symptoms will then depend on the extent of the area affected. The patient will sit up frightened, gasping in an effort to breathe, his colour will be grey and cyanosed and he may cough up some blood; he will complain of acute pain in his chest.

Treatment and nursing. The *first-aid or immediate treatment* is important, and this is usually carried out by a nurse, who must keep quite calm and not appear flurried while she reassures the patient, supporting him in a sitting position until she can maintain him in this position by means of pillows; she should advise him not to move and must loosen any tight bands of clothing round his neck and waist, open an adjacent window so that he gets plenty of air, give intranasal oxygen if it is available, and press her hand against the patient's side in an attempt to relieve the pain; she may apply a hot-water bottle or some antiphlogistine or other hot application. She should hold the sputum cup for the patient, but must try not to let him see any blood he brings up; she may moisten his lips and give him small sips of water. She should prepare morphia which the physician will order when he arrives.

Subsequent nursing measures aim at keeping the patient as quiet as possible and maintaining the blood pressure comparatively low; the physician will order sleeping draughts so that the patient sleeps at night, but the nurse should see that his days are uneventful, visitors who might excite him not being admitted; he should not be allowed to read newspapers or exciting literature, his diet should be light, and it should be given cool; fluids ought to be limited to 3 pints; the bowels should be kept acting twice a day, by the use of saline aperients at first, and after the first week by means of liquid paraffin.

A careful record of the temperature and pulse and respiration rate should be kept, and the patient's colour should be noted. The portion of lung which has been deprived of its blood supply is not acting, and is called an infarct—if it is large, the degenerative changes which must of necessity follow may give rise to septic pneumonia.

When *embolectomy*, or removal of the clot, is performed, it requires to be carried out immediately, but this operation has not been extensively used in this country. Instruments for this emergency are shown on p. 675.

Chapter 24

Diseases and Disorders of the Organs of Digestion

Dyspepsia—Peptic ulcer—Haematemesis—Inflammatory conditions of the alimentary tract: stomatitis, gastritis, enteritis, colitis, diverticulitis—Diarrhoea, infective enteritis—Constipation—Worms—Pylocic stenosis—Hirschsprung's disease—Visceroptosis—Disease of the liver and gallbladder: jaundice, cholecystitis, cirrhosis of liver, liver abscess, acute yellow atrophy

Food poisoning is dealt with in Chapter 34, *p.* 495.

The digestive tract extends from the mouth to the lower part of the small intestine; many substances enter it, and various parts of it secrete digestive and lubricating fluids which act on its contents, and the secretions of other organs are received by it, notably the salivary, pancreatic and bile fluids.

Loss of appetite, nausea, vomiting and indigestion are the symptoms commonly met with when the functions of this group of organs are impaired. The causes of disorder of digestion are manifold—the secretion of the digestive fluids is disorganized in all diseases associated with a rise of temperature, in diseases of the heart and circulation, and in many functional and organic nervous diseases. (The note on indigestion as a symptom of disease, on p. 345, will suggest the number of diseases and conditions in which it may occur as a symptom.)

Dyspepsia may be acute or chronic, and it may be mild, severe or very severe. In the mild forms the symptoms commonly met with include discomfort after meals, nausea, heartburn, dryness of the mouth with thirst, a dirty flabby tongue, a disagreeable taste in the mouth with offensive breath, and in some instances salivation is increased. Nausea may continue for days and be accompanied by headache, constipation and vomiting.

When the condition is more severe, indigestion may be accompanied by a rise of temperature and a more marked degree of malaise, the patient feeling ill enough to remain in bed; the abdomen may be very tender, distended and painful, and the pain intermittent and colicky in character.

The *treatment of dyspepsia* aims primarily at the relief of the symptoms; the cause should then be investigated and treated; a diet which is suitable for each individual case is ordered, any foods which irritate or give rise to symptoms of indigestion being studiously avoided. The general condition of the patient's health should be investigated and it should be maintained at a high level. Adequate fluid should be given, the bowels regulated, and the patient should endeavour to obtain a normal amount of rest, sleep, recreation and exercise.

During an acute attack of indigestion it may be necessary to keep the patient in bed; when vomiting is persistent it will be necessary to omit food; but fluid starvation should be watched for (see dehydration, p. 268), and an adequate amount of fluid given, with some glucose added if possible.

In *chronic dyspepsia* the patient often becomes so much afraid of the distressing symptoms of the condition that he will not eat enough and consequently loses weight. He will then become anaemic and is in danger of developing an abnormally small appetite.

In the medical treatment of dyspepsia it is usual to examine the secretions and the functions of the stomach by means of test meals and X-ray investigation. The preparation for, and the manner of assisting at, a test meal is described on p. 172.

PEPTIC ULCER

The term peptic ulcer implies the presence of an ulcer on the parts of the stomach or duodenum which are exposed to the presence of the acid gastric juice. Whatever may be the cause of such a lesion, once present, constant contact with the gastric juice serves to keep it from healing and will probably cause it to spread.

The **symptoms of peptic ulcer** are those of dyspepsia or indigestion; as a rule a patient has attacks of this, he is sometimes better and sometimes worse, and usually notices that the attacks become more frequent—he then consults a doctor. The doctor proceeds to make a diagnosis, examines the general condition of the patient, takes his history, investigates the presence of pain and tenderness in the epigastrium and has the stomach contents examined by means of a test meal, and the movements of the stomach and duodenum investigated by means of a barium meal and X-ray examination.

The symptoms vary slightly according to the position of the ulcer. In *gastric ulcer* pain is experienced near the cardiac end of the stomach, coming on very soon—about 20 minutes—after a meal. It may be relieved by taking sodium bicarbonate or by vomiting. The patient becomes afraid to eat because of the pain he will suffer and consequently loses weight.

In the case of *duodenal ulcer* the pain is to the right side rather than in the middle line; it does not begin until some time has elapsed after taking food—in some cases not until about 2 hours after; the patient may say that he wakens with pain after he has been in bed for an hour or two. This pain is relieved by taking food or drink and a patient will often say that it is relieved by taking a glass of milk and soda or a couple of biscuits. It is also relieved by alkalis. These patients do not lose weight as consistently as do those with gastric ulcer, as they are probably taking small frequent meals.

On examination pain and tenderness will be found to be present over the region of the duodenum.

Treatment of peptic ulcer is mainly dietetic and each hospital has a detailed diet regime. The *principles of treatment* include the provision of rest, by limiting the movement of the stomach and its functional activity; by avoiding large meals and long spaces between meals, giving small liquid meals at short intervals of 1½ to 2 hours; providing substances such as belladonna before meals in order to reduce spasm and so allay irritability of the stomach and to inhibit the secretion of gastric juice.

Olive oil is also employed as the oil inhibits the movement of the organ. Alkalis are given between meals, in order to reduce the acidity of the contents of the stomach, and if possible prevent acidity.

Complications. The complications of peptic ulcer include bleeding, which may be slight or severe; in some cases oozing of small quantities of blood occurs, though the amount may be so slight that the presence of melaena in the stool is not obvious. In these cases a special test may be made and the nurse will be required to send a specimen of the stool to the laboratory for this purpose. (See special care in preparation of a patient for this, as noted on p. 79.) A small quantity of hidden blood, known as '*occult*', is such as can only be discovered by careful examination and cannot be suspected by the naked eye.

Melaena (altered blood) may be observed as black 'tarry' stools. The blood may be unaltered when bleeding is rapid and severe, and the stools passed may be well coloured by the large quantity of blood in them.

Haematemesis is the vomiting of blood from the stomach, and when copious it may be very little altered; but when the blood has remained even a short time in the stomach it becomes acted upon by the gastric juice and altered, and the characteristic appearance of this vomited blood is described as being of coffee-grounds consistency and colour.

Adhesions may form as the result of a long-continued inflammatory lesion in the vicinity of an ulcer or ulcers, and these may result in fastening the stomach or duodenum firmly to its adjacent structures, either to the liver, pancreas, colon or peritoneum. In such a case, movement of the organ will be limited and contraction may occur.

Scarring and contraction. When an ulcer occurs on one wall of the stomach, the irritation set up tends to produce spasm, which results in contraction of the muscle fibres and approximation of the opposite wall, and in this way an ulcer on the stomach wall may set up a contraction sufficiently marked to divide the stomach into two chambers—an hourglass stomach. An ulcer at the pyloric end of the organ may result in stenosis, and give rise to a very dilated stomach.

Fistula. In some cases where the stomach has been firmly attached to the wall of another organ a communication (fistula) may be made between them. The commonest type of fistula occurs as an opening between stomach and colon—a gastro-colic fistula.

Malignant disease may complicate peptic ulcer, but this rarely happens.

Nursing care. Many patients with peptic ulcer are cheerful and optimistic; others, having suffered discomfort in the epigastrium, off and on, perhaps for many years, with the irksomeness of always having to consider what they may or may not eat, become introspective and fidgety; others develop some irritability of temper and many are thin, and feel the cold very much, and often feel generally out of sorts and miserable. The nurse must therefore be able to visualize the state of life that has brought about the mental attitude of any given patient to his surroundings, and be prepared to encourage and help him.

The bed should be comfortable and the personal clothing warm, and as the patient will have to spend several months in bed in many instances, any recreation he likes should, if possible, be provided. At first his diet will be limited to small quantities of fluids at regular intervals, and as far as she can the nurse should consider the patient's taste as to whether he likes things hot or cold, and allow him to have any little flavouring he fancies, if permissible. His feedings should always be brought punctually and the empty vessel removed at once; it is apt to depress patients to have an empty feeding cup or glass left at the bedside, apart from being bad bedside technique.

Later, as the patient is allowed fuller diet, he should be encouraged to look forward with pleasure and without apprehension to the new dishes until the day comes when a poached egg may be allowed for breakfast.

It is very important to encourage the patient to adhere exactly to his diet and to avoid eating anything that is not allowed, and to abstain from eating between his times for meals. Smoking is usually forbidden.

The bowels should act regularly every day. A difficulty may be met here because the diet, at first, is so very limited, but to obviate this some physicians give their patients liquid paraffin, others order the administration of a small olive oil, or glycerine and plain water, enema daily. The alkalis the patient is taking vary slightly in type, in many instances the powder is a mixture of bismuth and magnesium carbonate. Bismuth tends to produce constipation, but magnesia counteracts this as it is a laxative; sometimes a patient may react to bismuth and become very constipated, in other cases he may be affected by magnesia and have diarrhoea; it is important therefore for the nurse to co-operate with the physician and endeavour to find whether, by altering the mixture in order to regulate the bowels, the use of aperients may not altogether be avoided, which is very desirable.

Whilst a patient is on milk feedings his mouth will require care, the hygiene of the mouth being a very important point in the care of all cases of disorder of the digestive tract. The patient is often thin, and great care must therefore be exercised in the prevention of bedsores.

When the patient begins to get up, this must be carried out carefully; he should be warmly dressed and lifted on to a couch at first; and should only be out of bed for half an hour; in a few days he may feel strong enough to stand by his bedside for a few moments and after ten days or so he may be permitted to walk a few steps. He has probably been ill for some time, and his muscles will be flabby, so that he will tire easily and should be encouraged to go very slowly; if allowed to get tired he will become depressed and discouraged, and this should never be permitted to happen.

HAEMATEMESIS

Haematemesis as a complication of peptic ulcer has already been referred to (see p. 381). A patient with a peptic ulcer may be admitted because he has had a severe and serious attack of haematemesis, and a nurse must be prepared to deal with this emergency. She should be familiar with the symptoms of severe bleeding, and expect such a patient to be blanched in colour, with a subnormal temperature and cold clammy skin, a rapid, weak pulse and respirations that are sighing and shallow. In appearance the patient will be shrunken, because his body is dehydrated from loss of fluid, his eyes will be sunken and his face looked pinched; he will be restless and anxious unless the degree of shock which accompanies the condition is severe enough to render him unconscious.

The **treatment of haematemesis**, like the treatment of any other case of severe bleeding, is by rest, and this will be obtained by placing the patient flat in bed, and reassuring him so that he does not worry;

the physician may order a hypodermic of morphia to be given as this will depress the central nervous system and so prevent anxiety, and it will also help to arrest bleeding by lowering the blood pressure. On the other hand if the haematemesis is due to cirrhosis of the liver, morphia is contraindicated as the liver cannot detoxicate the blood.

Fortunately very few patients die of haematemesis, as the bleeding usually stops when the blood pressure is low enough; a few cases continue bleeding and in these the prognosis is very grave. An hourly pulse chart should be kept. The blood pressure and haemoglobin percentage should be taken every 12 or 24 hours.

The *rest* which a patient must have if a case of serious haematemesis is to be properly cared for by nurses cannot be over-estimated or exaggerated. All the routine nursing treatment which is so usual on the admission of a new patient must be omitted, as in this case the patient must lie totally undisturbed, covered by enough blankets to keep him from getting cold. He should not be washed, and no movement of his limbs should be permitted. If a sheet is soiled it may not be changed as this would necessitate moving the patient. In order to avoid moving him for the purpose of inserting a bedpan, should he need one, pads of brown wool and tow should be placed on the bed beneath his buttocks, and fresh pads can be reinserted as these pads are soiled without disturbing him. If a divided mattress is obtainable, it should be employed, as then the middle portion can be removed for sanitary purposes and for attending to the patient's back. This patient cannot be moved to have his back washed and rubbed, and he most certainly cannot be turned on his side until all danger of immediate bleeding has passed.

The bed should not be made for at least 24 hours; the top bedclothing might then be rearranged, but the bottom sheet should not be removed—it may be untucked and tightened and tucked in again. After 24 hours, if the patient's condition is considered to be improving, his face and hands might be sponged; but his arms should not be moved and further washing should be postponed until he is safely better.

His mouth will be very dry and he may suffer severely from thirst; for the relief of this his mouth should be cleaned frequently and his lips and tongue moistened with water, or glycerine and borax and water. Ice should not be sucked.

With regard to the *administration of fluid*, the body may not show signs of diminished fluid until 24 or 36 hours after the attack of vomiting; but by this time the physician will probably have ordered the administration of fluid other than by mouth, either in the form of rectal or subcutaneous saline, or in more severe cases by intravenous infusion of fluid, either saline or blood.

After one or two days provided bleeding has ceased, shown by absence of haematemesis and improvement in the general condition, four to five ounces of half-strength normal saline are given by mouth every four hours for the first day. Then milk feedings are given beginning with one ounce of milk and one ounce of water, combined with an alkali, every two hours. The amount may be gradually increased up to five ounces every two hours. Tincture of belladonna (in 10–15) is given *before* three feeds alternatively with ½ ounce of olive oil before three other feeds. A teaspoonful of an alkaline powder such as magnesium hydroxide or chalk and bismuth carbonate is given *after* all feedings. The last dose at night is a double dose. Aludrox, which is a preparation of these alkalis, is alternatively used.

The bowel should not be opened for five to seven days when a small enema may be given.

Professor Meulengracht of Copenhagen has introduced an alternative method of treatment. He considers the provision of a diet of high calorie value and rich in vitamins will produce more rapid healing of a bleeding ulcer. In a series of over 200 cases he has given a liberal diet from the first day in haematemesis and obtained great success. Dr. Witts has modified the original dietary for use in this country. It includes tea and bread and butter, porridge and cream, milk and eggs, cream cheeses, cooked fruits and vegetables provided these are passed through a fine sieve, pounded fish and chicken, and light milk puddings.

INFLAMMATORY CONDITIONS OF THE ALIMENTARY TRACT

Stomatitis is inflammation of the mucous membranes of the mouth, it may be due to a variety of causes, including indigestion, bad teeth, pyorrhoea, or the presence of septic foci in other parts of the alimentary tract. It occurs in infants when scrupulous cleanliness is not observed in the care of feeding utensils; one infantile form which is specific is described as 'thrush', and is due to a vegetable parasite.

A similar type of stomatitis is described as *catarrhal*, while more severe types may be *ulcerative* or *gangrenous*. *Cancrum oris* is a severe type.

The treatment of simple stomatitis consists in careful attention to the hygiene of the mouth and teeth, and cleanliness of feeding utensils; mild antiseptic mouthwashes are employed; the mouth should be cleaned in the usual routine manner, with glycerine of borax. Potassium chlorate is given.

Since eating is painful when the mouth is sore, non-irritating fluids should be given during this stage, but as improvement takes place the patient may be given soft foods and then have solid food when he is ready to take it.

Cancrum oris is a very serious ulcerative type of stomatitis which is only met in debilitated patients, and it requires constant attention to keep the parts irrigated and clean; liberal nourishing fluids should be given. The aim of treatment is to prevent toxaemia as much as possible and to raise the resistance of the patient in order to overcome it. This condition is very serious but it responds well to penicillin and/or sulphonamides.

Pyorrhoea is infection of the epithelium lining the parodontal sulcus usually associated with *gingivitis* or inflammation of the gums. It may lead to septic osteitis of the jaw. Scaling the teeth and effective oral hygiene help. Gingivectomy may be necessary combined with penicillin treatment. Extraction of the teeth when considered necessary is preceded by penicillin treatment.

Pharyngitis has been dealt with in discussion of the respiratory tract.

Tonsillitis is described in the section dealing with inflammatory conditions of the ear, nose and throat.

GASTRITIS

Gastritis is here considered as an inflammatory condition of the stomach such as may be due to infection or irritation by means of infected food, highly irritable food, or to some form of poisoning. *Dyspepsia* has been described on p. 379.

Gastritis may be acute or chronic. The best example of acute gastritis is gastric influenza, the symptoms of which are pain in the epigastrium, accompanied by nausea and vomiting and sometimes by diarrhoea; there is a rise of temperature to anything from 101° to 104° F. The mouth and tongue are dry and dirty and the patient complains of severe thirst; all the symptoms which usually accompany the febrile state are present and the patient is considerably prostrated by the combination of discomfort, toxaemia and loss of fluid from which he is suffering.

The **treatment** adopted is to rest the stomach by omitting all food and fluid by mouth, until the nausea and vomiting have ceased and then to give fluids, very carefully at first so that vomiting may not be induced, and afterwards more liberally, in order to make up for the loss of body fluid. The diarrhoea which accompanies the onset of the inflammatory condition will subside as the patient improves, though the constipation which may be present later will require the administration of carefully chosen laxative aperients for its relief.

During the acute attack the symptoms complained of should be relieved, and applications of heat may be tried to relieve the abdominal pain, while for the headache a small dose of aspirin may be given and the application of an ice compress to the head may also help.

ENTERITIS

Enteritis is inflammation of the enteron or intestine; either the small or large intestine may be affected, and the term *colitis* is applied to inflammation of the large intestine, or colon, exclusively.

Acute enteritis is most commonly due either to bacterial infection or to irritation of the intestine by unsuitable foods, infected food or food poisoning.

The **symptoms** are abdominal pain, which is colicky in nature, accompanied by nausea and often by vomiting and by the passage of frequent stools which usually contain bile, mucus and undigested food and, in very severe inflammatory lesions, blood and mucus in varying quantities.

Sooner or later, in fairly marked cases as early as 24 hours after the onset, the patient will present the typical picture of dehydration, owing to loss of body fluid—his face is pinched, eyes sunken, mouth and tongue parched and dry, the tongue is furred, and thirst is marked; the pulse is rapid, the blood pressure low, and the temperature subnormal except in cases due to a very acute bacterial infection when it may be very high.

The **treatment** aims at the relief of the dehydration and of the other symptoms which are present; hot applications are applied to the abdomen in an attempt to relieve the pain; in many instances the physician will order morphia; the patient is kept in bed as warmly clad as possible and, as he rolls about in pain, it is necessary for a nurse to stand at the bedside constantly covering him with the bedclothes.

The *administration of fluid is important*, and yet this may be impossible by mouth or by rectum in cases where vomiting and diarrhoea are marked symptoms, and sedative drugs will be used to allay the restlessness which is due to pain, starch and opium enemata being employed to lessen the number of stools. If the patient is very prostrated it may be necessary to give saline by the intravenous route.

As soon as the attack begins to abate water can be given by mouth then albumin water, glucose and whey, giving as much as the patient can take and keeping him on similar fluids until the inflammatory condition can be considered to be improving; he may then be given diluted milk and gradually allowed milky foods and light diet when all symptoms have disappeared.

The mouth should be carefully and frequently cleaned throughout the illness, and kept as moist as possible as this will help to allay thirst.

In cases where diarrhoea and vomiting are present the use of aperients is contraindicated; the stomach and intestine are already irritated and the administration of an aperient will only increase the irritation. There is such a tendency to administer castor oil to patients with gastro-intestinal disorder that this cannot be too emphatically stated. The only occasion when castor oil or any other aperient may reasonably be employed is when an attack of enteritis is known to be due to the taking of some unsuitable food, as when a tiny child eats too many green apples; but even in this case the child will suffer pain, and should therefore be put to bed and kept warm until the aperient has acted, and during this time his stomach should be kept at rest—later, when he is better, he may be given diluted milk and water.

Chronic enteritis may occur. This type is often tuberculous in origin, and is associated with intermittent attacks of pain, malaise, loss of weight and a varying degree of pyrexia.

COLITIS

Ulcerative colitis is an acute inflammatory catarrhal condition of the large intestine, due to bacterial infection or occurring as the result of a severe toxaemia.

It is characterized by a rise in temperature, marked wasting, distension of the abdomen and the passage of frequent watery, offensive stools, containing blood and mucus. This disease may last for many weeks, the patient becoming more and more prostrated and the toxaemia more marked.

The *treatment* adopted is complete rest in bed; these patients require very careful nursing as they are often emaciated and therefore liable to bedsores; the frequent passage of stool necessitates constant attention and, as the prostration becomes very marked, it will be found that the patient passes fluid stool involuntarily. The *medical treatment* consists in the administration of non-residue bland diet (see p. 284); in some cases local treatment in the form of colonic lavage is undertaken (the method of administering this is described on p. 141).

Another form of colitis is described as **muco-membranous colitis** or **mucous colitis.** It occurs in persons who have led a worried life and ossibly have a tendency to neurasthenia, and is characterized by constiation, though in some cases this alternates with attacks of diarrhoea. 'he stools frequently contain large shreds of membrane or even casts of he colon—hence the name, muco-membranous colitis.

The alimentary tract of these patients is disordered and they suffer from ɔss of appetite, nausea and indigestion.

The *treatment* is the administration of a bland diet. The bowels are kept cting by the careful use of bland laxatives such as liquid paraffin or senna ea. Strong or irritating aperients must be avoided. Colonic lavage is mployed. An important part of the treatment may be to discover the ause of any underlying neurasthenia such as the existence of a septic ocus and then to try to treat this.

DIVERTICULITIS

Diverticulitis is inflammation of little sacs which lie in the walls of the olon, particularly at the lower end, and when these become infected r irritated the resulting inflammatory changes in the colon are quickly ransmitted to the peritoneum when the infection is an acute one, and this ives rise to symptoms similar to those of appendicitis. *The treatment of the cute type of diverticulitis is surgical.*

Chronic diverticulitis may also occur, characterized by constipation and y the passage of mucus, accompanied by colicky pain. Medical treatnent employed consists in the use of a bland diet, the administration of axative and lubricating aperients, and colonic lavage.

DIARRHOEA

Diarrhoea is the term used to describe the condition present when an excessive number of stools are passed; 4 or 5 stools a day would constitute a state of diarrhoea, whilst 8 or 10 would be considered very excessive.

The *causes of diarrhoea* are very numerous, and in addition to epidemic diarrhoea, which is described below where inflammatory conditions of the alimentary tract are dealt with, diarrhoea is present in some cases of typhoid fever, and in cholera and dysentery and in most inflammatory conditions of the intestine (see also enteritis).

In infants it may also be due to unsuitable feeding, or either over or underfeeding. In adults the number of causes include dietetic errors, partaking of decomposed food, and food poisoning; it occurs as a symptom in mercurial poisoning, and may also occur under conditions of emotional stress.

The *treatment of diarrhoea* is to investigate the cause and then to direct treatment towards its removal; in the meantime, as the patient is losing a good deal of fluid, he should be kept at rest, preferably in bed, and should be kept warm and comfortable. Any pain which accompanies the passing of stool should be relieved by applications of heat to the abdomen; the patient's mouth should be kept clean and his lips and tongue as moist as possible; if he is not vomiting, he may be given water, or half-strength saline containing glucose to sip; his drinks should be warm, neither hot nor cold, as extremes of temperature may stimulate peristalsis and result in his passing a stool immediately after taking a drink. It is important to note whether this happens, as, if it does, it may indicate that there is irritation of the gastro-colic reflex, causing the ileo-colic valve to ope and allow some of the contents of the small intestine to pass through an so set up peristalsis in the large intestine each time fluid enters th stomach; in such a case the administration of fluids would have to b arranged at regular intervals only, either every 3 or every 4 hours.

Patients who are having frequent stools soon become very tired; the get thin and the pressure of a bedpan on the skin of the lower part of th back predisposes to soreness—some means should therefore be taken t pad the pan and make it soft. The patient should be washed and powdere locally after the use of the pan and observation made to see whether th stools are making the skin sore; if so, it should be protected by an applica tion of some slightly greasy preparation—carron oil, which is a mixtur of linseed oil and lime water, is excellent for this purpose, and the ski might be cleansed with this instead of with soap and water when th stools are very frequent and the skin tender and reddened.

The general appearance of the stools must be carefully observed.

INFECTIVE ENTERITIS (*Cholera Infantum*)

Infective enteritis, *epidemic diarrhoea* or, as it is also termed, *summe diarrhoea*, is an acute infective inflammatory catarrhal condition of th intestine due to several organisms. It affects infants and young childre and is most commonly met with during the hot months of the yea when flies and dust are present in great quantities and when infection o food, particularly milk, is therefore most likely to occur.

The onset is sudden with diarrhoea, vomiting, toxaemia and dehydration. An infant admitted in this condition will be very seriously ill The temperature may be high, the pulse rapid, weak, running, thread and compressible; dehydration is indicated by sunken eyes, boat-shape abdomen, sunken fontanelle and inelastic skin; thirst, prostration, toxaemia and collapse are marked. Coma and convulsions may occur. Unless relie can be obtained the infant will die.

The **treatment** adopted is *absolute rest*, *applications of warmth*, and the *administration of fluid*, either by the peritoneal or intravenous route. When danger of death is more remote, the stomach may be gently washed out and the bowel irrigated; then, when these organs have had a little rest, some non-irritating fluid may be given—small sips of water at first by mouth, then whey, albumin water, glucose and water, and—by rectum—saline with glucose.

In the nursing care of this tiny infant great gentleness is necessary; and he should be kept warm, and it is a good plan to nurse him on a water cushion, containing water at 120° F., and to wrap him in cotton wool, or light warm woollies. When fluid is given by the mouth it must be administered very slowly and at frequent regular intervals. His mouth should be kept moist by applications of boroglycerine.

Isolation is very important, as this disease is highly infectious and the excretions and vomited matter are potent sources of infection. The nurse's hands must be carefully washed after handling infected articles, especially napkins. In some hospitals certain nurses are responsible for the babies' feedings; others deal with the washing of the babies and the care of the cleanliness of their buttocks and napkins, and thus any possibility of infecting the feeding utensils is prevented.

CONSTIPATION

In this condition the output from the bowel is diminished. Normally, the amount of faeces passed by an adult is 4 ounces once a day. In constipation the action may be rare, occurring only once in several days, or, occurring daily, it may be small in quantity.

The causes are numerous. The diet may include insufficient fat, or it may not contain enough fresh fruit and vegetables and water, or it may be too rich in meat. Sometimes a patient omits the use of valuable fats and cereals because he is afraid of 'putting on weight'.

Any neglect of the regular emptying of the bowel will result in failure of the reflex to act and in time this will lead to constipation. If the impulse to defaecate is ignored on one day, it may not occur until the same time next day and, if ignored again, irregularity may be set up. The training of children to have their bowels opened at the same time each day is of very great importance in the formation of a good bowel habit.

The taking of aperients or the administration of enemata regularly is another cause of constipation since, as the result of these, the bowel may not function without the artificial stimulation provided.

Other causes include atony of the bowel wall; weakness of the abdominal muscles; spasticity of the muscle of the wall of the bowel which gives rise to tight contracted bands, damming back the contents; any form of indigestion which is caused by decrease in the normal digestive fluids may cause constipation. The presence of any obstruction such as might be caused by the existence of a tumour in the pelvis or lower part of the abdominal cavity; or by a strangulated hernia, or intestinal obstruction will result in constipation. When the obstruction is complete there is constipation of flatus also.

The *treatment of constipation*, apart from the removal of any definite cause such as indigestion, aims at providing the type of diet which will be effective in producing a normal action of the bowel each day. This dietetic treatment is described in detail in the section dealing with diet on p. 284.

WORMS

Intestinal worms. The worms which most commonly live in the human intestine are threadworm, roundworm and tapeworm.

The threadworm or *Oxyuris vermicularis* is small, being less than half an inch in length; it lives in the caecum and migrates to the lower end of the colon at night, where it causes intolerable itching about the anus; it is visible to the naked eye and similar to a tiny piece of cotton thread.

The round worm or *Ascaris lumbricoides* is several inches long, lives in the upper part of the small intestine and causes considerable abdominal discomfort, pain and diarrhoea.

The tapeworm most commonly found in the intestine of man is the type described as *Taenia mediocanellata*, which is conveyed by eating encysted beef, and the *Taenia solium* by eating encysted pork. These worms are both from 10 to 40 feet long, segmented, with a tiny head by which they burrow into the intestine and attach themselves to the wall thereof. As the result of infection by tapeworm the patient suffers malaise and discomfort, loses weight and becomes anaemic.

Treatment. These worms are parasites, living, that is to say, on and at th expense of their host—in this case, man. The principle of treatment is t rid the body of the worms by using some drug which will stupefy them an then to remove their surrounding medium by purgatives and so rende them uncomfortable; further purgation will usually result in the expulsio of the worms. The substances which will help to get rid of worms ar described as *anthelmintics*.

In the treatment of tapeworm, extract of male fern or filix mas is used, but th patient requires to be specially prepared for this, and the treatment i carried out as follows—The patient is admitted and, as the treatmen is apt to be very severe, he is kept in bed. His diet consists of weak tea an beef tea only; on the second day the administration of purgatives is begun the patient being given 2 drachms of magnesium sulphate three times a day; this is repeated on the third day and on the morning of the fourt day one dose is given in the early morning. Two hours later the extrac of male fern is administered. It is a fluid extract, 15 minims are given, an repeated every quarter of an hour until 1 or 1½ drachms have been ad ministered. Two hours afterwards the patient is given another purgativ usually in the form of 1 ounce of black draught which contains magnesiun sulphate, liquorice and senna.

After this treatment the patient may be expected to pass tapeworn and the stools must be very carefully inspected; at first considerabl quantities of segments will be passed; the smaller segments are nearest th head end of the worm; it is important to search diligently for the head, an it can be recognized as a tiny triangle, almost as small as the head of a ordinary pin.

In order to be able to inspect the worm easily, it is advisable to put a little tepid or warm water in the bedpan, as this prevents the separatio of the segments and so makes it easier to see the head of the worm shoul it be passed. The stools should all be passed through a fine hair sieve, black crape having formerly been used for this purpose—in either case th material is fine enough to prevent the head of the worm from passing through it.

If this treatment is not effective and the head of the worm is not re-covered, the patient will have to return home and wait for three month before it can be undertaken again.

Another drug which is used in the treatment of tapeworm is *pelletierine tannate*; preliminary starvation and purgation is employed as before, one dose of the drug, from 2 to 8 grains, is given, and the final purgative administered 2 hours after this.

Santonin is used in the treatment of roundworm and in some cases of *thread-worm*, when the condition is persistent. The patient is given very light diet for a day or two, a dose of castor oil is given on the last evening and the dose of santonin, from 1 to 5 grains, is given next morning whilst the stomach is empty and before any food or drink is taken. If the bowels are not thoroughly opened, a dose of magnesium sulphate is given later in the day. The stools are inspected for the worms which will usually be passed.

An alternative method of treatment for threadworm in children is by gentian-violet. No starvation is necessary, for five days the drug is given daily, after meals, in doses of one-sixth of a grain for each year of age, then five days rest and then repeat for five days. The drug is given in gelatin capsules.

The adult dose is about two grains a day.

It is important to apply germicidal ointment, such as a preparation of mercury, to the anus in order to destroy worms that migrate during the night. Means should be taken to prevent the patient, who is usually a child, from reinfecting himself by putting his hands to his mouth after handling the area of his anus as he may do by scratching.

PYLORIC STENOSIS. HIRSCHSPRUNG'S DISEASE. VISCEROPTOSIS

Congenital hypertrophic pyloric stenosis is a rare condition which occurs in tiny infants, and it is very important that a nurse in a general hospital should know how to deal with this infant, as such cases may be admitted either for medical or surgical treatment.

It is thought that the condition is probably present at birth, but it does not usually produce any symptoms until the baby is several weeks old. The fibres of the pyloric end of the stomach then become tightly contracted.

The *symptoms* are—vomiting which becomes forcibly projectile in character, meaning that it is projected on to the floor beyond the cot; the baby is ravenously hungry and sucks his fist continuously; he whines and cries, his urine becomes scanty and he presents the appearance of a baby who is extremely dehydrated. On examination of the abdomen peristalsis may be visible as a ball, about the size of a golf ball, passing from left to right. The contracted pylorus can sometimes be felt.

Medical treatment consists of gastric lavage, with saline solution, once or twice a day, or every 4 hours. Feedings should be given in small quantities at regular intervals, expressed mother's milk being used. The nurse should use her ingenuity to try and get some milk retained in the stomach; giving a second feeding immediately after one the baby has vomited may succeed and thickening the milk sometimes helps. Small doses of atropine may be ordered to relax the pyloric sphincter and small doses of mildly sedative drugs, such as bromide, may be useful to assist relaxation and diminish the neuromuscular irritation which may be producing the condition.

Surgical treatment is by means of Rammstedt's operation, the fibres of the sphincter being partially divided.

Preparation of an infant for the performance of Rammstedt's operation when a local anaesthetic is used. Sixty cubic centimetres of normal saline are administered by the intraperitoneal route four hours before the operation is to be performed, and the infant is given a warm bath two hours later. The stomach is washed out with normal saline 1½ hours beforehand and then the infant is bandaged on to the fixation splint, as shown in the illustration, and kept very quiet for at least an hour before being taken to the operating theatre.

A feeding of glucose and water ready prepared in an infant feeding bottle, but with a piece of sterilized linen inserted in place of the ordinary rubber teat, is taken to the theatre. The infant is allowed to suck this during the operation; it helps to keep him quiet; he may vomit what he has taken on return to the ward, but does not usually vomit during the short time he is in the theatre.

The cot is prepared for the reception of the infant immediately after the operation, the foot of it being elevated on low blocks; a water pillow is filled with water at a temperature of 118° F. and placed in the bed, covered

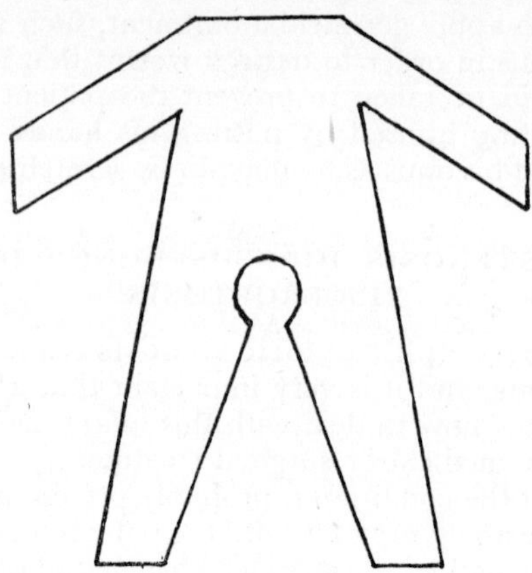

FIG. 171.—FIXATION SPLINT ON WHICH A TINY INFANT IS PLACED, AFTER FIRST BEIN WRAPPED IN COTTON WOOL, DURING THE PERFORMANCE OF RAMMSTEDT'S OPERATION UNDE A LOCAL ANAESTHETIC.

by a blanket; an electric cradle is placed on the bed, under the uppe bedclothes and the electricity is turned on.

The *post-operative treatment* commences immediately—when performec under a local anaesthetic the operation takes less than five minutes. Th infant is lying on the fixation splint, wrapped up in cotton wool, a surgica dressing is placed on the operation wound, covered by a pad of wool, anc this is retained in position by a many-tailed binder. The infant is placec in his cot, and the electric cradle is generally removed as the bed is ready warmed and the infant does not usually suffer from shock. The danger t be feared is *hyperthermia*; the pulse and temperature are taken ever hour for the first 12 hours; after two hours the infant's temperature ma be expected to be 100° F. When the temperature has reached this poin the bandages and wool may be removed and the use of the fixatior splint omitted; the dressing on the wound is now secured by an abdomina binder made to fit the infant and his clothing may be put on. If th temperature continues to rise, when it reaches 102·5° an icebag may b applied to the head; if this fails to relieve the condition of pyrexia the bed clothes covering the infant may be removed, and if the temperature stil continues to rise his body may be sponged with tepid water.

Post-operative feeding commences 4 hours after the operation; expressec breast milk should be given. For the first 20 hours, small quantities ar given—from the 1st to the 3rd hour, 1 drachm is given each hour; at th 4th and 5th hour, 2 drachms each hour; from the 6th to the 9th hour 3 drachms each hour; at the 10th and 11th hour, 4 drachms each hour from the 12th hour, 6 drachms may be given every 2 hours; and fron the 16th to the 20th hour, 1 ounce every 2 hours.

The end of the first 24 hours has now been reached, and during th second 24 hours the infant is given 1½ ounces every 2 hours for the firs 12, and 2 ounces for the second 12 hours. The return to normal feeding i now gradually made until, by the 5th day, the normal routine should b established.

Pyloric stenosis sometimes occurs in adults, but it is then most often due to the formation of adhesions, scarring and contraction which may complicate a peptic ulcer.

Hirschsprung's disease or megalocolon is a hypertrophic condition of the colon which is probably congenital although it may not be noticed for a number of years. It is due to functional derangement of the nervous control of the colon, and is characterized by marked dilatation and distension; *the treatment adopted* is sympathetic ganglionectomy, meaning that certain nerve ganglia are removed in order to cut off the passage of nerve impulses to the part affected, in an endeavour to relieve spasm and permit the dilated colon to return to its normal size.

Visceroptosis is a dropping of the viscera—most often of the hollow organs such as the stomach and large and small intestine—but the solid organs can be displaced also, the displacement of the kidney giving rise to the condition described as *floating kidney* is an example.

When the stomach or intestines have dropped lower down in the abdominal cavity than they should normally lie, the symptoms of the condition are dyspeptic in character. The patient is easily tired, he is languid and incapable of exertion; in many cases he is thin and wasted and feels the cold severely. In some cases of gastroptosis acute attacks of vomiting occur at intervals.

Treatment is directed to improvement of the general condition of the patient; his weight should be increased, he needs rest and should be advised never to overtire himself, particularly he should rest before and after his meals; he should try and discover the foods which agree with him and have regularly spaced meals, and his bowels should be kept open by laxatives.

DISEASES OF THE LIVER AND GALLBLADDER

Jaundice is a term used to describe a condition in which the skin is tinted and the conjunctiva discoloured yellow, due to retention of the bile pigments in the blood, and is usually brought about by congestion, or obstruction, of the bile capillaries and ducts. This condition exists in catarrhal and obstructive jaundice. In the former, an inflammation which may be of an infective character causes congestion of the lining of the biliary tract and results in an acute attack of jaundice, lasting about 3 weeks, which in addition to the symptoms of jaundice detailed below is characterized by a rise in temperature. In *obstructive jaundice* the bile is dammed back and, as it cannot escape into the duodenum, it gets into the blood, and this may be due to the presence of gallstones in the duct or to obstruction due to pressure upon the duct, such as would happen in the case of a tumour at the head of the pancreas.

Jaundice is a condition due to the retention of the bile pigments in the blood, and this may also happen in certain diseases, and in some conditions of poisoning, when the red blood cells are disintegrated in the blood stream, without the intervention of the liver and spleen. This state occurs in *haemolytic jaundice* or *acholuric jaundice* which is due to a disease of the spleen. It may also occur by the introduction of poisons, particularly when these have a destructive action on the tissue of the liver. Examples of such poisons are snakebite and tetrachlorethane, the latter being used for painting the wings of aeroplanes and the subject poisoned by inhaling the fumes from this. Trinitrotoluene (TNT), used in munition factories, is another similarly poisonous substance.

Homologous serum jaundice is a type which is seen after the intravenous injection of blood serum and plasma, after the injection of yellow fever vaccine prepared from human serum, and after injections of arsenic. It is considered to be due to a virus.

Epidemic catarrhal jaundice or *infective hepatitis* is due to a filter-passing virus. The *incubation period* is variable. The *onset* is characterized by lassitude, headache and nausea. Vomiting and abdominal pain follow and jaundice appears.

Weil's disease or *leptospiral icterohaemorrhagica* is due to the *Leptospira icterohaemorrhagiae*. The *incubation period* is six to twelve days or longer. The *onset* is abrupt with prostration and high fever; jaundice appears by the fourth day of disease. After the tenth day the fever declines by lysis. Remissions are common. Cases of either of these types of jaundice should be isolated. *Treatment* consists in the administration of penicillin combined with measures for the relief of the symptoms which are enumerated above and a diet as described below.

The symptoms of jaundice. *Tinting of the skin* and *conjunctiva*, which may vary from pale to bright yellow or even, in severe cases, to olive green, is the most characteristic symptom. The skin is irritable owing to the retention of bile salts.

The *urine* and other secretions, except the stools (see note below), are coloured by the bile. The urine varies from a slight greenish-yellow tint to deep mahogany colour. When shaken up the froth looks multicoloured in bright daylight.

The *stools* are pale and are described as putty or clay colour; the faeces are dry and crumbling in consistence and offensive in odour, and they may contain undigested fat.

Owing to the absence of bile the functions of the digestive tract are disorganized, there is loss of appetite and nausea, particularly at the sight or even sometimes the thought of fat, and vomiting may occur. Constipation is usually present.

The patient is lethargic and often depressed, and this is due to the action of the bile salts on the central nervous system. He feels the cold easily and yet, when he gets warm, his skin often begins to itch intolerably; thus he is faced with being alternately cold and itchy—both very uncomfortable states—and consequently he finds it difficult to sleep. The temperature, except in infective catarrhal jaundice, is usually subnormal, and the pulse is slow, as the bile products depress the circulation.

Treatment and Nursing. In the routine care of a case of severe jaundice a nurse will find her resources severely taxed; she has to deal with a depressed difficult patient, one who is constantly irritated by the itching of his skin and in many cases one in whom the sight of food causes uncontrollable nausea—patients sometimes cannot bear to see or consider drinking even skimmed milk. In her care of this patient the nurse will bear constantly in mind the distressing symptoms from which he suffers, as the medical treatment employed for the relief of these will be largely in her hands, and will require constantly applied intelligent thought and consideration.

The *diet* will be as free from fat as possible and, during the stage when nausea is acute, bland fluids containing glucose may be all that the patient can take; he may, however, be persuaded to try fresh fruit, appetizingly prepared, and fresh green salads; these may be dressed with a little black pepper and vinegar, oil and salad creams being omitted. A patient may be induced to take some toasted breadcrumbs, a little of the specially prepared breakfast toasties or a small piece of dry toast with his salad. As he feels a little better, he may be willing to take cooked fruit and, as sugar can be added to this, it becomes a valuable source of food for him. During serious nausea and vomiting, water, or alkaline drinks, should be given as freely as the patient can be persuaded to take them.

As the condition improves the diet may be increased, but it is important for some time to eliminate fats and eggs, as the latter contain fat and cholesterol. Fluid may be given in abundance, and the patient should be encouraged to drink plenty of water, lemonade and grapefruit drink or any other fruit drink he fancies.

It is important to *inspect the stools* for any undigested food, especially fat. The *bowels* should be kept acting regularly, and it may be necessary to use aperients.

Saline aperients will be found most acceptable; some physicians order mercury in the form of calomel, but nausea would be considered a contraindication to the use of calomel and a saline aperient would then be substituted.

Other drugs which may be ordered include hexamine and salol, both of these acting as biliary antiseptics. Various alkalis and bismuth may be employed for the relief of vomiting but bismuth causes constipation. Sometimes, when the irritation of the skin is very marked and is causing undue distress to the patient, a physician may order a diaphoretic; pilocarpine is an example of this, the dose being from $\frac{1}{8}$ to $\frac{1}{4}$ of a grain administered by hypodermic injection. It is a powerful diaphoretic and the skin will act freely, thus bringing some of the irritating bile salts away in the perspiration. Hot sponging should follow in order to get the best result, by removing the products of perspiration.

Other means of relieving the irritation of the skin are by sponging with weak carbolic, a solution of 1–100, or a solution of sodium bicarbonate, or borax, or calamine lotion may be dabbed on.

Jaundice is occasionally, but not invariably, associated with gallstones, and when due to this cause attacks of biliary colic may ensue; it is necessary to be on the watch for pain over the region of the gallbladder because, apart from the presence of stone, viscid thick bile may act as an obstruction.

Attacks of biliary colic necessitate the use of heat and counterirritants in an attempt to relieve the pain; but morphia will usually be ordered for this, as the pain is severe and very prostrating in its effects (see also colic on p. 343).

CHOLECYSTITIS

Cholecystitis is inflammation of the gallbladder, and it may be either acute or chronic. **Acute cholecystitis** gives rise to symptoms of an acute abdominal condition, very like those of appendicitis, only that in this case the inflammation affects the upper, rather than the lower portion of the abdominal cavity. It is thought in many instances to be due to infection by *Bacillus coli*.

The **symptoms** are abdominal pain, nausea and vomiting accompanied by a rise in temperature; the abdomen is tender, particularly over the right upper quadrant; pain passes round the epigastrium and up to the right shoulder.

Medical treatment, if it should be decided to adopt this, consists in the administration of morphia to relieve the pain and counterirritants and hot applications applied over the region of the gallbladder; the patient is kept in bed and plenty of water is given when vomiting ceases and he can retain it. When the attack of acute pain has subsided, biliary antiseptics are ordered to dilute the bile, and a small dose of concentrated magnesium sulphate is given each morning in an endeavour to drain the gallbladder.

The *diet* consists of mild, non-fatty foods and plenty of fluid containing glucose, fresh fruit and green vegetables.

Chronic cholecystitis usually occurs about middle age, and it may follow acute attacks or begin more insidiously with recurrent attacks of indigestion.

The usual *history of a patient with chronic cholecystitis* is of this nature—indigestion, characterized by a sense of fullness after meals, which is more marked towards the end of the day and particularly after partaking of tea, pastry, foods cooked in fat, sardines, herring and salmon; the patient is often fat and heavy, and suffers from constipation; he has attacks of pain on the right side and suffers from frequent headaches; he may have acute attacks of pain due to biliary colic and he may, though this is rare, say that he has sometimes been jaundiced.

Treatment is on the lines indicated in acute cholecystitis. *Cholecystography* is usually undertaken in order to investigate the function of the gallbladder. This test has been described in the section dealing with investigations on page 168. In persistent cases, and because an inflamed gallbladder is always liable to be the cause of an acute abdominal catastrophe, *surgical measures* are commonly undertaken. The care of a patient on whom cholecystectomy has been performed is described on p. 717.

CIRRHOSIS OF LIVER. LIVER ABSCESS. ACUTE YELLOW ATROPHY

Diseases of the liver more rarely seen are cirrhosis, liver abscess and acute yellow atrophy. The liver is one of the sites of *hydatid cyst*, a condition due to infection by means of the tapeworm of the dog; in this type man becomes the intermediate host and the parasite develops in his tissues, a hydatid cyst sometimes growing to a very large size. The treatment is removal of the cyst.

The liver is also a common site for metastatic growth in cancer—*secondary carcinomatous lesions*. This is easily understood when it is remembered that the liver receives the portal blood; secondary growths in the liver may lead to marked interference with its function, resulting in jaundice as the result of obstruction, and also in ascites.

Cirrhosis of the liver is a type of degeneration which is due to toxaemia and is known to be frequently associated with taking excessive alcohol, though this is not an invariable cause of the condition.

The *symptoms* are those which result from obstruction of the portal circulation, such as chronic indigestion; attacks of haematemesis occur, melaena is present in the stools and, as time passes, the patient becomes wasted, anaemic, jaundiced, ascites occurs, and the prognosis is considered to be serious.

Treatment is palliative; the limitation of spirits is important and the diet should be light and easily digested. Rest is essential.

Liver abscess is usually associated with amoebic dysentery, and it is characterized by pain and tenderness over the liver, with rigors, a rise of temperature and marked prostration.

Acute yellow atrophy of the liver is a very rare condition which is thought to be due to severe forms of toxaemia. The patient becomes seriously prostrated.

TESTS OF HEPATIC FUNCTION

The Van den Bergh reaction is employed in cases of jaundice and suspected jaundice as by means of it the character of the bile in the blood is investigated, and from this the type of jaundice present, whether obstructive or non-obstructive, is determined.

Graham's Test (cholecystography) used to test the function of the gall-bladder is described on p. 168.

Lyon's Method of collecting specimens of bile is used to investigate the contents of the duodenum and determine the character of the bile passing into it (see p. 169).

Chapter 25

Diseases and Disorders of the Organs of the Urinary Tract

Nephritis, acute and chronic—Uraemia—Infections of the urinary tract: pyelitis and cystitis—Disorders of micturition; frequency, incontinence, enuresis, retention, dysuria

NEPHRITIS

Nephritis, which is also known as Bright's disease, is inflammation of the kidneys, and it may be either acute or chronic. Acute nephritis affects the entire organ; of the two forms of chronic nephritis usually described, one—*chronic interstitial nephritis*—affects the interstitial tissue between the tubules, and the other type, *chronic parenchymatous nephritis*, which is also described as *chronic tubular nephritis*, affects the tubules. Another form results in a degeneration of the substance of the kidney and is known as *nephrosis*, in order to distinguish it from nephritis—kidney inflammation.

There are many **causes of nephritis**, but the acute form is most commonly due to bacterial infection and may be associated with infectious fevers, such as scarlet fever, or with influenza; it is also caused by toxic bodily conditions, so that a badly infected focus anywhere in the body may cause nephritis; it occurs as a complication of pregnancy when toxaemia is present; it is sometimes due to very intense irritation of the kidney, as may occur when certain irritant poisons—such as carbolic acid or turpentine—have been taken and the kidney, trying to eliminate the poison from the body, becomes inflamed and a state of acute nephritis results.

Of the two examples of chronic nephritis given above, *chronic tubular nephritis* may follow the acute type, or the condition may have been chronic from the outset; in this case the onset is insidious rather than rapid. *Chronic interstitial nephritis* is often caused by slow poisoning of the system by toxins or poisons, as by chronic constipation, gout, rheumatism, syphilis, chronic alcoholism and chronic lead or arsenical poisoning. It is also very closely associated with arteriosclerosis and with a raised blood pressure.

The *nursing of nephritis* is very interesting. It is necessary to know the symptoms of this disease, but it is even more necessary to remember the important functions of the kidneys—man cannot live without a reasonable amount of healthy kidney tissue—and when the functions of the kidneys are understood by a nurse she can do much by her general care of a patient with nephritis to relieve the work of the kidneys by stimulating the skin to free action and so help to rid the body of urea and other nitrogenous waste products. Stimulation of the large colon to eliminate water, by giving aperients which will result in watery stools, combined with a limitation of the intake of food which would leave waste to be got rid of by the kidneys and, within reason, a restriction of the intake of water, are the principles which underlie the nursing cases of nephritis. It requires intelligence to apply these principles, but for that very reason the work can be profoundly interesting, and often very satisfactory.

ACUTE NEPHRITIS

Acute nephritis is usually characterized by a fairly rapid onset, in which the temperature rises, the pulse quickens, the skin becomes hot and flushed, there is furring of the tongue, loss of appetite, nausea and vomiting, headache, marked malaise and in some cases sore throat is present.

The urine is very characteristic; it is small in quantity, and contains albumin and blood; the urinary output may be seriously diminished, and the patient who passes only several ounces a day is threatened with complete suppression.

Complete suppression of urine is also termed anuria, as urine is entirely absent and the function of the kidneys in abeyance; this condition cannot last long, it will prove rapidly fatal as the urinary waste products are in this case being stored up in the blood and will lead to uraemia. *Partial suppression,* in which the quantity of urine may be seriously diminished, even to 6 or 8 ounces during 24 hours, is a condition through which good nursing may carry a patient safely, even over many days, provided his resistance and strength can be maintained.

A patient with acute nephritis is seriously ill and is threatened with uraemia; his skin is dry and it is difficult to make it act freely, though this is necessary; his mouth is very dirty, and his breath is often offensive; continued nausea and headache render him very uncomfortable; oedema may or may not occur, but when it does happen it usually begins in the loose subcutaneous tissues about the eyes and of the scrotum; later, it occurs in dependent parts as the ankles and over the sacral region and if it spreads ascites occurs.

Acute nephritis remains an acute illness for about 3 weeks; in a satisfactory case the symptoms begin to abate about this time, the urine becomes clearer, containing less blood, then very little blood, and finally the amount of albumin begins to abate; more urine is passed and in about 5 or 6 weeks from the commencement of the illness the urine may be quite clear.

Treatment and Nursing. The principles of nursing have been mentioned; a patient with nephritis requires a blanket bed, he should wear light warm woollen clothes and have some form of artificial heat in the bed —all this in an attempt to make the skin act. For the same reason the skin should be washed or sponged with really hot water (from 116° to 120° F.) twice a day; this helps to remove waste products, the treatment should be carried out fairly rapidly and briskly, taking care to see that chilling of the patient does not occur. After he has been washed, the patient should be cosily tucked up, all his wants being attended to at the same time; if he is given a hot drink, covered up and allowed to lie, resting, there will be some hope that his skin will act, and in this way excretion of water will be obtained and the function of the kidney assisted.

As a patient with acute nephritis is very ill, and suffering from marked malaise, the usual nursing attentions necessary for the prevention of bedsores must be carried out; special care will be needed if oedema occurs, as then the skin is stretched and so deprived of its normal supply of blood, and bedsores may easily occur.

The *diet* will be carefully ordered by the physician; as very little urine is being passed and much blood and albumin are being lost, showing that the kidney is highly inflamed and incapable of functioning, he may go so far as to eliminate all protein, even diluted milk, for the first 7–10 days of illness, giving only 1½–2 pints of lemonade and from 6 to 8 ounces of glucose in order to supply the patient with some nourishment during this time. In this case the physician will begin to order a little milk at the end of 10 days, taking care not to give it undiluted, and he will not usually increase the amount of fluid given beyond two pints until the acute symptoms begin to abate and the urine to clear.

As the patient improves he will be given less-diluted milk, then Benger's food, and other milk foods and drinks and gradually be allowed milk pudding, bread and butter and other cereals, and when the urine has become quite clear and the temperature is normal and the mouth clean, a little fish or chicken may be allowed. As a rule salt is not given, and very little protein allowed, red meat being altogether prohibited until the patient is beyond the convalescent stage. Bearing in mind the necessity for keeping the patient warm and encouraging his skin to act freely, all fluid food will be given as hot as he can be persuaded to take it throughout his illness.

Bowels. One of the principles of nursing mentioned above is the necessity of keeping the bowels acting regularly, and it is desirable to obtain at least two fairly fluid stools a day. In many cases aperients will usually have to be employed for this purpose, and either saline aperients, jalap, or liquorice powder may be found effective. When attending to the needs of the patient in this respect another valuable nursing opportunity arises—the bedpan should be thoroughly warmed. When the patient is washed locally after the use of the bedpan, the water used must be hot, and he should then be given a hot drink and tucked warmly up again.

Mouth. The condition of the mouth needs constant attention when the patient is acutely ill, and it should be kept as clean as possible.

Drugs. Very few drugs will be employed in the treatment of acute nephritis; practically all drugs have to be eliminated by the kidneys and for this reason are contraindicated. The necessary aperients have been mentioned; in some instances *diaphoretics* will be employed to make the skin act freely; the most powerful one is pilocarpine, from $\frac{1}{8}$ to $\frac{1}{4}$ grain administered by hypodermic injection; ammonium acetate is another, but this drug is mildly diuretic also in its action and *diuretic drugs* which will stimulate the work of the kidneys are definitely contraindicated in the treatment of acute inflammation.

Whenever pilocarpine is ordered as a diaphoretic in the treatment of acute nephritis, it is primarily the business of the nurse to see that her patient is so prepared that the very best effect is obtained; and, as this drug is a cardiac depressant, she must also be on the look-out for any symptoms of this.

Before the drug is administered, since when given it will act in from 10 to 15 minutes, the patient should be wrapped in hot blankets and artificial heat applied, either several hot-water bottles or an electric cradle being used; a small basin should also be provided, as pilocarpine also acts as a silagogue, increasing the activity of the salivary glands, and the patient should be encouraged to allow the excessive secretion to run out of his mouth. Hot drinks should be given a few minutes after the pilocarpine, all treatment being aimed at getting the very greatest amount of diaphoresis. A nurse should stand by the bedside and be prepared to wipe perspiration from the brow and face, using a warm towel for this. It is useful to sponge the body with hot water, about 1½–2 hours after the drug is first given—thus ensuring that the patient is not disturbed whilst it is acting—and the hot sponging afterwards may induce further diaphoresis.

Other treatments which may be ordered for the production of efficient action of the skin are hot air and vapour baths, and hot wet or hot dry packs.

CHRONIC NEPHRITIS

Chronic parenchymatous nephritis, or chronic tubular nephritis is characterized by slightly diminished urinary output; the urine contains a great deal of albumin, and casts and sometimes blood. As the end products of protein metabolism are not retained in the blood, there is no reason for limiting protein in the diet: on the other hand, the patient is constantly losing valuable protein in the form of albumin in his urine, and his blood becomes poor and he is anaemic, therefore a high protein diet is indicated, such as that described in the section dealing with dietetics on p. 276.

In *the general nursing care* of these patients they need rest, and may require to be kept in bed until the general condition and the anaemia can be improved; the skin tends to be dry, and they should therefore wear light woollen clothing and sleep between blankets and have a hot-water bottle or two in their beds. Their *diet* should contain *liberal protein* material. In many instances *oedema* is present, and this necessitates a limitation of fluid and salt, but as the general condition improves the oedema often gets less or disappears. Diuretics and diaphoretics are frequently employed.

As patients with this type of nephritis are subject to intercurrent infections—colds, influenza and bronchitis—they should be protected from chills and not allowed to become tired or worried or be harassed in any way.

Chronic interstitial nephritis is a more serious condition; the urine is often much increased in quantity and, although it may only contain a trace of albumin, the function of the kidneys is definitely and often seriously impaired. The large quantity of pale urine which is being passed has a low specific gravity because it is not concentrated, demonstrating that the kidneys are failing to concentrate their secretion, as they should do. Nurses are often questioned as to the seriousness of kidney disease, and they must remember that patients speaking to them about this disease should be advised to consult a physician. One point they should recollect is that disease of the kidney may have far-reaching and serious effects on the heart and other organs of the circulation.

In chronic interstitial nephritis, for example, the waste products of protein metabolism are not being excreted, but are retained in the blood. This type of chronic nephritis is associated with degeneration of the blood vessels (arteriosclerosis) and with a high blood pressure, and consequently, sooner or later, the heart will suffer strain, it will become enlarged and hypertrophied, and cardiac failure will eventually occur. In the meantime, because the arteries are degenerated, rupture may occur, cerebral haemorrhage may take place (for example), or epistaxis, haematuria or retinal haemorrhage.

A patient with chronic interstitial nephritis does not usually discover that he is ill until the condition is fairly well advanced, when he may complain of nausea and loss of appetite, or headache and noises in the head, or that he has to get up a number of times in the night to pass urine.

Treatment. At the outset the function of kidney and heart will be investigated; the possibility of the existence of any toxaemia or septic focus which might be a contributory cause will be considered, and for a time the patient may be kept in bed; but, once his general health is established at a reasonably high level, he will be taught to live a quiet, rather uneventful life. The advice given him will be similar to that for a case of hyperpiesis (see p. 358), he should rise late and retire early, have a day in bed each week, and rest for 2 hours every afternoon; his diet should be light, red meat ought not to be taken, alcohol and coffee avoided and weak tea taken only in moderation. He should have at least one good action of the bowels each day and take a mercurial purge or saline aperient once a week.

URAEMIA

Uraemia is a condition of poisoning due to the retention of the waste products of protein metabolism, because the kidney is unable to eliminate them; it is called uraemia, although urea is not poisonous, because the quantity of urea in the blood can be taken as an estimate of the amount of other, more poisonous, nitrogenous waste products.

Uraemia may arise whenever the tissue of the kidney is inflamed or degenerated, provided that its function of eliminating waste products is impaired; it may come on rapidly, as occurs when it complicates acute nephritis or poisoning by carbolic acid, or it may come on more gradually as when the function is being gradually interfered with because the urinary output is obstructed as in cases of prostatectomy, partial blockage of the ureters or hydronephrosis.

Oliguria is the term used to describe deficient urinary secretion characterized by very infrequent micturition.

The **symptoms** may occur gradually or more suddenly; those which characterize nephritis may be present, such as a hot dry skin, rise of temperature, nausea, vomiting, headache, and malaise; the urine may be loaded with albumin and blood, or diminished, or entirely suppressed; the pulse may be rapid, it may also be full and bounding, there may be dyspnoea and stertorous breathing, or the Cheyne-Stokes type of breathing.

Other symptoms more directly affecting the nervous system include twitchings, fits and convulsions, paralysis, stupor and coma, insomnia, delirium and mania. There is no rule about these symptoms, as in some instances a patient may be in stupor, while in other cases he may have fits and convulsions.

Treatment and Nursing. The nursing care in uraemia is similar to that described in acute nephritis. In addition, any other symptoms which arise require treatment. The general lines of treatment aim at relieving the blood of poisons by making the skin and bowels act more freely; diuretics are rarely employed and, when used, mild ones are preferred such as ammonium acetate and potassium citrate; in cases with a marked degree of suppression pilocarpine is ordered.

The *diet* is similar to that ordered for acute nephritis; cases of marked plethora and cyanosis are temporarily relieved by venesection; lumbar puncture may be valuable in relieving oedema of the brain and so decreasing intracranial pressure, and it is also employed occasionally for the prevention of uraemic fits. During a fit or convulsion it is essential to protect the patient from injury, and a gag or wooden wedge should be put between his teeth to prevent him from biting his tongue; frequent convulsions become prostrating and may be controlled by morphia or inhalations of chloroform. Cheyne-Stokes's breathing may be relieved by inhalations of carbon dioxide 7 per cent in oxygen.

Local treatment in the form of applications of heat or dry cupping the loins over the kidneys may relieve congestion in those organs, and *general applications of heat* may be ordered to assist the action of the skin.

Restlessness and twitchings may respond to sedatives such as bromide and chloral. Inhalations of oxygen may be useful in relieving restlessness.

INFECTION OF THE URINARY TRACT

Pyelitis and *cystitis* are the conditions most commonly met. Either condition may be acute or chronic.

The commonest *cause* is infection by *Bacillus coli* but urinary infection may be associated with chronic suppuration of the kidney, renal tuberculosis, calculus, obstruction to the urinary output and malignant disease.

In the care and treatment of infection of the urinary tract careful investigation of the urological system is very important. This includes X-ray of the tract, pyelography and cystoscopy, and the various tests of renal function, such as the urea clearance and urea concentration tests. (For full information see investigations and tests on pp. 169–71.)

PYELITIS

Inflammation of the pelvis of the kidney is usually due to infection by *Bacillus coli* though it may accompany other conditions.

In **acute pyelitis** the *onset* is sudden with a rise of temperature and marked toxaemia; the patient suffers considerably from malaise, the temperature runs a continuous course and rigors are not uncommon; the tongue is dry and covered with brown fur, there is marked thirst and loss of appetite.

Local symptoms may be very indefinite, as a rule there is aching pain in the region of the loins—when the right kidney only is affected the condition may be mistaken for appendicitis. There may be some frequency of micturition, but this is not invariable.

The *urine* is highly acid and has a characteristic shimmering opalescence; it has a slightly fishy odour, usually contains some albumin and has a deposit of pus cells and casts. On bacterial examination it is found to contain quantities of *Bacillus coli*.

The **medical treatment** of this infection includes rest in bed, the administration of bland fluids, the provision of a very light diet, only diluted milk being given whilst there is pyrexia; and, as long as the inflammatory condition persists, low protein diet with easily digested carbohydrates should be administered, unless the diet is a special feature of the treatment as in the administration of a ketogenic diet, mentioned on p. 286.

The pyrexia present, and the symptoms associated with this, need treatment for their relief. The urinary output should be measured and the urine tested for the presence of albumin and pus; bacteriological tests should be employed at regular intervals, in order to estimate the rate of progress of recovery.

Any special treatment carried out aims at destroying or inhibiting the growth of organisms in the urine, and to raising the resistance of the patient. *Many urinary antiseptics are employed*, and hexamine may be given in doses of from 5 to 15 grains, three times a day; it is usually combined with acid sodium phosphate in 15-grain doses, as hexamine will only be effective as an antiseptic in an acid medium.

Pyridium, pyridine and acriflavine are other examples of urinary antiseptics.

Another plan made use of is to render the urine alternately acid and alkaline; the patient may be given potassium citrate for 10 days or so and then, when the urine is alkaline, he is given the mixture of hexamine and acid sodium phosphate previously mentioned. This method is employed by those who consider that the *Bacillus coli* thrives least well in a changing medium.

Mandelic acid treatment is an alternative method. It can be used in acute and chronic cases. Three grammes of mandelic acid combined with a dose of 1½ grammes of sodium bicarbonate in solution is given three times a day. The amount of fluids taken is limited to 2 pints a day in order to obtain the concentration of mandelic acid in the urine which is known to produce the best effects.

The urine is kept at a definite degree of acidity (about *p*H 5·4) by the administration of ammonium chloride, 2 grammes, three times a day. In many instances it has been found most successful when the mandelic acid is given before and the ammonium chloride after meals. The amount of ammonium chloride given in the day is regulated by the acidity of the urine, and the nurse in charge of the patient must be prepared to make the *necessary test* as follows :

Two cubic centimetres of urine are put into a test tube, five drops of methyl red are added, when a slightly pink colour will show that the urine is of the correct acidity; if too acid, the colour will be deep pink, but if too alkaline it will be pale yellow.

The nurse should know that large doses of ammonium chloride may irritate the kidney, and if she discovers albumin in a previously normal urine, this should be reported at once. She should notice whether the patient complains of nausea, vomiting or diarrhoea.

In the majority of cases the nurse will note that improvement occurs after a few days, or between 10 and 14 days from commencement of the treatment, that the frequency of micturition is less and that the discomfort disappears. Bacteriological examination will demonstrate the improvement in the condition of the urine.

Sulphadiazine is very effective in the treatment of pyelitis. Penicillin is not employed.

In *chronic pyelitis* vaccines are employed in addition—either stock or autogenous—in order to try and raise the resistance of the patient to *Bacillus coli* infections.

CYSTITIS

Inflammation of the urinary bladder may be due to infection by the *Bacillus coli*, staphylococcus, streptococcus, gonococcus, tubercle bacillus and bacillus typhosus.

Predisposing causes are a chill, and retention of urine or incomplete emptying of the bladder as occurs in enlargement of the prostate gland in men and in some gynaecological and obstretric conditions in women.

In **acute cystitis** there is severe pain over the bladder in the hypogastric region, and the frequent passage of small quantities of urine—a drachm or two every five minutes, accompanied by pain—is a most distressing symptom.

The *urine* is thick and contains large quantities of mucus and pus; it is acid when the condition is due to *Bacillus coli* but alkaline when due to other causes. There may be a rise of temperature but this is not invariable and in many cases the constitutional symptoms are slight. As the days pass the patient becomes tired and weary because of the pain and the inability to sleep owing to the marked frequency of micturition.

Treatment. The patient is kept in bed and hot applications are applied over the bladder. The diet should be light and plenty of bland fluids should be given; the bowels must be regulated. When the urine is acid the treatment by drugs is the same as described in pyelitis; when it is alkaline acid sodium phosphate is given to reduce the alkalinity. When infection is due to penicillin-sensitive organisms this drug is employed.

In *chronic cystitis* similar measures are taken and in addition the bladder is irrigated with a mild antiseptic, and vaccines are employed.

DISORDERS OF MICTURITION

Disorders of micturition may be dealt with under the following headings —frequency, incontinence, enuresis, retention and dysuria.

Frequency of micturition is usually attributable to some disorder or disease of the urinary tract, and in some cases to lesions outside the tract which are irritating it. In a great number of conditions it is due to an irritable urine, and in others to polyuria. Examples of conditions of the urinary tract giving rise to frequency are pyelitis, cystitis, and urethritis.

Incontinence means the involuntary expulsion of urine from the bladder. This must not be confused with an urgent desire to pass urine, which will cause urine to be involuntarily passed if the patient has to wait long. Another condition allied to incontinence is the passing of a few drops of urine under conditions such as stress and strain, as when intra-abdominal pressure is increased; this may happen when sneezing, laughing or coughing.

True incontinence, which is entirely involuntary, may mean that the sphincter muscle is completely relaxed, the urine dribbling away as it is secreted and the bladder remaining quite empty.

In some cases, however, there is spasm of the sphincter urethrae and urine is retained in the bladder which is always distended, only the overflow dribbling away. This occurs in injuries to the brain and spinal cord, and is best described as retention with overflow.

Stress or orthostatic incontinence (in women) is a condition in which urine escapes from the bladder on any exertion. Orthostatic means, causing to stand erect, and escape of urine occurs when standing or on sneezing, coughing, laughing, straining and so on; and the patient, usually a middle-aged woman, 'wets her clothes'. She lives in constant dread of this happening and often fails to consult a specialist until she has suffered for many years.

The condition, whatever may be the contributing cause, is one in which the sphincter of the neck of the bladder is stretched.

Many treatments have been advocated without success until Terence Millin planned the *sling operation* described on page 731, which is proving successful in a great many instances.

Enuresis is the term used to describe incontinence which may be *diurnal* (by day) or *nocturnal* (by night)—it usually occurs in children, and is due to the incomplete establishment of voluntary control. It may be that control once established has been lost; but in most cases the history will be that the child or adolescent has always been incontinent.

In considering the treatment of enuresis it is essential to look for other factors which may be contributory causes such as the presence of worms, a highly acid urine, the existence of enlarged tonsils or adenoids, or any other condition which causes a child to sleep lightly.

The nurse is very intimately concerned with the treatment of this type of incontinence. The diurnal type is easily dealt with by getting the child to empty his bladder every two hours, or every hour if necessary. *Nocturnal enuresis* is more difficult to treat, but it is very important that all commission should pass unnoticed, uncommented on, and all omission be highly praised. Some recommend the use of a hard mattress, waking the child say at 10 o'clock to pass urine, limiting any fluid intake after 5 p.m.; but in many cases these measures have not been found of any use. The child usually grows out of the condition, and in the meantime psychological treatment indicated above is probably the best to use. Belladonna may be ordered to help control the activity of the bladder.

Retention of urine means that urine is retained in the bladder, which becomes distended and on examination can be felt above the symphysis pubis. This condition gives rise to discomfort and pain, and it is very important that the nurse should not confuse it with suppression of urine as described on p. 399.

The causes of retention are numerous. There may be interference with the nervous mechanism; nervousness and hysteria may cause spasm of the sphincter of the urethra; organic lesion of the brain and cord, especially when this occurs as the result of an injury, may have a similar effect; interference with the sympathetic nerves following operations on abdominal and pelvic organs, depression of the micturition centre following general anaesthesia, the use of certain sedative drugs, shock—which depresses all the vital centres, including those governing micturition—pain, as in urethritis and cystitis, when the patient inhibits micturition, and eventually the reflex is interfered with and retention occurs—any of these may be a cause. Decrease of intra-abdominal pressure may arise when the abdominal muscles have been recently stretched, and this may occur immediately after childbirth, or after the removal of a large quantity of intraperitoneal fluid by tapping, or after the removal of a large ovarian cyst. Diminished tone of the musculature of the bladder may be associated with debility, severe anaemia and senility. Pressure externally on the urethra or neck of the bladder, as may arise from the presence of tumour, or be due to enlargement of the prostrate gland.

The nursing treatment for the relief of retention. From the list of causes given above, it can be seen that in the majority of instances the nurse may be able to effect relief without resorting to catheterization. The point to remember is that the distention of the bladder has probably suppressed the normal impulses of micturition, so that this reflex is temporarily out of control.

The following measures may be tried—the giving of hot or cold drinks which, slightly altering the tension by adding quickly to the contents of the bladder, may stimulate the reflex; altering the patient's position in bed, encouraging him to try to micturate while lying on his side, if he cannot do so while lying on his back; and a male patient may be allowed to kneel in suitable circumstances upon the bed to pass urine.

The addition of a little warm water to the bedpan, or pouring a little warm water over the vulva in the case of a woman—it is important to measure the amount of any water put into the bedpan in order to ascertain how much urine has been passed—turning on a tap in the vicinity may act by suggestion; applications of warmth over the distended bladder—any of these may perhaps give relief.

The patient's feet should be quite warm, and he might be allowed to wash his hands, as moving them about in the water may assist in relaxation. The administration of a hot bath, if the patient is allowed to go to the bathroom, has been found particularly useful in male cases, especially when retention is due to some painful condition, as in orchitis.

The administration of an enema may be effective. This acts because it makes the patient empty the bowel, and it is most valuable in the case of women patients, since, in the female, contraction of the pelvic diaphragm by the act of defaecation causes movement of the other sphincters opening into it.

Dysuria, or difficulty of micturition, is a term used to indicate the fact that pain accompanies the act; it may be due to some diseased condition of the bladder and uretha which leads the patient to attempt to inhibit the desire to micturate. In such instances, allowing the patient to sit in a hot bath and pass urine in the water is often very efficacious. The administration of liberal amounts of bland fluid, by diluting the urine and so possibly rendering it less irritating, is another way in which the nurse may help.

Chapter 26

Diseases and Disorders of the Nervous System

Introduction: Symptoms of an upper and lower neurone lesion—Hemiplegia—Paraplegia—Disseminated sclerosis—Infantile paralysis—Bell's palsy—Neuritis—Syphilis of the nervous system—cerebral syphilis, locomotor ataxia, general paralysis of the insane—Inflammation of the brain and meninges—Meningitis, epidemic encephalitis—Infections of the spinal cord: transverse myelitis—Functional disorders—Neuralgia—Hysteria—Paralysis agitans—Chorea—Anorexia nervosa—Psychoses and Neuroses—Fits and convulsions—Epilepsy—Hysterical fit—Apoplexy—Coma

Diseases *of the nervous system* may be divided into: (1) those affecting the central nervous system, the several parts of the brain and the spinal cord, and (2) those affecting the nerves given off from the central parts, the peripheral nerves. They are said to be *organic* when a definite lesion exists, and *functional* when no changes take place in the organ.

Nervous diseases are also very commonly classified according to the neurone affected—a *neurone* is a nerve with its cell, dendrons and axon; some of these neurones function in the central part where they are called *upper* motor or sensory neurones; others in the peripheral portion are called *lower* motor or sensory neurones.

A nervous disease which affects the function of the muscular system is characterized by changes in the behaviour and functions of the muscles supplied by the disordered or diseased nerves, and it has therefore been found convenient in describing some of the nervous diseases to classify them as upper or lower motor neurone lesions, according to the symptoms which are manifest.

Symptoms	*In lesions of the upper motor neurone*	*In lesions of the lower motor neurone*
Wasting of Muscle	Very slight, and only so far as due to disuse of the muscle	Very marked, so much so that in children the limb will cease to grow
Rigidity of Muscle	The limbs tend to be very rigid	None—but complete flaccidity present
Reflexes	Deep reflexes exaggerated, knee and ankle jerks very brisk; the plantar reflex gives an extensor response (Babinski's sign)	Reflexes abolished
Electrical reactions	No change, the reactions are present as in a normal muscle	Reactions always modified. In complete lesion the muscles fail to react to faradism and react only sluggishly to galvanism. (This is called the reaction of degeneration)

ymptoms (continued)	In lesions of the upper motor neurone	In lesions of the lower motor neurone
eformities	Rigidity of muscle is accompanied by contractures; the arm becomes flexed and adducted and the leg flexed at the knee and adducted at the hip joint	Deformities occur owing to the unopposed action of healthy muscles

The articles shown in illustration (fig. 234, p. 678) are those which will e required for the examination of the nervous system.

The best examples of disease of the upper motor neurones are hemilegia, paraplegia and disseminated sclerosis.

HEMIPLEGIA

Hemiplegia is paralysis of one side of the body, face, arm and leg. It is ue to a lesion of disease, injury or cerebral haemorrhage on one side of ıe brain which produces paralysis of the opposite side of the body.

The *onset* may be sudden with an apoplectic seizure in which the patient ecomes immediately unconscious and lies breathing heavily with a full ounding pulse, noisy respirations and flushed face (see also p. 431); r the onset may be more gradual, when signs of paralysis come on slowly. 'he paralysed parts are limp and flaccid for the first day or two, and then he symptoms characteristic of an upper motor neurone lesion are maniested by rigidity of muscle, exaggerated reflexes and a tendency to ontractures. If the patient protrudes his tongue it will be inclined toyards the paralysed side; he may have difficulty in speaking and in exressing what he wishes to convey, and this is termed dysphasia. The peech area may be involved on the left side of the brain in the case of a ight-sided hemiplegia, and the patient be unable to speak, which is ermed *aphasia*.

Treatment and nursing. The patient should be put to bed, with the ıead of the bed slightly elevated; a cold application may be applied to ıis head and his feet should be kept warm. A four-hourly record of the emperature, pulse and respiration rate should be kept; the temperature nay rise. The bowels should be kept active by the use of aperients which vill produce several watery stools for the first few days; then two soft tools a day. The urine should be tested, and the bladder watched for any endency to retention of urine.

The patient is usually an elderly person, and there is therefore coniderable danger of hypostatic pneumonia; the position in which he lies ›ught to be changed at least every 2 hours in order to obviate this. As a 'ule his breathing will be fairly deep; but, when he is moved, he should be vell disturbed in order to make him breathe deeply and so ventilate his ungs; this requires caution, as injudicious handling may cause a recur'ence of the cerebral haemorrhage which may have caused the hemiɔlegia.

The skin requires regular attention in order to prevent the formation ›f bedsores; the patient's mouth should be kept clean, and as it is likely to be dry, it should be moistened frequently. As soon as he wishes l may have small drinks of bland fluids but, for fear of raising the bloo pressure in cases of an apoplectic character, the quantity given should l less than 3 pints during each 24 hours. When the patient is able to tak food, light diet will be given—but red meats, soups made from mea stimulants, including tea and coffee, should be avoided. The patie may require to be fed; if one side of the face, including the movemen of the tongue, is paralysed, he may have difficulty in mastication an swallowing, and this must be taken into consideration when feedin him.

The patient should be kept quiet and not allowed to get excited, t indulge in attacks of violent coughing, or sneezing, to move himse violently about in bed or perform any other action likely to cause eve a slight rise in blood pressure.

The position of the limbs in bed should be observed and deformiti prevented from occurring; the affected arm should be abducted from th side of the body by means of the insertion of a wedge-shaped pillow in th axilla. The forearm should be extended and supinated and the wrist e tended a great many times a day, in order to prevent the deformities c flexion and pronation of the forearm with flexion of the wrist which s easily occur in cases of hemiplegia. The affected lower limb should b kept in good alignment—not too straight. The tendencies to be counte acted here are flexion of the knee, plantar-flexion of the ankle and ex ternal rotation of the thigh. Splints or sandbags may be used to correc the position in which the limb lies.

As recovery takes place the affected limbs will be massaged and passiv movements of the joints carried out, encouraging active movements a soon as possible.

A nurse should keep in mind any cases of hemiplegia she may have see walking in the street with the characteristic gait and attitudes which ar apt to persist unless care is taken in the prevention of deformity and th re-education of the weakened groups of muscles to overcome the con traction and rigidity of stronger groups.

The typical gait and attitude mentioned are, that the patient carrie his afflicted arm closely adducted to the side of the body, with forearn flexed and pronated. As he walks, in order to avoid tripping over th affected leg, he leans over towards his sound side and throws the affecte limb out in a circle in order to bring it to the ground in front of him. Thi necessitates great effort, in addition to being a deformity and attractin notice in the street.

PARAPLEGIA

Paraplegia is paralysis of one half—the lower half—of the body. It i usually due either to pressure from an injury as in the case of a fracture spine, haemorrhage into the spinal cord, the presence of a tumour on th cord, or collapse of the diseased bodies of the vertebrae in Pott's disease

As the result of this pressure the lower limbs are paralysed and th sphincters of the urethra and anus are involved; there may be retention or incontinence of urine, and incontinence of faeces is frequently present though the patient is usually constipated.

In the nursing care the aims of treatment are to prevent bedsores an infection of the bladder; the details of the care of a similar case will b ound in the account given on p. 615 of the nursing of a patient with a actured spine, which is one of the causes of paraplegia.

DISSEMINATED SCLEROSIS

Disseminated sclerosis is a fairly common organic disease of the central ervous system. It occurs in persons, of both sexes, between the ages of 8 and 35, and is characterized by scattered patches of degeneration over ne brain and spinal cord—hence the term disseminated.

Symptoms. There is usually some paralysis with rigidity of the muscle, xaggerated reflexes, and a tendency towards occurrence of contractures; t first the paralysis may be temporary, as one of the chief characteristics f disseminated sclerosis is that it is marked by remission and relapses, but n the majority of patients the spastic paralysis will, eventually, become ermanent.

Other characteristic symptoms include tremor of the hands, and unteadiness in walking—in some cases a subject will consult a physician ecause he falls down in the street for no apparent reason. Eye changes vill sometimes occur and the patient may complain of double vision or be ound, on examination, to have some degree of nystagmus—which means hat there is an involuntary twitching of the eye, which may consist of ither coarse or fine oscillating movements.

Subjects of this disease have a particularly happy temperament; they re obliging, cheerful members of the community and smile a great deal.

Treatment and nursing depend, as far at least as the latter is conerned, on the condition of the patient when he is seen; a badly paralysed case will be nursed in bed and the precautions against bedsores be taken; it is customary, however, in all cases to use massage and re-educative exercises in order to keep the patient an effective member of society for as long as possible. Apart from this, the patient should be advised not to get overtired and, if he suffers from intercurrent infections such as colds and slight influenza, he should remain in bed and take a long rest as convalescence. In many cases, remissions occur and the patient can keep well for long periods together, while less fortunate ones will have more frequent relapses.

A course of arsenic is usually prescribed. Treatment by protein shock therapy and by malarial therapy has been tried.

The best examples of disease of the lower motor neurones are *infantile paralysis*, *Bell's palsy* and *neuritis*.

INFANTILE PARALYSIS

Infantile paralysis, called also *acute poliomyelitis*, is an acute lower motor neurone disease which affects the motor cells in the anterior horns of the spinal cord and results in destruction of some of the nerve cells and serious injury to others. It is due to a specific organism, which is carried in the nasopharynx. It affects children and young people but adults also may be affected; the disease is sporadic in this country, though epidemics of it have occurred.

The *onset of the disease* may be severe with a great deal of pain, a rise of temperature, severe headache, and marked malaise; or it may be more gradual, when slight paralysis is first noticed.

Treatment and nursing. The disease is infectious, it may be conveyed to others or contracted by those attending to the patient, and to avoid these tragedies the simple methods of bed isolation, described on p. 463, are usually considered advisable for the first three weeks of illness.

At the outset the patient may have a great deal of pain and resent any handling of his limbs; if this is so, they should be wrapped in cotton wool and very gently touched. The limbs must be kept in such a position that deformities cannot occur, though it may be difficult at first to determine which groups of muscles are affected, and it is advisable to keep the limbs in a fairly neutral position for a time, so that neither one group nor another will be unduly stretched. The patient should be nursed lying flat in bed, or on a plaster of paris bed, in order to keep the muscles of the trunk at rest. Very gentle movements only are permissible during the early weeks, months in severe cases, as increasing pain and tenderness must be avoided. The hot local packs recommended by Kenny are useful at this stage. Lumbar puncture may relieve headache. A mechanical respirator may be needed when the muscles of respiration are affected.

The duration of rest in the treatment of infantile paralysis is long, and in adult patients particularly this is found very trying and as much as possible should be done to keep the patient cheerful during this irksome wait, when he is moreover troubled by uncertainty as to whether he may or may not recover completely.

As soon as possible some light splint will be adapted to the affected parts and the patient encouraged to get up and move about; massage and electrical treatment will be prolonged for as much as two years, as recovery often takes place after a very long time. Later, when the resultant recovery is not complete, surgical measures may be considered for the sake of securing better functioning by the fixation of joints and the transplantation of healthy muscles to take the place of, and perform the offices of, some which will not recover.

BELL'S PALSY

Bell's palsy was described by Sir Charles Bell, the founder of the Middlesex Hospital Medical School. It is a lower motor neurone paralysis —affecting the facial nerve, the seventh cranial, which supplies the muscles of expression of the face. It may be due to exposure to cold.

Symptoms. At the onset slight pain may be complained of behind the ear and down the side of the neck; the affected side of the face is limp and quite expressionless; but, as the muscles on the other side of the face have no opposing muscles to balance their action, the latter—the sound side—is drawn up in a most grotesque manner. The eyelids on the paralysed side droop, the corner of the mouth is relaxed and saliva dribbles out of it; the folds and creases and wrinkles are all obliterated.

Treatment and nursing. The eye should be bathed and kept covered, the corner of the mouth supported by means of a silver hook placed inside the corner of the mouth and fastened up over the ear to prevent the muscles from being constantly dragged down by the weight of gravity. This hook must be kept very clean and the mouth should be cleaned;

eating may present some difficulty, but the actual muscles of mastication are not included in the paralysis since these are supplied by the fifth and not the seventh cranial nerve.

Massage and electrical treatment will be employed when the initial inflammatory stage has passed; as soon as active movement is permitted the patient should be taught to use his muscles by trying to smile, whistle and frown, in front of a mirror.

NEURITIS

Neuritis is inflammation of a nerve fibre and its covering. The condition is described as *polyneuritis* or *multiple peripheral neuritis* when it exists on both sides of the body, affecting a number of nerves. *Alcoholic neuritis* is an example of this type.

In *interstitial neuritis* one or two nerve trunks only are affected; examples of this variety are *sciatica* and *brachial* and *intercostal neuritis*.

The **symptoms and signs** of neuritis include pain, tenderness and swelling over the affected nerve trunks, alterations in sensation—such as tingling and numbness—wasting of muscle with loss of tone, and diminished tendon reflexes and paralysis.

The **treatment** includes investigation for any possible cause—the presence (for instance) of a septic focus in the body, such as septic tonsils, teeth, gallbladder, appendix, or the existence of colitis. These factors should be treated.

Meanwhile the distressing symptoms of neuritis require *local measures* for their relief. During acute pain rest is necessary, applications of heat may give relief and soothing analgesic preparations may be employed for this purpose also.

In the *nursing care* of a neuritis case it is essential to discover the position in which the patient can lie most comfortably, and also to observe the effect of the various local treatments employed, and to find out which gives most relief and which may be contraindicated since it seems to irritate the condition.

The patient should be very gently moved; the bed should be free from creases and the weight of the clothes should not rest on the painful parts. Wrapping the painful parts in cotton wool will sometimes be found soothing, at other times supporting them on pillows or splints or between sandbags may bring relief; in a few instances, where no relief seems to be obtainable, elevation of the foot of the bed and the application of slight extension to a painful lower limb may help.

The diet will as a rule be specially ordered and it is the duty of the nurse to make it as appetizing as possible; a patient who is in pain is disinclined to eat, he is depressed and every little surprise and change of any kind will, by awakening interest, help to relieve the painful monotony of his present existence.

Diseases of the sensory neurones cannot as readily be classified into upper and lower as are those of the motor system just described. Three relays of sensory nerves convey impulses from the periphery to the brain. One of the best examples of disease of sensory neurones is *locomotor ataxia*.

SYPHILIS OF THE NERVOUS SYSTEM

Syphilis is described on p. 529. One of the most serious results of thi disease, and the one which is most disabling, is manifested in the disease of the nervous system which are due to it. These are *cerebral syphilis, locomotor ataxia* and *general paralysis of the insane*.

Cerebral syphilis may be manifested by inflammation of the coverings of the brain—the meninges—or the arteries which supply the brai with blood may be affected.

A variety of symptoms may be present including severe headache epilepsy, hemiplegia, double vision, general mental changes characterize by loss of memory and irritability of temper. This type of case is treate with the usual antisyphilitic remedies, novarsenobillon (arsenic) an mercury.

LOCOMOTOR ATAXIA

Locomotor ataxia is a disease of the sensory neurones. It is also describe as *tabes dorsalis*. This disease occurs some years after syphilitic infection in what is known as the tertiary stage of syphilis.

Symptoms. Locomotor ataxia is characterized by shooting pains i the limbs and by lack of co-ordination of voluntary movement; the diseas does not affect the motor nerves, sensation is affected and in the late stages of the disease the patient loses the sense of the position of his bod in relation to other things, such as the floor or his chair, and fails to be abl to co-ordinate his movements even so far as to touch some part of his body, his nose for example, without groping over his face with his hand in order to find it by feeling for it.

Other symptoms and signs include smallness of the pupils of the eyes and their failure to react to light. As the sensory portion of the reflex arc is not functioning there is loss of deep reflexes. The patient's gait becomes very characteristic. He behaves like a high-stepping horse and lifts his leg high and then bangs his foot forcibly on the floor, swaying from side to side as if drunk. This is called the stamping or *tabetic gait*.

As the disease progresses all these symptoms get worse. *Tabetic crises* may occur. A gastric crisis is characterized by attacks of abdominal pain and vomiting; a vesicle crisis by attacks of acute retention of urine. *Charcot's joint* may develop; this is a form of arthritis characterized by laxity of the ligaments of the joint affected which renders it weak and flail. The knee joints are most commonly affected.

Treatment. Penicillin is employed, even in late syphilis, often combined with arsenic and mercury. Pyrexial treatment also is used (see p. 415).

The ataxia and inco-ordination can be very much improved by re-education by means of Fraenkel's exercises, which aim at improving the movements, by making the patient use his eyes to see where he is putting his hands or feet; he is taught to walk along a strip of floor, on which footmarks are placed, and he is expected to put his feet exactly on these as he walks along.

Massage will improve the general tone of the muscles of the limbs; e patient should be warned not to allow himself to get tired; his diet ould be nourishing and he should live an easy comfortable life, and get much rest as possible but he should not stop in bed, as surrender to his sability in this way will allow the disease to progress, and he will then iite quickly become a very helpless member of society.

GENERAL PARALYSIS OF THE INSANE

General paralysis of the insane, which is an inflammatory lesion affecting e nerve cells in the brain, is due to syphilis and occurs in the tertiary age of the disease, except in those comparatively rare cases which are ongenital. As a rule this disease occurs between the ages of 40 and 60.

Symptoms. The onset is characterized by mild mental symptoms, ight loss of memory, apparent loss of interest, inability to concentrate, aking mistakes at work, and attacks of depression. If the disease is not eated, all these symptoms will become worse and the patient will evelop delusions of grandeur—he may order expensive articles for which e cannot possibly pay and imagine he is somebody very great. As the isease progresses mental failure occurs, the patient wastes and eventually ies. A fit or stroke may occur during the course of the disease.

Treatment. Penicillin and other antisyphilitic drugs, and in addition yrexial treatment, usually by means of an induced attack of malaria, re all employed in the treatment of G.P.I.

The malarial treatment of G.P.I. The patient is infected with benign ertian malaria either by allowing him to be bitten by infected mosquitoes, or by infected blood given intramuscularly. After a short incubaion period he develops malaria and is allowed to have eight or nine rigors —these occur on alternate days in the benign tertian type of malaria— nd the disease is then arrested by the administration of quinine.

Nursing duties during this period are observation of the patient's general ondition. As soon as he has been infected with malaria his temperature hould be taken every four hours; when malaise is complained of the atient should be kept in bed.

The time of the first rigor should be noted; at first the patient will be ery cold, and during this period his temperature will begin to rise and hould then be taken every 15 minutes; it will reach its maximum in a hort time, and, if it rises above 105° F., the patient should be sponged with tepid water, as such a very high temperature may be accompanied y delirium and will be followed by marked prostration. Apart from this recaution the nursing care of the patient during rigors is as described n p. 47.

The physician may require the nurse to take a blood film when the emperature is at its maximum, in order that he may note the number of malarial parasites in the blood, which indicate the severity of the infection.

The general condition of the patient must be carefully observed, as he will be weakened and rendered anaemic by this treatment; if he suffers from vomiting and diarrhoea or from delirium, during the course of his malarial treatment, it may be necessary to stop the treatment before he has had the number of rigors usually permitted.

After the treatment he will probably be very anaemic and will need liberal nourishing diet and some weeks' rest before any improvement noticed.

INFLAMMATION OF THE MENINGES (MENINGITIS)

The principal types of meningitis are meningococcal, tuberculou pneumococcal and streptococcal.

MENINGOCOCCAL MENINGITIS

Meningococcal meningitis is also described as *cerebrospinal fever*. It is due to specific organism, *Neisseria meningitidis* or *Neisseria intracellularis*. The disea is of the nature of an acute infection. The organism is carried in the nas pharynx; the disease is sporadic in distribution in this country bu epidemics do occur, particularly under conditions of bad general hygier and overcrowding.

The *onset* of the disease is usually short and acute, and the *course* mor rapid than that described in tuberculous meningitis.

The **symptoms** also are similar, but more acute. There is a severe head ache, and the patient lies curled up on his side with head markedl retracted; he is extremely sensitive to the slightest irritation by touch, c sound, and also to light. His mouth is very dry and his tongue coated, h temperature is high and pulse rapid at first; there may be paralysis, th pupils may be unequal and squint may be present. The mind wande and the patient is delirious. Rigidity of the muscles is very marked an Kernig's sign is present—this means that when the thigh is flexed th marked rigidity of the flexors of the knee prevents the knee joint from bein extended. Wasting is marked, the patient passes urine and faeces involun tarily and rapidly reaches the stage of coma. There is increase of in tracranial pressure manifested by deepening coma, slowing of the pulse deepening of the respirations and, unless adequate serum treatment ca be obtained, death may occur after several weeks. Some cases recover an are left with a permanent disability, which may be mental or physica in character; a few make a slow, uncomplicated recovery.

Treatment. Sulphonamides and penicillin are now used with grea success and as a result the period of acute disease is shortened and th prognosis is favourable.

Nursing. The nursing of meningitis is difficult, because the patient i acutely ill and liable to become worse and, as cerebral irritation is marked it needs keen observation and great gentleness and patience on the par of a nurse who is to deal successfully with such a case.

As the disease is infectious the principles of bed isolation should b employed, and all swabs used and all discharges from the nose and mout should be destroyed by burning.

A well-ventilated room is necessary but the patient should not face the light. As he lies curled up in bed, sensitive even to the slightest touch, which in this case acts as an irritation, great care must be taken in moving this patient; he must not be touched by a cold hand, and should be grasped firmly but not roughly, the hand being imposed gently and the hold firmly nd evenly maintained; all movement performed should be as slow as ossible and should not be jerky but rhythmical in character. The head ust not be moved as the slightest attempt to flex it is accompanied by vere pain which increases the irritation.

As the patient is emaciated and incontinent the skin requires the reatest care and attention if bedsores are to be prevented; he may lie ith a ring air cushion under his side to prevent sores from forming over e great trochanter; he can be turned to alternate sides but should not be laced directly on his back, though he may lie partially over on his back r definite periods provided he is supported by pillows.

He should be sponged twice a day, and the nurse must notice whether arm or hot water proves least irritating to him, and use whichever seems ost acceptable.

The mouth requires constant care to keep it clean and moist; secretion hich dries in the nose should be moistened and removed; in the stage of oma the patient will lie with his eyes open and they should then be bathed egularly in order to prevent the occurrence of conjunctivitis. As already entioned, all swabs used for these purposes should be burnt.

The bladder must be watched for fear of retention, and it is advisable o measure the urine, so that any diminution in quantity does not go nmarked; it should be tested regularly. The bowels must be kept acting y the use of aperients or enemata if necessary. The method adopted of eding the patient will depend on his condition; if conscious he will be ble to swallow; even when in a state of stupor it may be possible to rouse im to take sufficient fluid; but when in coma he will have to be fed rtificially and as he requires nourishment to combat the wasting that is haracteristic of this infection, it is advisable to use the nasal tube for this urpose. The temperature, pulse and respirations should be the subject of onstant and frequent observation. Slowing of the pulse and deepening of he respirations, when accompanied by headache, drowsiness and in-reasing unconsciousness, indicate that there is increase in intracranial ressure. A nurse should learn to recognize this; in a case such as that nder discussion, in which lumbar puncture will be frequently performed, areful observation of the changes which occur in the patient's pulse and epth of respiration as the pressure is relieved by removal of fluid from he theca, should demonstrate this effect to her. Icebags are frequently rdered for the relief of headache, and it is advisable to get permission to ut the hair short.

The special dangers which are to be avoided in nursing a patient in the tage of coma are pneumonia, which may be brought about by his in-haling saliva; hypostatic pneumonia, because he is not turned and moved ften enough; infection of the bladder, should retention of urine be eglected; bedsores and hot-water bottle burns, and infection of the con-unctiva when the corneal reflex is abolished, if the eyes are open.

Tuberculous meningitis occurs most often in children, though any age may be affected; in adults it may arise as a complication resulting from spread of the disease from some other lesion in the body.

The *onset* in tuberculous meningitis is gradual with headache, malaise, loss of appetite, and a slight rise of temperature.

The stage of irritability. As the disease progresses the symptoms of cerebral irritation becomes manifest—the patient lies curled up in bed with head retracted and the muscles of his neck are rigid. He will cry when touche and resents being moved; paralysis may now be present or convulsions delirium occur.

The next stage of the disease is manifested by *coma*; unconsciousne gradually becomes deeper, and retention of urine will very likely occu Many cases terminate fatally in about 6 weeks.

The **treatment** is largely palliative but streptomycin is at prese being employed with success in some cases. Lumbar puncture is pe formed to relieve pressure; the cerebrospinal fluid is always clear i tuberculous meningitis; in other types it is turbid.

Other types respond to sulphonamides and/or penicillin depending o the causal organism.

EPIDEMIC ENCEPHALITIS

Epidemic encephalitis or *encephalitis lethargica* is an infectious diseas affecting the brain and in some cases the spinal cord. It is often associate with epidemics of influenza and may occur in epidemic form; sporadi cases are invariably present in this country and each case is notified to th Medical Officer of Health.

Infection is considered to be carried in the nasal mucous membrane, an it is due to a virus. The *incubation period* is from a few days to twenty-on days.

The **onset of the disease** varies from a rapid, sudden onset in acut cases, which often terminate fatally in a week or two, to a slow onset of subacute type in which either lethargica, diplopia, headache, restlessnes and delirium or persistent hiccup may be the only symptoms present.

The **symptoms present in the course of the disease** are as variabl as those of the onset. When lethargy is present the patient lies inert unheeding anything which is passing around him, and passes his urin and faeces in the bed. This state may last for some weeks and then th patient may slowly recover or he may develop Parkinsonism.

It is generally considered that the more acute the onset the graver is th prognosis and, conversely, that the slower the onset and the fewer th symptoms the more likely is the patient to recover completely. Many case of epidemic encephalitis who recover are found to have a complete chang of character, mischievous lads may develop quite saintly characters though, conversely, previously well-behaved children sometimes develo habits of lying, stealing and teasing. Adults frequently become unable t sustain effort and find themselves unable to concentrate and persever in their former employments, and become careless and slovenly in habit.

Other mental symptoms include restlessness, delirium and mania the patient is unusually wakeful at night and in many cases is quite insane Even mild cases often develop a reversed sleep rhythm, and the mischievous boys wake at night and prowl about annoying other persons i the same ward, or in the same house or street.

In a case with an acute onset there is a rise in temperature, the mout is dry and the tongue furred, incontinence of urine and faeces is present.

Parkinsonism is the name used to describe a group of symptoms—th nmon sequelae of epidemic encephalitis—which are frequently seen adults, but rarely occur in children.

The attitude the patient adopts is of flexion of the trunk with stooping oulders and head projecting forwards; his elbows are held to the sides of body and his fingers are constantly employed in performing rhythmical ovements. When he walks he progresses by short mincing steps and takes le runs forward and sometimes backward; the knees are slightly bent, d the general attitude as described makes the patient look much older an he really is.

The face is characteristically masklike and remains expressionless; the eech is monotonous and slow and the patient frequently repeats his ords. In severe cases salivation is troublesome.

Nursing and treatment. Very little is known about the treatment of is disease, though in some cases intravenous infusion of a solution of llosol iodine or of sodium salicylate has been found of value. Anti-asmodic drugs including hyoscine and belladonna have proved useful; art from these measures treatment aims at relief of the symptoms.

With regard to the nursing care more can be said. If the patient is acutely with a high fever, dirty mouth and incontinence, the same careful ursing as described in the care of cases of cerebrospinal fever cases on 417 will be required.

When lethargica is present the patient should be moved frequently in der to prevent hypostatic pneumonia; he should be roused to take fficient fluid. Feeding may be difficult, as keeping the patient roused ng enough to swallow is often a problem; moreover, he may have fficulty in swallowing and in mastication, and may persistently refuse en to attempt to take either food or drink. In such cases he may have be fed by means of a nasal tube or by rectum.

The *prevention of bedsores* is important; the patient should have sanitary tention at regular intervals and if possible be persuaded to use the vessels pplied at these intervals; if he will not, he should be cleaned as soon as s bed is soiled and should always be provided with pads of wool and tow nder him so that faeces can be absorbed, and he should have a urinal in e bed, so that bedwetting is avoided.

The bladder must be observed lest retention of urine should occur, and e bowels kept acting regularly by the use of aperients or enemata if ecessary.

When the patient begins to recover he should be given interesting occupa-ons and encouraged to take an interest in everything going on around im; the nurse should watch carefully for alteration in character and do er best to train the patient in good habits—in eating, cleanliness and ressing for example. He should be taught to take an interest in his ersonal appearance and in his accomplishments. It is important to member that if the patient's behaviour is ill favoured, he probably grets this as much as the nurse, but the tendency to be tiresome may be pressing and his will so weak that he needs all the help she can give him nd she should never let him see that she is annoyed, but should make im understand how pleased she is when his behaviour is kind and ourteous.

Children should never be punished, but they must be carefully per-uaded, rewarded when they have tried and succeeded, and merely allowed to realize that they are not interesting to others when th behaviour is abnormal.

INFECTIONS OF THE SPINAL CORD

Myelitis is inflammation of the spinal cord; *infantile paralysis*, which described on p. 411, being an example as it is definitely a disease of t lower motor neurones. The object of this note, however, is to describe t condition knows as acute transverse myelitis.

Acute transverse myelitis is an acute inflammation of a comple section of the spinal cord; it is thought to be an infective condition, a may follow acute nephritis and influenza, but in many cases it cann be attributed definitely to any known cause.

The *onset* may be very sudden; there may be a slight rise of temperatu accompanied by malaise, when the patient notices he has lost the use his legs and may be unable to pass urine, retention having occurred.

The first effect of the inflammatory lesion is to produce softening of t cord, with the result that spinal shock is manifest; and there is total flacc paralysis below the level of the lesion. If examined, the reflexes will missing and sensation will be impaired; retention of urine is present.

This condition persists for a few days—ten or more—and the impair sensation gradually improves and the tendon reflexes return. Eventual the character of the paralysis is that of an upper motor neurone lesion, occurs in pressure on the spinal cord, spastic paralysis is present, t tendon reflexes are exaggerated and the extensor plantar respon (Babinski's sign) is obtained.

The **nursing care** is as described in the case of fracture of the spine. transverse myelitis the recovery made may be partial or complete, and depends to a great extent upon good nursing. The use of a water bed essential. The skin must be carefully tended—the patient should nev be moved by one nurse, and he may not be rolled over but must be lifte while great care is necessary to prevent injury to the skin of the ba when using the bedpan. Hot-water bottles should be carefully guarded a owing to diminished sensation, burns occur very easily. The helpless paralysed patient is unable to move away from the vicinity of a hot-wat bottle or any other source of possible injury.

Catheterization will be necessary for the relief of retention and t danger of bladder infection must ever be remembered. It is unlikely th a nurse will, even inadvertently, fail to use proper precautions regardi the aseptic technique of passing a catheter, but since the bladder is not ab to empty itself, owing to the absence of the normal reflex, infection ma occur. Part of the nursing care which will help to prevent this is the a ministration of bland fluids in large quantities which act as a mild urina antiseptic. Some urinary antiseptic may be ordered by the physician.

The prevention of deformity, especially footdrop, is important; a lig rectangular footsplint is suitable for this purpose, and the bedcloth should not be drawn tightly over the feet. The use of mackintoshes may b considered necessary in order to prevent soiling of the mattress; but in patient with retention this is unlikely and mackintoshes are very unsui able for use in the beds of paralysed patients—however carefully attende they tend to collect moisture, which is a potent cause of bedsore. When nackintosh is employed, the precaution should be taken of covering with a blanket, placed between it and the bottom sheet, which will sorb moisture.

FUNCTIONAL NERVOUS DISORDERS

Functional nervous disorders are those in which no organic lesion is esent, such as *major epilepsy*, *neuralgia*, *hysteria*, *paralysis agitans*, *chorea*, d a large number of conditions which are described as *neurasthenia*.

Neuralgia is pain in a nerve, and it may either be due to a number of uses—including local pressure, inflammation, toxaemia—or be a manitation of debility or anaemia.

Trigeminal neuralgia is a very painful type which occurs in the fifth anial nerve and is characterized by acute attacks of agonizing pain companied by tenderness and swelling of the skin over the course of the rve.

The *treatment* carried out at first is to apply heat to the painful area and ght counterirritation; at the same time the general health should be nsidered and attempts made to improve this and also to discover and eat any underlying or contributory cause. In some very persistent ses it becomes necessary to inject alcohol into the nerve or to remove e ganglion from which it arises.

HYSTERIA

Hysteria is a functional nervous condition which produces many varieties symptoms. An hysterical fit and its treatment are described on p. 430.

The **symptoms** manifested by a person with hysteria may be motor, as ralysis or spasticity or rigidity; or they may be *sensory*, as loss of sensation hyperaesthesia. They may show a mental tendency such as melancholia, nd many other symptoms may be complained of, including headache, digestion and palpitation.

The **treatment** should be in the hands of a good neurologist, but in the eantime the nurse must remember that the patient may not be able to elp himself and that he is ill, though not in body. The attitude the nurse ight to adopt is to suggest that the physician will effect a cure, and that the meantime it is necessary to be cheerful and not speak of the mptoms but rather try to forget them. If the patient displays emotion e should be brought to reason by a sharp command.

PARALYSIS AGITANS

Paralysis agitans is also described as Parkinson's disease, because Dr. arkinson first described it. The characteristic symptoms which are corded here are also seen in the chronic stage of encephalitis lethargica, hen they are known as Parkinsonism or Parkinson's syndrome—a ndrome being a collection of symptoms which manifest some characteric features.

Symptoms. Paralysis agitans is characterized by tremors and loss power in the muscles, and for this reason it is sometimes called 'shaki palsy'. The tremors tend to cease as the patient attempts to perform a action. The arms are held close to the sides of the body and the thun and fingers of both hands are constantly moving as if rolling a pill betwe them. The body is slightly bent, and the head is poking forward betwe stooping shoulders; the patient takes mincing steps and little runs as progresses in walking. The face is expressionless, the skin smooth and fr from wrinkles, and the speech is slow and deliberate.

Treatment aims at relief of the symptoms, and attempts are ma to re-educate the patient in the performance of his movements. He shou not be kept in bed, but rather encouraged to do as much as possible f himself; as all his movements are slow and deliberate, he may take sever hours to get up and dress himself, even with help, but he should be allow to do so. Massage is employed to keep the muscles of the body in ton and the patient should be taught to perform active exercises under dire tion. The disease is progressive, but a cheerful companion can do much make the patient's last years more interesting. When eventually the patie is confined to bed, very careful attention is necessary in order to preve bedsores.

CHOREA

Chorea, or St. Vitus's dance, is described in this section of the wo because the manifestations of it are largely nervous in character. It however, a disease associated with rheumatism and tonsillitis and frequently complicated by a heart affection which likewise is due to t infection which provides the underlying cause of the condition. It is m with in children and young adolescents, more often in girls than in boy and it may occur during pregnancy. An attack of chorea may last for month or two.

The **manifestations of the disease** begin gradually; at first the chi is noticed to be fidgety and nervous, he drops things and cries easily; time goes on he becomes subject to constant involuntary movement jerky in character and quite purposeless. In slight cases the involunta movements cease during sleep; in severe cases they disturb the patient rest and sleep very seriously.

The *mental aspect of the child* is altered; he is emotional, subject to ou bursts of crying and of temper; speech is often difficult, being hesitant an jerky, and as he is very conscious of this he often refuses to attempt speak.

Feeding becomes a great difficulty in severe cases as the child cann masticate; he bolts his food when it is retained in his mouth at all, but it so often lost in transit from plate to mouth that marked emaciation occur The constant movements of the child's limbs, head and trunk, caus injuries to the skin from the bedclothes and bedsores occur easily.

Chorea may be complicated by endocarditis and pericarditis, and it this danger which has to be avoided if possible; its association wit rheumatism and tonsillitis must not be forgotten, mania may occur i severe cases, hyperpyrexia is also a complication to be feared, and relaps are common in children who have had one attack.

Treatment and nursing. *Rest* is ordered in the treatment of chorea, ad it is the business of the nurse to see that this is applied as thoroughly possible, having ever in her mind the danger that heart disease may cur. The *drugs* employed will be probably aspirin and salicylates, ad sedatives such as bromide and chloral, chloretone and sometimes rertin.

In severe cases, when the movements are violent and constant, it may e necessary to nurse the patient on the floor, in a pen made of mattresses that he cannot either fall out of bed, or hurt himself as he is thrown bout the bed by the violence of the movements over which he has no ontrol; or a padded bed with sides may be used. The patient's clothing ould consist of light warm woollens of a shape that will not be easily moved; a sleeping suit and bedsocks might be used; the buttons should e removed as the patient will only pull them off, and the suit should be stened by stitches, the bedsocks being sewn to the legs of the sleeping it. The bedclothes should include a blanket placed next the patient, nd a low pillow is given as it is desirable to keep the patient lying as flat s possible in order to avoid strain on the heart.

The mouth should be cleaned regularly and drinks of water given etween feedings and, as there is danger lest a patient with chorea should ot receive enough fluid, a record should be kept of the amount given and, nce he will be able to take only a little at a time, a drink should be epeated often. The diet should be light, carbohydrates being mainly mployed, but it should be sufficient to avoid wasting. In feeding a child ith chorea great patience is necessary; his head will be constantly moving, nd he should be given small mouthfuls of food at a time which has een well broken up or minced; if a metal spoon is used, it should be one ith a very blunt edge—though a wooden spoon would be preferable— nd a fork ought not to be employed for fear of injuring the mouth. A ooden or blunt metal cup should be used for drinking, as the patient nay break a china one with his teeth. He should be fed slowly and given rinks at intervals during the feeding; any sensation of choking must be voided as this tends to raise the blood pressure, and is an effort for the atient which causes strain on the heart.

The skin should be washed once or twice a day, and the nurse must ecide whether warm or hot water is less irritating or more soothing for his purpose, and then use what she finds by experience to be best in ach case. The routine measures for the prevention of bedsores will need o be frequently employed; if parts of the body seem to be predisposed to oreness, from either pressure or friction, these parts should be protected y applying ring wool pads to them, or by their being wrapped in cotton vool.

The patient should be placed on a bedpan regularly as he will usually ass urine and stool when this is done and soiling of the bed will thus be voided. The amount of urine should be measured and compared with he amount of fluid taken, and it should be tested daily for the presence of lbumin. The bowels must be kept regularly acting, since constipation hould never be allowed to occur.

Sleep is often disturbed by the involuntary movements; this should be oted as the physician, knowing rest to be essential, will order some form f sedative drug for the control of the movements and to secure for the hild sleep that is less disturbed.

The temperature, pulse and respiration rate should be taken an charted every four hours; the pulse should be taken oftener in sever cases, and any change reported.

As the disease begins to abate a child patient will need some amuse ment, and this should be carefully chosen; he might have a soft toy to pla with, but for her own sake the nurse will take the precaution of tyin this to his bed, as otherwise she will be required to pick it up from th floor even very much oftener than she will for most children. Voluntar movement must not be permitted for some time, because of the tendenc to disease of the heart, and the nurse must be prepared to sit by the be of the child, constantly but quietly amusing him in very gentle ways. Sh ought also to use the opportunity for teaching him to speak slowly an distinctly, but she must not tire or bore him; his little efforts should b encouraged and repeated at intervals and failure should never be laughe at. When he is allowed to use his hands, placing little articles in definit positions, such as is involved in a game on a board, may be useful i training him to co-ordinate the finer movements performed by the hand:

When the child gets up, he may only be allowed out of bed for a fev moments at first, and the process of getting him up should be slowly an deliberately carried out; when he first walks, a little game might be mad of this, the nurse making him place his feet near hers as when teaching a infant to walk for the first time. He should not be allowed to feed himse until he is getting up, and then his movements must be guided for som time, as either he will develop the habit of bolting his food or he will nc get enough.

ANOREXIA NERVOSA

Anorexia Nervosa is a functional disorder in which loss of appetit is manifested, the patient being very wasted and having lost all desir for food. The patient is often a young woman and it is very sad to see he playing with food and taking an hour or more to eat one piece of thi bread and butter.

PSYCHOSIS AND NEUROSIS

Since the passing of the Lunacy Act of 1930, fewer cases of insanity ar certified and therefore many insane and borderline cases of mental diseas may come into the hands of the general trained nurse, particularly i private practice. Many of these cases will be neuroses, some will b psychoses and a few possibly dementia, either dementia praecox or senil dementia.

Cases of *psychoses* may have delusions and hallucinations.

Manic depressive psychoses are most commonly met. These case are depressed and cannot concentrate; this state may pass off and the will be normal for a time, then they may become excitable and talkative rushing from one subject to another and then becoming destructive an breaking things up. At this period they will be overwhelmed by a sense o their unworthiness, and will lose appetite and weight; they are restles and anxious and cannot sleep, and as they are convinced they will neve get better, and may commit suicide, they cannot be left alone. They wi usually recover in from 2 to 6 months.

When the patient becomes noisy and destructive the nurse must not le him think she is afraid, and she should not argue with him but agree, i this is possible. As soon as she goes off duty the nurse should go over in her mind the behaviour of her patient, and make notes of anything like a delusion and in doing this she should write down the patient's exact words.

Schizophrenia (*dementia praecox*) occurs in young persons, from 15 to 30. It is characterized by hallucinations and delusions; the subjects of this condition are incapable of rational thought, and become so apathetic that they will neither eat nor speak. For years schizophrenia has been considered hopeless, but recently two physicians have established treatment by *cardiazol* and *insulin* respectively. When cardiazol is used large doses are given to cause epileptiform convulsions; in treatment by insulin coma is produced. In both cases the patient requires observation and care to treat emergencies which may arise.

Senile dementia usually occurs in persons over 50 years of age, and it is sometimes associated with arteriosclerosis. In these cases the patient's memory begins to fail, and he becomes suspicious of friends and relatives whom he formerly trusted, imagining that they are talking adversely about him. He gets worried about his money problems and thinks he is becoming poverty-stricken and broods over this.

As the disease advances cases of dementia lose all interest in their personal appearance and become dirty in their habits.

In the treatment and care of them it is necessary to try and get them interested and to keep them as cheerful and happy as possible.

NEUROSES

A neurosis is a manifestation of symptoms without the foundation of any organic disease, and neuroses occur in persons who are unable, for one reason or another, to adapt themselves to the conditions which they meet in life.

The *typical picture of such a patient* is one who is always worrying about some problem; he is anxious and sleeps badly, is unable to concentrate and is quite certain that he is suffering from some serious organic disease. He may present all kinds of symptoms, including palpitation, indigestion, constipation and even colitis, rapid action of the heart, headache, aches and pains of all descriptions, sweating, especially of the palms of the hands, his hands may tremble when performing movements, and if asked to put out his tongue this is tremulous. He gets thin and looks very anxious and worried.

Such a patient will go from one doctor to another until he may meet one who may tell him something which pleases, such as the fact that his heart may be overacting a little; the patient is pleased and broods on this and imagines himself a very ill person indeed and his state of neurasthenia goes from bad to worse.

In the treatment and nursing care of a patient suffering from any neurosis the nurse must remember that, although not organically ill, the patient is ill, and requires just as much care as a serious case of heart disease, though in a different way. The physician does not tell the patient there is nothing the matter; he listens most sympathetically, talks over the patient's symptoms with him and tries to show him how they have arisen and in what ways they can best be dealt with in order to effect a cure. Such patients are very anxious to help themselves, they will receive suggestion willingly and can be encouraged to do as the physician suggests.

SPECIAL POINTS IN THE NURSING OF NEUROLOGICAL CASES

In the *nursing of neurological cases* certain points have to be considered. Some neurotic symptoms are associated with all organic lesions and allowance must be made for this; it is probably due to the fact that the disease from which the patient is suffering and the mode of life he is forced to live because of it, is undermining the mental resistance of the patient as well as his vitality.

Again, a neurosis may be present in conjunction with some organic disease; or the neurosis may be the only condition present.

Neuroses may be present in hysterical form, as an anxiety state or as an obsessional condition. The symptoms which are manifested depend usually for their existence on some emotional conflict; the patient is not aware, nor does he want to be, that this conflict exists.

All illness has a mental aspect, no sick person can be considered normal; in the nursing of neuroses the mental symptoms will be most obvious; in the care of a patient who has sustained a fracture, the condition may appear to be entirely physical; but, as people consist of both mental and physical parts, one part cannot be disorganized or diseased without the other's being affected. There is no subjective symptom which cannot be produced by the mind; conversely the mind can act upon every symptom and effect some relief.

The **nursing of neurological cases** does not differ from other branches of nursing in that the highest qualities of mind and body are required in a nurse. The mental aspect of the care of a patient is of very great importance in cases of disease or disorder of the nervous system. This depends on the ability of the nurse to get into contact with the mind of another, and to do this she must be interested enough to learn facts about the patient, his ordinary life and surroundings. She will gain influence over her patient only in so far as she realizes that the relationship between them is that of one human being to another.

It would be ideal if every nurse in training could attend a number of lectures on elementary medical psychology and that this should be followed up by clinical instruction on the mental symptoms manifest in patients in a medical ward. This should be carried out and supervised by a mentally qualified practitioner or trained mental nurse.

In handling neurological cases it is wise to develop a quiet confident attitude; a nurse should be transparently honest with her patients, answer their questions with directness, and never tell a patient a lie. The nurse who can forget herself and think first of her patient is invaluable; her generosity will react on his behaviour, and help him to recovery more than could anything else. There need not be any display of sentiment, and the nurse must never abandon her authority, but this attitude will inspire the patient with the trust, confidence and hope he needs.

If the patient wishes to talk about his symptoms it is advisable to allow him to do so, but only in so far as it will help. A nurse should learn to be a good listener; she will be, if she is really anxious to help. As the patient elates his symptoms the nurse must remember that a number of causes ıay be contributory, and that if she can discover a possible cause, and get er patient to see this also, she may help in his cure.

Palpitation, rapid action of the heart and headache, may all be due for example) either to anaemia, fatigue or irritability. If the patient has ttacks of palpitation (for instance) the nurse should try and notice what onditions precede the attack; if she can discover that it was provoked by rritability she might try and get the patient to see this; she may have to et to work in a very roundabout way to reach the end she has in view, xplaining to the patient how the mind reacts on the body, showing how ear will make the pulse beat more rapidly, that hurrying up a hill might ıave the same effect, and so eventually bring him to be interested in inding the possible cause of his own attack—in this case, of palpitation—ınd so try and get him to avoid the display of irritability which may ıave been a contributory cause.

In many cases a patient will be pleased and will be found willing to help y trying to find the causes for and to cure his own condition.

On the other hand, some patients will think they know better, and will ılways find some reason for not doing what the nurse may require; it is a ood plan to try and strike a bargain with such a patient as this and, iving in to him in small matters such as the way in which his bed is made r his lunch tray arranged, getting him in exchange to carry out the wishes f the physician in regard perhaps to what he is to eat or drink, the time e is to take medicine, the hour at which he is to retire, and other similar letails which are far more important than those in which he is being ıllowed to please himself.

Other patients always want to please themselves, finding it difficult to lefer to a nurse, and it is advisable in dealing with a patient of this type to efer all the important points to the physician in the presence of the patient, o that, when the time comes for any treatment to be suggested, the patient nows the doctor said exactly this or that and will submit more readily.

The nurse may find the patient's relatives difficult, but she must treat hem also in a quiet confident manner, hoping that they may follow her example, so that when in the sickroom they may avoid giving the patient any disturbing news, telling him any distressing tales, moving about in a way which will irritate him, speaking in loud tones, and so on.

FITS AND CONVULSIONS

Convulsions in infants are likely to occur whenever the nervous system is either directly or indirectly irritated. In infants and young children convulsions occur during teething as the result of gastro-intestinal disorder, particularly constipation; owing to the presence of intestinal parasites; because the infant is debilitated, particularly when the calcium content of the blood is abnormally low—it is because of this, that convulsions are sometimes seen in cases of rickets. They also occur as the result of irritation from the circulation of toxins of disease in the blood; they are met at the onset of many diseases such as measles, scarlet fever, broncho-pneumonia and meningitis; they may occur during the course of these diseases, particularly the two last mentioned; they may occur at the end of a severe attack of coughing, in whooping cough; they are also seen in uraemia, in any condition where asphyxia is present and will frequently be seen when an infant is dangerously ill and very near death. Convu sions also occur in infants as a symptom of disease of the brain, such a cerebral haemorrhage. Sometimes convulsions occur in infancy and n apparent reason can be discovered, and in many instances these childre will be found to develop epilepsy in later life.

A typical fit. The infant becomes rigid and pale, twitches slightly an his eyes become fixed. After a moment or two pallor gives way to cyanosi and the infant loses consciousness. This usually lasts for a few moment and then he regains consciousness, but is left weak and falls into stuporous sleep.

The immediate treatment is to loosen all clothing, see that breathing is nc obstructed and hold the infant's head over to one side; if the teeth ar erupted and there is any tendency to bite the tongue, a pad of material or spatula should be held between them. *In the case of a prolonged convulsion* th infant should be kept warm and have a cold-water compress applied t his head. A sedative drug such as paraldehyde may be ordered per rectum Bathing in hot water or mustard and water is rarely employed except i healthy infants when a fit may be due to teething.

The nurse should observe the duration of the fit and the manner of it starting, and note which muscles twitched and in what order, whether th pupils were dilated, and whether the eyes remained fixed or squinting, o moved in any way. She should also note whether consciousness was com pletely lost, and for how long the condition continued, and whether th infant passed urine and flatus or faeces.

Subsequent treatment. The occurrence of a fit will be reported to th physician who will try to discover its cause; if constipation is present a enema will usually be given, followed by a dose of grey powder or casto oil; if cerebral irritation is suspected a sedative may be ordered, such as a small dose of bromide, which may be given rectally or by mouth.

Fits or convulsions in adults may arise from a number of causes, fairl common ones being uraemia, epilepsy, apoplexy, cerebral tumours, anc other organic disease of the brain; they may also arise in cases of tetany when the calcium balance of the body is disturbed; they occur in tetanus, and may be met as a complication of pregnancy in eclampsia. An hysteri- cal fit may also arise as a manifestation of functional nervous derangement.

EPILEPSY

Epilepsy may be of various types, major, minor and Jacksonian epileps being described.

In **major epilepsy** the actual fit is commonly preceded by a warning or *aura*, which takes the form of some sensation, such as discomfort, smell, taste or sound.

The *next stage* is described as *tonic*, and in this the patient falls, is stif and rigid, his eyes are fixed, his teeth and hands are clenched, the muscles of his chest are not moving, and he becomes deeply cyanosed. This lasts for about half a minute, but to the onlooker the time seems interminable. The patient then relaxes, and passes into the next stage of the fit.

The *clonic stage* is characterized by convulsive movements, the limbs jerk and the tongue may be bitten in the convulsive muscular movements of the jaws. Urine and faeces may be passed involuntarily.

The patient will now probably come round, but he is dazed and scarcely recognizes his surroundings; he is tired and weary and will usually fall asleep and when he wakens he may not even know that he has had a fit.

Care of a patient in a fit. The clothing should be loosened about the neck and chest; note should be taken that the breathing is not obstructed, if the tongue tends to fall back it should be pulled forward, either by taking hold of it with a clean handkerchief or with tongue forceps if these are available. All nurses should be clearly instructed that a patient will not die whilst he is having a fit, provided a clear airway is maintained and he is not allowed to turn over on to his face and suffocate. Knowing this a nurse will be able to act promptly, calmly and with confidence; further, she should be told that, having seen to the point just mentioned, her most important duty is to observe exactly what happens during the fit and write this down at once; otherwise in half an hour's time she will not be sure whether the movements began on the right or on the left side.

The patient should lie where he has fallen, provided he is not in danger, and any firm article such as a rubber ring or a spatula should be held between his teeth to prevent his biting his tongue during the convulsive movements of his jaws. If, however, the patient is in bed, he should be prevented from falling out.

The *following points should be noted:* The mode of onset of the fit, whether sudden or gradual; whether it began with a scream; the character of the movements, whether tonic, or clonic; the part of the body where movements began, and the exact order of spread and whether the tongue was bitten. The colour of the patient, as to whether his face was flushed or pale, and the condition of his pupils, whether dilated or not. The presence or absence of the corneal reflex, the condition of the pulse during the attack, and whether the patient passed urine or faeces involuntarily. The duration of the attack should be noted and any symptoms which followed observed, such as headache, drowsiness or vomiting, whether the patient immediately went to sleep or whether, alternatively, he performed movements automatically (see note on automatism below).

Dangers of epilepsy. There is always danger that the patient will be injured during a fit, as he may fall in a dangerous place, under a moving vehicle, from a height, into water or on to a fire, and it is for this reason that persons who are subject to epilepsy should not follow dangerous occupations, such as working on a high building, in a factory where machinery is used or driving a vehicle.

Status epilepticus is a condition associated with epilepsy in which fits follow one another in rapid succession. The treatment is medical and the physician will as a rule order an enema to be given. He may order sedative drugs such as luminal, paraldehyde, potassium bromide and chloral hydrate.

The physician will expect the nurse to obtain a specimen of urine and test it for albumin as soon as possible, as repeated epileptiform seizures may be caused by uraemia and an early diagnosis is important. The pulse and the character of the tongue should be observed in elderly persons, the pulse may be found to be tortuous, full and bounding, or slow; in some cases of severe heart block seizures very similar to epilepsy sometimes occur. Stimulants should never be given in status epilepticus.

Automatism is a condition in which a patient performs movements and carries out, in some cases, very complicated performances, without having the least idea of what he is doing or any memory of it afterwards. A patient in this state is not responsible for his actions, even should he commit violent injuries to other members of society. He needs careful watching and should not be left alone, even for a moment.

The mode of life and general care necessary in cases of epilepsy. An epileptic should lead a quiet, fairly uneventful life; he should sleep well and, if unable to do this naturally, the physician may order small regular doses of some sedative drug—luminal ½ to ⅓ of a grain is commonly given twice a day or one dose of 1½ grains may be ordered to prevent an attack. More recently epanutin or alepsin has been employed to prevent fits or lessen the frequency and severity of them. The diet should be nourishing but not stimulating, and the bowels should be kept acting regularly. If the patient has any idea when a fit is likely to occur he should regulate his life in order to try and avoid having a fit.

Petit mal, or minor epilepsy, is a form in which only very slight attacks occur, but this form of the disease unfortunately tends to become worse as time goes on and is difficult to treat.

In an attack of petit mal there may be a slight momentary lapse of consciousness; should it occur in a nurse she might be seen to stand rigidly still for a moment or two, perhaps when making a bed, and then continue the work as if nothing had happened; she might be making a report and suddenly stop speaking, continuing after the lapse of a few moments; if she was holding something she would probably drop it. The colour of a person having an attack of petit mal may change, and he may become pale with fixed staring eyes during the momentary lapse of consciousness.

The *treatment* in the first instance consists in trying to discover any cause, and then in keeping the patient on some sedative drug; either bromide or luminal in small doses several times a day is frequently employed for this purpose. A fairly long rest from occupation should be advised at the beginning, and it is very obvious that if the subject is a nurse she will not be able to follow her occupation, as during even a short lapse of consciousness she might be the cause of serious injury to a patient.

The prognosis of petit mal varies; some patients tend to recover, others do not; some develop major epilepsy and many of those who do not recover become subjects of automatism following an attack, are difficult to handle and behave in a dangerous manner.

Jacksonian epilepsy is considered to be associated with some organic lesion of the brain, whereas the types of epilepsy already described are of a functional nature. One cause of Jacksonian epilepsy is a cerebral tumour, and it is therefore most particularly necessary in this type to make accurate observations of the happenings during a fit, since what the nurse can tell the physician or surgeon about this will go far in helping him to decide the exact localization of a tumour. In attacks of Jacksonian epilepsy consciousness may not be lost.

HYSTERICAL FIT

A nurse should be familiar with the differences between the condition of a patient in a true epileptic fit and that of one in an hysterical fit. The main points may be outlined as follows:

(1) An hysterical fit never occurs when a patient is alone or during sleep.

(2) The order of events described in epilepsy does not occur in hysteria.

(3) The movements which are made during an hysterical fit are not involuntary; they are wild and spectacular in character and if attempts are made to restrain the movements their violence is increased.

(4) The patient does not hurt himself in falling, and he does not bite his tongue.

(5) Incontinence of urine is not present—unless the patient happens to know a great deal about epilepsy, in which case he may pass urine during the attack, wishing to complete the picture he desires to convey.

(6) The corneal reflex, which is lost during the clonic stage of true epilepsy, is present in an hysterical attack.

The *treatment of a patient in an hysterical fit* is to give a sharp command to be still, and then to ignore the attack. One point, however, must be considered: an hysterical fit may follow an attack of petit mal, so that the history should be investigated when the patient is behaving normally again.

APOPLEXY

Apoplexy is the term used to describe a seizure characterized by sudden loss of consciousness, accompanied by noisy stertorous breathing, flushing of the face, a full bounding pulse and paralysis of one side of the body (see also hemiplegia).

Apoplexy is due to cerebral haemorrhage in most cases, although in other instances it may be brought about by cerebral thrombosis or cerebral embolism.

The *symptoms of onset* may occur suddenly as instances above; or the condition may come on gradually. When the cause is thrombosis—that is, a blockage of one of the blood vessels—the onset may be gradual, as the clot gradually forms in the vessel. In such a case the onset of paralysis may precede the other symptoms; later, as the blood vessel becomes completely blocked, the typical picture of a patient in a state of apoplexy will be seen.

The *immediate treatment* of a patient who may (for example) have had an attack of apoplexy either in the street or at his work is to put him to lie down, with his head raised, and the clothing about his neck and chest loosened; his head should be placed to one side and means taken to see that his breathing is not obstructed. A cold application should be placed on his head and he may have a hot-water bottle at his feet; he should not be given any stimulant and a doctor should be informed at once.

The *subsequent nursing* will be that described for a case of hemiplegia on p. 409.

(**Eclampsia.** This is a complication of pregnancy in which epileptiform seizures occur; it is described on p. 561.)

COMA

Coma is a state of deep unconsciousness from which a patient cannot be roused. It may be brought about by a number of causes. It has been mentioned in connexion with injuries to the skull. It may also arise from pressure caused by a cerebral tumour or abscess; and in cerebral haemorrhage, and meningitis. Other causes include toxaemia of disease, uraemia, diabetes, poisoning by the abuse of alcohol or hypnotics, and sunstroke.

The **most important observations** to be made in the case of coma are:

(1) Any irregularity of the temperature, pulse and respiration; a half hourly note should be made for the first few hours.

(2) The degree of coma, whether this varies at all, and whether the patient is able to swallow.

(3) Any movements of the limbs; if these occur only on one side, this fact should be noted in particular; any movements of the eyes should also be noted—if the eyes are being constantly turned to one side, it is important to know which side.

(4) The pupils should be observed for irregularity in size; the eyes should be examined for the presence of the reaction of the pupil to light and also for the presence or absence of the corneal reflex—this is only lost when coma is deep.

(5) A specimen of urine should be obtained as soon as possible, and tested. The bladder should be watched for distension; any incontinence of urine should be noticed.

(6) Any retraction of the head should be noted.

Treatment and nursing is similar to that described in the care of a fractured base of the skull (see p. 610). Cases of coma should be nursed on a water or air bed, and the area on which the patient lies should be attended to every four hours as there is danger of bedsores; the head should be kept turned to one side in order to obviate the danger of the tongue's falling back and so obstructing the breathing; the mouth, nose and the eyes, when these are open, should receive regular attention and be kept clean and healthy. The bowels should be kept open; if the patient does not recover from coma within from 36 to 48 hours he will be artificially fed by the rectum or by means of a nasal tube.

Chapter 27

Diseases and Disorders of Metabolism

Deficiency diseases: rickets—scurvy—beri-beri—pellagra—Diabetes mellitus—Acidosis—Alkalosis—Gout—Obesity

Metabolism is a series of chemical and physical changes which are constantly going on in the body, upon which its well-being depends.

Metabolism is disturbed in most diseases and disorders but certain diseases and conditions, particularly associated with disturbances of metabolism, can be classified as Diseases of Metabolism.

DEFICIENCY DISEASES

These disorders include rickets, scurvy, beri-beri, pellagra and a short account of each is appended. The dietetic treatment of these conditions, both preventive and curative, will be found on pp. 286–88—where mention will also be found of other deficiency disorders such as night blindness and xerophthalmia.

RICKETS

Rickets is a constitutional disease affecting children. It occurs from the sixth to the twenty-fourth month of life, and manifests itself in general constitutional disturbances and in bone lesions. It is caused by absence of fat-soluble vitamin D in the diet, excessive carbohydrates, absence of sunlight and deficiency of calcium in the bones. It is most commonly met amongst the poor, where generally bad hygienic conditions prevail.

Symptoms and signs. As a rule a rickety child is fat and flabby; he is irritable, sweats at night, especially about the head; his sleep is restless, teething is late and irregular; the fontanelles close late and the child is backward in walking. The teeth may be small, badly formed and decay early. He has a large abdomen described as a *pot belly*, due to enlargement of the liver and spleen; he is liable to bronchitis, convulsions, and enteritis.

The *changes* in the size and shape of the bones are the most characteristic manifestation of rickets. They may be described as an increased preparation for bone formation and a diminished completion thereof. Thus the bones are soft, with enlargement of the ends due to extensive growth of cartilage and cessation of ossification processes; this improves later, and the bone ossifies in its enlarged condition, this enlargement being most marked at the ends of the bones. If weight is borne on the soft bones, deformities occur. (The deformities which result from rickets are described on p. 783.)

Treatment. It is important to improve the general hygienic surroundings of the rickety child. The general tone of the health should be improved; massage will assist the nutrition of the muscles; the child should be warmly but lightly clad, and the recumbent position and complete rest are essential whilst the bones are soft. The child should be out in the air, reasonably exposed to sunlight, when possible.

Dietetic treatment is all-important. Fat-soluble vitamin D is essential; it should be given to infants in the form of small doses of halibut-liver oil or cod-liver oil, and they should be suitably fed on fresh milk, cream being added. Fresh orange juice should be given or, alternatively, rose-hip syrup or black-currant purée, as there is often a tendency to scurvy associated with rickets. Older children should have in addition a fairly liberal protein diet, red gravy of beef, underdone meat (minced), lightly cooked eggs; also bacon, butter and cream. Green vegetables should be given and fresh fruit juice and fruit pulp. Carbohydrates should be limited, and cakes and sweets should as far as possible be avoided. (For details of dietetic treatment see p. 286.)

Sunlight is also important. Natural sunbaths should be given when possible, and note taken of pigmentation, as, unless this occurs, there is danger of burning. Artificial sunlight may be used during the sunless months of the year.

Irradiated ergosterol, which contains vitamin D, is also useful.

The *prevention of deformity*, during the stage when the bones are soft, is important; to effect this, the child must not be permitted to walk or crawl until the bones have hardened.

INFANTILE SCURVY

(*Barlow's Disease*)

Scurvy is a disorder of nutrition due to deficiency of the antiscorbutic vitamin in the diet. The disease occurs in infants between the ages of six to eighteen months, and is most often met with when the infant has been for some time fed on sterilized food.

Symptoms. The infant ceases to gain weight, cries when touched and does not move his limbs about as he should; there is tenderness to touch and on movement; the bones are very tender, due to subperiosteal bleeding; in some cases the ends of the bones appear to be enlarged. The infant becomes very debilitated and anaemic; the gums are spongy, the mouth sore and ulcerated and, if the teeth have erupted, they become loose. In severe cases, bleeding occurs into the skin and from the bowel. The infant lies on his back with his limbs relaxed and his thighs separated and outwardly rotated.

The *specific treatment* is the administration of the *antiscorbutic vitamin* in the diet. The infant should be fed on cow's milk, and should be given orange and lemon juice, tomato juice and potato cream. The mouth should be kept clean, care being used in handling it, and, when feeding by mouth is painful, the nasal tube may be used for a day or two. The infant should be gently and carefully handled in order to avoid giving him pain. The condition is usually cured in a few days.

ADULT SCURVY

This condition only occurs when people are deprived of all sources of vitamin C. The treatment is the administration of large doses of ascorbic acid.

BERI-BERI
(Epidemic polyneuritis)

Beri-beri is a peripheral neuritis which occurs mainly in rice-eating natives when the rice is polished and so deprived of the husk which contains vitamin B.

The *symptoms* are numbness and partial loss of power in the hands and feet. In *dry beri-beri* there is wasting of the affected muscles and the tendon jerks in the affected parts are absent. *Wet beri-beri* is characterized by dropsy, the patient is markedly oedematous, and ascites is also commonly present, being superimposed on the muscle weakness and wasting.

Treatment. In common with the musculature of the body, the cardiac muscle is affected so that rest in bed is essential. No exertion should be allowed, no aperients should be given except those specially ordered by the doctor. The bowels must be kept open by enemata or liquid paraffin, straining at stool being avoided. The urine should be measured and tested for albumin; the passing of large quantities of urine in those cases recovering from dropsy is to be expected when the water collected in the tissues is removed and excreted.

In addition to rest, which is merely treatment directed towards the weakness of heart and muscle, dietetic treatment effects a cure. The diet should include vitamin B, therefore such foods as fresh green vegetables, tomatoes, eggs, peas and beans, yeast and Marmite, and in the case of rice-eating natives meals of unpolished rice are given (see p. 287).

Fluids may be given liberally except in cases in which there is dropsy, when they should be limited to two pints a day, and in some of these cases salt also should be restricted.

PELLAGRA

Pellagra is a disease which is characterized by leg dermatitis, ulceration of the mouth and gastro-intestinal symptoms and a tendency to mental confusion. The *treatment* is dietetic (see p. 287).

DIABETES MELLITUS

Diabetes is a disease characterized by serious disturbances of metabolism due to deficiency of insulin; the use of all three foods is affected.

Carbohydrates. Insulin is necessary for the utilization of sugar in the body and its conversion into glycogen. In diabetes the resting blood sugar is higher than normal and after a carbohydrate meal glucose appears in the urine.

Fat. Sugar must be available in the tissues for the complete oxidation of fat. In diabetes fats are imperfectly broken down, the fats produce acetone bodies and a condition of acetonaemia or ketosis is the result.

Protein. Metabolism of protein is also disturbed because in a starving diabetic the carbohydrate stores in the tissues are soon used up and then tissue protein is broken down, and amino-acids which are the end products of protein metabolism are converted into glucose and excreted as glucose.

When planning the dietetic treatment of diabetes (see p. 275) the physician must consider that all the carbohydrate taken, a large percentage of the protein and a small proportion of the fat must be regarded as materials capable of being converted into sugar.

Diabetes occurs at all ages but less often at the extremities of life; the majority of patients when first seen are over forty years of age.

Contributing causes include mental and physical strain, worry and anxiety, the presence of septic foci in different parts of the body, and certain infective diseases such as influenza; diabetes is also sometimes associated with gout and with obesity when brought about by overfeeding.

The **symptoms of diabetes** are the passing of a lot of urine—up to several hundred ounces in severe cases—which contains a varying amount of sugar (*glycosuria*) and of acetone and diacetic acid. Urine is frequently passed because of the excessive amount and the rate at which it is excreted, but this symptom, *polyuria*, is only nature's way of dissolving the sugar so that it can be excreted, and it is an attempt to lessen the abnormally high percentage of sugar in the blood. Normally the amount of sugar contained in the blood is about 0·1 per cent, but in diabetes it may be as high as 0·5 or 0·6 per cent.

Thirst is another symptom which is due to the serious loss of water from the body by the kidneys, and the tongue is characteristically dry, red and raw.

Muscular weakness and *loss of weight* occur because the sugar cannot be used unless insulin is also present in the blood. In some cases the patient is thin (*diabetic maigre*) and in other instances the patient is well nourished (*diabetic gras*).

Hunger is more or less marked. *Constipation* is usually present.

There is a tendency to bedsores, partly because of the emaciation, and partly due to the impoverished condition of the skin. *The skin is dry*, as perspiration is diminished because of the loss of water in the excessive amount of urine passed.

A form of *dyspnoea* described as air hunger occurs (see below).

Acidosis is present, and if untreated will lead to coma.

Sugar, which is necessary for the combustion of fat, cannot be stored in the muscles, and heat and energy are therefore lacking and the patient is weak and listless and very easily fatigued.

Complications and dangers of diabetes which accompany the symptoms in severe cases include *itching of the skin*, *pruritis* and *eczema*, *septic spots on the skin*, and *boils*, *carbuncles*, *abscesses* and *coma*; the patient is subject to any infection, especially *bronchitis* and *pulmonary tuberculosis*; diabetic patients often get *neuritis*, which is thought to be due to lack of proper nourishment for the nerves; and for the same reason they are subject to *retinitis* and *cataract*. In very severe cases *gangrene* of the extremities, particularly the toes, occurs; and, owing to the excessive sugar in the blood and the consequent difficulty of healing, diabetic patients are considered bad subjects for surgical operation.

Coma. The most serious and immediately fatal danger is of diabetic coma, which is due to the presence in the blood not of sugar, but of diacetic acid and acetone (*acetonaemia*), which occurs owing to the defective metabolism of fat.

The *symptoms of threatened coma* are diacetic acid in the urine, complaint of headache, and vague abdominal pain; the patient begins to be drowsy, his breathing becomes gasping, which demonstrates '*air hunger*' and there is a sweetish odour in his breath due to acetone and eventually coma ensues.

The *immediate treatment of coma* is essential, or the patient will die; he is kept warm in bed and given glucose and saline and large doses of insulin intravenously; if he is not comatose but only drowsy he is given insulin hypodermically, and glucose in lemonade to drink; fluid is given freely and he may be given a saline purgative or an enema; it is always important to remember that diabetics should never be allowed to become constipated. The urine should be tested for the presence of diacetic acid. The tests for sugar, acetone, and diacetic acid are described on p. 72.

A patient with a history of diabetes may be admitted to a hospital in coma, and it may be necessary to decide whether the condition is diabetic or insulin coma. If the patient is accompanied by a relative or friend it may be possible to obtain a history which will aid the diagnosis; if diacetic acid is found in the urine the coma can be treated as diabetic. Before a specimen is obtained it may be possible to make an accurate diagnosis by detecting an odour of acetone, by the presence of gasping breathing, and by the dry hardness of the tongue, since the tongue of a patient in insulin coma will usually be moist.

The treatment of diabetes. This consists in the first place of *stabilizing treatment* including if necessary the *administration of insulin.* A blood sugar estimation is made to confirm the diagnosis. The patient is put to bed, he is kept on a standard diet for a few days; during this time his urine is tested for sugar and acetone and the blood sugar is estimated. If the diabetes is found to be severe he is given insulin at once but if it is not severe he is then given a period of starvation for 24 to 48 hours until the urine is sugar free. He may have fluids such as weak tea, lemonade and water but no sugar or milk may be given. The patient is then given a series of graduated diets until he is having sufficient food to enable him to live his normal life and perform the work he has to do without undue fatigue or loss of weight. During this period his urine is tested at regular intervals and the necessary amount of insulin is prescribed to enable the patient to take the requisite diet and maintain his urine sugar-free.

Insulin was discovered by Banting and Best in 1922. Since then there have been modifications. *Soluble insulin* was the first employed. It acts rapidly and the effect wears off quickly. *Protamine zinc insulin* acts slowly and *globin insulin* has a duration of effect between soluble and protamine zinc insulin.

Insulin is prepared in different strengths and all brands are packed with distinctively coloured labels so that everyone can recognize the type and strength of the insulin he is using.

The dose of insulin is a matter of prescription. In some cases one type and in another a different type is ordered. In certain cases soluble insulin only is

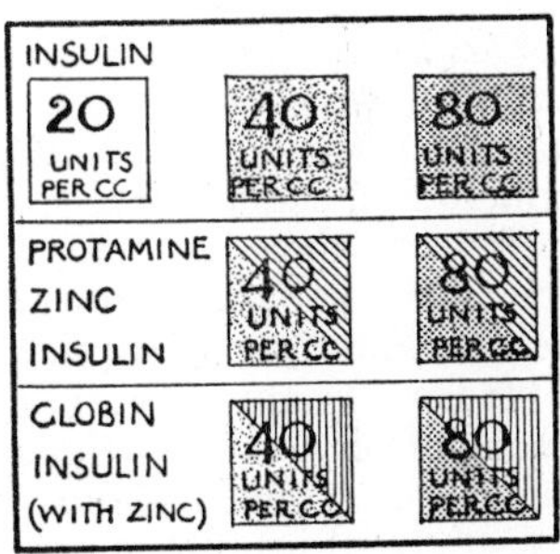

FIG. 172. CHART OF TYPES OF INSULIN.

employed. In others it is found that one injection a day of protamine zinc insulin will take the place of two or three daily injections of soluble insulin and in some cases two brands of insulin are combined. When a dose of zinc protamine is given, the effect of this will last for 15 to 60 hours, but only begins to act 3 hours after injection, therefore in conjunction with this a small dose of soluble insulin is given which, acting quickly, will prevent the blood sugar rising immediately after a meal containing carbohydrate.

In cases where the blood sugar rises very much between the doses of insulin, three doses a day may have to be given, and this occurs most often in very severe cases and in children.

Insulin coma is brought about by deficiency of sugar in the blood—*hypoglycaemia*. The normal blood sugar is 0·1 per cent; if it falls below 0·08 per cent the patient will feel ill; and if it falls as low as 0·05 per cent he will become comatose. (See fig. 31, p. 175.)

It is important for the patient to realize that hypoglycaemia will be likely to occur if a carbohydrate meal is not taken within half an hour after the injection of insulin, and if an adequate meal is not taken symptoms may arise about 3 or 4 hours afterwards. The *symptoms* of hypoglycaemia begin with lightheadedness, sweating, trembling, feeling cold and shaky and faint, while the pulse will become weak and rapid. As a rule such symptoms will be present for from 10 to 15 minutes before there is immediate danger of coma, and the patient should be warned to carry lumps of sugar always with him, and to eat two as soon as he experiences any of these symptoms, or he may eat an orange—if there is no improvement he should repeat this—and he should keep quite still, resting if possible, and keeping warm. Because of the danger of insulin coma all diabetic cases are permitted to experience these symptoms and so learn to recognize them before they leave hospital. These signs mean that either the amount of insulin should be reduced or the food intake increased; they may occur, however, because the patient has been unusually vigorous and active, or because he did not eat all of his ration allowance, and therefore any food a patient leaves should be carefully weighed and the amount recorded.

TRAINING AND EDUCATION OF THE PATIENT

Testing the urine. The patient should be expert in testing his urine for sugar and acetone bodies before he leaves hospital, and he should be taught under what conditions sugar may appear in the urine without much significance. For example, in all severe cases, it will be present before the morning dose of insulin and it may be present also before the evening dose; but if present less than 4 hours after the injection it may be serious and the patient should consult his doctor.

It is very important that the patient should be trained in the management of his own diet, in testing his urine and knowing when to expect sugar and when it should not be present, and also in giving himself his injections of insulin, and if all this is not done the nurse has so far failed in her care of him, since diabetic patients cannot be constantly under the eye of doctors and nurses and it is important that they should be able to take care of themselves.

On leaving hospital a patient should be provided with the following—

Enough insulin to last for a specified time; some reserve insulin in case of emergency; two syringes and four needles; a receptacle for keeping the syringe in spirit (as shown in fig. 151, p. 290); methylated spirit to replenish this jar or tube every 3 or 4 days, when the spirit gets cloudy. He should also have a small spirit lamp for testing urine, and either Fehling's solution or Benedict's solution for the sugar test.

He should be taught to record each day the presence or absence of sugar in the urine.

He should know exactly how much insulin he is to take and should have a copy of the 'line ration' diet scheme or other dietary table prescribed and know what he is to have and how to read and vary this.

In addition to the principles of treatment of diabetic patients already outlined, it is important that certain other minor points in regard to their general health should have attention, as the standard of health should be maintained at as high a level as possible—every diabetic will be worse when his health is poor and vice versa.

He should have adequate rest and sleep and never be fatigued; dental hygiene is important; he must have a regular action of the bowels every day, as constipation lowers his vitality; his skin should be well cared for, kept free from spots and well dried after washing because of the tendency to sepsis; a diabetic having two doses of insulin a day (morning and evening) should take his exercise in the middle of the day, midway in the 10 hours which intervene between the doses; this precaution helps to prevent the possibility of hypoglycaemia brought about by injudicious exercise; if the midday meal is taken before the exercise this further excludes such a possibility.

He ought to know that he should report to his doctor or to the hospital if, after his urine has been sugar-free, sugar is present for several days; frequent attacks or even warnings of hypoglycaemia should also be reported, and both these conditions necessitate that a blood sugar test should be taken. He must be warned also that it is necessary to exercise considerable will power under temptation to be lax in regard to diet, and difficult as this will be, especially when away from home, he must remember that his health depends upon it.

ACIDOSIS

Acidosis is a condition in which there is decrease of the alkaline reserve (bicarbonates) in the blood. It is due to faulty metabolism of fat, and healthy persons taking a well-balanced diet do not suffer from it. In the normal person, the fat when digested reaches the blood stream in the form of fatty acids and glycerine, and eventually reaches the liver via the bloodstream. The liver changes the chemistry of the digested fat, and in the presence of glucose (digested sugar) the fat is safely used by the body, but in cases such as diabetes, where sugar is deficient in the tissues, partially changed fat acts as a poison, and the condition of acidosis is thus produced.

Symptoms of Acidosis. The sickly sweet odour of the breath of a patient with acidosis is characteristic of the condition. Every nurse should be trained to recognize this odour, which is present even in slight cases before other symptoms have developed. Other persistent symptoms are headache, nausea and vomiting; visual changes may occur and acetone bodies will be present in the urine.

Children are ready subjects of acidosis, and any nausea, headache and malaise should be investigated by testing the urine and, if acetone bodies are present, the condition treated by the administration of glucose and absolute rest for a few hours. Diabetic coma has been described in the section on diabetes (see p. 436). Migraine with vomiting in children may, unless treated, result in acidosis of a nature sufficiently severe to produce stupor and even coma, and should be treated by the administration of glucose, intravenously if necessary.

The general *treatment* of acidosis is the administration of glucose and the reduction of fat in the diet. The symptoms which have arisen may be treated, such as cold compresses for the headache, etc. Sodium bicarbonate, 10 to 20 grains given every 4 hours, will assist in maintaining the alkaline reserve of the blood.

ALKALOSIS

Alkalosis is the condition opposite to that of acidosis. In it the available alkali in the blood is increased. The condition may be induced by the administration of large doses of alkali, such as sodium bicarbonate; it may also arise after severe vomiting.

Symptoms. At first there may be merely a disinclination to take milk, some degree of anorexia and nausea, headache and malaise. If the condition is not treated drowsiness may occur, or twitching and tetany, and in very severe cases the condition may terminate in coma.

Treatment. Whenever the earliest symptoms are noticed, the diet and medicine should be investigated and any alkalis that are being given should be omitted; this may be sufficient to relieve the condition. If, however, the symptoms are marked, and the condition has persisted for any length of time, calcium, saline and glucose are given.

GOUT

Gout is a constitutional disease due to defective protein metabolism which is characterised by excess of uric acid in the blood. Gout in the foot is called *podagra* and in the hand, *cheiragra*.

Little is known of the true cause. Predisposing factors include excessive alcohol, and the overeating of meals rich in meat and nitrogenous foods. It may also be associated with overwork and bad hygiene and the presence of septic foci. It is sometimes brought on by poisoning, such as by lead.

The patient is usually a middle-aged man with a tendency to digestive disorders. The attack is ushered in with acute pain and signs of inflammation in the joint, which is red, tender and swollen; so tender that the patient cannot bear the least touch and dreads the approach of others near his bed or near the stool on which he rests his foot. There is usually a rise in temperature and shivering may occur. The patient passes scanty and very high-coloured urine, depositing urates, and containing uric acid in excess, which may be seen deposited on the glass as cayenne-pepper-like crystals. The attack gradually subsides, and the joint returns to almost its normal size. There is a deposit of biurate of soda in the joint which may work out through the skin, or be seen on the dressing.

The condition may become chronic, in which case the joint becomes deformed, and stiff. The disease may be complicated by a high blood pressure, or by chronic interstitial nephritis, neuritis and eczema.

Treatment. During the acute attack the joint is fomented, or wrapped in wool and raised on a pillow. The diet is attended to and a suitable low diet with absence of alcohol insisted upon. The kidneys and bowels should be kept active. Diuretics are of value.

Drugs used are *colchicum* and *potassium iodide*. *Atophan* is used between the attacks, but it is only given at intervals and always combined with alkalis.

Dietetic treatment is mentioned on page 278.

OBESITY

As in the case of Pharaoh's lean and fat kine, so humanity is disposed to variations of weight. Obesity or the excessive deposition of fat in the body may be due to several factors.

(1) A family tendency to obesity.

(2) Disturbances of nutrition and lack of exercise.

In those with a tendency to increased weight a sedentary life, excessive meals and quite moderate quantities of alcohol tend to produce obesity. Sometimes there is retention of water in the tissues and some people seem either to absorb more food than others or to receive more nourishment from their food.

Internal secretions control mental and physical activity to a very great extent, and thyroid, adrenalin, and ovarian secretions, led by the pituitary body which may be looked upon as the brigadier-general of the force, play a very active part in the physical well-being of each of us. It is well known that some disturbance of the pituitary gland results in the deposit of fat in the tissues. The fat boy in Pickwick probably had deficiency of secretion of the anterior lobe of his pituitary gland. The decrease which takes place in the production of internal secretions controlling ovarian and uterine functions at the menopause also causes a tendency to obesity and in many women nutritional changes take place in the early sixties.

On examination the patient will be found to be several stones above the normal weight for age and height. The patient may seek treatment because of the alteration in her personal appearance and discomfort from the excess fat. She may complain of dyspnoea and cardiac embarrassment. The basal metabolic rate should be estimated in order to exclude myxoedema; sugar tolerance and water elimination tests should be made.

Treatment. Dietetic restrictions on the lines indicated on p. 275 should be carried out and increase in exercise is recommended. When obesity is due to hypothyroidism, thyroideum gr. ½ to 1 may be advocated. When fluid is retained in the tissues, limitation of fluid and salt is advocated and in resistant cases mercurial diuretics are sometimes indicated.

Chapter 28

Diseases and Disorders of the Endocrine Glands

Introduction—The thyroid gland: cretinism, myxoedema, and thyrotoxicosis—The suprarenal glands: Addison's disease—The parathyroids, tetany and von Recklinghausen's disease—The pituitary gland: functions of anterior and posterior lobes, gigantism and acromegaly, Simmonds's disease, The ovarian and testicular secretions—Diabetes insipidus—The intrinsic factor of Castle—The pancreas. diabetes

The importance of the endocrine system, its association with the central nervous system, and the necessity for the perfect regulation of the mechanism by which the chemical messengers or hormones are sent out from the endocrine glands to the blood stream, to exert their action on the physical and mental wellbeing of the body, are the subject of great interest and much research today. Many of the organs producing internal secretions have a dual function—the pancreas (for example) makes an external secretion which it pours into the duodenum, and a hormone which it sends into the blood—this is known as *insulin*, and it controls the use of carbohydrates in the body and a deficiency in its supply gives rise to diabetes mellitus.

In the *nursing care* of patients with disordered endocrine conditions, particularly perhaps in disorders of the thyroid and pituitary glands, the nurse is faced with difficulties very similar to those with which she meets in the care of neurological cases, for it is the disturbance of the emotions, so common in such patients, that gives rise to difficulty.

DISORDERS OF THE THYROID GLAND

The thyroid gland produces the thyroxin which regulates metabolism. Lack of this substance—*hypothyroidism*—causes *cretinism* in infants and *myxoedema* in adults.

In **cretins** the baby is born apparently normal and the symptoms begin to develop in from three to six months; the child then becomes lethargic, the skin is dry, and the hair brittle; he is constipated, and dentition and talking are delayed. He makes no attempt to move, but sits lazily about, his abdomen becomes prominent and, if this condition is not treated, he will grow up an imbecile cretin with undeveloped sex characteristics.

Myxoedema arises in adult life—the patient gets fat, the skin and hair become dull and dry, the hair falls out, the subcutaneous skin becomes thickened, giving the patient a gross bloated appearance, great bags of skin lie under the eyes, the mentality is dull, lethargy proceeds to idiocy and the patient is inattentive to his surroundings and consequently appears to be deaf. Constipation is present. In women amenorrhoea occurs. Both myxoedema and cretinism respond to the administration of thyroid extract.

HYPERTHYROIDISM

Hyperthyroidism is due to *overactivity* of the gland, which causes it to roduce an excessive secretion. In some cases the secretion is definitely hought to be abnormal in character, and it then produces symptoms of yrotoxicosis. There are several forms of this condition, but the one which ost seriously disturbs the patient's mental balance, and which requires finite tact, patience, observation and thoughtfulness on the part of the urse is *Graves's disease*, or *Basedow's disease* or *primary thyrotoxicosis*. In these ses the sympathetic system is overactive and a train of emotional mptoms arises, accompanied by a number of other symptoms due to efective control of metabolism.

The **symptoms** most commonly met with are protrusion of the eyes xophthalmos), tachycardia and other forms of irregularity of the heart; ere is usually some enlargement of the gland, the skin is moist, the mperature is usually raised a little; the patient may have a normal petite, but owing to defective metabolism he loses weight. In many ses diarrhoea is present, and insomnia, irritability and general restssness are all exceedingly troublesome symptoms. Such patients are in state of high nervous tension, they are apprehensive and critical, sensitive nd introspective, and they require to be frequently reassured and must ot be worried or frightened. If nursed in a general ward they should placed in a quiet part of it and not in the vicinity of very ill patients, ut if possible near to happy cheerful ones.

In *secondary thyrotoxicosis* or *toxic adenoma* the symptoms are the same cept that eye signs are not present.

Treatment and nursing. When a patient is admitted with thyroxicosis the physician has to decide whether *thiouracil* is indicated or hether thyroidectomy should be considered. The reception of this patient important, and he should be made to feel that he is expected and that is bed is ready for him.

The rapid action of the heart is due to toxaemia from the abnormal cretion of the overactive gland, and the primary treatment is rest. *The lministration of this rest* must be considered in all its phases, both as regards hysical rest in bed and also regarding the avoidance of mental excitement, such as might be brought about by injudicious visitors or the reading unsuitable exciting literature. Observation of the rhythm of the pulse very important, and the physician will usually order some form of dative drug, together with some drug to control the action of the heart. e will also investigate the presence of any septic focus in the body, and careful record of the basal metabolic rate (B.M.R.) will be made.

Thiouracil. Before this drug is given, the weight of the patient, the rcumference of his neck, pulse rate and blood pressure, white cell ount and basal metabolic rate will be carefully noted. Thiouracil is iven in tablets by mouth. During its administration the white cell count taken twice a week as there is danger of agranulocytosis (see p. 361). Vhen the B.M.R. is falling satisfactorily the dose of thiouracil is gradully reduced until the dose which is to be maintained for a period of veral months is reached. The initial dose of thiouracil is 200 mg. 3 times

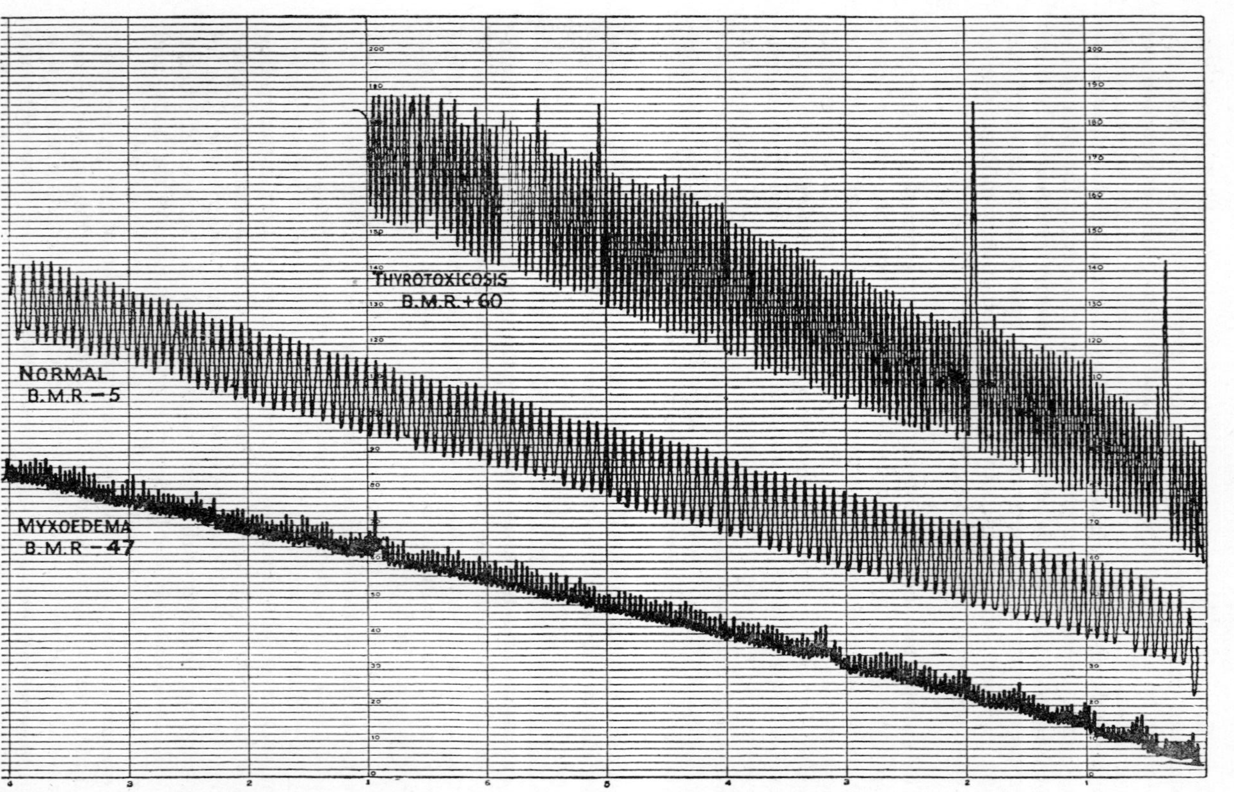

Fig. 172.—Diagram of Respiration of a Normal Patient, a Patient with Myxoedema and a Patient suffering from

a day and the average maintenance dose 100 mg. 2 or 3 times daily. *Overdose* is shown by increase in the size of the thyroid, excessive fall in the B.M.R., malaise and depression.

The *diet* is very important, and should be nourishing and easily digestible; stimulants should be avoided and red meat given only sparingly. The patient may have plenty of fish and eggs, and a little chicken, plenty of milk, cream and butter, milk puddings and fruit and green vegetables in order to try and overcome the wasting due to toxaemia. In patients having thiouracil, yeast tablets will be given in order to prevent agranulocytosis.

When *thyroidectomy* is considered the patient will question the nurse as to the necessity of an operation, and she should make it her business to know what the physician in charge advises and, if he advises operation, she should talk quite naturally and simply to the patient about the benefits to be obtained. She might say, for example, that patients recover very rapidly, that the symptoms disappear quite quickly, and that one reassuring feature is that, because the gland has been removed, there is no fear of any return of the condition. She should never tire of reassuring these patients, and should not forget the mental strain they are undergoing, realizing that the patient's co-operation is very necessary for a good recovery, and that she herself can help him to face the immediate future, and in so doing ensure a happy, confidently accepted, more remote future, looking forward to the time when the patient can again take his place in the world, in a fit state to face the difficult problems of life.

The *preliminary iodine treatment* is the administration of Lugol's solution. The condition of the patient including the B.M.R. is noted. Ten drops of the solution are given three times a day in milk; the effect, which is only temporary, is an improvement in the symptoms and reduction in the B.M.R. The maximum effect is obtained as a rule in ten to fourteen days. (The preparation and post-operative nursing care are described on pp. 713–15.)

THE SUPRARENAL GLANDS

The suprarenal glands produce two secretions, one from the medulla, which is known as *adrenalin*, and the other from the cortex—*cortin.*

Addison's disease. In the disease described by Dr. Addison the function of the suprarenal glands is disordered and, as there is deficiency of adrenal secretion, the disease is therefore characterized by a low blood pressure, and the pulse is poor and of low volume; the patient is incapable of exertion, attacks of fainting occur and he feels the cold severely. There is usually marked wasting, and in many cases there is discoloration of the skin, the patient is subject to frequent attacks of nausea and vomiting and in some cases diarrhoea occurs.

The disease is progressive, and if untreated the patient becomes very anaemic, and gets gradually more emaciated and weaker, until he is unable to leave his bed. The disease is characterized by attacks of syncope, and may end fatally in an attack.

Treatment. Quite good effects are being obtained from the administration of *cortin* which is an extract of the cortex of the gland.

THE PARATHYROID GLANDS

The parathyroid glands produce a substance which has been isolated and is called *parathormone*. It is concerned in maintaining the calcium content of the blood, and deficiency or *hypoparathyroidism* produces many conditions including tetany, osteomalacia and severe chilblains.

Tetany—due to hypoparathyroidism and brought about by deficiency of calcium in the blood may occur in infants and adults. In infants it is associated with rickets, laryngeal spasm and convulsions. It may be associated with marked diarrhoea and vomiting, with removal of the thyroid gland, and occurs as a complication after removal of a parathyroid tumour (see below) and is sometimes seen in pregnant women.

The *onset of tetany* is manifested by tingling in the limbs and stiffness and rigidity. *The characteristic carpo-pedal spasms* are painful contraction of the thumb across the palm of the hand and adduction of the feet and flexion of the toes. Convulsions and twitchings may also occur.

The *treatment* consists in the administration of calcium daily; in some instances parathyroid extract is employed. If the spasms are frequent and distressing, chloroform inhalations may be necessary for immediate relief. Sedatives such as bromide and chloral are employed. The provision of a diet rich in calcium is necessary and it should therefore include milk, eggs and cheese. Constipation must be prevented and the bowels should be kept acting regularly.

Hyperparathyroidism. Acute hyperparathyroidism is rare. Von Recklinghausen's disease or chronic parathyroidism is thought to be due to tumours of the parathyroid glands. It is also described as *osteitis fibrosa*. Owing to the excessive activity of the parathyroid glands the calcium content of the blood is abnormally high, but the skeleton is deprived of calcium, and consequently the bones are brittle and fractures occur easily—a bone may be broken by simply turning over in bed—and as the result of numerous fractures the skeleton becomes seriously deformed.

The *treatment* adopted is removal of a parathyroid tumour if one is present. Before operation the patient is admitted for observation; his diet is regulated, and he is given at first a low calcium diet, the intake and output of calcium being measured and the blood calcium content estimated, and the skeleton is X-rayed to note the condition of the bones.

The *post-operative care* is complicated by anxiety for fear lest tetany should develop. The calcium content of the blood falls rapidly once the over-acting glands have been removed.

The nurse must watch for any signs of the development of tetany; she may notice that the patient becomes irritable; if he complains of sensations as of pins and needles in his limbs she may know that tetany is imminent, and these symptoms will soon be followed by spasms. The physician usually orders the patient to be given calcium gluconate by the intramuscular route sufficiently often to prevent attacks of tetany.

THE PITUITARY GLAND

The **anterior part of the pituitary gland** produces a number of hormones, and it is now considered that these play a very important part

THE PITUITARY GLAND IN CONTROL OF THE ENDOCRINE SYSTEM

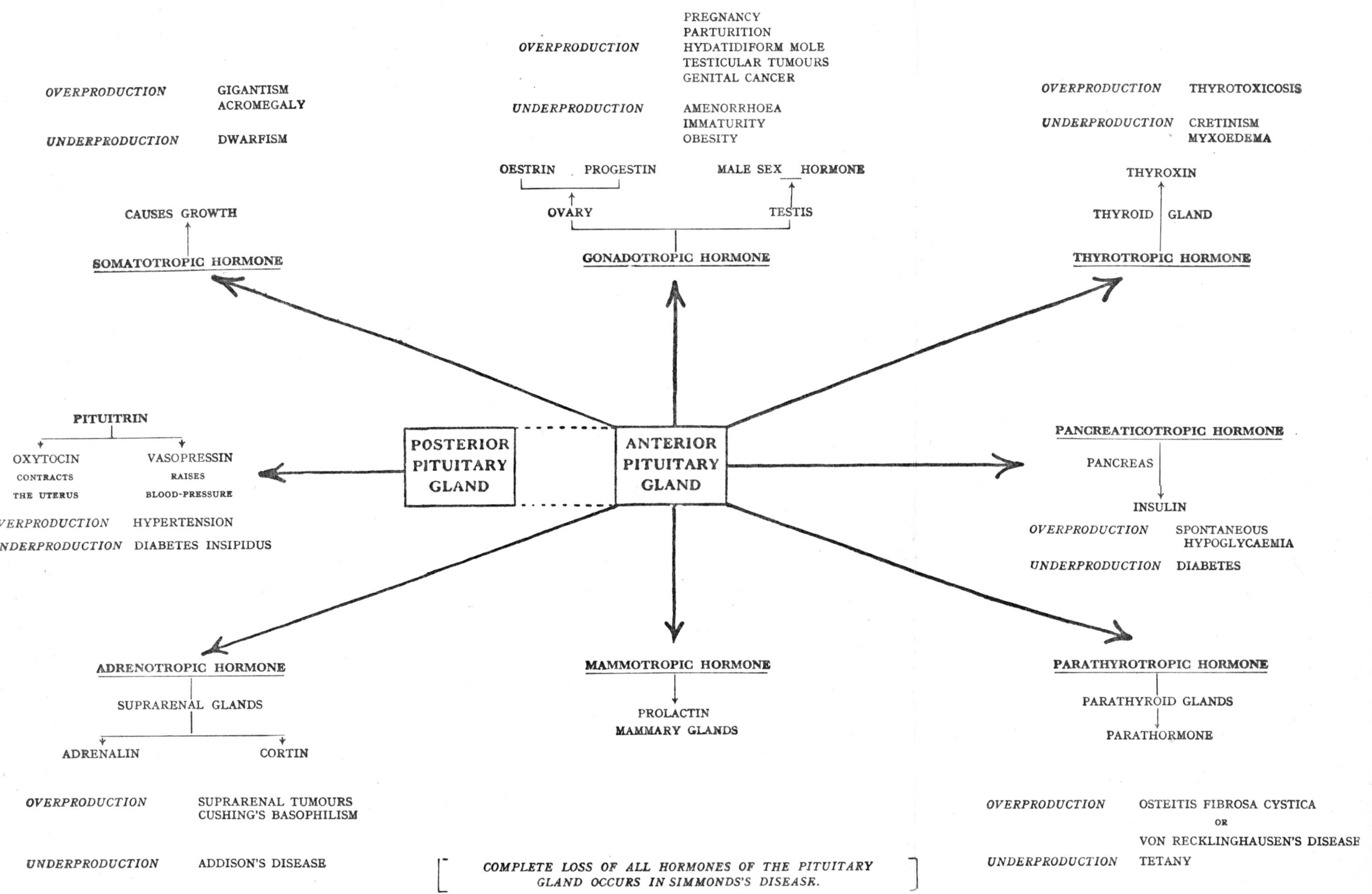

[*COMPLETE LOSS OF ALL HORMONES OF THE PITUITARY GLAND OCCURS IN SIMMONDS'S DISEASE.*]

To face page 446

n the control of the general wellbeing of the metabolism of the body, promoting the regulation of all physical activity, the growth of the body and the activity of the sex glands; one of these secretions controls the activity of the ovarian hormones, and is thought to play a great part in he control of emotions, and to be intimately concerned with the control of leep. Disease or disorder of the pituitary gland gives rise to a long train of ymptoms many of them affecting the sympathetic nervous system and being characterized by emotional disturbance. Other hormones from the anterior lobe of the pituitary gland are concerned with the control of the breasts and the secretion of milk during lactation, and with the control of the activities of the thyroid, adrenal and parathyroid glands (see accompanying chart).

Gigantism and acromegaly arise as the result of hypersecretion of the somatotropic hormone, which controls growth. *Gigantism* occurs when the condition is present before growth has ceased. *Acromegaly* is seen in adults, of middle age; it is characterized by enlargement of the lower jaw and malar bones, the nose is broad and the skin thick and coarse, the feet and hands are large and the fingers spatulate in shape.

It is thought that this condition is produced by the presence of a pituitary tumour, a danger of this being that pressure on the adjacent optic nerves may cause loss of sight. The tumour is sometimes removed; in other instances the condition is treated by the administration of thyroid extract and also by extract of antuitrin.

Dwarfism is retarded growth due to undersecretion of the somatotropic hormone.

Simmonds's disease is characterized by cachexia and premature senility due to deficiency and loss of all the hormones of the anterior lobe of the pituitary gland, as the result of degenerative changes which have taken place in it.

The **posterior lobe of the pituitary gland** produces a secretion called *pituitrin*. It contains two hormones: *vasopressin* which raises blood pressure and *oxytocin* which stimulates contraction of the uterus.

Overproduction of pituitrin causes hyperpiesis (see p. 357) and *underproduction* gives rise to *diabetes insipidus*.

In **diabetes insipidus** the balance of water in the body is upset and the patient passes large quantities of pale-coloured urine with a low specific gravity of 1,002 or 1,005. As much as several hundred ounces may be passed in 24 hours. This marked polyuria is accompanied by thirst and constipation, wasting occurs owing to deprivation of the body of fluid and, because he is frequently disturbed at night to pass urine, the patient becomes tired and weary from loss of sleep. He is unable to carry on any ordinary occupation owing to frequent interruptions.

In some cases the condition is relieved by pituitrin.

The ovarian and testical secretions. Two ovarian hormones are described: one, *oestrin* or *folliculin*, is thought to control sex development and the activity of the uterus during the menstrual cycle, and a preparation of this hormone is employed in the treatment of a number of symptoms occurring at the menopause; the second ovarian hormone, prepared in the corpus luteum and usually described as *progesterone*, is thought to be concerned with the control of the periods of rest of the uterus.

The *testes* also produce internal secretions which are thought to control sex characteristics in men.

THE INTRINSIC FACTOR OF CASTLE

Pernicious anaemia is now known to be associated with lack of an anti-anaemic principle, comprised of an 'extrinsic factor' present in protein food and of the 'intrinsic factor' of Castle in the gastric juice, which is a hormone. In the treatment of pernicious anaemia, either liver or extract of desiccated hog's stomach is given (see p. 360).

THE ISLETS OF LANGERHANS IN THE PANCREAS

Diabetes is a disease which is now known to be due to deficiency of an internal secretion produced by the beta cells of special areas in the pancreas, known as the islets of Langerhans. The secretion produced by these cells is called *insulin* and when it is deficient in quantity, owing to disease or disorder of the function of these cells, there is an excess of sugar in the blood and sugar is then excreted by the kidney, and by this characteristic the condition of diabetes is recognized. The disease is described in Ch. 27, p. 435.

Chapter 29

Examples of Diseases of the Skin

Introduction—Characteristics of skin lesions—Examples of non-specific conditions: Urticaria—Eczema—Psoriasis—Diseases due to microbic infection, vegetable fungi and animal parasites—Impetigo—Pemphigus—Lupus—Seborrhoea—Sycosis—Scabies—Pediculosis—Ringworm—Athlete's foot—Favus—Herpes

The skin has many functions. It covers and protects the supporting structures of the body, prevents the entry of micro-organisms and assists in the regulation of the temperature of the body. It has a slight respiratory action, eliminating a small quantity of CO_2, and is an important excretory factor in that it eliminates water and salts in solution, fatty acids and cholesterol. It has slight absorptive faculties.

The skin has also an important psychic function; developed, as it is, from the same elements as the nervous system, it responds to emotional states, and expresses emotions of fear, shame, anger, pleasure, etc., and it is this intimate association of the skin with the functions of the nervous system that makes the care of patients with diseases of the skin so very important as well as so particularly interesting.

These patients need very careful consideration in order to make them feel that they are really wanted, and that they are going to be cared for and helped to overcome that dreadful attitude of mind in which they imagine themselves to be deformed, and think that people consider them infectious, with consequent development of a tendency to hide not only their disability but themselves, and often to refuse to appear in public.

Patients with diseases of the skin are always very thoughtful and grateful and make a display of gratitude for even the slightest consideration which is almost embarrassing to the recipient of it.

The **symptoms of diseases** of the skin are divided into *subjective*—which the patient complains of—such as burning, itching, tingling, heat and, more rarely, pain. The *objective* symptoms are those which can be discovered on examination. The lesions most commonly seen in skin diseases are divided into primary and secondary lesions.

The **primary lesions** are:

A *macule,* which is a slight discoloration of the skin, an example being seen in the rash of measles. A freckle is a macule—it is not raised above the level of the surface of the skin.

A *wheal* is slightly raised; it may be a blotchy patch, or a line or streak; it is raised because the skin is swollen. An example of this is urticaria.

A *papule* is a little raised elevation, like a pimple. A *nodule* or tubercle is a large papule, as seen in lupus and in the tertiary stage of syphilis.

A *vesicle* is a tiny sac of fluid, which may surmount a papule or appear on the skin independently of any other lesion. A *bulla* is a large blister or bleb containing fluid.

A *pustule* is a similar little sac filled with pus.

A *scale* is produced when air gets between the layers of the skin, causing it to separate as do the scales on fish. This lesion is seen in ichthyosis and psoriasis.

The **lesions** described as **secondary** are produced by the irritation of some discharge or exudate or by injury to the skin, often by scratching. These lesions include:

Crusts, such as arise during the healing stage of a papule; and (in the case of the other examples below) when the top has been knocked off a lesion or when it has been made to bleed. A crust consists therefore of dried serum, blood or pus.

Excoriation is usually due to scratching. *Pigmentation* may be due to the same cause; or it may be produced by the presence of constant moisture, or may be left after crusting has occurred.

Ulceration and *erosion* are due to destruction of the superficial tissues.

Scars are left as the result of healing by the formation of fibrous tissue.

Rhagades or *fissures* appear as splits or cracks in the epidermis, exposing the dermis which lies beneath. These are often the result of excoriation either by scratching or from constant contact with an irritating discharge or exudate.

Examination of the skin. Examination should take place in good daylight; artificial light is not to be recommended. The whole of the patient's body should be exposed for examination so that both sides of it can be seen at once. The *area of distribution* of the lesion should be carefully observed and note taken as to whether it is symmetrical or asymmetrical and also where the lesion is most marked, and whether it exists only on certain parts, such as the flexor or extensor surfaces of the limbs. The *type of lesion* should be determined, as to whether it is composed of wheals, papules, macules and so on; or whether the condition seen is multiform in character. The colour of the rash and of the remainder of the skin should be considered and the condition of the hair follicles and the pores. The lesion should be felt to discover whether it is hot or cool, and whether the skin is swollen.

The **history** is important and should include the patient's age, address and occupation. For example, a nurse may get a skin reaction from using antiseptics, and bakers develop a well-known trade dermatitis.

The patient should be asked whether he has any relatives who are similarly afflicted, as in the case of some of the non-specific skin diseases there may be an hereditary tendency to such. In the case of the specific skin diseases there may be a history of contact for example with cases of scabies or impetigo.

Another series of questions includes those which would elicit the existence of any emotional stress or strain, anxiety, or nervous tension. The patient should also be asked whether he is taking any medicine, and the prescription should be looked at to note whether it contains any drug which might cause a rash. For example, potassium bromide may produce a pustular rash, particularly on the face and shoulders; sulphur may cause a local or general dermatitis while both arsenic and belladonna may cause an erythematous rash.

The urine should be tested, as eczema may be associated with glycosuria or albuminuria. The general condition of the patient should be observed—he may be fat or thin, may appear nervous and fidgety or be phlegmatic.

The patient should be asked what he complains of, and if he says 'itching', he should be asked whether this is worse when he gets into bed.

He should also be asked whether the partaking of any particular foods or any special set of circumstances makes the lesion worse and whether he has noticed any treatment or other conditions which may have seemed to relieve it.

The **causes of skin diseases** are numerous, and may be divided into specific and non-specific conditions. The majority will be found to be in the group described on pp. 453–8.

POINTS IN THE NURSING OF DISEASES OF THE SKIN

Treatment and nursing. A patient with a skin disease—let it be repeated—must be made to feel that he is going to be cared for. It is a very good plan, if the physician will permit it to be done, to bath the patient at the outset in some emollient bath, such as oatmeal; by this means the whole of the patient's skin can be thoroughly examined and he will feel he is really being well attended to. He can then be put to bed and should be given a hot drink and tucked up and made to feel happy, cheerful and contented as he looks forward to his future treatment.

A nurse requires to be tactful and gentle always; she considers the feelings of her patient in the nice way she performs routine nursing duties for him; she must stress this attitude even more in caring for patients with skin diseases, as they are so sensitive about their condition, and may conjure up convictions that people are being impatient with them, or think they see a flicker on the face of the nurse which, though it really means no more than that she is preoccupied for the moment, makes them imagine that she feels disgust at attending to them. In these instances particularly she must develop that habit of attending only to one patient at a time, and of giving him all her thoughts as well as her actions, for the time being.

In the treatment of skin diseases rest is just as important as it is in the treatment of a broken leg. Rest in bed is usually ordered at the commencement of treatment; but, even if this is not so, means will be taken in an ambulatory case to protect, and prevent irritation of, the affected area.

Speaking generally penicillin is useful in those skin diseases in which some secondary infection due to penicillin-sensitive organisms is present. Penicillin can safely be applied locally in the form of a cream or solution in impetigo, eczema, sycosis barbae, and infective dermatitis. Skin conditions which are deep seated such as boils, carbuncles and abscesses require systemic treatment with penicillin.

Other forms of local application include cooling lotions for hot tense lesions or alternatively a bland powder may be used. Powders or pastes are employed for moist lesions. Calamine liniment which is soothing and protective is employed for subacute cases.

A *scaly lesion* must be freed of scales; crusts and scabs have to be removed before treatment can effectually be applied to the lesion which lies beneath.

Chronic skin diseases require stimulating dressings; but very mild preparations will be used at first, and observation of the effect will be made before the strength of the application is increased.

Cleansing the skin is important at all times; but the use of water is in some cases questionable. It is used for removing scales in psoriasis; but, when the skin is hot and inflamed, soap and water act as an irritant, except in so far as water is applied in the form of some evaporating lotion.

Weeping lesions are usually cleansed by means of paraffin or olive oil, though in some instances normal saline is employed for this purpose. In most chronic skin lesions, or those which are covered with crusts and scabs, either olive oil or starch poultices are used.

The baths which are commonly employed in the cleansing of subacute and chronic skin cases are *emollient baths*, containing either a pound of borax, from 2 to 4 pounds of bran or oatmeal, or from 1 to 2 pounds of starch to a bath of 30 gallons of water.

Antiseptic baths employed are from 2 to 4 ounces of sulphur, used in parasitic conditions, such as scabies; a weak solution of Condy's fluid is employed; it should not be strong enough to discolour either the patient's skin or the bath.

Observation is very important. It is impossible to state how this can be carried out, and it must be sufficient to say that a nurse, who is handling a patient daily, should be the first to note whether a treatment is suiting a lesion or not, and that she should be able to formulate and express what she has observed, and to report fully to the physician as soon as possible.

General treatment. Enough has already been said to help the nurse to realize that the wellbeing of a skin lesion may depend to a very great extent on the absence of nervous tension, anxiety and emotional disturbance. A patient's mind must be at rest, whether it is considered necessary to rest his body by keeping him in bed or not. Any indigestion, constipation, sleeplessness, renal disorder or disorder of menstruation should be investigated and treated, as it may have a bearing on the cause of the disease. The presence of septic foci should be considered and treated.

The bedclothes must be smooth and even, and non-irritating; the clothing the patient wears next to his skin may be of silk or cotton, but not of wool.

The bowels should be kept acting regularly; but if aperients have to be employed these must be judiciously chosen. Unless a nurse knows exactly what a particular doctor prefers in certain cases, she had better refer this matter to him.

When drugs are employed the nurse must observe their effects, and the same applies to the administration of vaccines and glandular extracts.

Diet may not have to be considered in many cases, but in some it will be an advantage to avoid all highly seasoned foods, stimulants such as alcohol and coffee, excessive use of sugar or heavy protein food. Plenty of bland drinks and water should be given, and careful note is always to be made of the effect any particular food is found to have on a patient.

EXAMPLES OF NON-SPECIFIC DISEASES AND INFLAMMATORY LESIONS OF THE SKIN

Urticaria. This condition is usually acquired, because the patient has some idiosyncrasy to a given set of circumstances—to the pollen of some plant, or to some particular food, e.g. shellfish, or any other fish, sometimes being the determining cause of an attack of urticaria. The administration of horse serum in the treatment of disease is very frequently followed by a reaction which is characterized by an urticarial rash.

Acute urticaria is characterized by wheals and swollen patches which are red at first, the vesicles afterwards becoming blanched and the patch turning white. If this occurs on the mucous membrane of the throat it may be dangerous, as asphyxia may be caused. As a rule, this form of urticaria can be relieved by the administration of from 5 to 10 minims of adrenalin, given by hypodermic injection.

The acute form of urticaria tends to become *chronic*. The patient is constantly covered with nettlerash, and this is so irritable that it prevents his sleeping. He may have a few days of freedom from the irritating condition, but it recurs and may continue at intervals for months or even years. It is difficult to find a cause for this type, which sometimes seems to be associated with distress or emotion, though frequently there is no such apparent association. Treatment is very difficult.

Eczema occurs in many forms, and *trade dermatitis* is one of these which is usually produced by some external irritation. *Baker's dermatitis* is due to handling flour; surgeons and nurses may get dermatitis from the use of antiseptics. The use of irritating clothing and soaps is another cause, and it may also be associated with disorders of the endocrine glands or with disorders of metabolism.

Eczema is described in three main forms—acute, subacute and chronic. It may be extensive or localized and it may be present in an acute form on one part of the body and in a chronic form on other parts.

The **symptoms present in eczema** are various—The part may be *red and hot* to the examining hand, and this is due to dilation of the blood vessels. As a rule this symptom passes on to *swelling* of the affected area and the skin may pit on pressure.

Weeping is the term used to describe the presence of an exudate; blood from the vessels, which passes into the epidermis and dermis, separates the epidermal cells, and lakelets of fluid collect between the cells. This forms vesicles on the surface of the skin, and serum oozes out—a condition known as weeping eczema.

Crusting occurs when fluid which contains debris rests and dries on the surface.

Scaling is due to heaping up on the surface of imperfectly formed epidermis. This is quite different from crusting.

In the **treatment of eczema** the symptoms which are present are dealt with. If a cause is known it should be considered. The main points in the treatment as regards local applications are: First to protect the skin so that it can have rest, and to see that all aggravating substances, including soap and water and the use of any irritating coverings, are eliminated. The next point is to relieve the skin of all irritation—patients must not be allowed to scratch and some means should be taken to prevent this.

The following substances are included amongst those which will often be ordered.

In *acute eczema* lotions which cool and relieve congestion will be employed, such as lead and glycerine. The affected part should be kept wet, a fairly thick layer of material being used which will retain moisture; the nurse should keep wetting this, but she must take care that the part undergoing treatment does not become chapped. If this happens, calamine cream or paste will be used instead.

In the *subacute forms*, pastes will be employed. Lassar's paste is an ointment with a good deal of powder in it; it contains zinc and starch, salicylic acid and some ointment base, such as vaseline. The amount of powder that is present permits the paste to take up the exudate from the surface of the lesion and allows it to pass through the paste instead of being confined underneath the dressing as it would be if an ordinary ointment were used. As a rule an application of paste is made twice a day, but it is important to clean off one application by means of liquid paraffin or olive oil before a second application is made; if this is neglected, it means that paste will be put upon paste and a mass will accumulate on the surface of the lesion.

In *chronic eczema* stimulating applications are employed. Ointment or paste may be used. Coal tar preparations are applied and X-ray treatment used in order to help the cells to return to their normal character.

Infective eczema or *dermatitis* is treated with penicillin.

Psoriasis forms a rather large percentage of the non-specific skin diseases. It tends to run in families, and it may begin early in life and the patient never again be free. He may have one attack, be treated, find it clears up and never have another. It may commence in middle age or old age; no age is free from the onset of psoriasis. The cause is not known.

The *lesion* and the *distribution* is characteristic; in most cases the knees, elbows and scapulae are the sites commonly covered. The lesion begins as a red patch with a heavy scaly surface; the scales split and air between them gives the silvery appearance which is so well known.

Many forms of *treatment* are tried, in some cases with success. Before treating the lesion it is necessary to remove the heavy silvery scales by warm baths, containing lysol, using a nailbrush and coal tar soap to scrub the scales off. They will reform, but in the interval treatment can be applied. Amongst the substances used are wood tar, oil of cade, salicylate ointment, chrysarobin, ultra-violet light and X-rays.

SOME OF THE COMMONER SKIN DISEASES WHICH ARE DUE TO MICROBIC INVASION, VEGETABLE FUNGI AND ANIMAL PARASITES

Impetigo is a very common affection of the skin in the case of children, due to the presence of pus-producing organisms, staphylococci or streptococci, and characterized by blisters on the skin, the fluid in the blisters becoming pus which in a few days dries up and forms into crusts. The lesions occur most commonly on the face, head, arms and legs.

Impetigo frequently occurs as a complication of scabies and pediculosis, and may begin by septic infection of a scratch or abrasion of the skin. The disease, which usually terminates within a fortnight, is very contagious, especially amongst children, and care must be taken to prevent spread of infection. When a child with impetigo is first seen, his face may be covered by blisters, pustules and scabs.

Treatment. When staphylococci predominate sulphadiazine and sulphathiazole are given and when streptococci are present sulphapyridine is the drug of choice.

All *crusts* must *first* be removed by bathing them with borax and water, or by applications of olive oil or starch poultice. When soft they can be picked off with forceps and the area cleansed with a weak antiseptic lotion and gently dabbed dry. Watery solutions used as local applications include aniline dyes such as acriflavine, gentian violet, brilliant green, and mercury. Ointments are not used, but Lassar's paste, which contains zinc and to which 2 per cent ammoniated mercury may be added, can be employed.

Sulphonamides such as M & B 693 may be given orally for a week, and sulphathiazole may be applied locally.

All fresh scabs which form must be removed before each fresh application. As a rule the condition clears up in a week to 10 days. Slight discoloration will be left but this will disappear in a few weeks.

The child's feeding and toilet utensils should be kept separate, and he should not be allowed to play with other children unless the affected parts are covered. It is important to try to discover any underlying cause of impetigo, and if the subject is debilitated a good nourishing diet and a change of air will be beneficial. Impetigo may be complicated by adenitis of the local lymphatic glands, and in a severe case suppuration of the glands might occur.

Pemphigus is a skin disease characterised by the formation of blebs and bullae, which become purulent and rupture, and form crusts. It is due to several organisms including staphylococci and streptococci. It may be present in the newly born, when it is thought to be a manifestation of syphilis. An acutely infectious form may occur in adults or a more common form, which is less infectious and is described as *pemphigus vulgaris*. The treatment is similar to that described for impetigo.

Lupus vulgaris is a skin affection produced by the tubercle bacillus. It begins early in life and usually appears first on the cheeks and nose as small red patches which spread very slowly until they form a reddish scar.

The *treatment* is selective, in order to damage the bacillus. Ultra-violet light treatment is employed both locally, and generally to the whole body.

In addition any lesion such as suppuration of the glands of the neck, which may be giving rise to infection of the skin of the face, should be treated. The general treatment described in the case of pulmonary tuberculosis is also applicable to cases of lupus.

The result of lupus may be extensive scarring and contraction of the skin as the result of tissue destruction.

Septic infections of the skin, occurring as boils and carbuncles, are mentioned under the heading 'infection' on p. 570.

Seborrhoea is inflammation of the sebaceous glands, which are most numerous on the scalp, resulting in excessive secretion of these glands. It usually responds to cleansing of the surface and keeping the head free of scurf. In some cases salicylate and sulphur preparations are employed.

Sycosis is infection of the hair follicles by staphylococci, and it occurs in children on the scalp and in men on the chin. In a few cases infection is general and the axillary and pubic hairs and eyebrows are affected.

Epilation of the infected hair is carried out, and great care must be exercised to prevent reinfection. Men have to be particularly careful, when shaving to cleanse the skin with spirit and to sterilize the razor carefully. Penicillin is effective.

Scabies is due to the presence of a tiny parasite, the itch mite—*Acarus scabiei*. The female burrows into and eats her way through the horny layer of the epidermis. She is a cold-blooded animal and works best when the skin is warm and the patient is in bed at night. She lays her eggs as she burrows and also secretes an acrid fluid which irritates the skin and keeps the patient awake and scratching.

The burrows are about ½ inch long, and the margins are rough and may collect dirt, so that they often appear as dark streaks. The eggs hatch in about 3 days and become adult mites in a week. The young emerge when the body is warm, which is another cause of irritation and scratching.

Scabies affects the skin of the hands and wrists, at the sides and webs of the fingers, the axillary folds, backs of the knees, elbows and buttocks. The lesions are papules, vesicles and pustules. Scratching may result in impetigo.

A *history of severe itching* which is worse at night would always suggest the possibility of scabies. The *cure of scabies* is quick and sure—the eggs and insects are susceptible to benzyl benzoate and sulphur.

Treatment consists in (1) *breaking up the roofs of the burrows* to expose the itch mite's eggs, by washing and scrubbing with soft soap and (2) the *application of an ascaricide*, either benzyl benzoate emulsion or sulphur ointment may be used.

The patient is soaped all over with a green soft soap rubbing it well into all parts which itch, he gets into a hot bath and continues to rub and scrub with a soft brush for twenty minutes. The skin is dried and an emulsion of benzyl benzoate, 25 per cent made up in water with 2 per cent lanette wax, is either rubbed in or painted on all over the body, except the face and head, paying special attention to the itching areas. During this time the patient's underclothing is steam-disinfected ready for him to put on again. The local sanitary authorities disinfect his bed clothing and return it to the house before night. Some authorities consider one thorough treatment is effective, others recommend two treatments.

Prevention of infection and *reinfection* is very important, and all members of a household in which a case of scabies occurs should be questioned about itching. Anyone who has shared the same bed as the patient should be treated at the same time.

Pediculosis may affect the head, body and pubes, axillae and eyebrows. *Pediculosis capitis*. The head louse or *Pediculus capitis* is a small grey parasite; it infests the hair of the head and the female lays about 50 eggs, called nits, which are deposited on the hairs close to the scalp, by a sticky film. These eggs hatch in about a week. The movement of lice in the hair is irritating and the patient scratches his head in order to obtain relief. Sores may be produced by scratching and these may be infected which in a serious case would result in enlargement of the lymphatic glands in the suboccipital region of the head.

The *treatment* has been described in the cleaning of a verminous head on p. 61.

Pediculosis corporis. The body louse or *Pediculus corporis* is slightly larger than the head louse. It lives in the seams of the clothing which lies next to the body. This condition is met in dirty people and those who are debilitated and neglected. The female louse lays her eggs in the seams of the clothing; they hatch in from 2 to 3 weeks. The lice biting the skin cause itching but when examining the patient they are not found on the skin, but on the clothing.

Treatment. Lice are destroyed by D.D.T. but in addition clothing, bedding and blankets should all be disinfected.

Pediculosis pubis. The *Phthirus pubis* or crab louse is shaped like a ladybird. It is a dirty grey colour. It has claw-like processes attached to some of its legs by which it clings closely to the pubic hairs. The female lays about 15 eggs. This parasite may spread to hairs on the skin of the abdomen and also to the eyebrows and eyelashes.

It is very unlikely that a nurse will see pubic lice, but the presence of little greyish spots over the pubes and the skin of the lower part of the abdomen should arouse her suspicions and then she should get some more experienced person to look at the patient.

Treatment. The hair of the affected parts should be shaved off and burnt; an ointment containing 10 per cent mercury should then be rubbed well into the parts. After some hours the patient may have a bath or be bathed.

When the eyelashes are affected the parasites must all be picked off with forceps and yellow oxide of mercury 2 per cent applied.

The clothing should all be disinfected.

Ringworm is due to a vegetable organism of a similar class to that which forms fluff on jams, etc. Ringworm attacks the skin and its appendages, the hair and nails.

Ringworm of the scalp or *Tinea tonsurans* is a fairly common and very highly contagious disease in children. The fungus attacks the hair, which breaks off; the skin of the affected area of the scalp is covered with debris and scales, and it may be slightly reddened. The area is often circular in outline, and the disease spreads until a large area may be affected.

The modern *treatment* is by means of a carefully graduated dose of X-rays. The skin of the scalp should be well washed with soap and water, the hair cut short for an area around the affected part, and the scalp cleared of debris and scales. The X-ray treatment is then given, and the patient is afterwards kept under observation; his head is washed with soap and water daily, and after the eighteenth day the affected hairs fall out. The hair will grow again in from two to three months.

Isolation of the patient is necessary, particularly from other children, and when nursed in a ward his toilet and feeding utensils should be kept separate, and his head covered by a clean linen cap.

Another modern treatment of ringworm is by the administration of *thallium acetate*, a very carefully graduated dose of the drug being ordered as it is highly dangerous.

Ringworm of the body—Tinea circinata—and *of the groins—Tinea cruris*—attacks the skin. A red patch appears which spreads until a fairly large oval lesion is formed; it may be surrounded by a ring of vesicles. Lesions occur on the forearms and neck.

As the lesion is on the surface of the skin it is easy to cure and will respond to antiseptics such as aniline dyes, mercury and iodine. The patient's toilet articles should be kept separate until the condition is cured. The patches should be covered, so that the patient's clothing is not infected.

Tinea barbae requires the same treatment as ringworm of the scalp.

Athlete's foot is contracted from swimming pools, baths, and the floors of gymnasiums, contaminated by infected feet. It is a form of ringworm. The lesion, which appears as white skin between the toes, very quickly responds to cleansing with a mild antiseptic and painting with iodine.

Favus is also a vegetable fungus; it is rarely seen in England. It affects the scalp mainly and most commonly of children. The condition begins as little yellow follicles, and as it spreads large yellow honeycomb-like masses exuding pus form on the scalp.

The treatment consists in removing the masses by the use of spirit lotion and salicylate ointment. X-ray treatment is employed, as in the case of ringworm.

Herpes zoster is inflammation of the posterior primary division of one or more spinal nerves. It affects the intercostal nerves or any spinal nerve and in some cases the fifth cranial nerve.

The condition is thought to be due to a filtrable virus. It is considered to be associated with chickenpox though little is known about its exact relationship.

The *symptoms* in herpes zoster are pain and tingling over the course of the nerve affected, the area becomes tender and red and after a few days crops of vesicles appear along the course of the nerve which is inflamed. After several days the vesicles dry off and separate but the skin continues to be tender and painful and in some cases remains hypersensitive for months.

The *local treatment* is to keep the vesicles dry by applications of slightly astringent powders or to keep them covered by collodion. It is important to prevent secondary infection. Any dressing used as a covering should be lightly applied because the skin is very tender. The affected part should be kept at rest; in the case of an affected ulnar nerve the arm might be supported in a sling. But in intercostal cases the patient should be kept in bed.

General treatment consists in rest in bed if the temperature is raised or if the patient is very uncomfortable and fatigued owing to loss of sleep. Aspirin is ordered for the relief of pain, and the diet should be nourishing and the bowels kept active. Considerable debility follows an attack of herpes zoster and therefore a good convalescent period should be arranged.

When the pain persists after the attack, painting the affected area with belladonna may help; applications of heat are useful in some cases, in others electrical treatment or X-ray treatment may be ordered.

Herpes simplex, although not associated with herpes zoster, is also considered to be due to a filtrable virus, which in this case is known to be of a kind that will produce encephalitis in rabbits.

An attack of herpes simplex often occurs on the face, and round the nose and mouth of persons who are subject to it, and one attack predisposes to others. It also occurs at the onset of some of the febrile diseases, as in pneumonia.

Herpes begins with tingling sensations in the affected part, followed by neuralgic pain and the eruption of a crop or crops of vesicles, which dry up in about a week. The eruption may be prevented by dabbing the parts with alcohol or with a mixture of tannic acid and methylated spirit every half-hour. If not so treated, when the eruption has formed, the vesicles should be kept dry.

Section 5

Communicable Diseases and their Treatment and Nursing Care

Chapter 30

Introductory

Terms used in describing communicable diseases—Control of communicable diseases —Notification of disease—The course of a communicable disease

A *communicable disease* is any disease or condition which can be communicated from one person to another. The terms *communicable* and *infectious disease* may be regarded as synonymous. Many medical and surgical conditions including the common cold, impetigo and other (but not all) skin diseases, surgical infections such as boils and carbuncles, are infective conditions and can be communicated from one person to another. But speaking generally the term communicable or infectious disease is reserved for the description of those diseases which are notifiable diseases or may be made so, and which if allowed to spread may give rise to epidemics and seriously and adversely affect the health of the community.

Epidemiology is the study of epidemic diseases.

An *epidemic disease* is one which suddenly attacks a great many people at the same time.

An *endemic disease* is one which occurs constantly in a particular area.

A *sporadic disease* is one in which a few cases occur from time to time. It is generally widely distributed.

A *pandemic disease* is an epidemic disease which is so widely spread that almost the entire world is involved, as happened in the influenza epidemic in 1918.

An *indigenous disease* is native to a particular place.

An *exotic disease* is one which is introduced from abroad.

Isolation is a measure adopted for patients and carriers who, under special circumstances and in given instances, are segregated in order to prevent spread of infection to others.

Quarantine is the term used to describe the period during which persons who have been exposed to infection require to be isolated, in order to prevent infecting others by themselves contracting the disease.

The period of quarantine is the longest-known maximum limit of the incubation period and if the contact does not show signs of disease during this period it may be assumed that he has escaped infection and can be released from quarantine.

Some physicians and some authorities add two days to the longest-known incubation period as a measure of greater safety.

In some cases, instead of insisting on segregating contacts during a period of quarantine, they are allowed to mix with the population but are kept under medical observation during the incubation period and promptly isolated should symptoms appear.

CONTROL OF COMMUNICABLE DISEASES

The public health authorities exercise an important function in taking steps to prevent the spreading of communicable disease in the community and the principles of the existing methods of the control of these diseases have originated during the past hundred years or more. *The methods adopted in the control of communicable diseases* have been aimed at eliminating the cause, but, as these diseases are caused by living micro-organisms and it is not possible to destroy all such organisms, progress in prevention has developed principally along two lines:

Reducing the prevalence of the organisms.

Increasing the resistance of the community.

The patient is dealt with by *notification* of disease, *isolation* of the patient, *disinfection* of all excreta and discharges from the patient and articles which have become infected, *treatment* of the patient and *terminal disinfection* when necessary after recovery.

Contacts, those who have been in contact with the patient, or, in the wider term, with recently infected articles, may be dealt with by *quarantine*, *close observation*, *exclusion from certain places and facilities*, such as from school and from the use of public transport, and by the closure of hospital wards, of schools and other institutions, though these measures are only adopted in certain rare instances.

The *source of the outbreak* or epidemic is investigated and when possible removed. For example an infected water supply would be cut off until rendered harmless, and the sale of infected food would be prohibited.

Prevention. All the above means deal with the control of disease when it has occurred but much more valuable measures are, *improvement in social conditions*, *immunization of the community*, *education by the teaching of general hygienic means* for preventing the spread of disease, and constructive intelligent *propaganda* aimed at inviting the co-operation of the general public.

Immunization. Immunity to infection may be *natural*, some degree of immunity is general; or it may be *acquired* by having an attack of disease, or immunity may be *conferred* by inoculation with bacteria or their toxins. See also the use of serum p. 322 and of vaccine p. 324 and the methods of immunization employed in the prevention of diphtheria, scarlet fever, smallpox and other acute infections.

NOTIFICATION OF DISEASE

When a group of communicable diseases are required by the local health authority to be notified these diseases are often spoken of as *notifiable diseases*. The following is a list of diseases which are notifiable in this country.

Smallpox	Scarlatina
Diphtheria	Typhus
Scarlet fever	Enteric fever
Relapsing fever	Puerperal fever
Erysipelas	Cerebrospinal fever
Poliomyelitis	Tuberculosis
Ophthalmia neonatorum	Polio-encephalitis
Encephalitis lethargica	Malaria
Dysentery	Trench fever
Acute primary pneumonia	Puerperal pyrexia
Acute influenzal pneumonia	Measles
Whooping cough	Plague
Cholera	

Chickenpox may be made notifiable when smallpox is present.

German measles is made temporarily notifiable when measles is prevalent.

Infective enteritis and diarrhoea are also frequently made notifiable.

Anthrax is notifiable in certain areas.

Food poisoning is notifiable in England and Wales under the Food and Drugs Act 1939.

THE COURSE OF A COMMUNICABLE DISEASE

Each communicable disease is caused by some definite organism and the course the disease will follow can with more or less degree of accuracy be anticipated. The course of a communicable disease is divided into several stages.

Incubation. A period of incubation *precedes the first symptoms* of the disease. It is the period that elapses from the *moment of infection* until the first symptoms appear. Each disease has its own particular length of incubation.

The prodromal period is a term used to describe a period immediately *preceding the appearance of the first true symptoms* of the disease. This period is marked in some diseases by special symptoms; in particular certain rashes are described as *prodromal rashes*.

The invasion or onset is really the first stage of the disease. It lasts from the appearance of the first true symptoms of the disease until the height of the disease is reached; and in the communicable diseases characterized by rashes, until the rash is fully developed.

The stage of advance, the height of the fever, the fastigium or acme, is that period during which the symptoms are fully developed and the temperature (if raised) usually remains elevated. This stage lasts until the symptoms begin to abate, which may be hours, days, weeks, or months.

The stage of decline or defervescence is that in which the symptoms abate and the temperature (if raised) falls.

The stage of convalescence begins when the temperature has reached normal, remains down, and the symptoms have mainly disappeared. During this stage the conditions gradually return to normal and the patient recovers his strength.

Chapter 31

The Nursing Care of Communicable Diseases (Fever Nursing)

General management of communicable diseases—Methods of isolation—Prevention of cross infection—Measures for the protection of the nurse—The nursing of a patient in a private house

GENERAL MANAGEMENT OF COMMUNICABLE DISEASES

In her care of a patient suffering from a communicable disease the nurse is called upon to consider:

The nursing care of the sick person,
The necessity of preventing spread of infection to others, and
The prevention of infection to herself.

The provision of good ventilation. Fresh air is very necessary; the more air available, the smaller is the risk of spreading infection. If possible each bed should be allowed 1,200 cubic feet of space. Provision should be made to prevent the rising of dust when sweeping; dust collected around the area of an isolated bed should be picked up at the foot of the bed and not swept down the ward. The importance of careful wet dusting of furniture and walls in a ward or room in which patients suffering from communicable disease are nursed cannot be overestimated.

The **diet** during the febrile stage should be limited to fluids; the patient must be given plenty of water and watery drinks, and these should be pressed upon him. A thirsty patient is usually willing to drink, but a patient with a bad sore throat may need a good deal of persuasion to take the fluid he needs. In most cases of communicable disease the febrile stage is comparatively short, unless complications occur; but, when it is prolonged, means must be found of giving plenty of nourishment in whatever form the patient can be persuaded to take it.

Rest. During the period of acute illness it is essential for the patient to be at rest in bed, and the ward should be quiet. The period of rest that is needed varies with each disease but, generally speaking, a patient should be kept in bed until all danger of serious complications is over. Cases of measles are liable to develop pneumonia up to the fourteenth day, and cases of scarlet fever are not out of danger of nephritis until after the nineteenth day.

The care of the **toilet** is important in all cases of communicable disease. The patient should be bathed night and morning; the mouth must be kept clean; the nose, eyes and ears will need careful treatment in special cases; and he should be washed locally after the use of the bedpan.

In otitis media and otorrhoea the auditory canal should be cleansed with peroxide of hydrogen followed by the instillation of glycerine and carbolic 5 per cent. The carbolic relieves pain and the glycerine is hygroscopic. In *cleansing the ear* padded ear sticks, carefully dressed with a fairly large pad of cotton wool at the end, should be used. These may safely be inserted from ½ to ¾ of an inch, if the canal is first straightened by pulling the pinna gently upwards and backwards. The frequency of the treatment depends on the amount of discharge, of which the canal should be kept free; the latter should not be plugged with cotton wool but left clear, and the ear may be covered by a pad of sterile wool lightly bandaged on. The pinna should be kept clean and free of discharge, as if this is neglected chronic eczema may ensue.

The nose. When rhinorrhoea is present the nose should be kept quite clean and dry, the margins of the nostrils being lubricated with white vaseline or liquid paraffin, or excoriation will result.

The eye. Whenever there is any conjunctivitis, however slight, the eyes should be bathed with a weak solution of boracic or saline; and they must be protected from exposure to light when photophobia is present. The presence of an exudate necessitates lubrication of the margins of the lids with yellow oxide of mercury ointment 2 per cent at night and the removal of any crusts by bathing with a solution of borax and water as often as necessary to keep the margins of the eyelids free.

METHODS OF ISOLATION EMPLOYED IN FEVER HOSPITALS

Pavilion system. In this plan separate blocks are provided for the care of each type of disease, some being set apart for measles, others for diphtheria and so on. Nurses working in these wards usually wear an overall over their dress when on duty and they share a house or home with other nurses, but when transferred from one block, to nurse another disease in a different block, they disinfect themselves by having an antiseptic bath, washing their hair and putting on fresh clothing.

Cubicle system. Each patient has a separate cubicle and, if the system is strictly adhered to, every article for the patient's use is kept in his cubicle. The doctor and nurse put on gowns when entering, and remove these, and wash their hands carefully before leaving the cubicle. Articles used for the patient are disinfected and replaced in his cubicle.

Barrier nursing is a system which was instituted when physicians began to consider that disease germs are not carried by the air, but on particles in the air and on utensils and articles used by, and persons who have been in contact with, infected persons and places. This system was first practised extensively in England at Plaistow by the late Dr. Biernacki. He isolated one or two patients, amongst others, not so isolated, in a general ward. A slight distinguishing mark was used to indicate the beds isolated and all the utensils and articles likely to be required by a patient were kept on or in a specially devised locker at his bedside. Two gowns hung by the bed for the use of doctor and nurse, and arrangements for washing the hands after handling the patient or any of his utensils were provided at each bedside.

Bed isolation was the next advance. This system was extensively used by Dr. Rundle at Fazakerley in 1918. This differed from barrier nursing in that it was considered that the majority of articles needed by a patient could be used in common with other patients, provided they were properly sterilized or disinfected after use. Gowns were provided at each isolated bed, and arrangements for washing the hands, preferably under running water, were supplied. All feeding utensils may be used in common provided that they are rinsed and washed in a sink kept specially for this purpose after use and then boiled for twenty minutes in a sterilizer in the ward kitchen. It is important to note that all feeding utensils handled by an infected patient, including the dinner knives, must be boiled. Sanitary utensils can be washed and disinfected or boiled after use.

Application of method. Before approaching the bed to perform any treatment of the patient, the nurse should roll her dress sleeves up well above the elbow, and put on the overall which is hanging at the bedside—this is made to fasten at the back of the neck by a button or tape, the waist being secured by a tape.

To put on an isolation overall it is important to avoid contamination of the dress or apron; therefore remove the gown from the peg by taking hold of the loop by which it hangs, hold it by the neck and put first one arm and then the other into the armholes, fasten the button and tie the tape. To remove it, unfasten the overall, grasp the outer side of the margin of the sleeves and pull off, drawing the hands through the sleeves gently to avoid contaminating the interior if possible; then, holding the overall at the shoulders, loosely so that the outer contaminated side is folded inside, return it to the peg and as it hangs the inner uncontaminated side lies outermost. This is important, as the other nurses in the ward may inadvertently touch the gown as it hangs, and moreover the nurse will handle this side in putting the overall on, thus rendering contamination of her dress and apron less likely to occur.

The nurse should remove the overall before washing her hands. She should not leave the bedside wearing the overall, *except* to remove and empty used sanitary utensils, in which case any doors through which she may have to pass should be opened for her so that they are not handled by the nurse who is infected.

The personal bed laundry from an infectious case which is being nursed in a general ward should be disinfected before being sent to the laundry. This may be done either by steam disinfection, or by soaking the linen in some efficient disinfectant solution, such as carbolic lotion 1–40, for two hours. It is then wrung out, put into a separate receptacle and labelled 'Wet, disinfected laundry'.

Excreta. The nurse empties the utensils wearing her overall, and then sterilizes them. Excreta from typhoid patients must be disinfected before it is disposed of, and this is done by receiving the excreta into a small quantity of disinfectant solution, such as 1–40 carbolic, covering it with 5–10 ounces of the lotion and allowing it to stand in an air cupboard, provided the receptacle is covered with a cloth wet with disinfectant, for from 2 to 4 hours before being disposed of.

Visitors. Whereas it would be ideal if one could arrange for visitors to view their infectious relatives from the ward door only, this is not always possible. When visitors are admitted, the nature of the infection should be explained to them and they should be advised not to touch the patient or his bed. They should wear an isolation gown with long sleeves to the wrists, and if infection is conveyed by the nose and mouth they should also wear a mask. On removing the gown, the face as well as the hands should be washed before leaving the ward premises.

The disinfection of a patient before discharge. The evening before a patient is discharged he should have a bath, and his hair should be washed. He should then be put into a clean bed if possible. All the articles which have been used for him will then be sterilized, and it is very important to see that such articles as the soap, the washcloth and toothbrush are burnt. The bed and bedding and floor should be dealt with as described on p. 31.

Relapse is comparatively common in some of the communicable diseases: the patient, when the symptoms of the first attack have subsided, entering upon a second course of the disease. This is usually less severe than the first attack; but, because the patient may be very anaemic and debilitated as a result of the first—particularly when relapse occurs after a long illness, such as typhoid fever—he may then be more seriously ill than during the first attack, because his powers of resistance are lower.

Return Case. This term is used to describe a communicable disease which occurs in a house or locality to which a patient has recently returned after hospital treatment for the same disease. For example, a patient who has had, and recovered from, scarlet fever returns home; within the incubation period—that is, within 10 days of his return—another person living in the same house contracts the disease and is taken to hospital. This is a *return case*, the infection being due, almost undoubtedly, to the fact that the patient who returned home was not free from infection.

PREVENTION OF CROSS INFECTION

(*See also Methods of Isolation, p.* 463.)

The term *Cross Infection* has been in use for many years to describe the contraction of a communicable disease or infection whilst a patient was suffering from another communicable disease. It has recently been extended to cover any infection acquired under hospital conditions.

Sources of cross infection in hospital. Any evident communicable disease or infective case; any infective case which may not have been diagnosed; any communicable disease which, during the incubation period (before the disease is diagnosed), is infectious, measles, for example. A carrier of disease.

Modes of conveying infection and control of infection. The skin, hair and nails of patients, staff, and hospital visitors are likely to be contaminated with infective secretions, excretions, discharges, and with dust from the floor, personal clothing and bedclothing. It is in order to avoid carrying infection in this way that nurses are provided with facilities for frequent and careful hand washing, and with lotion or cream for the care of the skin. The nurse's cap is not a badge of office, it is intended to cover the hair in order to protect it from contamination and from becoming a source of infection. The hair should be pinned up under the cap. The nails should be kept short and nail varnish should not be used. Wrist watches should not be worn when on duty.

Clothing. The personal clothing of patients becomes contaminated and that of nurses may do so. The handkerchiefs of those who harbour haemolytic streptococci in the nose and throat are serious sources of infection.

Bedclothing. When infection is disseminated, in particular from the respiratory tract and the skin, and to a lesser extent from gastro-intestinal infections and wounds, the bedclothing is heavily contaminated. Every possible precaution should be taken to handle bedclothes and pillows carefully so that dust is not raised (see also cleaning, below).

Laundry. Soiled linen is contaminated by secretions, excretions, discharges and dust. Very great care should be taken when handling it. Collection at the bedside should be into soiled linen canvas bags on wheeled frames. The bag should be sent to the laundry where it will be sorted and counted by porters or the laundry staff. Soiled linen should not be handled by nurses as this causes serious contamination of their dress and they thus become sources of infection to others. In certain cases of communicable disease soiled linen requires disinfection before it is laundered. Certain articles, such as handkerchiefs and pillow cases, from tuberculous patients should be boiled before they are washed. Infant's napkins should not be dealt with by nurses, they should be put into disinfectant fluid and sent to the laundry where they will be separately washed and they should always be boiled.

Furniture and Utensils. All articles used in a ward are contaminated. All ward furniture should be kept clean. All articles and utensils used should be sterilized between use. This necessitates having adequate equipment, which is a point that requires attention.

Food and milk readily grow bacteria, especially when not properly stored. All articles of food should be covered and stored in a cool place.

Flies are a serious source of spread of infection. Flies and their breeding places should be destroyed.

Toys, books and papers. Only washable toys should be provided. These should be tied to the head of the bed and the lead should not be long enough to allow the toys to fall on to the floor. Books and papers should not be passed from bed to bed.

Ward Cleaning. Bedmaking and sweeping raise dust and it has been shown that the air of the wards after these processes has a high bacterial content. The experience gained in the plastic surgical units has demonstrated the effective control obtained in this matter by the oiling of blankets and floorboards. But this measure is not always possible and a good deal can be accomplished by the use of scientific methods of sweeping and cleaning.

Dry sweeping should never be permitted. Damp sweeping and damp dusting are essential. Brooms, brushes and dusters should be soaked in disinfectant after use, then washed and dried. Nurses should not do the domestic work of a ward if they are responsible for patients' treatments and surgical dressings.

Floor dust and bedclothing are great sources of infection. Bedmaking disseminates organisms. Dry sweeping of floors fills the air with organisms. Bacterial examination of ward air taken after bedmaking and sweeping shows an increase of 150 to 200 times in the bacterial count.

Carriers of Disease. A 'convalescent carrier' is a person who is convalescent from a communicable disease or infection. A 'healthy carrier' is a person who harbours infectious organisms in his tissues in sufficient virulence to cause disease in others without himself falling a victim. These carriers are dangerous because they are not recognized and may pass unsuspected for a long time. Their danger can only be determined by bacteriological examination.

Both the segregation and the treatment of carriers has to be considered.

ersons who carry haemolytic streptococci in the throat should be sepa-ated from those liable to infection such as obstetric and surgical cases. arriers of diphtheria may be successfully treated by having the tonsils nd adenoids removed. But when the nasal mucous membrane is the ource of infection local applications of antiseptics may be tried.

In addition the general health of the person who is acting as carrier hould be attended to and any measures which will improve the condition dopted. During this period of treatment any test available will be made, om time to time, in order to ascertain when the individual ceases o be infectious.

MEASURES FOR THE PROTECTION OF THE NURSE

Control of droplet infection. Moist infective particles from the nose nd mouth may contaminate an object or surface directly by falling upon ; and less directly by being carried on particles in the air as in dust.

The patient who is suffering from an infection of the respiratory tract hould be taught to cover his nose and mouth when coughing and to void spraying moisture in speaking and laughing.

The nurse should develop a regime when nursing patients suffering from espiratory infections. She should not get her face near to the patient's ace, turn his head to one side when performing any treatments for him, isualize the range of droplet infection and avoid directly facing the atient. *Face masks* should be worn so that she does not spread infection om her nose and mouth when attending to babies and infants, when reparing feeds for infants, when preparing and performing surgical ressings, and when attending to the nose and throat of a patient.

Face masks must cover the nose and mouth, they must be of adequate hickness, they should be placed in disinfectant after use, and boiled and vashed. If possible they should never be used a second time; if this is ot possible then the inside of the mask should be clearly marked. Masks should *not* be kept in the pocket.

Ventilation and bed spacing. Free and good ventilation will go a long way owards preventing droplet-borne infection. Wards should be thoroughly ired after bedmaking, sweeping and dusting. The windows should be pen as much as possible. Thorough airing should precede closing down or the night.

Bed spacing is important, and if droplet-borne infection is to be pre-ented the distance between beds should not be less than 8 feet. In naternity units, hospitals receiving communicable diseases, and children's vards the space should be not less than the 12 feet recommended by the Ministry of Health. The distance is calculated from bed centre to bed centre.

The nurse has to realize that she may become infected, and then she is erself a source of infection to other people. It is for this reason she wears n overall when in the sickroom. She may move about the usual offices uch as the lavatory, w.c. and her own bedroom in her nurse's dress, but he should not go into the living room or the dining room or leave the ouse unless she is wearing her private dress. If she writes letters or does ny sewing in the sickroom, these articles must be disinfected before they eave the room. She could disinfect them by boiling some formalin solu-ion 1 per cent in a kettle in the room and holding the articles in the steam rom this until they are thoroughly saturated.

The nurse must maintain a high standard of general health. She mu take her meals regularly, and if possible elsewhere than in the sickroon It may not, however, always be possible to have a separate room at h disposal for this, but in that case she might have her meals in her ow room. She should attend to minor ailments when these occur, and kee her skin free from abrasions and cracks.

If the patient is suffering from typhoid fever or any other disease i which the excreta are known to be infectious, the nurse should be ver particular to wash not only her hands but her face before eating, and t handle her food as little as possible.

COMMUNICABLE DISEASE IN A PRIVATE HOUSE

It is interesting to note that the majority of nurses to be found on th private nursing staffs of hospitals and institutions have been drawn fror general hospitals and have had very little, if any, experience of commun cable diseases, and yet the first case to which a nurse will be called ma possibly be one of this nature. It behoves her therefore to consider ver carefully what she will do in these circumstances. The relatives and every body with whom she comes in contact will expect her to be a fount c information and resource in the difficulty in which they find themselve placed.

The *choice of a room* is important; if possible the aspect should be south west, and the room should be well lit and ventilated. A fireplace in th room is valuable, as by means of it waste food, dressings, letters, etc., ca be destroyed. The room should be as far as possible from the living room and near to a bathroom and w.c., and also near the nurse's bedroom. A little furniture as possible should be retained in the room and the wal should be equally bare. A bed will be necessary, one or two tables, a chai or two, a small chest of drawers and some shelves on which feeding uten sils, etc. can be kept. The patient's washing basin, toilet articles and sani tary utensils should all be kept in the sickroom, and a pail in which th nurse can carry waste water, disinfected laundry, and so on, from th room. Near the door, either just outside or just inside, should be place provision for the nurse and doctor to wash their hands. This provisio should include a bowl of disinfectant solution and a nailbrush. Coat should be provided for the doctor and nurse, and for visitors in case o necessity. A sheet hung outside the door may be found to give the relative confidence. In any case it acts as a reminder that the room is not to b entered and that its occupant is isolated.

In the nursing management of this patient it is an important point tha articles once in the room remain there and do not leave it—therefore, i receiving food from the kitchen the nurse might have a table just outsid the door on which the utensils are placed, then having removed her gow and washed her hands she could transfer the food from the kitchen utensil to the patient's utensils, without contaminating those from the kitchen.

The nurse will do all the domestic work required in the patient's bed room. She will sweep and dust it, attend to the fireplace, wash up all th crockery in the room, carrying the waste water to the lavatory and empty ing it as she would excreta. Unless excreta are a source of infection th nurse empties them into the w.c. pan, without soiling the sides more tha she can help. She pours some disinfectant round the sides of the basi fterwards and then pulls the plug. All discarded food and used swabs hould, if possible, be burnt in the room. The ashes from the fireplace, which he nurse attends to herself, she will collect in a piece of paper and transer to the dustbin. The nurse will be responsible that infection is not coneyed to the public through the medium of laundry. Soiled clothing from he patient's bedroom, including doctors' and nurses' gowns, should be oaked in some disinfectant, such as carbolic acid, 1–40, for several hours efore it is dispatched. The laundress should be notified that she is to eceive wet disinfected laundry, and that proper precautions have been aken to prevent infection.

Visitors. The same precautions will be taken regarding visitors as desribed on p. 464. It is always inadvisable to permit children to visit an nfectious patient.

Terminal disinfection. This is carried out as previously described see p. 465), the patient having his head washed, being bathed and put nto a clean bed, and if possible into a clean fresh bedroom.

The room he has occupied will then be available for disinfection. The edding should all be sent to be steam disinfected, including any other eavy articles such as pillows or rugs he may have used. Personal clothing nd bedclothes left in the room should be disinfected before going to the aundry. As a rule it is sufficient if the walls are swept and washed, the loor scrubbed, and all furniture washed with hot water and soap. All the tensils which have been used should be boiled, and all toilet accessories, f possible, burnt. In a few instances it is necessary to strip the wallpaper nd subject the room to fumigation; but as a rule this will be ordered by he doctor and attended to by the local sanitary authorities.

Chapter 32

Communicable Diseases (Particularly of Childhood)

Diphtheria—Scarlet fever—Measles—German measles—Whooping cough—Mumps—Chickenpox—Smallpox

Patients suffering with the diseases treated in this chapter are gene ally nursed in a hospital for communicable diseases or fever hospita but the nurse working in other types of hospitals may meet the also. A child, for example, may develop any of these diseases which mig necessitate putting a ward into quarantine. Every nurse should be awa of the symptoms of onset of each of these diseases and of the dangers an complications likely to result from an attack.

Many of the communicable diseases are responsible for a number the septic nasal and aural conditions, and the cardiac and rheumat diseases met with in general practice.

DIPHTHERIA

Diphtheria is diagnosed by taking a swab from the affected area an discovering the causative organism which is a rod-shaped bacillus—th *Klebs-Loeffler bacillus* or *Corynebacterium diphtheriae.*

Infection is direct or indirect. The disease may be conveyed by milk an by carriers. The *incubation period* is from 2 to 4 days, with extreme limits c from 1 to 6 days. The fauces are the part most commonly affected, an the disease may spread to the larynx or the nose; any mucous membran may be affected and diphtheria has been known to infect wounds.

Faucial diphtheria. The *onset* is short, but more insidious than that c scarlet fever, and the throat in diphtheria may not be very sore. Th patient suffers from malaise and may complain of headache, and ther may be a slight rise of temperature.

A *greyish-yellow membrane* forms on the fauces, and it is firmly adheren just as a slough would be. There is a little inflammation around the mem branous area and the lymphatic glands beneath the jaw may be enlarge and tender. The temperature may remain elevated for a few days, and i cases complicated by sepsis it is more marked.

In diphtheria the organisms remain at the site of the lesion, pourin their toxins into the blood stream, and this results in marked toxaemi characterized by a soft pulse of low volume since the blood pressure is low while the patient lies listless and pale, obviously uninterested by anythin that is going on around him.

It is in the *complications* which may occur during the course of diphtheri that the danger lies. *Spread of infection* downwards to the larynx and up wards to the nose increases the severity of the disease, and the gravity o the toxaemia which is depressing the heart may result in *cardiac failure, denitis* and *otitis media* may occur, and in the later days *post-diphtheritic paralysis* is to be anticipated in all severe cases.

The **treatment** is the early administration of the specific, antidiphtheritic serum. It is given in doses of from 3,000 to 100,000 units, an average dose is from 15,000 to 30,000 units. Penicillin in large doses is given in conjunction with serum treatment.

In the routine nursing care the danger of cardiac failure must be ever borne in mind. The patient should be nursed flat, with one low pillow or without a pillow; he may not move to do anything for himself. He should never be allowed to become constipated but only the mildest of laxatives, such as liquid paraffin, may be employed, or small lubricating enemata. It is necessary to be constantly on the watch for signs of muscular paralysis; *palatal paralysis* may be manifested by a slight catch on drinking, by difficulty in speaking certain words and by a slightly nasal intonation.

Either *ptosis* or *squint* may be observed, or the patient may be seen to have lost eye accommodation, and he may sometimes be seen to push an article farther away from him when he wants to look at it.

The slightest indication of paralysis suggests that the toxaemia has been severe and calls for greater and more prolonged rest, for fear lest the dreaded complication of cardiac failure should arise.

The rest necessary at the outset should be only gradually encroached upon as uncomplicated convalescence progresses. The patient may gradually be elevated from the recumbent position and allowed to sit propped up, and at the end of two weeks he may be allowed some little recreation in bed—reading, writing or playing a game.

Intubation and *tracheotomy* may be necessary for the relief of symptoms in laryngeal diphtheria, and these procedures are described on pp. 742–3.

Schick's test is used to determine the susceptibility of a person to diphtheria. A small quantity of diluted diphtheria toxin is injected intradermally into the skin, usually of the forearm, while a control injection, consisting of the same quantity of the solution, heated to about 160° F. in order to destroy the toxins, is injected into the skin of the opposite forearm. The result may be as follows:

(1) A *positive reaction*, which would indicate that the person was susceptible to diphtheria, would be an area of redness appearing within 48 hours and fading after a few days, to be followed by desquamation of the skin. The control arm remains unaffected.

(2) In a *negative reaction* both arms would be unaffected. If both arms are slightly and equally affected, the reaction would be due to serum proteins and not to the toxin. This is called a *pseudo-reaction.*

(3) A *combined reaction* sometimes occurs, and this is manifested by a pseudo-reaction as described above on the control arm, with a true reaction as described in the first instance on the arm on which the test was employed.

Diphtheria is a serious and too frequently fatal disease and nurses should do all they can to encourage the protection of children by immunization which can be performed by inoculation with one of the following.

Alum-precipitated-toxoid. (A.P.T.) A dose of 0·2 c.c. is given, followed 4 weeks later by a second dose of 0·5 c.c. But in cases which show undue reaction only the smaller preliminary dose is repeated. The injections are given into the deltoid muscle.

Toxoid-Antitoxin Floccules (T.A.F.) is a mixture of toxoid and antitoxin which results in a suspended precipitate, hence the inclusion of the term *floccules*. This prophylactic gives the very minimum of local reaction and it is therefore recommended for adults actively engaged in work. Three doses of 1 c.c. are given at intervals of 2 or 3 weeks.

Toxoid-antitoxin (T.A.M.) is also used for adults but much less often than T.A.F. Three intramuscular injections of 1 mil. are given at intervals of 2 or 3 weeks.

Active immunity takes several weeks or even a couple of months to develop, but alternatively passive immunity may be employed to protect those who have been in contact with diphtheria by the injection of 1,000 to 2,000 units of diphtheria antitoxin.

SCARLET FEVER

Scarlet fever is a very highly communicable disease due to a haemolytic streptococcus—*Streptococcus scarlatinae.*

Infection is direct or indirect. The disease may be conveyed by milk and by carriers. The secretions are infectious and so is any exudate or discharge from the body cavities or from cracks or abrasions of the skin. The *incubation period* is from 1 to 7 days, with an average of from 2 to 4 days.

Symptoms. The *onset* is sudden, with headache, sore throat, vomiting and a rapidly rising temperature up to 103° or 104° F., and marked increase of pulse rate, 120 or over. In adults there may be an attack of shivering, and in children convulsions may occur.

The tongue and the throat. The tongue is covered with a thick white fur and the throat is red and injected. On the second day red papillae show through this fur, giving the typical strawberry tongue. The tongue peels.

The *rash appears on the second day*, covering the sides of the neck and chest and spreading over the trunk and limbs. The face is flushed and the circumoral region characteristically pale. The rash is composed of minute points and is scarlet in colour; it is described as a punctate erythema and lasts from a few hours to a few days, being followed by desquamation, skin rubbing off from the sides of the neck like powder; at the end of a week little pinhole breaches occur in the skin over the front of the trunk; later, the skin separates at the tips of the fingers, and then larger pieces of skin come off from the hands and feet.

During the febrile stage the patient suffers from marked malaise, headache, loss of appetite, his urine is scanty and high coloured and constipation is present.

The *complications* of scarlet fever are adenitis, rhinitis, otitis media, arthritis, nephritis and endocarditis.

Treatment. The specific treatment of scarlet fever cases is the administration of antiscarlatina serum, which is given in doses of from 20 to 30 c.c., intramuscularly and in the more severe cases into a vein. Penicillin is given, combined with serum therapy. Complications are treated by penicillin and/or sulphonamides.

It is usual to keep the patient in bed for 21 days in order to avoid the complication of nephritis; he should be kept warm, and receive a liberal supply of fluid; and his urine should be tested daily for albumin. The symptoms are dealt with as they arise, complications are anticipated and treated should they occur.

Dick's test. This test is employed in order to determine the susceptibility of a person to scarlet fever. It is carried out by the intradermal injection of a small quantity of diluted scarlet fever toxin, in the way described in the case of the Schick test (see p. 471), a control area being similarly used.

The result may be:

(1) A *positive reaction*, shown as a patch of redness at the site of the injection, occurring approximately within 24 hours with no change on the control area.

(2) A *negative reaction* shows no change on either area. In a *pseudo-reaction* slight inflammatory changes occur on both areas due to protein irritation.

(3) In a *combined reaction*, as in the case of the Schick test, a pseudo-reaction occurs on the control arm and a true reaction on the test arm.

Schultz-Charlton's test. The Schultz-Charlton reaction, which is sometimes described as the *blanching test*, is used as an aid to diagnosis in suspected cases of scarlet fever in which a rash is present. A minute quantity of dilute scarlet fever antitoxin is injected intradermally where the rash is bright. A *positive reaction* would be demonstrated by the blanching of an area of the rash around the site of injection, and the area blanched may be the size of a two-shilling piece.

A *negative reaction* need not necessarily mean that the case is not one of scarlet fever—it is in its positive reaction that this test is valuable.

Immunisation to scarlet fever may be produced either passively or actively. A preliminary Dick test is performed to detect susceptible subjects.

Active immunity can be produced by the subcutaneous injection of graduated doses of streptococcal toxin at intervals of a week or longer. Several doses are necessary. Local and general reactions follow and it is thought that immunity is developed within a month and will last for from six months to a lifetime, with an average duration of two years.

Passive immunity can be produced by the injection intramuscularly of a small amount (5 to 10 c.c.) of streptococcal antitoxin. This immunity is believed to last from 10 to 14 days and is of value in persons who have been exposed to the infection.

Chemoprophylaxis is now recommended as producing better results as an alternative to passive immunization.

Repeated exposure to the disease helps to maintain immunity.

MEASLES

Measles or *morbilli* is a highly communicable disease which is responsible for a large percentage of deaths among infants and young children, and all nurses should realize that children must be protected from this dread disease; not every child has measles and the idea in the minds of some members of the lay public that a child had better have it and get it over is deplorable. A delicate child is very likely to develop broncho-pneumonia which is a serious and often fatal complication of measles.

Infection. The disease is spread by direct and indirect means, and, as the infectivity is high, few persons escape if they are exposed to infection. The *incubation period* is from 10 to 14 days, but it may be longer in those who have been immunized.

Symptoms. The *onset of measles* is manifested by catarrh of the upper respiratory passages; there is sneezing, running at the nose (coryza), watery eyes, intolerance of light (photophobia) and a tendency to conjunctivitis. The patient is hoarse and has a short dry cough, due to an inflammatory condition of the larynx which may spread down the bronchial tubes and give rise to bronchitis and broncho-pneumonia.

A *prodomal rash*, which is sometimes the only rash present, occurs during the catarrhal stage. It is known as *Koplik's spots*, which are bluish-pearly-white spots seen on the buccal surface of the membrane of the mouth.

The *typical picture of a patient with measles* is seen when the true rash appears on the fourth day, beginning at the roots of the hair and behind the ears and spreading over the face, trunk and limbs. The eyelids are swollen and heavy, the patient is very miserable, the heaviness of his eyelids is wearying and he is unable to tolerate any direct light upon his eyes.

The *characteristic rash* of measles is macular; it appears in irregular patches which give a blotchy appearance to the skin. It lasts 2 or 3 days and then fades, leaving the skin slightly stained but the staining disappears after about a week.

The *temperature* rises at the outset of the catarrhal stage, and then declines, to rise again when the rash appears, and eventually declines as the rash fades. The pulse is increased in rate, but not markedly so; it is the increase in the rate of respiration which is characteristic of measles, and this is due to the inflammatory condition of the respiratory tract. The patient is restless, tossing about in bed, and sometimes delirious during the febrile stage.

Complications. It is in the complications that the danger lies in measles. Some degree of *laryngitis and bronchitis* will be present in most cases; *broncho-pneumonia* may arise. A little *conjunctivitis* is invariably present, and a more serious degree may occur; *corneal ulcer* may complicate measles, especially in debilitated subjects. *Otitis media, enteritis and cancrum oris* are other possible complications.

Treatment. A *serum* is now obtainable which is taken from cases who are convalescent from measles, or from young adults who have had measles during recent years. It is used, partly as a prophylactic measure, but more particularly to protect delicate children who have been exposed to the disease and who may have entered the incubation period. Alternatively *gamma globulin* may be given. When given before the seventh day the attack may be prevented, when given after the seventh day, although the attack may not be avoided it will render it less severe.

In the nursing care of measles the room should be warm, from 62° to 65° F., and it should be well ventilated, the patient being kept very warm in bed, which should not be facing the light, and having his chest and back rubbed with warm camphorated oil at night, and wearing a warm woollen vest. In cases where bronchial catarrh is marked, it may be necessary to moisten the air in the room by the use of a steam kettle. The eyes should be bathed morning and evening, and oftener if there is any discharge. Care should be taken to prevent a child with measles from picking his nose, rubbing his eyes or irritating any part of his body where the rash is thick.

In most cases fluid diet will be given whilst there is a rise of temperature; afterwards the diet should be light and very nourishing; the patient ought to stay in bed for a week after the temperature has declined, and be kept in a warm well-ventilated room for several days after he gets up; he may then be allowed out of doors during the warmest part of the day provided he is warmly clad.

GERMAN MEASLES

Rubella, Rötheln or *German measles*, which is a much milder disease than measles, occurs most commonly after the age of ten and until the end of adolescence.

Infection is by direct contact with a patient, by means of *droplet infection*; it is rarely conveyed by indirect means. The *incubation period* is from 14 to 19 days (average 17–18 days).

Symptoms. The *onset of the disease* may pass unnoticed, or it may be that the patient has slight malaise, sore throat and headache. The *rash*, which is often the first sign noticed, occurs on the second day of disease and is rose coloured; it begins in the same way as the rash of measles, behind the ears and at the roots of the hair, but it differs from measles in being a much finer rash. It fades in about 24 hours and leaves no staining.

The other symptoms are not severe. The conjunctiva of the eyes is slightly injected, but the eyelids are not heavy as in measles. The throat is slightly sore and there may be a short dry cough for a day or two; the temperature may rise to 99° or 100° F., but rarely higher than this. One sign, which is characteristic, is enlargement of the suboccipital group of lymphatic glands, which lie above the nape of the neck, at the margin where the occipital bone can be distinctly felt. They may be felt as little hard roundish lumps, and it is worth remembering that these glands are also swollen in the case of a head infected with lice.

As a rule there are no complications in rubella, and ordinary nursing care is all that is necessary whilst the patient is in bed.

WHOOPING COUGH

Whooping cough or *pertussis* is a communicable disease which usually attacks children. It is caused by the *Bordet-Gengou bacillus* or *Haemophilus pertussis*.

Infection may be direct or less often indirect. It is most usually spread by *droplet infection* or infection by means of very recently used feeding utensils, handkerchiefs, and articles the child may have had in his mouth, such as a pencil, which will be covered with moist infective particles. The disease is infective from the moment the catarrhal stage begins, and the *incubation period* is from the moment of infection until the onset of the catarrhal stage, 7 to 14 days.

Whooping cough is divided into the catarrhal and the spasmodic stages, and the stage of convalescence. The *catarrhal stage* is manifested by a short dry cough, coryza and bronchitis. There may be a slight rise in temperature, the child's sleep is disturbed by coughing, and at the end of two weeks the typical paroxysms of whooping cough will usually be present.

Paroxysms of coughing may occur only once or twice in 24 hours, or they may occur frequently about every hour, though this is less usual. A *typical attack of coughing* begins with several short coughs following one another so rapidly that there is no time for the child to inspire. A forcible indrawing of air then occurs, which produces the characteristic whoop. The attack may be repeated, the child sits up in his cot, clings to the side of it, tears stream from his eyes, mucus runs from his nose and mouth and his tongue is protruded against his lower teeth. The child's face becomes deeply cyanosed and may become oedematous; he may pass urine and faeces involuntarily, epistaxis may occur or bleeding into the conjunctiva or into the tissues around the eye. In adults there may be cerebral haemorrhage. Rupture of the pleura may occur, causing spontaneous pneumothorax. The attack of whooping may end in vomiting. The child falls back very exhausted after a severe paroxysm.

Paroxysms occur with greatest frequency during the night, when whooping cough is always at its worst and, as this is when the first whoop is heard, in a suspected case the night nurse should be particularly observant. The attacks of coughing continue for several weeks, and in a case of moderate severity abatement may be expected after 6 weeks from the commencement of the illness. Improvement is fairly rapid when convalescence begins, and the child quickly recovers the ground he has lost.

Complications. *Laryngitis* and *bronchitis* occur in most severe cases, but *broncho-pneumonia* is the complication which is most dreaded, since it is as serious in its effect with whooping cough as it is with measles, and is the cause of death to many children. *Emphysema*, *asthma* and *pulmonary tuberculosis* may be sequelae of whooping cough.

Apart from the complications already mentioned, a large group of conditions may arise from mechanical causes. *Prolapse of rectum* may occur, and *umbilical hernia* may be caused by increase in intra-abdominal tension during a paroxysm of coughing. A *sublingual ulcer* may be produced by the sawing action of the tongue against the lower incisors when the tongue is protruded during coughing. *Convulsions* may occur during, or at the end of, a paroxysm. *Emaciation* due to wasting of the tissues is present in cases where vomiting invariably follows frequent attacks of coughing.

Treatment. *Vaccine treatment* is employed with success in many cases. *Belladonna* and *ephedrine* are used to reduce the spasm in the respiratory passages. *Luminal* is given to control the cough. *Penicillin* is given by injection and the use of a penicillin test is advocated. Sulphonamides will prevent complications.

The *nursing care* of a child with whooping cough is very important. The room should be warm and the child kept well covered because of the tendency to develop broncho-pneumonia. It is usual to keep the child in bed during the catarrhal stage, but later he may be allowed up. He should live in a well-ventilated room and may be taken out during the warmest parts of the day, provided he is properly wrapped up and does not get cold. The chest should be rubbed, back and front, with warm camphorated oil at night. Support of the child is essential during an attack of coughing, and a tiny infant should be lifted and supported, as he needs to be helped to get the mucus and expectoration from his mouth. An older child should be trained to support himself, and to use a bowl for his sputum and vomit. All secretion and vomit, as it is infectious, should be disposed of as quickly as possible. A binder round the abdomen will help to prevent an umbilical hernia, and the child should never be allowed to have an attack of coughing while sitting on a chamber, as this position would predispose to prolapse of rectum.

Feeding is very important, and diluted milk and glucose drinks should be given during the febrile and catarrhal stage. Subsequently the diet should be nourishing and easily digested. A child who vomits after frequent attacks of coughing will become very wasted unless the precaution of feeding him immediately after an attack is taken. The vomiting induced by coughing is not necessarily accompanied by nausea or by any disinclination for food; it is a mechanical result of a bad attack of coughing.

A child in whooping cough may be so fatigued and disinclined for exertion that he will not want to take his food, but he must be encouraged and coaxed, and even spoiled a little, and may be given anything he will take.

Isolation is necessary from the commencement of the catarrhal stage, and it should be continued until this has abated, and in most cases until the whoop is no longer heard.

MUMPS

Mumps or *specific parotitis* is a communicable disease characterized by swelling of the salivary glands, which is most noticeable in the parotid, because of its position in front of and below the ear. It occurs in adolescence but is rarely met with in infancy.

Infection is usually direct, from contact with a patient, but indirect infection can also occur. *Incubation period*, 12 to 30 days, usually 17 to 18 days.

Symptoms. The *onset* of the disease is accompanied by vague symptoms of malaise, and characterized after a day or two by the typical swelling of the parotid gland, usually on one side, the other side beginning to swell three or four days later. The skin over the swollen glands is tender, and there is difficulty in opening the mouth; the secretion of saliva causes pain, which would be accentuated on any stimulation, and for this reason acid fluids such as lemonade, which tend to increase salivation, are contraindicated. When both sides are very swollen great discomfort is experienced, and this may be accompanied by a slight rise in temperature.

Metastatic swelling of the sex glands and the pancreas may complicate mumps in adolescents and adults; *orchitis* sometimes occurs in males and *mastitis* and *ovaritis* in females.

Pancreatitis, which is very rare, is serious and accompanied by colicky abdominal pain.

Other complications include *suppuration of the affected salivary glands, otitis media, deafness, arthritis and meningitis.*

Treatment. The patient is isolated and kept in bed until the swelling of the glands has subsided and the temperature, if any, abated; 10–14 days in bed is the average time necessary. Keeping a patient in bed during this period should prevent the appearance of the metastatic swellings mentioned above.

Feeding is a little difficult; the patient can usually swallow if he can get the food into his mouth; he may have any food he can take but articles of diet likely to stimulate the flow of saliva should be omitted, and it is cruel to allow the patient to see or smell such things as oranges. The mouth should be kept clean and the glands wrapped in hot wool whilst they are tender. Any local application should be light as the least touch causes acute pain during the inflammatory stage. Ordinary routine nursing measures are all that will be required. The patient should be isolated for three weeks, and for one full week after the swelling has subsided.

CHICKENPOX

Chickenpox, or *varicella*, which is a most highly communicable disease, is one of the two examples in which the rash appears in successive crops—the other example being typhoid fever.

Infection is direct or indirect, and the disease is infectious from the commencement of the illness, before the rash appears, until the last scab separates. The *incubation period* is from 10 to 21 days, with an average of 14–18 days. Infection may also follow contact with a case of herpes zoster.

Symptoms. The *onset* may be so slight as to pass unnoticed, and the rash, as it appears after 24 hours, is often the first sign observed. The *rash of chickenpox* is vesicular, each vesicle containing inflammatory exudate, and when the vesicles first appear they are bright and shining, but after a few hours lose this shimmering effect and become dull. The rash appears first on the body, inside the mouth and on the scalp. In a day or two some lesions of the rash will be seen to have become slightly purulent, others have dried and scaled off; the purulent ones will form scabs, which will separate later. As the rash spreads, most of the body will be covered, and it is also seen on the face.

Crops of the rash appear daily for several days, so that it is quite usual to see clear vesicles, vesicles filled with purulent fluid, dried vesicles scaling off and scabs—all on the same area of skin.

The temperature may be raised a little, but this depends on the density of the rash and the amount of pus present. The rash is irritating and the patient is inclined to rub and scratch the irritable area, and this causes the scabs to be knocked off, delays healing and may result in scarring.

Treatment. The patient is kept in bed for the first week or two, and ordinary nursing measures will be necessary; in addition the precaution of having non-irritating clothing next to the skin should be taken. When the rash is very irritable bathing with weak carbolic lotion, or dusting with an astringent powder and applying an ointment containing a mild antiseptic may give relief.

Complications are rare; in debilitated children *gangrenous pocks* may develop, and *impetigo* may arise as a secondary infection.

SMALLPOX

Smallpox or *variola* is an acute very highly communicable disease, and as it is very likely to be confused with chickenpox a nurse should know how these diseases differ.

Infection is direct and indirect. One attack gives immunity for life, and it is considered that vaccination in infancy, repeated at the age of 12 years, will give complete immunity in most cases, while in others these precautions will considerably modify the attack should the disease be contracted. The *incubation period* is from 10–14 days, with an average of 12 days. If a person is exposed to infection, vaccination should be performed; within the first 2 or 3 days it will prevent the attack, and up to the sixth day it will afford some degree of protection.

Symptoms. The *onset of smallpox* could never possibly be confused with chickenpox, because in smallpox the patient is very ill, suffers from headache, pains in the back and limbs, vomits, runs a high temperature and is very seriously prostrated. This continues for 2 or 3 days, and then the *rash* appears. Unlike the rash of chickenpox, that of smallpox appears in stages. A papular eruption appears on the face, hands and feet on the third day of disease, whereas in chickenpox the rash appears first on the trunk and upper parts of the limbs and is centripetal in distribution, while that of smallpox, appearing on the face, hands, forearms and feet, is centrifugal.

Another difference is that in chickenpox the papular stage is so short that it is usually not noticed, whilst in smallpox the papular eruption which appears on the third day persists until the fifth or sixth day, when the papules become vesicles; these remain until the eighth to tenth day and then become pustular. After the twelfth day the pustules begin to dry up and form scabs.

In chickenpox the skin is clear around the rash, but in smallpox there is a surrounding area of induration.

The lesions in smallpox are round, and lie embedded in the skin; in chickenpox the lesions are oval, and lie on the skin. If a vesicle in chickenpox is pricked, it will be seen to collapse; in smallpox, collapse will not occur, as each vesicle is bilocular.

To recapitulate: *the rash of smallpox* appears in stages:

On the third day—papules.
On the sixth day—vesicles.
On the ninth day—pustules.
On the twelfth day—the rash begins to form scabs.

The scabs have usually all separated within about 6 weeks.

The *temperature in smallpox* is high at the onset of the disease, but declines when the rash first appears and then rises again, once again becoming very high when the pustular stage begins, as this is accompanied by serious prostration and toxaemia. This period is called the 'stage of secondary fever'. The temperature is high, 104° F. or over, the pulse rapid, and breathing usually distressed; in most cases there is some laryngitis and bronchitis. The patient becomes delirious, is unable to sleep, and lies plucking at the bedclothes, markedly prostrated and exhausted.

In cases terminating favourably the temperature declines, and the toxaemia grows less as the patient's general condition improves, but he now enters a very trying and difficult period of convalescence, as when crusts form, and the scabs gradually and slowly separate, this is accompanied by considerable irritation. The patient is faced with the knowledge that his skin will be pockmarked, and that it will be discoloured for many months. He requires constant encouragement to help him face the long isolation period which must pass before the last scab has separated.

Varieties of Smallpox. *Modified smallpox* occurs in those who are partly protected by vaccination, persons who have probably not been revaccinated. The symptoms in these cases are milder.

Discrete smallpox describes the mildest form of unmodified smallpox when the lesions, or 'pocks', remain separate.

Confluent smallpox describes the more severe forms where the rash is thick and the individual lesions coalesce. The accompanying symptoms are severe.

Malignant or *haemorrhagic smallpox* is very severe and is characterized by bleeding under the skin and from the mucous membrane. The rash is haemorrhagic in character.

Alastrim or *variola minor* is a form which becomes prevalent in countries where protective measures against smallpox are taken or where the majority of persons are immunized. This type may occur in epidemics, but the symptoms are mild.

Complications are numerous. *Laryngitis*, *bronchitis* and *broncho-pneumonia* are comparatively common. *Conjunctivitis* occurs in most serious cases, and really bad ones are complicated by *iritis* and *corneal ulcer*. Sepsis results in *otitis media*, *adenitis*, *boils*, *carbuncles* and *abscesses*. *Bedsores* are very common, especially if the parts of the skin on which the patient lies are covered by the rash. *Hyperpyrexia* occurs during the stage of secondary fever; *albuminuria* is present during the febrile stage and *nephritis* and *uraemia* may occur. *Abortion* occurs in pregnant women.

Treatment. The description of the serious degree of illness through which the patient passes when the disease is at its height, followed by the period of depression when the scabs are separating, suggests the lines of nursing care which are necessary. The possibility of each complication mentioned should be borne in mind, and means taken to keep the mouth, eyes, nose and ears as clean as possible; while keeping the skin free of exudate from the ruptured discharging pustules will go far to prevent the complications that might be due to sepsis.

The patient should be nursed in an airy, warm room; his diet should be nourishing and fluids given freely; his urine should be tested for albumin daily and his bowels kept in regular action. The application of an icebag will help to relieve the constant headache, and sponging will reduce fever and also help to keep the skin clean. The application of antiseptic fomentations to the discharging pustules will assist in clearing them; large pustules should be opened by incision with scissors, curved on the flat, followed by the application of fomentations. Frequent sponging and hot bathing is of value in assisting the scabs to separate. Sulphonamides and penicillin are used to prevent complications.

PROPHYLAXIS

Vaccination is the only efficient way of preventing smallpox. Edward Jenner of Gloucester observed that dairy maids who contracted cowpox from animals did not get smallpox, and from this observation routine vaccination with calf lymph was developed.

Vaccinia or *cowpox* is the disease or condition which is transmitted to man when he is vaccinated, by inoculation with calf lymph, in order to protect him from smallpox.

Healthy calves or alternatively sheep and rabbits are inoculated on the skin of the abdomen; 96 hours later a crop of vesicles appears, the exudate is collected and made into an emulsion with glycerine and put up in phials ready for use. Chick embryo suspension is also employed.

The operation of vaccination is carried out under strict aseptic technique. The skin of the area, arm or leg, is carefully cleansed; but care must be taken that antiseptics are not used; it should be well washed, cleansed with alcohol and washed again with sterile water, and then rubbed dry with a sterile towel.

The physician takes the capillary tube which contains the prepared calf lymph, breaks off each end and, by means of a small rubber blower, spreads the lymph on the prepared skin. He slightly scarifies the skin—through the lymph—but does not draw blood. When dry the area is covered by dry sterile gauze.

The course of vaccinia. An *incubation period* of three days elapses and then, if the vaccination 'takes', red papules appear; by the fifth day these change to vesicles, and by the eighth day the contents become purulent. At this stage there is a definite area of induration around the crop of pustules; this lasts a few days and the pustules then begin to dry. The scab separates in less than three weeks, a pink scar remains, which gradually fades to white. The surface of a vaccination scar is stippled.

Treatment. In the case of a vaccinated person it is all important to keep the area covered with sterile gauze, and to prevent the occurrence of any secondary infection. The vesicles and pustules should be protected against the possibility of being knocked and ruptured, and the best result will be obtained if they scab off, uninjured. If the whole arm is swollen during the stage of maturation it should be carried in a sling and hot fomentations may be necessary, and if a leg shows marked inflammation the patient should rest in bed for a few days. A saline aperient is given on the third day.

Complications are rare. The danger of *secondary infection* has already been mentioned. A mild degree of *adenitis* may arise in the neighbouring lymphatic glands. *Erysipelas* may occur.

Revaccination. *Primary vaccination* is usually performed at the age of from 2 to 6 months. *Revaccination* is recommended at the age of from 7 to 14 years. It is significant that in countries where revaccination is systematically practised smallpox has been entirely stamped out.

Chapter 33

Louse-borne Diseases

Introduction—Epidemic typhus fever—Epidemic relapsing fever—Trench fever

The three diseases described below are transmitted by lice, as the term *louse-borne infection* implies. They tend to occur when louse infestation of the population increases as happens under conditions of war. It would be ideal to prevent the conditions under which these diseases prevail, but whilst this is not always possible, prophylactic measures, which consist of thorough disinfestation or 'delousing' of the patient and as far as possible of contacts, and the use of protective clothing by doctors, nurses, and attendants, should always be employed.

PROPHYLAXIS

The measures which can be used should an epidemic occur include the following:

(1) The *disease is made notifiable* to the Medical Officer of Health.
(2) *Specially trained teams* to deal with an outbreak would be organized.
(3) The services of medical men well versed in the early recognition and treatment of typhus would be requisitioned.
(4) *Protective clothing* consisting of a one-piece garment closed by zip-fasteners, with gloves and gumboots would be available for the use of doctors, nurses and attendants handling patients prior to, and during, delousing.
(5) In conveying cases from house or camp to hospital it is recommended that the *patient should be enveloped in a sheet* over his own clothing, as lice do not move easily on smooth fabric and by this precaution infected lice may be immobilized.

Delousing must be thorough. The hair of axillae, pubes, and any other parts covered with hair such as abdomen, chest and limbs must be shaved, and in men the hair of the head is cropped. The eyebrows and eyelashes should be carefully examined for lice. After delousing an infested person the attendants strip, bath and put on clean clothing. Their infested clothing is disinfected and disinfested.

A synthetic preparation known as D.D.T. is employed both as a powder and in liquid form. It destroys insects at all stages of development and was successfully employed in preventing an epidemic of typhus fever in Naples in 1943. The use of D.D.T. has revolutionized and simplified the prophylactic measures recommended in louse-borne infections.

EPIDEMIC TYPHUS FEVER (*Jail fever*)

Typhus fever is conveyed from sick to healthy persons by the body louse, and also probably by the head louse. This disease has been epidemic throughout centuries, and tends to spread in conditions of famine and here there is overcrowding and lack of sanitation. It is due to one of e Rickettsia bodies—*Rickettsia prowazeki*, named after Drs. Ricketts and n Prowazek.

The **course of the disease** is of about 3 weeks' duration. The *in-bation period* is from 5 to 21 days. The *onset* is sudden with severe head-che and general pains, marked prostration and characteristic mental rpor. The *rash* appears between the 3rd and 6th days as red papules ver chest, abdomen and trunk, and spreads to the limbs. On fading a aining is left. In some cases there is desquamation. The rash may be aemorrhagic. The *tongue* is furred. The *temperature* is high—104° to 106° F. r more; this persists for about 12 days and declines rapidly. The *pulse rate* also increased, but not proportionate with the degree of temperature.

There are two characteristic features:

(1) The *blood pressure is markedly low*, so low that the circulation to the extremities may be seriously affected and give cause to gangrene.

(2) *Mental* changes are present. There may be torpor and lethargy, witchings, hyperasthesia, convulsions, or violent delirium.

Complications. The commonest are *bronchitis* and *epistaxis*. There is anger of *heart failure*. *Toxaemia* is grave. The possibility of *gangrene* has een mentioned.

Treatment and nursing. *Cardiac stimulants* and regular doses of *drenalin* are given to help to maintain the blood pressure. The *diet* needs o be very nourishing and should be supplemented by glucose. The disease s serious, the patient requires *good nursing care* and the nurse can do much y careful handling and frequent feeding to bring about a favourable ermination. In addition, the mouth should be kept clean, the tongue noist, the skin free from pressure, the bowels acting regularly, and the rine should be measured and tested for albumin. Tepid or cold sponging vill help reduce the temperature.

Recently *aureomycin* and *chloromycetin* have been used with success. *ulphonamides* and *penicillin* help in preventing complications.

EPIDEMIC RELAPSING FEVER

Louse-borne relapsing fever is conveyed by lice, as the name implies o distinguish it from the tick-borne relapsing fevers of the tropics. It is a lisease which spreads when the population is cold, starved and debilitated nd was formerly known as *famine fever*, typhus (see above) being desig-nated *jail fever*. The European type of relapsing fever is due to the *Spiro-haeta recurrentis*, it is conveyed by body and head lice and possibly also by he bed bug. The *incubation* period is *five to ten* days.

Symptoms. The *onset* is sudden with rigor and rise of temperature to 104° F. or more, headache and general pains. The pulse is rapid. The emperature remains high for about 6 days, during this time the patient s restless and thirsty, refuses food and may vomit. When the temperature alls he wants to eat, is sometimes ravenously hungry, and may feel well nough to get up, whilst in other cases he may be so prostrated by the period of high fever that he is in danger of collapse.

The chart is characteristic. After *a week of fever* there is a *fever-free period* of about a week or so, then up swings the temperature again and all the symptoms are repeated. After 4 or 5 days it falls rapidly once again unt the next relapse occurs. In untreated cases this sequence is repeated unt the fever wears itself out. The disease may be complicated by jaundic diarrhoea, haematuria and pneumonia.

Treatment and nursing. General nursing measures are necessar high fever may be reduced by cold spongings; perspiration at the cris must be removed by hot sponging, drying and changing the clothin Symptoms are treated as they arise, plenty of fluids containing glucos should be given during the bouts of fever, and nourishing diet during th fever-free periods; care must be taken not to set up diarrhoea by injud cious feeding as the patient being hungry will eat anything and every thing.

Arsenic is specific and an intravenous injection of neosalvarsan at th outset usually proves effective. The duration of the disease depends upo the early administration of neosalvarsan and the length of convalescenc depends on the general condition of the patient. Those who are physicall fit recover rapidly, but those already debilitated by starvation, such a those living under conditions which pertained in the occupied countri during the last war, will find convalescence long and tiresome and nee good nursing care until recovery is complete.

Prophylaxis is the same as for typhus.

TRENCH FEVER

Trench fever is so-called because it occurred amongst the men in th trenches during the war of 1914–18. It is a disease due to one of th Rickettsia bodies—*Rickettsia quintana*. *Infection* is conveyed by lice—not, it i thought, by the bite of the louse but by the excrement being rubbed int the skin in scratching. The *incubation* period is from 10 to 30 days.

Symptoms. The *onset* is characterized by headache, and genera pains, particularly of the shins, the pain is worse at night and prevent sleep. The spleen is enlarged. In a number of cases there is a papular re rash on the trunk. The temperature may be intermittent, resemblin relapsing fever to some extent, or low fever may persist for weeks. Th patient gets thin, he looks ill and anxious and becomes anaemic; he i very depressed.

Treatment lies in relieving the symptoms. Some analgesic such a aspirin is given for the aches and pains. Hot stupes may help. Rest tonics, and a good nourishing diet are necessary to relieve the state o debility to which cases of trench fever are liable.

Prophylaxis is the same as for typhus.

Chapter 34

Acute Infections

fluenza—Vincent's angina—Acute rheumatism—Typhoid fever—Undulant ver—Dysentery—Food poisoning (notifiable), salmonella, botulism—Cholera— Erysipelas—Anthrax—Tetanus—Glandular fever—Malaria—Plague

A*n acute infection* is due to some definite organism which results in an acute illness with marked prostration. In some instances, as in acute lobar pneumonia and erysipelas, the illness may be short and sharp, oducing great strain on the heart and calling for the most perfect lministration of absolute rest, and the immediate relief of symptoms. In her instances, as in typhoid fever and undulant fever, the illness may be rolonged, but the toxaemia is no less marked, and the wasting, exhaus- on and prostration present necessitate the greatest possible conservation the patient's energy, in order to bring him safely to the conclusion of e illness, and for the avoidance of complications.

Many of the acute infections are communicable diseases, but, not giving se to epidemics in all cases, are sometimes nursed in the wards of a eneral hospital provided the precautions described as bed isolation or arrier nursing can be carried out. For example, all the diseases described nder the heading of acute infections are communicable, and influenza is equently epidemic in distribution, but most of the others mentioned ccur only in sporadic cases in this country. It is doubtful whether acute ieumatism is communicable or not.

A number of diseases which are acute infections have been described other parts of the book, including pneumonia (p. 370), infective ndocarditis (p. 349), acute infection of the urinary tract, infective undice (p. 394). Acute infantile paralysis, cerebrospinal fever and ncephalitis are described in the section devoted to diseases of the central ervous system (see chapter 26).

INFLUENZA

Influenza is an acute infection of the respiratory tract, which may be light at first, but which, because of the marked degree of toxaemia and rostration accompanying it, lowers the patient's powers of resistance nd either leads to spread of the infection or results in very serious compli- ations. The causal organism is a virus.

Symptoms. The *onset is sudden*, with headache and general aching ains. The patient aches all over and there seems to be no part of his body —muscle, joint or nerve—that does not take part in this general ache.

The tongue is dry and coated, the mucous surface of the fauces red nd injected. There is a rise in temperature, and discomfort is so great hat sleep is practically impossible. In most cases of any degree of severity here is delirium. The skin is usually hot and dry, the urine scanty and the owels constipated.

Infection may spread to the larynx and trachea, causing laryngitis a tracheitis, and to the bronchi, causing bronchitis. A very severe form, whi is often fatal, is influenzal pneumonia, characterized by lobular infecti and accompanied by a usually severe and rapidly accumulating toxaemi On the other hand the infection may spread to the sinuses of the face a the mastoid antrum, giving rise to sinusitis, otitis media and mastoidit

Other types of influenza include the gastro-intestinal and the *febrile type*. In t febrile type the only symptom, apart from the dry tongue and inject fauces and general aching pains, may be a rise in temperature persisti for weeks, and followed by great wasting and prostration.

In the gastro-intestinal type the symptoms of nausea, vomiting a diarrhoea are prominent. This results in loss of fluid and conseque marked dehydration accompanied by toxaemia and prostration.

Treatment. Sulphonamides and penicillin are contraindicated. T treatment of influenza is considered under two aspects.

Prevention. Isolation of the patient is carried out. Effective ventilation essential, and the windows should be wide open several times a day order to ventilate the room; during this time patients should be warm tucked up in bed so that they may not feel the cold. During an epidemi effective ventilation must be insisted upon in the home and in the wor room. Travelling in crowded vehicles, and visiting places of amuseme which are crowded, should as far as possible be avoided. It is doubtf whether gargling, mouth-washes, nose sniffs, or saturating handkerchie in menthol and eucalyptus are of very much value; but, if during a epidemic they lessen the tendency to fear, they should be employed, an if a body of nurses think that gargling with 1–100 carbolic is a preventi measure they should be encouraged to do this. If a man thinks that di infecting the mouthpiece of his telephone receiver is just the one thir necessary to prevent his taking influenza, let him disinfect it. Fear lowe the resistance of the body, and everything possible should be done to giv the public confidence.

The *treatment of the patient* depends on the severity of the infection fro which he is suffering. The principles of treatment are:

(1) Isolation of the patient and of his feeding utensils and handke chiefs as far as possible.

(2) Confinement in a warm well-ventilated room. As he has a rise temperature he should remain in bed; when the infection is slight h should remain in a sitting-room provided with a comfortable chair, fire and whatever recreation he pleases.

(3) The bowels should be opened by an aperient; this depends on th amount of gastro-intestinal disturbance; if the tongue is coated, a dose calomel may be given followed by a saline aperient.

(4) The patient should be given large quantities of any fluid he wi drink—lemonade, barley water, aerated waters, milk and soda, tea. H should have about 6 pints each 24 hours. The patient may also have an diet he is willing to take.

(5) Many physicians order some antipyretic mixture, such as aspirin c sodium salicylate, in order to relieve the pains in the limbs and back, an so permit the patient to go to sleep.

The headache may be due to involvement of the sinuses, and for th relief of this inhalations or nose sniffs may be employed. The possibility complications must be remembered and these should be dealt with as they arise. The severity of the toxaemia produces strain on the heart and, as influenza is followed by marked debility, a change of air and fairly long convalescence with good nourishing diet should be recommended after an attack.

VINCENT'S ANGINA

Vincent's angina is an inflammatory condition with ulceration of the tonsils and fauces due to infection with two organisms; a fusiform bacillus and a spirillum, the spirochaete of Vincent (*Treponema Vincenti*). Both are anaerobic organisms. The infection may spread to the mouth and gums, giving rise to stomatitis. The *symptoms* are very similar to those of subacute tonsillitis, with sore throat, general malaise and slight fever. In some cases, however, the temperature may be considerably raised and the patient very ill. As a rule these cases are associated with streptococcal throat infection or diphtheria. The diagnosis of Vincent's angina is made by the examination of a throat swab for Vincent's organisms. In most cases the disease runs a short course except for a few cases which prove intractable and where the symptoms may be prolonged for several weeks.

Treatment. Antiseptic treatment of the local lesions is carried out. Hot gargles are given and swabbing and painting the affected parts with peroxide or iodine. In cases which do not respond, swabbing with a weak solution of salvarsan is employed. Nicotinic acid has recently been given with some success but penicillin is the drug of choice. It is given by intramuscular injection and as lozenges.

ACUTE RHEUMATISM

Acute rheumatism is considered to be due to a definite organism which is thought to be a haemolytic streptococcus. It occurs most commonly in children and young people, and is a disease of very grave severity. (It is also described as *rheumatic fever*.) Many children suffer from subacute rheumatism described as 'growing pains' which occur in the limbs and back. These should not be lightly dismissed but should be reported to the family doctor.

Symptoms. The *onset* is sudden with a high temperature, headache and sore throat, and pains all over the body and specially in the limbs and joints. The skin is moist as sweating is profuse, the urine is diminished in quantity and constipation is present.

The *great danger of rheumatism* lies in the tendency to disease of the heart; carditis is usually present and endocarditis and pericarditis may occur.

Treatment and nursing. The administration of *salicylates* is considered to be specific in the treatment of acute rheumatism. From 10 to 20 grains is administered every four hours, combined with a similar dose of sodium bicarbonate. This does not do any good to the heart infection which may be present, but by checking the disease may prevent the occurrence of such infection. Vitamin C is recommended.

Nursing. The patient should be kept in a blanket bed, and wear warm light woollen clothing. As *absolute rest* is essential, the patient must lie flat and keep quite still, and never be allowed to turn over or move himself about in the slightest. He should be moved by nurses, as all strain on a heart which is liable to become infected should be carefully avoided.

As a rule the pain will soon respond to the administration of salicylates; but, whilst the joints and muscles are painful, it must be remembered that this pain is very severe and that the slightest touch accentuates the discomfort; the weight of the bedclothes cannot be borne on the limbs, and neither can the patient turn his head without great pain. Such a patient will be seen to follow the nurses about with his eyes, which may dilate in horror for fear lest someone approaching his bed may touch or jar it. The greatest care should be taken in handling a patient who is suffering such pain and discomfort; the nurse must never move him quickly or hurry over any treatment she is carrying out for him. All her movements should be slow and gentle and rhythmical; her hand should be warm before she touches him, and she should hold him firmly but gently.

Sponging the skin once or twice a day with hot water will often soothe and give relief, and it will also remove stale perspiration. A patient with acute rheumatism is constantly perspiring, and the sodium salicylate which he is having greatly increases the action of the skin.

The *diet* should be very low whilst the temperature is high; diluted milk is given, citrated or flavoured with lemon, tea, coffee or any other flavour the patient likes. Whey made with lemon, and barley water slightly spiced, form valuable alternative drinks. In addition the patient may have as much water as he will take. When the temperature declines he should be given a fairly liberal carbohydrate diet, but protein should be limited until convalescence is reached.

The urine should be measured and tested daily for albumin, as nephritis may complicate acute rheumatism. The bowels should be kept acting by the use of mild laxatives in order to avoid constipation as the passing of a constipated stool is a severe strain on the muscular system and causes strain on the heart.

Local treatment may be ordered for the painful joints, which should be wrapped in warm wool and supported on pillows and protected from the weight of the bedclothes by bedcradles. Deformity must be prevented, by the use of sandbags and splints, and plaster of paris if necessary. Preparations of wintergreen and salicylate are employed as liniments and ointments; hot fomentations and alkaline fomentations are also employed.

Complications. *Acute rheumatism is the commonest cause of heart disease in young adults* (see pericarditis, p. 347). The results of rheumatic infection on the heart, particularly in children, are very serious, and the very small percentage of children thus affected, who reach adult life, are subject to chronic heart disease and so are unable to carry on their ordinary life and work. *Hyperpyrexia* may occur.

Erythema nodusum is a condition which is associated with acute rheumatism, and also chorea, particularly in children. Nodules appear over the surface of the subcutaneous borders of some of the long bones, particularly the ulna and tibia, and large patches of erythema are seen on the arms and legs. The condition is accompanied by pain and fever; the tongue is furred and the patient suffers from considerable malaise. The *treatment* is rest in bed, warmth is essential, salicylates are administered. The possibility of cardiac complications has to be considered, as in rheumatism.

When the patient is well the tonsils, if infected, should be removed.

ACUTE RHEUMATISM IN CHILDREN

Acute rheumatism in children. The type of acute rheumatism which is characterized by a sudden onset has been described on p. 487. Two other types must be mentioned—(1) in which chorea is the most marked symptom, and (2) in which the onset is very insidious.

The latter is the more commonly met with in children who are affected. The child may have growing pains, or complain frequently of sore throat. He may lose a little weight, be disinclined to eat, have a slight rise in temperature with some increase in the rate of the pulse, or it will be noticed that he is restless during sleep, or pale and listless, or slightly dyspnoeic or cyanosed.

The treatment of acute rheumatism is always on the same lines, that is, the administration of salicylates and rest in bed.

Preventive treatment is very important, and to effect this the earliest signs should be dealt with, a child in whom any of the symptoms mentioned above are manifest being at once examined by a heart specialist.

If acute rheumatism is suspected he should be kept in bed and treated; if no active signs of any cardiac lesion are present, he may be given gentle graduated physical exercises in bed, and then allowed to get up, for a short time at first, taking the same care as described when getting any patient up after he has had heart disease.

Special schools are available for the accommodation of children with rheumatism, in whom cardiac disease may be anticipated. At these schools they can be nursed, treated and educated at the same time, and they are protected from the full energetic life of a child in a house full of other children, or in a school where the routine is regular but rather strenuous.

See **Chronic Rheumatism,** p. 792.

TYPHOID FEVER

Typhoid fever is a communicable disease due to the *Bacillus typhosus*. It is one of a group—the enteric group—the others are known as para-typhoid fever, types A, B and C. The differences between these diseases are only bacteriological, as the symptoms and the course of all four of them are similar and one is not necessarily more or less severe than another. As far, therefore, as the nursing is concerned, each of them needs exactly the same careful attention. The disease is characterized by inflammation and ulceration of the Peyer's patches in the small intestine and caecum.

Infection may be direct or indirect, by means of food, or carriers of the disease, and the *incubation period* is from 11 to 15 days with limits of 5 to 23 days.

Symptoms. The *onset* is slow and insidious. The patient suffers from malaise, loss of appetite, abdominal discomfort and a severe frontal headache. There may be epistaxis. After about a week, he feels ill enough to stay in bed; his temperature rises, taking 4 or 5 days to reach 103° or 104° F., since it rises two degrees each evening and then falls one degree each morning. (See the illustration on p. 45.)

The disease is now advancing, the abdomen is large and doughy, and there may be diarrhoea, though constipation is more often a feature of the disease. The patient feels sick and may vomit, his skin may be dry or he may sweat profusely, and he suffers from considerable thirst, his mouth being dry and his tongue coated. By the seventh day the rash usually appears.

The *rash* is composed of discrete rose-coloured papules which disappear on pressure. There may only be two or three, or a number, 20 to 30, may be seen, and they appear on the abdomen, flanks and thighs. They last 3 or 4 days and then fade; successive crops may appear every 2 or 3 days for a week or so.

The patient is now well into the second week of the disease, and the symptoms become more marked. If there is diarrhoea, the stools will present the characteristic yellow ochre colour and pea soup consistence, being offensive and containing curds of milk and undigested fat. The urine is scanty and high coloured and may contain albumin. The pulse is soft and of low tension, and may become dicrotic.

Toxaemia is marked, the patient lying listless in his bed, flat on his back, with a colour suggestive of grave toxaemia and a hectic flush on each cheek. His mouth is very dry, the tongue covered with dry brown fur and the teeth and lips with sordes. He gets weaker and weaker and finally sinks into what is described as the *typhoid state*, characterized by low muttering delirium with constant involuntary plucking at the bedclothes. The eyes are held wide open, as if staring at the ceiling (*coma-vigil*).

The end of the second week has now been reached and the dreaded complications of haemorrhage, due to the erosion of a blood vessel by the deeply sloughing ulcer, or penetration of the wall of the intestine (perforation) may occur. At this period there may be remissions in the fever and gradually, if the illness terminates satisfactorily, the temperature declines and the toxaemia and other symptoms abate.

During the third week the patient begins to feel better and his temperature falls by a fairly long lysis. He is very weak and hungry, demanding food which will probably be denied him and possibly being very irritable and discontented in consequence.

The **complications** are numerous. *Haemorrhage* and *perforation* and *toxaemia* have been mentioned. *Severe abdominal distension* may be a complication. *Bronchitis* and *pneumonia* may occur. *Septic parotitis* may result from poor oral hygiene. *Otitis media*, *cholecystitis*, *periostitis*, and *osteomyelitis* and the formation of *boils*, *carbuncles* and *abscesses* may arise. *Phlebitis* and *thrombosis* of the veins of the legs may arise as the fever declines. *Abortion* occurs in pregnant women. Two rare complications mentioned in most textbooks are *typhoid spine*, which is a spondylitis, and *tender toes*, which is a sensitiveness of the skin over the toes, due possibly to neuritis.

Treatment and nursing. The principles of treatment are dictated by the length of the illness and the severity of the toxaemia from which the patient suffers and by the possibility that serious complications, perforation and haemorrhage, may occur.

Good nursing is essential, the patient being nursed in a sheet bed, and great attention paid to the skin for the prevention of bedsores and the removal of perspiration. Rest should be as definite as possible, the patient being nursed fairly flat, with his back and thighs—which ache severely—supported during the first ten days; footdrop must not be allowed to occur.

The patient should be moved every 2 or 3 hours, as movement helps to prevent the possibility of pneumonia, and also to prevent the retention of flatus which may result in very severe abdominal discomfort. It is essential, however, that the patient should not be allowed to make any effort himself.

The mouth needs frequent attention in order to keep it clean, and the swabs used should be destroyed at once; and, as retention of the urine may occur, it had better be measured to make sure that the patient is passing a normal amount.

The bowels require attention if they are constipated, and some physicians order liquid paraffin to be given in small doses, three times a day, while others prefer that the bowel action should be regulated by the administration of small, carefully administered, olive oil or glycerine and water enemata.

The *diet* will be definitely ordered, but in most cases the patient is kept on a limited amount of nourishment, 2 to 3 pints of milk—given diluted with water—and ½ to 1 pint of beef tea, or chicken soup. Unless instructions are given to the contrary the nurse should strain all feedings. (For the management of a fluid diet see p. 267.)

In addition, water and lemonade containing glucose may be given in quantity, and the patient should be encouraged to drink at least three pints of such fluid a day, in addition to his feedings.

The diet may require very much modification during the course of the illness; should there be excessive abdominal distension and diarrhoea it may be necessary further to dilute the milk, or even to citrate or peptonize it and it may become necessary to omit the meat broths. On the other hand, if the patient is less seriously ill, he may be able to have thickened (strained) food and jelly, and junket and custard even before his temperature has declined.

Drugs. Aureomycin and *chloromycetin* are giving good results. *Sulphonamides* and *penicillin* help to prevent complications.

Any symptoms which are distressing should be relieved as much as possible; an icebag or cold compress may relieve headache; restlessness may be obviated by sponging the skin, changing the position of the patient in bed, altering the arrangement of the bedclothes, shading a light and all the other little attentions a good nurse would instinctively offer.

As thirst is often intense, and the mouth very dry and sore, the administration of fluids will help, and a few sips every few minutes will help to keep the mouth moist.

The temperature should be taken every 4 hours and the pulse observed more frequently. Sleep is very necessary and the nurse should never waken the patient either to take his temperature or to give him a feeding; she should, however, be ready at hand with a drink as soon as he wakens, because on wakening from a sleep the mouth, in typhoid fever, is dry.

When the temperature declines the diet will be increased; a little fine bread and milk may be given; some thickened milky foods, jellies and custards are added at first, and then, after about a fortnight a little steamed fish, pounded chicken, potato and milk pudding may be added.

Disinfection and isolation are important points in the nursing of typhoid fever patients, and the method of bed isolation or barrier nursing is usually employed. Certain articles should be kept separate for the patient, including his washing, toilet and feeding utensils and articles, and a clinical thermometer.

The nurse or doctor will not handle the patient or his bed or utensils unless wearing a gown, and they must remove the gown and wash, scrub and disinfect their hands after touching him.

Everything that is removed from the patient's bed or used for him must be adequately disinfected, preferably by boiling; his excreta, secretions and discharges should be covered with disinfectant and allowed to stand in it for at least an hour before being disposed of. This also applies to bedclothing soiled with excreta—it must be soaked before it is sluiced. The bedclothes, all personal clothing, towels, etc., should either be soaked in disinfectant or steam sterilized before being sent to the laundry.

The nurse must spare no pains to prevent the spread of infection, either to others or to herself. She must take the greatest care in washing and scrubbing her hands; she should keep the skin soft, so that cracks and chaps do not occur. It would be ideal if she could be persuaded not to handle her own food, or any food, except the patient's, with her hands. She should eat with a knife and fork, using these for bread and butter, cake and everything she conveys to her mouth.

A point that nurses often forget is the long range of infection from a patient who is coughing, and the even greater range of one who may be vomiting. The greatest care should be taken whilst helping and supporting the patient during either of these acts to keep out of the range of droplet infection, as all secretions as well as excretions are highly infectious.

Convalescence is a very trying time for a patient who is approaching the end of a long illness. He may now be raised on pillows and should be encouraged to move his legs and arms. After his temperature has been down for about a fortnight he will be allowed to get up, for a very short time—about 15 minutes the first day—and gradually increase the effort he is allowed to make as he gets stronger. He must never be allowed to become tired as this might be followed by indigestion and sleeplessness which would further retard his recovery.

Complications will be treated as they arise. In the event of *haemorrhage*, which will be accompanied by a sudden drop in temperature, a weak, thready pulse and cold, clammy skin, the nurse should send for the doctor, and in the meantime elevate the bedclothes from the abdomen by means of a cradle, refrain from giving anything by mouth, continue to moisten the patient's lips, see that he is not cold, and give him a hot-water bottle or two if he feels cold. She should reassure him; but if he demands the bedpan she should avoid giving it as this would mean moving him, and she should arrange to receive any stool on pads of wool and tow.

In the event of *perforation*, the nurse should send for the doctor, give the patient nothing by mouth and unobtrusively prepare for taking him to the operating theatre. In the meantime his relatives should be sent for.

The Widal test. The Widal—or agglutination—test or reaction is used as an aid to diagnosis in typhoid and paratyphoid fevers, in some forms of dysentery and in cholera and undulant fever. It depends upon the known fact that the presence of agglutinating substances in the blood of patients suffering from either of these diseases will cause clumping or agglutination of the germs, if the blood serum and organisms are placed together.

A specimen of blood is taken and allowed to clot. The serum is diluted in a variety of different strengths; an emulsion of the germs is then added and the result watched by the aid of a microscope; the amount of dilution which will produce agglutination suggests the agglutinin content of the blood. It is important to note that the test is specific, since the serum of a patient with typhoid fever will not agglutinate any other bacteria, while the serum of a patient with paratyphoid 'A' (for example) will not agglutinate the organisms of paratyphoid 'B'. The serum of persons who have been inoculated against a disease will contain agglutinins, and consequently give a positive reaction to this test.

UNDULANT FEVER

Malta or *undulant* or *abortus fever* is a disease transmitted to man from infected animals—goats and cattle—by means of milk, butter and cheese. Abortus fever is due to *Brucella abortus* and Malta fever to *Brucella Melitensis*. The *incubation period* is 5 to 14 days.

Symptoms. The *onset* is insidious, and is accompanied by vague pains in the limbs and back, headache and a rise of temperature. The fever rises gradually, taking about a week to reach its maximum, as in typhoid fever, and then continues for two weeks; it is remittent in character.

During the *course of the disease* the patient suffers from exhaustion with great thirst, has no desire for food and his mouth is very dirty. He sweats profusely and is unable to sleep. He becomes very weak, wasted and anaemic.

Malta fever is depressing, debility is very marked and the inability to sleep renders the patient miserable. The temperature usually declines after two weeks, and there is then a period of freedom from fever, but it rises again and recurrences of fever may be expected for many months.

Treatment and nursing. Protein shock therapy by peptone or T.A.B. vaccine has been employed for some time. *Streptomycin* and *aureomycin* are undergoing trial. Malta fever requires exactly the same care as a case of typhoid, except that the diet need not be restricted. The patient should be given plenty of fluids containing glucose, and persuaded to take as much nourishment as he will, in whatever form he likes.

The infection is carried by the secretions and excretions and these should be disinfected before disposal. The patient must be kept in bed whilst he has a high temperature; in between the attacks of fever he may get up; he should be kept as happy and cheerful as possible and can be promised that he will get better eventually, and told that in the meantime it is wisest to try and make the best of the intermittent periods, when he is free from fever, in order better to conserve his strength against the recurrences that must be expected.

He should be brought to see that as he gets stronger the attacks seem to be shorter and that one of them will really be the last, and that then he will be free from the tiresome disease. He needs all the help that can be given him as a long tedious illness, characterized by prostrating bouts of fever, is trying even to the most courageous temperament.

DYSENTERY

Bacillary or *epidemic dysentery* is characterized by blood and mucus in the stools and is due to two organisms, Flexner's and Sonne's bacillus. Shiga's bacillus causes a tropical dysentery.

The *incubation period* is short, from a few hours to a week. There is acute inflammation of the lining membrane of the lower part of the ileum and the large intestine.

Symptoms. The *onset* is sudden, with abdominal pain and diarrhoea, a rise in temperature, rapid pulse, thirst and vomiting. Tenesmus or straining at stool is frequent and distressing; a small quantity of blood and mucus is passed each time and the stools are entirely devoid of feculent matter.

Bacillary dysentery may be acute, as described above, or a mild or a chronic form may be seen. In the acute form the patient becomes rapidly prostrated, dehydration is marked and he is cold and collapsed.

The **treatment** during this stage is to keep the patient warm in bed, make hot applications to the abdomen in order to try and relieve pain, while sedatives are given to help the patient to get some sleep, and starch and opium enemata are employed for the relief of tenesmus.

The *diet* is very restricted during the acute illness; milk should be omitted, albumin water, and watery drinks containing glucose are used as nourishment, and the patient should be given small drinks of water frequently in order to allay thirst and provide him with fluid.

The administration of a polyvalent serum is employed, but it must be given early in the disease or it is of little value.

In the *nursing care* of bacillary dysentery *isolation* is essential. This form of dysentery is carried in the same way as typhoid fever, and the excreta must therefore be covered with disinfectant and allowed to stand for an hour before being disposed of. The bed and personal clothing of the patient should be disinfected before being sent to the laundry. The doctor and nurses must wear coats over their clothing before handling the patient or his utensils and they should wash and carefully disinfect their hands afterwards.

The dry mouth and thirst is a distressing symptom which the nurse should attempt to relieve by frequently cleaning the mouth and giving small drinks of water. The skin of the patient must be kept clean and free from soreness; he will become very thin and must be protected from pressure of the bedpan if one is used. To prevent the area around the anus from becoming sore, it should be cleansed with soft wool and carron oil (equal parts of linseed oil and lime water) after stool, and the swabs burnt.

During the stage of acute illness in severe cases the patient becomes exhausted and collapsed and may sink into the state described in typhoid fever as the *typhoid state*, when he lies quietly muttering and plucking at the bedclothes.

Very acute bacillary dysentery runs a comparatively short course, and if it terminates fatally the patient will only live for a few days. When the disease terminates satisfactorily the stools will be seen, after a week or 10 days, to contain some feculent matter, and this is satisfactory as it will be accompanied by decrease in the frequency of the stool, decline of fever, improvement in the pulse and gradual abatement of the symptoms.

As soon as improvement is definite the diet may be gradually increased. Citrated or peptonized milk may be given, jelly, lightly steamed custard, a little crustless bread and butter and steamed fish pounded. Any return to the state of dysentery would indicate reduction of the diet.

Sulphapyridine and sulphaguanidine are used with success in the treatment of bacillary dystentery.

Amoebic dysentery—known also as tropical dysentery—is caused by protozoa, and spread by flies, contaminated water and carriers of the disease.

In acute amoebic dysentery the *onset* is abrupt, with abdominal pain and diarrhoea. Unlike the temperature in epidemic dysentery, that in this variety is not very high. In severe cases the disease may terminate fatally within a week, but in the majority of cases the condition becomes chronic.

Subacute or chronic amoebic dysentery may follow an acute attack or it may have commenced gradually with symptoms of indigestion, vague abdominal discomfort, listlessness and headache. Amoebic dysentery may be complicated by liver abscess.

The *treatment* of amoebic dysentery is by emetine which is an alkaloid of ipecacuanha.

Prevention of dysentery. The stools must be disinfected, and all precautions taken to keep the utensils used by the patient separate and to disinfect his linen before it is washed. Food must be protected from flies and, during an epidemic, very careful supervision should be made of persons who handle food. It is important also to safeguard the water supply from contamination.

FOOD POISONING

Food poisoning may be produced by eating *poisonous foods*, such as fungi in mistake for edible mushrooms, or berries such as those of the deadly nightshade (belladonna). Certain shellfish may cause symptoms of poisoning either because they are poisonous as mussels may be, or because they have been contaminated by bacteria as may happen where cockles and oysters are exposed to sewage contamination.

A number of people are allergic to shellfish and the symptoms which follow eating the fish are due to the sensitivity of the individual and not to infection.

Foods may be contaminated by *chemicals* which cause poisoning. Those which most commonly do so are tin and antimony which are part of the material of which cheap cooking utensils are made.

The *organisms* most commonly responsible for acute food poisoning are known as the salmonella group and *this form of poisoning is notifiable* under the Food and Drugs Act of 1939. The foods which may be contaminated include meat products, such as brawn, pies and sausage, fish pastes, artificial creams and custards, ice cream, and duck eggs. Dried egg which is not properly safeguarded after exposure to the air may also be a source of poisoning.

The *salmonella group of organisms* may be conveyed to the food by carriers. The infection is acute and most people who partake of the contaminated food will be affected.

The symptoms may come on within two hours or up to forty-eight hours after partaking of the infected food. In *acute cases* the onset is rapid, there is high temperature and severe prostration and dehydration, abdominal cramp, diarrhoea and vomiting. Mortality is high. In *mild cases* the symptoms are less severe.

The **treatment** is to keep the patient warm and in bed; if seen early and his condition will permit, the stomach is washed out. Fluid is given by the intravenous route to replace water or salt and alkalis are given to relieve acidosis. Once the patient begins to improve fluids are given by mouth and subsequently food is judiciously increased.

Botulism is an acute form of food poisoning due to the *clostridium botulinum*. The symptoms come on immediately. There is headache, and diplopia. The mouth is dry and swallowing difficult, fluids may be regurgitated down the nose.

The *treatment* is as described for salmonella poisoning. The breathing must be watched as failure of the respiratory muscles may occur which would necessitate the use of a mechanical respirator.

Prophylaxis. The supervision and inspection of food, food utensils, and the preparation and storage of food is important. The care of the health and hygiene of those handling food and the recognition of carriers of disease and their treatment is a duty of those entrusted with the care of the health of the community.

CHOLERA

Cholera is an acute epidemic tropical disease due to *V. cholerae* or the cholera bacillus. It is spread by carriers and by infected food, water, milk and also very largely by flies. The *incubation period* varies from a few hours to several days.

Symptoms. The *onset* is sudden. Diarrhoea and vomiting are present and even in the early hours of the disease in severe cases the patient is passing copious watery stools. These contain little flakes of epithelium from the mucous lining of the intestine which give to the pale watery stools the appearance of 'rice water'.

The patient becomes rapidly dehydrated and very collapsed, the temperature is subnormal and the pulse weak. In many instances the patient is pulseless. This condition persists for 24 to 36 hours when improvement may be seen. The stools become less continuous and less frequent, the skin improves in colour and the temperature rises to 101° or 103° F. In a few cases hyperpyrexia occurs.

The *complications* which occur are cardiac failure, suppression of urine, pneumonia and septic conditions of the mouth.

Treatment and Nursing. The patient should be kept quiet and nursed flat in bed. He must not be allowed to do anything for himself, all exertion must be carefully avoided because of the danger of heart failure. External applications of warmth, blankets, cradles and hot bottles will help to treat the severe collapse from which the patient is suffering. Hot stupes to the abdomen will relieve the cramplike pains. It is important to note and measure the amount of urine passed so that any tendency to suppression may be observed without delay.

The *administration of fluid is important*. Saline and glucose are given by parenteral routes. As soon as vomiting abates the patient may be given fluids such as water and glucose, whey, and later when the diarrhoea ceases he may have diluted milk. *Diet* can only be very judiciously introduced, arrowroot is a good beginning and the patient can then be given light carbohydrate diet. Protein should be given with caution until renal function appears to be normal.

Convalescence is fairly rapid. The patient should be careful for some time as any sudden movement may result in heart failure.

Medicines and Drugs. Kaolin is given in large doses as long as diarrhoea persists.

Precautions against spread of infection. The patient should be isolated and the precautions taken in nursing typhoid fever should be applied to cholera.

In countries where cholera is prevalent and in any country where an epidemic occurs very great care should be taken in the preparation of food, water and milk should be boiled before use, green salads and uncooked fruit and vegetables should not be eaten unless they can be peeled. Cleanliness and the importance of washing the hands before eating should be stressed. All food should be protected from flies, and flies should be eliminated as far as possible.

ERYSIPELAS

Erysipelas is an acute communicable disease characterized by swelling and redness of the skin and mucous surfaces, and accompanied by a very high degree of temperature. It is due to a haemolytic *streptococcus*.

Infection occurs by inoculation of a wound or abrasion of the skin, though this may be only microscopic. It is highly infectious to wounds and obstetric cases, and therefore has to be strictly isolated whenever it occurs in the wards of a general hospital. The *incubation period* is from 1 to 7 days. Erysipelas may attack any part of the body, but the face, in which the skin is exposed, is most often the site of inoculation. The disease frequently commences at the inner canthus of the eye, or the margin of the nose, where the mucous and skin surfaces meet.

Symptoms. The *onset* is sudden, there may be rigors and shivering, headache, sore throat, vomiting and a high temperature, 103° or 104° F., with a rapid pulse.

The *rash* is a dull red colour; the skin is tense, swollen and shining, with a raised margin which denotes the area of rapidly spreading rash. The surface of the rash may be covered with blebs and bullae. When the face is affected, if the rash begins at the margin of the nose, it spreads over the face, butterfly fashion, and up over the forehead and on the scalp. The whole of the scalp may be invaded. The eyes are closed, the lids swollen, the ears thick and the face so disfigured by swelling that the features may be unrecognizable.

Headache is very severe, and there is usually delirium; the pulse is rapid, the temperature remains high, and the patient is unable to sleep because of the severe headache and great discomfort he is suffering. The temperature usually persists for a week or 8 days. During this time the patient is passing through a very serious illness, his heart may fail, cyanosis is a serious sign, and prostration becomes more and more severe as the patient becomes weaker and is unable to withstand the toxaemia and discomfort from which he suffers.

The temperature declines fairly rapidly at the end of the illness, in an uncomplicated case, usually by crisis or a short lysis; when suppuration occurs, the temperature becomes intermittent in character and persists for longer.

The **complications of erysipelas** are *suppuration*, *sloughing*, and *cellulitis* of the tissues, *adenitis* of the local lymphatic glands, *toxaemia* and *pyaemia; broncho-pneumonia* may occur, especially in elderly persons, and *mania* may follow severe delirium.

Treatment and nursing. The sulphonamides are specific treatment in erysipelas. Within 48 hours symptoms and fever abate, improvement is rapid.

Isolation of the patient is necessary, and great care must be taken to avoid transmission of the infection to surgical and obstetric cases. A nurse looking after a case of erysipelas should not touch surgical cases. She should be warned against infecting herself, she should not touch her face and must guard against cracks and abrasions on her hands. If these occur she should report the fact.

The patient is kept in bed, in a warm quiet room, and his headache may be relieved by aspirin, his temperature by sponging, and his thirst by the administration of fluids. The diet should be fluid, up to 3 pints of nourishing fluids being given daily and, in addition, several pints of watery drinks containing glucose. The mouth should be cleaned, the urine measured and tested for albumin and the bowels kept acting regularly; the usual attention for the prevention of bedsores is necessary, and elderly patients should be moved fairly frequently in order to obviate the danger of hypostatic pneumonia. As the disease is severe and exhausting, stimulants are usually given and sedatives employed to induce sleep.

Some *local treatment* may be needed but many physicians prefer to keep the skin dry and order it to be dusted with a mildly astringent powder; others like it to be painted with a weak solution of iodine.

Convalescence. Once the temperature has declined and the rash disappeared, the patient will make rapid strides towards convalescence. He should have a change of air, a good nourishing diet, and a little stimulant such as whisky or port wine to increase his resistance and hasten his recovery from the anaemia and debility which follow this short serious illness.

The skin will be tender and delicate for some time, and should not be exposed to the injudicious use of strong soaps or to biting winds. It is better to teach the patient to cleanse his skin with olive oil, or oatmeal and water, and it must be well dried and any abrasions or cracks treated with healing ointments.

It is important to remember that one attack of erysipelas predisposes to others—immunity is lowered, not raised.

ANTHRAX

Anthrax is a disease due to a spore-forming organism, the *Bacillus anthracis*. It is transmitted to man from infected animals in hides, wool and hair. Men unloading hides and wool at the docks may be infected. The *incubation period* is short, from 1 to 3 days.

There are two *varieties* of the disease—external anthrax or malignant pustule, which is the result of inoculation; and internal anthrax, when the organism is inhaled. The latter may be characterized by acute pulmonary or abdominal symptoms, accompanied by severe prostration, and usually terminates fatally within 48 hours.

External anthrax or *malignant pustule*, which is the type most commonly seen, usually appears on the exposed parts of the body, face, neck and arms.

It begins as a pimple surrounded by an area of inflammation; in a few hours the pimple is encircled by an area of induration which is covered by yellow blebs and surmounted by a black scab from which the name malignant pustule is derived. The skin for a considerable area around the lesion is livid, tense and swollen.

The constitutional symptoms present demonstrate the severity of the toxaemia from which the patient is suffering; in a day or two from the onset, in an untreated case—and because of the cardiac failure and asphyxia which accompany the severe toxaemia—the temperature is high, the pulse rapid and the patient lividly blue, delirious and gasping for breath.

Treatment and nursing. The only treatment of any use is the early administration of Sclavo's anti-anthrax serum in sufficiently large doses. This is followed by decline of the local inflammation and abatement of the constitutional symptoms. Serum is repeated until the temperature has declined. Sulphapyridine and arsenical preparations are given in conjunction with serum. Penicillin is valuable in the most acute cases.

In the *nursing care* the high degree of infectivity must be taken into consideration. A nurse attending a case of anthrax should not have the care of any surgical case. She must protect the skin of her own hands by wearing rubber gloves; if her skin becomes abraded she should be removed from the case. Infection will be transmitted to her from any slight abrasion on the patient's skin or from any article, such as a hypodermic needle, which may have been used for him. She must keep her nails short and neat, and wash and disinfect her hands carefully for fear of inhaling or ingesting the organism with her food.

As far as possible old bedding and clothing, which can be destroyed after use, should be provided.

The symptoms will be treated as they arise, and the patient requires constant care during the acute stage when he is livid, dyspnoeic and delirious. Oxygen is administered continuously, and fluids should be given liberally by whatever channel is convenient. In very severe cases continuous intravenous infusion of fluid is employed.

TETANUS

Tetanus, like anthrax, is a disease due to a spore-forming organism. This organism lives in the intestines of grazing animals and is deposited in their droppings, so that man may be infected by road dirt, and also by the intestine of the sheep in prepared catgut and by animal wool. The length of the *incubation period* depends on the virulence of the infection, it varies from 24 hours to several weeks, with an average of 7–14 days.

In tetanus the organism, having gained entrance to the body by inoculation, multiplies and pours its toxins—which have a selective action on the central nervous system—into the blood stream, and this is manifested by rigidity of the skeletal muscles.

Symptoms. At first the patient complains that he finds it difficult to open his mouth—this is why tetanus is sometimes called lockjaw. The facial muscles are contracted in a grin, described as *risus sardonicus*. As the condition becomes worse, spasmodic contractions of the muscles occur and the patient's body is contracted, his head retracted and back arched. The intercostal muscles are also contracted and this results in dyspnoea. These muscular spasms cause great pain, the patient is very cyanosed, his skin is covered with a cold sweat, and he becomes rapidly exhausted. Death occurs from heart failure in untreated cases.

Treatment and nursing. The only treatment of any value is the early administration of antitetanus serum, in large doses. Penicillin is given in conjunction with serum. This treatment will prevent further damage to the central nervous system but will not repair the harm already inflicted.

The administration of antitetanic serum is employed as a prophylactic measure in all cases admitted to the casualty department of a hospital with injuries or wounds which are contaminated by road dirt, and as a prophylactic it is considered invaluable.

In the *nursing care* of a patient with tetanus, *isolation* is essential and the nurse attending him should not have charge of any surgical case.

The patient should be nursed in a quiet well-ventilated room and, as even slight external stimuli will provoke a muscular spasm, the bed should be approached quietly and the patient touched gently, allowing him to become accustomed to the weight of the nurse's hand very gradually. Her hand must be warm, not cold, and the grasp should be gentle, even and firm. All moving of the patient should be slow and rhythmical, but he should be moved as little as possible and must not be overnursed. He should be washed only as much as is absolutely necessary and, although it is most desirable to prevent the formation of bedsores, yet here again the least possible handling and treatment should be employed.

Most physicians will order sedatives in sufficient quantity to keep the patient in a stuporous condition, and in some instances avertin is employed for this purpose. When spasms arise in these circumstances, they are controlled by inhalations of chloroform.

It is very important to get as much fluid as possible into the patient, and when he is kept in a stuporous state this is usually managed by means of continuous rectal administration and in severe cases fluid is given intravenously.

The nurse must watch the patient's colour and pulse, measure his urine and compare the output with his fluid intake. His bowels should be kept acting, and his tissues must be watched for oedema, as this would indicate failure in the circulation of his body fluids—probably because his heart had begun to fail.

When death occurs it is due to toxaemia and cardiac and respiratory failure. As already stated, the only treatment of value is the administration of antitetanic serum, but a nurse can assist the patient throughout the course of this serious disease by helping to avoid muscular spasm, by maintaining him in a state of rest and quiet and by the liberal administration of fluids.

GLANDULAR FEVER (*Infective mononucleosis*)

Glandular fever is an acute infection, but the causative organism is not known. The *incubation period* is from 5 to 14 days. *Infection* is due to droplet infection and close contact with the patient. Three types of the disease are described:

An *angiose* type characterized by sore throat.

A *febrile* type in which fever and a rash occur, and

The *glandular* type characterized by painful swellings of the lymphatic glands. This is the commonest type.

In the glandular type the *onset* is marked by malaise, headache, general pains and a rise of temperature. In some cases tonsillitis occurs. Epistaxis is occasionally seen. The spleen is enlarged. The disease runs a *course* of about two weeks during which the temperature remains elevated, ranging from 101 to 102, or even 104 degrees Fahrenheit in some cases, and then declines, but relapse may occur and in many instances there is a rise of temperature in the evening for some weeks after decline of the initial fever.

Diagnosis is made on blood counts and special blood tests. There is an increase in the white cell count with a high percentage of monocytes (monocytosis). The *Wassermann reaction* is positive in about 50 per cent of the cases and therefore the possibility of syphilis has to be excluded. A special blood test—the *Paul and Bunnell test*—is based upon the known fact that the blood serum of a patient suffering from glandular fever will cause sheep's red blood cells to agglutinate.

Treatment and nursing. The patient is kept in bed during the acute stage and should be isolated for about two weeks, or until the temperature has declined. Ordinary nursing measures are necessary, the diet should be fluid and the bowels kept acting regularly. A fairly long convalescence is necessary, and debility should be counteracted by tonics and nourishing diet.

MALARIA

Malaria is a disease which is conveyed from man to man by an anopheles mosquito. This insect sucks the blood of its host and at the same time injects the malarial parasite into the blood stream. After an *incubation period* averaging from ten days to a fortnight but which may be considerably longer, the *onset* of the disease occurs with a rigor.

Types of malaria. The simplest form and the one which is used in the malarial therapy of general paralysis of the insane (see p. 47) is *benign tertian*. This variety is characterized by a rigor on alternate days.

Quartan malaria is characterized by a rigor every third day.

Malignant tertian is a more serious type and one which may present a variety of symptoms. In some cases there is continuous high fever with delirium and prostration. In others it may take the form of algid collapse again accompanied by severe prostration. A cerebral type of malaria is also met. The patient complains of headache, he becomes rapidly prostrated with marked hyperpyrexia and lapses into unconsciousness.

Treatment. The successful treatment of malaria is of comparatively recent date. Patrick Manson in 1878 discovered that an embryo filaria from a man could develop in a mosquito; Ronald Ross in 1898 discovered that malaria was spread by an anopheles mosquito and he taught the necessity of eliminating the mosquito by destruction of its breeding places if the incidence of malaria was to be reduced.

Treatment by cinchona bark is several centuries old and preceded the use of quinine which is a pure alkaloid of cinchona. Until recently, in fact until 1939, quinine was the only drug used in the treatment of malaria, but a great deal of research was done during the recent war and the following *anti-malarial drugs* are now in use. They are employed for cure and prevention. The *treatment dose* is larger than the *suppressive dose*. The latter term implies that manifestations of the disease will be suppressed by the drug and although the patient has been infected with malaria he will not have an attack. Children require proportionately smaller doses.

Anti-Malarial Drugs

Name	*Treatment Dose*	*Suppressive Dose*
Quinine	15-30 grains daily	5-10 grains daily
Mepacrine (Atebrin)	0.3-0.6 grammes daily	0.1 grammes daily
Paludrine	0.3-0.6 " "	0.1 grammes twice or three times a week
Aralem (Diphosphate)	0.3-0.6 " "	0.5 grammes twice a week
Pamaquin (Plasmoquine)	0.3 " "	

The treatment of malaria is always accompanied by microscopical examination. The result of the initial examination of the blood will assist the physician in deciding on his method of treatment. In order to prevent relapse, treatment is continued for a week or more after cessation of fever. *Chronic relapsing malaria* may be the result of failure to observe this precautionary measure.

A patient suffering from malaria is given a dose of calomel at the outset, followed by a saline aperient. The bowels should be kept acting well during the time that quinine is required. Any symptoms due to quinine (see p. 298) or any other anti-malarial drug should be noted. Headache may be treated by aspirin. When the temperature is so high that it is causing grave restlessness and discomfort the patient may be tepid or cold sponged to relieve this.

After an attack of malaria the general state of health will be low, the patient becomes anaemic, he loses his appetite and gets thin. Arsenic and liver preparations are given to treat the anaemia. The appetite should be tempted and good nourishing food supplied. Convalescence should be long and effective, if this is not attended to there is danger that relapse will occur.

Prophylaxis. *Anti-malarial measures* should be insisted upon for those who are resident in a malarial infested country. Nurses working in the tropics should do all they can by their own example, which is the best form of propaganda, to teach the importance of:

Avoidance of litter and destruction of the breeding places of mosquitoes

The importance of maintaining a high standard of health and a very high state of anti-malarial morale

The necessity of using mosquito nets and protective clothing, such as mosquito boots

The value of anti-malarial drugs as a suppressive measure and the need for persevering with the use of the drug chosen.

PLAGUE

Epidemics of plague have spread over Europe during several centuries; the last epidemic in this country was the Plague of 1665.

Plague is due to the *Pasteurella pestis* or plague bacillus which is carried by rats. The fleas which infest the rats carry the organisms in their stomach. When the rat dies of plague the fleas leave its body, and it is by the bite of these infected fleas that plague is conveyed to man.

There are several types of plague. *Bubonic plague* has an incubation period of about 3 days; it is characterized by swollen lymphatic glands (bubos), malaise and fever. *Pneumonic plague* has an incubation period of from 2 to 8 days. This is a very fatal type, and a healthy person can be infected from inhaling the patient's breath. A *septicaemic type* is equally severe and fatal.

Cases of plague are seen in some of our communicable diseases hospitals from time to time, as they may be admitted from ships docked in our ports. A patient with pneumonic or septicaemic plague is extremely ill and is unlikely to recover. Fever and toxaemia increase in severity during the early hours of the illness, the tongue is black, there is great thirst, pyrexia, prostration and delirium. Death in untreated cases occurs in 24 to 48 hours.

Treatment. The use of chemotherapeutic drugs has superseded all other treatment. Sulphonamides, particularly sulphadiazine is given by the intravenous route. Intensive treatment should be given early and once an effective concentration of the drug is established in the blood the general condition of the patient improves. Penicillin is sometimes given in addition.

Prophylaxis. In order to prevent plague being admitted into this country, the Port Sanitary Authorities are constantly on the watch. An officer boarding a vessel arriving in this country makes searching enquiries regarding any cases of sickness aboard, and 'any rats?' Metal rat-guards are attached to hawsers to prevent rats getting ashore from ships. Rat proofing is taken into consideration when building ships, and also in house-building by provision of concrete foundations and properly protected drains.

A *campaign for the destruction of rats* is undertaken at intervals; some local authorities institute a rat week, when special measures are taken to exterminate rats, not only because they destroy buildings and contaminate food, but because they are carriers of disease.

Strict *isolation* of plague patients is necessary. All articles used by the patient, including the bedding should be destroyed, and it must be remembered that the dead are infectious.

Nurses and attendants on cases of plague require adequate protection by wearing gowns, gloves and special boots, and in the case of pneumonic plague adequate masks should be used.

Chapter 35

Pulmonary Tuberculosis *(Sanatorium Nursing)*

Introduction—Predisposing factors—Sources of infection—Varieties—Changes in the tissues—Resistance of infection—Preventive measures—Diagnostic procedures—Modes of onset—Symptoms—Complications—General treatment and nursing—Special nursing care—Treatment for relief of distressing symptoms—Collapse therapy—Monaldi drainage—Hints on hygiene to nurses

(See also Thoracoplasty, p. 721)

Tuberculosis in so far as it is due to a micro-organism is a communicable disease. It is the commonest communicable disease in this country but differs from many of the others because the *onset* is insidious, often passes unnoticed and moreover the course of the disease is long and chronic in character.

The *incidence of tuberculosis* rises and falls with the state of the health of the community and this depends to a great extent on suitable food and good social conditions of living. A century ago tuberculosis had a high death rate. During the past 80 years the death rate has progressively fallen, from 1860–1900 it fell by over 40 per cent. This improvement was due principally to amelioration of social conditions, it began before the discovery of the tubercle bacillus by Koch in 1882 and before the establishment of Sanatorium treatment.

There has been a progressive decline in the incidence of tuberculosis from 1860 to the present day. Conditions of war usually result in some increase. During the last war there was a slight rise in the number of deaths from pulmonary tuberculosis. This occurred in 1942, but since then the incidence has declined again and with the present determination in the country to control tuberculosis it is hoped that it will be possible to eradicate this disease.

Tuberculosis in the occupied countries and amongst prisoners of war where in both cases food has been in short supply and the conditions of living have been poor have resulted in an increase in this disease.

Early Recognition. At the present time the tuberculosis service is developing in some parts of the country and the facilities required for early recognition of the disease, i.e. X-ray examination of chest, laboratory examination of sputum and Mantoux's test are available. Physicians and nurses are being specially trained to deal with early cases, to teach the importance of prophylaxis in the home and workshop, to encourage the regular examination of certain groups, to educate the public to eliminate their present fears of the terms 'tuberculosis', 'consumptive', 'sanatorium' and such-like terms and to understand the importance of the early recognition of symptoms and early treatment of the disease in order that the source of infection being found it may be removed and that disease in the individual may be arrested. When doctors, nurses, patients and the public all work together then, and not till then, will tuberculosis be effectively controlled.

Prevention. The tuberculosis service began by considering *treatment* but in its development prevention is now assuming its proper place. Prevention of disease should precede treatment; so it is with nursing, caring for the patient, sick and in bed, is a great work, but preventing that illness is much more important, and helping a patient back either to perfect health or to rehabilitation is second only to prevention. In tuberculosis it is important to teach the public what this disease is and how it is transmitted.

Cause. Tuberculosis is due to a germ, the *tubercle bacillus* or *mycobacterium*, which because it is enclosed in a very resistant capsule is difficult to destroy. The covering membrane is weakened by exposure to sunlight and heat, and then the germ is more easily killed.

The tubercle bacillus may settle in several parts of the body and cause changes there; for example it may settle in the lungs, bones, joints, lymphatic glands, abdomen, urinary tract, skin and meninges. There are two types of tubercle bacillus which chiefly affect man—the 'human' which originates usually in a lesion in the lung, and the 'bovine' which is found in tuberculous cattle. Two other types which infect birds and fish are described as the 'avian' and 'cold-blooded' types.

Predisposing Factors. *Hereditary.* Tuberculosis is not hereditary in that, except very rarely indeed, babies are not born with it, but babies who are born into a family where there is a case are in contact with and subject probably to massive infection and they tend to develop pulmonary tuberculosis. The infection in these cases is usually a severe one, and where a primary infection of this type is contracted during infancy it is generally fatal. A baby born of a tuberculous mother will not, unless it should come into contact with some other source of infection, develop tuberculosis if it is removed from its mother and brought up away from its dangerous environment.

Race. Tuberculosis is a disease of civilization. It has already been pointed out that where there is no tuberculosis there is no immunity. For example those who lived in country districts are found to be Mantoux-negative which shows that they have never been infected and have not therefore developed any immunity. Whereas 80 per cent of town dwellers are Mantoux-positive demonstrating that they have been infected and have therefore developed some immunity. Immunity thus developed is a safeguard. The Irish, Welsh and Scottish Highlanders living in country districts are particularly vulnerable to tuberculosis and a number do contract the disease when they come into contact with it for the first time.

Another popular theory is that certain types of individuals have a greater tendency to tuberculosis than others. Those with a fine skin, milk and roses colouring, long eyelashes, long narrow chest and winged scapulae are spoken of as having a *tuberculous diathesis*. But with the tendency to develop an open air life and the increase in outdoor games the general health of the population has improved and this type of person is extremely rare.

Age Incidence. When children under two develop pulmonary tuberculosis it is generally fatal and when acquired between the age of from 2 to 5 years it is very serious. Adolescents and young people between 15 and 25 years form the majority age group in which tuberculosis occurs and in these the disease assumes a chronic course. It is essential that the disease should be recognized early, when, in the majority of instances, it can be arrested. If neglected the disease will progress and enter the advanced stage when there will be little hope of return to anything approaching a normal life. It should be remembered that the first 'strain of life' is taken at the age of 15 to 20. The individual begins then either to earn his living or to take seriously some aspect of work or study. He is of an age in which he is still developing and is therefore very vulnerable to tuberculosis and it is essential that his resistance should be maintained by good food and healthy living. He should make sensible use of his leisure time for rest and recreation, should spend some of his time in open air occupations and obtain sufficient sleep under healthy conditions. Any persons in this age group such as nurses should be given all the help they need to enable them to maintain resistance to infection and all the protection which is available for the prevention of infection if and when they may be brought into contact with tuberculosis.

Sources and modes of Infection. The human tubercle bacillus is the most dangerous organism. Pulmonary tuberculosis is caused almost entirely by this type; the bovine type being mainly the cause of infection of the abdomen, bones, joints and glands.

The principal sources of infection by the human bacillus are *droplet infection* from those suffering from pulmonary tuberculosis and the inhaling of *infected dust* and *dried sputum* carried on particles in the air.

The *tubercle bacillus* taken in as food is usually the 'bovine' type which is swallowed principally in milk and also in eating butter, cheese and the meat of infected animals. The 'human' tubercle bacillus, however, may, and not infrequently does, gain access to any type of food and it is therefore most important to have control exercised over those who handle food in the home, restaurant, and provision store, particularly with regard to milk. Organisms may enter through the mucous membranes and through the abraded skin by inoculation, and probably most cases of skin tuberculosis are contracted in this way.

Living tubercle bacilli are to be found wherever people group together as in places of entertainment, public conveyances, restaurants and air raid shelters. Eighty per cent of the adults in towns are infected. The majority are unaware of it; either there are, or were, no symptoms, or the disturbance is, or was, so slight that no notice was taken of it. The initial dose of infection passes unnoticed therefore because the power *of resistance of the individual* is sufficient to overcome the strength, or virulence, of the invading germ, and so the disease does not develop. But in a few cases, a very few indeed, resistance is low, the micro-organisms increase and multiply and pulmonary tuberculosis is established.

Varieties. Pulmonary tuberculosis may be an *acute* condition with a rapid onset which is a type most often met with and tends to run a short course in children; or it may be *subacute* as are the majority of cases. The latter form is seen in young adults between the age of 18 to 30 and in the average case particularly when the disease is diagnosed early this form of tuberculosis can be arrested. *Miliary tuberculosis* is an acute form when areas of disease arise in a number of organs, including the lungs, at the same time. These minute areas or tubercles resemble millet seeds. In the majority of instances miliary tuberculosis runs a rapid course, ending fatally, though chronic cases do arise and the disease in these can be arrested.

Changes in the Tissues. When tubercle bacilli invade the tissues certain characteristic changes occur which lead to the formation of a primary lesion or tubercle.

A *tubercle* begins by the presence in the tissues of a little colony of tubercle bacilli. These become surrounded by some giant cells formed from mononuclear cells and layers of epitheloid cells enclosed by a zone of lymphocytes. In this way the tubercle bacilli are imprisoned and, according to the changes which take place in and around the tubercle so formed, the disease progresses, remains quiescent or heals. Tubercles are visible to the naked eye and vary in size from a pin's point to a pin's head.

A number of terms have been used in describing the type of tuberculosis from which a patient is suffering. Laennec's original classification is as follows:

Consolidation. Inflammatory changes occur and the lung becomes airless and solid.

Softening or *caseation.* As the result of changes which are the beginning of ulceration, the centre of the mass or tubercle softens. The contents are at first of the consistence of a cheesy mass, later liquefaction occurs.

Cavity formation. Ulceration progresses until sufficient tissue has been destroyed to result in the formation of a cavity. This becomes filled with infective material. When the cavity remains closed the patient is described as having a 'closed tuberculosis', but when the cavity involves a bronchial tube the secretion gets into the tube and is coughed up as sputum. This state of affairs is described as an 'open tuberculosis'.

Sputum from a cavity is expelled by the lashing movements of the cilia which line the tube carrying the secretion onwards and upwards towards the larynx; by the constant movement of the bronchial tubes which helps to keep the secretion moving, and by coughing which by the expulsive expiration involved forces air out of the tubes and carries with it any secretion or other foreign body contained in the bronchial tubes.

Fibrosis. This occurs when the tissues are resisting the invading organisms. After an initial inflammatory reaction cells multiply round the infected area and a barrier of fibrous tissue is formed. So long as this is complete the disease does not spread. This fibrous tissue contracts and forms scars and cicatrices which are intended by nature to close or shut off the cavity but do not always produce that effect. Sometimes these fibrous bands act as *adhesions* which may fasten the lung to the chest wall and so prevent movement, or they may exert a pull in different directions and prevent the closure of a cavity which might otherwise heal. In this way the period of incapacity of the patient may be prolonged until these adhesions are dealt with surgically.

Calcification. Sometimes lime salts become deposited in a tubercle which hardens and becomes separated from the lung tissue. It may remain in the lung or it may be coughed up as a 'lung stone'.

These various stages representing the changes taking place in the lung after invasion by the tubercle bacillus may all be present in the same patient. For example there may be areas of caseation, cavities and fibrosis in the same lung.

Resistance to Infection. Two factors are principally concerned in all infections (a) the virulence of the invading organisms and (b) the resistance of the individual. Both these factors are concerned in tuberculosis and in particular the resistance of the individual plays a very important part.

The *virulence of an organism* depends on the conditions under which it has lived or existed. The tubercle bacillus, for example, will have a low virulence if the conditions under which it has lived are unfavourable, but if favourable, such as those existing in an advanced progressive case of pulmonary tuberculosis, then the organisms will be very virulent and likely to cause active disease if inhaled in any numbers, particularly when the individual infected by these organisms is tired, run down and overworked or anxious.

Factors which lower resistance include exposure to infection, particularly frequent exposure such as occurs when living with a tuberculous member of the family, working in a confined space with a tuberculous colleague. When a teacher has tuberculosis infection is rapidly spread to the children. Nurses need all the precautions that can be taken by them and on their behalf when nursing cases of pulmonary tuberculosis in order to avoid infection, particularly when nursing patients with advanced disease who are too ill to take ordinary precautions against spreading the disease by means of droplet infection and by sputum.

Malnutrition. There is no better example of the ravages which malnutrition can make and the increased incidence of, and mortality in, pulmonary tuberculosis than that occurring in the enemy occupied countries in the last war. War brings a world shortage of food. During the 1914–18 war it was observed that deaths from tuberculosis increased in the neutral as well as in the belligerent countries.

Overcrowding means that people are congregated together so that infection is more easily conveyed.

Poor housing. This means that there is probably overcrowding and a low standard of hygiene and sanitation. There is also insufficient income to ensure enough food.

Low Standard of living. Poverty may exist in good as well as in poor houses. It means that there is insufficient food and added to this there is anxiety as to how the next supplies will be obtained.

Dirt and neglect usually go together. They may be the result of bad housing, overcrowding and a low standard of living, or they may be the result of apathy, produced by the depressing conditions under which the poor live, which should never be allowed. Apathy and indifference may be due to ill health and/or mental deterioration, and this may result in serious neglect of health.

Certain Occupations are accepted as a specific hazard such as those in which silica is inhaled. Silica dust injures the lungs and so predisposes a subject to tuberculosis.

Long hours and Fatigue. Long hours, particularly when the span of day is long, are fatiguing and lower the resistance. A day spread over beyond 12 hours, to 13 or 14 hours for example, is not compensated by off duty time no matter how liberal this may be. Irregular hours of work and irregular meals also lower the resistance to infection.

Mental Factors, such as worry and anxiety, tend to lessen the ability to eat and sleep, and these also play their part in lowering the resistance to infection.

Pregnancy. A pregnant woman is usually very fit and well, it is in the early weeks and months following parturition that pulmonary tuberculosis does, in some cases, appear and therefore everything that could be done both during pregnancy and after the birth of the child to prevent this lowering of the resistance of the mother should be carried out.

Slimming. Happily slimming is not in fashion at present. Nevertheless there is many a girl suffering from tuberculosis because she thought more of her 'line' than of her health.

Diabetes. There is an increased incidence of pulmonary tuberculosis in diabetes probably because this is a disease which affects nutrition and also because a majority of young persons who get diabetes do so between the ages of 15 and 20, which is the age when the body is most vulnerable to attack by the tubercle bacillus.

Preventive measures. If spread of infection could be prevented and the resistance of the individual adequately maintained then tuberculosis would be controlled. Enough has been said (above) about the factors which lower the resistance of the body to indicate how it may best be maintained.

Immunity. As already mentioned, about 80 per cent of adults in towns have been infected with tuberculosis, though not clinically infected. Soon after Koch discovered the tubercle bacillus in 1882, he discovered also the important fact that a primary infection rendered the subject sensitive to the tubercle bacillus. This discovery was called Koch's phenomenon, it demonstrated that the subject previously infected became sensitive. To this phenomenon the term *allergy* is now applied, and the test most commonly employed to determine its presence is the Mantoux test.

Tuberculin Tests and Mantoux's Test. For this purpose a preparation of tuberculin which is made of dead tubercle bacilli in glycerin, known as old tuberculin (O.T.), is used. Tuberculin is standardized by its action on guinea pigs which are sensitized by previous infection with tubercle bacilli. The dilutions in sterile saline generally used for Mantoux's test are:

1—10,000 (0·01 mg. tuberculin in 0·1 c.c.)
1— 1,000 (0·1 ,, ,, ,, 0·1 c.c.)
1— 100 (1·0 ,, ,, ,, 0·1 c.c.)

The test is made by intradermal injection of the most dilute preparation into the skin of the forearm. If no reaction follows the next dilution is employed. A positive reaction is demonstrated by a swollen indurated area which appears after 2, 3 or 4 days, persists for 48 hours and then fades rapidly. Healthy infants and persons who have lived protected lives in the country and at the sea give no reaction. They are Mantoux-negative which shows that they have not yet received their primary infection and it would be unwise to expose these individuals to contact with cases of tuberculosis until they have, in the normal way, by mixing with the community in a populated area, received their first dose of infection and developed some degree of immunity. They would then show a positive reaction and become Mantoux-positive.

Patch Test. For this test a preparation of dried tuberculin is taken and a piece of filtering paper is saturated with it. These pieces of paper are each one square centimetre in area. They are fixed on to a piece of adhesive tape in the following arrangement: **Human—Control—Bovine.** One square carries *human tuberculin*, one *bovine* and a central square is a *control* saturated with glycerine broth.

When using the test, in the case of children the patch is applied over the sternum; in infants over the upper spine and in adults over the inner aspect of the forearm. The skin is cleansed with acetone. Antiseptics should not be used. The strip is left in contact for 48 hours. It is then removed. The result is read 48 hours later. A *positive reaction* is indicated by an infiltrated reddened area, the control patch remaining pale. In a *negative reaction* all the areas are pale.

The patch test is considered as reliable for infants and children as the Mantoux test is in adults.

Other tests such as those of Calmette, Moro and Von Pirquet are not employed at the present time.

Immunization. It is not possible at present to produce either a known degree or a protective degree of immunity to tuberculosis such as can for example be procured in smallpox, diphtheria, scarlet fever and typhoid fever. Experiments have been made both by using virulent tubercle bacilli and killed bacilli. Tuberculin is a preparation of killed bacilli which is used for the tests mentioned above. Tuberculin given as a series of injections has also been tried in the treatment of tuberculosis but the results of this method of treatment have been difficult to assess.

Prophylactic Treatment (Bacille Calmette-Guerin, B.C.G.) is a means which was first developed by two physicians in Paris of giving attenuated bovine tubercle bacilli to new-born infants. The organisms are rendered avirulent by 280 passages over a number of years on potato-glycerin. Unfortunately, owing to an accident at Lübeck, when the vaccine used was contaminated by virulent tubercle bacilli, a number of infants died of tuberculosis. B.C.G. vaccine has been used in the Scandinavian countries for twenty years and British medical opinion is now in favour of making use of B.C.G. vaccine in this country under careful supervision.

Pasteurization of Milk is essential to eliminate the bovine bacillus.

Voluntary segregation of patients in a sanatorium for treatment until a tuberculosis lesion has closed, and the danger of spread of infection to the community is minimized, should be taught and encouraged.

Widespread propaganda in which nurses can play a great part is essential, and the public must learn:

That tuberculosis is an infectious disease and the ways in which it may be spread, that it is not a disgrace to have, or have had tuberculosis, and that there is no stigma attached to having been treated in a sanatorium, that tuberculosis, though one of the greatest social evils of our day, is preventable and taken in the early stages is curable, and that everyone should be familiar with the means of detecting this disease at its very beginning.

Diagnostic procedures. The history of the diagnosis of tuberculosis is of interest. Physical examination of the chest by auscultation was recommended by Laennec who invented the stethoscope. A physician named

Williams paid great importance to the excursions of the diaphragm and found that these were diminished on the diseased side in pulmonary tuberculosis. *Physical examination* includes percussion, auscultation, palpation and observation. The two last are applied particularly to noting the movements of the chest wall and the excursions of the diaphragm.

The lesions found in the port-mortem examination of patients who died of tuberculosis were shown to contain small nodules which were called *tubercles*. These lesions were thought by many physicians to contain living germs even before Koch made his *discovery of the tubercle bacillus in* 1882. The discovery by Röntgen of X-rays in 1895 which were employed comparatively soon in the diagnosis of pulmonary tuberculosis was the next step in diagnostic procedure. *The tuberculin test*, also elaborated by Koch and at present employed by means of Mantoux's test, followed.

At the present time the means available for the early diagnosis of pulmonary tuberculosis include:

X-ray examination of the chest now developed to so fine a means of scientific investigation that the earliest signs of disease can be detected.

Mass miniature radiography has recently been employed for the examination of groups of persons who, by reason of the nature of their work, the stress and strain with its resulting fatigue to which they may be exposed, or who by virtue of their particular age-group might, under certain given circumstances, be suspected of a tendency or liability to contract the disease. The results of this measure are satisfactory.

Bronchoscopy is employed under special circumstances as an aid in diagnosis.

Examination of sputum. Facilities for laboratory examination of sputum are now available to all physicians who care to make use of it.

Blood examination. The sedimentation rate of red blood cells is estimated because in acute tuberculous infections there is a considerable increase in sedimentation rate. Special serological tests are also employed.

Modes of onset. It is very important to be familiar with the modes of onset in tuberculosis. Many of these symptoms will be common to a number of other conditions but their cause should be investigated. The *symptoms of onset* will occur in one of two different forms. Either *general symptoms* will be set up, due to the toxins circulating in the blood stream. These include malaise, a tendency to be easily fatigued, anaemia and breathlessness, amenorrhoea, loss of appetite, indigestion, nausea, palpitation, repeated colds in the head, sweating, particularly at night, increased pulse rate, rise of temperature in the evening and gradual progressive loss of weight.

Local symptoms associated with the respiratory tract may arise. There may be *cough*, a little irritating cough which does not improve, or an attack of coughing may occur on waking each morning. *Sputum* may or may not be present. *Haemoptysis*, this may be a little staining of sputum, occasional slight spitting of blood or a severe attack may occur. *Pleurisy* is a fairly common mode of onset. The subject may have had an attack of pleurisy some years previously or the first attack may be the onset of tuberculosis. An attack of pleurisy should never be ignored.

Symptoms. A very great variety of symptoms may occur in most cases of pulmonary tuberculosis, the following group may be considered fairly characteristic:

Cough, which is dry and hacking at first, later loose and, in severe cases, paroxysmal in character.

Sputum, at first scanty and mucoid, then copious and muco-purulent; in all cases it may be blood-stained and, in cases with cavity formation, it is nummular in character (see p. 75).

Dyspnoea is present in all acute cases, and in chronic cases which are not responding to treatment.

Pain may be present either as the result of pleurisy or of pleural adhesions.

Temperature. All cases with toxaemia show a rise in temperature, and acute cases run a high temperature which may be either constant, intermittent or remittent. In some cases the fever is inverse in type (see p. 42); this is considered to be a serious sign.

Wasting is marked when the disease is progressive.

Sweating is very troublesome, and so-called *night sweats* are disturbing to the patient's rest as his clothing becomes soaked with sweat and has to be changed frequently.

Clubbing of the fingers occurs in most cases of advanced pulmonary tuberculosis.

Complications. Many of the distressing symptoms met with in pulmonary tuberculosis may be regarded as complications; *laryngitis* may be catarrhal or tuberculous, *pleurisy* may be dry or with effusion, *haemoptysis* may be slight or severe. Less common complications include *spontaneous pneumothorax*, *bronchitis*, *asthma*, *bronchiectasis* and *empyema*.

Spread of infection to other parts of the body may give rise to intestinal tuberculosis, fistula-in-ano, meningitis, tuberculous infection of the lymphatic glands, bones, joints and urinary tract.

Treatment and nursing. *Rest* is of importance, and febrile cases will be ordered absolute rest, until the temperature has been down for several weeks, then graduated movements will be permitted.

The *aim of the treatment* is to relieve toxaemia, and therefore rest is maintained until signs of toxaemia have abated. Another important point in treatment is to help the patient to build up a resistance to the disease, and this is carefully carried out by giving him short periods of graduated exercise. Each time this exertion acts as a slight stimulus to the patient's body and a certain small amount of toxin is poured into the circulation, and by this means he is actually being given a dose of his own toxin in much the same way that vaccine treatment would act. This form of treatment is described as *graduated exercise and work*, and it is important for the nurse to realize that the success of the treatment throughout depends on a progressive increase, provided that the temperature remains normal and the weight stationary, and that untoward symptoms can be avoided, such as increased cough and sputum. Should either of these conditions arise, a return to a quieter life and in some cases to a further period of rest would have to be considered.

In the care of a patient with pulmonary tuberculosis, food, fresh air, observation of weight and observation of sputum are very important. The *diet* will be of high calorie value, as described on p. 285, but in many cases the nurse will find her resources taxed to the utmost to persuade the patient to take the amount of food he really requires. As far as possible the patient should sleep in the open air day and night; if he is indoors the windows should always be open and his bed should face an open window. When patients are nursed indoors there should be 12 feet of wall space between the beds in the ward if possible.

The *weight* should be carefully charted and the patient weighed every week, at the same time of day, and wearing exactly the same clothing each time.

With regard to the *sputum*, the quantity and character should be carefully noted. It is definitely infectious in cases of open tuberculosis and it is best to consider it so in all cases. It may be received in sputum cups or flasks, which should be sterilized every day. The patient should use only paper handkerchiefs which must be burned after use, and he should be provided with a calico pocket in which to keep this handkerchief to avoid soiling either his personal clothing or the bedclothing. This calico pocket should be boiled or steam disinfected before it is washed.

Special nursing care. A patient with pulmonary tuberculosis may be only slightly ill or he may be confined to bed suffering from many distressing symptoms and marked weakness and prostration. The nurse who undertakes sanatorium work should be able to adapt herself readily to the physical state and temperament of her patients.

A patient on *absolute rest* has to be helped to be helpless. It will help him to rest if he is treated skilfully, if his bed is carefully and well made and he is cleverly handled when being washed, so that he feels he is being attended to by one who cares for the work she is doing and who, whilst being businesslike about it, can at the same time spare a moment to speak and smile and keep him interested so that the treatment, which might otherwise be dreaded, becomes a pleasure to be anticipated.

When absolute rest is ordered, a patient requires to be fed because he must be spared all exertion. To many, it is very irksome to have another person put food into one's mouth, and to avoid irritation this must be done with care and tact.

Patients who are very ill, and running a temperature, may not be able to take solid food and may be fed on fluids and semi-solids and jellies. Care should be taken to see that the patient takes the amount of food in calories that is ordered. In all cases it is possible to disguise cream in soups and sweets, and cases have been known where patients who had been fat-shy all their lives have taken their allotted portion disguised in this way.

Most cases of pulmonary tuberculosis even when allowed up will be on definite periods of rest; these are usually planned to be taken before and after meals. The importance of rest before the two main meals, dinner and supper, should be impressed on the patient and he should have a good rest after the midday meal also. Patients must be taught that these rest periods must be real rest and no work or recreation which can be performed when lying down should be permitted. They ought not to read but relax, and as the art of relaxation can be taught, the nurse in a sanatorium who makes one, or even two rounds amongst her patients during the rest hour, showing her interest in each, and encouraging by a cheerful word that will inhibit any restlessness she may notice, will do much to help her patients to bear what might be irksome, until as habit forms they may perhaps come even to enjoy their rest.

Advice may be given about personal clothing. Many patients wrap up too much; in a number of instances cases of pulmonary tuberculosis tend to perspire a good deal and excess of clothing increases this. If a patient can be brought to see that he is in more danger of being chilled by this than by the movement of air he notices when sleeping out of doors, in a shelter, or in a room with all the windows open, this would be an advantage. The nurse might point out how few persons living habitually in the open air get colds. But this must not be done at the expense of comfort and all cases of pulmonary tuberculosis should always be warm enough. When in bed in the open air in winter they should wear clothing which comes well up round the neck, the hands should be protected from chapping, and the feet kept warm by properly protected hot-water bottles.

Painful and distressing symptoms may depress and weary a patient. *Haemoptysis* is a dreaded complication, many patients being frightened by tiny streaks of blood in the sputum, and even the slightest sign of haemoptysis should always be reported to the doctor, who will decide whether what is seen suggests a threatened attack of haemoptysis or is comparatively unimportant, and the nurse must try and help the patient to have absolute confidence in his decision and should take all steps to see that the patient does not worry, and if the doctor has decided the occasion is of no importance the patient must not be permitted to act as an invalid by staying in bed and refusing food.

When a patient has a *severe attack of haemoptysis* the nurse must remain by his side, send for the doctor—an emergency tray is usually ready in a sanatorium, containing the remedies the physician is in the habit of ordering. Keeping the patient still the nurse should reassure him, clear his mouth of bloodclot, keep the blood he has brought up out of his sight and remove all traces of blood from his mouth and clothing. She must be encouraging, as the patient will be frightened; feeling his pulse, she should nod her head or make some other movement indicating her satisfaction with her findings; then, wiping the sweat from his brow and putting his head on the pillow he may relax and rest, reassured.

After an attack of haemoptysis the patient will be kept in bed, his diet will be light and absolute rest may be ordered. He should be watched for any recurrence of the symptom.

Breathlessness is apt to be distressing, and the patient may have to be propped up in bed. The doctor will order any drugs necessary. The nurse should see if support of the chest gives relief, and she might support the patient's head during an attack of dyspnoea; even if it does not relieve the condition, which is unlikely, at least it lets the distressed patient realize that she is willing and anxious to help him and the proximity of a sympathetic nurse gives mental relief.

Pain in the chest may be due to pleurisy or it may be muscular in origin. The doctor should be informed of the onset of pain and in the meantime the nurse might rub some liniment gently in and cover the painful part with a pad of warm cotton wool or hold a lightly filled warm water bottle to the painful area. Strapping the chest will usually give relief; but this is better left until the doctor has been, as he will want to examine the chest first.

Nausea, indigestion, vomiting and *diarrhoea* are symptoms which so very commonly accompany pulmonary tuberculosis and increase the difficulty of feeding a patient. These symptoms necessitate altering the diet and making experiments to try and discover when the patient can eat and, if he is vomiting, what he can retain. In cases where vomiting is marked, only small quantities of beef extracts, champagne and glucose may be tolerated during an attack.

Diarrhoea often indicates infection of the small intestine—tuberculous enteritis. The doctor will order medicines and perhaps suggest trying peptonized foods, arrowroot and Benger's food until the attack may abate. As in serious attacks of vomiting, very little of anything can be taken during a bad attack, and the provision of foods and fluid acceptable to a patient in these distressing circumstances taxes the resources of a nurse to the utmost.

Pharyngitis, laryngitis and *loss of voice.* An alkaline mouth-wash is an excellent remedy for the slight mucoid secretion many patients with pulmonary tuberculosis complain of first thing in the morning. When the larynx is affected the voice is usually affected also, and the only way to rest this organ is to rest the voice.

To be forbidden to speak is very trying, and keeping silence often makes a patient depressed; the nurse must adapt herself to the new conditions and chatter pleasantly and agreeably, never expecting to be answered or using conversation which might provoke, or tend to provoke, an answer from a patient bidden to be silent. She may tell cheerful stories of what is happening amongst the others; recount items of interest she has read, describe the last picture she saw, if this is a suitable subject, and so on. The patient may be irritated at not being able to tell her of his interests, but if she has only one or two patients she might try to read the same newspaper and say 'did you see this?'—she could be answered by a nod or shake of the head—and then go on to say what in it has interested her. The patient will read and think and perhaps write a note for the nurse to consider, and talk about on her next visit.

When there is pain and difficulty in swallowing, the diet may have to be modified, and irritating or hard foods omitted. Local treatment or inhalations may be ordered, the nurse may have to encourage a patient to persevere with an inhalation, or in the use of an inhaler he dislikes.

Sleeplessness and night sweats. Sleeplessness and its treatment have been described on p. 338. Nightsweats may be the discomfort keeping a patient awake. In a mild form night sweats may be induced by excessive bedclothing; sweating may occur in a patient with even a slight rise of temperature as the temperature declines during the early morning hours and the skin acts profusely. In the majority of instances night sweats occur most frequently in acute cases and in others towards the last stages of illness.

The sweating is usually severe enough to cause the clothing, bedclothing and mattress to be thoroughly wet. In some sanatoria the patients sleep on rush matting, the sweat being absorbed by the matting, which dries quickly. The patient should be rubbed down, or sponged if necessary, and if it will not waken him so thoroughly that he may not sleep again. He should have dry clean clothing and be given a drink, and if his feet are not warm he should have a hot-water bottle.

Some physicians order a patient small doses of belladonna for the relief of night sweats.

Fever. A rise of temperature usually occurs in most cases of pulmonary tuberculosis. In some the type of fever is inverse, in others the patients have a high temperature at six o'clock in the evening but intermissions occur in the early morning.

When the temperature is very high, tepid sponging may be ordered. When in charge of a patient who is having a rise of temperature each evening the nurse will find he complains of headache, malaise and feels hot and uncomfortable, and she can help to relieve these distressing symptoms by performing his evening bath and toilet with care, aiming at reducing the heat of the body, and increasing his comfort so that he may obtain rest and perhaps go to sleep.

In a patient with pulmonary tuberculosis even a slight rise of temperature, 100–101° F., is usually due to an increase of toxaemia and indicates the need for rest.

A patient who is having a marked rise of temperature each evening may be unable to take his usual amount of food for supper, and this will necessitate a rearrangement of the diet so that more food is taken at the other two meals during the day.

Getting up. When patients with pulmonary tuberculosis are getting up out of bed, great care must be taken to see that they do not exert themselves excessively, and that they understand thoroughly the necessity for leading a comparatively quiet life; they should rest conscientiously for half an hour on their beds before each of the two main meals of the day, and after the midday meal they should rest, and if possible sleep for an hour to an hour and a half.

On *discharge from hospital* it is important that patients should be able to continue the mode of life they have learnt to follow during their hospital treatment, particularly with regard to the prevention of infection to others, and this should be their guide on returning home. The nurse should take the opportunity of impressing on the patient the need for having a comparatively early bedtime, and a fixed time of rising; the necessity of having good regular meals; and that, with regard to recreations, excessive exertion and excitement should be avoided, as well as anything which might lead to the infection of other people, such as dancing, the use of playing cards and so on. The occupation a patient chooses on leaving hospital should, as far as possible, enable him to live the type of life that he has grown used to.

A number of supplementary treatments are employed during the treatment of cases of pulmonary tuberculosis in hospital and sanatorium including various forms of collapse therapy, monaldi drainage of lung cavities, sanocrysin and vaccine therapy.

Collapse therapy. The operations which are undertaken in the treatment of pulmonary tuberculosis, are based on the principle of collapsing the lung in order to bring the walls of cavities into such approximation that healing may take place. This treatment results in expelling, in open cases, the secretion contained in the cavities, so that it is coughed up. In this way improvement is brought about in the general condition of the patient because the pus and secretion which is causing toxaemia is first diminished and finally removed. The healing of the cavity allows the wound in the lung to close and therefore the source of infection to others, i.e., an open tuberculosis, is removed (see below). At the same time the lung is rested because it is put out of action.

Artificial pneumothorax is employed when thin-walled cavities are present and when the disease is mainly affecting one lung, although bilateral pneumothorax is also employed in selected cases. In early cases this may be employed at the beginning of treatment. In other cases it is used when a period of rest in bed does not result in a fall of temperature to normal. When an artificial pneumothorax can be adequately established it is maintained for an indefinite period. Failure to establish an artificial pneumothorax may be due to adhesions which prevent the lung from collapsing; failure to maintain it may be due to complications, the commonest being pleural effusion.

Pneumoperitoneum. Passing air in to the peritoneum is employed in cases which may not respond to pneumothorax probably because the cavity in the lung lies deep. A phrenic crush usually precedes pneumoperitoneum in order to ensure that the diaphragm is as high as possible.

Before operation the patient's bladder must be emptied as otherwise it may be perforated. A needle is passed into the upper part of the peritoneal cavity, above the level of the umbilicus, either in the middle line or a little to the right. Air is then introduced by means of the Lillingston-Pearson apparatus. The amount introduced varies, and is determined by the pressure shown on the manometer and subsequent X-ray examination. Refills are required more frequently than in the case of pneumothorax.

Oleothorax is the injection of oil into the pleural cavity. This measure is not often used as the oil is not absorbed and sepsis may result.

Apicolysis is the injection of paraffin wax between the chest wall and the parietal pleura. This measure aims at collapse of the apex of the lung. As it may be attended by complications it is not often used.

Phrenic Nerve Paralysis. The nerve which supplies the diaphragm may be crushed (phrenic crush), or it may be divided (phrenic avulsion). A phrenic crush paralyses the diaphragm for about six months and the diaphragm rises about two inches.

A small incision is made at the side of the neck, the nerve is steadied by means of a hook and crushed between the blades of a pair of forceps. In avulsion the nerve is divided and drawn out from its attachments in the thorax.

Thoracoscopy for pneumolysis. A small incision is made in the wall of the chest and an endoscope consisting of lamp and telescope is introduced into the space provided by a pneumothorax. The presence of adhesions is investigated. If adhesions are present an electro-cautery is passed in through a second cannula and the adhesions are divided.

The small wound is closed by one stitch. A pad is strapped over the opening and the patient is advised to press on the pad when he wants to cough, otherwise air, from the pneumothorax, may be forced out of the chest and, by entering the subcutaneous tissues, this air would cause a mild surgical emphysema. Subcutaneous emphysema is characterized by a crackling sensation beneath the skin around the wound.

After the division of pleural adhesions the patient should be kept fairly quiet. There will generally be a rise in the temperature and an increase in the pulse rate if the operation was more than slight. The reaction to be watched for and which may cause distress is pleural effusion. A collection of blood or pus severe enough to displace the trachea and heart would probably be accompanied by dyspnoea and a rising pulse rate.

Thoracotomy is an open operation performed for the removal of dense adhesions which cannot be dealt with by thoracoscopy. A small piece of rib is resected and the adhesions are divided.

Extrapleural pneumothorax is performed by resection of a short length of the back part (usually) of the fourth rib. The lung and the adherent parietal pleura are stripped from the endothoracic fascia, air is then introduced under pressure to fill the space created and keep the lung from expanding. Coughing may be frequent both during and after the operation, and as this increases pressure in the space which has been formed, air may be forced out of the chest into the subcutaneous tissue causing surgical emphysema. Firm pressure of the hand over the wound whilst the patient is coughing will help to prevent emphysema spreading.

In a few cases an emphysema may quickly spread up over the neck and side of the face. This may seem alarming but it is not dangerous. Another complication is that serum, blood or pus may collect in the space created. If this happens the fluid must be removed by frequent aspiration. In some cases this complication, particularly where pus collects, will be accompanied by symptoms of fairly severe toxaemia.

After this operation the patient needs the same care as after thoracoplasty (see below) but the shock is less severe.

Thoracoplasty is a major operation performed in pulmonary tuberculosis. It consists in removing ribs so that the lung can fall inwards, thus providing permanent collapse. The operation is divided into stages so that the shock inflicted at any one stage is not more than the patient can bear. Blood grouping is carried out because the patient will probably require a blood transfusion. The type of patient selected for this operation usually has cavities in the upper part of the lung which have not responded to treatment by other forms of collapse therapy. The general condition of the patient must be as high as possible, but it must always be remembered that the patient upon whom this operation is to be performed is already debilitated by his disease. For details of the operation and nursing care, and for operations performed for removal of lung tissue include *lobectomy* and *pneumomectomy*, see chapter 46.

Monaldi Drainage of lung cavity. During the last two to three years a closed suction drainage (monaldi drainage) of cavities filled with secretion has been developed. It has proved useful in relieving toxaemia in cases which have not responded to artificial pneumothorax. It is also of value in reducing the size of cavities, thus modifying the extent of the operation should thoracoplasty afterwards need to be performed.

A narrow tube is introduced into the cavity through a cannula. The free end of the narrow tube or catheter is attached to a suction pump which is kept working continuously and is connected with a glass bottle into which the secretion from the cavity is drawn. If drainage can be established the cavity will be reduced in size. It may even disappear altogether. The secretion which would otherwise be coughed up is removed by suction. In some cases drainage is continued for many weeks, with progressive improvement in the patient's general condition. As far as *nursing* is concerned, the chief point is to see that the catheter is attached to the skin of the chest and cannot be pulled out of the cavity. The amount of secretion collected should be measured and charted. The nurse should be familiar with the apparatus and know how to adjust it in order to keep it working effectively. If blood appears in the secretion it is usual to stop drainage for 2 to 3 days though the appearance of blood does not denote danger. The size of the cavity is watched by regular X-ray examination and the gradual reduction in size is noted. When all the benefit that can be expected from the treatment has been obtained the tube is removed. As a general rule the tube track heals without difficulty though in a few cases tuberculous granulation tissue forms and then healing takes longer.

HINTS ON HYGIENE TO NURSES

Tuberculosis is a preventable disease. Most hospitals and sanatoria have their own carefully-thought-out measures to prevent infection, which should be loyally observed. One of the functions of a sanatorium is to teach patients how to prevent spreading infection and how to live safely within certain limits. Instruction regarding the spread of infection and how this may be avoided is given to all grades of staff employed in a sanatorium.

In pulmonary tuberculosis infection is conveyed by droplet infection, secretions from nose and mouth, handkerchiefs, sputum, and dust which contains bacilli from dried sputum and secretions. Patients should be taught to avoid spraying droplets from nose and mouth in speaking and laughing, to cover the nose and mouth with a large handkerchief when coughing and to use a sputum cup or flask for expectoration.

When performing treatments at the bedside a nurse should see that the patient's head is turned away from her, to one side; she should stand on the same side of the bed as the physician when he is examining a patient; avoid touching patient's handkerchiefs or sputum cups except when wearing gloves, handle bedclothing and patient's personal clothing carefully so that dust is not raised, and wash the hands immediately after handling anything likely to be infected. (The application of white oil to blankets and spindle oil to floor boards is employed in some hospitals to reduce dust.)

When collecting sputum cups, gloves should be worn. Sputum is generally dealt with by a porter or orderly. It is sterilized before it is emptied into a drain. The cups are sterilized and returned to the ward. If any sputum is upset it should immediately be wiped up with swabs wrung out of a strong antiseptic. Receptacles for specimens of sputum should be labelled *before* they are handed to the patient.

Patient's handkerchiefs. Paper ones should be collected into a paper bag and burnt. Cotton ones are collected into a pail containing disinfectant. These are then taken to the laundry where they soak for some hours and are boiled before being washed.

Hospital Rules. Nurses should make themselves familiar with the hospital's rules for the proper method of collection and disposal of soiled dressings, dust sweepings, ward refuse and waste food; for the special treatment of all articles used such as thermometers, instruments, utensils, linen and bedding; the routine care of all fixtures and fittings including sinks and drains; and for the care of domestic appliances such as brooms, brushes and dusters. These rules should be conscientiously kept, they have only one object—the prevention of infection.

Ward maids and other domestic workers employed in a sanatorium should be taught scientific methods of sweeping, dusting and cleaning and the proper care of all the articles they use. They should understand how infection is conveyed and the measures laid down for the prevention of spread of infection.

Nurses' Health. Nurses undergo a physical examination before they are accepted for training in a sanatorium. This examination includes an X-ray examination of the chest, and Mantoux's test (see p. 509). Further to this the nurse will be expected to report minor ailments such as colds without delay so that she may be excluded from duty if the physician considers this advisable. She should attend for record of her weight at regular (usually monthly) intervals, and she will be submitted to regular periodical X-ray examination of her chest.

The maintenance of the general health of the individual is of primary importance in resisting infection to tuberculosis. Nurses will find that they are provided with good food—three meals a day with snacks in between meal times will be so planned that nurses are never on duty on an empty stomach. Nurses must eat their meals and never go on duty fasting. They must always wash their hands before meals and not eat anything in the wards.

Good living conditions, airy bedrooms, pleasant dining rooms and sitting rooms, recreational facilities, provision for adequate rest and good teaching and studying facilities will all be provided. Leisure should be wisely used for healthy recreation and occupation and nurses should keep reasonable hours. Friendships with patients should be avoided.

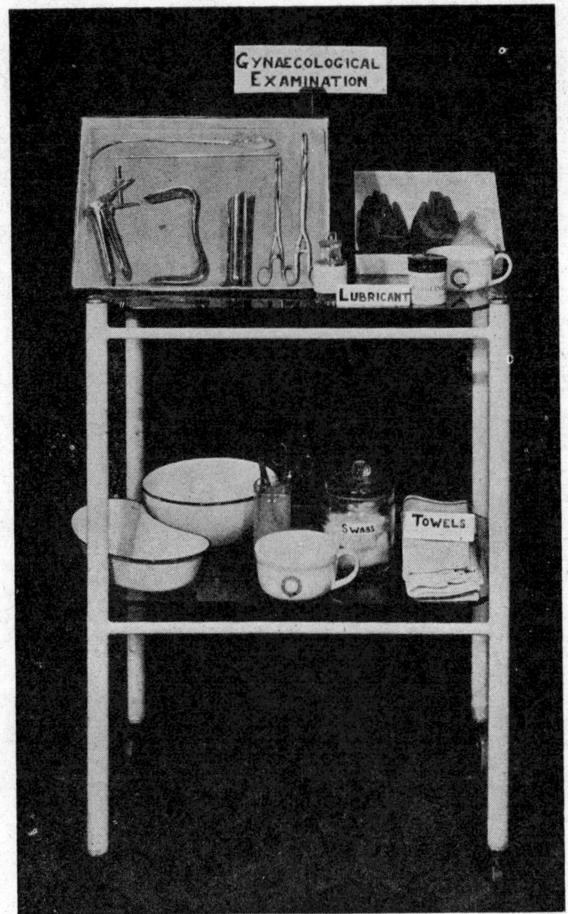

FIG. 174.—*see page* 545.

UPPER SHELF. Gloves, lubricant, swabs and instruments. Reading from Left to Right: Cusco's, Sims' and Fergusson's specula, two pairs of swab-holding forceps. At the top of the tray: Playfair's probe and uterine sound.

LOWER SHELF. Towels to protect the bed. Swabs, forceps and lotion for cleansing the vulva. Receptacles for soiled swabs and used instruments.

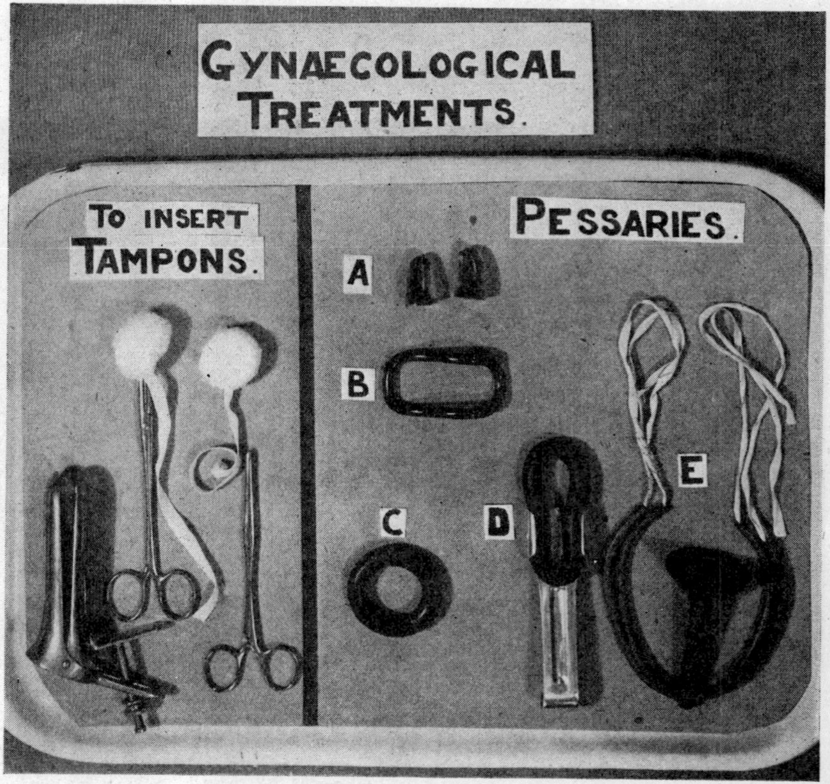

FIG. 175.—*see pages* 546–48. For the insertion of tampons Cusco's vaginal speculum and long forceps will be needed. The pessaries shown are: (A) medicated ones. (B) Hodge's pessary. (C) ring pessary. (D) shows a ring pessary in a pessary introducer. (E) is Napier's cup and stem pessary.

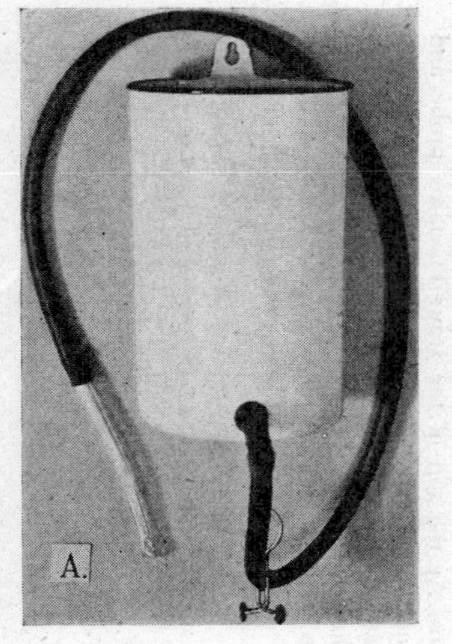

FIG. 176.—SIMPLE TYPE OF VAGINAL DOUCHING APPARATUS.
Can, tubing with control clip and nozzle. (*See also Fig.* 67, *page* 206.)

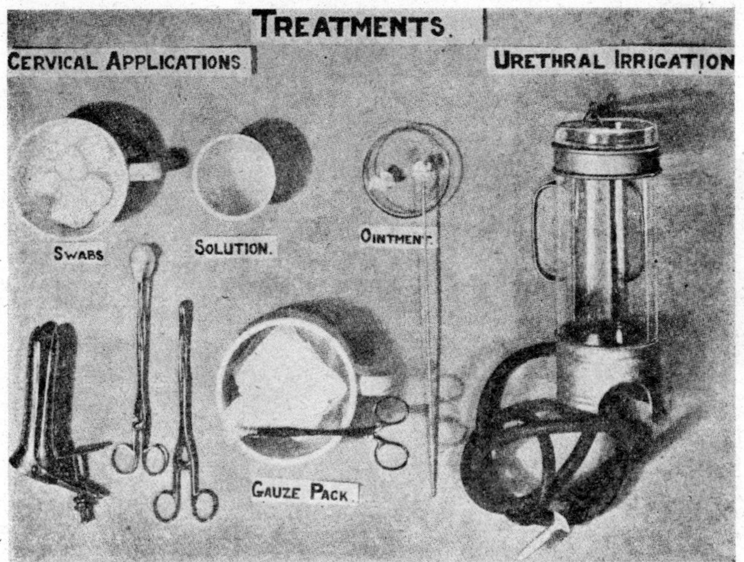

FIG. 177.—*see page* 546. Articles required for the local treatment of gonorrhoea in female patients. An irrigation can with tubing and nozzle is supplied for urethral irrigation. Reading from left to right: Cusco's vaginal speculum, forceps for holding swabs and for the insertion of gauze packing and an applicator for ointment.

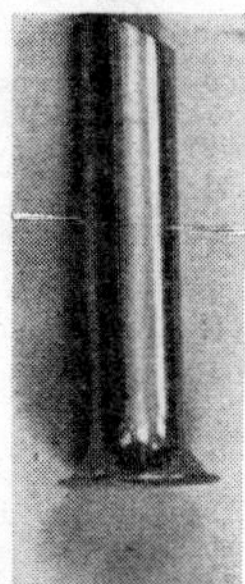

FIG. 178. Fergusson's vaginal speculum may alternatively be employed particularly for the purpose of applications to the cervix.

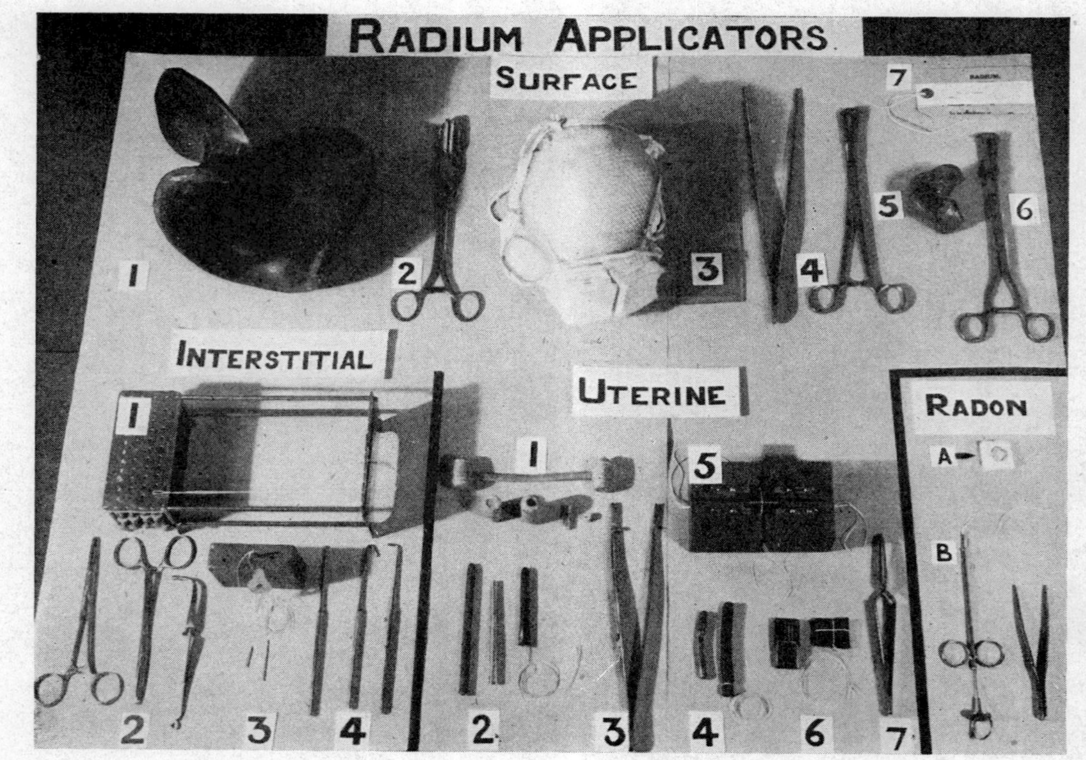
RADIUM APPLICATORS
SURFACE
1
2
3
4
5
6
7
INTERSTITIAL
1
2
3
4
UTERINE
1
2
3
4
5
6
7
RADON
A
B

FIG. 179.

FIG. 179. A VARIETY OF ARTICLES USED IN THE DIFFERENT METHODS OF RADIUM APPLICATION.

Reading from left to right, the articles on the upper row, for surface application, include:—

(1) Columbia paste collar for application to the neck;

(2) forceps, fitted with rubber for handling applicator;

(3) nedros applicator, which is lighter than columbia paste—the example shown is on the plaster cast on which it was moulded to fit the patient;

(4) long forceps for holding radium needles when charging applicators;

(5) dental applicator, and (6) special forceps for handling it;

(7) label, this is attached to the bed whilst the patient is wearing radium—during interstitial radiation it remains there until the radium is withdrawn—when applicators are employed the label is removed from the bed and attached to the carrier in which the radium is removed.

The name of the patient, the number of needles used and the date and duration of the application, are written on the label.

INTERSTITIAL APPLICATION.

(1) A special stand in which radium needles are sterilized—a needle threaded with silk is shown in position;

(2) forceps or holders for handling radium needles;

(3) lead block, for retention of needles whilst threading—a needle is shown threaded by means of a small needle threader;

(4) instruments called 'needle pushers' for projecting the loaded needles into the tissues.

UTERINE APPLICATIONS. For the *Paris method* articles 1, 2 and 3 are required.

(1) Colpostat composed of two hollow corks, one placed at each end of a flexible spring—below this the hollow corks can be seen; one has been charged and the other has the silver screen, containing radium, lying beside it;

(2) the blunt end of a gum elastic catheter (size 14), a strip of thin platinum is used to line the catheter and acts as a screen, and the catheter is shown ready charged, and threaded with strong silk.

(3) forceps, provided with a strong clip, for handling radium.

The *Stockholm method;* articles 4, 5, 6 and 7 are required.

(4) A silver screen fitted with caps, and rubber bag containing the silver screen which is holding radium—the bag is shown with silk thread ready in position for insertion into the cervix and uterine canal;

(5) lead box used for loading silver screens;

(6) square silver screens, grooved for the reception of radium-filled needles—beside it lies a closed screen in the rubber bag, tied round with silk, in which it is introduced;

(7) long forceps for handling radium-charged screens.

RADON.

(A) Radon seeds placed on a piece of elastoplast felt, ready for application to the surface of the skin;

(B) radon introducer showing seed in position, for insertion into the tissues of the body. Dissecting forceps are used for handling the radon seeds when charging the introducer.

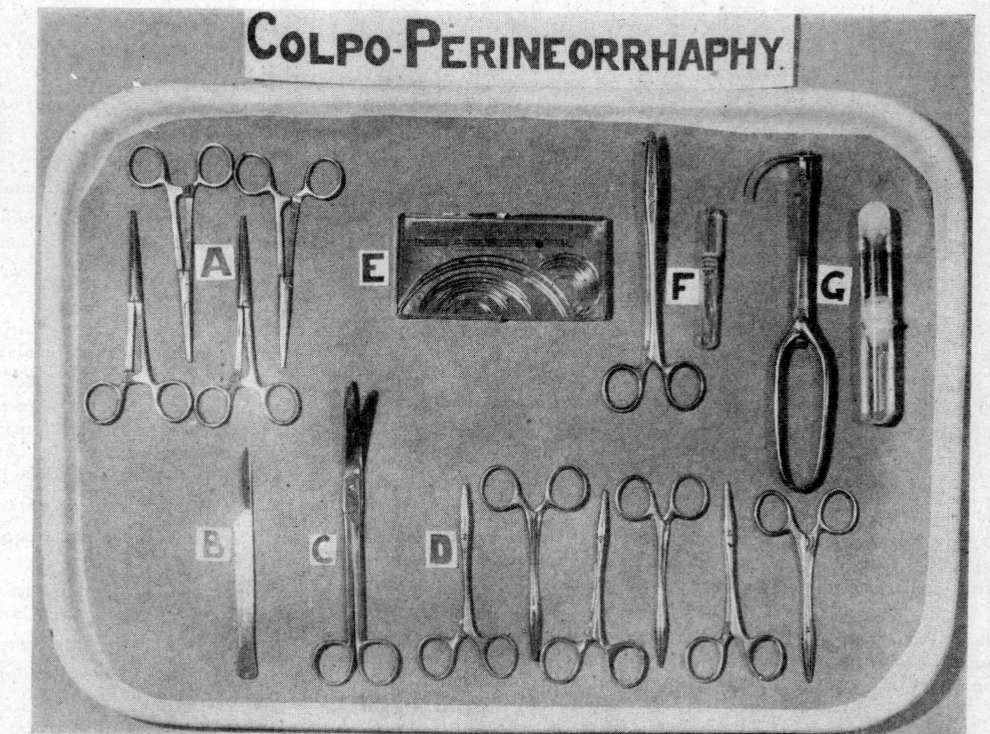

FIG. 180.—*see page* 537.
(A) Four pairs of Kocker's artery forceps. (B) scalpel. (C) angular round-point scissors. (D) six pairs of Spencer-Wells's artery forceps. (E) needles. (F) Bonney's needle holder and a tube of catgut. (G) Bonney's modification of Reverdin's needle and a tube of 'chorda' catgut.

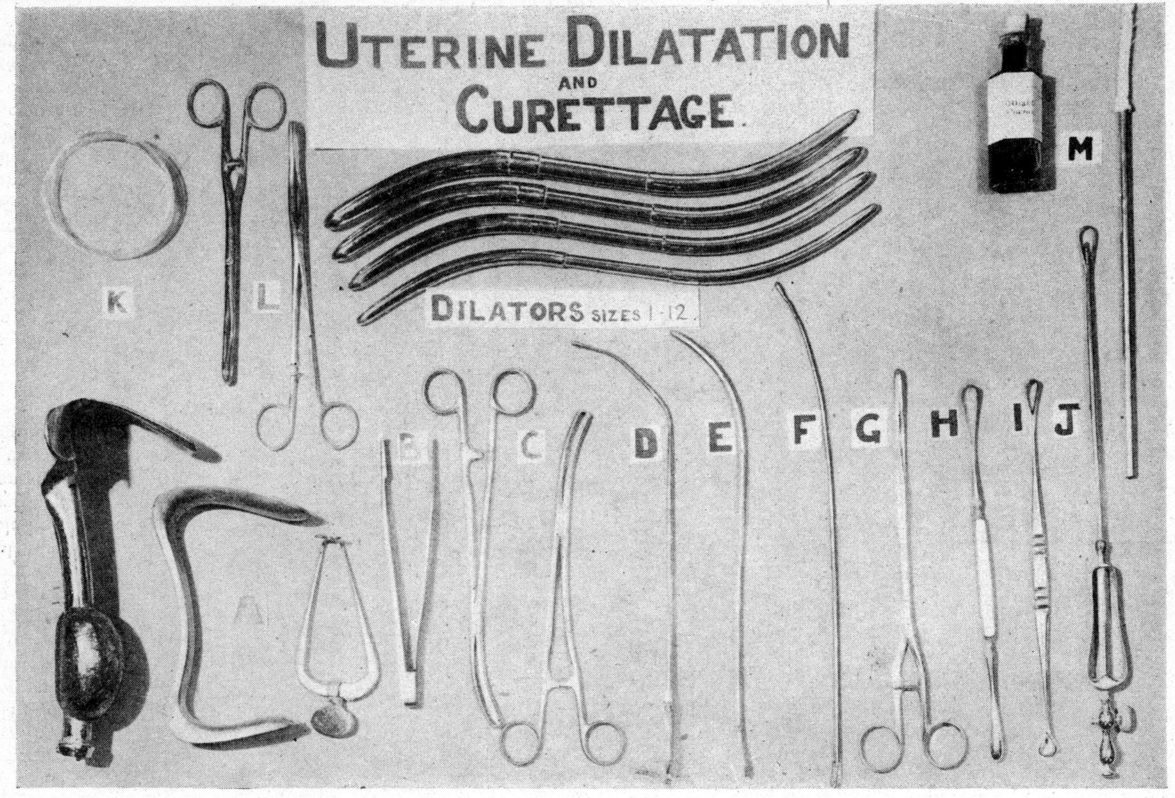

FIG. 181.—*see pages* 537–39. Reading from left to right: (A) Auvard's and Sims' vaginal specula and Berkeley's vulva retractor. (B) Bonney's dissection forceps. (C) Two pairs of vulsellum forceps. (D) Uterine sound. (E) Bladder sound. (F) Long probe. (G) Miscarriage forceps. (H) Large spoon. (I) Curette. (J) Flushing Curette. (K) Glass slides. (L) Two pairs of ovum forceps. (M) Iodized phenol and a Playfair's probe. In the centre sample sizes of Fenton's uterine dilators are shown.

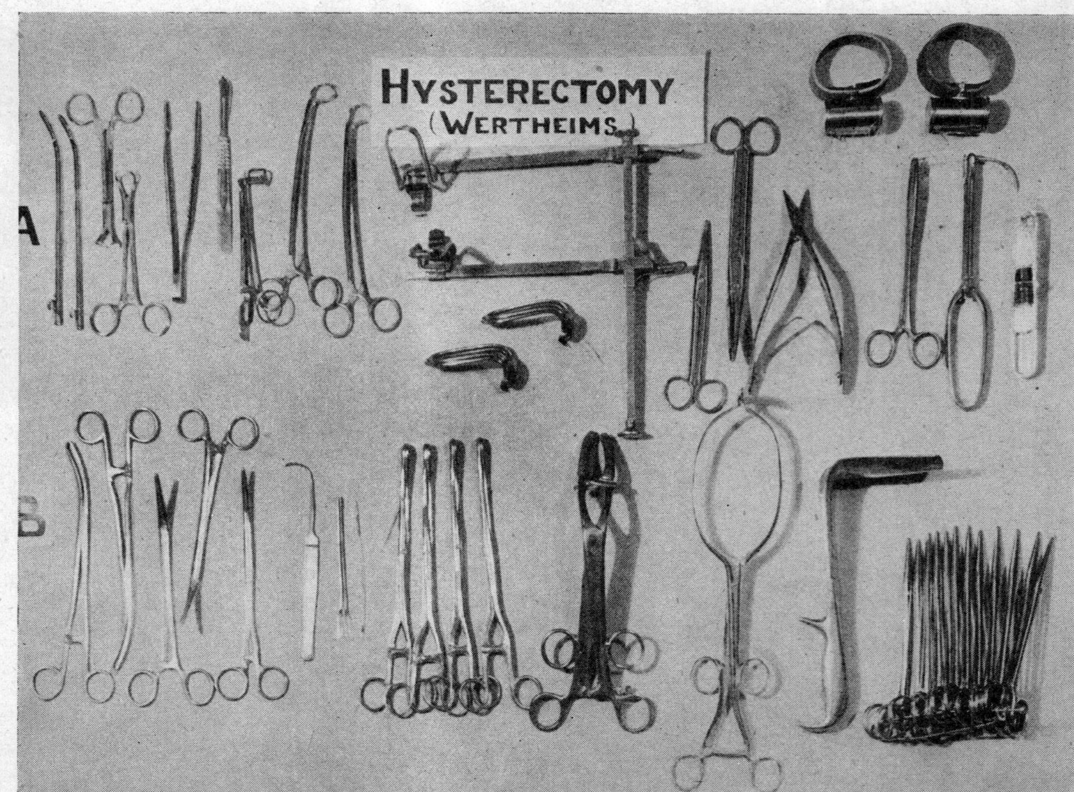

FIG. 182.—*see page* 542. Reading from left to right: UPPER ROW. (A) two silver catheters, two pairs of Mayo's towel clips, Bonney's toothed dissecting forceps, Bard-Parker's knife (large size), Gray's modified towel clip, Moynihan's tetra-towel clips (two pairs), Bonney's self-retaining abdominal wall retractor (with extra blades), Mayor's dissecting scissors, Wertheim's scissors, Bonney's (third hand) scissors, needle holders, catgut, and ligature carriers.

LOWER ROW. (B) Vulsellum forceps (two pairs), Kocker's angular artery forceps (two pairs), Berkeley-Bonney's round ligament forceps, aneurysm needle, probe director and probe, ovum forceps (four pairs), Bonney's myomectomy clamp, Berkeley-Bonney's special clamp for Wertheim's operation, bladder retractor and Spencer-Wells's artery forceps (one dozen pairs). *All the articles shown except the special Wertheim's clamp would be required for other types of hysterectomy.*

Chapter 36

A Short Outline of Venereal Diseases and their Management

A short account of syphilis and its treatment—The mode of infection in gonorrhoea, acute and chronic stages, treatment—Gonococcal vulvo-vaginitis—A note on soft sore and poradenitis

It is desirable that every nurse, however junior she may be, should have some idea of venereal disease and the types most commonly met with.

It is sufficient to say in description that a venereal disease is one acquired in a venereal manner. There are three diseases described,

(1) *Syphilis,* due to the *Spirochaeta pallida,* which was described by Schaudinn and Hoffman in 1905. Since that date the term 'Treponema pallidum' has been adopted by the International Committee on nomenclature, and this is now the only correct name for the organism of syphilis.

(2) *Gonorrhoea,* due to the presence of *Neisseria gonorrhoea* (the diplococcus of Neisser) discovered in 1872.

(3) *Soft sore,* due to Ducrey's bacillus, discovered in 1884.

Prevention of venereal disease. The only sane approach to the prevention of venereal disease is by education, and not by compulsion. Education may take longer but it will be more effective. Venereal disease is contracted principally by sexual promiscuity and what is needed to deal with this evil is a higher standard of the ideal of sex. At present the moral stigma attaches to those unfortunate victims of disease and not to those who have escaped! When public opinion *hates the evil* without judging the victim of disease then a standard will be reached and progress in the prevention of venereal disease may be expected.

As nurses we treat the individual patient without asking how or why. Early and adequate treatment is essential if success is to be attained. Treatment may be long, and the patient will require all the help and encouragement we can give in order to persevere until a cure is established. The following notes contain some idea of how far reaching in its disabling effects syphilis, for example, can be.

Nurses are a large section of the community and one which can contribute a great deal towards teaching the public what is the right attitude to adopt towards the prevention of venereal disease.

SYPHILIS

Syphilis is a disease which runs a definite course passing through several phases. The length of the *incubation period* is from 3 to 4 weeks, with extreme limits of from 10 days to 3 months. *Infection* is conveyed by sexual intercourse, and in addition in a few cases it may be transmitted by kissing. In these cases the mouth and lips are the site of infection. It may also be contracted by doctors, nurses and midwives handling infected material.

Syphilis may be prenatal (congenital), or acquired. The *first clinical sign* of acquired syphilis is, usually, the occurrence of a *primary sore* or *chancre* at the site of inoculation, in men on the penis, and in women on some part of the genital area. The lesion is described as *extragenital* when it occurs on some other part, as for example, in the case of a doctor or midwife, when it may occur on an infected finger.

The *treponema pallidum* enters the body at the site of inoculation. It causes a local reaction which results in the appearance of the chancre and possibly also of some adenitis of the neighbouring lymphatic glands. But the organism, or parasite of syphilis not only invades the tissues, it also invades the blood stream so that a general as well as a local infection is established.

Classification. The phases or stages of syphilis were formerly described under the Ricordian classification as:

Primary. The appearance of the chancre.
Secondary. Appearance of rash and constitutional symptoms.
Latent. A period during which no symptoms were present.
Tertiary. The stage when symptoms of the cardio-vascular system, viscera and nervous system appeared.

But this classification has been superseded by the more useful one elaborated by the late Dr. E. T. Burke in his work on Venereal Diseases in which syphilis is divided into two stages, acute and chronic, each containing a number of degrees.

Acute Syphilis	First degree,	primary stage, Wassermann	negative
	Second ,,	,, ,, ,,	positive
	Third degree,	secondary stage, Early	
	Fourth ,,	,, ,, Late	
Chronic Syphilis	Fifth degree,	Endosyphilis	
	Sixth ,,	Tertiary with visceral changes	
	Seventh ,,	Neurosyphilis	
	Eighth ,,	Prenatal (Congenital)	

Dr. Burke also described the significance of considering syphilis in the age group in which it occurs:

(1) Before the age of 20 years. In these cases the gravest and most irreparable damage occurs in the tissues because the body is still developing and the tissues are very vulnerable to attack by the *treponema pallidum.*

(2) From 20 to 50 years. This is the age when man is at his prime and the tissues are more resistant, so that although the effects of syphilis are severe they are not as devastating as when the disease is contracted before the age of 20 or after the age of 50.

(3) Over 50 years. Man is now past his prime, his body is less resistant to disease and if syphilis is contracted great damage is likely to ensue.

The *primary phase* (first and second degrees) is characterized by the initial reaction and appearance of the chancre 3 to 4 weeks after infection. Towards the end of this phase the Wassermann reaction is positive.

The *secondary phase* (third and fourth degrees) occurs some 3 to 4 weeks later or about 2 months after the initial infection, it is characterized by a rash and constitutional symptoms. The *rash* appears on the trunk and arms, face, palms, and soles, and over the anal, perineal and genital regions. It may be pinkish, dull red, macular, papular or pustular. When on the anal and genital regions it may take the appearance of patches, or wart-like or cauliflower growths. All nurses should be warned that small erosions, sores, or wart-like growths over the genitalia should not be touched, the matter should be reported to the head nurse or ward sister without mentioning the fact to the patient. These lesions are teeming with the parasites of syphilis and are a source of infection by contact.

The *constitutional symptoms* may be slight, mild or severe. In the majority of cases they may be described as mild, and include sore throat, hoarseness, headache, malaise, general pains and some rise of temperature. The throat may be red or ulcerated—*a snail-track ulcer* is characteristic of syphilis.

Malignant syphilis. This type is rare. The term malignant is used to describe cases in which there is definite ulceration of the skin. The patient becomes very toxic, is anaemic, emaciated and extremely ill, and usually dies after several weeks' illness.

Chronic syphilis or the *third phase of the disease* includes what was formerly described as the 'latent' period followed by the symptoms of the tertiary phase. But the valuable work of Professor Warthin of Michigan has shown that *syphilis is a progressive disease*, and is never latent. The term *endosyphilis* is used to describe the period during which clinical signs of disease are not evident. Endosyphilis implies that active pathological changes are taking place within the tissues, changes which will result later in serious disablement. Lesions characteristic of chronic syphilis are numerous and may be classified as follows:

Cutaneous lesions such as syphilitic ulcers and gummatous tumours of the skin.

Lesions of mucous surfaces such as leukoplakia of the tongue and fauces, ulcers, gummatous tumours and erosion of the palate with perforation.

Lesions of bone and muscle include gummatous tumours, periostitis, osteitis, osteomyelitis and dactylitis. *Joints* may be the site of synovitis and arthritis.

Cardio-vascular syphilis is one of the most serious forms because any part of the circulatory system may be affected causing great disablement. These diseases may be classified as affecting:

The *heart*. Endocarditis, pericarditis, and myocarditis may occur. Degeneration or tumour may arise in the bundle of His causing heart block. Arteritis of the coronary vessels will cause angina pectoris.

The *aorta* may be affected by aortitis, tumour, dilatation and aneurysm.

The *blood vessels* by arteritis and ateriosclerosis giving rise to hypertension. Raynaud's disease may be due to syphilis. Gummatous tumours may arise in the walls of any of the blood vessels and in the lymphatics.

The *blood*. A primary pernicious anaemia may occur during the stage of chronic syphilis.

Neurosyphilis. Syphilitic meningitis may occur. Endarteritis of the cerebral vessels may result in thrombosis, aneurysm, or cerebral haemorrhage causing hemiplegia, diplegia or monoplegia. Gummatous tumours may arise in the brain or spinal cord. Locomotor ataxia (tabes dorsalis) and general paralysis of the insane (G.P.I.) or a combination of these, taboparesis may occur.

Visceral syphilis. The nose, larynx, bronchi, lungs and pleura—the salivary glands, oesphagus, stomach, intestine and rectum—the pancreas, spleen and liver—the kidneys and bladder—any part of the male and female genital tract—some of the endocrine glands—the optic nerve, eye and eyelids—the pinna, middle and inner ear may all be sites of syphilitic lesions.

Prenatal (*Congenital*) *syphilis* is subdivided into early and late manifestations. The parasite of syphilis causes very destructive changes in the developing foetus and the result may be abortion, a macerated foetus or stillbirth. When the child is born alive, if premature he will have the appearance of a little wizened old man; if born at term symptoms of syphilis will develop within the first 2 weeks of life—the earlier the symptoms appear the more serious is the condition of the infant.

Early signs of prenatal syphilis include rashes, snuffles, cracks and fissures about the mouth, and characteristic lesions of the mucous surfaces. The child may cry a great deal and scream when handled. He probably has some bone lesion, osteochondritis or epiphysitis, and handling causes pain. Many of these infants do not survive for long.

Signs of late prenatal syphilis. The classical signs include the saddle-shaped nose due to ulceration of the nasal bones; Hutchinson's notched or peg-shaped teeth which occur in the second dentition; eye lesions include interstitial keratitis and choroiditis. There may be thickening of bone and swelling at the joints. Juvenile neurosyphilis takes the form of mental deficiency, epilepsy, juvenile tabes dorsalis and general paralysis of the insane.

Tests used in syphilis. Microscopic *examination of blood serum* from the chancre, or from one of the infected glands is carried out on a dark background slide. The T. pallidum is seen as a delicate white spiral. The Wassermann or *complement-fixation test* is performed on blood serum and on cerebrospinal fluid. The Kahn modification of *the flocculation test* is performed on blood serum.

Treatment. Antisyphilitic treatment must be adequate and effective. *Penicillin* has revolutionized the treatment of both gonorrhoea and syphilis. Penicillin has been used in the treatment of syphilis since 1944 and the results have been satisfactory in both primary and secondary syphilis. During the war, sixty injections of 40,000 units were given three hourly until a maximum of 2,400,000 had been received, in thousands of cases. In civilian life it is practically impossible for all patients needing treatment to be admitted to hospital and it is now the practice to give eight daily injections of not less than 500,000 units of penicillin in a beeswax-arachis oil suspension. The simultaneous administration of a standard course of an arsenic-bismuth compound also is recommended.

It is necessary to keep in touch with all patients treated for two years. Several blood tests should be made during the first six months, followed by tests at intervals of three months.

The treatment of late syphilis by penicillin cannot at present be assessed but good results in neurosyphilis have been reported. The treatment of general paralysis of the insane by fever therapy is still considered necessary but it is now combined with penicillin treatment.

Prenatal syphilis needs to be treated with vigour in order to ensure the birth of an infant free from disease. Some authorities consider penicillin suitable and adequate, others say that if the mother has not previously had treatment for syphilis it is safer to give arsenic and bismuth preparations in addition to penicillin.

Congenital syphilis. Penicillin is well tolerated even by small infants. Here again some authorities consider penicillin adequate, whilst others consider that it should be used in addition to other forms of treatment and not entirely as a substitute for them.

More recently aureomycin has been shown to have a curative action on syphilis.

GONORRHOEA

Gonorrhoea is a highly communicable disease characterized by an acute inflammation at the site of infection with widespread suppurative catarrh of the affected mucous surfaces. The *incubation period* is from two to three days, and this is followed by an acute stage during which the inflammation is marked and the discharge copious, and after a time a subacute period follows during which the disease becomes chronic.

Infection is usually conveyed by means of sexual intercourse, but it may be acquired also by contact with infected clothing and utensils such as lavatory seats or the splash from a lavatory pan. Infection is very easily conveyed to the eyes of attendants, and the eyes of an infant may be infected during its passage through the birth canal.

The glands of the affected genital tract become involved—in the male the glands are the Cowper, the prostate and urethral glands; in the female the cervical and uterine glands, Bartholin's glands, and the para-urethral glands are easily infected. In addition the disease spreads to the urethra and rectum and in the female to the uterine tubes and pelvic peritoneum also.

Treatment. The use of the sulphonamide drugs and penicillin have revolutionized the treatment of *acute gonorrhoea.* Penicillin is the drug of choice and some advocate a single injection of 100,000 units followed by a similar dose 6 hours later. Others consider that the best results are obtained by giving smaller doses over a period of time. Five injections of 20,000 units at 2-hourly intervals, until a maximum of 100,000 units have been given is one method of administration.

In giving penicillin in the treatment of gonorrhoea it must be remembered that the same patient may be incubating syphilis, and to ensure that this is not the case, as penicillin may mask the symptoms, the patient should be examined at reasonable intervals and have serum tests for syphilis carried out during six months after treatment by penicillin.

Acute gonorrhoea in the female is frequently characterized by vulvitis, urethritis and cervicitis. Bartholinitis, vaginitis, cystitis and proctitis may also occur. In some cases there is a good deal of local inflammation and copious discharge, in other cases the local symptoms are mild, and the infection tends to pass unnoticed with the result that the condition becomes chronic and may give rise to a good deal of ill-health later. The degree of local infection and the amount of discharge present necessitate frequent cleansing, swabbing, and in some cases local irrigation and treatment in order to keep the affected areas clean and free from discharge.

Chronic gonorrhoea in the female. Any of the acute infections such as urethritis, Bartholinitis, vaginitis, and cervicitis may become chronic.

The uterine tubes, ovaries, uterus, and pelvic peritoneum may be affected and any of these may necessitate operative treatment.

Tests used in gonorrhoea. Microscopic examination of *smears* are taken from the various sites in the genital tract where the gonococcus may be present. *Cultures* of the organism are also grown and examination of the blood is made for the specific antibodies by means of the *gonococcal complement-fixation test*. *Diagnosis* is made by means of these tests when *positive* and *cure* is demonstrated when they prove *negative*. In all cases of gonorrhoea the Wassermann and Kahn tests for syphilis are also performed as a double infection, syphilis and gonorrhoea, may be present. Penicillin may mask the treatment of syphilis and serum tests for syphilis should be carried out for six months.

Tests of cure are most important. These should begin one month after treatment and be continued for as long as is considered necessary. The urethral and cervical secretions in women and the vesicular fluid in men should be examined.

Gonococcal Vulvo-vaginitis in children. Little girls may be infected directly by indecent assault, or indirectly by the use of contaminated towels, sponges, by sharing a bed with an infected person or from contaminated lavatory seats.

The *symptoms* are inflammation and swelling of the vulva, vaginal discharge, and pain on micturition.

The condition is *treated with penicillin* but unfortunately relapse is frequent as re-infection occurs. Whenever possible the patient should be admitted to hospital and kept in bed. The strictest precautions should be taken to avoid re-infection by contaminated personal clothing, bed-clothing and towels.

The *local treatment* consists of swabbing the vulva with weak antiseptic solutions and the applications of protargol ten per cent to the cervix and urethra. Vaginal douches and hot sitz baths are also used. The vulva should be carefully dried after each treatment and powdered, and a sterile pad should be applied.

SOFT SORE OR CHANCROID

In distinction to the hard chancre of syphilis a soft grey-white ulcer acquired in a venereal manner but being non-syphilitic in origin and character is described as *soft sore*.

It is difficult to heal and the surface is covered with a purulent offensive discharge. In women this sore occurs on the vulva on both sides. A number of sores are usually present.

Treatment consists in the administration of one of the sulphonamide drugs, either sulphadiazine or sulphathiazole, and keeping the affected area clean and covered by an antiseptic dressing. Streptomycin is suggested as a means of treatment in patients who do not tolerate sulphonamides. Ducrey's bacillus is resistant to penicillin.

PORADENITIS

Lymphogranuloma inguinale or poradenitis is another venereal infection. It appears as a small sore or ulcer, usually on the external genitalia, and from there the infection is carried to the inguinal lymphatic glands where adenitis occurs; the condition may disappear or the gland may suppurate and break down.

An intradermal test—'Frei's Test'—is used to establish a diagnosis.

Treatment may be either by penicillin or one of the sulphonamide drugs. The latter is the drug of choice as administration of penicillin might mask the symptoms of syphilis should that disease be present. The local area should be kept clean and dry.

Section 6

Gynaecological Conditions and their Treatment and Nursing Care. A Short Account of Pregnancy, Antenatal Care and the Puerperium

Chapter 37

Gynaecological Nursing, Preparation for Operation, and Post-Operative Care

Introduction—Common gynaecological operations; dilating and curettage of uterus, perineorrhaphy, hysterectomy, ventrofixation, the Millin sling operation for stress incontinence—Notes on preparation and post-operative care in vaginal and abdominal cases—Examination of a patient and some special treatments including the toilet of the vulva, insertion of tampons, packing the vagina and the use of pessaries.

There are certain points to be considered in the nursing care of gynaecological patients both as regards the general condition of the patient, and in regard to the organs affected, which include the vulva, perineum, cervix, uterus, uterine tubes and ovaries. It is essential that nurses should have some idea of the anatomy and physiology of these organs and also of the relation of the bladder to them, which accounts for the fact that micturition is so commonly affected in these cases.

The majority of the gynaecological cases met with in the wards of a general hospital are wives and mothers, and in this dual capacity they have often led self-sacrificing lives and may have put up with some abnormal condition of the organs of generation, and suffered painful and otherwise distressing symptoms for a considerable period, and have only consented to leave their homes and families for the necessary treatment after considerable persuasion and at a time when they are in a very low state of nervous tension.

In many cases the general condition may be poor, with repeated bleedings and profuse menstruation, giving rise to anaemia; in many more instances these patients will be found to be losing their courage, they will be apprehensive and introspective, they cry easily, and are very readily upset by even the slightest imagined unkindness or slight. They are inclined to talk a great deal about their own symptoms and take a morbid interest in the symptoms of others; another point is that in some instances they may have been in hospital before and are apt to be exacting and talk quite openly about what they were accustomed to, they say, elsewhere, and what they think they should be having as treatment now and are not having. This type of patient will be found to take advantage of a junior student and work on her feelings, whereas a more senior nurse would treat her sensibly, and gently laugh her out of her imagined grievances.

The treatment of gynaecological patients must be kind and sympathetic, yet at the same time cheerful and happy and confident and firm. Many patients will tend to relax, and behave as if they are more helpless than they really need be in the circumstances; but the nurse should remember that when a patient acts like this and perhaps demands first one thing and then another and behaves in an unduly exacting and selfish manner, she is often a long-suffering woman who up to now has had to carry on, unrelaxingly and uncomplainingly, in her service of others in her own home. The nurse who reflects thus will at once appreciate that the attitude she notices in her patient is not the woman's true self, but an inevitable reaction following the anxiety which has preceded her admission into hospital, and that the best way to meet this attitude is, by kindness and generosity of service, gradually to encourage the patient to become more and more self-reliant.

GYNAECOLOGICAL OPERATIONS

In *the preparation of patients for operation* steps are taken to prevent shock, breathing exercises are taught and chemotherapy is generally employed.

The **operations performed** in gynaecology are divided into two groups, (1) the perineal and (2) the abdominal group.

The **commonest vaginal or perineal operations include:** *Dilatation of the cervix* such as may be performed to cure one form of dysmenorrhoea;

Uterine curettage, or the scraping of the endometrium, which is sometimes performed for the relief of menorrhagia due to an unhealthy endometrium, and also to clear away the retained products of pregnancy after an incomplete miscarriage, or to obtain a specimen of the endometrium for examination;

Amputation of the cervix may be performed for chronic inflammation of this part of the uterus, in order to relieve profuse leucorrhoea, or to treat cervical erosion or cervicitis. This portion of the uterus bleeds very easily and very freely and, in order to prevent post-operative haemorrhage, the vagina is frequently plugged with flavine before the patient leaves the theatre.

Colporrhaphy and *perineorrhaphy*. Colporrhaphy is repair of the vaginal wall and the surrounding structures and perineorrhaphy repair of the perineal body. The operations are frequently combined. When limited to the perineum it is described as perineorrhaphy, and the more extensive operation is called *colpo-perineorrhaphy*; this may be combined with ventral fixation, and it is for this reason that the skin of the abdomen, and the skin over the buttocks at the back, is prepared in addition to shaving and preparation of the skin of the vulva and perineal region.

Vaginal hysterectomy. In this operation the uterus is removed through the vagina, the advantage being that there is no external abdominal wound and there is said to be considerably less shock and disturbance to the patient. As a rule a vaginal packing is inserted and left in for the first 48 hours. The skin of the abdomen is prepared and the vagina is prepared by douches before operation.

Other operations include some on the vulva, such as those performed (*a*) to enlarge the vaginal orifice, (*b*) to open or remove Bartholin's cyst or abscess, (*c*) to excise the vulva and (*d*) to remove urethral caruncle.

Abdominal operations. These include *abdominal hysterectomy* which is removal of the uterus. There are a number of degrees of this:

(1) *Sub-total hysterectomy*, in which the uterus is removed above the cervix when the latter is healthy. This operation is commonly performed for the removal of the uterus when it is the site of a number of small fibroid tumours.

(2) *Total hysterectomy*. The removal of the whole of the uterus including the whole of the cervix.

(3) *Pan-hysterectomy*. The removal of the uterus together with the tubes and ovaries. This operation is performed in cancer of the body of the uterus.

(4) *Wertheim's operation*. Wertheim was an Austrian surgeon of Vienna. In this operation the uterus is removed and also the ovaries, tubes and the whole of the vagina, all the tissue on each side of the vagina and all the glands on the wall of the pelvis. It is performed in cancer of the cervix of the uterus.

Other operations on the uterus include *myomectomy*, the enucleation of fibroid tumours from the wall of the uterus, when the uterus is stitched up again; *ventro-fixation*, in which the uterus is stitched to the anterior abdominal wall, performed in cases of prolapse and in the correction of retroversion; *shortening of the round ligaments*, performed for retroversion, a pleat being put in the ligaments and by this means the uterus is pulled forward and the retroversion corrected.

Operations on the ovaries and tubes include *ovariotomy*—removal of an ovarian cyst; *oophorectomy*—removal of an ovary; *salpingo-oophorectomy*—removal of one tube and one ovary; *salpingectomy*—removal of a tube, and *salpingostomy*—the opening of a tube in order to make a new orifice.

The preparation for operations on gynaecological cases may be similarly divided into preparation for (*a*) vaginal and (*b*) abdominal operations.

In *preparation for perineal operations*, it is particularly important to bear in mind these facts—the rectum must be empty, and it is important to note that the administration of an enema five or six hours before the operation usually ensures that it will be full. In order that it should be empty an aperient may be given 48 hours before the operation followed by an enema 24 hours before and, if time does not permit of this, the enema *may* be given the night before the day of operation so that it has been administered well over twelve hours beforehand, in order to be at all safe. If given later the lower part of the bowel may be full of fluid which will be evacuated as soon as the surgeon begins to manipulate the perineum.

In preparing cases for *vaginal operations* in some instances douches are ordered, particularly when any vaginal discharge is present; douching may be followed by painting the interior of the vagina with some aniline dye, and in some instances packing with an antiseptic is also employed. The douche given for these cases is a cleansing treatment, and some mild antiseptic is usually employed; it is important that, if this douche is to be effective, the whole of the cervix should be reached. A nozzle that will reach these parts should be used and it should be moved about, in order to direct the fluid on to every part, including the vault of the vagina. A further point to be considered is that the bladder must be empty.

The *abdominal group* includes operations on the uterus, tubes and ovaries, and these do not differ regarding preparation, theatre technique and post-operative nursing care from ordinary surgical abdominal cases, except in one point—the fact that a mid-line incision fairly low down the abdominal wall is employed necessitates that the bladder should be quite empty.

In order to ensure effective emptying of the bladder in all major operations, the patient should be catheterized just as she leaves the ward for the operating theatre and it is advisable that the catheter should be left in, having a spigot placed in its free end, so that the bladder can be drained after the patient is anaesthetized and before the surgeon makes his incision or begins to manipulate the parts.

SHORT NOTES ON THE PREPARATION AND POST-OPERATIVE CARE

Dilating and curettage of uterus—Insufflation of uterine tubes.

Preparation. An aperient is given two days before, the vulva and perineal area are shaved, but no skin preparation is necessary. The patient may go to the bath after shaving, and there is no need to pass a catheter provided the patient passes urine before she is anaesthetized.

Post-operative care. The patient may be given two pillows and an air-ring cushion as soon as she comes round from the anaesthetic. A sterile pad should be worn and careful watch made for any bleeding. The toilet of the vulva should be carefully performed whenever the patient passes urine and faeces. It is particularly necessary to dry both perineum and vagina *before* a pad is applied. In many hospitals it is routine practice for the patient to be given 30 minims of ergot twice a day for 48 hours or until bleeding ceases. Provided bleeding is not excessive, the patient may have a bath 24 hours after the operation. She may be given an aperient on the second day. She may wash herself and sit out of bed on the day after operation and may go home as soon as she wishes.

Perineorrhaphy and amputation of cervix. These operations are of a rather more serious character.

Preparation. An aperient is given two nights before the operation, and the patient is shaved over an area extending from the sternum in front to the same level at the back, shaving right through the whole of the perineal and vulval regions. The same area is treated by an antiseptic, one of the aniline dyes being most commonly used. A catheter is passed just before the patient is taken to the theatre, and left in position until the patient is in the theatre, when the bladder is emptied by removing the spigot.

Post-operative nursing care. On receiving the patient back to bed she is given a knee pillow and a sterile pad is kept in position by a T bandage. She is nursed in the semirecumbent position and may have as many as three pillows for her head and shoulders and an air ring under her buttocks. The temperature is recorded morning and evening. Until she is round from the anaesthetic it is advisable to have her knees tied together to prevent any separation of the legs by violent involuntary movements with consequent strain upon the perineal region. *The most important point in the post-operative care of a case of perineorrhaphy is keeping the sutures dry* and so preventing sepsis. This may be secured by frequently changing the dressing and catheterizing the patient until she can pass urine without discomfort; then, when she is able to pass urine, the perineal dressing must be attended to each time (see note below).

After the operation the patient is usually allowed to sleep off the effects of the anaesthetic. Early on the morning following the operation the *perineal dressing* is performed for the first time and the patient is catheterized. The gauze dressing or sterile pad which is kept in position by means of a T bandage is removed, the parts are gently cleaned by swabbing with perchloride or mercury 1–3,000. It is very important that, in cleansing the labia of patients whom it is necessary to catheterize over a period of a few days or a week or so, the nurse must never *wipe* the parts with the swab, as this removes the surface epithelium and results in marked soreness which may give rise to sepsis. Swabbing should be performed by dabbing movements and not by rubbing or wiping. The catheter is then passed, the stitches are dabbed quite dry with a little alcohol or spirit lotion or by using dry swabs, and a clean dressing is applied. Before the bandage is reapplied, the patient is turned over and the routine treatment of the back—washing, rubbing and powdering—is performed. When regular catheterization is employed it is usually performed every 8 hours; and when the patient is able to pass urine voluntarily it is a good plan if she can be persuaded to do so at regular intervals—every 4 or 6 hours—and then the routine treatment as described above is carried out each time. The interior of the vagina should be dried carefully as in patients lying in bed it forms a cul-de-sac where urine can collect. The same careful treatment is necessary after the patient has had her bowels moved. Some surgeons like their patients to have a urinary antiseptic such as hexamine, or a mild diuretic such as potassium citrate. In some cases both treatments are employed.

This particular toilet of the perineum is carried out for from 7 to 10 days or until the stitches are removed. When catgut stitches have been employed, this material becomes absorbed during the course of a week or so; but when silkworm-gut stitches are used they are generally taken out between the seventh and tenth days.

Retention of Urine. It is important that the bladder should not be distended; the collection of more than 12 ounces of urine may affect the tone of the bladder for a week.

Another very important nursing point is the management of the action of the patient's bowels.

Control of the action of the bowels. Most surgeons consider that it is advisable if the bowels can be kept from acting until the third, fourth or fifth day after operation, some surgeons going so far as to ensure this by limiting the diet to fluids and jellies, avoiding foods which would produce a bulky stool, and also giving cool fluids rather than hot in order to avoid exciting peristalsis. Other surgeons allow the patient to have any diet that she fancies, but in order to ensure that the stools should be soft, and easily passed when they do occur, liquid paraffin is administered, either with or without the addition of a small dose of phenolphthalein two or three times a day as soon as the patient has ceased to feel the nausea resulting from the anaesthetic—if the bowels have not acted by the fourth or fifth day it is usual to give an aperient such as cascara evacuant. If the patient finds difficulty in passing stool she must be warned against straining for this purpose, as this will tug at the stitches, and advised to wait quietly until the aperient produces its action—if she is unduly worried, or if for any other reason the nurse considers it advisable to obtain a bowel action more rapidly, a warm small olive oil enema may be administered.

Patients usually get up after perineorrhaphy about the fourteenth day and are able to be discharged from hospital about the twenty-first day.

Vaginal hysterectomy. This operation is occasionally performed today and a nurse should know how to prepare the patient. An aperient is given two days before the operation and vaginal douches are administered twice a day; some mild antiseptic such as acriflavine 1–1,000 being employed. The area of skin prepared is as for an abdominal operation, from the sternum to the pubes, the vulva and perineal region also being shaved and prepared and the skin of the back as far as the top of the sacrum. Some surgeons like the vagina to be packed with gauze soaked in flavine in addition to having the skin prepared.

In the *post-operative nursing care* the patient is received back to bed recumbent, she has a knee pillow, and her knees are tied together, and she may subsequently be nursed in the semirecumbent position as described in the post-operative nursing care of cases of perineorrhaphy. It is important that the pulse should be observed every half-hour for the first few hours after operation, and subsequently a four-hourly chart of the temperature and pulse should be recorded for the first two or three days. After removing the uterus the surgeon fills the vagina with gauze packing, and he or his assistant will remove this after 48 hours, the nurse preparing the necessary appliances and utensils, and arranging the patient in a modified lithotomy position on the bed. Once this plug is out the surgeon may order douches twice a day or perhaps only one occasionally for cleansing purposes. The patient will probably have difficulty in passing urine until the vaginal plug has been removed and she may have to be catheterized, and this must be carried out with the same care and attention as described in the post-operative nursing of perineorrhaphy.

The patient will usually be allowed to get up about 10 days after operation and she may be discharged from hospital after 14 days.

ABDOMINAL OPERATIONS ON GYNAECOLOGICAL CASES

The preparation and post-operative care is very similar to that of any abdominal operation. In the following notes special mention will be made of ventro-fixation and Wertheim's hysterectomy, and Millin's operation for the relief of stress incontinence.

Routine preparation. All abdominal cases are given an aperient two nights before operation. A complete shave is carried out from the sternum in front over the skin of the abdomen through the vulval and perineal regions up to the region of the waist behind. The skin is carefully prepared, and an aniline dye is employed as an antiseptic. Brilliant green is a good one to use as it is powerfully antiseptic and non-irritating, though it has the disadvantage of staining the skin. The bladder should be emptied by catheterization before the patient is taken to the operating theatre. The catheter is usually left in so that the bladder can be evacuated on the operating table. A rubber catheter should always be employed for cases of Caesarean section.

In the *post-operative nursing* care of abdominal cases, it is usual to insert a knee pillow and to give the patient a sterile pad on return from the operating theatre. As soon as she has recovered from the anaesthetic she may be propped up on two or three pillows and given an air-ring cushion. In the opinion of many gynaecologists Fowler's position is inadvisable as it keeps the patient too rigidly still in bed, thus provoking a tendency to the formation of thrombosis. Free movement is better. In the majority of cases a four-hourly record of the pulse and respiration is kept for 36 hours. Fluids are given liberally as soon as the patient has recovered from post-anaesthetic nausea. An aperient is usually given on the second, third or fourth night, except in the case of Wertheim's hysterectomy when it is delayed for a day or two longer. The knee pillow and ring cushion are only permitted for the first few days after operation and should be removed not later than the fifth day in order to encourage free movement of the legs. Many gynaecologists consider that the provision of a dressing after an abdominal operation is not absolutely essential beyond the protection of the stitches by means of a sterile towel or a layer of folded gauze which can be maintained in position by elastoplast. Other gynaecologists employ a gauze and wool dressing maintained in position by a binder. When clips are employed these are removed about the fifth day and, as usual when removing clips, half are taken out on one day (alternate clips) and the other half the following day. When skin stitches are employed these are usually removed about the eighth day.

Getting up. In the majority of cases, excluding Wertheim's hysterectomy and cases in which complications may have arisen, the patient is allowed to sit out on a chair whilst her bed is being made on the eighth or ninth day after operations. She is allowed to get up for half an hour on the following evening and may have a bath the next day, and from then onwards she is allowed to get up to go to the lavatory until she is discharged from hospital between the twelfth and sixteenth day.

Ventro-fixation. This operation is performed in order to correct prolapse and retroversion of the uterus, when this cannot be satisfactorily secured by simpler measures. An incision is made in the anterior abdominal wall and the uterus is brought up and stitched to this wall. In addition to the routine preparation, the vagina should be douched and plugged with gauze soaked in some antiseptic, and a perineal compress applied as well as a compress over the skin of the abdomen.

In the *post-operative nursing care* the patient is received back to bed and placed in the same position as any other abdominal case. Care must be taken of the toilet of the vulva and perineum whenever the patient passes urine. The nurse should watch carefully the amount of vaginal discharge present on the pads which the patient is wearing. In all other points the post-operative care is the same as that described above.

Wertheim's hysterectomy. The patient is usually admitted at least a week before the operation, the bowels are maintained in activity by the use of aperients, and the patient is frequently given a full nourishing diet augmented by the administration of 4–6 ounces of glucose a day during this time. If she is not sleeping well the gynaecologist will order mild sedatives to be employed. The patient's blood will be grouped and arrangements made for blood transfusion.

The *skin preparation* and the *preparation of the vulva and perineum* is carried out as for any other abdominal case. In addition, the vagina is douched with a mild antiseptic before the operation and in some cases daily during the week the patient spends in hospital. Before the operation the vagina is plugged with gauze soaked in some antiseptic. In many instances this is performed when the patient is under the anaesthetic and catheterization is deferred until this time also.

In the *post-operative nursing care* the patient is carefully carried back to bed and the bed is maintained in Trendelenburg's position by putting the foot of the bed on chairs for the first 4 hours after operation. These are then replaced by 12-inch blocks, and by midnight of the day the operation has taken place—provided the operation was in the morning—the foot of the bed may be lowered to the floor.

The degree of post-operative shock from which these patients suffer is very serious, and for this reason all movement should be as gentle and infrequent as possible. If the patient is returned to bed on a stretcher she should not be rolled for the canvas to be removed—it should be left in for some hours and it will do no harm, provided that it is straightened and that the patient is not lying on creased canvas.

Every possible care will be taken to assist recovery from shock; the head of the bed should be screened in order to avoid draughts, and some sisters arrange a little shawl, cowl fashion, around the head to help prevent loss of body heat. In many instances the water pillow which is provided in the bed contains water at a temperature of 118° F. A pillow is placed flat against the bedrail at the top—in addition to providing a buffer, it helps to maintain warmth as would an eiderdown over the patient. The pulse is taken half-hourly during the first 36 hours, and then a four-hourly record is kept for several days.

Routine nursing measures. In addition to the observation of the degree of shock and the administration of any treatment that may have been ordered such as continuous saline, the patient is left undisturbed until the early hours of the morning following operation. At about five or six o'clock she is usually catheterized for the first time, the toilet of the vulva is carefully performed, the patient is gently turned, the routine treatment of the back is carried out and the stretcher canvas which has been underneath her is carefully rolled out and the upper part of the bed is remade. The patient may now be nursed in the semirecumbent position with three pillows to support her head and shoulders, a knee pillow under her knees, and an air ring beneath her buttocks.

The bladder is stripped of its normal attachments during this large extensive operation and, as it will be paralysed for some days, it is important that it should be emptied by catheterization as soon as 10 ounces of urine have accumulated and it should thereafter never be allowed to become overfull. It is routine practice to catheterize these patients every 6 hours for as long as necessary. When the bladder begins to regain its tone the patient will pass urine voluntarily, but for a considerable time she will never empty the bladder completely, and therefore, immediately after she has passed urine, the patient should be catheterized—and by *immediately* is meant within 5 minutes, in order to remove the *residual urine*. At first the residual urine may amount to 5 or 6 ounces, but as the tone of the bladder improves this will decrease in quantity, and only when the quantity has become quite minute is it safe to omit catheterization. All this time the nurse continues to observe her patient frequently and any indication of pain associated with micturition would necessitate the need for catheterizing her. *Cystitis* is a complication which may very readily arise owing to the irritability sustained by the bladder during and after the operation and for this reason some gynaecologists like their patients to have a urinary antiseptic, such as hexamine, and a mild diuretic, such as potassium citrate. In addition they should have plenty of bland fluids as soon as they are able to take them.

Dressing. In addition to the wound in the abdominal wall these patients are returned to the ward with a packing in the vagina. The gynaecologist or his assistant usually removes this after 24–48 hours. The patient continues to wear a vaginal pad and the nurse must very particularly note the amount of bleeding. As before mentioned, in performing the toilet of the vulva whenever the patient is catheterized it is very important to dry the interior of the vagina, as with patients lying on their backs this forms a cul-de-sac where moisture can collect.

The diet should be as liberal as possible and, as soon as the patient is able to take fluids, nourishment should be freely given and the diet increased as the patient is willing to take it. The bowels are kept active by the administration of liquid paraffin and phenolphthalein two or three times a day, and if this is not efficacious a slightly more drastic aperient such as a small dose of cascara is given on the fourth or fifth day.

Clips and stitches are removed on the fifth and eighth days respectively, and the patient is usually allowed to get up after 3 weeks and is sent home a week later. The *complications* which may arise are cystitis, bleeding and sepsis.

Stress or **orthostatic incontinence** in women is often serious and disabling. Up to the present many treatments have been tried without success, anterior colporrhaphy (see p. 537) has been performed in some cases but it has not proved entirely successful in all of them. Recently Terence Millin has devised an operation by which the neck of the bladder is raised and supported by slings of fascia, the *Millin sling*, taken from the anterior abdominal wall the free ends of which are attached to the rectus muscles.

The result of this operation is that:

(1) The neck of the bladder is raised, consequently the position of the urethra is raised also, and

(2) Any movement such as sneezing, coughing and straining which causes contraction of the anterior abdominal wall no longer causes urine to be voided involuntarily. Conversely, because the free ends of the fascia supporting the neck of the bladder are attached to the rectus muscles, any contraction tautens the muscle and further elevates the bladder neck so that the difficult and painful circumstances under which the patient previously lived no longer exist and she enjoys life without fear of incontinence.

In *preparing a patient for this operation* a rubber Malecot catheter is passed into the bladder and a flexible stilette is introduced. This enables the surgeon to feel the position of the neck of the bladder. The vagina is packed with gauze soaked in flavine. A transverse retropubic incision is made and the operation is performed. The wound is closed but a corrugated rubber drain is inserted. The catheter is left in position but the stilette is withdrawn before the patient leaves the operation room and the catheter is irrigated with a bland fluid just to see that it is not obstructed. The vaginal pack is removed.

Some surgeons, particularly when there is any possibility of bladder infection insert a suprapubic tube in order to provide for a period of post-operative continuous bladder drainage.

In the *post-operative nursing care* observations, similar to those described on page 732 after retropubic prostatectomy, are made. Drainage of the bladder through the catheter must be maintained; as a rule this catheter is retained for 5 days and then the patient passes urine normally. If the catheter should escape before this minimum period it must be replaced.

In exceptional cases where suprapubic leakage follows removal of the catheter, this indicates injury to the bladder neck or urethra, and will need a further period of indwelling catheter drainage.

The patient should be given liberal fluids and a chart of fluid intake and output should be kept. In all other respects the patient will be treated as after any abdominal operation.

THE EXAMINATION OF A PATIENT AND SPECIAL TREATMENTS

Preparation of the patient for gynaecological examination. This examination is divided into the following parts:

(1) *Abdominal*, in which the patient lies on her back with knees drawn up.

(2) *Vaginal*, in which inspection of the vulva and vagina is made, followed by manual examination and if necessary examination using a speculum.

(3) In *bimanual examination* two hands are employed, one with which to palpate the abdomen while the other hand is in the vagina or rectum, and in this way the position of the pelvic organs may be manipulated between the two hands.

(4) *Recto-vaginal examination* is made in order to ascertain the condition of the tissue between the vagina and rectum. One examining finger is in the vagina and the other in the rectum.

The articles which should be provided for a gynaecological examination are shown in fig. 174, p. 521.

These articles include towels to protect the bedclothing and forceps and swabs for cleansing the vulva. Rubber gloves, a lubricant, a bowl of antiseptic lotion and some swabs should be provided. Instruments which may be required are a vaginal speculum, long forceps for holding swabs with which to cleanse the vagina, and a long probe.

In **preparing a patient for this examination** it is important that the bladder and rectum and also the lower part of the colon should be empty. The vagina should not be douched, as this would remove any discharge present which the gynaecologist might want to investigate. The external parts of the vulva and perineum should be very clean. The position in which the patient is placed may be either the *dorsal recumbent*, the *left lateral* or *Sims's semiprone position* (see fig. 38, p. 186). A hassock should be provided at the bedside or the side of the couch in case the examining gynaecologist wishes to kneel.

Shaving a gynaecological patient. The ordinary articles required for shaving are prepared. The vulva and perineum cannot be properly shaved unless a good light is provided; the nurse must be able to see what she is doing and shaving should not be attempted under the bedclothes.

The order of procedure is rather important. When a 'through' shave is carried out, the hairs on the abdominal wall should first be removed, then those on the mons veneris and vulva; and after this the patient should be turned on her side and the hairs on the perineum should be removed, and those over the buttocks and lower part of the back as well.

It is quite usual for the patient to have a bath immediately after shaving to remove all the short cut hair, but if it is not advisable for the patient to go to the bathroom the parts should be thoroughly well washed to remove all the bits of hair, and then dried and powdered, unless a skin preparation is to follow the shaving.

GYNAECOLOGICAL TREATMENTS

The toilet of the vulva. A nurse will be frequently required to perform the toilet of the vulva, particularly after operations on the vagina and perineum, and whenever catheterization is employed, and with many bed cases who are unable to wash themselves.

The bed should be protected by a drawsheet and mackintosh, in some cases a special mackintosh and towel being provided. The patient should lie on her back in a semirecumbent position, the bedclothes being carefully folded, so that the upper part of her body is protected from chilling and her legs covered to above the knees. The nurse then washes the vulva and all the surrounding parts, with soap and water, also the inner sides of the thighs, paying special attention to the groins. Sterile swabs should be used for the internal labia and the inner aspect of the vagina; in some cases these parts are irrigated, not as described in the vaginal douche, but by allowing the saline or lotion used to flow gently over the different parts. Great care must be taken to dry the inner aspect of the labia by gently swabbing and not by rubbing as the latter might remove the surface epithelium and produces soreness. It is very important in the case of patients who are nursed on the back that the vaginal orifice be kept quite dry, as urine tends to collect in the posterior part of it and decomposition quickly gives rise to sepsis.

After the front parts have been attended to the patient should be turned on her side and the surface of the perineum and the area all round the rectum carefully washed, dried and powdered. If there are stitches in the perineum the case will be dealt with as described in the post-operative nursing of perineorrhaphy on p. 540.

Insertion of tampons. Tampons may be balls of absorbent wool tied up in gauze (see fig. 175, p. 522) and saturated with some antiseptic, astringent or other substance; or the substance may be prepared ready in gelatine pessaries.

To insert a tampon the patient should lie on her back or in the left lateral or in Sims's semiprone position; the bed should be protected and the patient adequately covered to prevent exposure and chilling. The vulva and the internal aspect of the vagina are swabbed and rendered quite free of discharge; a vaginal speculum is lubricated and inserted; or, alternatively, it may be sufficient for the nurse to retract the anterior part of the vagina with the first two fingers of her left hand. She then swabs and dries the interior of the vagina as far as she can reach, using sterile swabs on sponge-holding forceps. The tampon is taken between the blades of a pair of long forceps and inserted into the posterior fornix of the vagina as far as possible. If there is a tape or string attached to the tampon this should be left just inside the vaginal orifice, at the margin of the vulva, so that it can be easily reached when the tampon is to be removed later.

Packing the vagina. In many instances this treatment is performed by the gynaecologist or house surgeon. The occasions when a nurse will be asked to pack a vagina will be (1) as an emergency measure in the treatment of severe uterine haemorrhage when the help of a doctor cannot immediately be obtained, and also (2) when the gynaecologist requires the vagina packed with gauze soaked in some antiseptic previous to an operation on the vagina or uterus. In the latter case the vagina should only be lightly packed, and it is a very simple procedure and can be rendered quite painless. Having the roll of gauze in a bowl the nurse takes hold of the end of it with a pair of forceps and, either using the spatula or retracting the anterior vaginal wall with her fingers, gently plugs the cavity.

In packing the vagina in the treatment of serious uterine haemorrhage much firmer pressure is necessary. There may not be time to permit the patient to empty her bladder but if possible she should do so as she will be unable to pass urine afterwards. When blood is pouring from a patient's uterus there is usually no time to give an anaesthetic, but a $\frac{1}{4}$ grain of morphia is sometimes given. As a result of the shock the patient is rendered comparatively immune to discomfort, and it is only when the condition is as serious as here indicated that a nurse would be called upon to insert the pack.

In this case the gauze, soaked in some antiseptic, should be folded in three and packed firmly into the posterior fornix, continuing to pack firmly until the whole cavity is tightly packed and if necessary applying manual pressure on the pack until help can be obtained and the patient given an anaesthetic and the packing more tightly applied.

Pessaries. These are solid substances, frequently medicated, which are similar in shape to suppositories and may be described as *vaginal suppositories*. They are larger than the suppositories used for insertion into the rectum, and they are inserted in a very similar way to that described for the insertion of tampons (see fig. 175, letter A, p. 522). Pessaries of rubber or composition are sometimes used in the treatment of uterine displacement.

Hodge's pessary (see letter B) is used to correct retroversion of the uterus after childbirth. The obstetrician inserts the pessary which helps to keep the uterus forward. This simple means may be sufficient to correct the condition permanently; if it does not do so, three months later an operation will be undertaken for correction of the condition.

A *ring pessary* or watch spring consists of springs enclosed in rubber. It is used in the correction of slight prolapse of the uterus. In some cases a nurse is asked to insert this. She should have the woman lying in the left lateral position. The pessary is sterilized either by boiling or by standing in perchloride of mercury 1/2,000 solution for an hour. It is taken in the right hand and compressed, passed into the vagina and then allowed to expand. The cervix can be felt through the ring when the pessary is in the correct position—around the cervix, impinging on the walls of the vagina, and so correcting the tendency to prolapse. It is necessary to ascertain that the pessary is not displaced by coughing or straining before the woman is allowed to get off the couch. The patient should have a vaginal douche every day whilst wearing a pessary and must be seen by the gynaecologist or obstetrician every three months. If this treatment is not effective within a reasonable time, operative treatment will be undertaken. No woman should be condemned to wear a pessary for an indefinite time. (Letter D in fig. 175, p. 522, shows a watch spring pessary introducer; this is employed when the fingers of the operator are not strong enough to compress the pessary efficiently.)

Napier's cup and stem pessary (see letter E) is employed for the relief of prolapse of the uterus in very elderly women, in whom, for one reason or another, operative treatment may be contra-indicated. The pessary is prepared by soaking in mercury, it is inserted with the woman lying on a couch or in bed—it is usually inserted daily before she gets up in the morning. The cervix is supported on the cup; the pessary is maintained in position by tying the tapes—two behind and two in front—to a belt worn round the waist. It is removed at night, washed to render it free from mucus and then placed in a solution of mercury when it will be ready for use next morning.

Catheterization and **vaginal douching** are described on pp. 143 and 148.

Chapter 38

Inflammatory Conditions, Diseases and Disorders of the Female Generative Organs

Ascending inflammation of the genital tract: vulvitis, vaginitis, cervicitis, endometritis and salpingitis—Ruptured ectopic gestation—Disorders of the uterus: amenorrhoea, dysmenorrhoea, menorrhagia and metrorrhagia—Displacement of the uterus—Diseases of the uterus (including cancer) and diseases of the ovaries

In addition to the conditions dealt with in the previous pages on gynaecological nursing, the following short notes on some conditions and diseases of the reproductive organs with which a nurse should be familiar may be found useful.

Ascending inflammation of the genital tract is most commonly due to some pus-producing organism such as streptococci, pneumococci, bacillus coli, staphylococci and more rarely to the presence of gonococci. Any part of the tract may be infected.

The vulva (vulvitis). This is usually a simple inflammation due to an abrasion which has been infected by staphylococci. In some instances streptococci may be the causative organism and in such cases the condition is more severe, the vulva becoming red, dry and swollen, and possibly ulcerated. In severe cases *infection of Bartholin's gland* occurs and a Bartholinian abscess may be formed. This is manifested by a painful swelling distending the labia majora.

Vulvitis is treated by cleanliness, by frequent hot baths and by irrigation of the vulva with antiseptic solutions. *A Bartholin's abscess* usually requires to be incised, drained and packed, allowing it to heal from the bottom, and the parts should be kept as clean as possible during the process of healing.

The vagina (vaginitis). This condition is due to the same cause as vulvitis and may be combined with it in *vulvovaginitis*. The vagina resists sepsis fairly well, but infection of the vagina usually spreads to the vault where the cervix of the uterus lies, resulting in *cervicitis*; the inflammatory condition of the cervix gives rise to a profuse discharge which, passing over the surface of the vagina, is a contributory factor in causing reinfection thereof. In many cases vaginitis tends to become chronic, simple vaginitis does not usually spread very much—it is the more acute varieties which spread up the tract and give rise to infection of the fallopian tubes (*salpingitis*).

The uterus. *Cervicitis* is infection of the neck, and *endometritis* of the body, of the uterus. The term '*endocervicitis*' is also employed to indicate inflammation of the inner part of the cervix. Cervicitis is usually a mild infection, and it may follow childbearing or occur as a result of vaginitis. It is characterized by a vaginal discharge which is most marked during the days immediately preceding and following menstruation, and is accompanied by backache and some degree of general malaise. The inflammatory condition of the cervix may be a cause of cervical erosion.

In *cervical erosion* the surfaces of the cervix become red and raw, and they may be ulcerated or lacerated. Erosion means eating away, and it may be the result of chronic infection in which an irritating discharge is destroying the surface tissue, or it may be due to gonorrhoea, or follow lacerations of the cervix as the result of childbearing. In some cases the operation of amputation of the cervix is employed to cure the condition when local applications of antiseptics and astringent substances have failed to produce relief.

Endometritis is inflammation of the lining of the uterus which becomes very congested; this condition is associated with excessive menstruation, and a persistent vaginal discharge which is thin and watery in character results from it. The operation of uterine curettage may be necessary to relieve this condition.

Metritis, which results in thickening of the walls of the uterus, may be due to spread of the inflammation from the endometrium, or it may follow puerperal sepsis. It is accompanied by excessive menstruation which occurs in women who have borne several children and who are in a state of chronic ill health. It is usually treated by hysterectomy and in some cases by applications of X-rays and radium.

The uterine tubes (salpingitis). Inflammation of the uterine tubes may be due to ascending infection from the vagina, or to descending infection from the peritoneal cavity such as occurs in appendicitis, and the condition may be simple, in which it is catarrhal, or suppurative, when pus-producing organisms are present. The former may be due to staphylococcal infection and in this case the distension of the tube by serous fluid is described as *hydrosalpinx*. When pus-producing organisms are present the condition is designated as *pyosalpinx*; infection frequently spreads to the ovaries, giving rise to a pelvic abscess and pelvic peritonitis.

The condition is usually bilateral, and it may be either acute or chronic. In the chronic variety there is a serous vaginal discharge which is a characteristic greenish offensive fluid, most profuse during the days preceding menstruation. The patient has a slight rise of temperature—99° to 100° F.—accompanied by a varying degree of malaise, with pain in the back and sides. *This chronic form may be treated by medical measures*. The patient is kept in bed to rest, a light nourishing diet is administered, the bowels are kept regularly active, applications of heat are made to the lateral abdominal wall, hot vaginal douches and antiseptic tampons such as glycerine and ichthyol are employed.

Acute salpingitis is suppurative in character and the symptoms in a patient admitted with this condition are those of general peritonitis. The *onset* is usually sudden, accompanied by a rigor and a rise of temperature. The patient has acute abdominal pain, with tenderness and distension, the pulse is rapid and there is nausea and vomiting. The patient looks very ill.

The *treatment* of this condition is laparotomy, with removal of the infected tube (*salpingectomy*), and drainage of the peritoneum; if the ovaries are infected the operation of *salpingo-oophorectomy* is performed.

It is important to remember that a mild degree of salpingitis may become chronic. The chronic type may be tuberculous in origin.

Tubal gestation is growth of the fertilized ovum in the uterine tube. It may also be called *ectopic gestation*, and *extra-uterine gestation*. Abdominal gestation and even ovarian gestation may also occur.

When tubal gestation occurs, in a very short time the ovum burrows its way into the wall of the thin tube, and usually causes it to rupture. In a few cases of abdominal gestation the pregnancy may go on to term, but it is dangerous, owing to excessive bleeding which follows the separation of the placenta. In others cases the foetus dies and becomes calcified. It is then described as a *lithopaedion.*

Ruptured tubal gestation. This is an emergency with which a nurse will have to help to deal. The usual history obtained is that the patient has missed one or two menstrual periods. The present attack has come on suddenly, and is characteristic of an acute abdominal catastrophe. The patient collapses and is extremely pale, being blanched in appearance. There is acute abdominal pain, the abdomen is tender and there is usually nausea and vomiting. In other cases the symptoms may be very slight and may pass unnoticed.

The *treatment* is to open the abdominal cavity and remove the blood which has poured into it. Pending the operation palliative treatment for shock in the form of blood transfusion and saline infusion is carried out. A serious case of ruptured ectopic gestation presents the most dramatic degree of shock that a nurse will ever see—and as this is due to the haemorrhage that has occurred, combined with irritation of the peritoneum resulting from the presence of blood in it, in her *post-operative nursing care* she has therefore primarily these conditions to take into account.

As soon as possible the patient will be placed in Fowler's position in order to assist drainage from the vagina. The vaginal discharge will be collected on sterile pads and will be very carefully inspected. A careful record of the temperature and pulse must be kept, fluids should be administered freely, the bowels must be regularly active, and the patient requires to be as well nourished as possible as, owing to the lowering of her vitality, the complication to be feared in the later days of the illness is abdominal sepsis.

DISORDERS OF THE UTERUS

Disorders of menstruation are frequently met with in abnormal conditions of the uterus. **Amenorrhoea** or absence of menstruation, is normal before puberty and after the menopause; its absence during the menstruating period is most usually due to pregnancy, though absence may also occur as a result of general ill health, particularly associated with constitutional disease of the heart, lungs and kidneys, and diseases of the ovaries; and it also occurs as a result of emotional disturbance, disease of the endocrine organs, and is an inevitable result of hysterectomy and bilateral oophorectomy.

When the condition is brought about by some disease or ill health the cause has to be dealt with, otherwise no treatment need be suggested. The condition will right itself, and the fortunate woman might, in the meantime, consider herself a favoured individual.

A condition which is described as *apparent amenorrhoea* is due to an abnormality of the hymen, when the latter is not perforated (*imperforate hymen*). In these cases menstruation occurs, but the discharge cannot escape and remains pent up in the vaginal cavity until the hymen is divided.

Dysmenorrhoea is the term used to describe any difficult or painful menstruation. A number of types are described. *Spasmodic dysmenorrhoea* is the type which occurs in young women 2 to 3 years after the onset of menstruation; the pain, which coincides with the onset of the period, is in the lower part of the abdomen and in the middle line, and lasts from 5 to 6 hours and in some cases for a whole day and may be very disabling. As the subject grows older it may improve—if not, it may have to be treated by dilation of the os uteri. This type of dysmenorrhoea is usually cured by a first pregnancy.

Congestive dysmenorrhoea, occurs in older women, and is more common in those who have had children. The pain in these cases precedes menstruation for a day or two and is accompanied by severe backache.

Obstructive dysmenorrhoea is the type in which the pain is colicky. It is also described as 'clot' dysmenorrhoea, because it is thought to be due to the forcible contraction of the uterus on a clot in an endeavour to remove it—after a clot is passed the pain seems to be relieved.

Menorrhagia is excessive loss at the menstrual period, and **metrorrhagia** is bleeding between the periods.

It is important that a nurse should be able to help a woman to estimate the amount of menstruation, and this may be arrived at by considering the number of diapers she uses—over eighteen would be definitely excessive. The duration of the menstrual period and its frequency should also be noted, as in some cases it may occur at fortnightly intervals instead of monthly, also the number of clots passed, as clotting is definitely abnormal. The degree of anaemia from which the woman appears to be suffering, indicated by pallor of skin and mucous surfaces, would also suggest an excessive loss.

Displacements of the uterus. The commonest displacements of the uterus are retroversion and prolapse. In *retroversion* the uterus is lying backwards instead of forwards. It is due to weakness of the ligaments which normally hold the uterus in the correct position of anteversion. This weakness is most commonly brought about by childbearing, but any laxity of muscle tone indicates laxity of ligaments also, and in the case of growing girls any sudden strain may jerk the uterus out of its normal position and cause retroversion.

The condition is accompanied by backache, excessive menstruation and leucorrhoea. The treatment adopted is surgical, either ventro-fixation or shortening of round ligaments being performed.

Uterine prolapse. In this condition the vaginal walls become stretched; it may be brought about by lack of support owing to injury to the perineum, the vaginal wall begins to evert, bringing the uterus down with it. The condition is frequently accompanied by some degree of *cystocele* or *rectocele*.

The condition of *cystocele* is due to protrusion of the bladder into the anterior vaginal wall owing to the stretching of that wall. It frequently accompanies tearing of the perineal body.

The condition is rectified by anterior colporrhaphy. The preparation and post-operative nursing is similar to that described on p. 539, except that the patient is nursed as flat as possible when repair of the anterior vaginal wall is carried out. She will usually have difficulty with micturition, and catheterization may be necessary. Copious fluids are administered and urinary antiseptics employed. It is important to measure the intake of fluid, and to compare it with the output of urine as the nurse must be very careful not to allow residual urine to be retained. As a rule a vaginal packing is inserted and removed 24 hours after the operation. In performing the toilet of the vulva the interior of the vagina must be carefully dried. As catgut stitches are employed these should be expected to slough away after about a week and the increase in discharge which accompanies this process would necessitate frequent swabbing of the vagina.

Rectocele. In this case there is prolapse of the posterior vaginal wall, with the rectum protruding into it. It is due to the same cause as described in the case of cystocele. In repair of this condition, posterior colporrhaphy is frequently combined with perineorrhaphy, as the condition is commonly associated with tearing of the pelvic floor and perineal body.

DISEASES OF THE UTERUS AND OVARIES

Fibroid tumours of the uterus. The non-pregnant uterus is a canal with a strong muscular wall, lined with endometrium and covered with peritoneum. A fibroid tumour is a *myoma*, or a tumour of the muscular wall of the uterus. When it occurs in the wall it is described as *intramural*, and when near the outer aspect projecting under the peritoneum, as *subperitoneal*, and when it is nearest the inner lining of the uterus projecting under the mucous surface, it is described as a *submucous* tumour. A fourth variety is *polypoid* in character, and in this case the whole tumour projects into the uterine cavity. This type usually bleeds very easily.

The *symptoms* of the presence of a fibroid tumour are due to enlargement of the uterus. There is excessive loss at the periods, and, when the tumour is polypoid in character, bleeding occurs between the periods also. The presence of fibroid tumours results in delay of the menopause, which instead of beginning at the age of 48 may not occur till the woman is well over 50. Large tumours give rise to swelling and cause pressure on the adjacent organs producing difficulty of micturition, predisposing to haemorrhoids and varicose veins, causing constipation and in some cases giving rise to sciatica.

Treatment. When the tumours are small, and the woman is young, *myomectomy* is performed. If the tumours are large and the woman is over 40, *hysterectomy* may be performed or radium treatment may be employed.

Cancer of the uterus is usually carcinomatous in type. It may affect the body of the organ or the cervix. It is comparatively uncommon but very serious in its effects, particularly carcinoma of the cervix.

Carcinoma of the body of the uterus rarely occurs until after the menopause, at the age of from 50 to 60 years; it begins in the lining, endometrium, and ulcerates through on to the outer wall of the uterus where it extends to the peritoneum. This is spread by infiltration of the tissues as described by Mr. Sampson Handley, who also described the spread of cancer by lymphatic permeation. In cancer of the uterus the disease spreads by the lymphatics which pass out from the uterus in the broad ligaments to the sides of the pelvis; these then join up with the lymphatics passing up from the lower limbs and track along the course of the iliac vessels to the front of the aorta where numerous lymphatic glands lie; these then become infected and enlarged. Later, the disease tracks along the lymphatics to the glands in the thorax which also become infected.

The *chief symptoms of carcinoma of the body of the uterus* is post-menopausal bleeding; the usual history is that a woman had her menopause say at 49 or 50; then, 2, 3 or 4 years later she noticed slight bleeding; this was only a spot or two at first, but it increased and in a short time became continuous. Bleeding continued for several months and then she noticed that the character changed and became a discharge, which after a little further period of time became offensive in odour.

If these symptoms are neglected she will then have pain, difficulty of micturition and frequency, and later will notice that her abdomen becomes enlarged as ascites sets in, owing to infection of the peritoneum.

Carcinoma of the cervix has a wider age distribution, but is very rare indeed; most cases seen occur between the ages of 30 and 50, though some may occur earlier and others later than this.

The disease starts at the cervix, and spreads by infiltration of the tissue in this region and, as the cervix of the uterus is closely related to other organs, the disease rapidly spreads; from the front it reaches the bladder, from the back it spreads to the pouch of Douglas and the rectum, spreading laterally it infiltrates the cardinal ligaments and involves the ureters and, spreading downwards, infiltrates the vagina.

It also spreads by lymphatic permeation in much the same way as described in cancer of the body of the uterus.

The chief symptom is bleeding. A woman of from 40 to 50 years of age should have regular menstrual periods; in carcinoma of the cervix she will also bleed between her periods and this will go on, till after a comparatively short time she is never free from bleeding. Bleeding between the periods begins as an irregular spotting, after a time there is a continuous flow which changes in character, and after quite a short time becomes an offensive discharge.

Pain occurs considerably later when the bladder and rectum are involved; it is a dull aching pain, complained of about the lower part of the abdomen and vagina.

In a serious untreated case the picture presented is of a debilitated woman, weakened by continued bleeding, poisoned by an offensive discharge, irritated by discharge escaping by the bladder and rectum, both of which are by now involved in the disease. The ureters become obstructed and suppression of urine occurs.

Both in cancer of the body of the uterus and the cervix secondary deposits may arise in distant organs, carried there by lymphatic permeation, and reaching the organs in the blood stream. Those most commonly affected are the lungs, brain and bones.

Treatment. *Carcinoma of the body* is treated by pan-hysterectomy, that is removal of the uterus, with the ovaries and uterine tubes. Many gynaecologists consider that *cancer of the cervix* needs the performance of Wertheim's operation for successful treatment. In this operation the uterus, with the vagina, ovaries and uterine tubes and all the ligaments and lymphatic tissue in the pelvis are removed.

Treatment by radium and X-rays is undertaken in some cases. It depends n the condition of the growth and the choice the surgeon who is consulted makes, as to the type of treatment adopted.

Other forms of cancer may also affect the uterus.

Sarcoma begins in connective tissue, such as muscle, and may occur as he result of cancerous degeneration of a uterine fibroid. As a rule panysterectomy is performed in these cases.

Chorio-carcinoma is an interesting but extremely rare form of cancer which may arise in the uterus. It is the result of abnormal behaviour of the rophoblastic cells which form the chorionic villi which become engrafted on to the wall of the uterus to form the placenta. Normally, when the organ through which the interchange of nourishment is to pass from the mother's blood to the foetus is established, the growth of the placenta ceases and pregnancy proceeds. If it does not cease cancerous changes occur, the cancer cells rapidly invade the lymphatics and, passing on to he blood stream, result in secondary carcinomatous growths in various organs. Operative treatment is necessary as soon as this rare condition is diagnosed.

DISEASES OF THE OVARIES

Ovarian abscess has already been mentioned in connexion with pyosalpinx.

Ovarian tumours may be cystic or solid, the commonest being an *ovarian cyst*, which may reach a very large size, and be either unilateral or bilateral, and unilocular or multilocular. A *simple cyst* contains pure fluid; a *glandular cyst* is filled with mucoid glairy fluid; a *papillomatous cyst* contains watery growths; a *blood cyst* is due to effusion of blood into the ovary; and a *dermoid cyst* contains particles of skin, hair, teeth, etc.

The *symptoms of ovarian cyst* depend upon its size, and are due to discomfort from pressure, giving rise to indigestion, constipation and difficulty of micturition. Dysmenorrhoea and excessive menstruation may accompany the condition. The usual ovarian cyst consists of a body and a pedicle, and *the dangers of the condition* are rupture of the cyst, torsion of the pedicle giving rise to gangrene and infection of the cyst. The *treatment* is removal of the cyst.

Chapter 39

Pregnancy, Antenatal Care, and the Puerperium

Ovulation, menstruation and fertilization—The symptoms and signs of pregnancy— Antenatal care—The toxaemias and complications of pregnancy: vomiting albuminuria, eclampsia, miscarriage, antepartum haemorrhage, pyelitis—Labou and the puerperium—Puerperal sepsis—Nursing care in septicaemia

The changes which take place at puberty in the female organs o generation make it possible for a woman to conceive. The men strual life occupies about 35 years, from the age of 12 or 13 to 4 or 50 depending on climate and race, and this is followed by the meno pause, which is the cessation of activity of the female sex glands.

The *ovaries* are the female sex glands and the centre of the whole se mechanism; if an ovary is cut across it is seen to contain holes, like Gruyère cheese; these are the *graafian follicles*, the spaces in them contai fluid, and minute cells line the walls of these follicles, amongst which i one larger cell, the *egg cell* or *ovum.*

Ovulation is the ripening of a graafian follicle and discharge of the egg cell from it, which occurs once every 4 weeks, midway between the periods during the menstrual life of a woman. The graafian follicle increases ir size and is brought to the surface of the ovary; it bulges on the surface and eventually ruptures, the fluid in it which contains the hormone oestrin or folliculin flows out and the ovum or egg cell is carried out with the fluid into the peritoneal cavity and eventually reaches the uterine tube.

The funnel-shaped end of the uterine tube lies in close vicinity to the ovary; it is lined by ciliated epithelium which is constantly moving and exerting a current directed outwards—that is, along the tube to the uterus. By this movement the ovum is attracted into the external ostium of the tube, and it is conveyed along into the tube where, should the ovum be fertilized, this normally occurs.

Once the graafian follicle has ruptured, it becomes filled with blood and a number of cells grow out from its walls into this blood; these cells contain a yellow pigment and the mass is called the *corpus luteum* which produces the hormone progesterone.

Menstruation is the term generally employed to describe the loss of blood from the uterus which occurs as part of the menstrual cycle every 4 weeks, from puberty to the menopause, and which is brought about by changes in the endometrium resulting in shedding of the old, followed by the formation of a new, membrane. The structure of the endometrium is peculiarly soft, in order that it may form a comfortable resting place for the fertilized ovum during the early development. The uterus consists of unstriped muscle, lined by columnar epithelium; dipping into this structure are tubular glands, and between these glands is a stroma of soft cellular tissue; this stroma is the softest tissue in the body—so soft that it is similar in consistence to jelly just about to set. It is from this soft tissue that bleeding takes place in menstruation.

The *menstrual cycle* of 28 days consists of:

(1) A period of 4 days' *rest* which follows the menstrual loss.

(2) An *interval* of 10 days when the developing graafian follicle is pproaching the surface of the ovary. During this time the hormone oestrin active and stimulates the proliferative changes in the endometrium.

(3) A *pre-menstrual period* of 10 days when, ovulation having occurred, he corpus luteum hormone takes over the work of preparing the endome-rium for the fertilized ovum and progesterone stimulates the formation of ecretory cells in the endometrium.

(4) A *destructive period* follows, if the ovum is not fertilized, all the pre-aration of the endometrium ceases and the carefully prepared lining broken down, blood escapes from the congested capillaries, the epithelial ells disintegrate and the *menstrual flow* which lasts about 4 days is estab-ished.

After this, the cycle begins again and the endometrium is once more repared for the next ovum, which if fertilization does not occur will gain come to nought, but, when an ovum is fertilized, the corpus luteum evelops and continues to produce the hormones which stimulate the hanges which go on in the uterus, including the formation of the placenta pon which the development of the foetus depends.

The *control of menstruation* is dependent on the activity of the ovary, nd the function of the ovary is controlled by hormones produced by the nterior lobe of the pituitary body—two hormones known as Prolan A nd B govern the ovarian cycle of activity which consists of the ripening nd rupture of a graafian follicle and the formation of corpus luteum fterwards. Prolan A controls the changes occurring in the follicles during vulation and stimulates the production of oestrin in the ovary. Prolan B timulates the formation of the corpus luteum and the production of rogesterone from this organ.

The ovary produces two hormones which control menstruation:

(1) *Oestrin* which is produced whilst the follicle is enlarging and pre-aring to rupture. This hormone stimulates the proliferative changes of he endometrium.

(2) *Progesterone* is the hormone produced by the corpus luteum after upture of the follicle. It stimulates the secretory changes in the uterus reparing it for the reception of a fertilized ovum.

Fertilization is the fusing of the male element of reproduction, the *permatozoon*, with the *ovum* or egg cell. This usually takes place in the terine tube, the ovum, which is non-motile and is a round cell, being ransmitted through the tube by the action of the ciliated epithelium which asses it from the external ostium, on to the internal ostium, through which it reaches the uterus. The spermatozoon is a motile cell, shaped like tadpole with a head and a tail, and it passes up through the uterus and ights its way along the uterine tube against the stream of activity of the ilia which is bringing the ovum along, down the tube, to meet it. On neeting, the head of the spermatozoon penetrates the ovum and the tail drops off; the two cells fuse, but no change takes place in the ovum until growth commences.

Cell division commences and the fertilized ovum passes along the uterine tube into the uterus, which is prepared with its soft lining to receive it. Various changes now take place and different cells are formed, some going to the construction of the foetus while from others the placent and membranes are formed.

THE SIGNS AND SYMPTOMS OF PREGNANCY

A woman is said to be pregnant when she has conceived; the uteru will retain the growing foetus for 10 lunar months or 280 days, which the duration of pregnancy. To calculate the date the baby may b expected to be born, add 9 calendar months and 5 days from the last da of the last menstrual period. This reckoning is correct within 2 or 3 week

The **symptoms and signs** by which pregnancy may be determine are divided for convenience into those which appear during the first months, and those seen later.

During the first 12 *weeks*, *amenorrhoea* is considered to be a sign of preg nancy, provided the woman has previously menstruated regularly an that there is no other cause of amenorrhoea, such as the onset of th menopause, anaemia or other illness.

Morning sickness. This usually occurs from the sixth to the sixteent weeks, and is thought to be due to chemical changes in the materna blood owing to the passing into the maternal circulation of waste product from the foetus and the placenta. It may be relieved by taking a cup c tea and a biscuit before rising in the morning.

Breast changes commence about the sixth week, when the breasts are fu and tender. By the twelfth week the breasts are firmer and some mucu secretion is present. The nipples become erect and the areola, dark in tin with visible veins, appears beneath the surface of the skin. By the sixteent week, little nodules, called Montgomery's follicles, appear around th area of the nipple and by the twentieth week the secondary areola appears

Progressive *enlargement of the uterus*. The uterus can first be felt above th symphysis pubis at the sixteenth week. Before this time examinatio would reveal softening of the cervix and a little later the cervix and vagin become discoloured blue.

Frequency of micturition is complained of during the first 12 weeks o pregnancy.

Intermittent uterine contractions may be felt, after the sixteenth week *Quickening* occurs from the eighteenth to the twentieth week, when th mother feels the child moving. A number of other signs can be determine on examination of the patient by a doctor or midwife; foetal heart sound can be heard after the twenty-fourth week.

The *Aschheim-Zondek test* is positive from a time which may vary fron the fourth to the sixth week. The urine of a pregnant woman contains substance not present in non-pregnant women. If a small quantity of th urine is injected into immature white mice, after a few days develop mental changes will be found to have taken place in the generative organ of these animals, and these changes, if they are found, are diagnostic o pregnancy.

The Friedman Test is similar. It is performed on young rabbits.

ANTENATAL CARE

Antenatal care is undertaken in order to assist a woman throug pregnancy and to avoid and treat any diseases or abnormal condition which may arise in order to ensure a normal uncomplicated labour and puerperium. Every married woman should be advised either to consult her own doctor or to attend one of the many excellent antenatal clinics provided, as soon as she knows she is pregnant, for examination, observation, advice and treatment.

The date of her first attendance will be recorded and the *date of her last menstrual period*, and the *possible date of the expected confinement* will be estimated.

History. If previous pregnancies have occurred, she will be questioned as to whether these were normal or complicated, and whether she has ever had premature labours or miscarriages; she will also be asked whether she has had any serious illnesses, scarlet fever, tonsillitis, rheumatism and chorea being specially mentioned—and she will be asked whether she has ever had any surgical operations or met with any serious accidents.

Examination will follow, the condition of the heart and lungs being investigated and her blood pressure taken; she will be asked whether she has any vaginal discharge, and, if so, smears may be taken in order to determine the cause of this. A specimen of urine will be tested. As regards the patient's general condition, she will be closely inspected and questioned; her mouth, teeth and tonsils will be examined; the temperature, pulse and respiration rate, and her weight will be recorded; the colour of the skin and of the mucous membranes will be considered in order to note whether there is any indication of anaemia; she should be asked whether her ankles swell at night and whether she gets breathless on exertion or easily tired; she will also be asked about her appetite, and whether she has her bowels open regularly, and how she sleeps. Her breasts will be examined and particular note made of the condition of the nipples.

The midwife or doctor will examine the abdomen and vulva, but a vaginal examination is not usually undertaken early in pregnancy unless some abnormal condition is suspected.

Frequency of examination. At the first visit the patient is instructed how often she is to attend; it is usual for attendance to be made once a month during the first 6 months of pregnancy, once a fortnight during the next 2 months and every week during the last month. At each visit the urine should be tested for albumin, the blood pressure taken and recorded and in certain cases the weight, and the patient carefully questioned with regard to her general health and comfort.

Antenatal advice. Many books are procurable on this subject and it is treated in great detail; the main points on which it is essential that a woman should be clearly advised are as follows:

Diet should be light but nourishing, plenty of fish and some chicken may be taken, and all dairy produce, including a pint of milk a day. Red meat should be taken but sparingly—if the woman feels that she would miss this very much she may have a little once a day, but it would be better if she could have one day a week without taking red meat. Highly spiced foods, hot sauces and stimulants, and strong tea and coffee are inadvisable, though she may have a little weak tea or coffee twice a day. If she is in the habit of taking alcohol and it would be a privation to give it up entirely, a little may be taken once a day. Plenty of green vegetables and fresh fruit should be taken also; and at least 3 pints of such fluids as lemonade and orangeade each day, in addition to the ordinary drinks at breakfast and tea time.

Action of bowels. A pregnant woman must have a good action of the bowel every day. She should not take aperients except laxatives and lubricants such as senna tea and paraffin, or one of the petrolagar preparations.

Rest and sleep. As far as possible fatigue should be avoided—a pregnant woman should always have from 8 to 9 hours in bed at night and she should also rest for 15 minutes before the two main meals of the day and for one or two hours after the main meal.

Exercise. Moderate exercise is valuable but the patient must not get tired and she should avoid sudden strains and violent jerky movements. Open air exercise is to be recommended, but every woman will have to consider this question for herself—for example, a woman who does most of her own housework, and walks about doing the shopping, does not need a 3-mile walk every afternoon as well.

Clothing should be light and warm, tight bands round waist and breast being avoided, and a pregnant woman will find it most comfortable if her clothing is suspended from the shoulders as far as possible. High heels should not be worn, as they throw the body weight forward, with the result that the woman develops a lordosis in an attempt to balance her own weight and this causes backache.

A *bath daily* is advisable, and the patient should be told to wash her breasts and nipples thoroughly whilst in the bath and to train her nipples to be erect if they are at all inclined to retraction, though her handling of them should never be painful. She should be taught that the nipples contain the openings to all the milk ducts and that the surface should be gently rubbed free of old epithelium and wiped dry with a slightly rough towel to stimulate the circulation.

It should always be impressed on a pregnant woman that if she feels unwell, gets a bad headache, feels sick and disinclined for food or has any other symptoms of malaise, or any loss of blood, she should visit her doctor at once and not wait until the next visit is due.

THE TOXAEMIAS AND COMPLICATIONS OF PREGNANCY

In pregnancy, a number of complications may arise, some of these known as toxaemias are thought to be due to the passing by the child of all its waste products through the placenta into the maternal circulation, so that the excretory organs of the mother have a double load of waste matter to eliminate.

The *three most serious toxaemias* are pernicious vomiting, pregnancy albuminuria and eclampsia.

Morning sickness, if excessive, is abnormal and should be considered a complication.

Neurotic vomiting. In these instances, although the woman vomits a great deal she does not appear ill, and does not lose a great deal of weight, nor become dehydrated. The cause of this type of vomiting is not known.

Pernicious vomiting, though serious, is fortunately rare. When it occurs it is during the early months of pregnancy. The patient vomits frequently and does not retain any nourishment or fluid, and consequently becomes gravely ill.

Pregnancy albuminuria. When this toxaemia occurs, it arises during the latter half of pregnancy. It is far more common than pernicious vomiting. The *symptoms* include *albuminuria*; the urine may be loaded with albumin, the *quantity is diminished* and the urine may contain casts.

The *blood pressure rises*, the systolic pressure may rise to 170–180 and the diastolic to 90 or over.

The patient is *anaemic*; she is pale and puffy as *oedema* occurs; the eyelids, ankles, hands and vulva swell first. There is headache, and usually *sleeplessness;* sometimes visual symptoms arise, such as diplopia, dimness of vision, flashes of light before the eyes. If jaundice and vomiting occur, these symptoms are considered as indications that the liver is becoming affected by the toxaemia.

Medical treatment. Pregnancy albuminuria is a pre-eclamptic state (see below), but if medical treatment is carried out early the danger of eclampsia may be averted. Such a case is often admitted to the medical wards of a hospital for suitable treatment.

Absolute rest is of first importance. A *preliminary period of starvation* is carried out, and only fluids containing glucose are administered for the first 24–36 hours. *The bowels should be well opened* with salines and jalap in order to produce watery stools and so relieve the oedema and also facilitate the work of the kidneys. Large doses of *alkalis* are administered, as pregnancy toxaemias are thought to be associated with decreased alkalinity of the blood. *Drugs* are ordered for the relief of headache and sleeplessness.

If improvement takes place the patient may be given a little food; the diet should be light, bread and butter, a little fruit and green vegetables may be given, and this treatment should be continued for several weeks.

The nursing duties include keeping a strict record of the fluid intake and urinary output, testing a specimen of urine each day, and taking and recording the blood pressure twice a day—morning and evening.

Eclampsia is the name given to fits which occur during the latter half of pregnancy, and also during the puerperium. The condition is associated with raised blood pressure and albuminuria and is thought to be due to absorption of toxins from the placental site which injure the kidneys, as in pregnancy albuminuria, and also injure the brain cells, resulting in fits.

A patient admitted with eclampsia will usually have a history of the symptoms already described above. In pregnancy albuminuria, her urine will be markedly diminished and contain a lot of albumin, and oedema will be present. She may have had several fits.

An *eclamptic fit* is epileptiform in character and occurs in similar stages —(1) A *premonitory stage* lasting perhaps 15 seconds; (2) a *tonic stage*, lasting about 30 seconds, when the muscles are rigid; (3) a *clonic stage* when convulsive movements occur, beginning at the face and passing to the body; this stage may last for 1 or 2 minutes. The fourth stage (4) is of *coma* accompanied by stertorous breathing which may either last a few minutes or go on for many hours or days.

Treatment. Eclampsia is a very serious condition, the mortality being high, and the patient needs the same care as described in epilepsy, during a fit. *Medical treatment* is similar to that described for pregnancy albuminuria; the urine should be frequently tested and the blood pressure taken during the illness. The patient must be kept quiet in a darkened room, sedatives such as morphia and bromides being given, and the severity of the fits when they occur lessened by the administration of chloroform inhalations.

Miscarriage is the premature termination of pregnancy any time before the twenty-eighth week. The termination of pregnancy after that period is called premature labour; the child is viable after 28 weeks, but the longer labour can be delayed after this date the better chance the child has of living. A premature baby of 32 to 34 weeks has a better chance than one of 28 to 30 weeks.

There are a number of natural causes of miscarriage, and it is a fairly common complication of pregnancy—for example, a woman who has had 5 or 6 children may quite ordinarily have had one miscarriage.

Amongst the causes mentioned are—fibroid tumour of the uterus; the formation of bloodclot in the uterus: an unhealthy endometrium; the presence of a dead ovum. Any foreign body in the uterus will cause it to contract and probably result in expelling the foetus.

A dead ovum may be caused by certain diseases of the mother such as chronic nephritis, or any pyrexia or acute illness.

Symptoms of miscarriage. A miscarriage is really a miniature labour, and it may occur a few days, some weeks or several months after pregnancy began. A very usual history is that the woman has missed menstruation for 2 or 3 months; she then begins to bleed from the uterus, and this is accompanied by abdominal pain, followed by a stronger flow of blood, and the products of pregnancy are expelled from the uterus.

Treatment depends on whether the miscarriage is complicated by bleeding or not. If it is not, the duties of the nurse are to keep the patient in bed, to see that she remains quiet and that all pads are preserved for inspection and to note whether any of the products of pregnancy are discharged and to save them. If there is bleeding it may go on quietly for hours, resulting in marked anaemia, and in such a case the patient must be treated for shock and the nurse should make all preparations for taking her to the operating theatre.

The after care includes observation of vaginal discharge, and observation of the temperature and pulse for fear sepsis should complicate the miscarriage.

Antepartum haemorrhage means that there is bleeding from the uterus after the child is viable, that is during the latter part of pregnancy; haemorrhage occurring earlier is described as a threatened miscarriage. Antepartum haemorrhage, which is very serious, occurs when the placenta becomes separated from the wall of the uterus and there are two main reasons to either of which it may be due—(1) *the placenta may be unhealthy* and therefore not firmly attached to the uterine wall, so that it comes off and bleeding occurs into the uterus; (2) is described as *placenta praevia*, meaning that instead of the placenta being on the upper part of the wall of the uterus, as is normal, it is situated on the lower part, below the foetus; and, as the lower part of the uterus widens and spreads towards the end of pregnancy, it tends to cause separation of the placenta, resulting in serious bleeding.

The *treatment of antepartum haemorrhage* requires the services of a skilled obstetrician, but if a nurse is present she may, before his arrival, try to keep the patient very quiet, elevate the foot of the bed on which she lies on a chair or bedblocks, and prepare for giving a douche and for plugging the vagina.

Other complications which may arise include *carneous mole, vesicular mole, retroverted gravid uterus, chorea* and *insanity*. Less serious complications are *constipation, cramp-like pain in the legs, oedema of the legs, varicose veins, pruritis* and *pyelitis*.

Pyelitis occurs about the fifth month; it is fairly common and is thought to be brought about by pressure of the uterus on the ureters, occurring at the period during pregnancy when the uterus fills the pelvic basin, and before it rises out of the pelvis. It is thought that the pressure on the ureters causes stagnation of the urine in the pelvis of each kidney and gives rise to pyelitis; it is commoner on the right side than on the left. The *symptoms and treatment of pyelitis* have been described on p. 403. The prognosis in pregnancy is good, the condition responding to treatment and usually clearing up in a week or two.

LABOUR AND THE PUERPERIUM

The stages of labour. The nurse in training in a general hospital will not be expected to attend a woman in labour, but she should be able to recognize the symptoms of the onset of the first stage as she may have to nurse women who are pregnant in the medical and also in the gynaecological wards.

The *first stage of labour* begins with the onset of labour pains and lasts until the cervix is fully dilated. The pains are due to the contractions of the uterus, and dilation of the cervix is brought about when the uterus squeezes its contents down against the cervix.

The onset of labour is indicated by pain in the back, associated with hardening of the uterus under the anterior abdominal wall. Other points to note are—that labour pains are intermittent, not continuous, and that they tend to become stronger and more frequent. In addition there may be a blood-stained mucoid discharge from the vagina which begins with the onset of the pains, and if there is an escape of fluid from the vagina there is no doubt about the onset of labour. Nurses should not attempt to treat the symptoms mentioned, but should observe the character of the pains and send for a doctor at once and be able to give him a lucid account of the woman's condition.

The *second stage of labour* lasts from the time the cervix is fully dilated, to the birth of the baby.

The *third stage* is from the birth of the baby, until the placenta, which separates, is expelled from the vagina.

Dangers and complications. *Obstructed labour* is probably the most striking danger to be feared, and it may result either because the brim of the bony pelvis is too small for the head of the child to enter the pelvis, or because the head of the child is abnormally large.

A *contracted pelvis* may be due to rickety deformity, or to some developmental error less easily diagnosed.

Malposition of the child in the uterus is another cause of difficult or obstructed labour. The normal position is with the child's head down, fully flexed on the sternum, and the spine lying against the mother's anterior abdominal wall.

Post-partum haemorrhage is another serious complication of labour, and it is due to bleeding from the placental site after a portion of the placenta has separated. Normally, after the child is born, the uterus which has been contracting powerfully to expel the child rests for a little and then contracts again to expel the placenta. The blood vessels of the placental site are closed by the uterine contractions after separation of the placenta. If the uterus does not contract sufficiently to close these vessels the patient may bleed to death in a few minutes.

Post-partum haemorrhage is described as *primary* when it occurs immediately after the birth of a baby and *secondary* when it occurs hours, days or even weeks later. At the time primary post-partum haemorrhage occurs the midwife will be in attendance, but it may sometimes happen that a nurse who is not a midwife may have to deal with a patient suffering from secondary post-partum haemorrhage. In such a case bleeding may not occur in alarming quantities but as a continuous steady loss; the nurse should send for doctor and midwife and in the meantime, if she has pituitrin at hand she should give 5 units hypodermically; if not, and she has any preparation of ergot, she should give this, though it will not act as rapidly as pituitrin. The foot of the bed should be put on high blocks; shock relieved by applications of heat, fluid should be given by mouth and saline per rectum; if bleeding continues and the doctor and midwife do not arrive the nurse should give a hot vaginal douche. The patient must be reassured and kept lying quiet and still.

Ectopic gestation, tubal gestation or **extra-uterine pregnancy** may occur. The commonest site for this is the uterine tube, and the pregnancy can proceed here for from 2½ to 3 months, provided that it is lodged in the outer part of the tube, which is the widest part—the tube is stretched by the growing foetus and in the generality of cases it ruptures, and this is the danger to be feared.

Symptoms and signs of ruptured ectopic gestation. As the result of rupture of the tube, bleeding will occur and the symptoms present depend on (1) whether the bleeding is slight, when it may go on continuously for hours, until the woman notices she is getting weaker and probably has some abdominal pain; or (2) whether it is serious and sudden, and the appearance of the woman that of an acute abdominal catastrophe. When bleeding is very serious the patient becomes faint and collapsed and the skin is blanched. Her pulse is rapid and temperature subnormal. On examination the abdomen will be found to be tender but not much distended. Blood is discharged from the uterus. This patient is dying of loss of blood, and she requires immediate blood transfusion for relief of anaemia and an operation to stop the bleeding, the injured tube being either stitched up or removed according to the degree of damage found on opening the abdomen.

Many less serious cases are seen, but in all cases it is necessary to note the character of the discharge and to inspect all pads for any portions of membrane as these may be the decidua.

PUERPERAL SEPSIS

The **puerperium** is the period which follows labour during which the wounds left by the separation of the placenta, lacerations of the cervix and possibly tearing of the perineum, heal. Although the raw surface left after separation of the placenta closes a good deal by subsequent contractions of the uterus, there is nevertheless still a considerable surface left which has yet to heal.

Causes. A variety of organisms may give rise to puerperal sepsis, either staphylococci, streptococci or *Bacilli coli* may be the cause. *Streptococcal infection of the placental site* is the most serious type, accounting for 50 per cent of the cases of maternal mortality in this country. Efforts are constantly being made to prevent it, and one of the greatest difficulties is to know how the organisms reach the site.

At the present time in hospitals labour is conducted like a surgical operation: the labour room is like an operating theatre; everything used is aseptically prepared; the obstetrician and nurses prepare themselves as if about to assist at a major operation and wear sterile gowns, gloves and masks; the vulva and skin round the perineum is shaved, the skin of the patient's buttocks and thighs being specially prepared. All these precautions are taken in order to prevent the possibility of infection from those in attendance, and to prevent the conveyance of germs into the vagina from the patient's skin by the hands of the operators or from the utensils used. In spite of all precautions, however, a comparatively large percentage of women do become septic, and it is thought that the causative germs must be from the woman herself, either on her skin or in her tissues in the form of some septic focus, or from some person with whom she has been in contact—such as a child with a chronic nasal discharge or someone with septic tonsils—and it is particularly important that the pregnant woman should not be in contact with anyone who has an infected throat or nose during the weeks immediately preceding her delivery.

Similar precautions continue to be carried out after delivery, the woman being nursed with aseptic precautions and even the bedpans sterilized in hospitals.

In addition to the type of organism, its virulence and its mode of access to the placental site, certain predisposing causes must be remembered, including lowered resistance of the patient for any reason, and antenatal care aims at preventing this. The resistance of the woman may be lowered by an abnormal or protracted labour in which her liability to infection is further increased by the necessary handling and possibly by the use of instruments. Bleeding during and after labour, the retention of clots or of placenta, anything that causes delayed or incomplete involution of the uterus—any or all of these may lower her resistance to the invasion of sepsis-producing organisms.

VARIETIES OF PUERPERAL SEPSIS

Any rise of temperature occurring during the puerperium is considered to be an indication of sepsis. **Puerperal pyrexia** is a term used to describe the condition which exists whenever the woman's temperature rises to 100·4° F., or reaches that degree twice within 24 hours.

Sapraemia. Puerperal sepsis gives rise to a toxaemia, more or less grave according to the virulence of the infection. At first the condition usually remains local, but the organisms multiplying at the site of infection and pouring toxins into the blood stream give rise to *sapraemia.*

The *onset of sapraemia* usually occurs about the third day, the temperature rising from 101° to 103° F. and the pulse rate increasing proportionately. The symptoms which usually accompany the febrile state are present, such as thirst, a dry mouth, scanty output of urine and constipation; there is general discomfort with headache, malaise and sleeplessness. The lochia becomes profuse and is offensive.

(*Lochia* is the term used to describe the discharge from the vagina, due to drainage of the uterus following labour. Lochia is at first red and bloodstained, then becomes paler and pinkish, until at the end of about 9 or 10 days it clears altogether. There should never be any offensive odour, and the lochia should always be watery in character.)

Local treatment which will be employed consists in drainage of the uterus by the injection into it of glycerine. This treatment was introduced by Remington Hobbs. A graduated uterine terminal-eyed catheter is inserted into the os uteri by means of an introducer, a record syringe is attached to the end of the catheter and glycerine slowly injected. The patient is nursed in Fowler's position.

Septicaemia is a more serious form of puerperal sepsis, and is described as puerperal septicaemia. The onset is sudden—the most serious cases begin on the first or second day—with a rise in temperature of from 103° to 104° F., rigors occur, the skin is hot and there is often profuse sweating. The pulse is rapid. The mouth is dry and parched, the tongue furred and sordes collect on the teeth, the lips become cracked and sore. The appetite is poor, but the patient may ask for special dishes saying, for example, she would like a boiled onion or some bacon and eggs. There may be nausea and vomiting.

The urine is scanty and high coloured, diarrhoea or constipation may be present. Headache is usually present and the patient finds it impossible to sleep, she becomes more and more prostrated and develops delirium. The milk is suppressed and the lochia may be scanty and offensive or even entirely suppressed. As the days pass the patient becomes very weak and emaciated and has a tendency to develop bedsores.

In appearance her skin is grey and toxic, she has a malar flush and her eyes may be bright. A characteristic feature of the most severe cases is that they declare they are all right and do not feel ill—they are unduly cheerful.

Serious signs are persistent vomiting and marked diarrhoea, rigors occurring frequently, hiccup and jaundice, intractable insomnia and weakness of the pulse.

The prognosis is grave, and the earlier the appearance of the symptoms the graver is the condition. Very serious cases begin to be ill on the first or second day of the puerperium; milder cases on the third, fourth or fifth day.

Pyaemia may succeed septicaemia. In this condition the blood is liable to clot in the veins and portions of this friable infected bloodclot, breaking off, pass through the circulation and becoming arrested in various organs give rise to the formation of abscesses. In grave cases multiple abscesses form in the subcutaneous tissue, and in the joints, liver, lungs and brain.

The condition of pyaemia is characterized by very grave prostration and symptoms similar to those of septicaemia; the occurrence of rigors is frequent. The prognosis is grave.

Localized spread of infection may also occur. *Pelvic cellulitis* is due to spread of sepsis to the tissues and organs in close relation to the infected uterus and cervix. This does not usually happen until the second week of the puerperium.

Spread of infection upwards from the uterus may give rise to *salpingitis, pyosalpinx, ovarian abscess,* and *pelvic peritonitis.*

Thrombo-phlebitis of the femoral vein, which is also called *white leg* and *phlegmasia alba dolens,* is due to spread of infection from the pelvis. The lymphatics are infected, and this results in blockage of the passage of lymph, which exudes into the tissues so that the limb becomes swollen, with a characteristic marble-white shining appearance. There is pain over the affected vein, a rise of temperature and increase of pulse rate. This acute condition lasts about 2 weeks, but the swelling of the limb will persist for from 5 to 6 weeks.

Treatment is to immobilize the limb, which should be elevated on a pillow, carefully supported and protected from the weight of bedclothes by a cradle. Applications of glycerine of belladonna and fomentations are ordered for the relief of pain and swelling.

The diet should be low and the bowels active, the patient being kept as quiet as possible, free from anxiety and not allowed to move more than is absolutely necessary as there is danger of a pulmonary embolism, particularly during the first two weeks when the condition is acute.

THE NURSING CARE AND TREATMENT OF SEPTICAEMIA

The nursing of a case of puerperal septicaemia does not differ from that of any other case of septicaemia, except in so far as vaginal pads must be carefully inspected for the amount and character of any lochia, and it is advisable to have the patient in Fowler's position so that drainage from the uterus is made easier.

The *aim of nursing care* is to raise the resistance of the patient by the provision of a good liberal nourishing diet, with plenty of drinks containing glucose in addition, so that easily assimilated nourishment is readily available and that plenty of fluids may be provided in order to maintain the balance of fluid in the body and so lessen the toxaemia.

The patient should be nursed in the open air, and made as comfortable as possible, so that discomfort is minimized and relieved, and in this way rest is obtained and the maximum of sleep made possible.

Drugs. Sulphonamides are given when the infection is a streptococcal one. Large doses of either sulphapyridine or sulphathiazole are employed but patients need watching for signs of intolerance. Patients who do not respond to sulphonamides are given penicillin.

Diet. In many instances a case of puerperal septicaemia particularly is found to have a very dirty mouth when admitted to hospital for treatment. The best way to deal with this condition is to give the patient fluids for 2 or 3 days—lemonade and barley water sweetened with a little glucose, plain water and soda water and a little beef tea; as the condition of the mucous lining of the stomach improves the mouth becomes cleaner and the diet may be increased by adding jellies, clear soups, tea and dry toast, and after a day or two fish and chicken cream and stewed fruit, gradually introducing a fuller diet with the addition of a little white wine or other stimulant.

A four-hourly temperature record should be made and the pulse noted frequently; watch must be kept for the onset of rigors. During a rigor the temperature should be recorded every half-hour at least so that its rate of rising is noted, and the patient should be sponged if the fever reaches 105° F., or earlier should the symptoms of toxaemia, indicated by headache, restlessness and delirium, be straining the resources and lowering the resistance of the patient.

The skin will act profusely after a rigor and the patient should be sponged with warm or hot water as the temperature declines; a warm drink and a dose of stimulant may be given as the patient will be considerably weakened by having a rigor, and careful nursing may induce the sleep which is the best mode of rest.

Throughout the illness the nurse must remember the necessity of sleep. Patients with septicaemia are at times bright and talkative, and so inclined to develop restlessness and delirium, and she should do all in her power to keep these patients contented and peaceful, free from the sense of worry and anxiety, which is so readily contributed to by irritation and discomfort. In many cases hypnotics will be ordered.

The skin should be sponged night and morning, as this is soothing; in some instances the nurse will find the use of hot water most soothing and helpful, in others the patient will be made most comfortable by sponging with cooler water. The emaciation which exists tends to predispose to the formation of bedsores, but these must be prevented; frequent passage of stools makes the skin around the anus tender and sore. Using olive oil or liquid paraffin swabs to clean the patient after the use of a bedpan may be necessary.

Many cases of puerperal septicaemia are found to have *retention of urine*, and it is most important to observe the slightest fullness above the symphysis pubis indicating this condition; it should be relieved by catheterization. Some patients thought to be incontinent may be found to have a full bladder, the apparent incontinence being a dribbling of overflow from a very distended bladder.

Section 7

Surgical Nursing and Elementary Surgical Technique

Introductory

Surgery is described as a branch of medicine; it deals with the treatment of conditions brought about by malformation, deformity, tumours, injury, infection and inflammation. Surgery is both an art and a science; it is a very old art, but the science of surgery is of comparatively recent development. Dexterity in manipulative and operative surgery in the middle of the last century could not make up for the lack of anaesthetics and antiseptics, and skill in the performance of an operation had no relation to its ultimate success as the life of the patient was imperilled by serious shock and dangerous sepsis, known and described as hospital gangrene.

By means of these two important discoveries of the nineteenth century—anaesthetics and antiseptics—a surgeon can undertake and bring to a successful conclusion operations and manipulations which would otherwise have been impossible.

The *principles of the practice of surgery* include the provision of rest and treatment by passive and active movement; the application of soothing and stimulating remedies, the provision of free drainage in septic conditions, manipulative and operative technique, and the difference between domestic and surgical cleanliness. In his care of injured and diseased tissues a surgeon requires to be familiar with the normal processes of repair as he is constantly called upon to make decisions as to whether rest or manipulation is indicated and the necessity for operative interference. The effect on the patient of the tissues to be handled during operation is most carefully considered, pre-operative care and treatment can now practically eliminate post-operative shock, and chemotherapy is increasingly employed in order to prevent complications formerly due to sepsis.

Nursing is closely allied to surgery, and has developed alongside of it. Florence Nightingale first recognized the need for cleanliness in surgical wards, and the nurse of today puts Miss Nightingale's teaching into practice. She must understand the meaning of rest, passive and active movement; attempt to see what a surgeon is aiming at when he applies healing remedies, splints, plaster, or extensions, or incises and drains septic tissues, the effect he desires to obtain by manipulative surgery, and to follow the procedure he adopts in an operating theatre and be able to assist, by her intelligent nursing care, the recovery of the patient after an operation.

Surgical nursing provides a vast field of interest and wide experience in the general care and treatment of sick persons, including as it does acute infections, chronic states of illness, accidents and emergencies, and in addition in the complications of surgical conditions includes grave cardiac, respiratory and renal disease and disability.

Chapter 40

Infection—Inflammation—Haemorrhage—Ulcers —Tumours and Cysts

Surgical infection—Gas gangrene—Inflammation: symptoms, terminations and treatment—Haemorrhage: causes of bleeding, general classification, symptoms associated with bleeding, means used in treatment—Ulcers—Tumours and cysts: classification of tumours, differences between simple and malignant tumours

Infection is the successful invasion of the body by disease-producing organisms. The commonest modes of infection are (1) *pulmonary*, by droplets in moist air; (2) *intestinal*, when bacteria are swallowed with food and water; (3) *inoculation*, either through a mucous surface or an abraded skin, or by means of some biting insect.

Surgical infection is described as local or general. Examples of local infection include *boils*, in which inflammation occurs in the hair follicle; this becomes surrounded by dense tissue which deprives the centre of its circulation, resulting in a slough, commonly known as the 'core' of the boil.

Carbuncles are areas of localized inflammation in the deeper parts of the skin and subcutaneous tissue. The back of the neck is a common site for carbuncle. It is more serious than a boil, as ulceration occurs and large sloughs are formed, and infection may spread by means of the lymphatics, giving rise to general septicaemia.

Small subcutaneous abscesses may occur as the result of infected insect stings, infected abrasions and infected haematoma. An abscess is a collection of pus in a cavity. Common sites of abscess are the tonsils, appendix and mastoid cells.

Cellulitis is inflammation of the connective tissue and fascia lying beneath the skin and separating the different layers of muscles. It results in a brawny swelling, there is a very diffuse area of infection and septicaemia may result.

The organisms which commonly give rise to surgical infection are those which are always present on the skin, staphylococci, streptococci and bacilli coli. The organism producing erysipelas comes from one of the streptococcal groups. Other rarer surgical infections due to spore-forming organisms include anthrax, gas gangrene and tetanus.

Syphilis and gonorrhoea also come under the heading of surgical infections (see ch. 36).

The use of penicillin in surgical infections is general. It is employed by the systemic route in adequate dosage and over a sufficient period of time. It is also used locally where possible either as penicillin spray, powder or cream.

GAS GANGRENE

As the name implies, this acute surgical infection is characterized by gangrene or necrosis accompanied by the formation of bubbles of gas in the affected subcutaneous tissues.

The causal organism belongs to the *Clostridium group* which are spore-forming anaerobic organisms and include the *Cl. welchii*, *Cl. septique* and *Cl. oedematiens*. Infected wounds, such as war wounds, provide an ideal medium for the growth of these organisms.

The onset of gas gangrene is that of an acute, rapidly spreading infection. Muscle tissue is most commonly involved, the wound becoming covered with an offensive exudate having a characteristic odour, which is likened to the smell of acetylene gas. Local swelling of the tissues occurs, and when a limb is involved the entire limb becomes oedematous. Crepitation due to escape of gas into the subcutaneous tissue is present. In advanced cases the skin over the infected area is mottled dusky-brown, and purplish-black patches appear which may be covered with blebs and bullae.

Treatment consists in the administration of adequate doses of antitoxin with penicillin given as an adjunct to this treatment. The local application of sulphonamides is employed and surgical treatment is undertaken when necessary.

General Surgical Infection. A general infection may be caused by saprophytic organisms giving rise to fermentation and putrefactive changes; or by parasitic organisms producing pyogenic infection, such as *staphylococci*, *streptococci*, *B. coli*, *pneumococci* and *gonococci*. The varieties of a general infection may be classified according to severity:

Sapraemia. When local changes brought about by the products of fermentation occur.

Septicaemia. When the causative organisms circulate in the blood stream and produce extensive general disturbance.

Pyaemia. When the character of the blood is altered, clotting takes place and infected blood clot gives rise to the development of metastatic abscesses in different parts of the body.

(For details of the nursing of a patient suffering from septicaemia, see p. 567.)

INFLAMMATION

Inflammation is the reaction of healthy tissues to injury, and the reaction is characterized by a series of changes upon which the symptoms depend.

Causes. Inflammation may be due to a variety of causes, but bacterial invasion may be considered the commonest cause, other causes including mechanical, thermal and chemical injuries, excessive heat and cold, and electrical injuries including exposure to high tension current and X-rays.

The **changes** taking place in the tissues are described as follows:

(1) *Hyperaemia*—the small blood vessels dilate, with resultant greater supply of blood to the part.

(2) *Stasis*—as the result of dilatation of the blood vessels the blood in them slows down.

(3) *Exudation of lymph* and migration of leucocytes. Owing to the increased permeation of the minute blood vessel walls, and the slowing down of the blood stream, the leucocytes escape through the walls and act as phagocytes, serum exudes through the thin walls and this serum contains fibrin and antitoxin, both of which are valuable in arresting disease—some red cells also escape.

(4) *Proliferation of cells.* As the result of the changes described, there is proliferation of connective tissue cells, particularly the endothelial and fibro-blastic. The endothelial cells form new vessels; the fibro-blastic cells result in the formation of fibrous tissue which contracts and forms a scar.

Symptoms of inflammation. The *local signs* of inflammation are (1) *redness*, which corresponds with the hyperaemia, (2) *heat*, partly due to hyperaemia and partly due to chemical changes going on in the affected tissues, (3) *swelling*, which is brought about by the exudation of lymph and depends to a great extent upon the looseness of the tissues. For example, in a whitlow, which is an inflammatory condition of the periosteum of the phalange of the finger at the base of the nail, very little swelling can take place as the tissues are dense; but in inflammation of the orbit, as the tissues round the eye are very loose and almost devoid of fat, considerable swelling occurs. (4) *Pain* occurs as the result of the tension in the tissues which exerts pressure on the nerve endings. As the result of pain and swelling there is (5) *loss of function*, which is the natural desire of the subject to rest and to avoid using the painful member.

The termination of inflammation. The result of inflammation depends to a great extent on whether the condition was an acute or a chronic one. Acute inflammation may terminate in resolution, or there may be too much destruction of tissue for this—most chronic inflammatory conditions, however, do not terminate by resolution because the tissue changes have been too advanced for this to happen.

(1) *Resolution.* The cells which have been destroyed in the neighbourhood of the inflammation by the action of phagocytes, or broken down by them, are absorbed by the lymphatics. Some scar tissue remains for a time, but it also may be removed by phagocytic action and, when this happens and no thickening is left, the tissues are in the same state as before the inflammation and are said to have 'resolved'. The best example of resolution in medicine and surgery is the return to normal of the lung after an attack of lobar pneumonia, but resolution can also occur in some surgical inflammatory lesions.

(2) *Cell destruction.* Because there has been considerable cell destruction, certain other changes must take place. The cells may be liquefied and broken down and, although a certain amount of this fluid is absorbed, more may be formed than can be dealt with and in this case an abscess forms. An abscess consists of these liquefied cells and broken-down bacteria and phagocytes. It may work to the surface and burst, but most surgeons prefer to incise and drain an abscess.

(3) *Sloughing and gangrene.* A slough is usually defined as a small mass of dead tissue; the core of a boil is a slough, so also is the mass of grey tissue which forms on the surface of an ulcer, or on a very bad trophic sore or bedsore. Gangrene is death of a mass of tissue; for example, gangrene of a whole limb may occur.

As the result of death of the tissues, cells are killed, but not liquefied, and the solid mass results in slough or gangrene. This slough becomes separated from living tissue by an area of inflammation which is described in the case of a limb as the 'line of demarcation'; in the case of a slough separating from the surface of an ulcer, healthy granulating tissue occurs beneath it, absorption of a portion of the slough nearest this tissue which becomes liquefied is then possible, and the dead part is cast off.

Treatment of inflammation. Whenever it is possible the *cause of the inflammation should be removed.* If a child has fallen on his knees and got some gravel in, take it out; if a maid has run a splinter in her hand, remove it. The next important point is the *application of rest.* An inflamed hand should be carried in a sling, an inflamed eye should be covered. A sprained ankle should not be used. The degree of rest employed will depend on the presence of any constitutional symptoms; and since the local inflammatory reaction may give rise to a fair degree of malaise owing to the absorption of toxins, the patient may be ill enough to remain in bed. It is quite usual to find a patient with a bad septic hand complaining of headache, loss of appetite, rise of temperature and inability to sleep.

Treatment both local and systemic is by the use of penicillin and/or sulphonamides. Penicillin is the drug of choice as when infection is present this drug will deal with the condition and when the cause of the inflammation is non-bacterial, such as injury, penicillin will act as a prophylactic and prevent infection occurring in the injured tissues. Other forms of treatment include applications of cold to limit swelling and applications of heat to increase the circulation and promote absorption when the drying is not seen until swelling has occurred.

In *chronic inflammatory conditions* counterirritants are sometimes employed. These include the application of liniments, iodine and mercury, according to the cause of the inflammation.

HAEMORRHAGE

Haemorrhage is an ugly word to use to describe bleeding but its use is time honoured. Slight bleeding will be arrested by natural means, severe bleeding will require treatment to help in its arrest.

Bleeding may be classified in a number of different ways:

Causes of bleeding. *Local causes* include injury which may be accidental or intentional—as an operation causes bleeding. Excessive vascularity of the membrane lining a canal or cavity may cause bleeding; this is most commonly seen in the case of nasal polypi, uterine polypi, and papilloma of the bladder. Disease in the vicinity of a blood vessel may cause it to be eroded, resulting in escape of blood—this occurs in cancer for example; or it may result in spontaneous rupture of a blood vessel as when cerebral haemorrhage occurs.

General causes of bleeding may include such diseases as *arteriosclerosis. Purpura* is characterized by bleeding into the subcutaneous tissue and into cavities and from organs such as when haematuria occurs in purpura. *Scurvy* is fortunately a rare disease today, but it also is characterized by bleeding under the periosteum of the long bones, from the bowel and into the gums. Some of the varieties of anaemia mentioned on p. 359 are characterized by bleeding. *Haemophilia* is another example of a disease in which bleeding is likely to occur.

Type of vessel. *Arterial bleeding* is bright red in colour; and the blood is pumped out with the contraction of the vessel. This type of bleeding is arrested by pressure applied on the proximal side of the bleeding vessel.

Venous bleeding occurs as a continuous stream of blood, which is darker in colour. It is arrested by pressure on the distal side of the vessel.

Capillary bleeding is a regular oozing of blood on to the surface, or welling up in a wound. It is usually stopped by pressure on the bleeding surface.

Sites of bleeding. Epistaxis is bleeding from the nose; it may be due to injury such as a blow or from constant picking of the nose; it may be due to excessive vascularity of the nasal mucous membrane as when polypi are present; it may be the result of small ulcers on the surface of the nasal cavity; it occurs in the general diseases which predispose to bleeding: purpura, scurvy, some forms of anaemia, high blood pressure, arteriosclerosis and haemophilia. It may be a symptom of onset of one of the infectious diseases or of influenza.

The *treatment of epistaxis* is to sit the patient up and hold a basin to catch the blood; cold should be applied over the bridge of the nose and over the upper lip—whence some of the blood vessels supplying the nose pass to it. The patient may gently rinse his mouth with water, and have ice to suck.

The nose should be pinched, as pressure applied to the front part will stop the bleeding there. If the bleeding continues it may be necessary to pack the nose with gauze soaked in adrenalin. If post-nasal plugs are needed these should be inserted by a surgeon.

The patient should be kept quiet, and when there is danger of recurrence of bleeding he should have a light diet, given cool not hot, and stimulants should be omitted for a few days.

In some cases, when considerable loss of blood has occurred and the patient is suffering from shock, he may not be able to be propped sitting up and he should then lie down; in this instance epistaxis is complicated by shock and both factors require treatment. When shock is severe, saline infusion and blood transfusion may be necessary.

Haemoptysis is bleeding from the lungs; the blood is coughed up, and as it is mixed with air it consequently often looks frothy, but it may also be mixed with sputum; it is usually bright red in colour. Haemoptysis occurs most often in pulmonary tuberculosis, but it may also complicate mitral disease of the heart, and aortic aneurysm. The *treatment* is described in detail on p. 376.

Haematemesis is vomiting of blood. As a rule it comes from the stomach but it may have first been swallowed as might happen in severe epistaxis, and it may also have regurgitated into the stomach when severe bleeding complicates duodenal ulcer.

Vomited blood, which has been some little time in the stomach, is mixed with gastric juice or maybe with food; it is of a characteristic colour and consistence—like coffee grounds—and is acid in reaction. The *treatment* is described on pp. 382–4 in which an example is given of a patient with a very severe haematemesis who is admitted to a medical ward.

Haematuria is blood in the urine; when a small amount is present the urine will be slightly smoky in appearance, and this renders it less clear than normal. When a lot of blood is passed the urine may be bright red and clots may be present. When the blood is well mixed with the urine it is usually from the kidneys; when passed at the end of the act of micturition it is probably from the bladder; and, if passed at the beginning of the act, it usually indicates that the urethra is bleeding.

Melaena is the presence of altered blood in the stool; it may be present in large quantities, rendering the stool dark like tar, or there may be only a trace.

Uterine bleeding. Severe uterine bleeding may occur in disease of the uterus, particularly if polypoid growths are present, when the cavity is enlarged by the existence of fibroids, and in carcinoma. Such a condition calls for immediate treatment, and if a nurse has to deal with it she should elevate the foot of the bed, give a hot vaginal douche, prepare articles for packing the vagina and also for the administration of an intra-uterine douche. The surgeon will give this, but the nurse must be prepared to pack the vagina. Ergot, ½–1 drachm may be administered pending the arrival of a surgeon, if bleeding is severe; or, alternatively, a preparation of ergot may be given.

Extravasation of blood is the term used to describe the condition when blood is poured into the subcutaneous tissues; the area becomes swollen, and often tense and brawny. A large localized collection of blood is described as a *haematoma*—this may, however, become absorbed in time; if not, aspiration of the tumour of blood is usually tried; but when complicated by sepsis it is incised and drained. A small collection of blood immediately beneath the skin may be *petechial* in character, just minute puncta of blood. A larger collection in the same situation is a bruise or *ecchymosis*.

A large amount of blood may be present, and the aim of treatment is to prevent further effusion—rest and the application of cold may help in this. Later, the aim is to help absorption and removal by lymphatic and blood vessels, and applications of heat and gentle massage around the bruised area will assist in this process. A black eye is a good example of a severe bruise.

The time at which bleeding occurs. *Primary bleeding* occurs at the time of injury; *reactionary* or *intermediate* bleeding occurs within 24 hours of it. This is due to the rise of blood pressure which occurs as a patient recovers; he may return to consciousness, and cough or vomit and just this slight movement may be enough to start bleeding. *Reactionary bleeding* may also be due to the injudicious use of stimulants, to a clot being forced out of a vessel or to the slipping of a ligature—but this is rare.

Secondary bleeding does not usually occur until a week or 10 days have elapsed; though the term is used to describe any bleeding which occurs after the first 24 hours after injury. It is practically always due to infection; the wall of the vessel is gradually weakened by this and finally gives way, resulting in bleeding.

Bleeding is also classified, or more correctly described, as being either *external* when it can be seen, as for example in cut throat; or *internal* or concealed when the symptoms of profound shock and anaemia suggest that the patient is bleeding internally.

The **symptoms associated with bleeding** should be well known and quickly recognized. The skin is cold, pale and clammy, the temperature being so low that the moisture is not evaporated from its surface, as it should be. The extremities of the fingers and toes, and the ears and lips are livid; the eyes are deeply sunken in their sockets and the pupils may be dilated; the face looks pinched; the patient gasps in breathing, as he is suffering from air hunger owing to the diminution of the haemoglobin content of his blood by reason of the loss of red cells in the blood which he is losing; his breathing is rapid and sighing. Owing to lowering of the volume of fluid in the blood vessels, the pulse is rapid, weak and irregular; the blood pressure is low.

The patient will complain of thirst, of feeling suffocated, and he will move about restlessly in his effort to obtain the air he feels he needs. If he attempts to sit up he will feel faint and may faint; he may also complain of buzzing noises in his head and dizziness.

When bleeding is very severe syncope may be immediate and fatal; when less severe there may be attacks of syncope, and between the attacks weakness and collapse will be very marked.

The provision made by nature to arrest bleeding consists of (1) *decrease of blood pressure* due to loss of blood and lowering of the activity of the nervous system—the heart will beat less forcibly and the blood fluid collects in the small vessels in the abdominal cavity.

(2) *The clotting of blood.* As mentioned on p. 582 bloodclot forms more readily in a torn or lacerated vessel than in one which is cleanly incised. The decrease of blood pressure prevents dislodgement of the clot from the open mouth of the cut vessel.

(3) *Retraction and contraction of the walls of the divided arteries.* A cut vessel shrinks slightly in size by contraction of the muscular and elastic tissue in its walls; in addition the middle coat—the intima—retracts, or curls in, and so helps to retain the clot in the vessel against the pressure of the blood behind it.

Mechanical measures which may be used in the arrest of bleeding are applied locally. These are *applications of heat and cold.* Examples of heat are the vaginal douche recommended for uterine bleeding; applications of hot wet towels employed in the treatment of bleeding during operations on the abdominal cavity. Examples of cold include the cold compress applied to the nose and lip in the arrest of bleeding in epistaxis, ice applied to the head for cerebral haemorrhage, and the natural tendency to put a cut hand beneath the cold-water tap.

The use of styptics. The application of adrenalin in surgery of the ear, nose and throat for example; other styptic agents commonly employed are tannic acid, perchloride of iron, peroxide of hydrogen and nitrate of silver in a weak solution.

By *elevation* of the *bleeding part*, which makes the blood flow upwards, against gravity, the loss may be slightly lessened pending the preparation of more useful measures.

The *application* of *pressure*, proximal to the bleeding point in arterial, and on the spot in venous, bleeding. Every nurse should be familiar with the main pressure points of haemorrhage; she never knows when she will want to apply this knowledge; moreover, a merely theoretical knowledge will not help her; she must practise applying pressure over these arterial pressure points either on herself or on her friends, and she can test her efficiency by trying to find the pulse below the pressure point—which should be obliterated, if her pressure is on the right spot. The principal pressure points and methods of applying digital pressure are shown in figs. 183 to 189, pp. 593 to 596.

Pressure may also be applied by means of a tourniquet. *Plugging a wound* or other cavity from which bleeding is taking place and *firmly bandaging a dressing* on may also be tried in certain situations.

The *application of ligatures* to bleeding vessels, once the points have been secured by means of artery forceps, is not usually within the province of a nurse.

The **general treatment** of a patient who is bleeding is as follows—he must stay in bed and be kept quiet and warm; his head should be low, as he so easily feels faint. He should be confidently reassured in order to set his mind at rest; morphia will be ordered as a rule and the nurse should prepare this as soon as possible, so that when the doctor comes, who can order it, it is ready to give and even a moment's delay is avoided. In no circumstances should any stimulant be given, but thirst should be allayed by drinks of water, or half-strength saline may be given. The replacement of the lost fluid is very important, and as the patient is thirsty he will be ready to drink and should be given as much as he will take. If he will take enough fluid by mouth other means need not be employed, but otherwise it may be given rectally, subcutaneously and by the intravenous route.

The replacement of blood. So much of the patient's discomfort and many of the symptoms present are due to the diminished supply of oxygen to the vital organs of his body, owing to the loss of red blood cells and consequent loss of the oxygen-carrying haemoglobin, therefore blood transfusion may be given.

ULCERS

Gangrene has already been described as massive death of tissue—ulceration may be described as molecular death of tissue, cell by cell. An ulcer is a sore on the surface, and it may be on the outside or inside of an organ as in the case of peptic ulcers (see p. 380). Ulcers are classified to some extent according to their cause, such as *traumatic*, pyogenic or trophic; *specific* when due to syphilis or tuberculosis and *malignant* when due to cancer. They are also classified according to their position, or some characteristic such as a *varicose* ulcer, *gastric* or *duodenal* ulcer, *corneal* ulcer, *rodent* ulcer.

When a nurse is called upon to apply treatment to an ulcer, she should have some idea of the state the ulcer is in at the outset, and should be able to describe whether its condition remains stationary, whether she thinks healing is taking place, or whether the ulcer is spreading.

An ulcer consists of a bed which is the floor or surface of the ulcer, of edges which form the margins of the ulcer, and it is usually covered by an exudate or discharge. A *healing ulcer* is free from discharge, it has a pink, regular granulating floor, and shelving edges, and the epidermis can be seen gradually encroaching on the surface of the ulcer. A healing ulcer is movable on the structures beneath it and its margins are quite free from any area of inflammation. In the treatment of such an ulcer, protection is required by means of a sterile dressing, and it should be kept very clean, and the surface free from any excessive granulations.

A *stationary ulcer* is frequently described as atonic or indolent. Its floor is covered by pale, irregular granulations, and its edges are usually hard and bound down to the structures beneath them. Such an ulcer requires stimulating. Zinc is one example of a stimulating and healing dressing;

a more recent form of treatment of callous indolent ulcers is by the application of elastoplast, which is a thick adhesive plaster containing certain antiseptic properties; by means of its elasticity it helps to improve the circulation of the part to which it is applied.

A *spreading ulcer* is usually covered by unhealthy granulations or a slough, and is surrounded by a zone of inflammation by which it spreads to the surrounding parts. In the treatment of this ulcer any discharge or exudate from it should be removed by applications of fomentations and then, when it has been cleaned, it should be treated by stimulating applications as in the case of an indolent ulcer.

Penicillin cream is applied to static, indolent, varicose and traumatic ulcers.

TUMOURS AND CYSTS

A *tumour* is a swelling; a *neoplasm* is a new growth in the tissues. A *cyst* is a sac of fluid, and the term is used to describe a cystic swelling—a *sebaceous cyst* for example, which is a little swelling produced by blockage of the duct of one of the sebaceous glands in the skin or scalp, and in this case the fluid contained in the sac is sebum.

A *dermoid cyst* is an abnormal development of structures pertaining to the skin. It consists of a sac, containing skin, hair and teeth, which is usually congenital in origin.

Tumours. The application of this term is confined to description of the solid swellings consisting of new growths of cells. It may be simple (benign) or malignant, and the differences in the structure, mode of growth and dangers of these two classes are outlined below:

Simple Tumour	*Malignant Tumour*
Composed of cells similar to the tissue in which it grows. The cells are therefore harmless.	Composed of cells unlike those of the tissue in which it is found. These cells are destructive.
Encapsulated, and so the growth is confined.	Has no capsule, but spreads into the surrounding tissue.
Of comparatively slow growth.	Grows fairly rapidly.
Usually painless, but may cause pain by pressure on nerves in its vicinity.	Painless at first, but by the time pain is experienced much damage has been caused.
Dangers. Pain, as above and inconvenience due to position or size.	*Dangerous to life*. Spreading locally by infiltration and also by the lymphatics and blood, with the result that secondary deposits occur in other organs. Locally, ulceration occurs, followed by blockage of the lymphatics and consequent oedema.

Classification of Tumours. In addition to being classified as either simple or malignant, simple tumours are described according to the type of tissue in which they occur. *Tumours of epithelial tissue* are described as *epitheliomata*, when on the surface of the skin; as *papillomata*, when projecting from the surface or into a cavity; and as *adenomata* when present in the tissue of a gland.

Connective tissue tumours when present in fat and composed of it are *lipoma*; of fibrous tissue, *fibroma*; of nerve tissue, *glioma*; of muscle, *myoma*; of bone, *osteoma*; or cartilage, *chondroma*.

The **treatment of a simple tumour** may be necessary because of the inconvenience it causes; for example, a small lipoma on the face will be removed because it is disfiguring; a large myoma may be causing pain by pressing on the nerves in its vicinity, and this would indicate that it should be removed. Any tumour in the breast should be removed, because the breast is one of the commonest sites of cancer and the irritation caused by the presence of a simple tumour might cause malignant changes to occur in the tissues, though it is not usual for a simple tumour to change its nature in this way.

A **malignant tumour** may be either *carcinoma* or *sarcoma*. Speaking very generally, carcinoma affects epithelial tissue and will therefore be most commonly found on the skin and mucous surfaces, and in the cavities of the organs of the body and also in the substance of the organs when these consist of ducts, tubules and glands and are therefore lined by endothelial tissue.

When the growth or tumour is present on the surface the term *epithelioma* is used to describe it; when in the substance of a gland it is known as *carcinoma*. Carcinoma is of different types according to the character of the cell of which the growth is formed; the more virulent types will have a graver prognosis than those of lower virulence; but it is not necessary for the nurse to be familiar with this mode of classification.

Carcinoma spreads by infiltration—that is, directly into the tissues; it is not confined by any surrounding capsule and its growth is consequently irregular and rapid; the area of tissue into which this growth extends is described as the *cancer area*. It is for this reason and in order to ensure the greatest possible success that a surgeon when removing a cancerous growth also removes a very large area of the surrounding structures.

Sarcoma is the term used to describe cancer when it affects the connective tissues of the body, such as bone, cartilage and muscle—though this use of the word is not invariable.

Sarcoma spreads by means of the blood stream; unlike carcinoma, which derives its nourishment from the surrounding tissues, sarcoma is very richly supplied with blood, by the formation of new blood vessels within the growth. It is because of this that secondary deposits so rapidly occur in sarcoma. The venous blood returning to the lungs to be purified, and carrying its load of disease, frequently results in secondary growths in the lungs; similarly the blood from the alimentary tract, being carried by the portal system to the liver, will give rise to secondary growths in this organ in cases of cancer of the stomach or intestine.

The treatment of cancer is either its earliest possible destruction by applications of radium, or removal of the growth by surgery. The nursing of cases of cancer is dealt with in chapter 54.

(In order to avoid repetition other causes of deformity have been dealt with in the chapter on orthopaedic nursing, see p. 774.)

Chapter 41

Injuries to Soft Structures

Burns and scalds—Wounds, contusions and bruises—Crush syndrome—The healing of wounds—Care of an infected wound—Injuries to tendon, muscle and nerve—Stings and bites—Foreign bodies in the tissues

BURNS AND SCALDS

A **Burn** is due to the action of dry heat such as contact with fire, flame or hot air; and a *scald* is due to moist heat, such as contact with steam, boiling water or other hot fluids. Burns produced by corrosive acids and alkalis, electricity, X-rays, radium, and ultra-violet light, are very similar as regards the destruction of the tissues but they are much slower in healing than the burns and scalds produced by heat. Burns produced by nitric acid tend to go on burning and penetrate deeper into the tissues and produce a more serious degree of injury than the amount of acid used would suggest at the outset.

The injuries produced by burns are divided into five or six degrees. The first two are *erythema*, or reddening of the skin, and *vesication*, or blistering. In the third degree the *superficial layers of the skin are destroyed* and the nerve endings are exposed. This is the most painful type of burn. In the fourth degree there is *destruction of the whole thickness of the skin.* The nerve endings are destroyed, but it is less painful than a burn of the third degree. In the fifth degree the tissues beneath the skin, including the muscles, are also destroyed, and in the last degree there is extensive charring, including that of bone.

Symptoms, dangers and complications. It is very important for a nurse to realize that when a patient is badly burnt the *great immediate danger is shock*, which is most severe in the more painful degrees; the severity of shock is also contributed to by the extent of the area affected, as destruction of the skin permits evaporation of the fluid from the soft tissues.

About 12–24 hours after the initial injury, in the case of a severe burn, the patient will become very prostrated, and this is described by some authorities as a stage of *secondary shock.* It is probably also contributed to by the liquefaction of the broken-down proteins and their absorption, giving rise to a certain degree of *toxaemia*, accompanied by fairly marked *dehydration.* At this stage the patient becomes increasingly restless, he suffers from thirst, his blood pressure is low, and his colour of an ashen grey tint. These symptoms are largely due to loss of fluid from the vascular system.

As the days progress, the *danger of infection* is present, partly due to the lowered resistance of the tissues, and to the coming in contact with dirt of a raw surface, which gives rise to more marked signs of toxaemia, and the patient may develop septicaemia. As a result of local sepsis, pockets of pus may be found under crusts of dead material.

The *danger of deformity* which results from severe scarring in the later stages of the illness must also be considered. As a result of destruction of the superficial tissues a good deal of contraction takes place as healing progresses and, unless care is taken to see that deformities cannot occur, this contraction, by drawing the parts together, will give rise to very disabling deformities.

Treatment. As regards treatment, burns are considered in two groups: those where the skin is partially destroyed, as in the first and second degree burns, and those where the skin is completely destroyed. In the treatment, prevention of shock, toxaemia and sepsis are of first importance. The actual treatment can be considered under first aid, hospital treatment and after care.

First-aid treatment. Morphia in liberal doses to relieve pain, and fluids and warmth to relieve shock are the first considerations. Any local applications must be quickly made. Warm compresses of Milton made by using equal parts of Milton and warm water, sodium bicarbonate, two teaspoonfuls dissolved in a pint of water, saline, prepared by dissolving one teaspoonful of salt in a pint of warm water, or even water can be applied to exposed surfaces and also over burnt clothing. Gentian-violet jelly can be smeared on exposed parts such as the face, neck and hands. It forms a protection and lessens pain.

Hospital treatment. Shock must be treated first. Warm coverings, an electric cradle, elevation of the foot of the bed, morphia, hot drinks, warm fluids by rectum, inhalations of oxygen and intravenous infusion of plasma may all be employed in relieving shock. *Local treatments* include penicillin and sulphonamides, coagulants, antiseptics, baths and packs.

Gentian-violet is a coagulant which is frequently employed. It may be used alone or combined with other coagulants—tannic acid or silver nitrate.

When coagulants are employed it is important to see that oedema does not occur beneath the coagulum causing pressure on tendons and joints, and interfering with the circulation as this may result in necrosis and limitation of movement.

Antiseptics. A mixture of acriflavine, brilliant green and gentian violet (*triple dye*) may be painted on or applied as compresses. These antiseptics are non-irritating and cause slight coagulation.

Saline baths or packs. Immersion of the affected parts or of the whole body in warm saline twice a day is a method advocated by some authorities. Between treatments the burnt areas are covered with tulle gras over which saline packs or compresses may be applied. These can then be floated off the areas during the next bath, and in this way painful changing of dressings is avoided.

Tulle gras is prepared by taking curtain net with a mesh of 2 mm. and cutting it into suitable sizes. These pieces are placed in a tin and covered with paraffin 98 per cent, balsam of Peru 1 per cent and halibut-liver oil 1 per cent. The contents of the tin are sterilized and the layers of tulle gras used as required.

Intermittent irrigation by weak solutions of *electrolytic sodium hypochlorite* (*Milton*) is a treatment recommended by some authorities (see fig. 195, p. 600).

A preliminary cleansing of the burnt area is effected by irrigation with a 10 per cent or 20 per cent solution. The affected parts are then encased in *Stannard's silk-coated envelopes.* These may be sterilized by boiling, by steam disinfecting at 220° F. or by soaking in a 10 per cent solution of Milton for 20 minutes. No other dressing is needed. The envelope gives protection, permits movement to be carried out, maintains the covered areas at normal body temperature and excludes the air, so preventing infection and acts as enclosure of the field for irrigation. Envelopes are made to fit any part of the body, head, limbs and trunk, or the patient may be enveloped entirely in an envelope bath. No clothing is worn beneath the envelope. Treatment is performed for three daily periods of 20 minutes each, a reservoir of fluid of an exact temperature of 100° F. is suspended above the bed, the solution is allowed to flow into the envelope, over the burnt areas, and drain from the envelope by an exit channel provided. After irrigation the envelope must be thoroughly well drained of fluid otherwise maceration of the parts would occur.

Penicillin is used both by the systemic route and locally. It is used locally as *penicillin solution* which is sprayed on the burned surface until a film is produced and then covered by the usual dressing. *Penicillin powder* may be insufflated on to the surface or *penicillin cream* may be applied.

WOUNDS, CONTUSIONS AND BRUISES

Wounds are injuries to the tissues of the body, and they are commonly classified according to the type of wound inflicted—such as an *incised wound* which is a clean cut, made usually by some sharp cutting instrument. Bleeding occurs freely.

A contused wound is bruised—that is, the tissues are crushed beneath the skin which may not be broken; blood exudes into the subcutaneous tissue as in a *bruise*.

In a *lacerated wound* the structures are torn and the edges frayed and jagged. Tearing of the tissues exerts torsion on the injured blood vessels and consequently the bleeding is very slight in such a wound. The *danger of a lacerated wound is sloughing and gangrene*, as the edges may be deprived of blood, by crushing; sloughing if extensive will result in septic infection of the wound.

A *punctured wound* is usually made by stabbing with a sharp instrument; as a rule it is a deep wound, and the injury to deep structures may be very grave. Dirt and particles of clothing may be carried into the wound with the instrument used, resulting in the grave danger of deep-seated septic infection.

Penetrating wounds of the walls of the cavities of the body are usually of the class described as punctured, and the organs contained in these cavities may be so seriously injured in this type of wound that danger of death is imminent. In a stab wound of the chest, the lung is most usually injured; this may give rise to serious bleeding, or to collapse of the lung, which is characterised by serious embarrassment of the breathing, accompanied by heart failure and surgical emphysema. In emphysema air from the punctured lung enters the subcutaneous tissues; this may be local at first, but in a serious injury there is a danger of generalized emphysema which, combined with shock and pulmonary embarrassment, may rapidly prove fatal.

In *penetrating wounds of the abdomen*, the liver, kidneys, spleen, stomach, intestine, or bladder may be injured, and in this case there will be considerable internal bleeding, accompanied by shock. Unless the bleeding is continuous the patient usually recovers from shock fairly rapidly; but if he does not respond to rest, and treatment for shock, it may be concluded that the bleeding is continuous; he will then get worse, become very pale and restless, complain of thirst, suffer from shallow sighing respirations and have a rapid running pulse of low volume.

When one of the hollow organs is perforated, the symptoms of this will be characterized by marked collapse accompanied by boardlike rigidity of the abdominal wall.

Either of the two conditions described above is considered to be an acute abdominal catastrophe which calls for early surgical treatment.

If the early symptoms arising after a penetrating wound of the abdomen are not as severe as those mentioned in the two instances given above, the wound will usually be cleaned as well as possible, either with the aid of a general anaesthetic or not, and the patient will be kept under careful observation in case peritonitis should occur later, which is the danger to be feared.

Bleeding is another complication to be feared from a deep flesh wound, or a wound in a cavity. When this happens, it will be necessary for the condition to be surgically investigated; if bleeding vessels are discovered, these will be ligatured. The wound will be packed, and as a rule this pack will be retained for from 24 to 48 hours. When it is to be removed it will first be saturated (preferably with some antiseptic agent which is also haemostatic, such as peroxide of hydrogen), in order to avoid injury to the walls of the cavity as the gauze is withdrawn. Another packing should be ready at hand in case bleeding occurs, and it is considered desirable to repack the wound.

The general treatment of a patient who is bleeding is the provision of absolute rest, the administration of morphia, and the judicious treatment of the shock which is invariably present; with, as far as possible, an avoidance of any stimulation of the circulation, which, by raising the blood pressure, would predispose to further bleeding. (See also p. 577.)

Scalp wounds bleed a great deal; they are usually clean, incised wounds. In the *treatment* of wounds of the scalp, the hair around the injury should be cut away and the scalp carefully shaved; frequent mopping will have to be employed because of the bleeding. The surgeon will then inspect the injury and, if he decides to suture it, will clean the wound with antiseptics, get the edges into apposition, and put in the necessary sutures; otherwise he may retain the edges in apposition by the application of strapping or strips of elastoplast. The wound is usually covered by a pad, firmly bandaged on. Penicillin may be employed, but for local application of penicillin to head wounds a very pure product, such as white penicillin, only may be used.

In the subsequent care of such a case it is very necessary to arrange for the patient to have rest; if the patient remains in hospital he will be kept in bed. Every probationer nurse should make herself familiar with the symptoms and signs of cerebral concussion and compression very early in her training; in this instance for example it is imperative to be on the watch for symptoms of these two conditions, which should be recognized and reported upon without delay. (See also care of a case of fracture of the skull on p. 611.)

Wounds of the face. These are usually superficial wounds which bleed readily; the facial structures are very mobile and the face is a difficult part on which to retain a dressing.

A wound of the face requires similar treatment to one of the scalp. A type of dressing often applied to the face is collodion which serves two purposes—it obviates the necessity of a bandage and it can be applied under slight tension, thus preventing movement of the margins of the wound with every movement of the skin of the face.

To apply a collodion dressing to the face it is absolutely essential for the part to be dry, as neither collodion nor Whitehead's varnish will adhere properly to a damp surface. The blood should first be cleaned away; presuming sutures are not being used, but that some slight tension is to be maintained by means of the collodion, the edges of the wound should be brought into apposition, the area blanched by grasping it firmly between thumb and fingers, the blood wiped away until the edges of the wound are quite dry, and the collodion then painted on, the parts being held together until it sets, when it may be gently released and a second layer of collodion applied. A filmy layer of sterile cotton wool, or a single thickness of gauze laid over the wound first, over which the collodion is applied, will make a slightly firmer dressing.

A wound of the lip bleeds very freely and usually requires stitching, the dressing should be applied under as much tension as can be obtained, as the lip is so freely mobile.

A wound of the nose will bleed very freely and serious epistaxis may result from it (for treatment see epistaxis, p. 574).

A wound of the ear is always serious as the drum may be ruptured, and if this occurs the injury may have been sufficiently serious to be complicated by fracture of the base of the skull.

Whenever a nurse is in charge of a patient who has had an injury to the ear, it is essential to keep him at rest, in bed if possible. The ear should be carefully swabbed out, using sterile swabs, aural forceps and weak peroxide solution or boracic lotion. A small piece of sterile wool should be kept in the meatus and whenever this is removed it should be carefully inspected to see whether the discharge on it is blood, serum or a watery fluid—if the latter is seen, it may be that cerebrospinal fluid is escaping owing to penetration of the dura mater, which is a very serious injury. The general condition of the patient should be observed, his pulse rate noted frequently and any signs of concussion or compression or cerebral irritation (see p. 612) reported at once.

Cut throat is an emergency with which a nurse may have to deal until the arrival of a doctor, and it is usually an attempt at suicide. When the gash is at the front of the neck—which is usual—the trachea has received most of the injury. The degree of injury must be the guide for treatment, when only the skin and superficial tissues are cut, these will bleed freely and the patient will probably be very frightened. If he is put to lie down and his head is pressed towards his chest, this position will cause pressure on the bleeding parts and so prevent some of the bleeding. If, however, the trachea is severed it is imperative (1) to maintain an airway, or asphyxia will occur, and (2) to prevent blood from getting into the trachea as this will result in inhalation pneumonia later.

A doctor should be summoned, the patient may not be left, the instrument he has used should be removed, out of his sight, and he should be covered and kept warm.

The *dangers of cut throat* are those already mentioned, bleeding, asphyxia, shock and, later, inhalation pneumonia, or pneumonia may arise as the result of exposure, and sepsis may also occur.

When the doctor arrives, if the wound is only superficial he will clean it, put in sutures if necessary, and apply a dressing. When the trachea has been incised a tracheotomy tube is inserted. For nursing care of tracheotomy see p. 743.

Crush syndrome is the term used to indicate the characteristic features of a condition arising as the result of the pinning down of a limb by some heavy object for some hours after the collapse of a building, for example. When rescued, the patient may seem quite well, but some hours later he suffers severely from shock, followed by haematuria and suppression of urine.

There are two schools of thought regarding the probable cause and treatment of this condition. (1) The cause is thought to be due to toxins by damaged muscle entering the circulation and causing nephritis. This school suggest as treatment: (*a*) amputation of the limb, and/or (*b*) giving intravenous infusion of blood, serum, or saline in an attempt to prevent the fall in circulating fluid. (2) The second school consider the condition of shock and reduced renal output to be due to release of the blood constituents into a limb which had been compressed, and in which the arterial circulation had for a time stopped; when the pressure on the limb is released, the blood rushes into the limb with consequent fall in the circulating blood volume and resulting shock followed later by decrease in renal output. This school consider that by bandaging the limb tightly, oedema with its attendant symptoms can be prevented and alternatively, that intermittent pressure applied by some form of mechanical apparatus may also help.

THE HEALING OF WOUNDS

Most wounds heal by what is commonly described as **first intention.** A clean cut, or incised wound, made on the operating table, is expected to heal in this way, and for this it is essential that the wound edges should be accurately approximated without undue tension. The cut edges bleed slightly, and the space between them becomes filled with blood and lymph and injured tissue cells. It is then invaded by leucocytes which ingest all this foreign matter. Little capillary blood vessels are given off from the blood vessels on each side and infiltrate the debris in the wound, and so bridge the gap and restore the circulation.

In the care of this type of wound, it is necessary to keep the surface dry by means of a sterile dressing, and to keep the part at rest until the edges have united. The approximated edges will be held together by clips or stitches. Michel's clips are usually removed before the fifth day by means of special forceps, and other skin sutures are taken out by the tenth day. In observing the condition of the wound edges as healing progresses, the nurse must always be on the look out for any irritation caused by the stitches. The edges of the skin around the stitches would be red if friction were permitted, and this might occur if a dressing were too loosely bandaged on. Mild infection of a stitch puncture might result in a small stitch abscess. In this case the first thing to do is to attempt, by keeping the area dry with powder such as aristol, to prevent the spread of infection to other stitches. If this is not possible, and the infection is more than very slight, it will be necessary to remove the offending stitch and to apply a moist dressing. A spirit dressing is very effective. When the infection is more marked, and invades several stitches, it may be necessary to treat the inflammatory area by hot applications.

In some instances the protection of stitches by collodion or Whitehead's varnish is employed; as for example in operations on the face where it is neither convenient nor practicable to apply either strapping or bandage.

Healing by second intention. This is the way in which an open, gaping wound heals—blood, lymph and injured tissue cells fill the cavity, and tiny little capillary loops of blood vessels are formed all over the area of the wound. These are very red in colour, easily injured and bleed when touched.

At this stage such a wound requires a protective dressing of a nature that does not dry, and so injure the tissue whenever the dressing is changed. In time a little fibrous tissue forms, and this strengthens the newly formed capillary buds, and also causes contraction of tissue, so that the wound becomes gradually smaller as the cavity becomes filled by granulated tissue and the surface of the wound is eventually covered by scar tissue.

Throughout this healing process the nurse will dress the wound daily, or oftener if necessary, and she must be able to decide whether it is healing or not. A healing granulating surface will be velvety in appearance and pink in colour. A sluggish wound might be pale and shiny in character, and this would require a stimulating dressing such as hypertonic saline compresses, one of the aniline dyes, or red lotion, containing zinc—a very healing substance. On the other hand excessive granulations, commonly called 'proud flesh', may cover the surface of the wound. This is an unhealthy growth and must be destroyed before healing can proceed. It is usual to apply either silver nitrate, or copper sulphate—'blue stone'—for this purpose. In both instances the whole surface of the excessive granulation is smeared with the caustic substance. As the surface of the wound is moist there is no necessity to wet the caustic.

In the subsequent dressing of this wound, a moist, not a dry, dressing should be employed, and it should be changed after 6 hours because the action of the caustic in destroying the granulating area will give rise to sloughing. If a dry dressing is applied the sloughing area beneath, covered by a pool of exudate, will be confined beneath the dressing as if corked up; but the application of a moist dressing will permit the exudate, formed by the destruction of the excessive granulations, to be absorbed by the dressing applied. The reason for changing the dressing within 6 hours is that the exudate may be removed and not kept in contact with the wound any longer than necessary.

Secondary suture is the passing of sutures through deep structures in order to take the strain off the skin sutures. A secondary suture is also described as a *tension suture*.

CARE OF AN INFECTED WOUND

(See also Gas Gangrene, p. 570)

When a wound is infected the surfaces are red and swollen and a discharge of pus is present; the surrounding parts are tender and painful.

Most accidental wounds are liable to become infected, as they may be contaminated by road dirt, and particles of clothing.

The aim in the care of all wounds is the prevention of infection. To this end certain points should be attended to at the outset, including:

(*a*) The removal of all foreign particles;

(*b*) Thorough cleansing of the cavity and the margins and edges of the wound, with the removal of any torn parts, which have probably been deprived of blood supply and will therefore slough;

(*c*) The provision of adequate free drainage of serum or other discharge from the wound; for adequate drainage the openings provided must be large enough to permit escape of discharge from the whole of the cavity of the wound;

(*d*) The affected part should be kept free from movement, so that all possible sources of irritation of the injured tissues are eliminated.

In a very septic wound some provision may have to be made for continuous douching, baths or irrigation. In many cases treatment is carried out by Stannard's silk-coated envelope (see p. 581). In addition, the general health of the patient should be attended to; a four-hourly record of his temperature and pulse should be taken; his excretory channels should be kept in regular action and his diet should be nourishing and liberal. He should have adequate rest and sleep.

Penicillin is employed in the treatment of all infected wounds both by the systemic route and locally. It may be used alone or in conjunction with one or more of the sulphonamide group of drugs.

INJURY TO TENDON, NERVE AND MUSCLE

Tendons, nerves and muscles may be injured by the various types of wounds described on p. 582. In a wound of the front of the wrist for example, the flexor tendons to the hand will probably be severed, and the median and ulnar nerves may be cut through.

In the *immediate treatment* of such an injury careful investigation would be made of the structures which had been divided and these would be brought together and sutured if possible.

Rupture of a muscle or tendon may arise as the result of a severe strain or a wrenching movement. A portion of triceps muscle is sometimes ruptured in vigorous movement of the elbow. Plantaris is the muscle most easily ruptured in the calf of the leg in violent movement in running and springing as practised, for instance, in a hard game of tennis.

The result of rupture of a muscle, even if only a few of its fibres are torn, causes pain which is accompanied by tenderness and swelling.

The *treatment* is rest by any means by which the affected parts can be kept in a position of relaxation. Strapping may be sufficient in some cases; in others a splint or plaster of paris will be applied. Rest must be maintained for from 10 to 21 days, according to the amount of injury, and it must be sufficiently long to allow the torn muscle fibres to heal.

Teno-synovitis, or inflammation of a tendon and its sheath, may be caused by an injury such as a blow, and may result in a mild degree of inflammation. It may also arise when injury by stretching occurs to the tendons in the vicinity of a joint, when the joint is dislocated or sprained.

The *symptoms of teno-synovitis* are pain and swelling, and a grating sound is heard on movement of the tendon. The condition is treated by applications of heat in the first instance, in order to relieve the pain, and the affected tendon must be kept at rest as described in the treatment for rupture of a muscle.

STINGS AND BITES

A **sting by a wasp or bee** often causes considerable local pain and swelling, and in some instances it is accompanied by shock. In treating this, it should first be ascertained whether the sting has been left in—a bee usually leaves its sting in the tissues, but a wasp extracts it.

Having removed the sting an alkali should be applied—either a soda or a magnesium sulphate compress is useful; if glycerine of ichthyol is obtainable an application thereof will relieve the tension and pain more rapidly.

The **bite of the adder** is about the only injury which need be considered as regards poisonous reptiles in this country. This needs treatment at once, or the poison will be absorbed and, entering the blood stream, will act by depressing the vital nerve centres controlling respiration and cardiac action.

In the *immediate treatment*, if the part bitten is a limb, it should be constricted above the injury to prevent the venous blood from returning to the heart with its load of poison; the skin should be incised with a sharp instrument and the blood squeezed out; the best application to make is permanganate of potash but, not expecting snake bite, persons do not carry this with them—many, however, do carry iodine and it may be employed instead. If any form of suction, other than sucking by mouth and spitting out the venom, is available, it should be used—it may be possible to improvise some form of cupping. Hot wet dressing may also be applied.

When the patient can be taken to the surgery of a doctor the bite will be incised and permanganate of potash applied, followed by hot fomentations.

The *general condition of the patient* must be observed, and he should be kept as still as possible (exercise and movement are contraindicated), and warm in order to minimize the shock. He should be given stimulants, such as whisky and brandy, and ammonia in the form of sal volatile; if his respirations become very slow, artificial respiration must be performed.

Bites of the dog are always accompanied by fear of hydrophobia, even though this is a very unlikely complication nowadays. If the skin has only been grazed no special treatment is needed; the abrasion will be dressed in the usual way with some antiseptic. If the dog has bitten into the tissues the wound should be carefully cleaned and cauterized with nitrate of silver.

Bites of other animals, such as cats and horses, may give rise to infection and therefore the wounds inflicted ought to be treated like any other wound which is liable to become infected.

FOREIGN BODIES IN THE TISSUES

A **needle** may penetrate the tissues, or a person may step on and get a needle in his foot, or he may sit on a needle and get it into his buttock.

Unfortunately the needle moves freely along the muscle sheaths once it is embedded in the tissues, and the only way to prevent this from happening is to keep the part at complete rest until help can be obtained. If the needle has not disappeared, it can possibly be withdrawn; and when it has disappeared, advise the patient to keep still and, if it is in a part which can be splinted such as the foot, some form of splint might be applied; this should control the knee joint as well as the ankle joint, as movement of the knee will cause movement of the muscles controlling the foot.

The position of the needle will be determined by special X-ray examination, and the surgeon will operate and remove it.

A **splinter** in the soft tissues requires similar care to that described above; it may not, however, be deeply embedded. When superficial, the tract made by the splinter should be opened and the foreign body removed.

A **foreign body in the eye** may take the form of a particle of dust or grit on the conjunctiva. The eyelids should be everted and the particle removed by means of a soft swab; if the particle is sharp and is pricking badly, a little castor oil should be inserted before an attempt is made to remove it.

When the foreign body is on the cornea, its removal requires much more care; the cornea is very sensitive, and the eye will have to be anaesthetized by the insertion of cocaine before any attempt can be made to remove the object. The average nurse should not attempt to do this; she should merely cover the eye with a pad and take the patient to a doctor at once. Having cocainized the eye he will inspect it carefully with the aid of a magnifying lens, and if the particle is on the surface of the cornea it may be possible to remove it with a small pad; if embedded in the cornea he will need a small instrument to dig it out; if the particle is metal, the use of a magnet may be tried. *The nurse who deals with a patient, after the removal of a foreign body from the structure of the cornea*, will be required to irrigate the eye with weak boracic lotion twice a day; to insert atropine in order to keep the eye at rest, and to keep it covered with a comfortable eye pad. The patient should be seen by his doctor at regular intervals for some time to ensure that the corneal abrasion is healing.

The **result of a foreign body in the ear** is usually pressure, inflammation and ulceration. Children often put beads, peas, nuts and other small objects into the ear. A nurse should not attempt to remove a foreign body from the ear, as any attempt will usually result in pushing the article farther in; if she syringes the ear, hoping to remove the object, she may only result in making it larger, and so increase the pressure, since if it is of a vegetable nature such as a pea it will swell when wet.

She should take the child to a doctor, reassuring both child and mother that there is no immediate danger. The doctor will examine the ear with a speculum and head mirror, and he may then remove the object either by syringing or by means of some small special instrument. When the foreign body has been removed he will inspect the drum to see that it is intact, and carefully cleanse the meatus with small swabs, leaving it quite dry and he may perhaps insert a tiny piece of cotton wool.

Nose. Similar foreign bodies may be placed by a child in his nose; the child then probably forgets all about it. Some weeks later, the mother notices a discharge from one side of the nose, due to the inflammation brought about by pressure of the foreign body, which if left will lead to ulceration of the lining of the nasal cavity. It would be unwise for a nurse to attempt to remove a foreign body from the nose in the circumstances suggested above—she should take the child to a doctor. He will insert a nasal speculum and see where the article is, and then, having first cocainized the membrane, he will pass some small instrument behind the obstruction and so attempt to remove it.

If someone actually saw the child put the foreign body up his nose, a nurse might attempt to remove it immediately afterwards; she must remember, however, that this can only be successfully done by means of pressure from behind; she should therefore get the child to blow his nose and she might give a nasal douche, via the opposite nostril, hoping the return flow down the obstructed side will bring the foreign body down with it. She should never attempt to remove it from the front by means of forceps, as the instrument will only slip off and push the obstruction farther up.

A **foreign body in the larynx** produces alarming symptoms of suffocation and asphyxia and the patient may become black in the face. In such a case a nurse should send at once for a doctor, and in the meantime put her finger into the patient's throat and try to dislodge anything which may be there—very often a piece of food. She might also slap the patient forcibly on the back hoping to dislodge any foreign body from the chink of the glottis. If these means are not successful she should collect the articles required for tracheotomy—these are always ready at hand in the casualty department of a hospital. The doctor, when he arrives, will probably perform tracheotomy at once. It is useless to attempt artificial respiration when the respiratory passages are blocked.

Foreign body in the oesophagus. The foreign bodies which most often get fixed in the oesophagus are either a fishbone or a dental plate. If the article is just behind the mouth, in the pharynx, it may be possible to remove it with the fingers. Apart from this, a nurse should not attempt to remove a foreign body from the oesophagus; the condition is very dangerous, the oesophagus is a fine tube, very easily ulcerated, and this will cause mediastinitis and pneumonia.

The doctor who is called in to deal with this case will require an X-ray examination to be made, and when the position of the object has been ascertained it may be possible to remove it by means of oesophagoscopy.

After such treatment the patient will be given a diet which can be easily swallowed, in order to prevent irritation and any resultant injury to the lining of the oesophagus.

Foreign body in the urethra. Children sometimes push pins or other fine objects into the urethra, or a glass catheter may be broken in it when a female patient is being catherized. The nurse should not attempt to remove a foreign body from the urethra; she should prepare some fine forceps and a good light which the doctor will require for this purpose.

Chapter 42

Injuries to Bones and Joints

Fractures: predisposing and exciting causes, varieties of fracture, symptoms and signs, healing and repair, complications—Fractures of the skull: symptoms of fracture of the base, treatment and nursing—Concussion, compression and cerebral irritation: observation, treatment and nursing care—Fractures of the spine: signs and symptoms, treatment and nursing—Fractures of the pelvis—Injuries to joints: sprains and dislocations

A *bone may be bruised or broken* and, when it is bruised, blood is extravasated into the periosteum, causing swelling, tension, and pain. Even a slight blow on a bone, especially in children, may be complicated by sepsis and, beginning with a little *periostitis*, it may progress to *osteomyelitis* and the child become exceedingly ill within 24 hours, with a high temperature, rapid pulse and marked prostration.

In such a case it is necessary to operate at once, incising the bone and draining the medullary cavity. This will prevent the danger of septicaemia with which the patient is threatened.

A kick on the shin which results in a bump is a *periosteal bruise*; the extravasated blood may either become absorbed or fibrous tissue may form which results in a hard lump persisting for some time. A *subperiosteal haematoma* may form, this being most commonly met with in the case of a blow on the skull.

An uncomplicated bruise on a bone will usually respond to applications of heat which will help to relieve the pain and promote absorption of the fluid under the periosteum.

Osteomyelitis and other infections of bone respond well to penicillin.

FRACTURES

For various types of fracture see figs. 196–208, pp. 601–8.

The causes of fracture may be divided into predisposing and exciting causes:

Predisposing causes. Many local diseases of bone and some general diseases predispose to fracture. Local diseases include tuberculosis, inflammatory lesions such as osteomyelitis, primary tumours of bone and secondary carcinomatous deposits in bone. Cancer of the breast, thyroid, kidney and prostate gland may be extended by means of the blood stream to bone, the commonest sites of secondary carcinoma in bone being the spinal column and pelvic bones.

General diseases of bone which most commonly predispose to fracture are rickets and Paget's disease. Paget's disease is characterized by erosion of the bone, nature attempts to replace the eroded bone, with the result that a large soft mass is formed with a tendency to bending of the bone—only later does hardening occur.

Certain nerve diseases also predispose to fracture, including general paralysis of the insane and locomotor ataxia. *Extremes of age* are another cause;

the soft bones of an infant give rise to the greenstick fracture; the brittleness which characterizes the bones of old persons also predisposes to fracture.

Exciting causes are usually described as being those of *direct violence* such as occurs in a crushing accident; or *indirect violence* when the force applied is transmitted along a limb. Pott's fracture, which happens when a person slips and the fibula is broken about three inches above the ankle joint, is an example of the latter. Another example is the breaking of a collar bone by falling on the outstretched hand; the force is then transmitted along the arm to the collar bone. A Colles's fracture, fracture of the lower end of the radius, sustained by falling with the hand outstretched, the force striking the palm of the hand, is yet another example.

Muscular violence causes a fracture when a large muscle forcibly contracting breaks a bone. The best example of this cause is fracture of the patella—a person may, for example, trip, and, in order to save himself from falling, forcibly extend his knee by contraction of the quadriceps extensor muscle, resulting in a transverse fracture of the patella, the bone being divided into two, one half remaining attached to the patellar ligament and the other to the quadriceps muscle.

Varieties of fracture. A fracture may be *simple* or *closed* or *compound* or *open.* A simple fracture is described as closed because there is no opening in the skin; the bone is not seen protruding through the skin as it is in a compound or open fracture, but a simple fracture may become compound by injudicious handling, if splints are not properly applied the bone may be forced through the skin.

A fracture may also be *complete* when the bone is broken right through, or *incomplete* when it is not completely divided. *Examples of a complete fracture* are described according to the shape of the break, which may be *T-shaped, spiral, oblique* or *transverse.* A complete fracture may also be described according to the type of damage done to the bone—when two or more breaks occur, it is said to be *comminuted*; it may also be *splintered.* When the ends of the broken bone are driven one into the other, the term *impacted* fracture is used to describe the break.

Varieties of incomplete fracture are the *greenstick* already mentioned, and in this type the bone bends, like a green twig, but is not broken right across. *Depressed* fracture occurs of the bones of the cranium and face; the bone is struck and indented like the injury done to a boiled egg when it is struck on top with the ball of a spoon. *Fissured* fractures also most often occur in the bones of the cranium and other flat bones—the bone is split and fissured, but the parts are not separated or completely divided.

Symptoms and signs of fracture. The signs and symptoms associated with local injury—*bruising, swelling, tenderness* and *pain*—will be present. *Blisters* may arise on the skin over the fracture. Other special signs of fracture are *deformity*, which varies and may be slight or severe; there may be overriding of the ends of the broken bone causing shortening of the limb and marked thickness at the site of fracture; angular displacement may also occur.

Abnormal mobility—the normal alignment of the limb is interrupted and therefore the part below the break can be twisted in any direction.

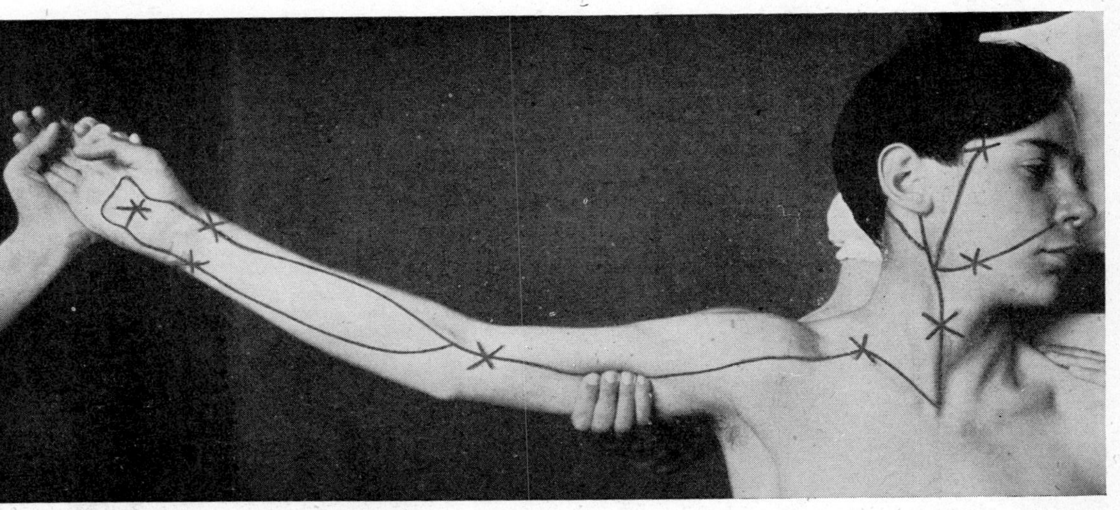

FIG. 183. THE PRINCIPAL PRESSURE POINTS OF THE HEAD, NECK, AND UPPER EXTREMITY. The fingers of the operator are shown compressing the brachial artery against the inner aspect of the humerus.

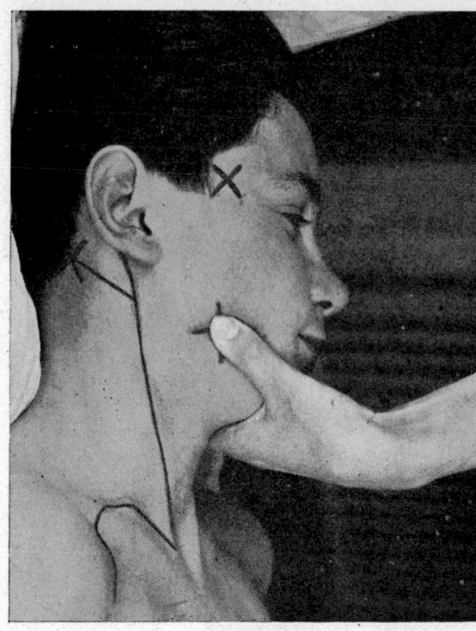

Fig. 184. Compression of th Facial Artery against th Mandible which it crosses t supply the Face.

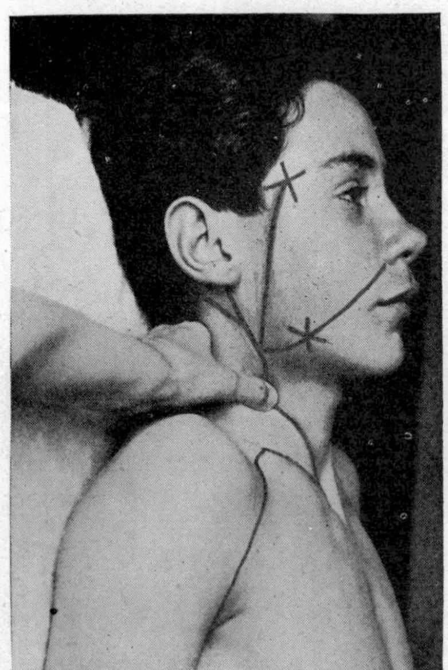

Fig. 185. Compression of Carotid Artery against the Transverse Processes of the Cervical Vertebrae.

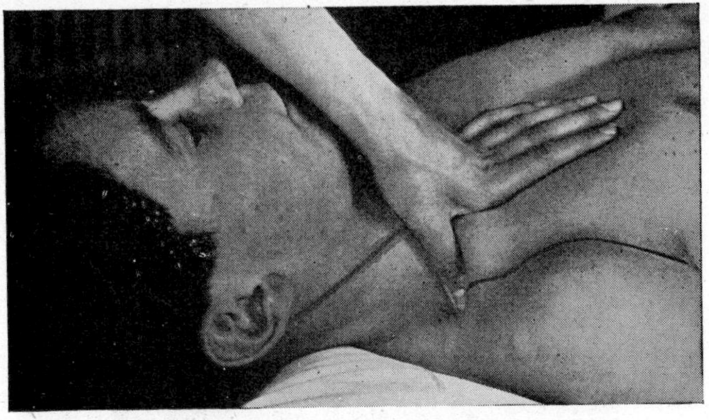

FIG. 186. COMPRESSION OF THE SUBCLAVIAN ARTERY BY PRESSING IT AGAINST THE FIRST RIB, BEHIND THE CLAVICLE. The patient is lying, the operator stands behind (*see also Fig.* 187 *below*).

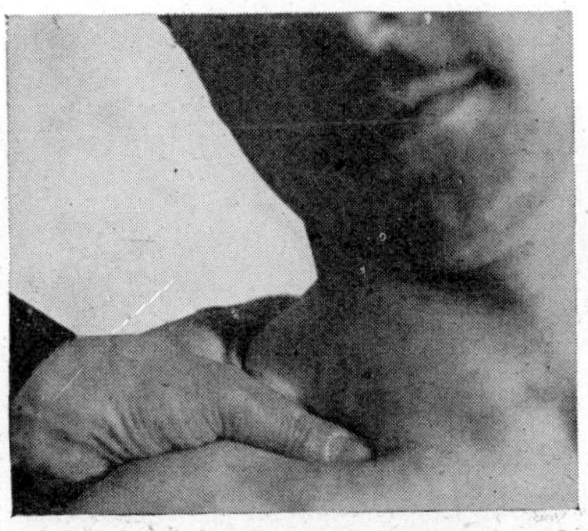

FIG. 187. ALTERNATIVE METHOD OF COMPRESSING SUBCLAVIAN ARTERY.

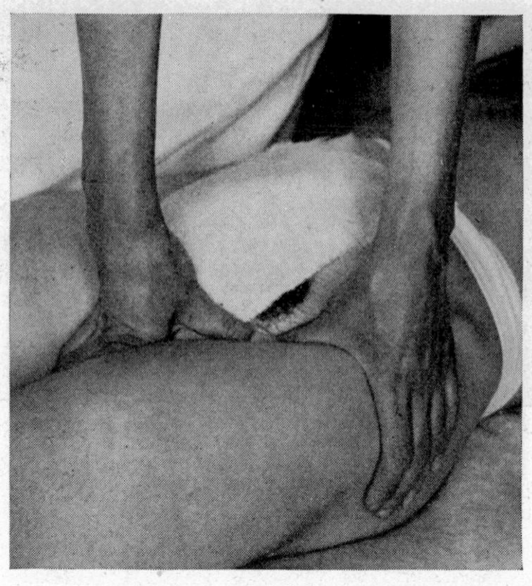

Fig. 188. Compression of the Femoral Artery by using both Thumbs and exerting Strong Pressure on the Artery as it passes over the pelvis.

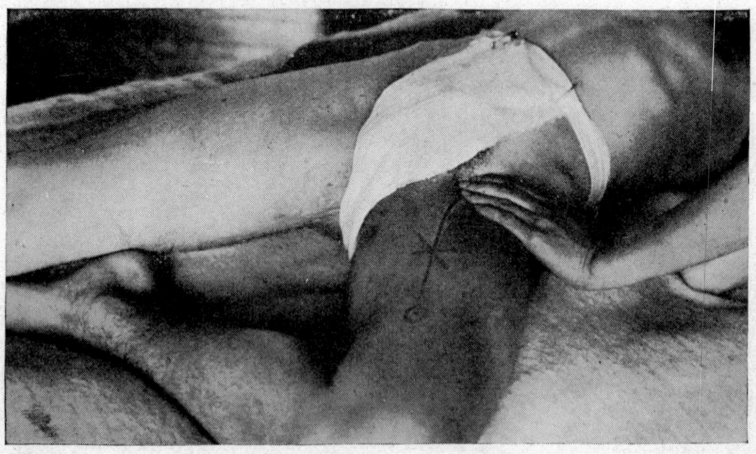

Fig. 189. By Flexing, Abducting and Rotating the Thigh outwards the Femoral Artery can be compressed against the Head of the Femur as it passes over the front of the Hip Joint.

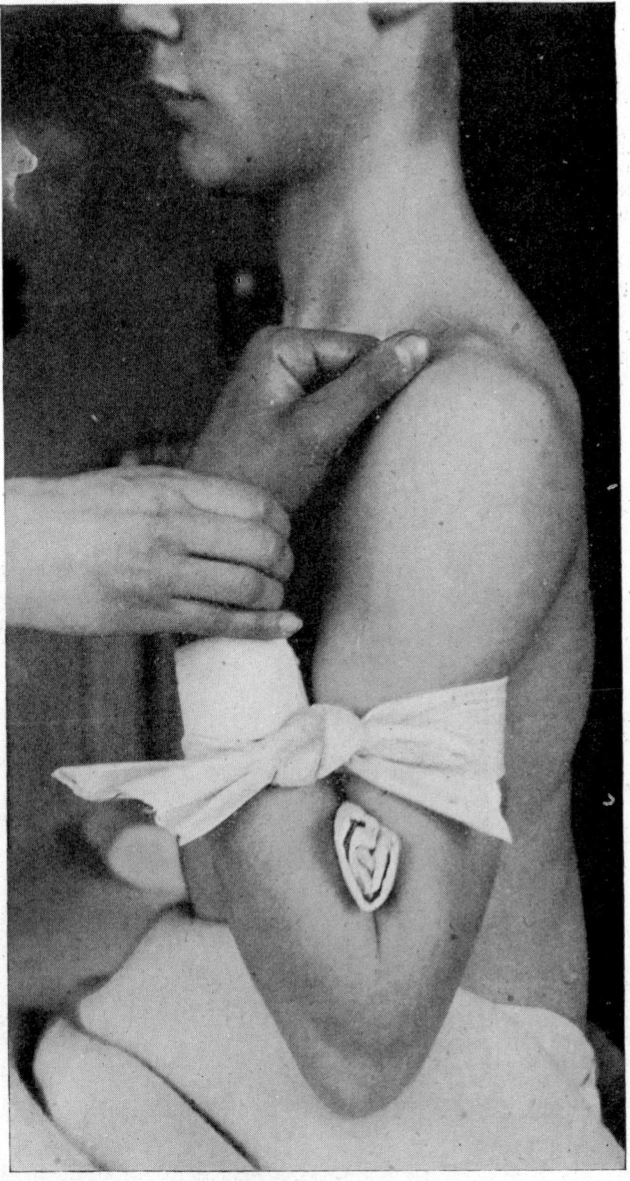

Fig. 190. Compression of the Brachial Artery.
By means of a pad at the bend of the elbow and flexion of the forearm. The fingers of the operator are seen on the radial pulse which is obliterated when the application is effective in compressing the artery.

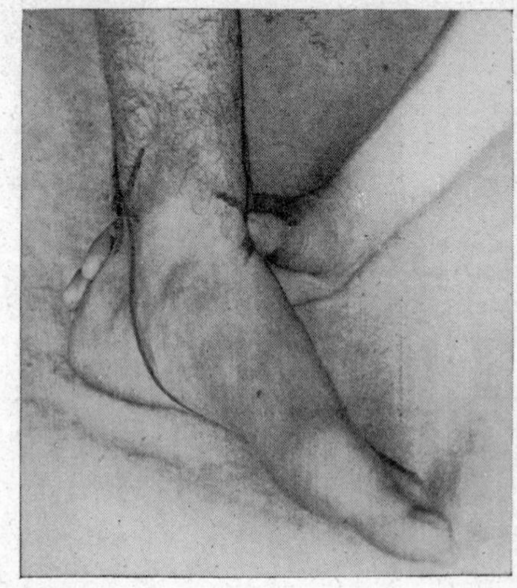

FIG. 191. TWO PRESSURE POINTS IN THE REGION OF THE ANKLE.
Of the posterior tibial artery as it passes behind the internal malleolus and of the dorsalis pedis as it crosses the bend of the ankle. The hand of the operator is shown using the thumb to compress the dorsalis pedis artery; counter pressure is made by the fingers gripping the back of the heel.

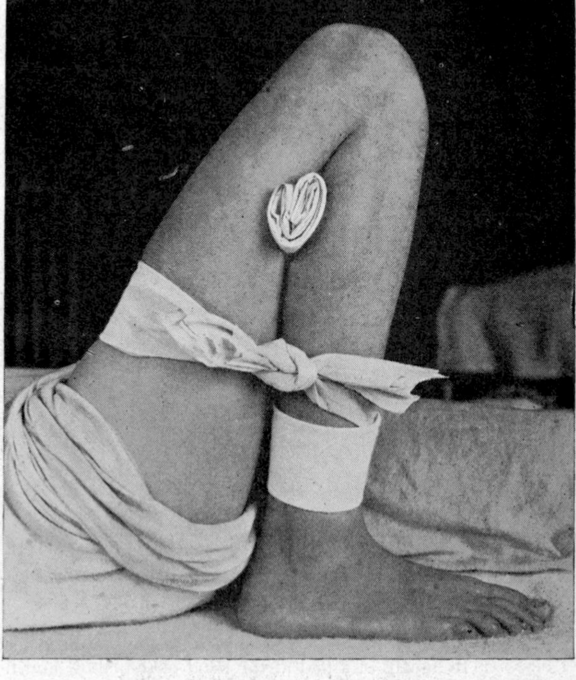

FIG. 192. PAD AND FLEXION APPLIED TO THE POPLITEAL ARTERY BEHIND THE KNEE, TO ARREST BLEEDING FROM LEG AND FOOT.

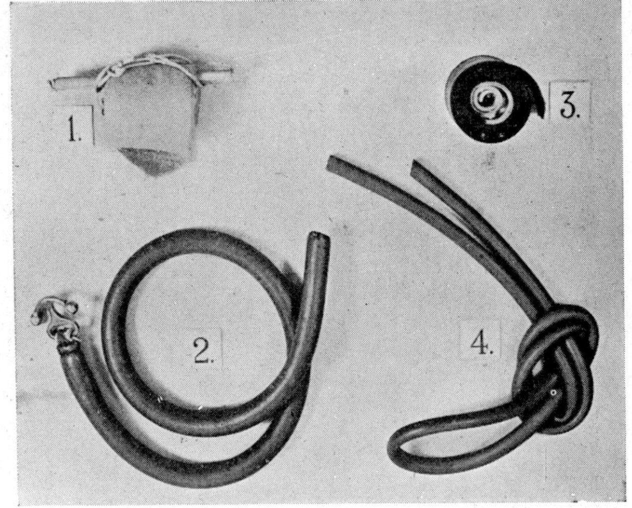

FIG. 193.
VARIETIES OF TOURNIQUET.
1. The field tourniquet.
2. Samway's.
3. Esmarch's bandage.
4. Strip of rubber tubing.

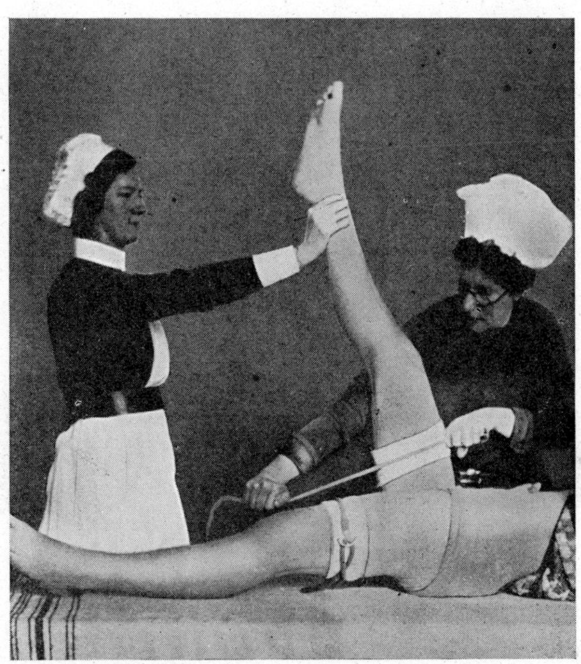

FIG. 194. APPLICATION OF RUBBER TOURNIQUET. Note the effort required to *stretch the rubber* before carrying the tourniquet round the limb. On the left thigh the tourniquet is shown applied.

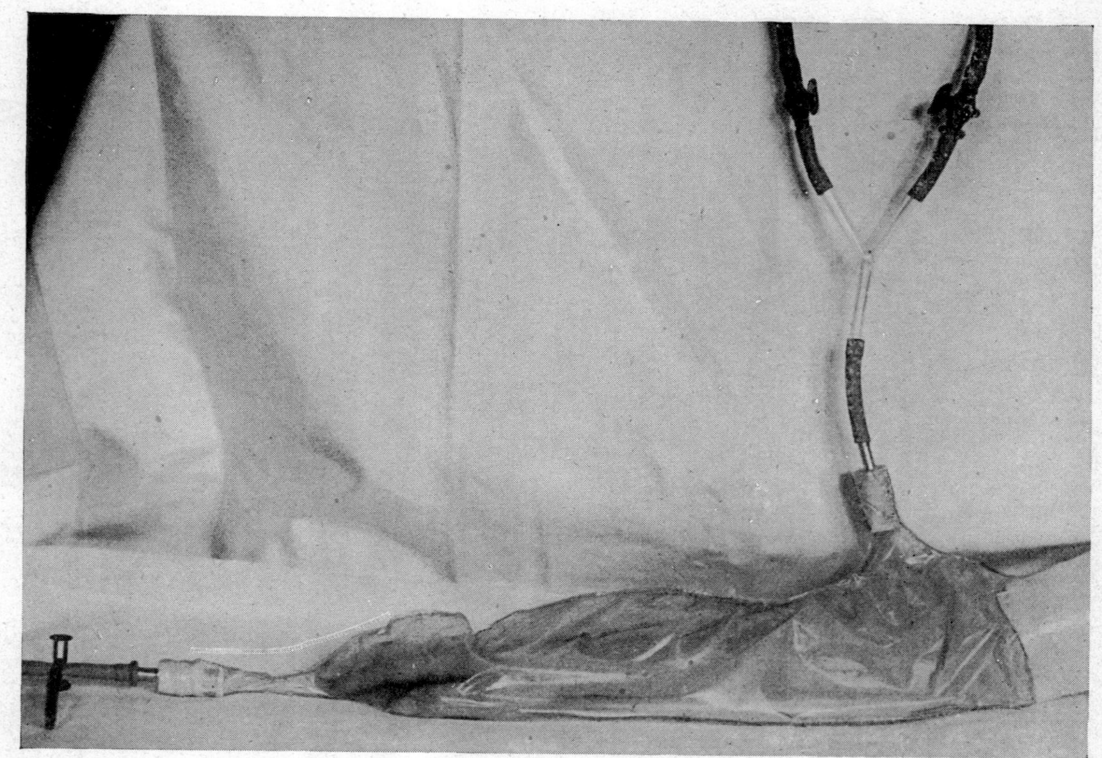

FIG. 195.—*see page* 581.
Stannard's envelope as used for the irrigation treatment of burns.

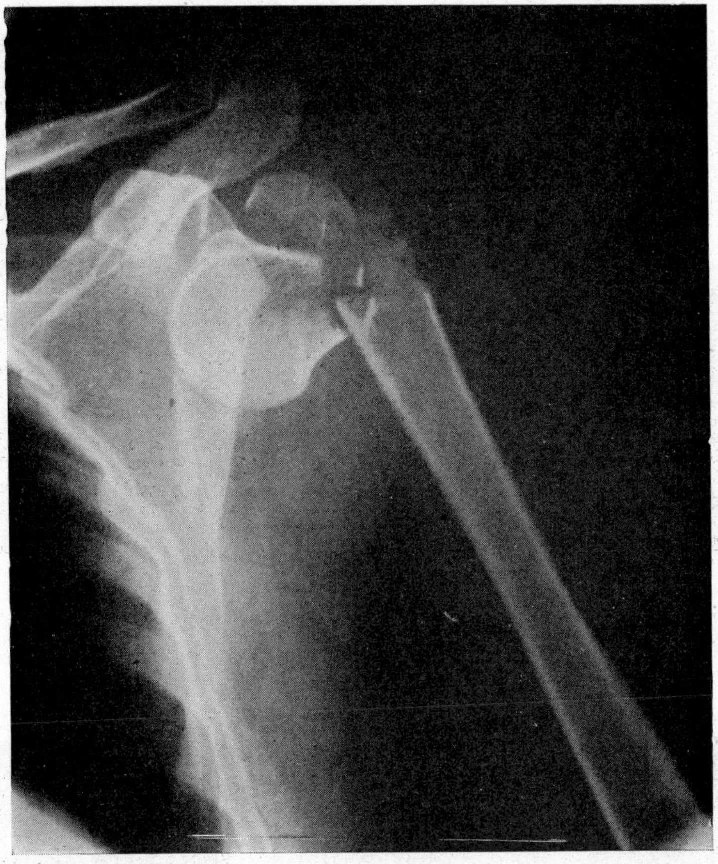

Fig. 196.

Dislocation of the Head of the Humerus as a result of a comminuted fracture of the surgical neck. The head of the humerus is seen displaced downwards. The great tuberosity of the humerus is separated and the bone in the vicinity of the surgical neck is broken into several pieces.

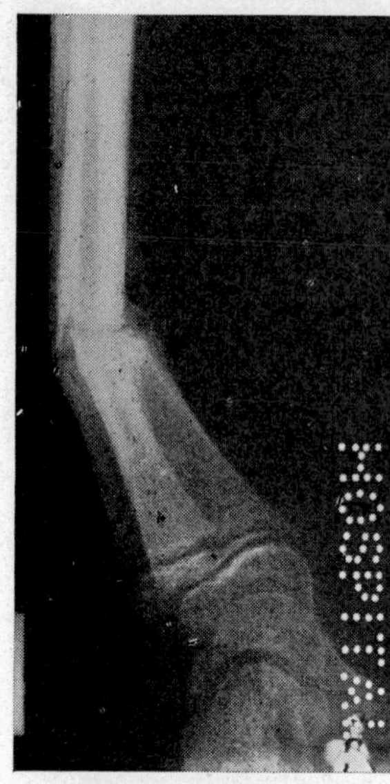

FIG. 197.
Greenstick fracture of both bones of forearm.

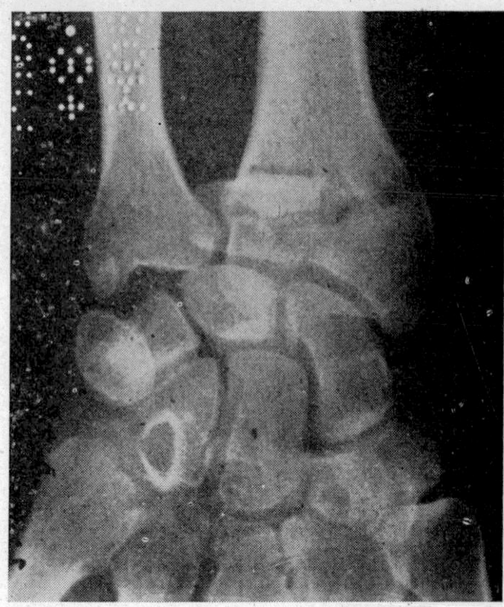

FIG. 198.
Colles's fracture of the lower end of radius.

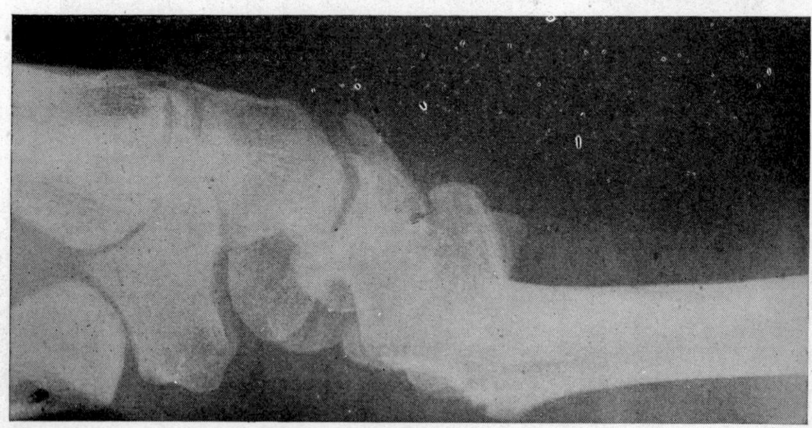

FIG. 199. COLLES'S FRACTURE.
Lateral view showing deformity due to displacement of bone.

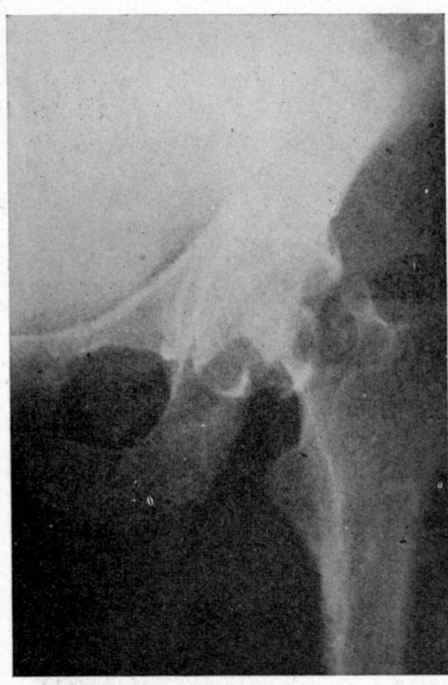

Fig. 200. Intracapsular fracture of the Neck of the Femur.

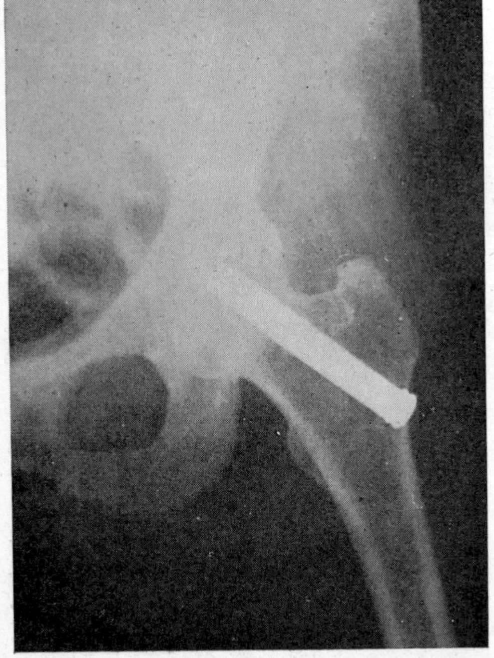

Fig. 201.
The same patient as in Fig. 200 after reduction of fracture and insertion of a Smith-Petersen pin.

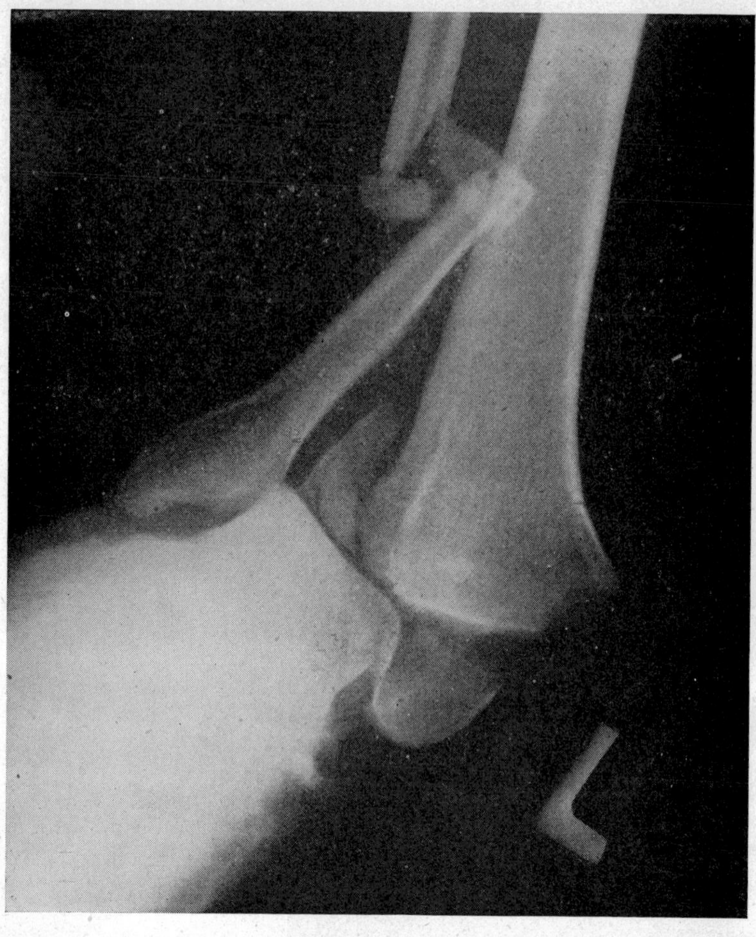

FIG. 202. POTT'S FRACTURE.

A badly comminuted Pott's fracture, i.e., a fracture of the lower third of the shaft of the fibula. In this illustration the tibia also is broken and the ankle is dislocated upwards and backwards (*see also Fig.* 203).

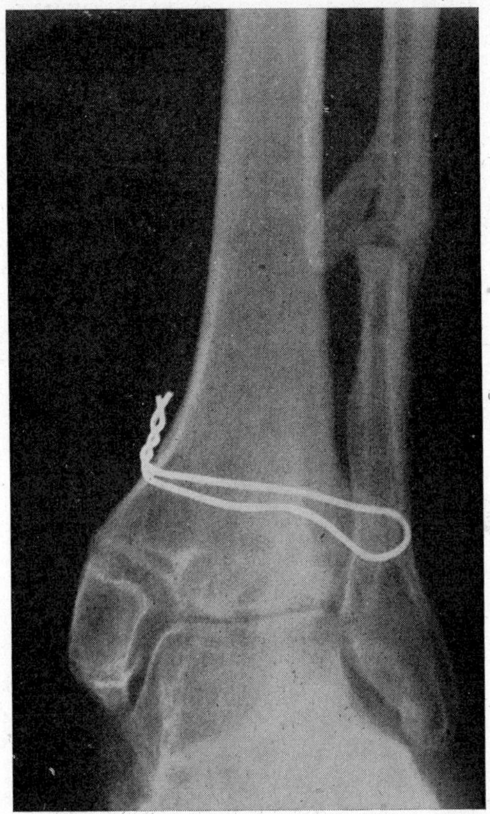

FIG. 203.
A severe case of Pott's fracture after operation for reduction which included wiring the fragments to maintain them in position.

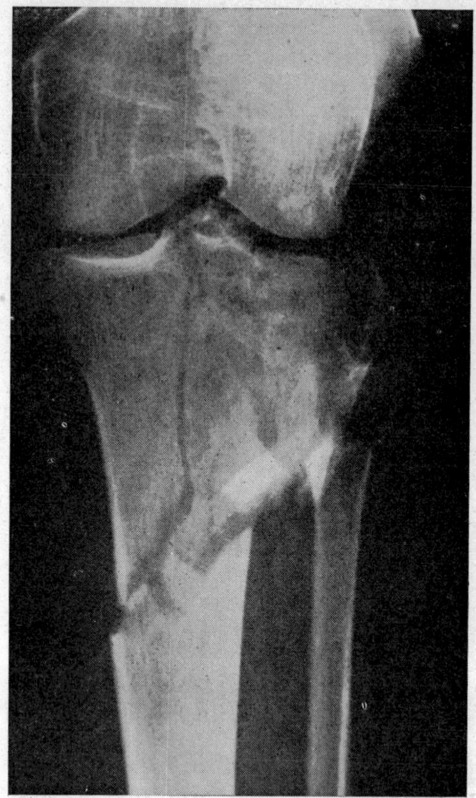

Fig. 204. Fractured Tibia and Fibula. A comminuted fracture of both tibia and fibula extending, in the case of the tibia, into the knee joint. Note that the breaks in the tibia are both oblique and longitudinal.

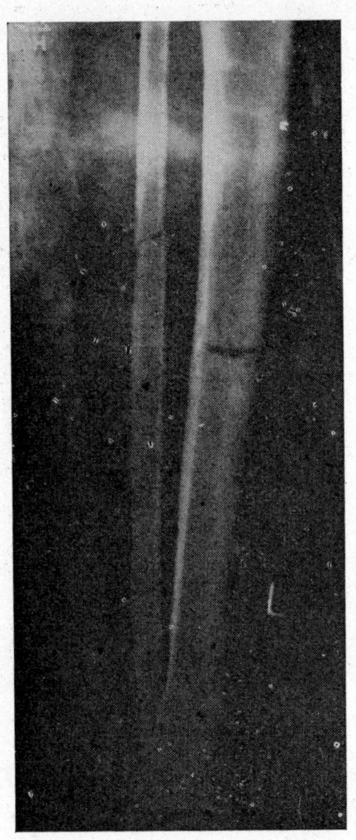

FIG. 205.
Transverse fracture of tibia and fibula.

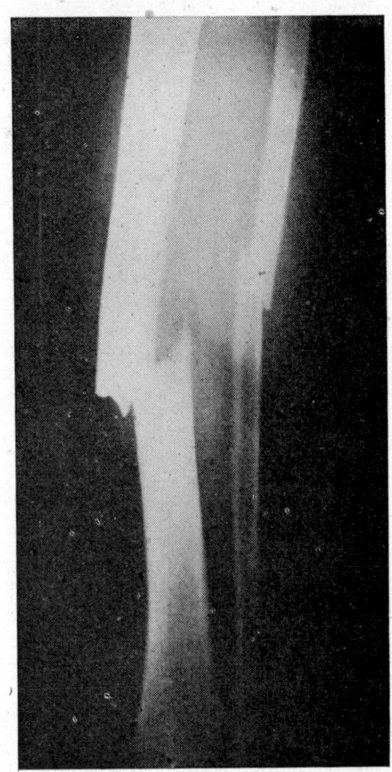

FIG. 206.
Fracture of tibia and fibula with slight displacement.

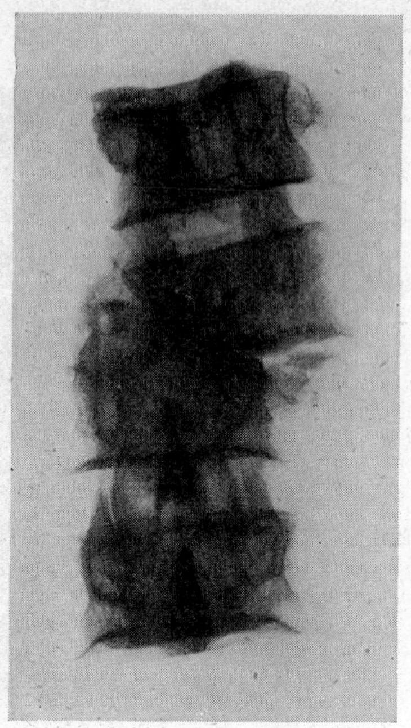

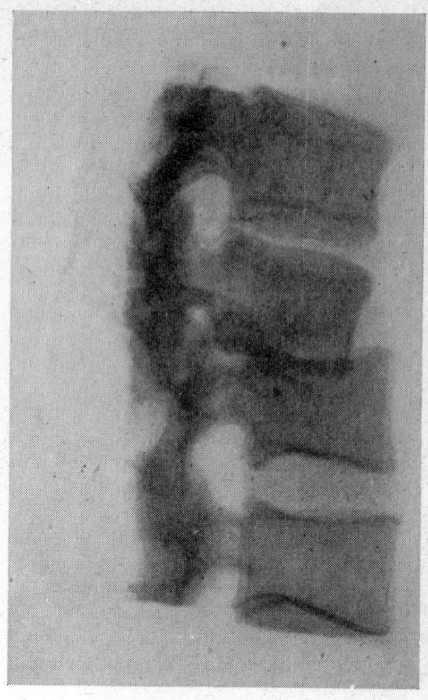

FRACTURE-DISLOCATION AFFECTING TWO OF THE LUMBAR VERTEBRAE.

FIG. 207.

View of the spine X-rayed with the patient supine. The front of the vertebral bodies is on view and the amount of lateral displacement can be seen.

FIG. 208.

Lateral view of the spine in the same patient as Fig. 207.

Crepitus is the grating sound produced when the broken ends of the bone rub together. Neither crepitus nor abnormal mobility will be present in an incomplete or impacted fracture.

The appearance of the fracture when exposed to X-ray examination will help to complete the information desired by the surgeon regarding the case he is examining.

Treatment. The *first-aid* treatment is important, as its efficiency may prevent a closed fracture from being changed into an open fracture. Some form of temporary fixation must be applied before the patient can be moved; any improvised splints that are used should control the movement of the joints both above and below the break. They should be firmly but not too tightly applied, and should be firm enough to prevent movement of the ends of the broken bone during transit from the site of the accident to the doctor's surgery, or to the casualty department of a hospital.

Reduction of deformity is carried out when the fracture is set and the ends of the bone are brought into apposition. A general anaesthetic may be necessary during this procedure.

Fixation of the position adopted is necessary until healing has taken place. This may be maintained by means of splints or plaster of paris. In some cases extension will be necessary in addition.

Healing or repair of a fracture. Healing is brought about by the formation of *callus*, which is granulation tissue of bone; it contains latent osteoblasts, and these cells take calcium from the blood and so bone is formed. At first the mass called callus is solid bone, but in time other cells, called osteoclasts—which are bone destroying—come into action and thus the canals and spaces necessary in bone are provided.

Factors necessary for good repair. The bone ends should be in fair apposition; there must be reasonable immobility in order to furnish the necessary rest; there must be freedom from infection; the patient's general health should be good and calcium should be provided if thought necessary.

For perfect success, restoration of the function of the limb, and of the joints near the break particularly, should be ensured by massage of the muscle and by passive and active movements of the joints.

Nursing care. It is necessary to understand the principles of treatment of fractures, as successful results depend on the correct application of these. The nurse will have to see that the splints or extensions that are used are maintained as they were intended in order to immobilize the fracture adequately. A patient with a fracture of the lower limb, for example, will be obliged to lie very still; he may be nursed on a firm unyielding surface, as when fracture boards are placed beneath the mattress on which he lies. This predisposes him to two possible complications: (1) *bedsores* because of the hard surface on which he is forced to lie, and (2) *hypostatic congestion of the lungs*, particularly if the person is middle aged or elderly.

A little *traumatic fever*, indicated by a slight rise in temperature, inability to sleep and loss of appetite, may be expected to arise after any serious injury. *Shock* may be present when the injury has been severe, and this will need treatment by means of applications of external heat, and the administration of fluids; the surgeon will usually order the patient to be given some morphia.

The patient may find it difficult to sleep, or to pass urine and faeces in bed in the very limited and unusual position in which he is probably forced to lie; the splints or extensions may be uncomfortable and, unless properly guarded, there is danger of pressure sores. Sleeplessness may give rise to wandering and delirium, while in chronic alcoholics delirium tremens may occur.

The digestion may be impaired for some days; the patient may suffer from flatulence and loss of appetite, and he should be given plenty of fluid and may have a light or a full diet as soon as he wishes to eat. His bowels should be regulated, if necessary, by some mild laxative such as liquid paraffin.

Complications of fractures. *Shock*, *traumatic fever*, *bedsòres*, *hypostatic pneumonia*, and *delirium* have already been mentioned.

Mal-union or *non-union* are probably those most dreaded by a surgeon. In *non-union* the bone does not unite, and this may be due to debility of the patient or to too little calcium in his blood. It may also arise as the result of faulty splinting, which allows movement and so prevents the repair of bone. It may be the result of sepsis, but may also be met when the gap between the ends of the broken bone is very wide, so that reasonable apposition is not possible.

Mal-union complicates, most often, fractures near a joint, particularly the elbow and the ankle joints, and it results in marked deformity.

Stiffness and rigidity following a fracture, particularly when near a joint, may be sufficiently marked to constitute a complication; treatment by massage and movement during the time the patient is under observation is employed in order to prevent the occurrence of this.

Paralysis and contracture. Sometimes, when a nerve is embedded in the callus which forms in the healing of a fracture, temporary paralysis may be met. As the excess callus is removed this will usually disappear; in the meantime, the affected part is treated by massage and electrical stimulation. *Crutch palsy*, which is paralysis of the posterior cord of the brachial plexus and therefore affects the muscles supplied by the musculospiral nerve, may be brought about by the injudicious use of badly fitting crutches but it never ought to occur. *Volkmann's ischaemic contracture* is due to the destruction of muscle and its replacement by fibrous tissue usually on the anterior aspect of the forearm owing to the too tight application of splints.

As interference with the union of a fracture and subsequent rigidity are usually due to infection, help can be given by the systemic administration of penicillin. When the fracture area is infected and/or where operative treatment is necessary the routine use of penicillin-sulphathiazole powder is recommended.

FRACTURES OF THE SKULL

Either the vault or the base of the skull may be fractured, or both parts may be involved in the injury.

Fractures of the vault of the skull may be *fissured*, *depressed* or *punctured*, and the treatment depends on the extent of injury to the brain. In a fissured fracture there may be few symptoms and but little injury; when a depressed fracture occurs the indented portion of bone presses on the contents of the cranium and gives rise to symptoms of cerebral compression (see p. 613).

Fracture of the base of the skull may be produced *directly*, when the blow falls upon the base, either as the result of an injury to the lower jaw, the nose or the roof of the mouth, or by an injury to the spinal column which forces it up against the base of the skull; or it may be produced *indirectly* as when a blow directed on the vault does not break one of the flat bones, but is transmitted to the irregular bones at the base of the skull, resulting in fracture of this region.

The **symptoms of a fracture of the base of the skull** vary according to the amount of damage done to the brain. The patient may be admitted in a stuporous or unconscious condition or he may be wandering and delirious. Compression of the brain will give rise to paralysis of the opposite side of the body, including in most cases the face; the breathing will be deep and stertorous in character and the pulse, unless considerable shock is present, will be full and bounding and slow. Certain eye changes may also be seen, including squint and inequality or irregularity in the size of the pupils. There may be bleeding into the conjunctiva, or around the cavity of the eye, or from the nose or ears. A discharge of watery fluid from the ears indicates that cerebrospinal fluid is escaping through an injured dura mater.

Treatment and nursing. The patient is placed flat in bed and kept in a quiet, slightly darkened room, in order to eliminate sound and bright light which would be sources of irritation to the injured nerve matter. A cold compress or icebag is usually placed on the patient's head and he may have some external heat applied over the lower extremities—such as an electric cradle—but, as he may be restless and is not responsible for his actions, great care should be taken to prevent the occurrence of burns.

A careful record, every half-hour at first, is made of the character and rate of pulse and respiration; the temperature is taken every 4 hours, unless it is found to be rising rapidly when it should be taken at one- or two-hourly intervals, as this is a very serious happening.

At the outset some drastic aperient is invariably ordered; if the patient is only stuporous and can swallow, he may either be ordered 3–5 grains of calomel or 1 minim of croton oil; it is advisable to place suitable wool and tow pads beneath the patient in order to avoid soiling of the bed if his bowels should act without warning. Even though a patient is apparently unconscious any slight movement which he may make after the administration of an aperient would probably indicate that it was about to act, and the insertion of a bedpan as soon as this observation was made would probably prevent the passing of faeces in the bed.

A specimen of urine should be tested as soon as one is obtained, and it is necessary to watch carefully for any indication of retention, since a patient who apparently has incontinence of urine may merely be dribbling urine away from an overloaded bladder. The bed of a patient with a fractured skull should always be adequately protected by mackintoshes, and care should be taken to prevent the formation of bedsores.

During the first 24–48 hours diet or even fluid is considered comparatively unimportant, but if a patient can be easily roused to swallow he may be given drinks of water or glucose in lemonade. Probably long before this time has elapsed the surgeon will have decided whether any surgical interference is called for and will carry it out if necessary. Alternatively, the patient may be doing well and by this time be able to take nourishment; if not, rectal saline containing glucose will be ordered.

During all this time the nurse should be observing her patient very carefully for any increase or decrease of the symptoms outlined above. It is necessary to attend to the mouth at frequent intervals, and the ears, nose and eyes should receive any attention they need; if discharge is present the character should be observed, and discharge from the ears particularly should receive very careful attention; in serious injuries to the dura mater, the nurse may notice tiny pieces of the grey matter of the brain escaping in the cerebrospinal fluid which is coming away. The amount of moisture escaping from the ears should be carefully reported upon.

In some instances bleeding occurs from the back of the nose and trickles down the throat; a conscious patient will be seen swallowing, but in the case of a patient who is unconscious this blood may be trickling into the respiratory passages where, in the lung, it will give rise to serious inhalation pneumonia in a day or so.

The nurse should be very familiar with the points to which attention must be paid in the nursing of any patient who is unconscious; these are described in more detail in chapter 50.

CONCUSSION, COMPRESSION AND CEREBRAL IRRITATION

When a patient is admitted with an injury to his head it may be difficult, at first, to ascertain whether the injury has only resulted in shock to the brain matter, or whether definite injury to it has been sustained, and it is very necessary that a nurse should be quick to recognize the symptoms of concussion and that she should be able to note the changes which will occur in the patient's condition should cerebral compression follow.

Concussion may produce only slight symptoms of nausea and dizziness, a vague inability to recognize the surroundings in which a patient finds himself, and slight confusion of mind; there may be a short interval of unconsciousness. When severe, concussion will be accompanied by unconsciousness, but usually the patient is only in a state of stupor and not in coma. He could be roused if shaken and spoken to, but it is not advisable to attempt this as there is always the danger of cerebral irritation following a state of concussion, which will be aggravated by any stimulation of the patient.

Signs and symptoms. When a patient is admitted with a diagnosis of concussion the nurse should expect to find him lying limp and flaccid, with a soft, fairly slow and rather small pulse, subnormal temperature, cold clammy skin and with rather shallow slow respirations. These symptoms, she will recognize, are very similar to those of shock, and this is because any serious shaking of the brain, described as concussion, gives rise to shock and, for the time being, the patient is in a cold, debilitated state.

Observations, treatment and nursing of concussion. The patient is received into a warm bed, but should not face the light; he should not be given hot-water bottles as he is likely to move involuntarily and may come into contact with one and be injured. He may have one low pillow under his head, and as a rule an icebag is ordered to be applied to the head. It is advisable to protect the bed with mackintoshes in case the patient passes urine involuntarily whilst in the state of flaccid passivity; the pillow should also be protected, as when the patient begins to improve he will invariably vomit.

A *period of reaction* occurs as a patient begins to recover from concussion; he has previously been cold, but his temperature now rises to 99° or 100° F. and his pulse improves in volume and rate; his colour, previously pale, improves and his face becomes slightly flushed. Hitherto he has been lying flat and limp in bed, but he now puts his hand to his head as it aches and turns over, curling his head down and drawing his knees up, and usually he vomits. From this time onwards he is restless, complaining of headache and slight nausea; as improvement continues he will ask for the urinal or bedpan and usually inquire the time, and ask for a drink. He may then be satisfied and apparently sleep at intervals, and it will now be most important to avoid all irritation, by touch, sound or light, as at this period the dreaded complication of cerebral irritation may make its appearance.

During the following days the patient should rest in bed, his bowels should be kept active, his urine be measured and tested and the bladder watched, as retention of urine may occur. He may have drinks at first and light diet if he is willing to eat.

Headache often persists and cold applications to the head are continued for its relief. Lumbar puncture may be performed with the same object, and analgesic preparations are sometimes ordered. The administration of hypertonic solutions of magnesium sulphate per rectum are also sometimes employed, as by producing dehydration this will relieve intra-cranial pressure.

During her nursing care of a patient with concussion the nurse must be on the look-out for any indication of either cerebral compression or irritation (see notes below).

Compression is more serious than concussion, because the brain is either pressed upon or injured, whereas in concussion it is only shocked or shaken.

The *symptoms and signs of compression* may come on gradually, or the injury may have been so severe at the outset that compression occurred immediately. In *severe compression* the patient is in a state of coma; his breathing is deep, stertorous and noisy; his pulse full and bounding and usually slow, and his temperature may or may not be raised; his face is usually flushed and he lies drawing his cheeks in and out with each deep act of respiration. On inspection of his eyes the pupils may be found to be unequal in size and there may be a squint; examination of the limbs may result in finding that one falls more limply than the other when raised from the bed and allowed to drop back again—indicating paralysis of one side. There may be incontinence of urine and faeces, or retention of urine may be present, and the abdomen may be distended by retention of gas in the intestine.

Observation, treatment and nursing care. The patient is received into bed and his head is kept flat, an icebag being applied to it; immediate observation is made of his condition which should be written down so that further observations can be made as they occur and any change accurately noted.

The nurse will make observations similar to those in the case of a fracture of the skull, watching the pulse, breathing and temperature, the eyes for certain changes, and the nose and ears for any discharge. *Dangerous signs which may arise* include alteration of the breathing, with increase in the irregularity and depth, or the breathing may become of the Cheyne-Stokes type. Any increase or decrease in the rate of the pulse should be observed, a rapidly rising temperature which may reach 105° F. or over being particularly serious.

Either a magnesium sulphate enema or a dose of one minim of croton oil will usually be ordered on admission, and a specimen of urine should be tested as soon as one is obtained. The mouth should be kept clean, bladder infection and bedsores prevented, and in cases of coma, the eyes—because they are sometimes widely open and the conjunctival reflex abolished—should be bathed regularly to prevent infection. (For further details of nursing care in cases of unconsciousness see chapter 50.)

Cerebral irritation may follow concussion or complicate compression. In this state the patient is conscious, though he may be very surly and refuse to rouse or move. Whenever any necessary treatment is performed as making the bed, washing him and so on, he shouts, and curses, and becomes very violent, even kicking and biting his attendants. This may go on for some time, and gradual recovery then takes place, leaving the patient mentally confused and dazed, with severe headache and in some cases loss of memory.

The *treatment* is rest, avoidance of irritation, and relief of intracranial pressure if this is suspected. A patient who has suffered from cerebral irritation needs a long rest during which he should have a nourishing but non-stimulating diet; his bowels should be kept in regular action by the use of a saline aperient each morning; he should not be subject to worry and anxiety and should be kept under observation for several months. It is inadvisable to allow him to go out alone for some time, as he may have a recurrence of loss of memory with very distressing results for himself and his relatives and friends should he wander off and be lost for a time.

FRACTURES OF THE SPINE

The *spine* may be fractured by *direct* violence, as usually happens in a serious crushing accident; or it may be fractured *indirectly*, as when a weight falls upon the head and shoulders—the spine, unable to adapt itself, snaps. In very many instances a fracture-dislocation occurs, and when this happens the cord may be crushed between the displaced vertebrae.

Signs and symptoms. At first there is spinal concussion; a patient admitted with a fractured spine will be pale and cold, with a small rapid pulse and shallow breathing; there will be total loss of power in the muscles of the parts below the site of fracture; sensation may also be completely absent, or it may be only impaired. In most instances at this stage there will be loss of power over the sphincters of the anus and urethra with total incontinence; in some cases, however, there may be retention of urine.

The higher up the spinal column the fracture occurs, the greater will be the disability and danger. In a *fracture of the cervical region* the arms, and the body below this, will be paralysed; the pupils of the eyes will probably be affected as the cervical sympathetic nerves are given off from ganglia in the cervical region; the phrenic nerves may also be injured; if badly, the diaphragm will be out of action and if the diaphragm is totally paralysed the prognosis is very grave.

Fractures of the dorsal region will result in paralysis of the trunk below the fracture and of the lower limbs. The intercostal muscles below the lesion will be paralysed so that breathing will be slightly interfered with. *Fracture of the lumbar region* will result in paralysis of the lower limbs with involvement of the organic reflexes controlling micturition and defecation.

The usual signs of injury may be present locally, and there will be bruising and swelling and possibly deformity also.

Treatment and nursing. On admission it is necessary to get the patient into bed as rapidly as possible, and to treat the degree of shock present. If possible he should be placed on the bed on which he will be nursed; some surgeons advocate a firm unyielding surface with fracture boards beneath the mattress; in this case a full-size air bed will usually be employed in order to prevent sores from forming as the result of lying on the hard surface.

The use of a sectional mattress makes it possible to attend to the patient's back and to put the bedpan in and out without moving him. Other surgeons immobilize the spine by means of a plaster of paris bed as soon as he has recovered from the initial shock from which he may be suffering.

The principles to be considered in the treatment of cases of fracture of the spine depend entirely on whether the spinal cord is injured or not. In cases where the cord has escaped injury the application of a plaster of paris spinal jacket with the spine fully extended will separate the crushed bodies of the injured vertebrae, prevent the occurrence of any injury to the cord subsequent to the fracture and lessen the period of complete rest in bed. A patient with a fracture of the dorsal region for example will have a spinal jacket applied to keep the spine extended and should be able to walk about, wear his ordinary clothes and follow his occupation, in many instances, a week or 10 days after the injury. Similarly a case of fracture of the lower cervical or upper dorsal vertebrae, uncomplicated by injury to the spinal cord, may have a spinal jacket applied with the head fully extended.

On the other hand when there is injury to the spinal cord the period of immobilization in bed is often very prolonged and the prevention of infection of the bladder, of bedsores and trophic sores and hypostatic pneumonia calls for very careful nursing throughout.

The bladder needs careful observation; there may be incontinence or retention of urine. The latter may be treated by regular catheterization or by inserting a self-retaining catheter or by one of the means described on pp. 145–8 of intermittent bladder drainage. The surgeon will usually order some form of urinary antiseptic to be given and he may also have ordered a mild diuretic at the outset; the nurse should provide her patient with plenty of bland fluids and see that he takes at least 6 pints in 24 hours, including barley water, lemonade and water. The administration of penicillin helps to prevent ascending infection of the urinary tract.

Constipation and abdominal distension may be very troublesome; partly because the patient is lying flat and partly because some of the nerves supplying the muscles of the abdominal wall may be involved. As a rule the bowel will be emptied by means of an olive oil enema; this may be repeated daily, or mild laxatives may be given in an attempt to keep the bowel active, supplemented by enemata as found necessary.

The *prevention of bedsores and abrasions of the skin* is also very important; at first sensation will be impaired. As a rule much of the impairment of sensation present at the outset may be associated with spinal shock and bruising of the cord which will disappear in time.

The trophic nerves to the skin may be impaired, and injuries to the skin will very easily occur; for this reason the patient should never be rolled or turned to have his sheet changed as this movement may be sufficient to abrade the surface of the skin—instead, he should be lifted.

If the pressure of the bedclothes appears to redden or injure the skin, or is likely to do so, either a bedcradle should be inserted to take the weight, or the parts affected should be wrapped in cotton wool bandages, but these ought to be taken off at least twice a day and the skin washed, dried and powdered before they are reapplied.

Deformity of the limbs should be prevented; if a paralysed foot is left unsupported, it will droop and footdrop may be the result.

Observation of the progress of the patient is made daily by the surgeon; but the nurse in attendance should take an intelligent interest in this, and note the findings at the first examination and the differences which appear later.

As already indicated, the shock sustained and the bruising of the cord will give rise to a flaccid or total paralysis; but as this passes off the lesion resulting from a fractured spine is that characteristic of an upper motor neurone lesion described on p. 408. The paralysed parts, from being limp and flaccid, become rigid and spastic; the tendon reflexes, lost at first, become brisk and exaggerated; reflex movements occur, and the patient may be seen to draw his legs up in response to any slight irritation. Spasm of the rigid irritated muscles may give rise to deformities due to the contraction of muscle, such as flexion and adduction of the hip, or contraction of the knee in flexion, or of the tendon of Achilles giving rise to footdrop. When any of these deformities are likely to occur the parts must be splinted in order to prevent contractures from arising.

Physiotherapeutic measures will be taken in order to prevent deformity and assist the patient to move without help, to balance and to walk.

FRACTURE OF THE PELVIS

The commonest cause of fracture of the pelvis is a crushing accident, and either the *true* or the *false pelvis* may be injured. Fractures of the true pelvis are very likely to be complicated by injury to the urethra, bladder and rectum.

The patient will usually sustain a great deal of shock, his lower limbs being temporarily paralysed. There will be considerable pain, and bruising and swelling may be present, depending upon the type of injury which caused the fracture.

Treatment and nursing. The first requirement is to keep the patient absolutely still, as if the urethra and bladder are not already injured they easily may be by injudicious handling. The patient will be gently put into bed, to lie on a firm even surface. He should not be permitted to pass urine; if he is able to answer questions it would be useful to know when he last passed urine, before the accident; the nurse will then have some idea how much urine to expect. He should be catheterized; if the patient is a female, and the nurse passes the catheter, she should use a rubber one and should notice whether any blood is obtained and, if this should come first, whether it is well mixed with the urine, or is obtained last. The quantity of urine should be noted. If any blood was present in the catheter specimen the patient should not be allowed to pass urine, but should be catheterized at regular intervals, the whole of the amount obtained each time being kept for the inspection of the surgeon. The area of the perineum, vagina and anus should be carefully examined for signs of bruising or laceration.

An X-ray examination of the pelvis will be carried out and the surgeon will decide whether the patient is to be put into a plaster of paris bed, or spica plaster of the hip, incorporating the trunk, or whether he is to be nursed flat on a firm bed, between sandbags with a firm calico binder applied around the pelvis in order to give some support. For nursing care see p. 615.

INJURIES TO JOINTS

Sprains and dislocations are the conditions produced when a joint is the site of injury.

A **sprain** is due to a forcible wrenching movement with sudden twisting of a joint which results in tearing the soft structures which surround it—ligaments, tendons and muscles.

The *symptoms* and *signs* are pain, swelling and difficulty in moving the joint. The *treatment* depends to some extent on the injury and also on the time which has elapsed since the injury.

When a sprain is seen immediately after it has occurred, applications of cold water or ice will prevent effusion into the joint structures; this is then followed by a bandage, either crêpe or elastoplast, firmly applied. The firm bandage will limit further swelling by preventing the effusion of fluid from the injured structures. This is of great value, as temporary and even permanent thickening of a joint may follow if treatment in the early stages is neglected or unobtainable.

If the injured joint is not seen for some time, and considerable swelling has occurred, the treatment is to apply heat in order to help absorption of the effusion which has collected around the joint, and this may be followed by gentle massage of the muscles above the injured area in order, by promoting the return of lymph and blood, to help removal of the waste products. A firmly applied bandage should then be put on. In both instances it is advisable to rest the joint until all pain has disappeared, and even when movement is permitted the patient should be advised to keep the joint elevated whenever he can, in order to assist the return of lymph and venous blood from it.

Dislocation. A dislocation is the displacement of two bones entering into the formation of a joint. Such an injury may be *congenital*, as in congenital dislocation of the hip which may be unilateral or bilateral; or it may be *pathological* when the bone ends become seriously eroded by disease and can no longer remain in an adapted position, one with the other—this occurs in Paget's disease and in tuberculous disease of joints.

A traumatic dislocation is dealt with here; it is the commonest type of dislocation, and is brought about by violence. The *shoulder* is most often dislocated by falling on the outstretched hand, as when falling down a flight of steps or off a bicycle; the *jaw* is also rather easily dislocated and *dislocations of the elbow and ankle* frequently complicate fractures of the bones in these situations.

The *signs and symptoms* are those of injury—pain, swelling, bruising, loss of function and deformity.

Treatment consists in *reduction of the dislocation* as soon as possible; the longer it is left, the greater will be the effusion and swelling, and the rigidity and thickening of the joint brought about by this will make the period of disability of function longer than it need be. *Fixation of the joint* is necessary for a variable time, but must be long enough to permit of repair of the capsule of the joint, which has been stretched, and possibly torn, by the force of the injury. Once this is established treatment is aimed at the *restoration of function* which should be as complete as possible. For this purpose the patient will be given massage; the joint will be passively moved and he will be encouraged to move it actively—gradually at first, and then within the whole range of movement possible. In cases where wasting is marked, electrical stimulation may be used as an adjunct to massage.

Penicillin is of value in preventing septic complications in all cases of injury.

Chapter 43

Operation Technique, including the Preparation for an Operation in a Private House. Examples of Anaesthesia and the Preparation of the Patient for Anaesthesia and for Operation, including Preparation of the Skin

Preparation of hands—Theatre dress—Sterilization of instruments, utensils and dressings—Lotions—Antiseptic powders and pastes—Sutures, ligatures and surgical needles—Preparation for an operation in a private house—Use of anaesthetics: general, local, regional, splanchnic, spinal and sacral—Use of basal narcotics with notes on post-anaesthetic care—Preparation of the patient for operation, including preparation of the skin—Value of breathing exercises

The vast subject of surgical technique can only receive an introduction in a book of this size, and the points given are those with which the nurse should be most familiar and will most likely have to deal.

The *antiseptic technique* introduced into surgery by Lord Lister has undergone many alterations and modifications up till the present day. He taught that organisms were destroyed by strong antiseptic substances which he used principally on the wound and dressings employed in order to destroy germs which had gained access to the wound. He made at the same time some attempt to prevent the access of organisms into the wound, and he was the first to teach surgeons to wash their hands before as well as after operating.

It is difficult and probably unnecessary to differentiate between antiseptic and aseptic technique as employed today, the main difference lying in the fact that the old antiseptic methods aimed at destroying organisms which had reached the wound, whereas the present *aseptic methods* aim at preventing organisms from reaching the wound. As organisms may reach the wound from the patient's skin, the hands of doctors and nurses, the expired air of those around the operating table, or the instruments, swabs and dressings used, the adequate sterilization of all articles in the vicinity of the wound is the principle involved in aseptic surgery.

Neither the patient's skin nor the hands of the surgeons or nurses can be rendered absolutely sterile, and the latter will therefore be covered by sterile rubber gloves. Instruments and swabs can be perfectly sterilized, and this is why as far as possible the surgeon always handles the tissues of the wound with instruments and swabs rather than with his hands even though they are gloved. A good nurse assisting at the operation in handling instruments and swabs will use forceps; she will also hold suture and needle in forceps when threading needles.

The **preparation of the hands of surgeons and nurses** is carried out as carefully as possible. Surgeons and theatre nurses should make a practice of protecting their hands from contamination by always handling contaminated or septic articles with forceps—they should *never* touch pus. Should their hands become contaminated they must wash them as soon as possible in water as hot as can be borne, using a nailbrush, soap and disinfectant, scrubbing the skin well, stretching the fingers and scrubbing the stretched skin between the fingers and knuckles, paying special attention to the papillary spaces over the pads of the thumbs and fingers. The nails should be kept well trimmed and should be short enough for the nailbrush that is used to get between the nail and finger bed. Nailbrushes employed for the preparation of hands before an operation should be boiled each morning for 20 minutes and placed in an antiseptic solution such as lysol 1 per cent, or perchloride of mercury 1–2,000 in which they will remain during the day.

The hands of nurses working in an operating theatre or surgical ward, maternity unit or infectious diseases block, should be kept free of rough skin, they should be well washed and cared for at night, the nails being attended to and any tags of cuticle removed, and the hands should be anointed with a healing lotion in order to keep the skin in good condition and as smooth as possible.

Immediate preparation of the hands. The preparation of the hands of surgeons and nurses varies with the wishes of the surgeon. Having the arms bare to above the elbow the first procedure is to wash them under running water as hot as possible, for 5 minutes at least, using a sterilized nailbrush and a liquid soap, paying special attention to the folds and creases of the skin, stretching the fingers apart to get between them, scrubbing well over the joints of fingers and knuckles and scrubbing the pads of the thumbs and fingers and paying special attention to the nails. The hands are next treated by an antiseptic such as biniodide in spirit 1–500, perchloride of mercury 1–2,000, or alcohol 70 per cent. This lotion is rubbed into the skin with a swab, using several pieces of gauze and discarding each in turn. Some surgeons like the hands to be soaked in the antiseptic solution for two or three minutes, the forearms being swilled with the lotion as the hands are kept in the solution.

The skin of the hands and arms is now considered prepared, and great care must be taken not to touch any non-sterile article. The next step in the preparation is to put on a special theatre dress and rubber gloves.

THEATRE DRESS (see fig. 211, p. 641).

It is usual to wear an apron of mackintosh similar in shape to a butcher's apron. This is put on first. Some surgeons like the nurses to wear canvas boots over their shoes and stockings; these are fastened round the legs with tapes, puttee fashion.

Cap. The cap is worn so that all hair is covered, and that there may be no risk that hair might fall from the heads of those around the operating table on to the articles in the vicinity of the wound. The cap should be put on by an assistant, as it is practically impossible for anyone to put a cap on his own head without contaminating his hands.

Mask. The mask, which should also be put on by an assistant, is used to avoid the danger of infection to the patient by the fall of moist infective particles from the nose or mouth of those working in the vicinity of the operating table on to the articles which will be used in and about the room. Droplets of moisture are carried a certain distance from the nose and mouth in speaking, and these are always a source of infection, more especially so when the speaker has a carious tooth, or a cold in the head.

The mask or veil should be of a material equal to the thickness of five layers of surgical gauze, and some surgeons have them made of several thicknesses of butter muslin or a fairly thick cotton material. The upper part should reach the bridge of the nose and the lower part extend below the mouth and chin where it hangs in sacklike fashion, the ends being tucked in beneath the neckband of the overall. If the person wearing a mask wishes to cough or sneeze his head should be turned away from the operating table and from all articles in the vicinity of it.

Gowns. The gown is put on next. A sterile drum is opened by an assistant and the person who is 'scrubbed up' takes a gown, which he finds folded up; holding it well out in front of him he unfolds it, taking care that it does not touch his own clothing or any other non-sterile article. He then puts his arms into the sleeves of the gown and extending them in front of him slips it on. As the gown is sterile, he may touch the front of it and so help to get it into position. It is usually fastened behind by tapes on the neckband, and at the waist, but he must not touch these as they may dangle against his clothing behind and so become soiled. An assistant will fasten these tapes; she takes hold of the ends, being careful not to touch the sterile gown, and ties them comfortably tight.

Gloves. Gloves are used as a protection; the impossibility of actually sterilizing the skin has been mentioned, so also has the necessity of protecting the skin of those who are to assist at surgical dressings from contact with septic matter and pus.

The gloves used for operation work should be thin rubber ones which will not interfere with the sense of touch; stouter ones may be used for the handling of surgical dressings. For preparation see fig. 212, p. 642.

Gloves may be prepared by boiling, in this case they will be wet, and placed ready in lotion; or they may be autoclaved, being packed in drums, and in this case they are dry and ready prepared in powder, packed up in pairs. Before applying dry gloves, the prepared hands should be dabbed dry with sterile talcum powder which is usually supplied ready in gauze packets. It is comparatively easy to put on dry rubber gloves (but see precautions mentioned below). Boiled gloves supplied wet require greater care. In this case the gloves are loosely tied in pairs, having been transferred from a sterilizer of boiling water to a bowl of cool lotion, but the gloves may contain some very hot water, and therefore the nurse who transfers them ought to hold them inverted in forceps long enough for this water to run out, otherwise the unwary may be scalded.

To put on the gloves. Take hold of the cuff and fill it with the lotion in which it lies. Holding the cuff with one hand insert the other hand into the glove, hold the glove fingers down over the pail or dish and *not over the lotion bowl* in which they were served. The hand will displace the lotion; having got the glove on raise the hand to allow the remaining lotion to drain out of the glove; this lotion should not be allowed to run over the surface of the gloved hand, as having been in contact with the skin of the hand it may be contaminated by staphylococci. When the glove is empty fold the cuff of the sleeve of the gown neatly about the wrist and bring the cuff of the glove up over it so that there is no space between glove and gown sleeve.

Precautions in the use of gloves. Gloves should be handled as little as possible. As already mentioned water or lotion from the interior should be drained out and not allowed to run over the glove. If the fingers of the glove are not properly on, they may not be handled with the skin of the bare hand but, when both gloves are on, they may be gently eased on the fingers; or a wet sterile swab may be employed to smooth the fingers down. If the ends of the fingers do not reach the ends of the gloves it is better to take the gloves off and put on another pair than to continue to wear them and so risk injury to the rubber. Gloves are easily pricked with needles and injured by rough handling; a punctured glove should be removed at once and a fresh one put on. Care should be taken not to injure the cuff in removing gloves.

After use gloves should be washed in cold water, turned inside out and washed again, boiled for ten minutes, hung up inverted in order to drain, and finally dried by blotting with a soft cloth and inflated to inspect them for minute punctures. *Small punctures may be mended*, but *mended gloves should never be used for operation work* though they may, with care, be employed for surgical ward dressings.

STERILIZATION OF INSTRUMENTS, UTENSILS AND DRESSINGS

Instruments used for operating work except sharp ones should be boiled for 20 minutes in a sterilizer with a closed lid in water containing 1 per cent sodium bicarbonate. They are then placed in sterile dishes, either lying on a dry sterile towel, or in sterile water or some antiseptic lotion such as carbolic 1–80.

Cutting instruments such as knives, scissors and needles have the edge blunted by boiling, and these are usually sterilized by placing them in pure lysol for 4 to 5 minutes and then in methylated spirit in order to remove the lysol which is injurious to the skin. A freshly sharpened knife is only used once; it is washed and boiled after use and then resharpened.

If an instrument slips off the operating table and is required again, it must be washed, and boiled for 10 minutes, and be cooled, before it can be handed to the surgeon again.

Rubber tubing is usually boiled for 20 minutes and then kept in carbolic lotion 1–60; any part removed from the jar which is not used should be boiled for 10 minutes before being replaced.

After use. Instruments must be washed in cold water after use, and all crevices and joints scrubbed with a nailbrush in order to remove blood and debris. Hollow instruments, such as cannulae, should be flushed with water after washing. The instruments are then boiled for 20 minutes before being put away. They are placed to drain on soft absorbent towels and polished with a soft dry cloth. Cannulae and hollow needles are syringed through with methylated spirit and well shaken to free them from moisture. The stilette is then replaced and removed over and over again, drying it each time until it has ceased to receive moisture from contact with needle or cannula. This instrument is then placed on a warm surface, such as a radiator, to finish drying. Large hollow instruments, such as flushing curettes, usually have a little rangoon oil poured in to prevent rusting of the interior. Needles and scissors are soaked in lysol and spirit after use.

Porringers, bowls, dishes, trays and receivers are all sterilized by boiling or by steam disinfection, and it is very important for the nurses to get used to handling these articles when sterile. It should never be permissible to lift a bowl or similar article with the thumb inside as one might take hold of a kitchen utensil. If the bowl or porringer has a handle it can readily be removed by one hand, but otherwise unless it is very small it will need the use of both hands. Again, bowls do not remain sterile just because they have been boiled, and once a bowl has, for example, been placed to stand on a non-sterile surface the outside is contaminated; if the bowl is inverted on this surface, then the inside is contaminated.

Care of syringes. A great many of the syringes used today are of the record type, which has a metal plunger and a glass barrel with metal ends. *It is necessary to take a syringe to pieces in order to sterilize it,* and afterwards it should be cooled in sterile lotion before assembling the parts again; and all parts should be quite cool because, glass cooling more quickly than metal, if the syringe were assembled before the metal had cooled, the glass contracting on the more slowly contracting metal would crack.

After using a syringe, it should be washed through in order to remove serum or any other substance containing coagulable protein; cold or tepid water should be used for this purpose. The syringe should then be taken to pieces and washed under running water. It should be shaken to dry it, or methylated spirit might be run through the syringe. When it is thoroughly dry it may be reassembled. The needle should be thoroughly dried by inserting, removing, drying and reinserting the stilette as often as necessary until no moisture remains on it.

Dressings. Materials used for surgical dressings must be sterile and should readily absorb moisture in order that the discharge from the wound will rapidly be collected by the dressing. Gauze is better than cotton wool as the latter becomes sodden, but the gauze readily evaporates the moisture it collects and thus encourages drying. By this means serum or other discharge is conveyed away from the wound, permeating a large area of gauze it rapidly dries, so that collection of fluid over the surface of the wound, which would provide a good medium for the growth of organisms, is prevented.

When the oozing of serum is profuse and the dressing, including the cotton wool covering the gauze, and perhaps even the bandage is permeated by it, it is important to cover the wet patch with dry sterile wool in order to prevent the entry of micro-organisms which will find the serum a suitable medium for their growth, and in the sodden wet dressing a rapid means of entry to the wound beneath. It is to prevent this from happening that operation wounds are carefully watched for the oozing of serum.

Materials used for surgical dressings, as those made of gauze and wool, gamgee tissue, and also such articles as jaconet bandages and safety pins may all be sterilized by steam disinfection.

Dabs and swabs. Dabs or swabs for ward dressings are often made of cotton wool wrung out of an antiseptic solution such as carbolic 1–60 or perchloride of mercury 1–2,000. Sterile wool is used, placed in a sterile towel across a sterilized bowl, the wool being folded into the towel as in the preparation of a fomentation, the lotion poured over and the wool wrung out. The wet wool is then separated into flakes of the size desired, and put into china or glass jars which have been prepared by washing in soap and water and rinsing with carbolic lotion. Similar swabs may be used for minor operation work, but as a rule sterilized gauze swabs are employed at all operations. These are made of gauze folded in different ways according to the custom of the hospital and the wishes of the surgeon. As a rule the precaution is taken of having all raw edges folded inwards so that frayed strands of gauze cannot catch in the wound or be caught by the instruments used. Swabs used in abdominal surgery are stitched to prevent this complication. Different sizes are put up in bundles of six and twelve. The gauze is folded into six or twelve thicknesses, the margins being stitched. Gamgee tissue may alternatively be used. The stitching is carried across from corner to corner, as in mattressing, in order to keep the shape better. For preparation see fig. 213, p. 643.

Abdominal swabs may be plain or taped, the latter having a length of tape sewn on one side or to one corner for use when the surgeon wishes to bury a swab deep in the abdominal cavity—the tape hanging out over

RECORD OF SWABS

Type.	Number available	Used swabs*	Unused	Total
Unstitched	3 dozen	IIIIIIIIIIII IIIIIIIII	1 dozen and 3	36
Abdominal 12 inch	6	IIII	2	6
,, 8 ,,	12	IIIII	7	12
,, 6 ,,	4 dozen	IIIIIIIIIIII IIIIIIIIIIII IIIIIIII	1 dozen and 4	48
Pieces of gauze cut from roll	2	I	1	2

*Each stroke represents one used swab.

FIG. 209.—ONE METHOD OF RECORDING THE SWABS USED AT AN OPERATION.

the edge of the wound and being anchored by a pair of artery forceps. It is very necessary that this tape should be securely stitched on. A roll of gauze may be required by some surgeons for packing into the abdominal cavity; the surgeon will cut off the length he needs, tuck it in and secure the free end by forceps as in the case of the taped swabs.

Some member of the nursing staff is usually in charge of abdominal swabs—it may be the theatre sister, theatre nurse or the ward sister. In hospital practice she is responsible to the surgeon and she should know how many swabs she has available at the beginning of the operation and check these numbers with her assistant. It is not sufficient to take it for granted that the specified number of swabs are contained in the different bundles—each bundle used should be counted, the swabs being handled by sterile forceps for this purpose. The number available at the commencement of the operation ought to be written on the slate provided.

The sister in charge of swabs should follow the movements of the surgeon and notice where he places them, the number of taped swabs and gauze packs he may insert into the wound. As soiled swabs are dropped on to the floor or into a pail, the assistant with a pair of forceps—which need not be sterile—picks them up and arranges them in bundles on a towel placed on the floor beside the swab table. When six or twelve have been used she catches the eye of the sister in charge, who watches her count them and place them in a bundle; taped swabs are similarly dealt with. All used abdominal swabs must remain in view until the operation is over. Before the surgeon begins to close the abdominal cavity he will usually ask the sister if the swabs are correct; she must be prepared to answer this question, and should one be missing the surgeon will search for it before he proceeds further. The swabs should again be checked when the operation is finished and the towels may then be removed from the area of the operating table.

LOTIONS

Various lotions are used in surgery, each surgeon having his own particular choice in the matter. Some of the common ones in use include the following: *Water, boiled for* 20 *minutes*, is used by some surgeons for rinsing the gloved hands during an operation and for the immersion of sterile instruments, but it is doubtful whether water exposed to the air remains sterile.

Normal saline solution 0·9 per cent sodium chloride dissolved in sterile water is used to moisten swabs for use on wounds and for irrigation of cavities and by some surgeons for swilling the gloved hands during operation.

Boracic lotion is a saturated solution which contains 5 per cent of boric acid in sterile water. The lotion is made with boiling water in order to obtain saturation and it is then allowed to cool before use. It is very slightly antiseptic and is used in strength 2½ per cent instead of saline, but it is more irritating to the tissues and to the lining of cavities.

A weak solution of one of the aniline dyes is a very favourite antiseptic lotion today. In addition to its antiseptic properties most of those solutions possess the power of stimulating the healing of wounds and some—particularly flavine—are moderately powerful styptics. *Flavine* is used in the strength of 1–1,000. Others include *scarlet red* which is employed as a stimulating dressing to wounds; *brilliant green* and *methyl violet* are used for their antiseptic properties in the preparation of the skin for operation.

Peroxide of hydrogen is prepared in strengths described as 5, 10 or 20 volumes. This indicates that the solution contains so many volumes of available oxygen. It is valuable in treating septic wounds and cavities, and is also a valuable styptic. It should be mixed with warm water as hot water lessens its usefulness. It always froths up when in contact with decomposable matter which is not necessarily septic or containing pus.

Alcohol is used for the sterilization of sharp instruments as *rectified spirit*, which contains 95 per cent alcohol, but as alcohol evaporates it is impossible to be sure of the concentration. A solution of *phenyl-mercuric-nitrate* 1–5,000, containing 1 per cent borax, in water, is alternatively used.

It is considered efficient for the sterilization of instruments, and the added borax helps to prevent the instruments rusting.

Iodine is used as liniment of iodine which is a 10 per cent solution—formerly known as tincture—for painting on the skin and preparing it before operation and also in repeated coats as a counter-irritant. To be effective the skin should be dry before the iodine is applied, and in order to avoid producing blisters the application should not be covered until it is dry.

Formalin. A 1 per cent solution is used for bathing wounds and as a lotion in preparing the hands before operation. It is, however, not very much used for these purposes but has by long use become invaluable for spraying the walls of rooms which have to be disinfected, and in solid form it is utilized for the production of vapour in the disinfection of such rooms and also in the sterilization of gum elastic and composition catheters and of certain surgical instruments and appliances.

Condy's fluid (permanganate of potash) is a very favourite household disinfectant for sinks, drains, etc., the crystals being dissolved in water until a pale purple colour is produced. The solution acts as a deodorant and also gives off oxygen; when in contact with decomposable matter it rapidly loses its antiseptic properties and then the colour of the liquid changes to a dirty brown. A weak solution, which may be indicated either by producing a very pale mixture, or by measuring it to produce a solution of 1–5,000 in strength, is used as a mouth-wash and for gastric, bladder and rectal irrigation, and for vaginal douches.

The **phenol group** are derived from coal tar by processes of distillation, and the one mainly in use is *carbolic*, or phenol. It is highly poisonous and corrosive in action. *Pure carbolic* is sometimes used by surgeons to touch up septic wounds or the stump of the appendix. A strong solution, 1–10 in spirit, is occasionally used to sterilize sharp instruments by immersion for 10 minutes; instruments so treated must be removed from the solution by forceps and washed in sterile water in order to remove the carbolic before they can be used.

Carbolic 1–20 *or* 1–40 is used as a stock solution in which to keep boiled rubber tubing and silkworm gut, etc. This also is the strength in which this lotion is used for disinfecting discharges and excreta from typhoid fever cases and others; and also for the disinfection of infected utensils and clothing which should be soaked in it for two hours. A solution of 1–60 is used as a lotion for disinfecting hands, a preparation of 1–80 or 1–100 for mouth-washes and gargles.

Other disinfectants of the *phenol group* include *izal*, *cyllin*, and *Jeyes's fluid*, *cresol* and *lysol*—the two last prepared with liquid soap and therefore, by reason of their soapy nature, useful for cleansing purposes. They are generally considered more valuable disinfectants than carbolic and less poisonous. *Pure lysol* is used for the sterilization of sharp instruments. Lysol in the strength of 1 drachm to the pint is used for vaginal douches and as a lotion for bathing septic wounds. A stronger preparation, usually a 1 per cent solution, is used for cleansing soiled ward utensils.

Picric acid is obtained by mixing phenol and nitric acid. It is used as a 2 per cent preparation in the treatment of burns and as a 3 per cent preparation in spirit for cleansing the skin before operation.

Chlorine group. *Eusol*, *Dakin's solution*, *chloramine-T* and *Milton* are examples of this preparation, *Eupad* is a mixture of bleaching powder and boracic acid in equal parts, and *Eusol* is a solution of these powders which is used as a wet dressing or for the constant irrigation of wounds.

Dakin's solution is a modification of eusol, and is a hypertonic solution employed in the Carrel-Dakin irrigation treatment of septic wounds. It was extensively used during the war of 1914–18. Being hypertonic, it encourages the free flow of lymph from the wound and results in the removal of dead tissue.

Milton (Electrolytic sodium hypochlorite) is used in from 1 per cent to 20 per cent solutions as treatment of burns and wounds. The use of hypochlorites is considered to dissolve and remove tissue debris. (See treatment of burns, p. 581.)

Mercury group. The mercury group contains *perchloride*, *biniodide* and *oxycyanide of mercury*.

Perchloride is also described as *corrosive sublimate*, and is the one most universally used. All mercurial preparations are unsuitable for the preparation of instruments as they discolour them. They may, however, be used for the sterilization of rubber composition and gum elastic catheters, in the strength of 1–1,000. Perchloride of mercury is most commonly employed as a hand lotion in the strength of 1–2,000; it is used for vaginal douches as 1–4,000 but the precaution is usually taken of following such a douche with one of sterile water to obviate any possibility of mercurial poisoning. A solution of 1–10,000 is used for bathing the eyes, but some surgeons prefer to use oxycyanide for this purpose as it is less irritating.

Biniodide of mercury is slightly less poisonous than perchloride and is used for similar purposes. A solution of biniodide 1–500 in spirit is used by some surgeons in the preparation of their hands before operation.

Silver salts. *Silver nitrate* is the most powerful but it is rarely employed. It will occasionally be used for irrigation of the bladder and rectum in solutions of 1–1,000 to 1–5,000.

Protargol and *argyrol* are used as antiseptics in the treatment of infective conditions of delicate mucous membranes—as of the eyes in purulent conjunctivitis—in ½–1 per cent solution, and in the treatment of acute cervicitis in 1–2 per cent solution.

Chlorocresol and Chloroxylenol. Some newer types of antiseptics are based on the chlorinated derivatives of the higher phenols, i.e. chlorocresol and chloroxylenol. These are powerful bactericides of relatively low toxicity. Chlorocresol 0·05 per cent is approximately equal to 0·5 per cent phenol as a germicidal agent.

Chlorocresol is used chiefly in the preservation of pharmaceutical preparations, such as those solutions which are put up in rubber-capped bottles for hypodermic injection.

Chloroxylenol is more powerful than chlorocresol, but it is less soluble in water and is usually exhibited in a saponaceous base, frequently mixed with aromatic and antiseptic oils. *Liquor Chloroxylenolis* N.W.F. meaning National War Formulary solution, and preparations such as Dettol, Kilsol, Zant, and Zenol are examples of solutions of chloroxylenol. These solutions may be safely applied to the skin, for a very short time, undiluted; a 5 or 10 per cent. solution may be employed for swabbing the skin around a wound and solutions of a drachm to the pint may be used for irrigation of the bladder, vaginal douching, etc. It is claimed that these preparations of chloroxylenol are non-irritating to the majority of skins.

ANTISEPTIC POWDERS AND PASTES

Penicillin and sulphadiazine powder is used for insufflating cavities, packing wounds or dusting on to surfaces. One gramme of the powder contains 5,000 units of penicillin.

Iodoform powder liberates iodine when in contact with warmth and moisture, as when it is applied to the surface of wounds, and is very largely used in the treatment of septic wounds and tuberculous ulcers.

Bismuth, iodoform and **paraffin paste** (BIPP) is a paste which may be applied to surfaces, packed into wounds or injected into sinuses.

Aristol is a proprietary preparation containing iodoform and is used for dusting wounds and ulcerated surfaces. It promotes healing.

Eupad is a preparation of eusol, and is a mixture of bleaching powder and boracic. It is sprinkled on to wounds instead of the solution.

Boracic powder, boracic and starch, or boracic, zinc and starch are all used as dusting powders, mostly for their drying effect and also for their slightly antiseptic properties.

SUTURES, LIGATURES, AND SURGICAL NEEDLES

(See fig. 221, p. 665.)

Materials used for sutures and ligatures are divided into absorbable and non-absorbable ones.

The most commonly used absorbable substance is catgut which is prepared by removal of the fat from the intestines of sheep by scraping and treatment in a preparation of sulphuric acid, and rendered sterile by means of soaking in iodine. It is then put up in different lengths and graded into different thicknesses ready for use.

Catgut may be 'plain,' when prepared as just described, in which case it is absorbed in about 7 days when buried in the tissues; or, it may be subjected to a hardening process by soaking in chromic acid for a certain time; it is then said to be 'chromicized' and, according to the degree of hardening produced, may last as long as 10, 20 or 30 days before it is absorbed.

Kangaroo tendon is also chromicized; it is very strong and hard and lasts from 6 to 8 weeks.

The **non-absorbable materials** include *silk* and *linen thread* used for buried tissues and *silkworm gut* and *horsehair* for suturing the skin. Coats's cotton, No. 24 and 40, has recently been recommended to replace catgut. These are all prepared by boiling.

Silver wire is used for maintaining parts of bone in apposition.

Michel's clips, which are used for the skin, are spiked clips applied by means of a special pair of forceps, and as a rule, when these are employed, tension sutures are inserted. Michel's clips are removed after 5 days, as if left longer they result in unpleasing marks on the skin; tension sutures are removed several days later.

Stitches used in surgery. These may be *approximation* sutures when used to keep the edges of the wound together, or *tension sutures* when intended to take the strain off the skin sutures. These are passed through the deeper structures. All surgeons do not use them, some claiming that they stitch up each individual tissue fibre so completely that tension sutures would be redundant.

Some of the commoner stitches used include a *continuous* one, which may be simple oversewing well spaced or a form of blanket stitch. An *interrupted* suture is one in which each stitch is tied separately, a reef knot being used. *Mattress stitch* is the form used when tension sutures are inserted.

To remove stitches. When interrupted sutures have to be removed, take hold of the knot with a pair of dissecting forceps and pull gently until a portion of the buried stitch is visible, cut this with sharp pointed scissors, then pull the stitch out by means of the dissecting forceps with which it is being held. Pull from the side of the wound opposite to that on which the stitch has been cut and, in this way, dragging any part of the dry suture material which has lain on the surface of the wound through the stitch puncture will be avoided.

Surgical needles. These are of various shapes, sizes and types. Those most commonly used are:

Half-circle. Curved. Straight.

Any of these shapes may be:

Round bodied, non-cutting needles, used for intestine;

Cutting needles with a 3-sided cutting edge and a sharp point;

Flat or *Hagedorn's needles*, with flat bodies and a bevelled edge which is fairly sharp (see fig. 221, p. 665).

PREPARATION FOR AN OPERATION IN A PRIVATE HOUSE

The amount of preparation depends upon the time available, the first and most important point being the avoidance of much moving of articles in the room with its consequent disturbance of dust—unless over 24 hours can be allowed for this to settle. The second point is to choose a room sufficiently large and if possible with a northeast aspect and a large window; a room near a lavatory or bathroom is preferable and if there is a fireplace in the room it can usually be employed for the burning of soiled dressings, etc. Some form of heat in the room must be provided.

Preparation when a reasonable amount of time is available— say 2–3 days. Take down curtains, windowblinds and pictures, remove carpets, rugs and ornaments, have all unwanted furniture carried out of the room; then cover the remaining furniture and sweep the ceiling and walls, windowframes, doorposts and all light fittings. As far as possible use damp brooms for sweeping and damp dusters for dusting. Open all doors and windows and leave the room for 12 hours. Then wash the floor with disinfectant and with a cloth moistened with disinfectant wipe doors and windowpanes and all woodwork, such as the wainscoting, and treat any heavy furniture that is being kept in the room in the same way. Then close and clean the windows and, if the room is overlooked, cover the glass with old muslin or old lace curtains stretched across the frame and secured with drawing pins.

Articles required. The furniture and other articles which might be provided in this room in which the operation is to be performed include a table suitable for the operation unless the nurse knows that the surgeon will bring his own. A small table, and a stool or high chair should be provided for the anaesthetist. Three or four small tables will be required for the surgeon's instruments, dressings and lotions, etc. Some means must be provided for boiling instruments; the nurse may have to provide a suitable utensil for this purpose, in which case she might choose a fish kettle; and she should have considered where this or other utensil can be boiled in case the surgeon does not bring his own sterilizer. A washstand with two basins, if possible two nailbrushes, ready sterilized, soap-dish and bowl for lotion, should be provided, unless the room contains hot and cold running water. Enamel or delf jugs which can be sterilized by flaming them with methylated spirit should be prepared; these will be used to contain quantities of cooled boiled water, and hot boiling water ready for making lotions, etc. One or two pails will be required for used lotion and either a small bath or several shallow enamel basins in which soiled dressings and used instruments can be placed. A number of basins and shallow dishes which can be sterilized by flaming if required should be at hand on which the surgeon might like to place his instruments and towels.

A number of clean blankets, sheets and towels and any mackintoshes the house can muster should be collected, also some old dustsheets to protect the floor. Hot-water bottles should be in readiness to be filled at the last minute and a change of clothing for the patient ought to be at hand in case what he is wearing during the operation becomes soiled.

The nurse should have ready any articles for which she is responsible, including some form of antiseptic, normal saline, bandages, and safety pins, razors and scissors. As a rule the surgeon will bring everything he requires —instruments, gowns, sterile towels and mackintoshes, swabs, gloves and dressings.

Emergency preparation. A nurse may be sent to a private house to make the necessary preparations an hour or two before the surgeon is expected. In this case her procedure would be very different. The room should be chosen as rapidly as possible, bearing in mind the points above mentioned. It is inadvisable to move anything excepting so far as to clear the centre of the room to make space for the operating table, and tables for instruments and lotions, etc., together with a table and chair for the anaesthetist. The articles moved to the sides are to be covered up with sheets or dustsheets; the carpet should be carefully covered with damped dustsheets in order to prevent dust from rising as the surgeon and others walk about. The windows should be closed and the curtains drawn gently to one side in order to prevent the displacement of dust, the blinds rolled up and if necessary some clean window muslin pinned across the glass. Dusting should be done with damp dusters. There should be an adequate supply of boiled water, and useful utensils should be collected and prepared.

THE USE OF ANAESTHETICS, AND THE CARE OF PATIENTS TO WHOM THESE HAVE BEEN ADMINISTERED

Before considering the care of a patient who has had an anaesthetic it is essential that the nurse should understand certain terms used in the administration of these.

General anaesthetics. For the induction of general anaesthesia, ether, chloroform, nitrous oxide gas, and gas and oxygen are amongst the drugs most commonly employed. The mode of administration varies—the *open* method indicates that the drug is dropped on to material stretched across a mask, such as Bellamy-Gardner's. The *closed* method means that the patient breathes in and out of a closed bag (see fig. 214, p. 644).

Stages of Anaesthesia. The degree of general anaesthesia which may be produced has, for convenience, been divided into four stages, although the margins which divide these stages are never very clearly defined.

First stage. This lasts from the commencement of induction until voluntary control is lost.

Second stage. Voluntary control is lost but the patient may continue to struggle involuntarily, and some of the reflexes are still present.

Third stage. This produces entire relaxation. It is described as full surgical anaesthesia. It is during this stage that operations are performed. The breathing is deep and regular, the conjunctival reflex is lost and the corneal reflex sluggish.

The *fourth stage* is that of overdose.

Local anaesthesia. This might more correctly be termed *analgesia*, as it produces loss of sensation to pain without loss of consciousness. Local anaesthesia may be produced in different ways (see fig. 215, p. 645).

(1) *By application of a drug to a mucous surface.* This method is used for operations on the nose, pharynx and larynx. In operations on the eye a number of drops of 4 per cent cocaine are instilled into the conjunctival sac.

(2) *By injection into the tissues.* This is termed *infiltration* anaesthesia, and paralyses the nerve endings in the part into which the drug is passed.

(3) *By injection into the vicinity of a large nerve trunk*, or into the nerve trunk itself (see also regional anaesthesia).

(4) *By freezing.* This is not very commonly employed. An ethyl chloride spray is used, the substance being directed on to the skin until, by the extremely rapid evaporation, the part is frozen hard. This takes place in a few seconds and only lasts for a few seconds and is therefore only available for operations of a very short duration, such as incising a septic finger. Freezing makes the tissues tough and difficult to incise.

Regional anaesthesia. This method of producing anaesthesia is an attempt to block all the afferent impulses passing from the operation area to the central nervous system. It may be carried out in two ways, either by injecting the drug into the area around a large nerve trunk—*paraneural*—or, more rarely, and very carefully, into the nerve trunk—*intraneural*.

Splanchnic anaesthesia. In this method, analgesia of the abdominal organs is obtained by regional anaesthesia of the coeliac plexus, which is the region where most of the sympathetic nerve trunks supplying the abdominal organs lie close together.

Spinal anaesthesia. This is a variety of regional anaesthesia employed to effect loss of sensation in the lower limbs. The needle is inserted into the sub-arachnoid space between the fourth and fifth lumbar vertebrae; cerebrospinal fluid is allowed to run out and, when flowing freely, the necessary drug is introduced by means of a 10 c.c. syringe (see fig. 216, p. 646).

Post-operative care. Nurses are sometimes worried as to the position in which a patient should be nursed after a spinal anaesthetic. The position he lies in whilst the anaesthetic is performed and during the operation depends entirely on whether the solution employed is denser than the cerebrospinal fluid as is stovaine, and some solutions of percaine, or whether it is less dense, as are the weaker solutions of percaine. This difficulty is dealt with by surgeon and anaesthetist; but, as the effect of the anaesthetic will be abating when the patient returns to bed, the position in which he is nursed does not depend upon the anaesthetic factor, though, since the drugs used may result in serious lowering of blood pressure, it is inadvisable to sit a patient up for fear of collapse; and it is for this reason that the foot of the bed is elevated on blocks for several hours after the spinal anaesthetic has been administered.

Sacral anaesthesia. This is similar to spinal anaesthesia and is similarly administered. It is used for operations on the perineum and its surrounding parts. The needle is introduced into the lower part of the spinal canal.

Basal narcotics. *Pentothal sodium* is given by the intravenous route immediately before the induction of general anaesthesia, in order to render the patient sufficiently unconscious to allow the subsequent deepening anaesthesia to proceed smoothly. Avertin, nembutal, pernocton and evipan are also sometimes used for a similar purpose.

THE PREPARATION OF A PATIENT FOR A GENERAL ANAESTHETIC AND OPERATION

An operation is a very serious matter; it is an ordeal which may be described as an injury to the general physical wellbeing of the patient. In many cases the ultimate result of an operation will be an improvement in health; nevertheless at the moment it is done it constitutes an injury. It exposes a patient to the condition of surgical shock which is largely brought about by repeated painful stimuli reaching the central nervous system. The patient may be anaesthetized and therefore does not feel this pain, but the stimuli produce their ill effects, and these are shown in the lowered blood pressure and the interference with the depth of respiration culminating in surgical shock.

The patient who is returned to the ward from an operating theatre is not just an operation case but a person who has been seriously hurt, and nurses should try to realize the injury sustained by cutting the skin and tissues beneath it, and, however gentle it be, the constant manipulation of delicate structures with knife, forceps and fingers, knowing that each injury which would cause pain in a conscious person is productive of almost similar exhaustion of the central nervous system in an unconscious person. The administration of a general anaesthetic helps a little; some forms of anaesthesia, such as local and regional, help considerably to prevent painful impressions from passing along the afferent nerves, with resultant injury to the central nervous system. The description of the various terms given above is intended to help nurses to know the value of the choice of the different forms of anaesthetization available.

The handling of certain tissues, particularly all nerve matter, serous membranes and the perineal region, results in a very rapid fall of blood pressure and consequently gives rise to a more serious condition of shock than does the handling of other types of tissue.

General preparation. The condition of the teeth, tonsils, heart and lungs and of renal efficiency will be investigated, and any treatment required will be performed some weeks beforehand. The patient should be made familiar with the conditions under which he is to live in the days immediately following his operation. In some instances it may be necessary for the patient to have complete rest in bed; in others it will be sufficient if he lives in the ward, getting used to sleeping in a ward with others, and becoming accustomed to the unusual sounds and so on. His temperature should be taken morning and evening so that any deviation can be noticed. He should have a daily bath, his urine should be tested, particularly for the presence of acetone, sugar, and albumin, and his bowels should be regulated if necessary by the use of an aperient to which he is accustomed. In some instances a special diet may be required, to improve the condition of the stomach, and in practically all instances fluids should be given freely. A woman should not be operated upon either immediately before or during her menstrual period.

The *prevention of fear* is highly important and it is avoided to a great extent by having the patient in hospital two days beforehand. Fear should not be mentioned, and the nurse who says 'Don't be frightened, you will be all right', is no psychologist. True peace of mind is induced by the confident, businesslike way in which surgeons, sisters and nurses perform their work in the preparation of the patient for operation, and such confidence can be drawn from the knowledge that they have successfully done the same for many others that the patient naturally comes to anticipate the same success in his own case. This attitude of complete confidence is conveyed to the patient by manner and by action rather than by words. If a patient asks questions about his operation he should be openly but carefully, thought not guardedly, answered.

More immediate preparation. During the two days of waiting a comparatively light diet is usually given; the bowels being regulated by a dose of a mild aperient 48 hours before the date of operation, thus leaving the night before operation free of anxiety with the possibility of obtaining restful sleep. It is essential for the patient to have a good night's sleep, and to ensure this some surgeons order a sedative.

The last meal should consist of bovril and toast, or tea and toast, and if the operation is at ten o'clock in the morning this may be given at 6 or 7 a.m. If the operation is in the afternoon this small meal may be given at 11 a.m.

Some surgeons give an alkali such as sodium bicarbonate and plenty of fluid with glucose several days beforehand in order to prevent the possibility of acidosis; and especially in the preparation for operations on the alimentary tract, when food may have to be restricted for some days after the operation.

Whenever the complication of sepsis is anticipated the systemic administration of penicillin is begun on the day before or in the early morning of the day of operation and continued afterwards as long as is considered necessary.

Immediate preparation. Half an hour before the anaesthetic is administered an injection of morphia or atropine or a combination of both is usually given. The dose of morphia may be $\frac{1}{6}$ to $\frac{1}{4}$ of a grain, and the dose of atropine $\frac{1}{120}$ or $\frac{1}{100}$. Morphia allays the patient's fears, and renders him drowsy so that he does not think or worry and is therefore less predisposed to shock. Atropine inhibits the secretions and limits the amount of mucus present in the respiratory tract.

Alternatively pre-operative medication includes omnopon $\frac{1}{3}$ grain and scopolamine $\frac{1}{150}$ grain.

Before this injection is given the patient should be made ready in the clothing in which he is to be taken to the theatre, and as chilling must be avoided this usually consists of a woollen jacket and leggings in addition to the nightshirt or nightdress—the latter should be cotton and of a shape that can easily be rolled up over the trunk when the abdomen is to be operated upon. The bladder should be emptied, but in operations on the lower part of the abdomen, particularly when a midline incision is to be made, a catheter should be prepared as it may be considered advisable to empty the bladder nearer the time of operation. A very large amount of urine may be secreted in a short time under conditions of fear such as a patient is to some degree experiencing in spite of all effort made to the contrary. Some surgeons like the patient to be catheterized and the catheter spigoted and left in the bladder so that the bladder may be emptied easily immediately before the first incision is made.

The patient's hair should be suitably arranged—in some instances it should be covered by a bandage or special cap; long hair is best plaited on each side of the head, all jewellery except the wedding ring should be removed. At the last moment, as the patient is placed on the trolley or wagon on which he is to be conveyed to the theatre, any dentures should be removed and put safely away in a bowl of antiseptic lotion. The patient now being ready for the theatre, the hypodermic injection is administered, and after this he should lie quietly and be disturbed as little as possible.

The nurse then collects the necessary bedcards and any X-ray photographs or other evidence of the patient's condition which may be required in the theatre.

The preparation of a patient who is to have an operation performed under a local anaesthetic is very important. He will naturally be apprehensive, and fear that he will be hurt or may have to look at unpleasant sights and that he may lose his nerve. No suggestion on the part of doctors or nurses should contribute to these fears, and if he speaks of them he should be gently but confidently reassured.

The patient should rest before the operation and have a good night's sleep; his bowels should be in regular working order, but he should not be given strong and unusual aperients. He need not be prepared by any preliminary starvation or purgation, and may have a meal which satisfies him a short time before the operation, but his stomach should not be over full.

For the hour or two immediately preceding the operation he should be kept as quiet as possible, undisturbed by noise or other sensory impressions. If necessary his bed should be placed in a quiet corner of the ward. About threequarters to one hour before the time of operation he will be permitted to empty his bladder and have a drink of water; he will then be put on to the apparatus on which he will be moved to the operating theatre. This may be a stretcher, and in this case the theatre canvas will be put beneath him as he lies on the bed; or it may be a special trolley or bed on which he will be gently wheeled to the theatre. When comfortably arranged he will be given the sedative ordered such as morphia gr. $\frac{1}{6}$ to $\frac{3}{4}$, omnopon gr. $\frac{1}{3}$ to $\frac{1}{2}$, or scopolamine $\frac{1}{120}$ to $\frac{1}{100}$. He must then be left entirely undisturbed, and should be advised to lie with his eyes closed. Some surgeons suggest that the patient's eyes be covered and a little oiled cotton wool put into his ears in order to prevent sensory impressions from reaching his brain. The reason for soaking the cotton wool with oil is that dry cotton wool is apt to move and make a gentle crackling sensation which is irritating. When the time comes the patient should be quietly and gently moved to the operating theatre, all talking must be avoided *en route*, and all unnecessary speaking avoided in the theatre. The movements of surgeons, doctors and nurses should be as noiseless as possible.

Preparation of the skin (see fig. 217, p. 647). The preparation of the skin has undergone a good deal of change since the days of Lister. He prepared it by washing with 1–20 carbolic and applying a lint compress of the same lotion.

At the present time it is usual to *shave the skin*, and for this the razor should be sterile. Either an ordinary or a safety razor may be used. When possible it is advisable that the patient should have a bath after the skin has been shaved, as this will render his body quite free from stray hairs.

Some surgeons do not require any further preparations, others like an *antiseptic preparation of the skin* to be carried out. Many different preparations are used, including the aniline dyes, iodine and picric acid. A common routine in practice is:

(1) To wash the skin thoroughly with warm water and liquid soap, then dry it with wool. Washing the area of the abdomen, for example, should occupy at least seven minutes.

(2) Taking a dry wool swab saturated with methylated ether, the skin should be well swabbed in an endeavour to remove grease and get rid of as much epidermic debris as possible.

(3) Swabbing with methylated spirit in order to dry the skin as thoroughly as possible should then be employed.

(4) Finally, the prepared area should be painted with the antiseptic chosen and, when it has dried in, the area covered with a sterile towel or cloth which should be securely bandaged on. This dressing will be removed in the operating theatre. Some surgeons consider that the use of antiseptics on the skin lowers its vitality, and only permit the employment of alcohol for this purpose.

In some cases certain modifications of the above method have to be considered to meet special needs. In the preparation of an acute abdominal catastrophe, for example, handling of the anterior abdominal wall is contra-indicated, as it would cause pain and so increase the tendency to shock later on. In this case the entire preparation might be delayed until the patient was under a general anaesthetic; in less severe cases the skin might be shaved and painted with an antiseptic and covered with a sterile towel.

Preparation of special cases. *For operations on the mouth* special care should be taken with regard to oral hygiene. Any necessary dental treatment should be undertaken first, and the teeth brushed and the mouth rinsed with an antiseptic thrice daily for a week or so before the operation.

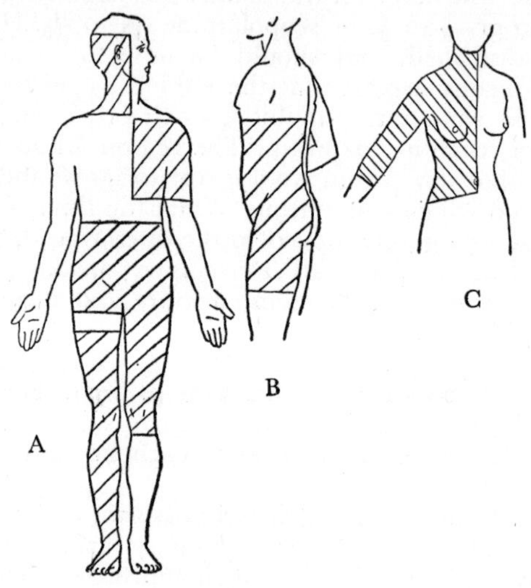

FIG. 210.

(A) Area of skin prepared for mastoidectomy, opening glands in axilla, Gallie's repair of hernia, and excision of semilunar cartilage. (B) Area prepared for an operation on the kidney. (C) For radical mastectomy.

Before operations *on the stomach* or *small intestine* the mouth should receive the same careful attention. It may be necessary to have the patient on a light diet for some days beforehand, and, in some cases of gastritis, or where there is accumulation of fetid fluid in the stomach, lavage will be ordered for two or three days beforehand.

Before operating on *the lower part of the alimentary tract*, particularly in the rectal or anal region, efforts are made to render the colon as free from food residue as possible. Aperients are usually given 4 or 5 days beforehand and repeated as necessary until 48 hours before the operation. Enemata may be used daily to clear the lower part of the bowel but an enema should not be given later than 24 hours before the time of operation. An enema given, say 6–8 hours beforehand, irritates the colon and causes spasm with the result that fluid is retained, only to be returned to the great inconvenience of the surgeon and the humiliation of the nurse as soon as manipulation of the parts is commenced. A non-residue diet may be given for from 5 to 7 days beforehand, the diet to include bland, non-irritating foods and cool fluids. In *cases of intestinal obstruction*, in which persistent vomiting is a marked feature, the stomach will be washed out before an anaesthetic can be given.

Before any operation by which the patient will be disabled during the days immediately following it, or an operation in which some specially rigid position will have to be maintained, it is most essential that the patient should be fully conversant with the conditions under which he will have to live. A case of cataract (see p. 765), for example, should be taught to use the bedpan lying flat in bed, and to take food from a vessel in the same position.

Moreover, when specially trying circumstances are to be anticipated, particular attention should be directed to the observation of the intelligence of the patient and the type of temperament he possesses, in order to note whether it is advisable to subject him to the necessary strain, or whether some less strenuous, even though it be a less useful, measure should be adopted. The responsibility is undoubtedly the surgeon's, but the nurse can do much by her observation to help him in arriving at a wise decision.

Before operations on the *genito-urinary tract* it is particularly important to test the renal function in order to determine the degree of efficiency. For this purpose the blood urea and urea concentration tests will be performed. In many of these cases the blood pressure will be raised. This also requires investigation.

In cases of low vitality and when *anaemia* is present it is important to estimate the haemoglobin content of the blood, and if necessary improve it by blood transfusion before operation. This is almost invariably carried out before operation for partial removal of the stomach where the patient has probably been subject to starvation for some time.

BREATHING EXERCISES AND PHYSICAL EXERCISES

Until comparatively recently post-operative chest complications occurred in over 20 per cent of the patients who underwent an abdominal operation, particularly after upper abdominal operations. The restricted movement of the abdomen due to pain and spasm, and the relaxation which accompanied shock tended to cause shallow breathing, and to reduce the normal range of lung expansion with resulting congestion and inflammation. Moreover patients who were getting up did not get dressed but tended to shuffle round the ward in dressing-gown and soft slippers with bent back and poking head, habits and attitudes not conducive to deep breathing.

All this is changed, because patients are now taught breathing exercises. They are taught that breathing out is important and that expiration should take longer than inspiration. Inspiration should be through the nose but expiration may be through the lips aided by a prolonged blowing sound which will help the patient to lengthen the act of expiration. The more the lung is emptied the more it can expand. General leg exercises and abdominal exercises are given as soon as possible, and should be taught in association with breathing to ensure that the patient does not hold his breath during the exercise.

Patients should be encouraged to get up and get dressed but they need to be interested and occupied; they should move, walk, work and play games. It needs very judicious handling to get some patients, who enjoy being ill, roused from this state and sufficiently interested to take their part in getting well with some degree of enthusiasm, but this is *a very important aspect of nursing*.

Chapter 44

Post-Operative Treatment and Nursing Care, including the Management of a Surgical Dressing

Post-operative nursing: position, prevention and treatment of shock, relief of discomforts following abdominal operations—Observations to be included in the nurse's report on the patient—Diet after abdominal operations—Action of the bowels—Care of the wound—Complications following abdominal operations—Management of a surgical dressing

The care of the patient after operation is a very extensive subject and will be considered under the following headings:

(1) Position of the patient.
(2) Prevention and treatment of shock.
(3) Discomforts that the patient may suffer during the first 24 hours.
(4) The report that one nurse going off duty will make to another, 6 or 8 hours after the operation. The report a nurse should be prepared to make to the surgeon 24 hours later.
(5) The diet and care of the bowels.
(6) Care of the wound.
(7) Complications.

Post-operative nursing care. After any operation performed under a general anaesthetic, nursing care includes observation of the patient's general condition and of his pulse, colour and respiration until he recovers from the anaesthetic; the arrangement of a suitable and as far as possible a comfortable position; the relief of minor discomforts which follow an operation, such as thirst and vomiting, and particularly with regard to whether the patient has passed urine; the administration of a fluid diet as soon as nausea and vomiting have ceased and the giving of a suitable aperient in order to obtain an action of the bowels as soon as convenient, usually about the second or third day. The condition of the tongue, particularly in abdominal cases, should be inspected daily; pain may need the administration of opiates; and complications should be watched for and recognized without delay.

The manner in which a patient is received back from the operating theatre is described in the routine preparation of an operation bed on p. 88. Until he is round from the anaesthetic he will be carefully watched as mentioned above, very particular attention being paid to his colour and the degree of body heat, the strength of his pulse and the depth of his respiration. Any increasing pallor or cyanosis, weakness or imperceptibility of pulse, diminution in depth and rate of respiration, or loss of body heat accompanied by the collection of beads of sweat on the skin, should be looked upon as danger signals, indicating an immediate need for restorative measures.

Position. The position in which a patient is placed as soon as he recovers from the effects of the anaesthetic depends upon the nature of his illness and the operation which has been performed. He may lie on his back in a *semirecumbent position* with a pillow under his knees after an abdominal operation. The foot of the bed may require to be elevated if shock is present. *Fowler's position* is used in cases of peritonitis, and in all other cases in which drainage of the abdomen is desirable; it is also used in the post-operative nursing care of cases of gastric and duodenal ulcer, and after other operations on the stomach, partly to relieve the operation area of the weight and pressure of adjacent organs, and partly because this position so materially helps to a general sense of wellbeing. The patient who is propped up and can see what is going on around him does not feel quite such an invalid as one who is obliged to keep quite still, lying flat in bed. Fowler's position is also adopted in cases of most elderly and stout persons in whom the development of pulmonary complications might be feared. The *prone position* is not often used, though it may have to be employed in some cases of laminectomy and is sometimes adopted for an hour or two at a time in the relief of flatulent distension of the abdomen.

Surgical shock is the complication which is so dreaded and which so much of the preparation of patients for operation is directed at preventing. The state of shock is due to depression of the vital centres, the blood pressure is low, the capillaries are dilated and even though the patient may not have bled, owing to blood stagnation the symptoms are similar to those associated with severe bleeding.

Symptoms characteristic of shock are a pale cold skin, feeble rapid pulse, subnormal temperature and shallow breathing, the face is pinched and pale, the eyes glazed and the mouth dry. The patient lies limp in his bed, he takes no interest in his surroundings, he may not be unconscious but he does not move when spoken to.

Prevention and treatment of shock. An acute abdominal catastrophe admitted for immediate operation often needs rest, warmth and blood or saline infusion as treatment for shock before operation. One of the chief considerations before any operation is to have the patient comfortable, warm, and free from fear and anxiety.

Care should be taken to prevent exposure of a patient after he has left his bed to wait perhaps in an anaesthetic room. He should be warmly clad and covered by warm blankets. He should not have to lie on a hard table but be placed on a sorbo mattress, folded blankets, or on a warm water bed. The nurse will do well to notice the high temperature of the operating theatre, and observe and imitate the care with which the anaesthetist inspects his patient before choosing the anaesthetic he will use, the gentleness with which the surgeon works and the care taken by all around the operating table to prevent exposure and unnecessary handling of the tissues under operation.

The nurse who prepares the bed to which the patient is to return (see fig. 36, p. 185), will provide materials for saline administration, and for the application of external heat and elevation of the foot of the bed in case of necessity; but the treatment for shock must often begin in the operating theatre in the form of administration of a blood transfusion or, alternatively, of intravenous saline infusion or infusion of glucose, 10 per cent. When the patient returns to the ward either of these treatments may be continued, or a less serious degree of shock may be treated by the administration of rectal or subcutaneous salines given either continuously or at regular intervals.

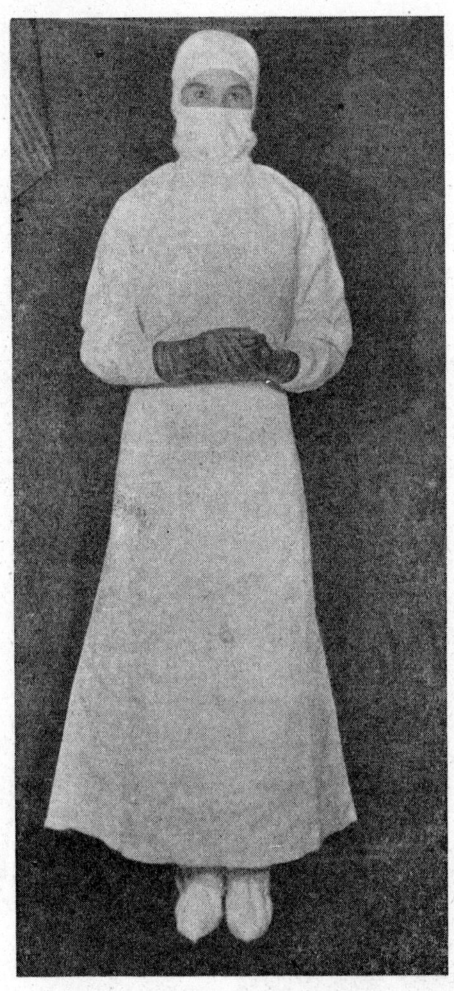

FIG. 211.—*see page* 620.
NURSE IN THEATRE DRESS: CAP, MASK, GOWN, RUBBER GLOVES AND CANVAS COVERS OVER HER SHOES.

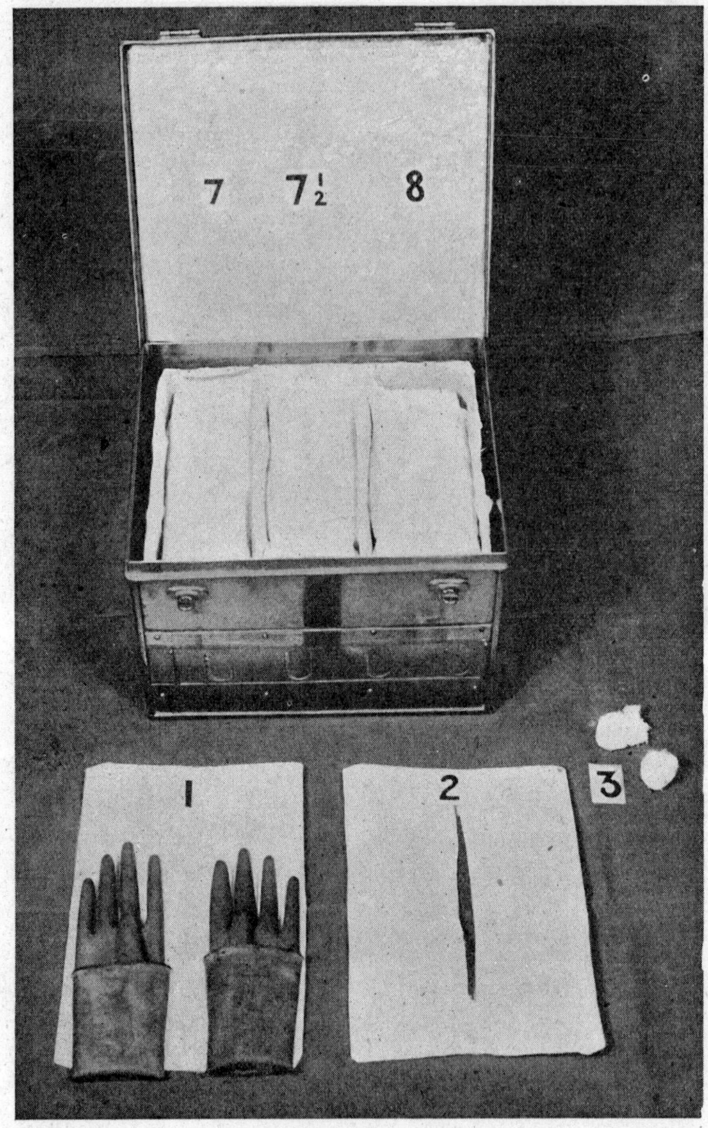

FIG. 212.—*see page* 621.

PREPARATION OF GLOVES FOR STEAM STERILIZATION.

(1) The cuffs are folded back. (2) They are placed in a glove sac. (3) A gauze packet of powder is placed in each glove sac. The gloves are packed in drums in sizes as shown.

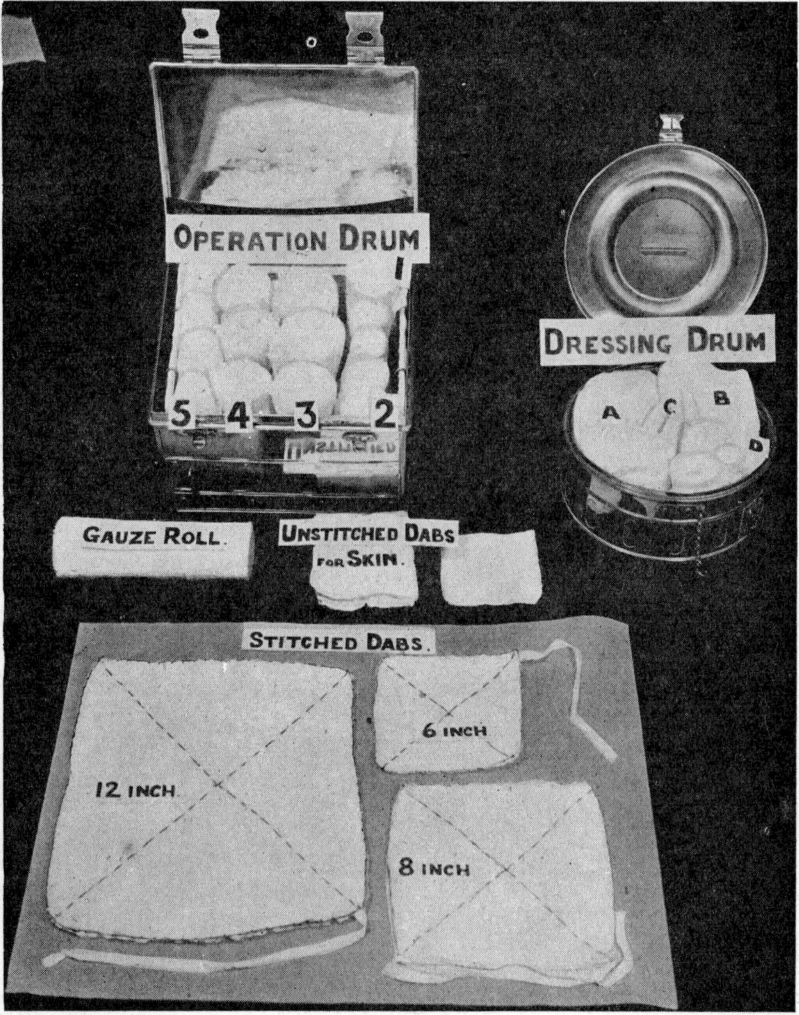

FIG. 213.—*see page* 624.

SHOWS THE CONTENTS OF AN OPERATION DRUM AND THE METHOD OF STITCHING THE ABDOMINAL SWABS OR DABS.

In the operation drum (1) gauze roll, (2) 6-inch stitched dabs, (3) 8-inch stitched dabs, (4) 12-inch stitched dabs, and (5) unstitched dabs for the skin.

The *dressing drum* contains (A) white wool, (B) gauze, (C) gauze packing, and (D) bandages.

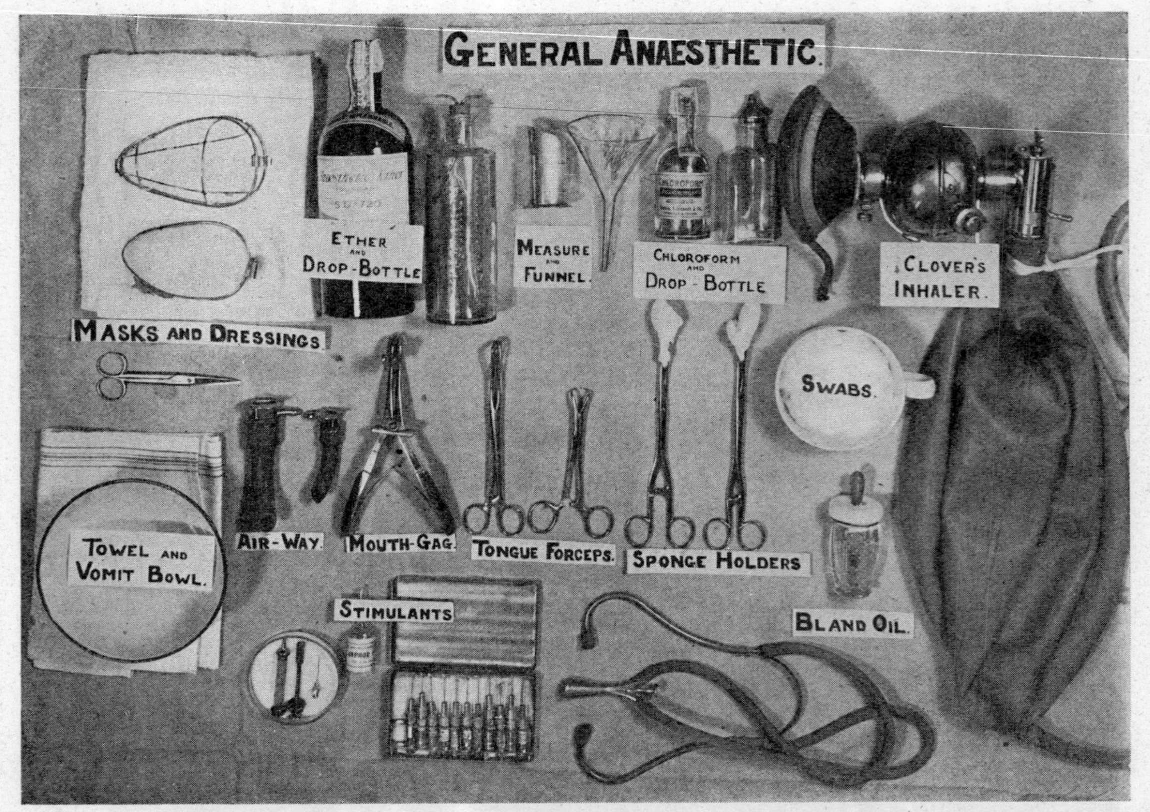

FIG. 214.—*see page* 631. ARTICLES REQUIRED FOR THE ADMINISTRATION OF A GENERAL ANAESTHETIC.

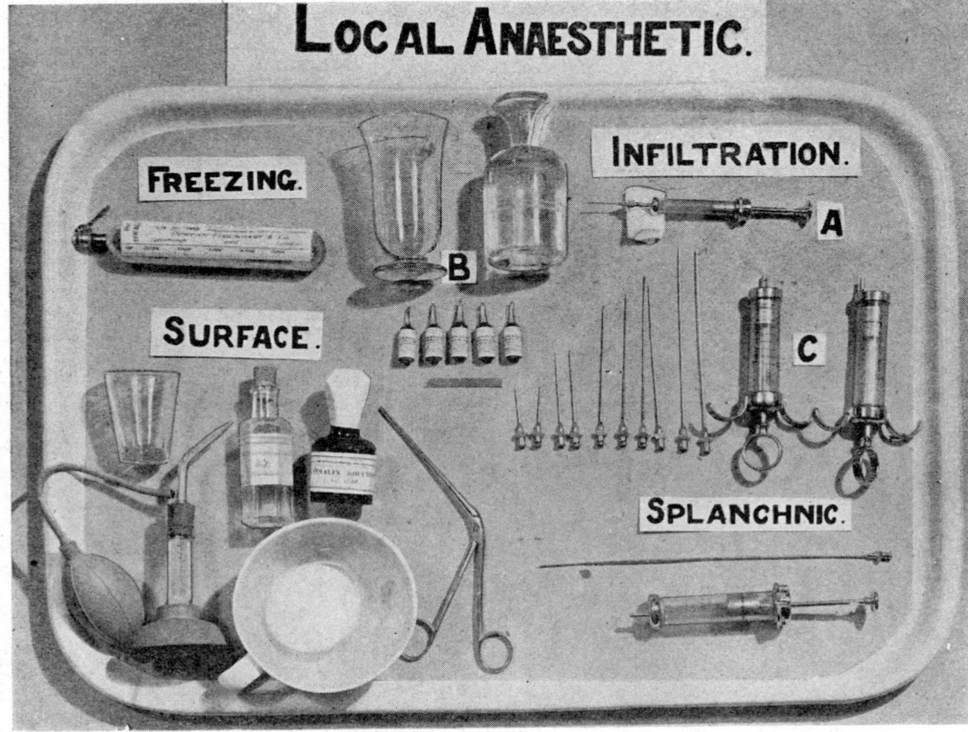

FIG. 215.—*see page* 631.
A local anaesthetic may be applied in a number of ways:
For *freezing*—ethyl chloride.
For *infiltration*—(A) a hypodermic record syringe. (B) local anaesthetic and measure. (C) two Hillman's syringes with a variety of needles of different sizes.
For *splanchnic anaesthesia* a 20 c.c. syringe and specially long needles are provided.
For a *local anaesthetic applied to the surface*—in this example to the nasal cavities and throat—the articles provided are cocaine 15 per cent and adrenalin 1/1,000, a throat spray, some ribbon gauze and a pair of nasal dressing forceps.

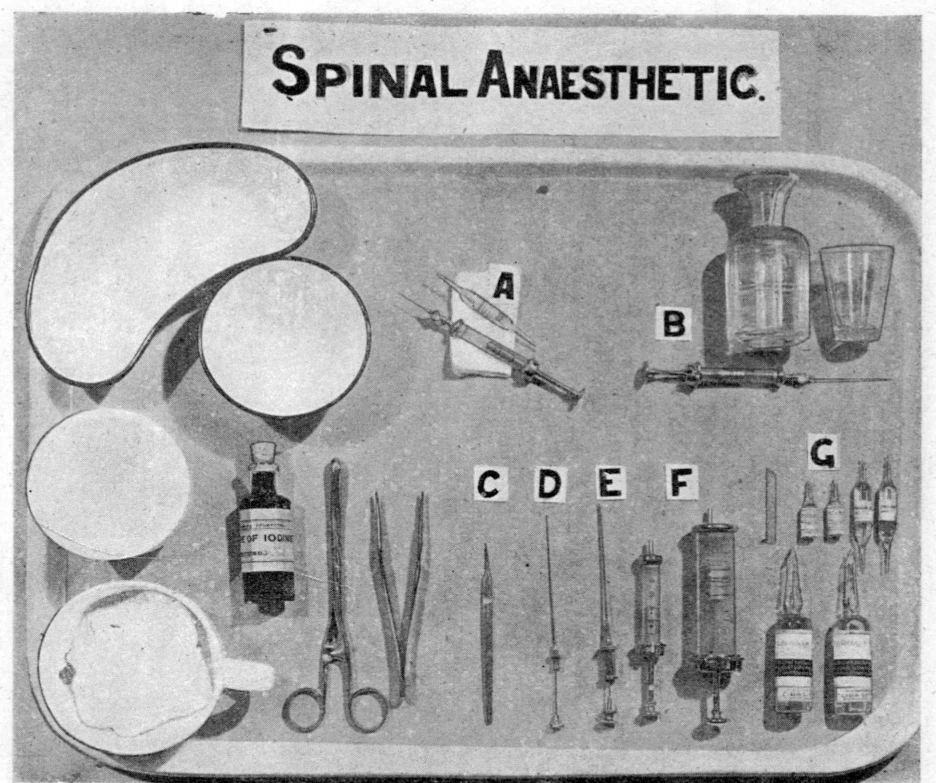

FIG. 216.—*see page* 632.
(A) a record syringe (2 c.c. capacity) and a phial of ephedrine.
(B) Record syringe (2 c.c. capacity), novocaine, 2 per cent, and a glass measure.
The special apparatus required: (C) tenotome. (D) Jones's spinal needle with stilette. (E) record syringe (2 c.c. capacity). (F) record syringe (10 c.c. capacity). (G) represents the anaesthetic used—in this instance, stovaine billon, stovaine with glucose and percaine are provided. In addition the articles needed for cleaning the skin are provided on the tray.

ARTICLES FOR SKIN PREPARATION

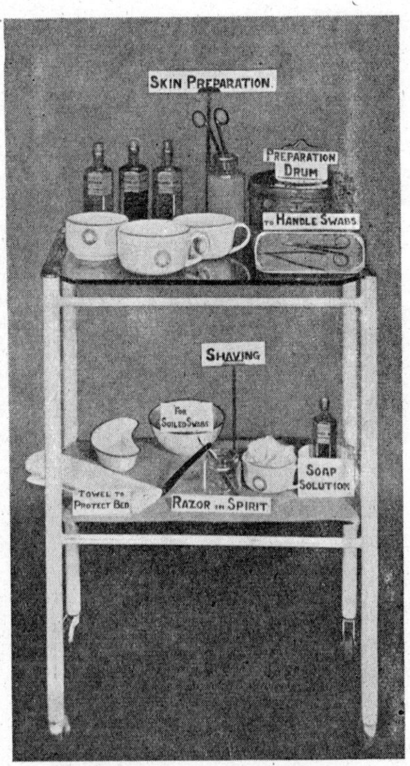

FIG. 217.—*see page* 635.

UPPER SHELF. Bottles containing methylated spirit, methylated ether and an antiseptic solution—three porringers—a preparation drum which contains sterile swabs, a sterile towel or pack for application to the prepared skin, and bandages. Forceps are provided to handle the swabs. LOWER SHELF. Towel to protect the bed and the articles needed for shaving the skin.

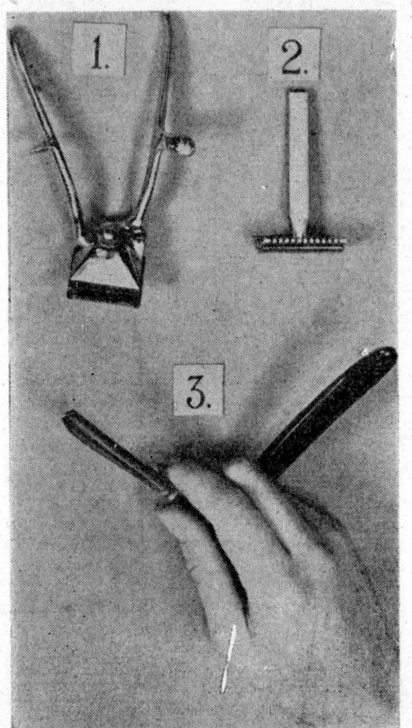

FIG. 218.

1. Pair clippers.
2. Safety razor.
3. Method of holding an open razor.

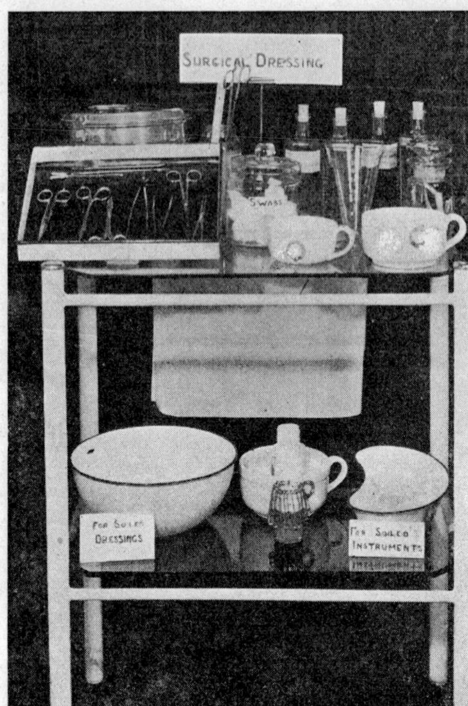

FIG. 219.—*see page* 66c The UPPER SHELF contains tray with instruments—scissors artery forceps, dissecting forceps sinus and dressing forceps, prob director and probes—also steril dressings and towels, antisepti swabs, sterile rubber tubing measure, lotions, porringers an lotion thermometer and Cheatle forceps.
THE LOWER SHELF contains band ages, safety pins and receivers.

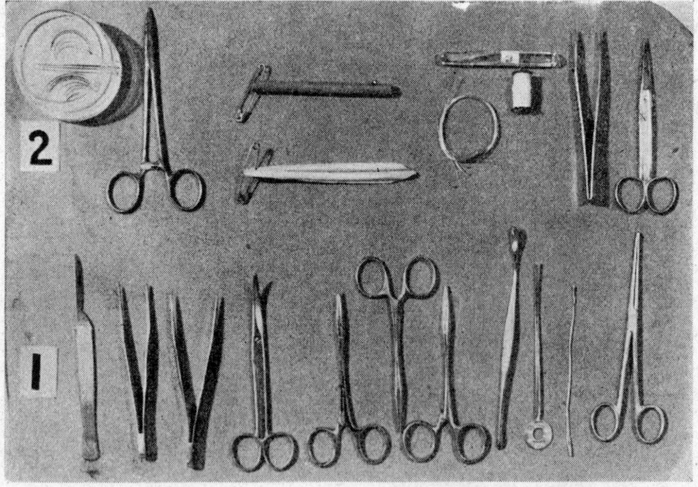

FIG. 220.—ARTICLES REQUIRED FOR OPENING AN ABSCESS.
LOWER ROW (1). Reading from left to right: Scalpel, dissecting forceps (plain and toothed), Mayo's curved dissecting scissors, several pairs of Spencer-Wells's artery forceps, Volkmann's spoon, probe director and probe, sinus forceps.
UPPER ROW (2). Surgical needles and Hegar's needle holder, drainage tubing (tubular and corrugated), silkworm gut, silk and catgut, small dissecting forceps and stitch scissors.

The nurse will wrap the patient in warm blankets, apply the electric cradle or hot-water bottles as soon as possible and when he comes round, provided that nausea and vomiting are absent, will encourage him to take small drinks, unless contraindicated, as shock is most successfully treated by increasing the volume of blood fluid.

The surgeon will order morphia which will relieve pain and discomfort and prevent painful impressions from reaching the nervous system and so may result in the induction of sleep. Cardiac stimulants, including strychnine, caffeine and pituitrin, are less commonly employed as there is the danger that they may stimulate the circulation without improving the condition of the heart and so, by whipping up a tired organ, may result in producing a more serious degree of shock.

Rest is another important nursing point. It applies to every circumstance in which a patient may be in danger of shock or already suffering from it. Movement should be limited to a minimum; when necessary it should be performed gently and as smoothly and rhythmically as possible, avoiding all jolting or jarring. Very careful consideration should always be taken before a decision is made to move a patient suffering from shock, even to change a damp drawsheet, as in the case of a patient who is beginning to respond to treatment the movement involved might very likely be sufficient to cause a relapse. Some palliative measures can be taken; for example, the insertion of a small mackintosh and towel might be made without disturbing the patient in order to prevent his lying on a damp sheet. Routine nursing measures must never be permitted to control the nursing of a seriously ill patient—each case should be individually considered.

DISCOMFORTS FOLLOWING AN ABDOMINAL OPERATION

Certain discomforts may arise after an abdominal operation which will naturally be less marked after an uncomplicated appendicectomy than after an operation for the relief of strangulated hernia, or in a case of appendicectomy complicated by peritonitis before operation.

Pain. A certain amount of pain will follow an abdominal operation because of the handling of the intestine and the incision made in the anterior abdominal wall. The nurse in charge should see that pain and discomfort are not in any way accentuated by restlessness or lying in an uncomfortable position. Every care should be taken to arrange pillows in order to provide adequate support, so that the patient's back, abdomen and thigh muscles are not strained to maintain the position. The bandage should not be too tight; the top bedclothes should be light and rather loosely arranged, pressure across the abdomen, thighs and knees or over the feet should be avoided. If a knee pillow is used it should be placed comfortably in order to support the thighs; if necessary a low bedcradle should be employed to take the weight of the bedclothes off the abdomen and in this case the patient should be provided with a light blanket next to him, *underneath* the bedcradle so that he is snugly wrapped up.

The patient should be carefully handled and the bed should never be jarred or shaken, as all such movements will cause the patient to contract involuntarily his abdominal muscles, and this movement would pull on the stitches holding the tissues together, and give rise to pain. As pain is likely to keep the patient awake, and this would delay his recovery from shock, the doctor will usually order an opiate on the first night.

Retention of urine. The abdominal wound will make the patient avoid all contraction of his abdominal muscles; the rigidly still position in which he rests in order to avoid this, combined with the fact that the nervous control of micturition may have been disorganized, partly by the depressing effect of the anaesthetic on the central nervous system, and partly because of the handling of organs adjacent to the bladder during an abdominal operation, all tend to give rise to disordered micturition and retention of urine is the form this most commonly takes. This complication may therefore be expected in many cases, and for this reason the nurse should always notice when a patient passes urine and how much he passes. A specimen should be taken and examined for any abnormality; most anaesthetics used are drugs which have to be eliminated from the body by means of the kidneys, and the renal efficiency may be slightly impaired during this process. Moreover, as before mentioned, an operation is an injury to the physical well being of the patient and is consequently a strain on the functional activity of all organs.

Treatment of Retention. The desire to micturate occurs normally whenever 8–10 ounces of urine have accumulated in the bladder; the desire may be acutely felt and yet the patient may experience difficulty because the sphincter muscle is in spasm. It is at this time that the nursing measures, described on p. 406, for the relief of retention should be applied. If the desire passes off it is probably because more urine has been secreted, and now considerable distension may occur before further discomfort is felt. It is important, therefore, to watch for distension of the lower part of the abdomen. A rapidly distending bladder should be relieved by catheterization. Most surgeons are agreed that overdistension is injurious to the bladder and prefer that it should be evacuated by catheterization.

Abdominal distension. Some flatulence will occur after every abdominal operation, due to the handling of the gut, and if inflammation is present the distension will be more marked. A very serious degree of abdominal distension will occur in cases complicated by peritonitis.

Treatment. The distension causes great discomfort, and results in tightening of any bandage the patient may be wearing; this should be loosened sufficiently to relieve the discomfort. Altering the position of the patient may give some relief. A patient who is in the recumbent position might sit up. Some surgeons allow a patient with abdominal distension to lie in the prone position for an hour or two in order to get relief. If the patient is not vomiting, some carminative such as peppermint water may be given by mouth, and in cases where the gut has not been involved in the operation an aperient may be given.

The passage of a flatus tube will relieve if gas has accumulated in the lower part of the bowel; for an accumulation higher up a turpentine enema is valuable, or some other carminative enema, including asafoetida, molasses and alum (see p. 136). *Applications of heat* to the anterior abdominal wall are sometimes employed but, unless the wound is covered by strapping and elastoplast, a hot moist application such as a fomentation would be inconvenient and might stimulate superficial bleeding.

Abdominal distension which is unrelieved by these measures is probably due to temporary paralysis of the gut. This is described as *paralytic ileus.*

It may occur in any part of the alimentary tract below the diaphragm, including the stomach. It gives rise to the symptoms of intestinal obstruction because the paralysed parts act as a block to the passage of the intestinal contents. The symptoms of this condition include marked abdominal distension, vomiting which may become persistently feculent, and absolute constipation of flatus and faeces. The pulse becomes rapid and compressible; the mouth dry and the tongue coated, and the patient is very soon in a gravely prostrated condition.

Drugs which may be ordered for the relief of distension include pituitrin, 5–10 units repeated as necessary, or eserine $\frac{1}{25}$ grain.

Hiccup. This complication is frequently associated with abdominal distension, particularly when an inflammatory condition of the gut or peritonitis is present. The diaphragm is irritated and spasmodic contractions occur, giving rise to the distressing symptoms of frequent hiccups. It is difficult to treat unless it responds to the treatment and relief of distension as described above. Sedatives may be ordered, and the administration of 7 per cent CO_2 in oxygen, five minutes in every hour, has been found of value.

Vomiting. Vomiting frequently occurs after abdominal operations, and is a cause of serious discomfort to the patient. It may be due to the anaesthetic, to peritonitis, or to paralytic ileus. *Anaesthetic vomit* is greenish in colour and smells of the anaesthetic. The patient has not swallowed anaesthetic but, because it is contained in the blood fluid, some of it reaches the stomach in its secretion. This irritates the stomach which rejects its contents.

Treatment. The treatment is to rest the stomach; food and drink, therefore, apart from small quantities of water, should not be given. Further treatment consists in attempting to neutralize and dilute the anaesthetic contained in the stomach secretions, and it is for this reason that a drink of half to threequarters of a pint of water containing sodium bicarbonate is sometimes given. Sodium bicarbonate is a gastric sedative, and sipping this solution may relieve the vomiting by settling the stomach; on the other hand it may induce a vigorous attack of vomiting as the stomach is so irritated that it rejects anything entering it, therefore the quantity given is rejected and so serves to wash out the stomach and relieve it of the irritating anaesthetic.

As vomiting is a source of loss of fluid to the body, whenever this complication arises a nurse should endeavour to administer fluid. Rectal salines are frequently administered, the provision of fluid diluting the anaesthetic in the blood fluid, increasing the quantity of urine secreted and so assisting in its elimination by means of the kidneys. Glucose is administered in all cases where vomiting is marked and persistent, as fluid starvation is likely to give rise to the condition of acidosis. Vomiting due to peritonitis or to paralytic ileus calls for special measures.

Thirst. Thirst is practically always complained of after an abdominal operation. It is partly due to dehydration owing to loss of fluid by bleeding and also to exposure of the subcutaneous tissues and abdominal contents during the operation. Thirst is accentuated by nausea and vomiting. It should be relieved as early as vomiting permits by the administration of small, frequent sips of water, by moistening the lips, swabbing the mouth and allowing the patient to rinse his mouth out and also by the administration of fluid by other routes as by means of rectal or subcutaneous saline. In the majority of cases milk or milky fluid should be avoided. Water and lemonade containing glucose may be given. A cup of weak tea will be gratefully received as it is most refreshing, and is frequently found to be more valuable in the allaying of thirst than any other means. The amount of fluid permitted will vary with the individual case.

THE NURSE'S REPORT

Presuming that the operation took place at eleven o'clock in the morning, the day nurses will have charge of the patient until eight o'clock in the evening and the report the day nurse will make to the nurse coming on night duty ought to include the following points:

(1) The drug used before the patient was operated upon, as to whether it was morphia, omnopon, or atropine and the amount given; whether a basal narcotic was given.

(2) Time and duration of operation and any untoward incident occurring at the time of operation.

(3) The time of return to the ward and the time the patient took to recover from the anaesthetic.

(4) The position in which the patient is to be nursed, and whether a knee pillow is to be allowed or not.

(5) Bearing in mind the discomforts previously described the nurse will report any *vomit*, whether this was excessive, and any treatment which was ordered for it and the effect of this. The amount of *thirst* complained of and how this was treated. Any *pain* the patient had and whether any treatment was ordered and whether the pain was relieved by this. Whether the patient has slept since the operation, the manner in which he came round and whether he was *restless*. Whether any sedatives have been employed since the operation. The time at which *urine was passed* and the amount passed and whether *any difficulty* was experienced. The presence of any *abdominal discomfort* or *distension*, and whether a flatus tube has been passed for the relief of this; any stool passed.

(6) The *temperature*, *pulse* and *respiration* are charted, and the character of the pulse whilst the patient was under the anaesthetic and coming round. Any diminution of respiration at this time, and whether the patient was a *good* or a *bad colour*. Any *cough* that may have been noticed.

(7) The *degree of shock* present at the time of operation and immediately afterwards; the response of the patient to treatment by warmth and rest. Whether any further treatment was necessary; if blocks were inserted, how long they were used and, if still in use, when they may be removed; whether any saline has been administered and if this is to be repeated and if other fluid has been administered otherwise than by mouth.

(8) Any drugs, including penicillin, that have been given in addition to the sedatives mentioned above. If penicillin is to be continued detailed instructions must be given.

(9) *The condition of the dressing*, particularly as to whether there has been *any oozing* and whether the dressing has been repacked, the presence of any drainage tubes and any orders that have been given with regard to the need for changing the dressing during the night.

(10) Any fluids that have been given, subsequent feedings that may be

used; if the patient is on a special diet the list should be given to the night nurse.

(11) Whether the relatives have inquired about the condition of the patient since the operation, and the reply which has been given to them. Indications should be given as to where the address or telephone number of the relative who is to be informed of any change is to be found.

Report to surgeon. The following are the questions the nurse should be prepared to answer and the information she should be prepared to give to the surgeon who visits the patient for the first time 24 hours after the operation.

The surgeon coming to the bedside will take in at a glance the general condition of his patient; the general attitude and position adopted in bed, the degree of interest the patient takes in his surroundings, the expression on his face, whether he is anxious and worried or calm and peaceful, the condition of the eyes, the dryness of the lips and tongue, and the state of the hands, whether they are tremulous or sweating, or lying quietly relaxed. This will tell him very much more than a chart at the bedside, although on reference to it he will see the temperature, pulse rate and respiration rate, and the action of the bowels and kidneys.

The nurse must be prepared to provide information regarding:

The degree of shock following the operation and how this was treated, and the response to treatment.

When the patient passed urine and the degree of *abdominal distension* and any treatment that has been used for this including the passage of a flatus tube —with result, and whether a turpentine enema has been employed.

Any pain and discomfort the patient experienced, and the *amount of sleep* he has had. If he had a sedative the amount and time should be stated, and the amount of sleep induced by it.

Whether the patient suffered very badly from *thirst*, and whether *vomit* was troublesome; the time when vomiting ceased and whether it was possible to give the patient fluids at the usual time, that is, about 4 to 6 hours after the operation. If vomiting has been persistent since the operation she should be prepared to specify the frequency with which it occurs, the character of the vomit, whether it is of the anaesthetic type, or whether it has become feculent.

With regard to the dressing, whether there has been oozing, and how this was dealt with; if tubes were inserted the dressing may have been changed and the nurse should be able to describe the amount of discharge present.

DIET

The diet after the administration of a general anaesthetic for whatever purpose it may have been given will depend upon the degree of nausea and vomiting present. In the nursing care of cases of general abdominal surgery, certain routine methods are adopted by most surgeons, but these should not be slavishly adhered to, and as far as possible the patient's likes and dislikes should be considered as well as his general condition.

In most cases the nurse should be sparing with fluid by mouth for 6–8 hours, allaying thirst by rectal salines, and by cleansing and moistening the mouth. Provided that nausea and vomiting have ceased she may then give small drinks, say 2–3 ounces every 1–2 hours.

Table of diet after uncomplicated appendicectomy.

As soon as the patient is able to take it, if nausea and vomiting have ceased, watery fluids, including weak tea, may be given in small quantities, for example 2 ounces every hour, or 4 ounces every 2 hours.

First day—fluids such as barley water, lemonade, soda water, weak tea, milk and water 5–7 ounces every 2 hours, with as much water as the patient will drink in addition.

Second day—very light diet such as bovril, or light soups, jelly, thin bread and butter, custard.

Third day—by this time the bowels have acted, and the patient will feel capable of taking a fuller diet; he may therefore have a little lightly steamed fish and potato, milk pudding, lightly boiled egg and fruit.

Subsequently, the diet may be increased, but large quantities of green salads or green vegetables and red meat should as a rule not be allowed whilst the patient is lying flat in bed.

Table of diet after an operation on the stomach, for example, partial gastrectomy.

As soon as he is able to take it the patient is allowed 1 ounce of water every hour, during the first day. This is increased to 1 ounce of milk and 1 ounce of water on *the second day*.

On the *third day* 3 ounces of milk and 2 ounces of water are given every 2 hours.

On the *fourth day* 4 ounces of milk and 2 ounces of water are allowed two-hourly and in addition a little jelly is given at lunch time and a beaten up raw egg at the time of the evening meal.

On the *fifth day* he is given a little light diet, including thin bread and butter and pounded steamed fish.

On the *sixth day* the diet is increased to white soup, minced chicken and baked custard.

Subsequently, the diet is increased by the addition of lightly cooked eggs, toast and butter, milk pudding, potato purée and so on.

OPENING OF THE BOWELS

If the alimentary tract is well prepared before operation, there is no need to consider the necessity of making the bowels act during the first 24–48 hours. If, however, the operation was an emergency one, the surgeon may consider ordering a small enema in order to empty a bowel which is overloaded. *In uncomplicated cases of abdominal surgery an aperient is usually ordered on the second evening following operation.* An aperient the patient has been in the habit of taking should, if possible, be used. It is important that one be employed which will not disturb the patient during the night—a small dose of cascara or infusion of senna pods is a suitable example. If a more rapidly acting aperient is used, or if the patient is likely to be disturbed by the knowledge that he has had an aperient, it should be given on the morning of the second or third day so that it will act in the day time. In either case the nurse should tell her patient not to worry about the action of his bowels or the effect of the aperient. If it does not act she should tell him it can be repeated, or a small enema may be given so that anxiety and straining at stool will be avoided. A number of surgeons order liquid paraffin three times a day from the second day until the bowels have acted, particularly after operations on the stomach or following resection of the gut, as in these cases considerably longer rest will be required. If the bowels have not acted by the fourth day a small enema is usually given. An enema is invariably ordered if there has been much distension.

CARE OF THE WOUND

A clean stitched incision usually heals by *first intention* (see p. 585). The wound is protected by a dressing of gauze and wool, but opinions differ as to the best means of retaining this in position, and incline to the use of elastoplast or Whitehead's varnish, omitting the use of a bandage or binder which so soon becomes tight and uncomfortable. The stitches will be removed between the 7th and 10th days—for method of removal, see p. 629. If there is the slightest threat of sepsis, penicillin powder will be applied.

Drainage of wounds. When a drain is employed, it is usually because infection is present, and it may be carried out by means of a gauze wick, rubber tube, or corrugated rubber tubing and, when the peritoneal cavity has to be drained, by the use either of long firm rubber tubes or perforated glass ones. The tubes should not extend very far beyond the level of the skin because, if pressed on by the dressing and bandage, discomfort will be caused.

The amount of discharge will determine the date of the first dressing, which may be done after the first 12–24 hours, the gauze and wool being changed, the tube inspected to see that it is acting effectively, and the surrounding area cleansed with antiseptic lotion. (For further details on the management of a surgical dressing see p. 660.)

COMPLICATIONS

In addition to shock and the discomforts described on p. 649–52, other complications which may follow an abdominal operation include:

Complications of a wound. Sepsis may occur in the following forms: A *stitch abscess* is infection of the puncture wound made by the needle in which the stitch lies; the treatment is to remove the stitch and either paint the inflammatory area with an antiseptic such as iodine, or apply a hot moist dressing, in the form of a fomentation. *Subcutaneous suppuration* may occur, especially in wounds in which large skin flaps have been made. This is usually due to a collection of serum and pus beneath these, which prevents healing. The treatment is to evacuate the fluid, and, if suppuration has occurred, to apply hot fomentations. *Haematoma* may occur, and when it does it is usually in the deeper tissues, where a collection of blood has been retained.

The use of *penicillin* either systemically and/or locally is always considered when sepsis may occur or does occur.

Rupture of stitches and escape of intestines. *This complication may occur early* owing to strain of the abdominal wall by coughing and vomiting, or by continuous restlessness in which vigorous movements are constantly made by the patient—wild throwing about of the legs, for example, is likely to strain the abdominal wall. In some cases the gut may escape through a small opening in the wound at the side of a large drainage tube. Gut is very slippery and elusive, and behaves rather like quicksilver once it escapes from the abdominal cavity.

When the wound gapes and the gut escapes *a week or so after the operation*, it may either be due to sepsis, or to the fact that repair of the tissues has not occurred by the time the deep catgut sutures have been absorbed. This sometimes happens in patients in whom the vitality is very low.

Treatment. Unless the nurse has experienced the care of a patient in whom this complication has occurred, it is difficult for her to visualize the degree of mental anxiety rapidly followed by prostration which the patient suffers. The first duty, therefore, is to reassure the patient, send for the doctor and, in the meantime, collect any intestines which may be lying around the patient in the bed, in sterile towels wrung out of warm saline solution. In no circumstances should the nurse attempt to undo the bandage or binder as by so doing she will permit the wound to open still more, and all the intestines will rush out. Instead, having collected all the escaped intestine in warm towels she should bring the drawsheet up against the patient's sides, in order to exert pressure on the sides of the abdominal wall and so make some attempt to help keep the wound in apposition. The surgeon will probably order morphia, and the nurse should prepare to take the patient immediately to the operating theatre. She should not attempt to get a specimen of urine, as the act of micturition is normally assisted by contraction of the abdominal muscles and this may give rise to a further escape of intestine, but she should prepare a catheter to take to the theatre.

Haemorrhage. Haemorrhage may occur. When this happens during the first twenty-four hours, it is probably due to the slipping of a ligature and will be treated by taking the patient back to the operating theatre and having the bleeding vessel tied. Bleeding may be visible—when it is easily recognized—or internal, and therefore a surgical nurse should be very familiar with the symptoms of internal bleeding (see p. 575) and so be able to recognize them before the patient is in serious danger.

Secondary haemorrhage may occur from about 7–10 days after the operation and is almost invariably due to sepsis. It also requires investigation and treatment of the bleeding vessels.

Cardiac and respiratory failure is usually preceded by *shock*, and is likely to occur mostly in seriously debilitated persons or those who have lost a lot of blood, or in whom for some other reason the haemoglobin content of the blood is low.

Paralytic ileus, as occurring in cases of intestinal obstruction, and after resection of the gut, has been previously mentioned on p. 650.

Pulmonary complications occur most usually after operations on the mouth, throat and chest, and also in elderly fat patients. *Bronchitis* is amongst the commonest. *Hypostatic pneumonia* is met in elderly persons. *Massive collapse of the lung* occurs after operations on the upper part of the abdominal cavity when the movements of the diaphragm are likely to be embarrassed.

The use of penicillin by inhalation has proved of great value in preventing chest complications.

Pulmonary embolism, which is a comparatively rare complication, is due to a clot from one of the small vessels in the vicinity of the operation area, which reaches the heart in the venous return, and is thence conveyed by the pulmonary artery to one of the lungs, where it passes along in the circulation until it reaches a vessel too small to carry it. It lodges there and the area of lung to which this vessel is passing is put out of action. This complication may occur at any time, either during the early days, a week or so later, or during convalescence. The *symptoms* of a slight embolism are dyspnoea and cyanosis; a more serious attack will seriously embarrass the heart and respiration. The symptoms may be very severe and sudden death occur.

Treatment. Dyspnoea causes the patient to sit up in order to obtain relief; he should be supported in this position by a nurse until pillows can be arranged to keep him erect. Oxygen should be administered in order to help the remaining lung to compensate for the inefficiency of the disabled part, and also to assist the work of the heart in maintaining the circulation. Morphia is given because it is essential for the patient to be kept at rest, and he must be quite still and free from restlessness and anxiety. It will also relieve the pain in the chest; in addition, hot applications are sometimes employed but, if they necessitate moving the patient, the nurse must remember that movement is definitely contraindicated.

Subsequent nursing and treatment will aim at keeping the patient quiet, and the blood pressure low. A light, non-stimulating diet and cool fluids may be given. Mild aperients should be used in order to keep the bowels acting freely or small enemata may be employed. All mental excitement must be avoided, and the nurse should therefore be very judicious in her choice of the visitors she permits the patient to have.

Lobar pneumonia is a rare complication, but *inhalation* and *aspiration pneumonia* may occur when blood and mucus have been indrawn during breathing, as may happen after operations on the mouth and throat. This variety of pneumonia is frequently of the type described as 'septic pneumonia', which is rather similar to broncho-pneumonia in which the patient runs an intermittent temperature, and has a very rapid pulse. The disease is prolonged over 2 or 3 weeks, results in marked prostration, and the temperature eventually declines by lysis.

Nursing care in preventing pulmonary complications. Even though penicillin helps to prevent chest complications it does not replace nursing care and the following points should be considered. It is very easy for the patient to be chilled, particularly when he is unconscious and anaesthetized as at this time his blood pressure is low. The special theatre clothing provided in many hospitals includes a warm bed jacket and long woollen leggings, and aims at the prevention of chilling. The patient should be warmly wrapped up as he is taken along corridors in transfer from ward to theatre and back again, and the nurse attending the anaesthetist should see that the patient's chest and the upper part of his trunk are covered before the sterile sheets and towels are placed across the table. As soon as the operation is over the nurses should remove any damp or wet clothing, replacing it by dry clothing, covering the patient and wrapping him up warmly before he is moved from the theatre.

During the days following the operation nurses must remember that the patient's vitality and consequent resistance to disease have been temporarily lowered; the strictest care should be taken to see that he is never exposed to chilling, particularly when his bed is made, when he is given the bedpan, and when the wound is inspected or the dressing changed. Every little treatment that is performed during these days and every movement of him should, if possible, be followed by the administration of a warm drink, with careful inspection of his extremities for coldness and applications of heat when necessary.

It is important to realize that the danger of pulmonary complications is increased by the presence of mucus in the respiratory tract during anaesthesia, and that the injection of atropine given beforehand is to combat this danger; but the danger does not end here, and nurses must not look on atropine as a mascot against pneumonia—the hygiene of the mouth, for example, requires very careful attention in order to prevent the inhalation of septic matter.

Uraemia may occur after any abdominal operation but more particularly so after operations on the genito-urinary tract, or when the patient has some renal disability. The *symptoms* are those of diminished urinary output, and the urine contains albumin. The skin is dry, the bowels constipated, the mouth dry and the tongue furred, the patient complains of headache and becomes drowsy and, if the condition is allowed to proceed, the patient will pass into a state of uraemic coma.

Thrombosis. Venous thrombosis of one of the veins of the lower limb may occur after operations on the abdomen and pelvis. Thrombosis may occur in a vein in the arm after radical mastectomy; sepsis is a predisposing cause of the condition, and so also is stagnation of the blood in the veins of the limbs which the patient tends to keep very still after an operation in their vicinity. In the case of the lower limbs this rigidity is often increased by the injudicious use of a knee pillow which renders the thighs immovable. When a knee pillow is employed, the knees should be extended whenever it is removed for nursing purposes.

The *symptoms* of thrombosis are pain, heat and swelling over the affected vein, accompanied by a rise of temperature and the other symptoms associated with the febrile state. The *treatment* is absolute rest to the limb, forbidding any movement, either active or passive. The limb should be elevated on a pillow and protected by a cradle bearing the weight of the bedclothes. The affected area is usually painted with glycerine of belladonna, the dressing being maintained in position by means of a many-tailed bandage made to fit the limb, which prevents any movement of the limb when the dressing is changed.

A portion of the clot may become dislodged by movement and so, travelling in the blood stream, give rise to pulmonary embolism (see also pp. 377 and 656). Therefore, in order to prevent the possibility of this complication, the patient must be nursed in a manner which would prevent any rise in blood pressure, so the diet should be light—it may be nourishing, but should not be stimulating—the bowels should be kept freely acting in order to avoid any straining at stool and the patient should not be permitted any excitement either of pleasure or anxiety.

Delirium tremens will only occur in patients who are in the habit of taking alcohol regularly, and who may be looked upon as chronic alcoholics. When an accident happens, or an operation is performed, and the system receives a shock and, at the same time, the patient is deprived of alcohol, a very serious type of delirium sometimes sets in. It is for this reason that a very careful history is taken, particularly of men patients when they are suddenly admitted to hospital, and that, if they are in the habit of taking alcohol, it is usually ordered in small regular quantities in order to try to prevent delirium tremens.

The seriousness of this complication cannot be overestimated as the prostration resulting from it is in many cases fatal.

A patient with delirium tremens begins by being unable to sleep, he then gets ill tempered and suspicious, and has hallucinations. The *treatment* as already mentioned includes the administration of alcohol; keeping the bowels acting freely by giving saline aperients; and the administration of sedatives, including bromide and chloral, hyoscine in doses of about $\frac{1}{100}$ of a grain, and morphia in doses of from $\frac{1}{4}$ to $\frac{1}{2}$ gr.

Post-operative mania. This complication is fortunately comparatively rare, but it is very serious when it does occur, as it usually necessitates removal of the patient to a mental hospital and the surgical treatment may have to be interrupted.

Sepsis. Sepsis of the wound has already been dealt with; sepsis predisposes to the complications of venous thrombosis and pulmonary embolism. In addition, *sepsis in the abdominal cavity* is a complication to be feared in all cases of abdominal surgery. The condition is accompanied by a rise of temperature and the symptoms which accompany the febrile state. In abdominal surgery the condition of the mouth and tongue are frequently inspected by surgeons and nurses; thirst, dryness of the mouth and a dirty tongue are very often the first signs of this complication.

A **pelvic abscess** or a **faecal fistula,** may complicate appendicectomy, particularly if the appendix is perforated or gangrenous. **Portal pyaemia** is infection of the liver which has reached it from an infected abdominal cavity in the portal circulation. This condition is very grave, the patient runs an intermittent temperature, intercepted with rigors, he has a very rapid pulse, sweating is profuse and there is grave collapse.

Subphrenic abscess may occur. It is to prevent the tracking of pus along the posterior abdominal wall to the diaphragm, that Fowler's position is adopted. Keeping the patient sitting as erect as possible when in this position is an important nursing point. Although a subphrenic abscess may follow appendicectomy, it is a complication most to be feared after operations on the organs of the upper part of the abdominal cavity, including the stomach and gallbladder.

Peritonitis is a very serious complication. It is most likely that infection was already present at the time of operation and, in spite of the care employed in the drainage of the abdomen, general peritonitis sets in. The *onset* is usually gradual, the *symptoms* not being very marked until the third or fifth day; the temperature then rises, the pulse rate quickens, the respiration rate increases, there is thirst, the mouth is dry and the tongue dry and dirty. Vomiting very soon follows, becoming faeculent in character and being brought up without effort. The abdomen becomes increasingly distended, painful and rigid. The patient lies with knees flexed in order to relax the abdominal wall. The arms are thrown above the head in an endeavour to help the respiratory movements which are thoracic in character, because movement of the diaphragm is restricted by the rigidly painful abdomen. Hiccup accompanies the condition, which is usually very troublesome and adds considerably to the patient's discomfort.

The *treatment* is surgical investigation of the state of the abdomen and free drainage of the cavity, the administration of rest and of fluids in order to help eliminate toxins from the body.

Nursing care. In dealing with a case of peritonitis the nurse is dealing with a very seriously ill patient, who is suffering from toxaemia and markedly prostrated; in addition he is inconvenienced by persistent vomiting, hiccup, and a painful, distended abdomen.

The administration of fluids becomes a difficulty as the stomach rejects anything that is put into it, and fluids must therefore be administered by various other channels. In some instances the surgeon will wash out the stomach in an endeavour to rest it, and enable fluids to be taken by mouth; in other cases he will provide some continuous drainage apparatus in order to keep the stomach empty. The patient may have constipation or he may suffer from diarrhoea—in the former instance the nurse should be prepared to empty the bowel by small enemata daily.

The persistent vomiting and the high temperature rapidly result in marked emaciation, thus enhancing the tendency to bedsores, which must be carefully prevented. The skin requires care as perspiration is profuse. Rigors have to be treated as they occur, the nurse keeping a careful record of temperature, pulse and respiration, and being constantly at the bedside of the patient who, by nature of his condition, is very restless and irritable, his senses are acutely active, and he frequently requires nursing attention in an attempt to obtain relief from the many discomforts he is suffering.

THE MANAGEMENT OF A SURGICAL DRESSING

In a surgical ward a dressing trolley is always in readiness and, as soon as it has been used, soiled articles are washed, sterilized and replaced, so that the wagon or trolley is always ready for action (see fig. 219, p. 648). It usually contains the following articles:

Sterile towels, dressings and antiseptic swabs.

Mackintoshes for protection of the bed.

Sterile bowls for lotions and swabs.

A sterile receiver in case a sterile specimen is required and non-sterile receivers for instruments, etc.

Instruments, ready sterilized and placed in spirit or some antiseptic solution, such as lysol. These instruments should include Cheatle's lifting forceps, Spencer-Wells's artery forceps, dissecting, dressing and sinus forceps, probes, directors and scissors.

Sterile rubber tubing or some other provision for draining.

Bandages of different types, some non-sterile ones, with safety pins attached, and others sterile in the dressing drum, with safety pins ready sterilized in the instrument dish.

Antiseptic lotions, and materials for cleansing the skin, including methylated spirit, methylated ether, ether soap and iodine. One or two glass measures.

Boracic powder.

A lubricant, such as sterilized vaseline or glycerine.

Sterile test tubes.

A receptacle for soiled dressings and another for used lotions.

The surgeon may wish to do some of the dressings himself, or on other occasions the ward sister may wish him to see some of them, but as a rule dressings are done by the sister or house surgeon who are attended and assisted by one or two nurses in training. Nurses are permitted to do simple dressings at first, and senior nurses, as they become proficient, will be allowed to do more difficult ones under supervision.

A patient usually and quite naturally dreads the first dressing, but the nurse as she makes the necessary preparation for it can do very much to relieve his mind and allay his fears. She should move quietly and without fuss, and thus by her manner inspire him with confidence—an occasional nod and smile and cheery word will probably succeed in setting him almost at ease.

In completing the preparations she will bring to the bedside everything likely to be needed, carefully explaining, if necessary, that they will not all be used on him. She will screen the bed so that the patient is not exposed to the gaze of others in the ward.

The bedclothes will then be arranged—if, for example, an abdominal wound is to be dressed, the top bedclothes will be turned down to the level of the upper part of the patient's thighs, leaving the pubes covered with a sheet and one blanket which can be turned over out of the way at the last minute. The patient should have some extra clothing on the upper part of his body which should be so arranged that it can be pushed up out of the way; the nightdress should be rolled up under the patient's arms or the pyjama jacket folded back.

The patient should be lying in the semirecumbent position with his arms by his sides. He should be comfortable and the nurse should question him as to whether a little support either 'here', or 'there', is not an improvement. The bandages should then be loosened or removed. When the surgeon or sister who is to do the dressing is ready to begin, the nurse will fold the lower clothes down and the upper ones back, and remove the already loosened bandage. She should lift off the top covering of wool with forceps, place it in a receiver, then hand the towels which the operator will arrange round the area to be dressed—partly in order to protect the bedclothes from being soiled and partly in order to ensure an aseptic surrounding of the part, and a place on which instruments or dressings can be placed if desired.

The nurse having collected everything necessary at the bedside, with knowledge of the details of the steps of the procedure, hands each article as needed. After the dressing the nurse will help to replace the bandage. She should then give the patient a drink if he is allowed one, and as she remakes the bed should note whether his feet are warm, and whether his hot-water bottle needs refilling. The articles used should all be quickly removed, and the things that the patient may have been using, such as reading materials, be placed within his reach.

Surgical Dressing Rooms. It would be ideal if all surgical dressings could be performed in a special room, adjacent to the ward, set apart for this purpose. This is not always possible and the following instructions entitled '*Routine for Surgical Dressings*' as carried out in Sheffield are repreduced here by the courtesy of Professor Price and the Matron of the Sheffield Royal Infirmary.

ROUTINE FOR SURGICAL DRESSINGS

Infection in wards is carried by:

(1) 'Droplets' from the nose and mouth.
(2) Hands, instruments, and utensils.
(3) Dust.

Therefore

(1) All the 'Dressing Team' must wear a mask.
This must be put on after the hands have been rendered socially clean by washing. Do not touch the face or mask again after it has been put on, and, when removed the mask must be put at once into the receptacle provided and not used again until it has been washed and re-sterilized.
(2) All dressings must be done with sterile forceps.
(3) The routine dressing round must not be commenced until at least one hour after the beds have been 'made' and the floors swept. Ward doors and windows are closed to prevent draughts during 'dressings'.

Order of Dressings:

(1) Clean wounds without drainage.
(2) Clean wounds with drainage.
(3) Infected wounds.

FIRST-TIME DRESSINGS SHOULD BE DONE FIRST UNLESS KNOWN TO BE ALREADY INFECTED

Technique. Sterile towels must be placed so that the dressing area is shut off from bed linen and blankets.

The Dressers wash their hands until socially clean and then rinse them in the solution provided.

The Dressing is done with forceps.

After the dressing, the used instruments and utensils are washed and boiled for two minutes before being used again.

The dressers again wash their hands under running water as hot as can be comfortably borne. They are dried on a sterile towel after being rinsed in the solution provided and then proceed to the next dressing.

STERILE GLOVES MUST BE WORN FOR ALL SEPTIC CASES

The Assistant places the patient in position, so that the breath and droplets from the patient cannot contaminate the wound. The superficial dressings are removed and later reapplied by the assistant after the dressers have finished.

The Trolley Attendant hands out the towels, instruments and dressings with Cheatle's forceps, and using another pair of forceps removes the dirty dressings into the receptacle provided. These dirty dressings are removed from the ward immediately the dressing of each case is finished.

NOTE. Plasters should not be removed in the ward.
Gloves and gowns should be worn when dirty linen is sorted.
Syringes and needles used for injection must be kept separately from those used for aspiration.
Sterile instruments should be kept in the solution provided.

MAKESHIFTS MAKE MORTALITY

Painful Dressings. In some instances an anaesthetic may be necessary for the performance of a dressing, as for example in children, in the first dressing after operation for mastoiditis and in the first dressing of an amputation. In other cases, pain may be lessened by the administration of a hypodermic injection of morphia, as for example, in the first dressing for the removal of a vaginal packing after Wertheim's hysterectomy has been performed, and in cases where a large area of bone has been gutted, as in the surgical treatment of osteomyelitis.

Large dressings with flaps and drainage tubes. Some cases such as amputation of the thigh or radical mastectomy will have large skin flaps which have been separated from the tissues beneath and turned back during the operation. These flaps have been deprived of blood for some time, and, when brought back over the surface which has been operated on, and placed in apposition, they may not adhere to the underlying tissues. It is important in dressing such cases to observe whether the flaps appear to be adhering or whether they are ballooning from the underlying surface—which would indicate a collection of serum. In most cases the surgeon will have inserted a drainage tube of some description, either a circular rubber tube, or corrugated glove tubing. The nurse should note whether the tube is acting as an effective drain, or whether the area into which it has been inserted has been blocked by clot. In this case she might move the tube gently, or if it is not stitched in she might take it out, sterilize and reinsert it, or it might have slipped out. In all cases where the nurse is dealing with large flaps, she should gently palpate the surface in order to detect the pocketing of serum and, by smooth even stroking movements, direct this fluid in the direction of drainage.

Another point is that in some instances a considerable area of superficial tissue may have had to be removed, and the amount left to form flaps may require considerable tension in order to bring the edges into apposition. In this case the nurse must watch carefully to see whether the tension stitches are exerting too great strain or pressure on the skin. If the edges are separating she might devise some means of easing the tension on the sutures. In some cases, the flaps are bound to separate and a skin-grafting operation will probably be performed later.

In other instances the flaps may have been considerably bruised. This renders them moist and sloughing may occur. It is a very important nursing point in these cases to keep the tissues as dry as possible, sulphathiazole powder is applied. Dry tissues being a less suitable medium for the growth of organisms, healing is more likely to take place.

With regard to rubber drainage tubes, it is always necessary to see that they do not become adherent to the tissues in which they are placed. In the case of amputation of breast, the tubing is for superficial drainage purposes and will usually be taken out in 48 hours. In the case of nephrectomy, the tubing is deeply placed in the tissues and can be slightly shortened, about $\frac{1}{8}$ or $\frac{1}{4}$ of an inch every day, until it can come out. After cholecystectomy has been performed, corrugated tubing may be placed between the muscles at the side, below the operation incision. In this way bile is prevented from collecting round the actual wound, and any bile will drain away between the muscles with less likelihood of the formation of a biliary fistula. When cholecystotomy has been performed it will be necessary to provide for the drainage of bile from the wound for some days. In this case Paul's tubing may be used and the bile conducted into a bottle at the bedside.

In cases of laparotomy for the relief of peritonitis, or the removal of a perforated appendix, several tubes will be inserted, both in front and at the side of the abdomen. Those at the side will usually be taken out and replaced each day, the one in the middle line probably being stitched in. In dressing the wound a syringe with rubber tubing attached should be placed through the tube in order to draw off fluid by suction. On the third or fourth day the stitch holding the tube will usually be cut and the tube moved and, once pus has ceased to drain and only serum is now being obtained, the tubing will be removed and a smaller one inserted.

Spirit dressings. An application of spirit covered by jaconet and wool is employed in the treatment of local septic conditions. It is used both in mild forms as when a septic finger may be imminent and by the antiseptic action of the alcohol or spirit this may be prevented from developing. It is also used in the treatment of serious and advanced septic conditions, as when employed as an application to a carbuncle for example.

The precaution of warning the patient of the danger of fire should be taken. A man with a spirit dressing on his face should not light a cigarette, as it may set fire to the dressing. A person with a spirit dressing on the finger should not, for example, approach near to a fire, or use matches.

Collodion dressing. Collodion is often used for the purpose of sealing small puncture wounds such as are made when performing lumbar puncture or exploration of the thorax.

Flexile collodion, which is composed of pyroxylin, castor oil, ether and alcohol, a very inflammable mixture, is the variety employed. As this will not adhere to a moist surface it is essential to dry it first, then the collodion may be painted on with a brush, or poured on to a circular piece of gauze or lint which is placed on the wound; sufficient collodion should be used to seal the edges of the cotton dressing and bind it to the skin all round. Collodion can also be employed to arrest bleeding from small cuts; in this case the skin on each side of the cut should be pinched up between the thumb and finger, wiped free of blood to dry it, and with the edges in apposition a collodion dressing is applied. When firmly set the tissues are released, and the firm collodion dressing maintains the parts in apposition and so arrests the bleeding.

Whitehead's varnish. This is another gluelike preparation which contains, in addition, iodoform. It is a very useful dressing for wounds on the face and whenever a wound requires protection from wetting or friction. To apply, a layer of cotton wool is placed over the wound and the varnish painted over this, taking care to seal the margins of the cotton wool down on to the surrounding skin where they will adhere.

For information regarding lotions, powders and pastes used in the treatment of surgical dressings see pp. 625–8.

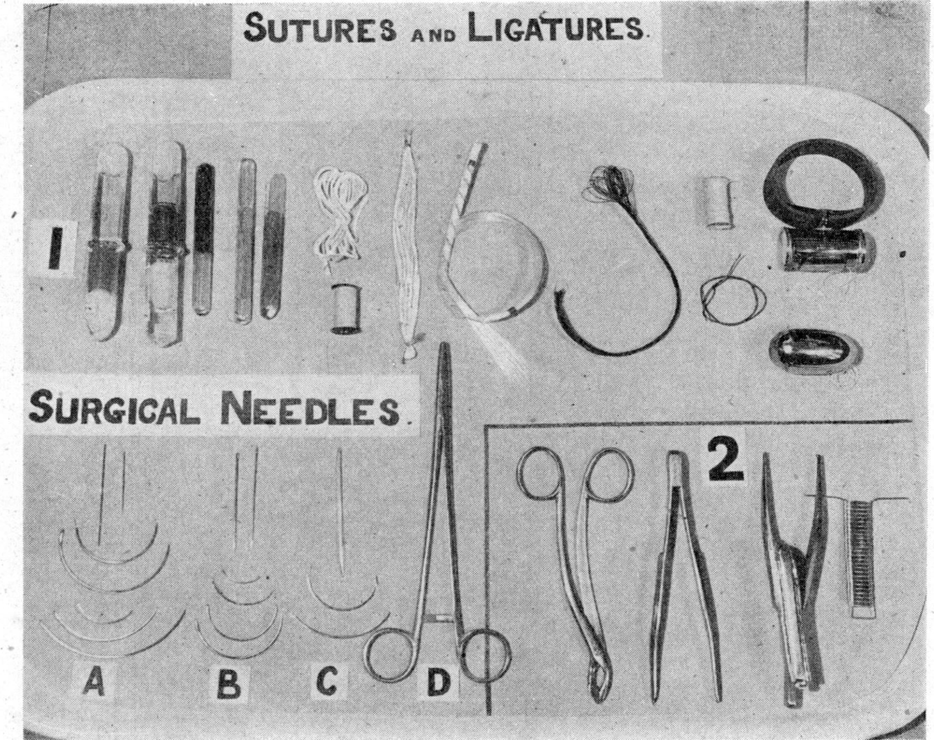

FIG. 221.—*see pages* 628–9.

Reading from left to right:—

UPPER ROW. (1) Samples of material. London hospital 'chorda' catgut, plain and chromicized, kangaroo tendon, plain and chromicized catgut, strong silk for fixation purposes, a reel of linen thread, lymphangio-plasty silk, silkworm gut horsehair, a reel of linen thread, silver wire. Two ligature carriers are shown at the end of this row—(*upper*) Bonney's wristlet and (*lower*) an egg-shaped carrier.

LOWER ROW. Surgical needles—(A) cutting needles, (B) round-bodied needles, and (C) Hagedorn's needles; (D) is Hegar's needle holder.

INSET, on the same row (2)—reading from left to right: clip removing forceps, Berkeley's clip forceps, Berkeley's clip galley charged with double Michel's clips and some single Michel's clips.

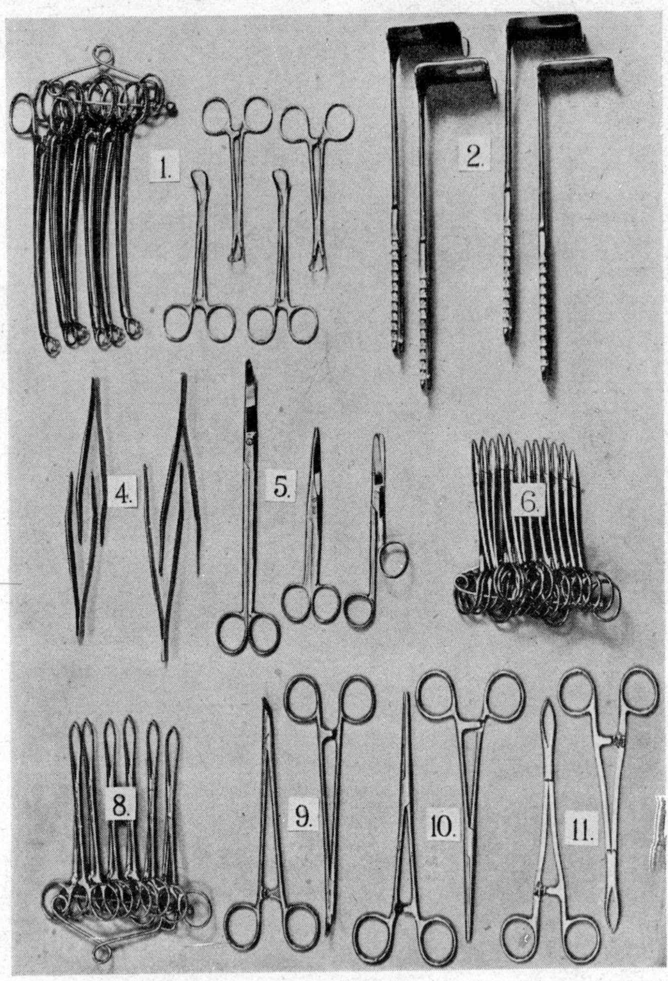

FIG. 222.

Reading from *left to right across both figures:*—

(1) Fagge's towel clips, 6 pairs; Backhaus' clips, 4 pairs. (2) Retractors: 4 Morris's, 2 Langenbeck's, 2 Mathieu's, and 3 pairs Durham's. (3) 2 Bard-Parker's knives. (4) Dissecting forceps, 2 plain and 2 toothed. (5) Thomson-Walker's, Mayo's and Kocher's scissors. (6) 1 dozen small and large Spencer-Wells's artery forceps. (7) Lane's tissue forceps: 4 small, 2 large. (8) 6 pairs Poirier's tissue forceps.

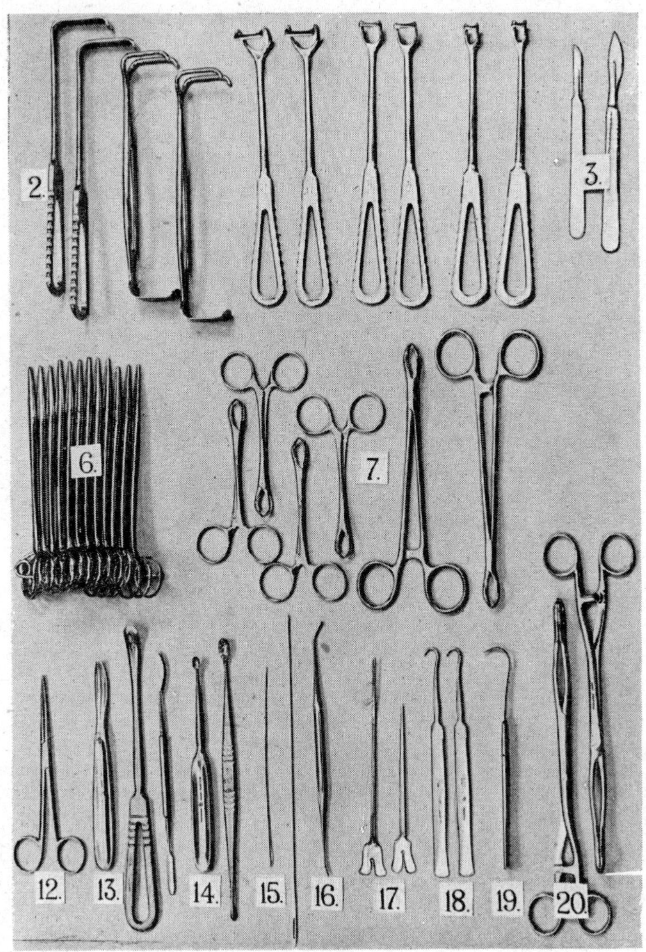

FIG. 223.

Reading from *left to right across both figures:—*

(9) 2 pairs Moynihan's gall bladder forceps. (10) 2 pairs Ochsner's compression forceps. (11) 2 pairs Littlewood's tissue forceps. (12) Sinus forceps. (13) Lane's, Syme's and Macdonald's raspatories. (14) Sharp scoops. (15) Slender probes. (16) Watson-Cheyne's probe. (17) Brodie's director and winged director. (18) Hooks. (19) Aneurysm needle. (20) Ovum forceps.

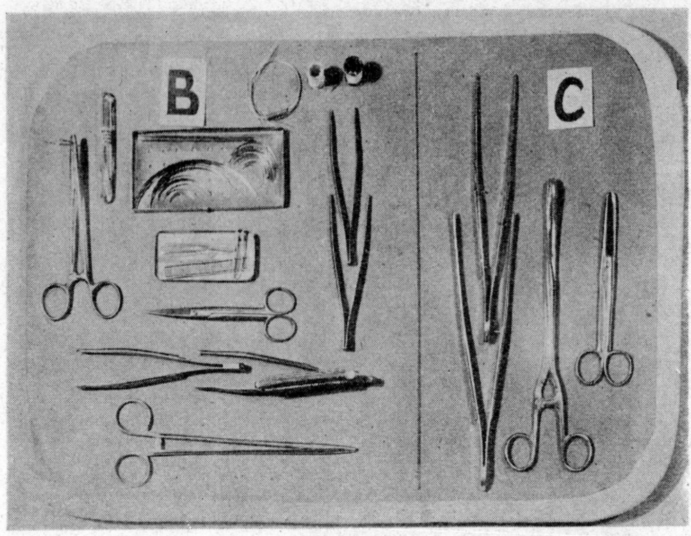

Fig. 224.—*see also Figs.* 222 *and* 223.
(B) Articles required by Theatre Sister
(C) Articles required by Ward Sister.

(B) The theatre sister may be required to prepare ligatures and sutures. Here she will need the following (reading from left to right):

Upper Row. Hegar's needle holder (*small size*), catgut, tray of assorted needles, silkworm gut, silk and thread and two pairs small dissecting forceps.

Below this Row. Reading from above downwards, are shown: stitch scissors, Berkeley's clip galley (ready charged) and clip forceps, and Hegar's needle holder (large size).

(C) The ward sister responsible for the patient will need large dissecting forceps, dressing forceps for handling dressings, dabs and swabs and scissors.

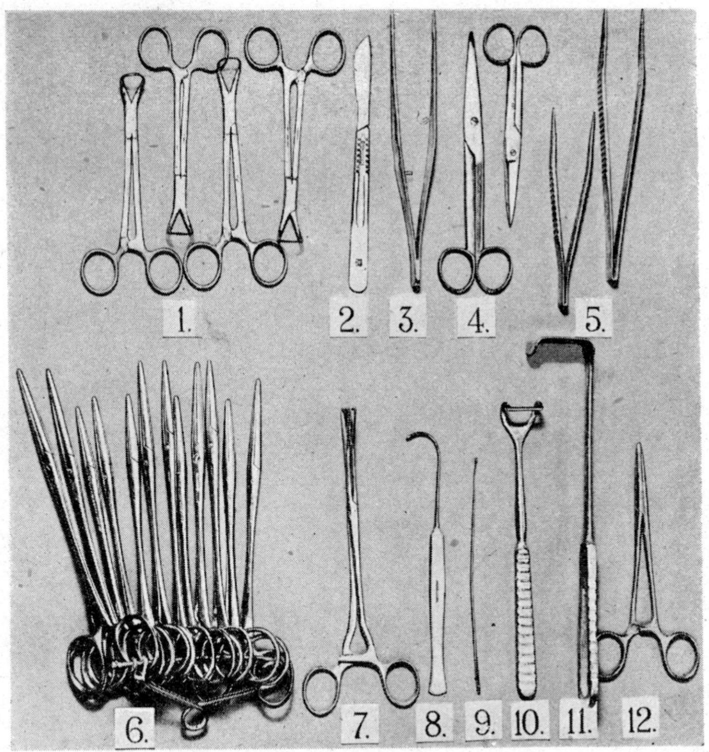

FIG. 225.

INSTRUMENTS FOR APPENDICECTOMY (*minimum requirements*).

(1) Four pairs Mayo's towel clips. (2) Bard-Parker's knife. (3) Toothed dissecting forceps. (4) Mayo's dissecting scissors. (5) Plain dissecting forceps. (6) One dozen Spencer-Wells's artery forceps. (7) Duval's tissue forceps. (8) Aneurysm needle with which to thread the appendix stump ligature. (9) Probe with which to touch the appendix stump with pure carbolic. (10) Durham's retractor. (11) Morris's retractor. (12) Hegar's needle holder.

In addition, materials for ligature and suture and needles must be supplied (*see Fig.* 221).

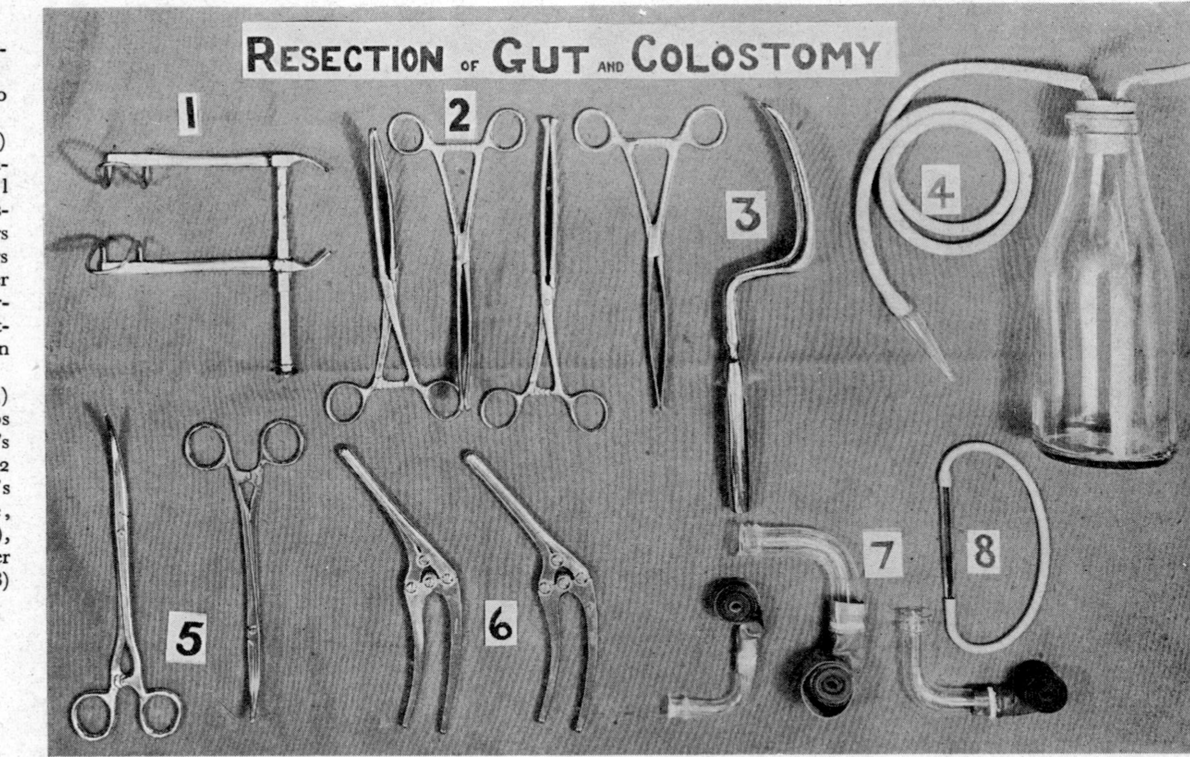

FIG. 226.—*see also general instruments, pages* 666–7. Reading from left to right:—

UPPER ROW. (1) Gosset's self-retaining abdominal retractor, (2) Intestinal clamps (2 pairs straight, and 2 pairs curved), (3) Liver retractor, (4) Aspirating bottle, for attachment to suction apparatus.

LOWER ROW. (5) Duodenal clamps (2 pairs), (6) Payr's crushing clamps (2 pairs), (7) Paul's tubing (large, medium and small), with tubular rubber tubing attached, (8) colostomy rod.

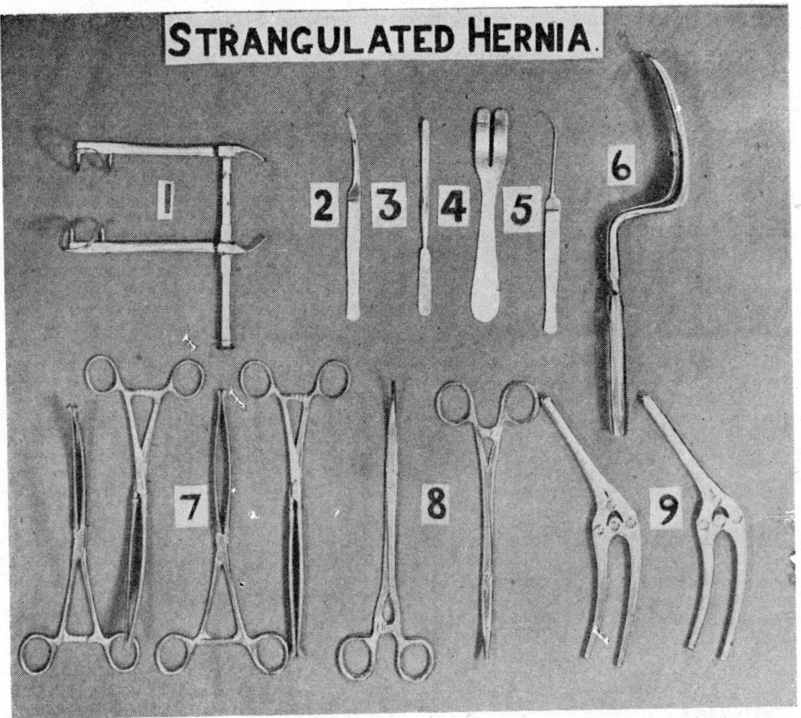

FIG. 227.—*see also general instruments, pages* 666–7.

Reading from left to right:—

UPPER ROW. (1) Gosset's self-retaining abdominal retractor, (2) bistoury, (3) hernia director, (4) hernia pusher, (5) hernia needle, (6) liver retractor. LOWER ROW. (7) Intestinal clamps (straight and curved) (2 pairs of each), (8) duodenal clamps (2 pairs), (9) Payr's crushing clamps (2 pairs).

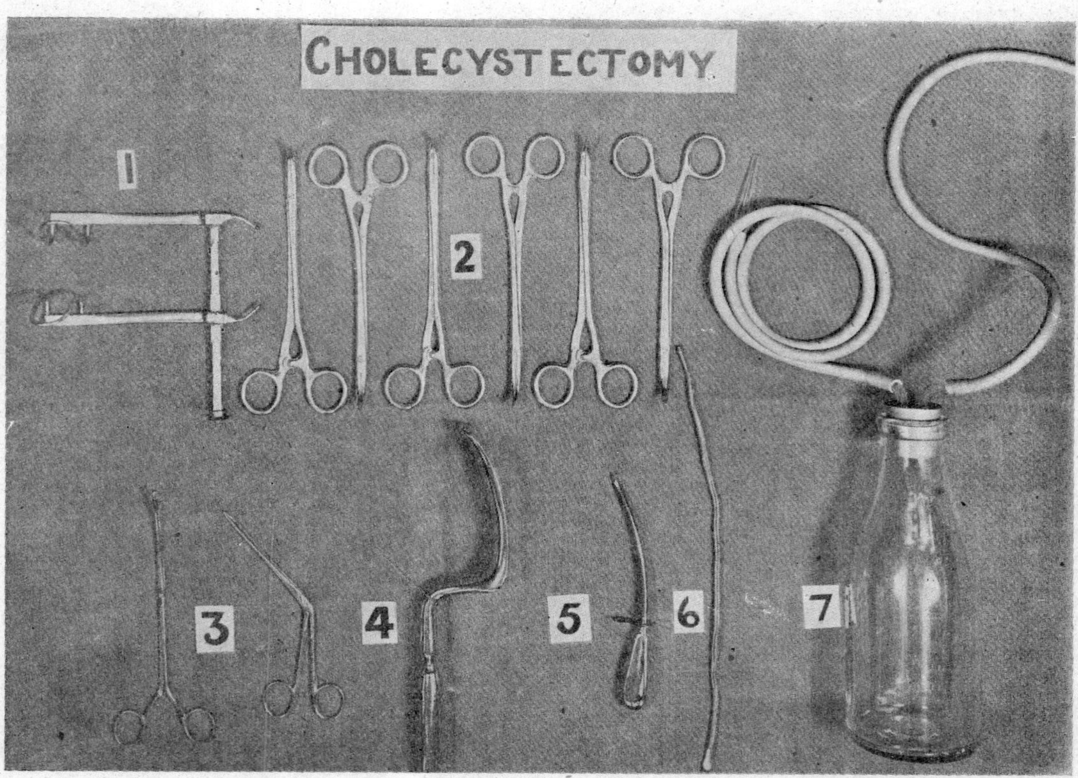

FIG. 228.—*see also general instruments, pages* 666-7. Reading from left to right:–
UPPER ROW. (1) Gosset's self-retaining abdominal retractor, (2) Moynihan's gall-bladder forceps (6 pairs).
LOWER ROW. (3) Stone forceps (2 pairs), (4) liver retractor, (5) trocar and cannula, (6) flexible lead probe, (7) aspirating bottle, for attachment to suction apparatus.

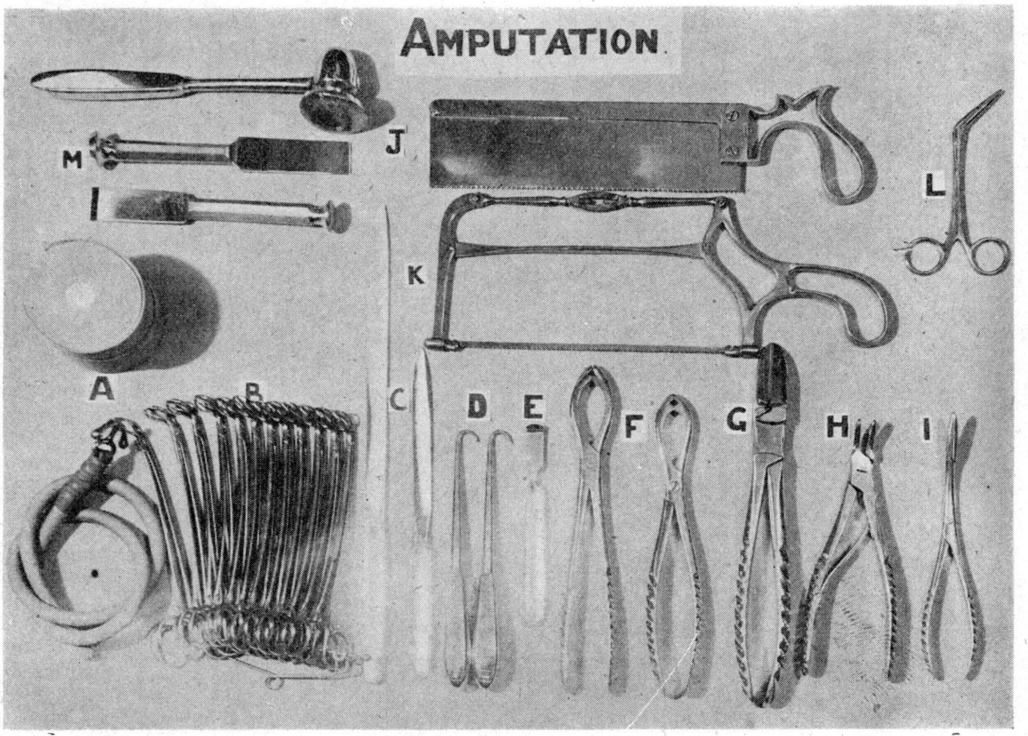

FIG. 229.—*see also general instruments, pages* 666–7.
Reading from left to right:—
LOWER ROW. (A) tourniquet and Esmarch's bandage, (B) twelve pairs of Fagge's tissue forceps, (C) two amputation knives, (D) two bone hooks, (E) rougine, (F) two pairs lion bone forceps, (G) bone-cutting forceps, (H) bone nibblers, (I) sequestrum forceps.
UPPER ROW. (M) Mallet, osteotome and chisel (various sizes would be required), (J) amputation saw, (K) butcher's saw, (L) Guy's ligature holding forceps.

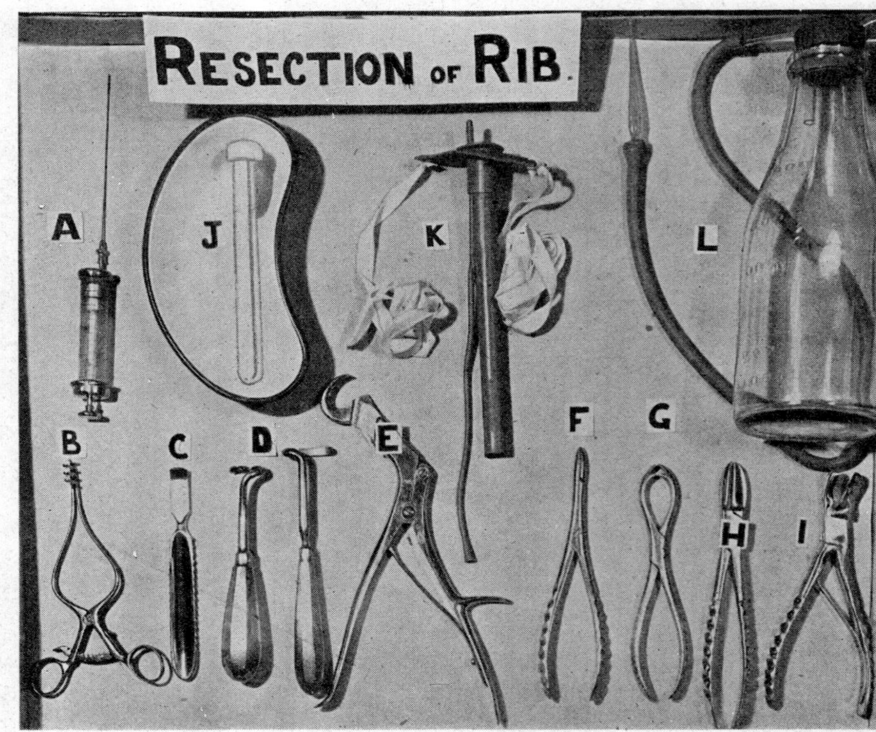

FIG. 230.—*see also general instruments, pages* 666–7.
Reading from left to right: (A) Hillman's syringe and needles, (B) Travers's self-retaining retractor (1), (C) rougine, (D) rib periosteal elevators (1 left and 1 right), (E) rib shears (1 pair), (F) sequestrum forceps (1 pair), (G) lion bone-holding forceps (1 pair), (H) bone-cutting forceps (1 pair), (I) bone-nibbling forceps (1 pair), (J) kidney tray, and sterile test tube, (K) Tudor Edwards's tube with tape attached, (L) aspirating bottle for attachment to suction apparatus.

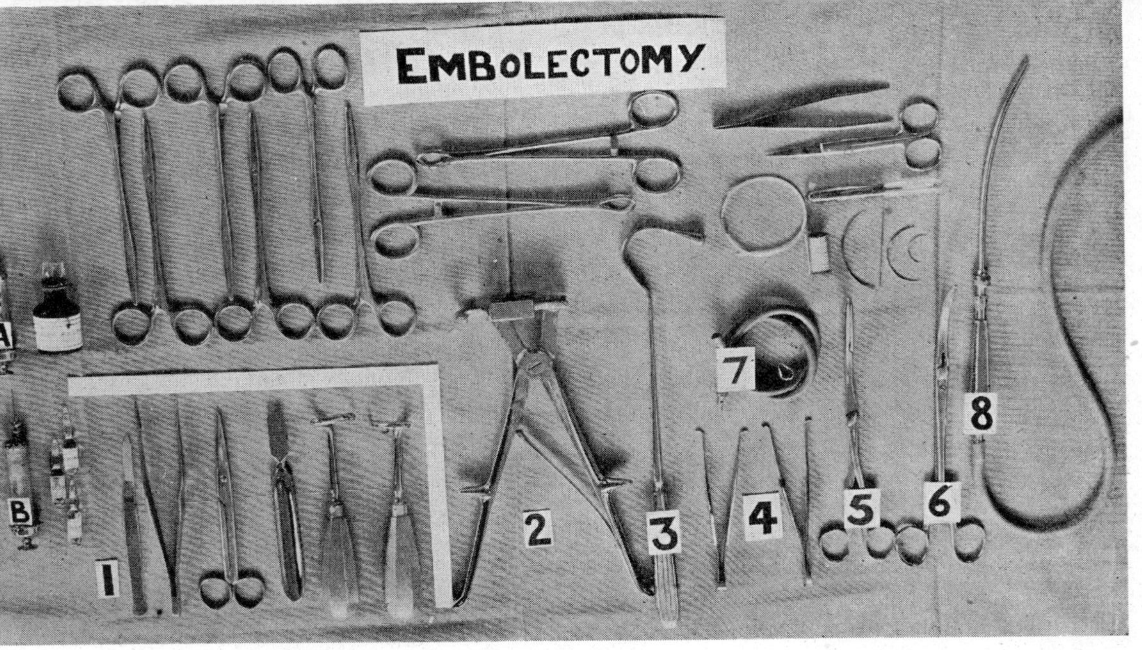

FIG. 231.—*see pages* 377–8. (1) Scalpel, dissecting forceps, scissors, rougine, and right and left rib elevators. (2) Rib shears. (3) Tension sound for use with No. 7 (stout sucker tubing). (4) Arterial dilatation forceps. (5) Thrombus forceps for removing clot. (6) Pulmonary clamp forceps. (8) Nozzle for connecting to suction apparatus employed to keep area clear of fluid. In addition on the *upper row* in illustration artery forceps, tissue forceps, and materials for ligature and suture are shown. The bottle and syringe with specially long needle marked A is for injecting adrenalin into the cardiac muscle if necessary, and that marked B is an ordinary hypodermic for administration of coramine.

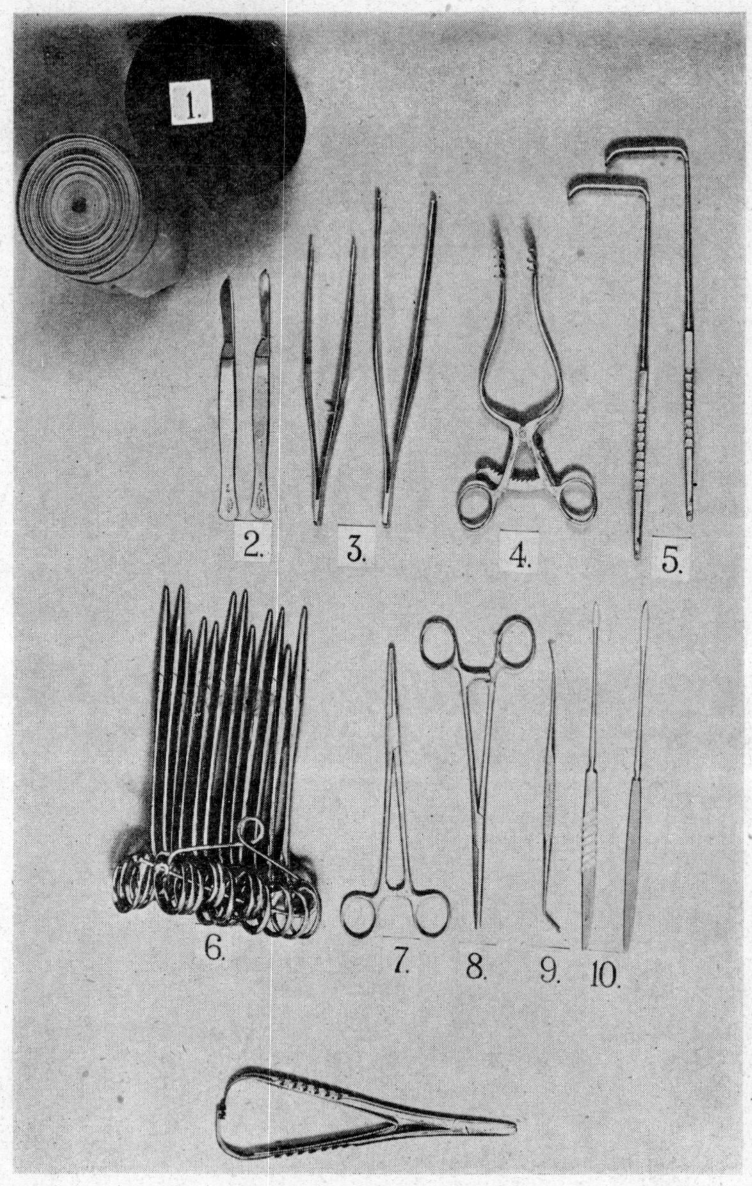

FIG. 232. REMOVAL OF SEMILUNAR CARTILAGE.

(1) Esmarch's bandage. (2) Scalpels, 1 for incising the skin and 1 for deeper tissues. (3) Toothed dissecting forceps. (4) Self-retaining retractor. (5) Deep-tissue retractors. (6) Spencer-Wells's forceps. (7 and 8) Mayo-Oschner's forceps. (9) Watson-Cheyne's probe. (10) Cleft palate knives for removal of cartilage. Alternatively a straight meniscotome may be employed which is the instrument originally made for the purpose of removing this cartilage.

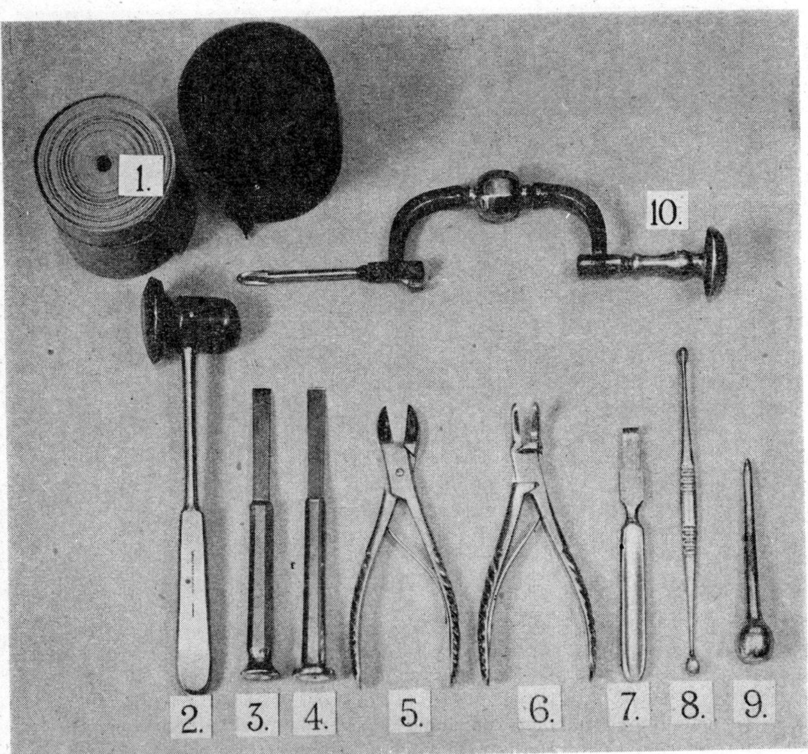

Fig. 233. Excision of Great Toe Joint.

The great toe joint may be excised in case of hallux valgus (bunion) or hallux rigidus. The instruments, in addition to the general instruments, which may be required include:—

(1) Esmarch's bandage.
(2) Mallet.
(3) Chisel.
(4) Osteotome.
(5) Bone cutting forceps.
(6) Bone nibblers.
(7) Rougine.
(8) Sharp bone scorp.
(9) Bone gouge.
(10) Bone brace and burr.

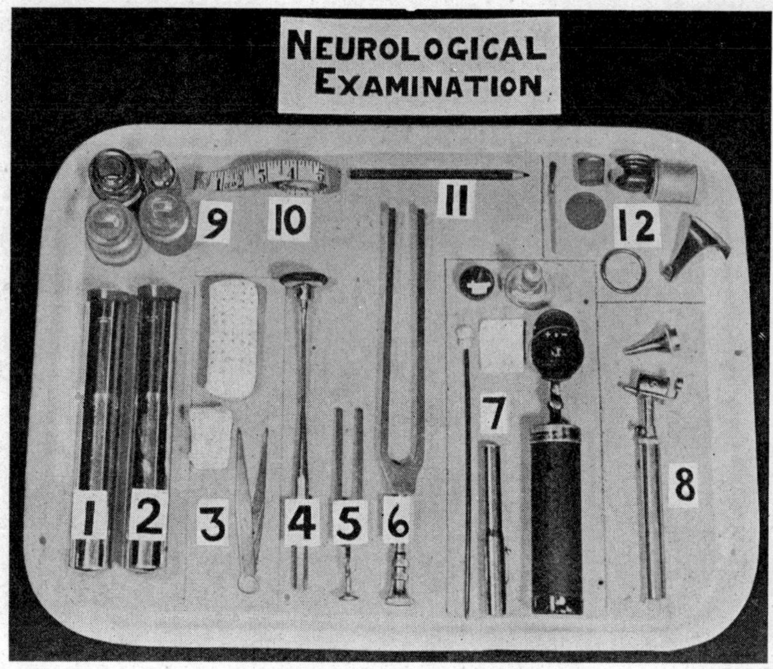

FIG. 234.—*see page* 408.

(1) and (2) are metal tubes containing hot and cold water for testing temperature sense. (3) Calipers for two-point discrimination, cotton wool for light touch and pincushion with pins for 'pinprick'. (4) Hammer for deep reflexes—tendon jerks. (5) Tuning fork for bone and air conduction tests. (6) Large tuning fork for vibration sense. (7) A group of articles for examination of the eyes, ophthalmoscope, eserine and atropine drops, rod with padded end for roughly testing the visual field, a square of fine lawn for corneal reflex and an electric torch for pupil reaction. (8) Auroscope and aural speculum. (9) Bottles containing different smelling substances to test the sense of smell. (10) Tape measure. (11) Skin pencil. (12) A group of articles of different size, shape and texture for stereognosis.

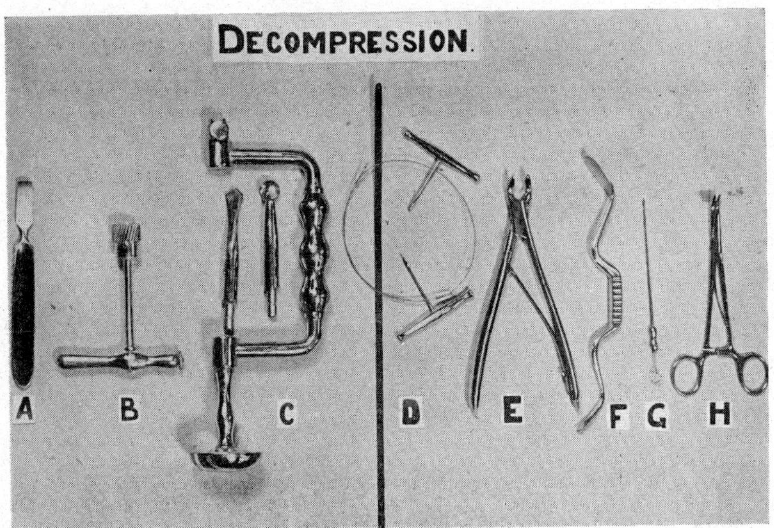

FIG. 235.

The instruments required for cranial decompression are numerous and varied. Cranial surgery is a highly specialized branch. The instruments shown above are of the simplest and include:—

(A) Rougine.
(B) Trephine.
(C) Burr and burr ends.
(D) Gigli's saw with handles and Martell's guide.
(E) Bone nibblers.
(F) Horsley's elevator.
(G) Brain needle.
(H) Silver clip forceps.

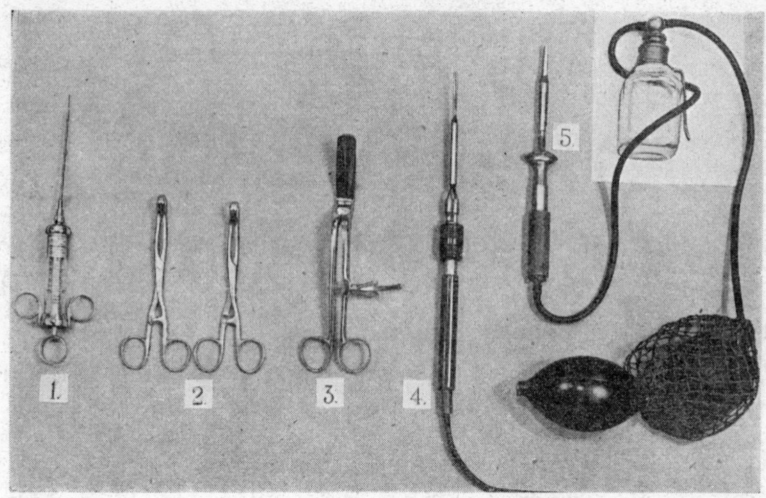

FIG. 236.

INJECTION AND CAUTERIZATION OF HAEMORRHOIDS.

The articles and instruments required include: (1) Haemorrhoidal syringe. (2) Haemorrhoidal ring forceps. (3) Haemorrhoidal clamp. (4) Electric cautery—this type is commonly employed. (5) Paquelin's thermo-cautery which may alternatively be used.

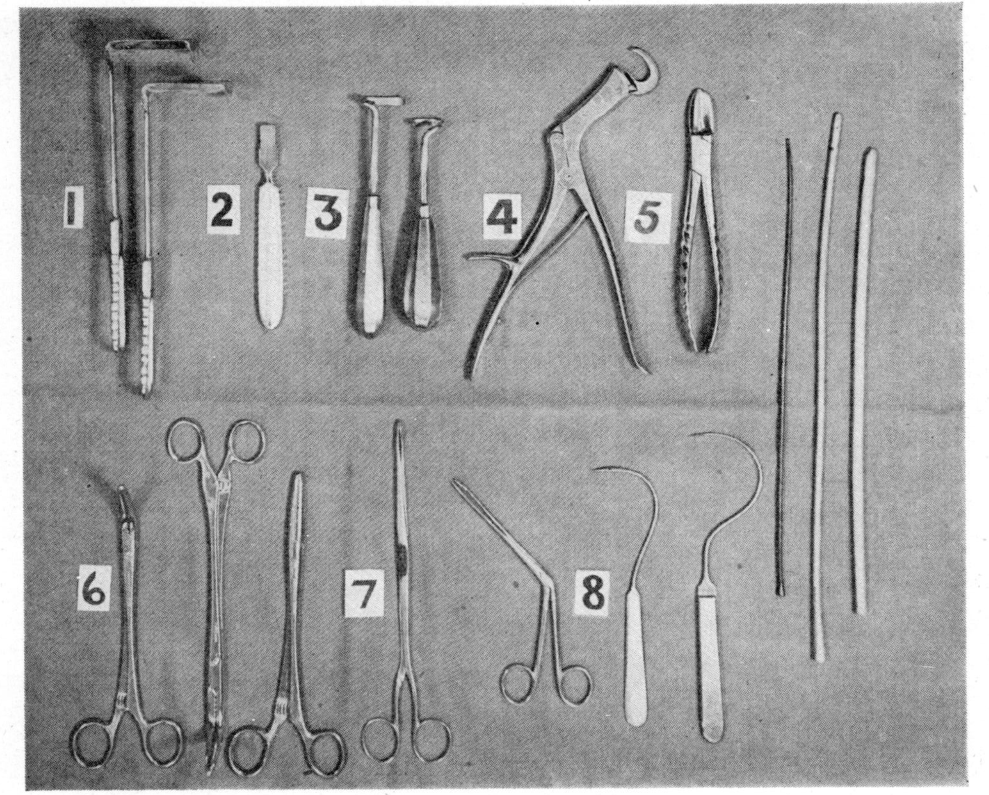

FIG. 237.—*see page* 729. (*See also general instruments, pages* 666–7.)

NEPHRECTOMY

Reading from left to right:—

UPPER ROW. (1) Two kidney retractors, (2) rougine, (3) rib periosteal elevators (1 right and 1 left), (4) rib shears, (5) bone-cutting forceps.

LOWER ROW. (6) Kidney clamps—angular and straight (3 pairs), (7) stone forceps (1 straight pair and 1 curved), (8) kidney needles.

In addition gum-elastic bougies, and catheters of various sizes and types should be provided.

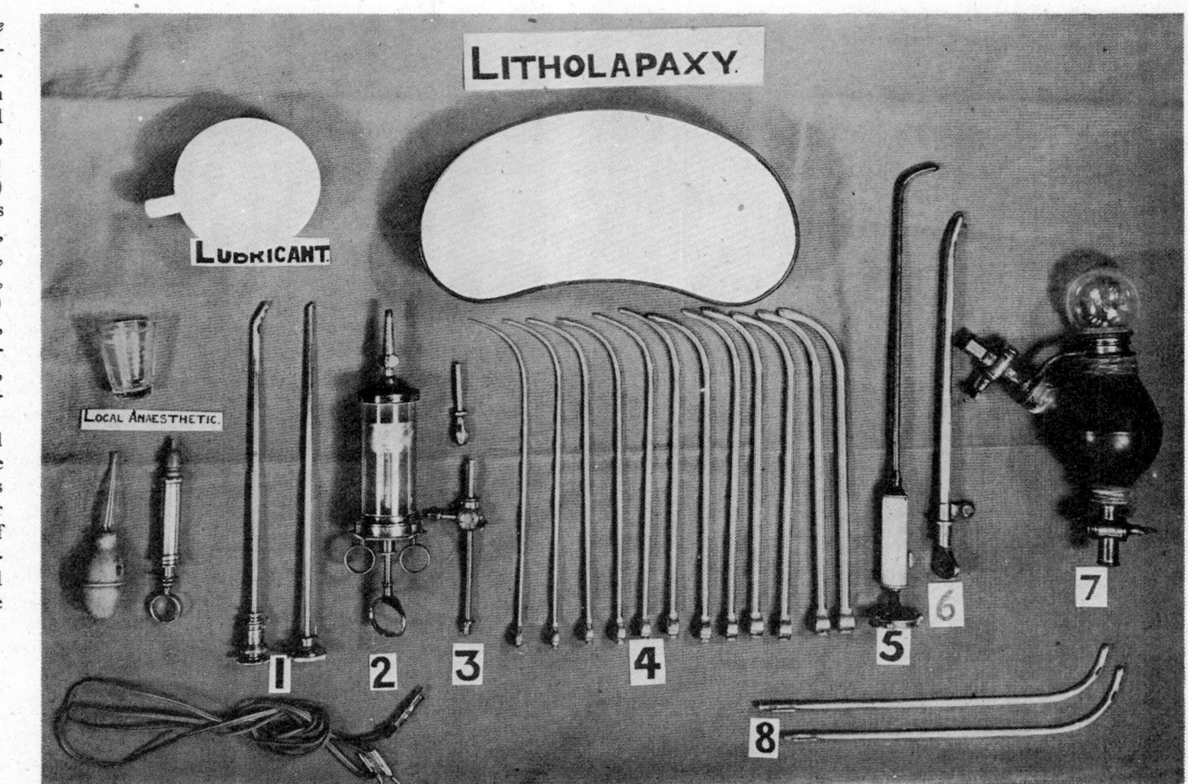

FIG. 238.—*see page* 730 (*also see general instruments, page* 666-7). (1) Cystoscope, in two parts with lead for connexion to transformer, (2) bladder syringe, (3) spigot attachments for cystoscope, (4) urethral bougies, of assorted sizes, (5) lithotrite, (6) evacuating cannula, (7) Bigelow's evacuation bladder bag, (8) prostatic catheters, different sizes. In addition, a local anaesthetic and male urethral syringes are supplied for anaesthetization of the urethra, a lubricant for bougies and a receiver for urine or fluid are shown.

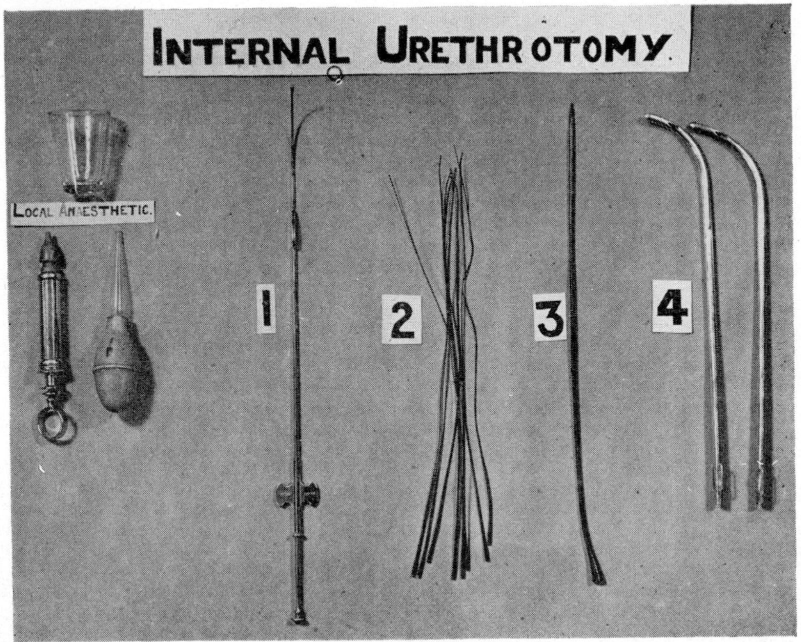

FIG. 239.—*see page* 731.

(1) Feevan's urethrotome with guide.
(2) Filiform bougies (various sizes).
(3) Guide with concealed screw for carrying filiform bougies.
(4) Prostatic catheters, different sizes.

In addition a local anaesthetic for the urethra, and male urethral syringes are shown.

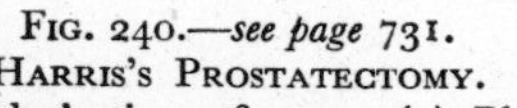

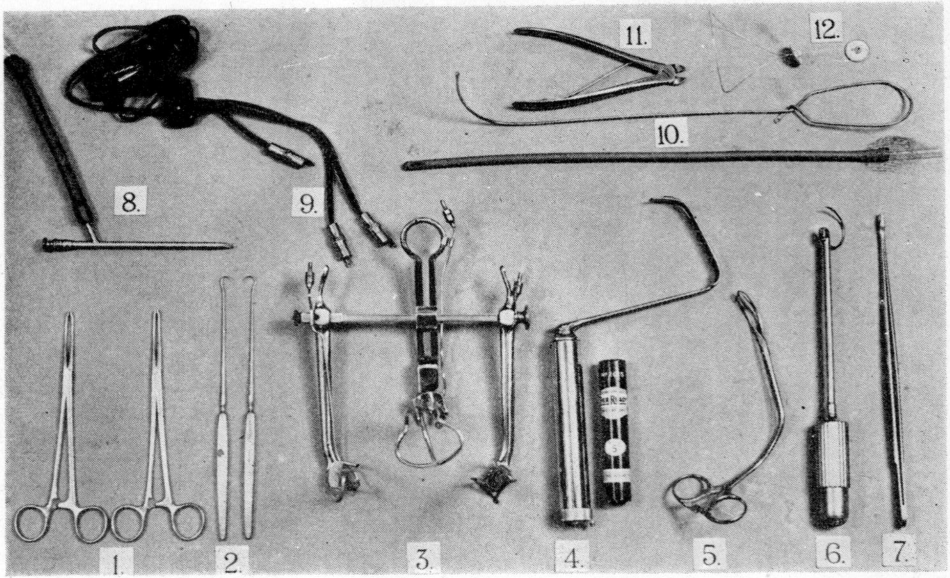

FIG. 240.—*see page* 731.
HARRIS'S PROSTATECTOMY.

(1) Taylor's tissue forceps. (2) Bladder hooks. (3) Harris's illuminated bladder retractor for back and sides. (4) Anterior bladder wall (illuminated) retractor, with battery. (5) Bladder capsule forceps. (6) and (7) Boomerang needle and ligature carrier. (8) Trocar and cannula for suction of bladder cavity. (9) Lead and electric attachment for Harris's retractor. (10) Harris's catheter with introducer. (11) and (12) Metal button for attachment of silkworm gut suture retaining catheter in bladder, and special forceps for closure of button.

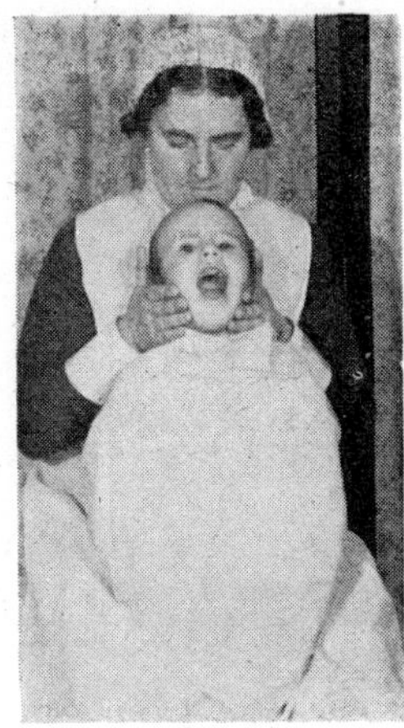

FIG. 241.—*see page* 733.
METHOD OF HOLDING A CHILD FOR EXAMINATION OF THE THROAT.

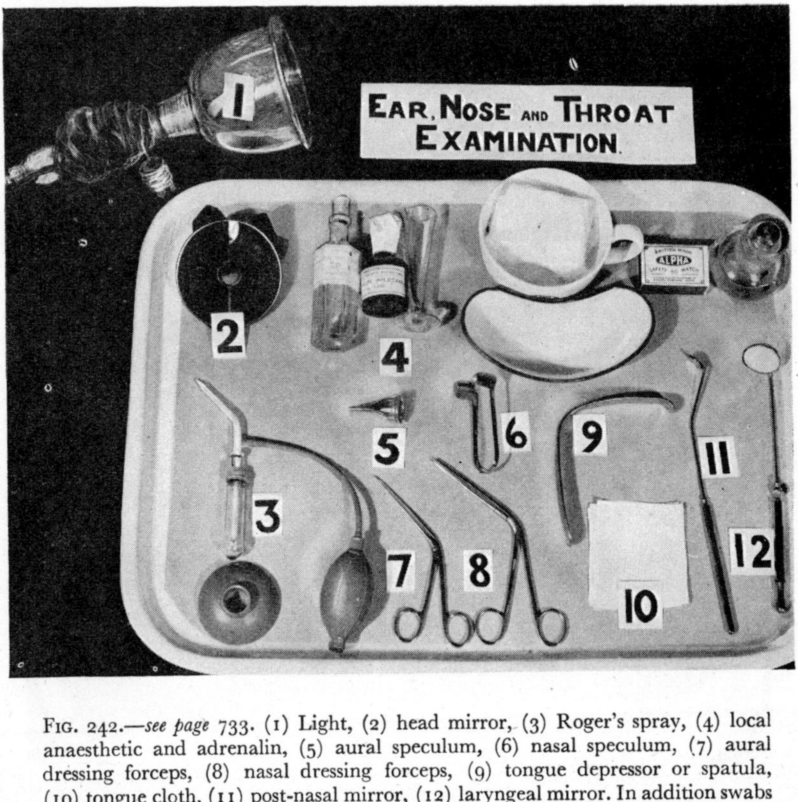

FIG. 242.—*see page* 733. (1) Light, (2) head mirror, (3) Roger's spray, (4) local anaesthetic and adrenalin, (5) aural speculum, (6) nasal speculum, (7) aural dressing forceps, (8) nasal dressing forceps, (9) tongue depressor or spatula, (10) tongue cloth, (11) post-nasal mirror, (12) laryngeal mirror. In addition swabs should be provided, and a spirit lamp for warming the mirrors; and matches.

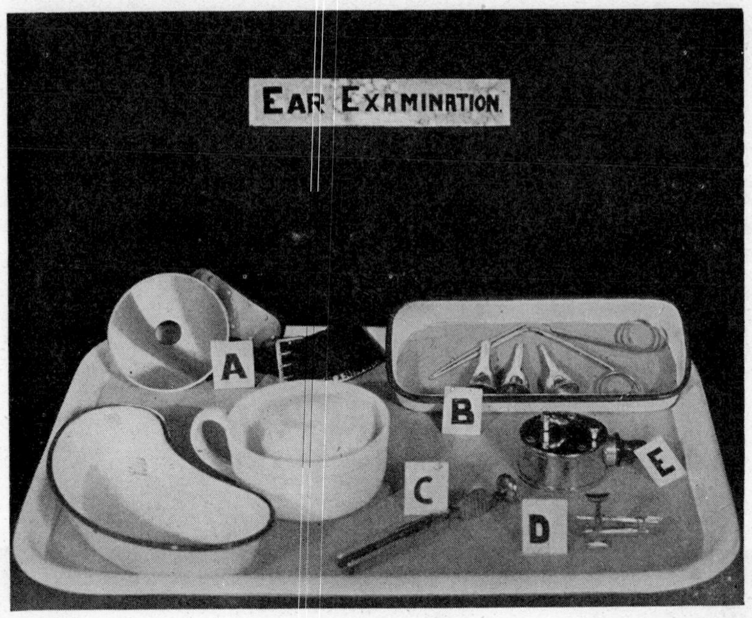

FIG. 243.—*see page* 734. (A) Head mirror, (B) tray containing aural specula and dressing forceps, wool in porringer for swabbing ear and receiver for soiled swabs.
Articles to test hearing are included: (C) tuning fork, (D) acoumeter, (E) noise box.

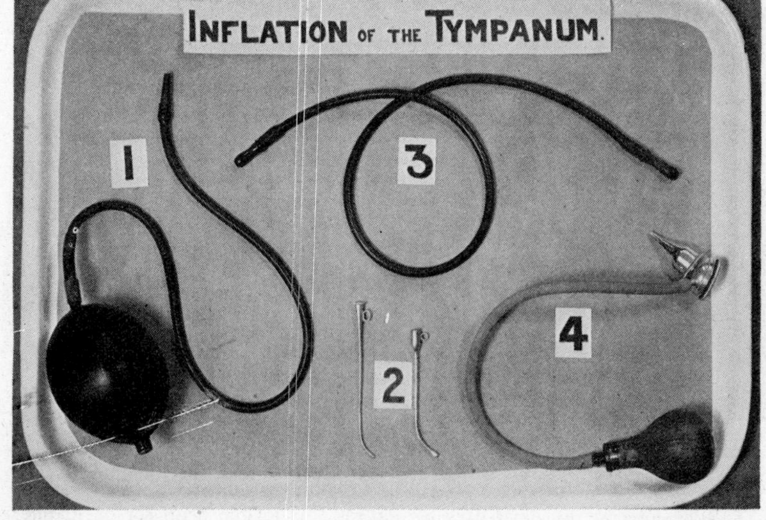

FIG. 244.—*see page* 734. (1) Politzer's bag, (2) Eustachian catheters, (3) auscultation tube for use with Politzer's bag, (4) Siegel's speculum.

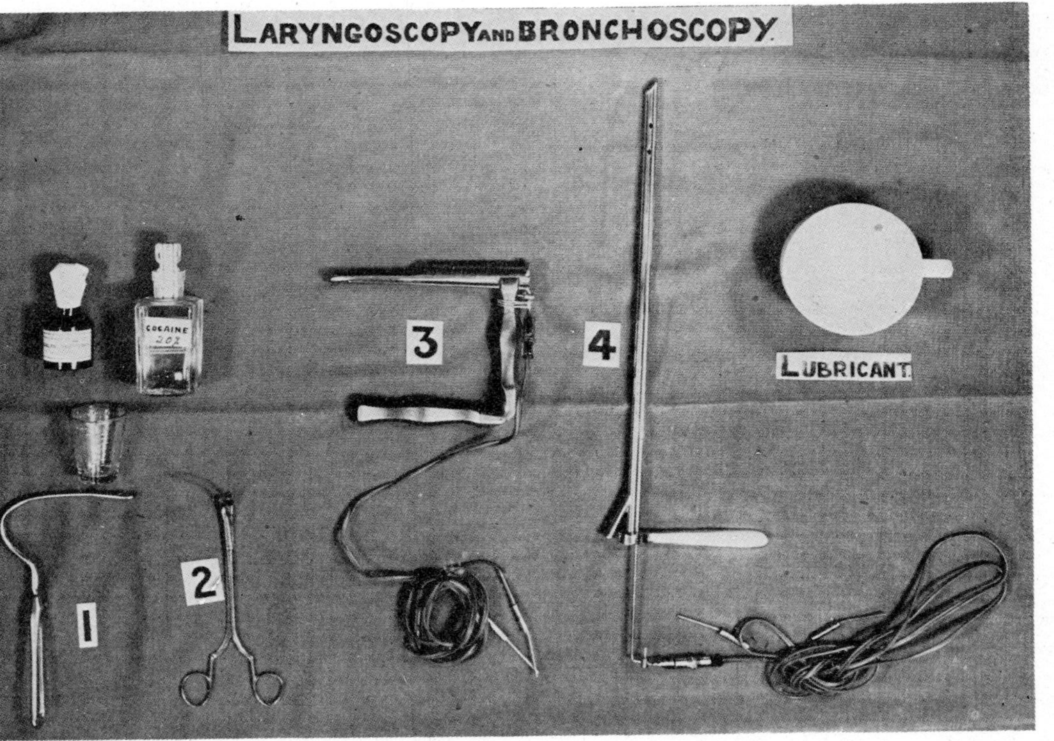

FIG. 245.—*see pages* 734–5. (1) Fränkel's tongue depressor, (2) oesophageal forceps, (3) laryngoscope with lead for attachment to transformer, (4) bronchoscope with lead attached.

In addition, a local anaesthetic and adrenalin are supplied and a lubricant for the bronchoscope.

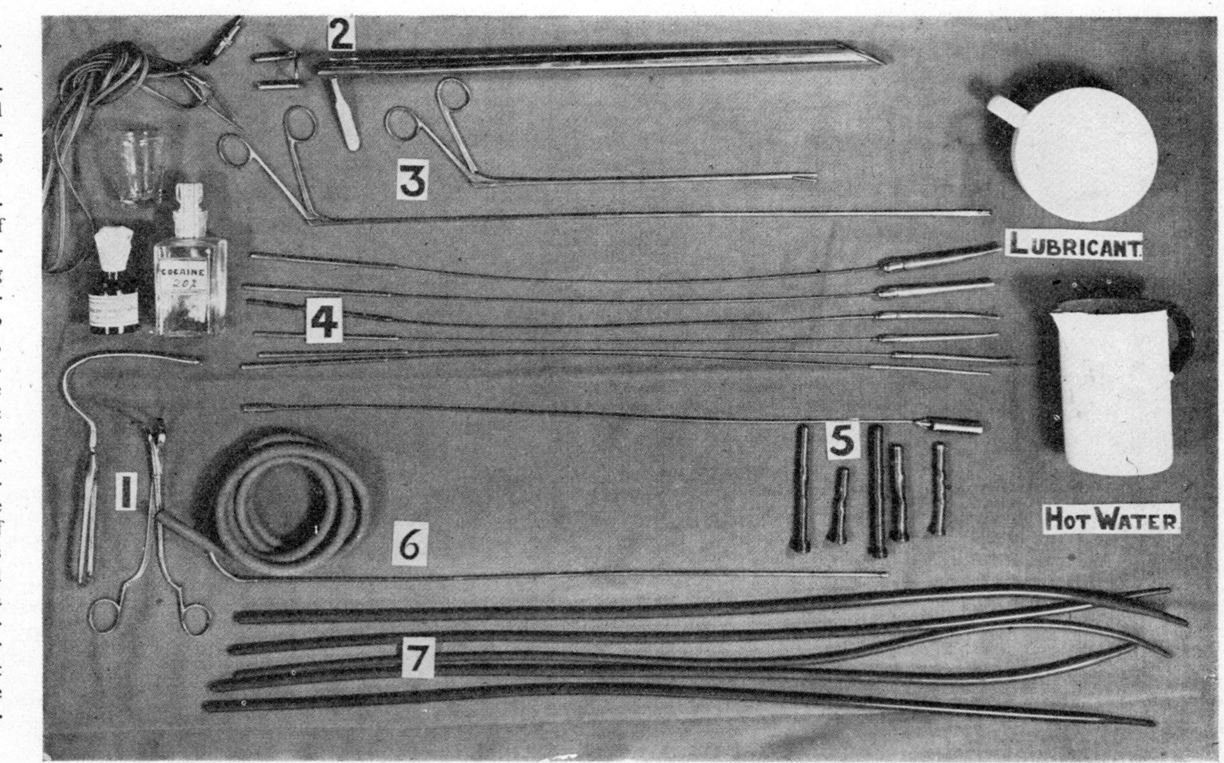

FIG. 246.—*see page* 734.
OESOPHAGOSCOPY.
(1) Fränkel's tongue depressor and oesophageal forceps, (2) oesophagoscope, (3) Paterson's forceps (1 long and 1 short pair), (4) oesophageal bougies of various sizes, (5) Souttar's tubes, (6) long metal sucker with tubing for attachment to suction apparatus, (7) Gum-elastic bougies. The oesophagoscope contains an electric bulb to illuminate the cavity; the lead for attachment to the transformer is shown in the top left-hand corner of the picture. Here also is shown the cocaine and adrenalin used as a local anaesthetic. A lubricant is required for the bougies, and hot water to render the gum-elastic more flexible.

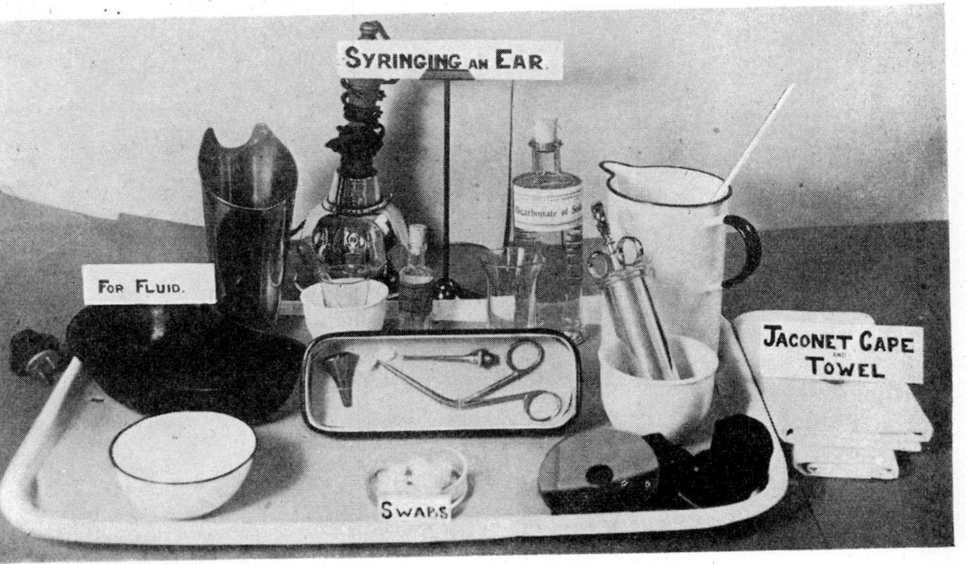

FIG. 247.—*see page* 734.
The tray contains: light and head mirror, special aural syringe with nozzle, aural speculum, and dressing forceps in receiver, small wool swabs, lotion and thermometer, special aural receiver and black kidney dish, ear drops and pipette, and bowl for used swabs. A jaconet cape and towel is provided to protect the patient's clothing.

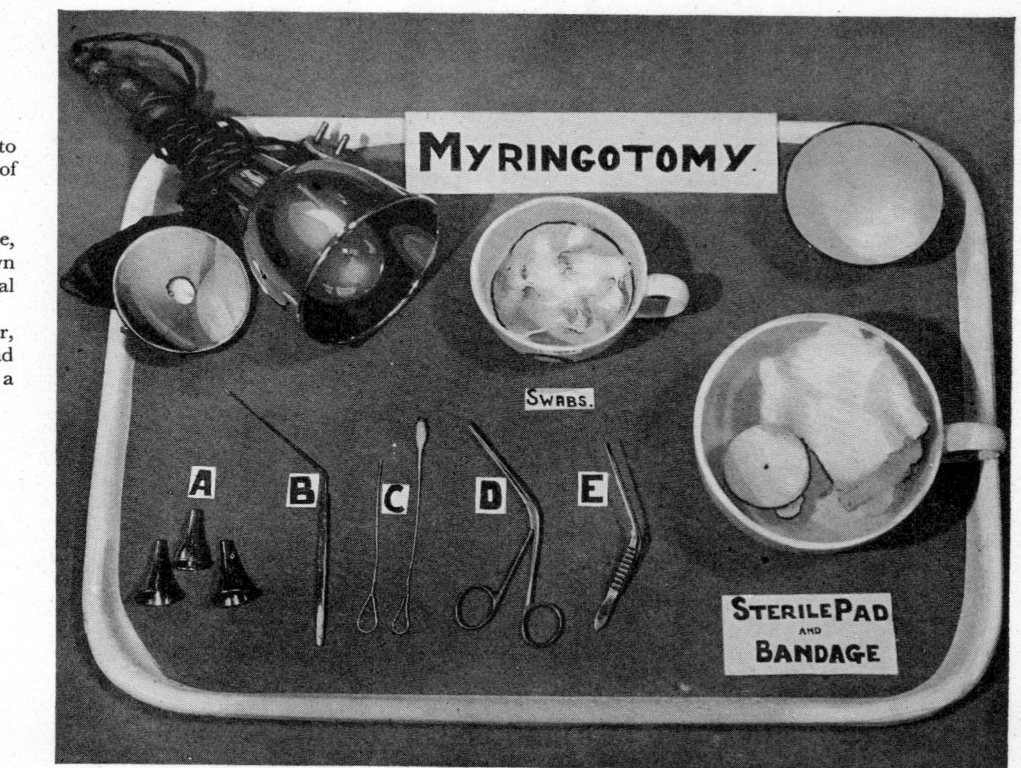

FIG. 248.—*see page* 736.

Myringotomy is an incision made into the tympanic membrane in cases of otitis media.

The articles required include:

(A) Aural specula, (B) myringotome, (C) cotton wool carriers, one is shown dressed with wool, (D and E) aural dressing forceps.

In addition light and head mirror, specially prepared swabs, a sterile pad and bandage to cover the ear, and a receiver for soiled swabs are needed.

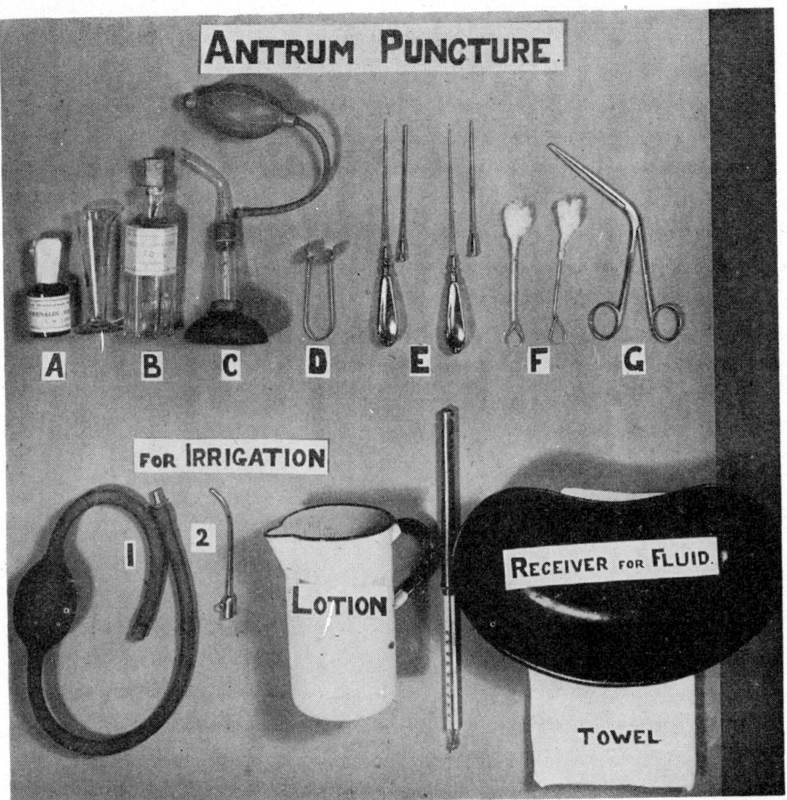

FIG. 249.—*see page* 739.

In antrum puncture an opening is made into the maxillary antrum. The articles required include:

(A) Adrenalin, (B) local anaesthetic, (C) Roger's spray, (D) nasal speculum, (E) trocar and cannula (2 sizes), (F) cotton wool carriers (dressed), (G) nasal forceps.

Articles for irrigation are shown below: (1) Higginson's syringe and (2) antrum cannula. A black receiver is supplied so that the presence of pus can easily be detected.

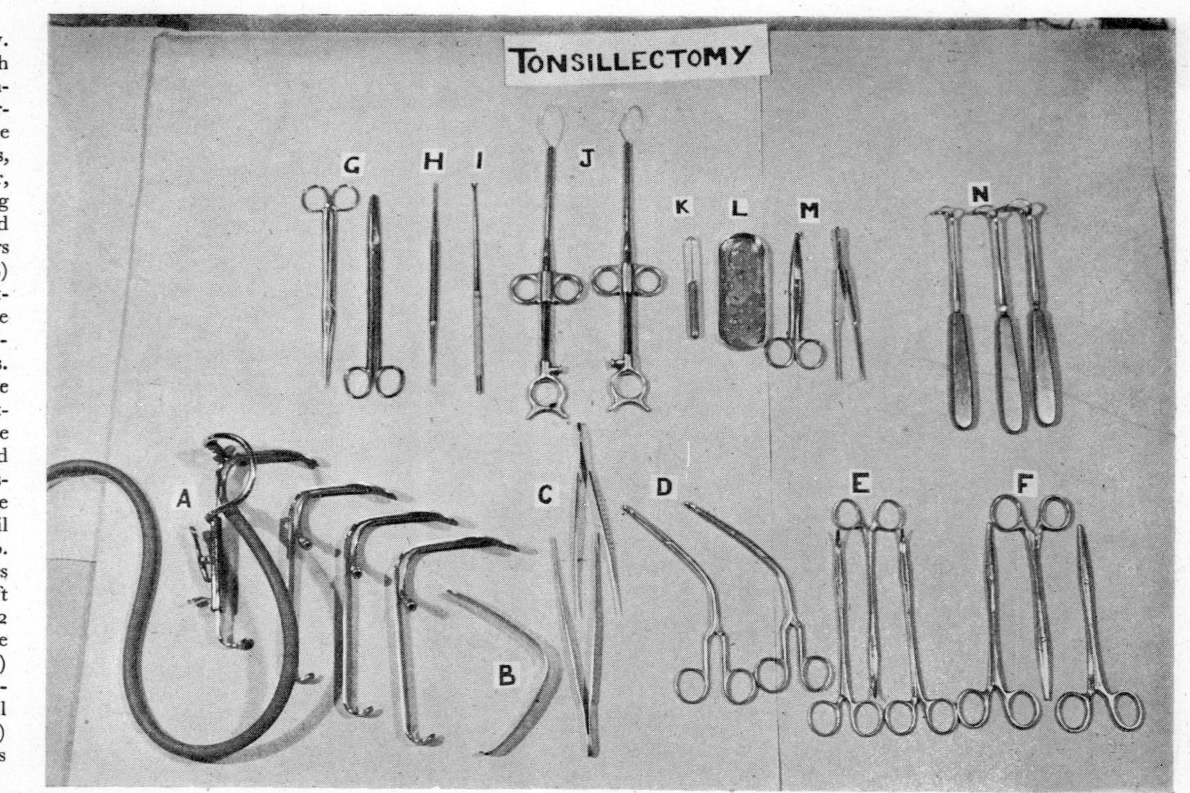

FIG. 250. LOWER ROW. (A) Davis's gag with rubber tubing attached for anaesthetic purposes and four tongue blades of various sizes, (B) tongue depressor, (C) long dissecting forceps, plain and toothed, (D) two pairs ethmoidal forceps, (E) three pairs curved artery forceps, (F) three pairs long Spencer-Wells's artery forceps. UPPER ROW. (G) One pair of tonsil dissecting scissors and one pair of round pointed scissors, (H) blunt dissector, (I) ligature pusher, (J) two tonsil snares, (K) catgut (No. 0), (L) tray of needles containing Lane's cleft palate needles Nos. 2 and 4 and half-circle cutting needles, (M) one pair of stitch scissors and one pair small dissecting forceps, (N) adenoid curettes, sizes 1, 2, and 3.

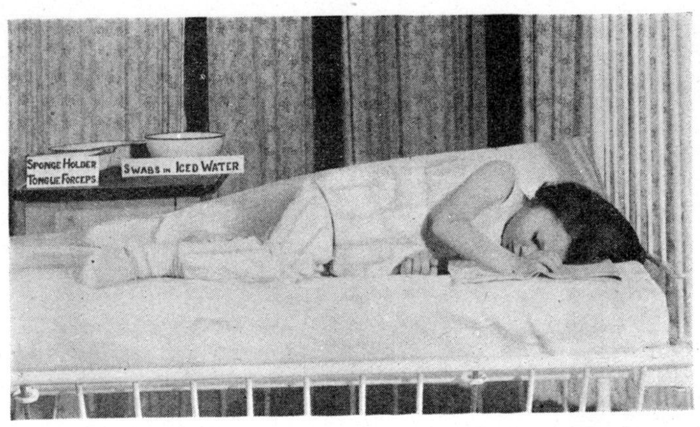

FIG. 251.—*see page* 741.
THE POSITION IN WHICH A PATIENT SHOULD LIE AFTER TONSILLECTOMY HAS BEEN PERFORMED.

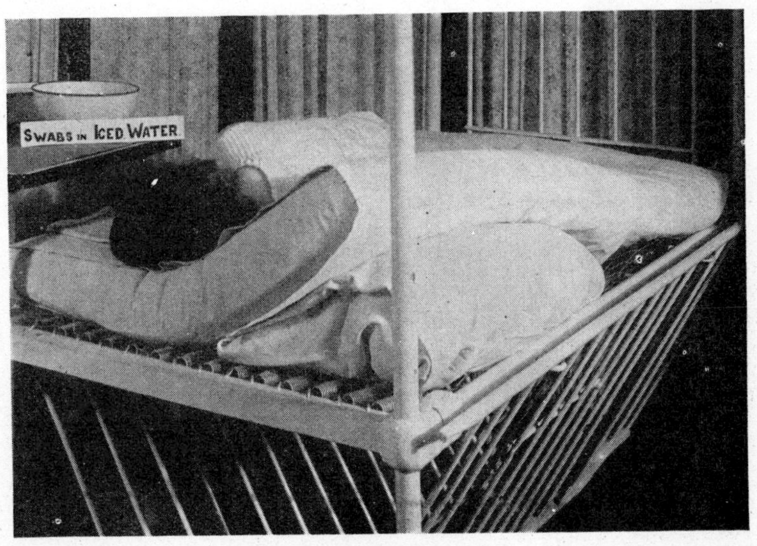

FIG. 252.—*see page* 741.
SHOWING HOW THE POSITION ILLUSTRATED IN FIG. 251 IS OBTAINED.

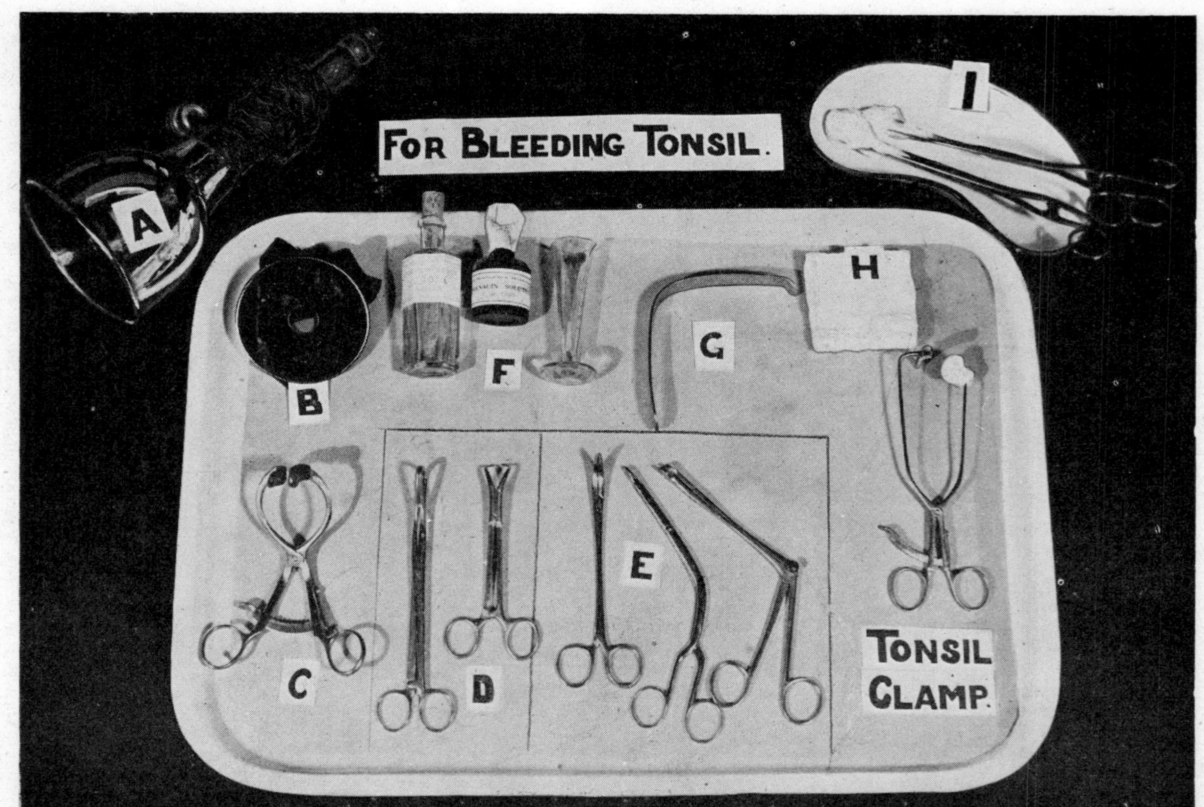

FIG. 253.—*see page* 741.
(A) Light, (B) head mirror, (C) mouth gag, (D) tongue forceps (two patterns), (E) from left to right: curved artery forceps, ethmoidal forceps, and tonsil tag forceps, (F) local anaesthetic and adrenalin, (G) tongue depressor, (H) tongue cloth, (I) sponge-holding forceps, ready dressed. The tonsil clamp is shown with the blade covered with a small pad.

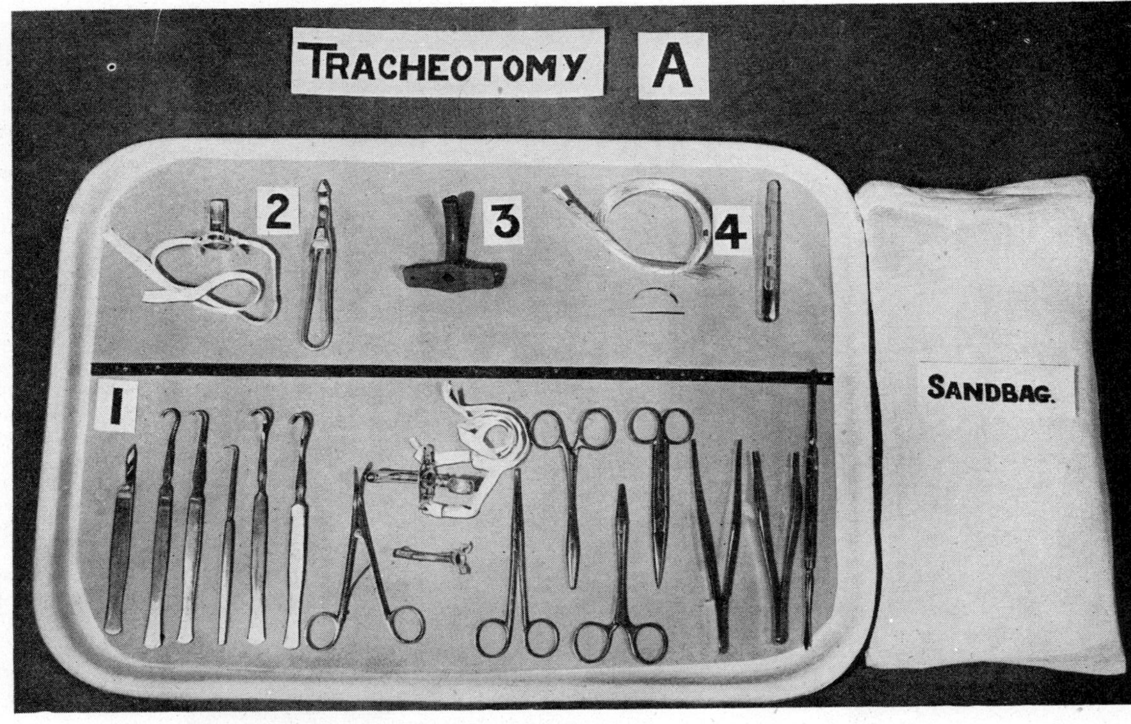

FIG. 254.—*see page* 742. The articles required for tracheotomy include: LOWER ROW. (1) reading from left to right: one scalpel, two blunt hooks, one sharp hook, two double hook retractors, tracheal dilator, tracheotomy outer tube, ready taped with pilot inserted, inner tube, one pair sinus forceps, two pairs artery forceps, scissors, two pairs dissecting forceps (one plain and one rat-toothed), one blunt dissector.
UPPER ROW. (2) laryngotomy tube, ready taped, pilot; (3) rubber tracheotomy tube; (4) silkworm gut, surgical needles and catgut. A sandbag is required to place under the patient's shoulders.

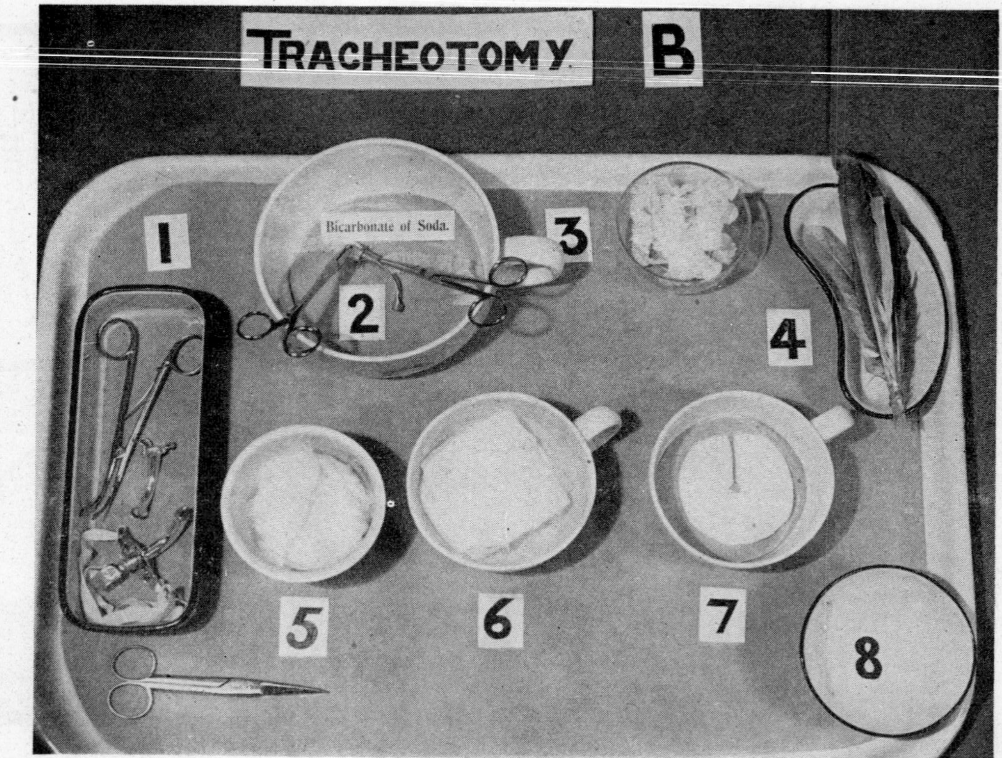

FIG. 255.—*see page* 743.

TRACHEOTOMY BEDSIDE TRAY

The articles which should be kept ready at the bedside of every case of tracheotomy.

(1) Tray containing tracheal dilators, tracheotomy tube ready taped and with pilot inserted, and inner tube. (2) Bowl of soda bicarbonate solution showing method of handling inner tube when cleaning with gauze wick. (3) Gauze wicks for cleaning inner tube. (5) Swabs. (6) Folded layer of gauze to place in front of tube. (7) Specially cut dressing for insertion between tube and the skin of the throat. (8) Bowl for soiled swabs. A pair of scissors should always be ready to hand with which to cut the tapes should the tube inadvertently slip out of the trachea.

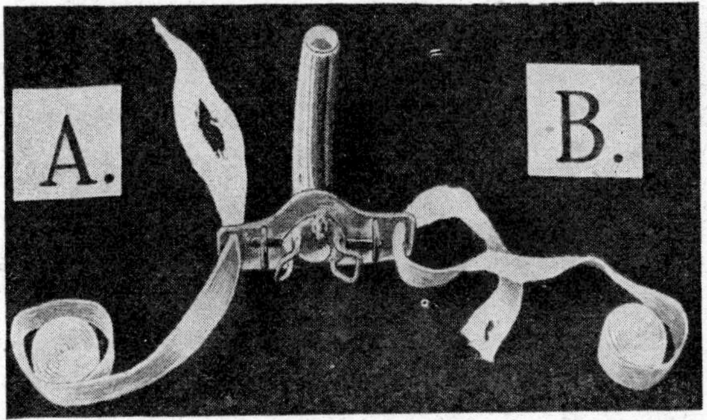

FIG. 256. Every tracheotomy tube should be securely taped. A shows the direction in which the end of a piece of tape, in which a slit has been made, is taken through the metal slot. B shows the longer end of the tape carried through the slot in the shorter end.

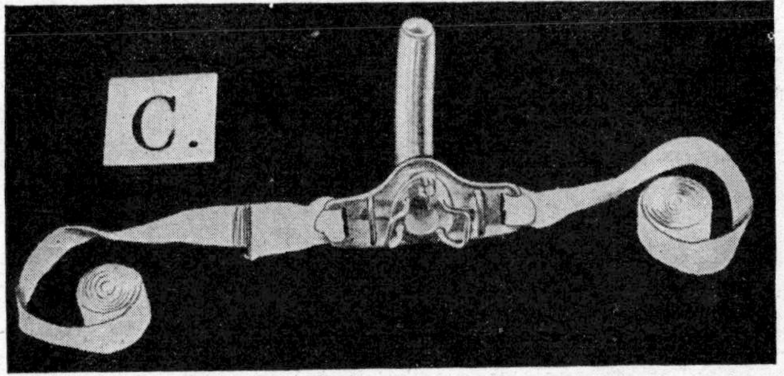

FIG. 257. C shows the tube taped and ready for use.

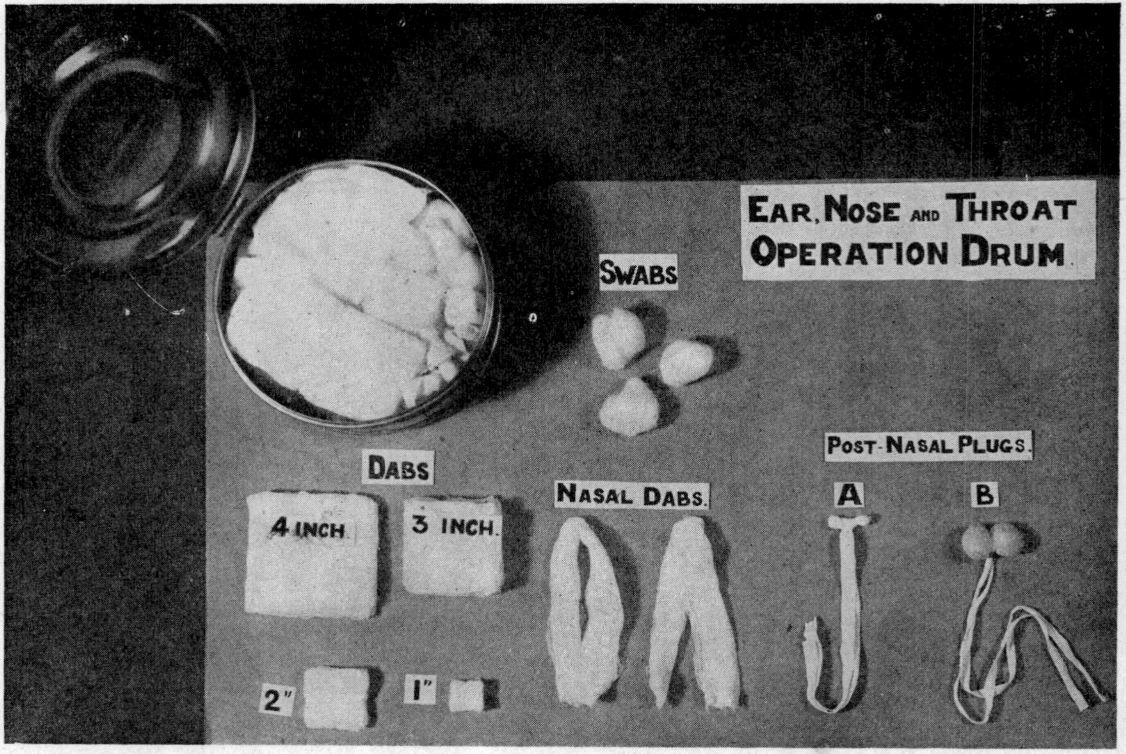

Fig. 258.
Contents of drum specially prepared for Ear, Nose and Throat surgery. The drum contains wool swabs for mopping, and gauze dabs of various sizes; the small 1 in. variety are used in cases of oesophagoscopy, the larger ones being employed for adenoid and tonsil cases.

The *nasal dabs* shown are used for operations on the septum and antrum; and the post-nasal plugs are inserted before all operations on the nose, except that for removal of the posterior ends of the turbinates.

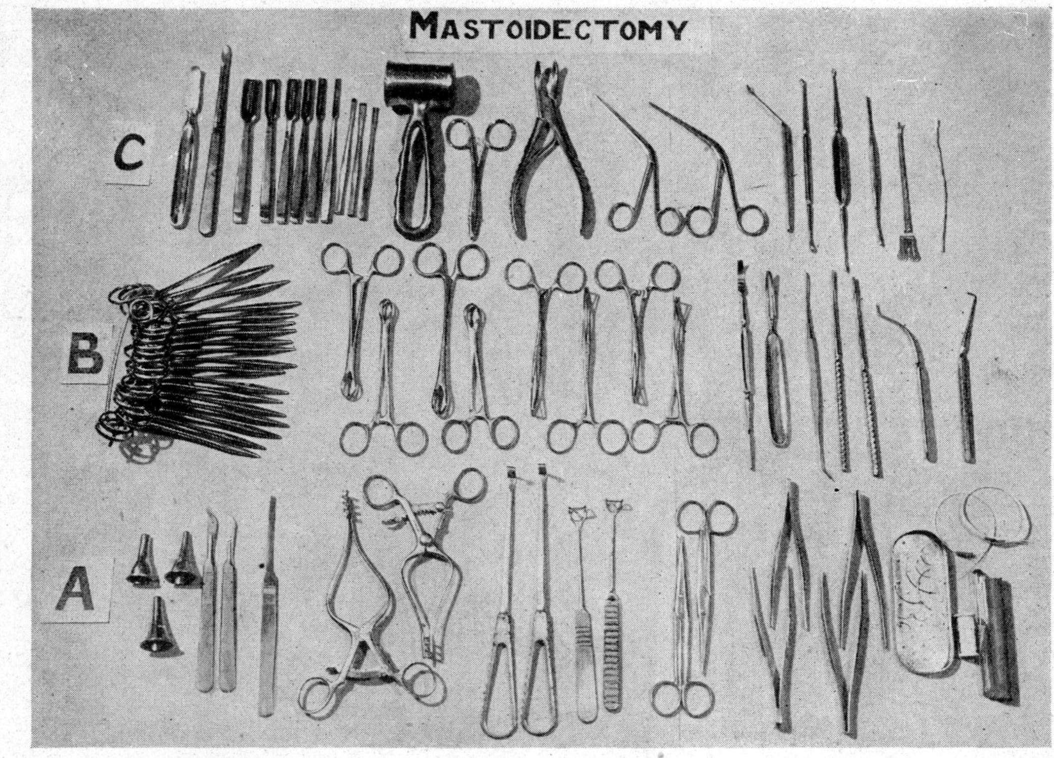

FIG. 259.—*see page* 736. Reading from left to right:—Row A. Three aural specula; two Bard-Parker's knives, No. 10 blades; one bistoury; two Travers's retractors; two hip retractors (small); two Durham's retractors (small); two pairs Mayo's dissecting scissors; two pairs plain dissecting forceps; two pairs rat-toothed dissecting forceps; tray of curved cutting needles (various sizes); silk-worm gut (medium size); reel of No. 4 silk; phial of No. 0 catgut; rubber drainage tube. Row B. One and a half doz. short Spencer-Wells's artery forceps; four short Lane's tissue forceps; four short Duval's tissue forceps; Macdonald's raspatory; Kocher's raspatory; Watson-Cheyne's probe; two eustachian burrs; Staeck's guide; Dundas-Grant's probe. Row C. Periosteal elevator; Lane's raspatory; set of mastoid gouges and chisels; copper mallet; one pair small bone-nibbling forceps; one pair Lane's bone-nibbling forceps; two pairs aural dressing forceps; three curettes (assorted sizes); small spoon; probe and director.

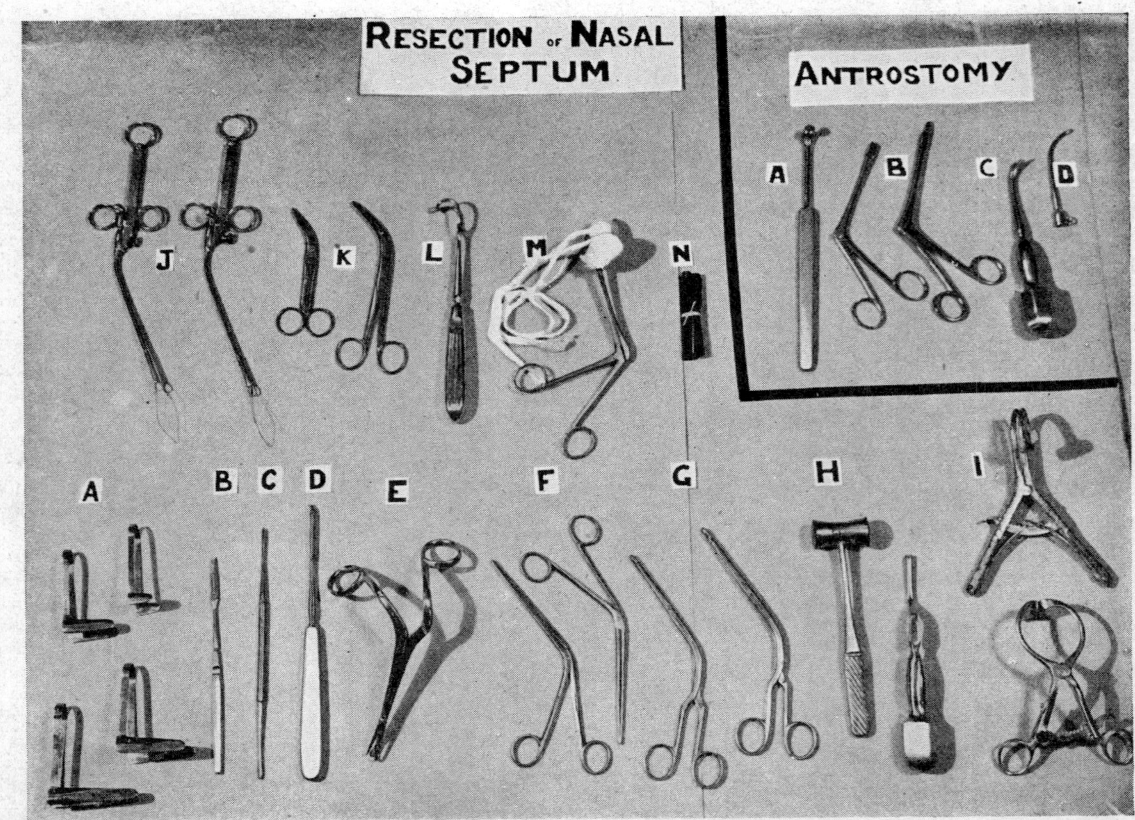

FIG. 260. — *see page* 737. LOWER ROW. (A) four nasal specula; (B) Bard-Parker's cleft palate knife, No. 15 blade; (C) blunt dissector; (D) Ballenger's swivel knife; (E) Heath's septum punch forceps; (F) two pairs nasal dressing forceps; (G) two pairs ethmoidal forceps; (H) mallet and chisel; (I) two types of mouth gag.

UPPER ROW. (J) two nasal snares; (K) Tilley's angular scissors and Beckmann's curved scissors. (L) blunt adenoid curette; and (M) tonsil holding forceps used for inserting a post-nasal sponge; (N) septum plugs, of rubber or oiled silk.

INSET. Instruments for intranasal antrostomy; (A) Antrum burr; (B) one pair of backward-cutting forceps; (C) Myles' retrograde trocar and chisel; (D) antrum cannula for irrigation (*see also Fig.* 249, *page* 691).

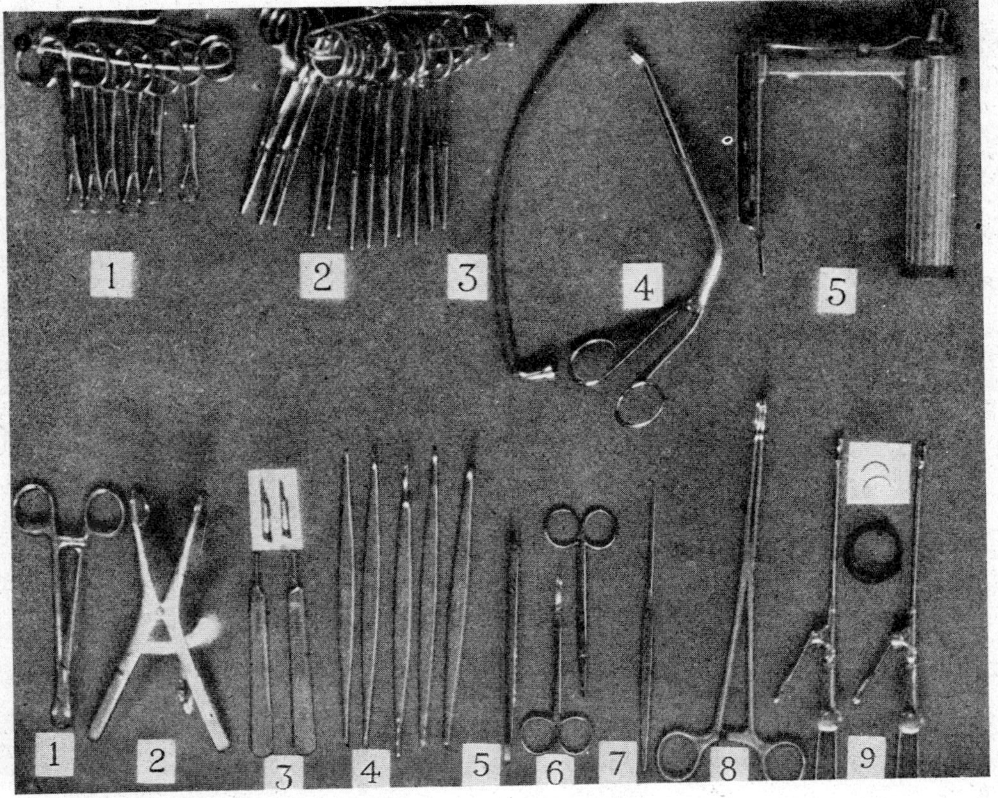

FIG. 261.—*see page* 746.

OPERATION FOR CLEFT PALATE.

UPPER ROW. (1) Towel clips. (2) Artery forceps. (3) Intratracheal catheter. (4) McGill's catheter introducer. (5) Laryngoscope.

LOWER ROW. (1) Tongue clip. (2) Mouth gag. (3) Bard-Parker's knives. (4) Cleft palate dissectors. (5) Waugh's fine dissectors. (6) Scissors (straight and curved). (7) Gillie's hook. (8) Sponge-holding forceps. (9) Lane's needle holders, fine needles and fine silkworm gut.

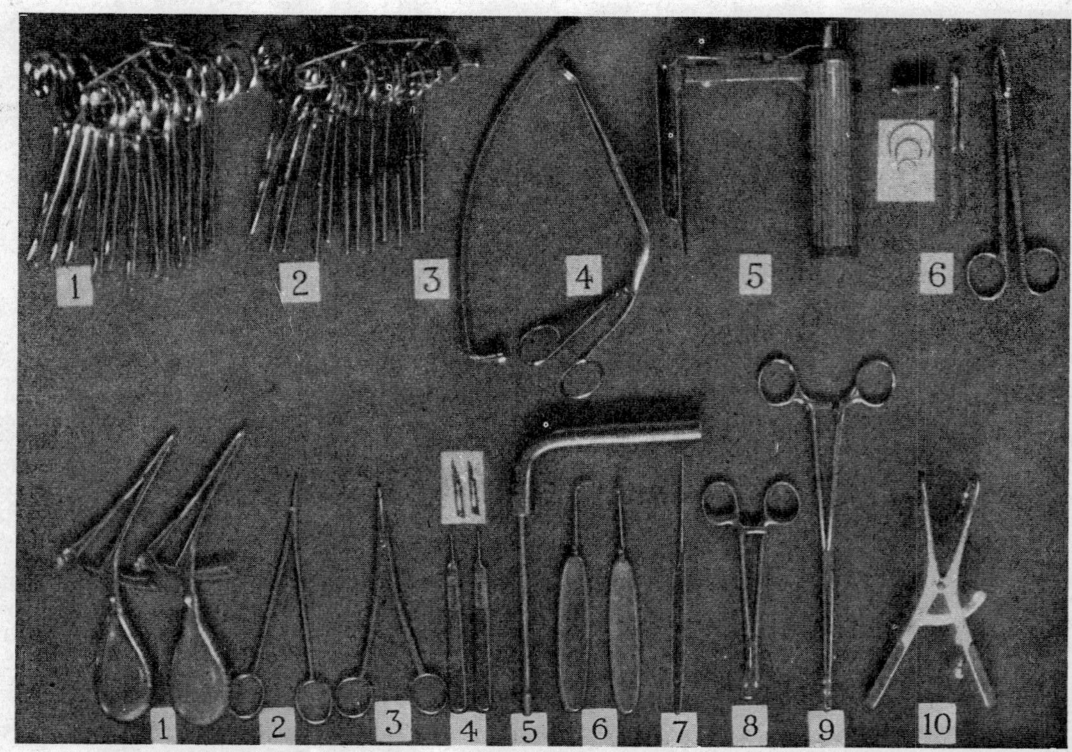

Fig. 262. Operation for Cleft Palate (including Mr. Denis Browne's instruments).
Upper Row. (1) Denis Browne's towel clips. (2) Spencer-Wells's artery forceps. (3) Intratracheal catheter. (4) McGill's introducing forceps. (5) Laryngoscope. (6) Needles, ligatures, sutures and catgut-tube breaking forceps.
Lower Row. (1) Denis Browne's needle holders. (2) Denis Browne's needle catching forceps. (3) Denis Browne's scissors. (4) Bard-Parker's knives. (5) Denis Browne's sucker. (6) Denis Browne's dissectors. (7) Gillie's hook. (8) Tongue clip. (9) Sponge-holding forceps. (10) Mouth gag.

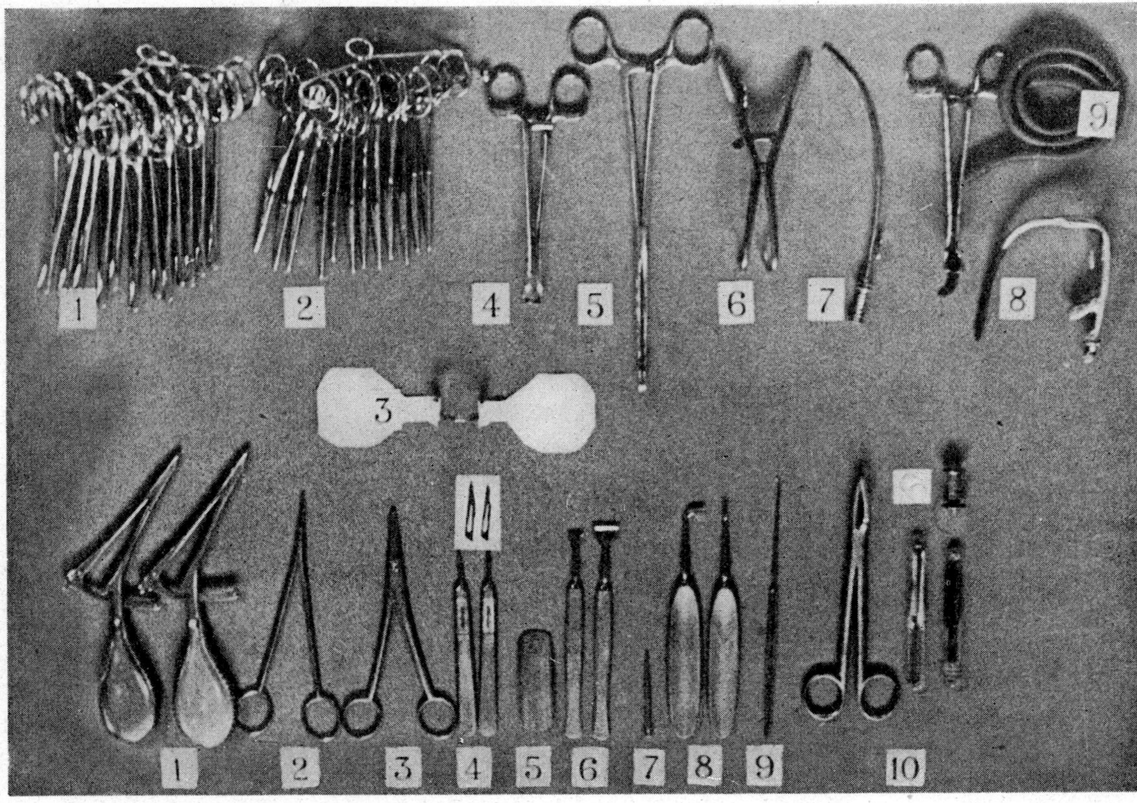

FIG. 263.

REPAIR OF HARELIP (including Denis Browne's instruments).

UPPER ROW. (1) Denis Browne's towel clips. (2) Spencer-Wells's artery forceps. (3) Logan's bow (Denis Browne's modification). (4) Tongue forceps. (5) Sponge-holding forceps. (6) Toothed mouth gag. (7) **Metal end of** sucker apparatus. (8) Apparatus for intratracheal apparatus (oral). (9) Birt's airway with tubing for attachment to anaesthetic apparatus.

LOWER ROW. (1) Denis Browne's needle holders. (2) Denis Browne's needle-catching forceps. (3) Denis Browne's scissors. (4) Bard-Parker's knives (Nos. 15 and 11). (5) Wooden wedge. (6) Denis Browne's harelip chisel and blunt dissector. (7) Trephine. (8) Denis Browne's dissectors. (9) Gillie's hook. (10) **Catgut-tube** breakers, needles, thread and **catgut.**

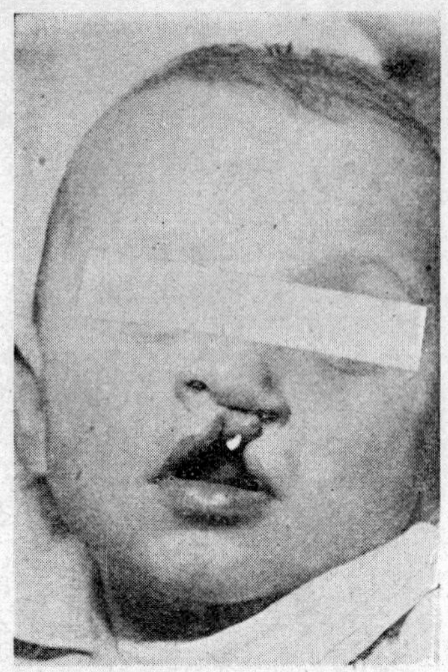

Fig. 264. Single (Unilateral) Harelip.

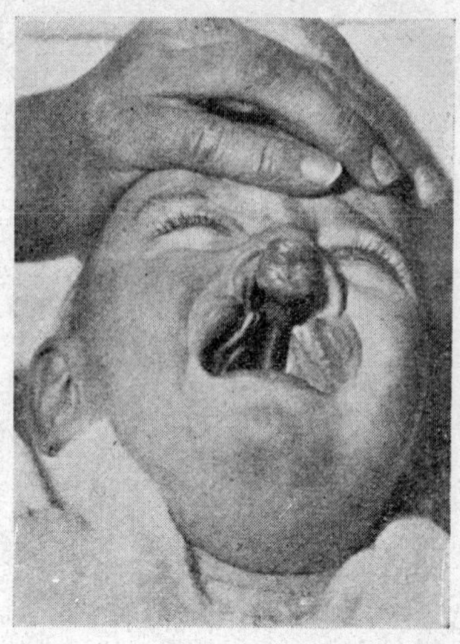

Fig. 265. Double (bilateral) Harelip with Cleft Palate.

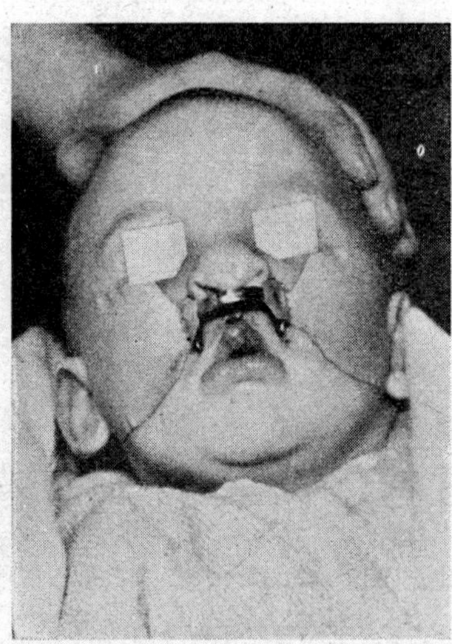

Fig. 266. Modified Logan's bow used as "Tension Bridge" after harelip operation.

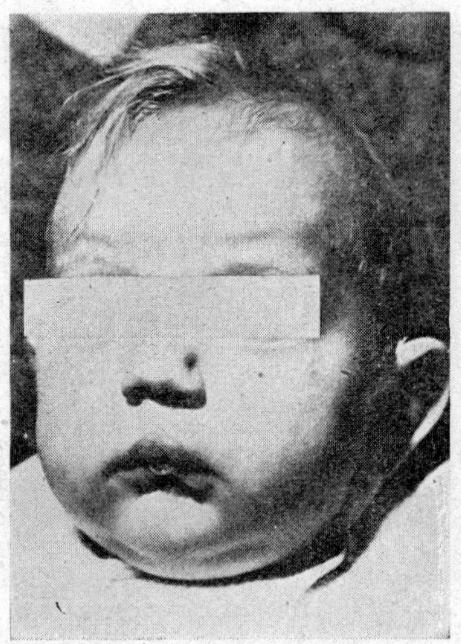

Fig. 267. A good result after operation for harelip. *Note the normal "pouting" position of the mouth.*

Harelip (*see pages* 746–7).

Chapter 45

Common General Surgical Conditions Treated by Operation, including Some Points in the Preparation and Post-Operative Care

Acute abdominal conditions: inflammation, obstruction and perforation—Appendicitis: symptoms, post-operative nursing—Operations on the stomach—Hernia—Haemorrhoids—Resection of colon, colostomy and excision of rectum with notes on post-operative nursing—Thyroidectomy: preparation and post-operative nursing care—Operations on the breast and post-operative nursing care—Operations on the gallbladder and post-operative nursing care—Amputation of a limb—Skin-grafting

ACUTE ABDOMINAL CONDITIONS

An acute surgical abdominal catastrophe will usually be due to one of the three following causes:

Some acute inflammatory condition
Acute intestinal obstruction
Perforation of hollow viscera.

The first thing the probationer nurse will probably notice is the similarity of symptoms complained of in each of these cases. *Pain* is invariably present, varying in intensity from a tiresome ache to an acute agonizing degree which renders the patient rigid and afraid to move. *Vomiting* is also varied, and most patients will complain of nausea; some will vomit once or twice, the material consisting of stomach contents, while others will suffer from persistent vomiting of a more serious character. Some degree of *collapse* will usually be present, varying from a mild degree of coldness to the acute condition described under shock on p. 640, in which the extremities are cyanosed, the skin is cold and clammy, the pulse feeble and the breathing shallow. The temperature, pulse and respirations may or may not vary; the temperature may be high in an acute inflammatory condition or markedly low in collapse; the pulse will vary with the amount of shock when pain is present, and the respirations with the extent to which movement of the anterior abdominal wall is interfered with as a result of pain or of abdominal distention.

(a) **Inflammation.** The commonest cases of inflammation admitted include those of appendicitis, acute cholecystitis, salpingitis and diverticulitis. The inflammation is at first local, but it usually spreads to the peritoneum and then gives rise to the characteristic symptoms of peritonitis.

(b) **Intestinal obstruction.** Any mechanical disturbance will give rise to some degree of obstruction, the causes including strangulated hernia, in which the obstruction may be partial or complete, volvulus, adhesions, tumours, intussusception, and impaction of the small intestine by gallstones.

The *symptoms of intestinal obstruction* are characterized by pain, which is intermittent and colicky in character and varies in intensity—this pain is due to the increased rate of peristalsis which occurs as the involuntary muscle contracts in order to try and overcome the obstruction and pass the obstructing body on. The abdomen is usually distended because, owing to the obstruction, both gas and fluid accumulate above it—the distension will therefore be most marked when the obstruction is low, and least marked when the obstruction is higher up. Vomiting occurs—at first the patient vomits stomach contents and then later, as the intestine becomes distended by the fluid accumulating in it above the obstruction, this fluid is regurgitated into the stomach and the stomach expels it by vomiting. When this happens the vomiting therefore becomes regurgitant in character; it is effortless and large quantities of brown fluid are brought up. Collapse is marked.

The *history* usually elicited is that the bowels acted at the beginning of the illness but not since, and if the patient has taken any aperients he will usually say that they either failed to act or that he vomited after taking them. The nurse should also try to discover whether the patient knows if he has passed flatus or not, as in complete intestinal obstruction flatus is not passed.

(c) Perforation. As a rule the stomach or duodenum is the site of perforation resulting from a peptic ulcer, but any part of the hollow viscera may perforate from other causes.

Symptoms. The pain in perforation is distinctly localized, sharp at first and frequently described as agonizing, and afterwards continuing as a severe burning pain. Vomiting may occur at the outset, probably induced by the severe pain. Collapse is very marked; the injury to the peritoneum following perforation, when the contents of the hollow viscera enter the cavity and irritate the membrane, gives rise to a profound degree of collapse and prostration; the temperature remains subnormal for several hours, then a reaction sets in, the temperature rises somewhat, the degree of collapse becomes slightly relieved and the patient is a little warmer or better. It is for this reason that surgeons may sometimes wait for an hour or so after a case of perforation has been admitted before they operate. In perforation the abdomen is characteristically rigid, it is not usually distended but on the other hand appears flatter than normal; the muscles are contracted and show a characteristically hard boardlike rigidity.

The **preparation for an emergency operation** should be as slight as possible, and it is important to remember that the first nursing duty is to provide the conditions which will tend to reduce the production of post-operative shock. The patient should be very carefully and gently handled, moved with care and quietly placed into a warm bed and lightly but adequately covered, be made as comfortable as possible, and reassured that his wellbeing is the first consideration of everybody. If, as so frequently happens, he tends to lie on his back with his knees flexed, a knee pillow should be inserted; if the bedclothes appear to lie heavily on his tender distended abdomen they should be supported by a low bedcradle. For coldness of the extremities, either an electric cradle or electric blanket or hot-water bottles should be used, but when the latter are employed they must be thoroughly well protected as a patient in a very severe state of collapse has lost a great deal of his ability to feel. If dyspnoea is present the patient should have several pillows, otherwise it is advisable to keep him as recumbent as possible.

Some patients, owing to the limited movement of the painful abdomen, tend to lie with the arms above the head in order to assist the movements of the chest in breathing. In this case a bed jacket with long sleeves should be employed to protect the arms and keep them warm.

Pending the arrival of a doctor the patient must not be given anything by mouth, but his mouth should be cleaned and his lips moistened. The nurse should use every available opportunity during the waiting period in order to promote the reaction which may be expected after the initial condition of shock, and a very large part of her preparation of the patient for operation is the improvement of his general wellbeing, which is best carried out by the provision of rest and warmth, maintenance of his general comfort and reassurance in order to avoid, or at least decrease the degree of shock which must of necessity follow the operation which is to be performed.

Handling of the patient as regards preparation should be as light as possible. In some cases shaving and preparation of the skin of the abdomen may be possible; in others, to whom the slightest touch gives pain, this must be left until the patient is under the anaesthetic. A specimen of urine ought to be obtained and tested for acetone, sugar, and albumin.

Aperients and enemata should never be given unless specially ordered. In some cases, where vomiting is persistent, the doctor may wish to wash the stomach out before an anaesthetic is given and the nurse will be expected to prepare for this. As a rule, a pre-operative injection of morphia or atropine, or of both drugs, may be ordered.

ACUTE APPENDICITIS

Symptoms. The symptoms of acute appendicitis include pain, usually of sudden onset, at first generalized over the whole abdomen, and later becoming localized to the characteristic site of appendicitis, i.e. McBurney's point, situated midway between the umbilicus and the anterior superior iliac spine. The patient complains of nausea and in some cases he vomits; the temperature may be slightly raised and the pulse rate quickened, though these are not invariable; the abdomen is rigid and tender, tenderness being particularly marked over the right iliac fossa.

The *pre-operative care* described on p. 632 is carried out as a routine measure. In emergency cases the full preparation is not possible as the patient may be taken almost directly to the operating theatre.

Post-operative nursing care. On return from the theatre the patient will be placed recumbent in bed with one soft pillow for his head and a knee pillow to support the thighs. If there is a fair degree of shock it is usual for a rectal saline to be given. If the patient has drainage tubes in the abdominal cavity, he is placed in Fowler's position as soon as he is round from the anaesthetic in order to facilitate drainage and to prevent the complication of abscess formation; otherwise, he will be nursed recumbent with two or three pillows supporting head and shoulders.

The ordinary routine care of a patient under an anaesthetic is carried out. As soon as vomiting has ceased he may be given fluids, light fluids being continued for two days followed by a light farinaceous diet. An aperient is administered on the second or third night, and after the bowels have acted the patient may have ordinary diet. A flatus tube should be passed whenever necessary to relieve abdominal distension. The knee pillow should be omitted by the fifth day and the patient encouraged to move.

Dressing. If the dressing is simple, it is merely necessary to keep it covered in order to protect it from the bedclothes either by means of elastoplast or by a bandage. On the fifth or sixth day any Michel's clips should be removed, and the rubber tubing which has been placed under the tension sutures should be cut, these sutures being removed about the tenth or twelfth day. When the dressing is complicated by the insertion of drainage tubes it requires to be attended to fairly frequently, the wound being redressed and repacked and the drainage tubes removed as soon as they cease to be effective. In a straightforward case they would be removed in two or three days.

An average case of simple appendicectomy will get up about the twelfth day and be discharged from hospital on the fourteenth day. Cases in whom a mid-line incision is necessary get up about the sixteenth or seventeenth day and are discharged at the end of 2 weeks.

The **complications to be feared** in the post-operative nursing care of acute appendicitis include peritonitis, abscess formation, faecal fistula, and pleurisy and empyema occurring on the right side.

OPERATIONS ON THE STOMACH

Gastrectomy, *gastro-duodenostomy* and *gastro-enterostomy*, are the operations commonly employed on the stomach. These are usually undertaken in cases where medical treatment has proved unavailing in extensive peptic ulceration; and also in cases where the patient has been the victim of repeated bleeding (haematemesis); in cases where perforation has occurred and in others where marked scarring and contraction has rendered the stomach unable to fulfil its normal function.

In *gastro-enterostomy* communication is made between the stomach and intestine; in *gastro-duodenostomy* it is between the stomach and duodenum; in *partial gastrectomy* the ulcer-bearing area of the stomach is removed, that is, the pyloric end and in total gastrectomy the entire stomach is removed. All these operations are followed by considerable shock; in the last-mentioned case shock is probably most serious.

Preparation. The usual preparation for operation is carried out; in addition, it is important for the stomach to be clean and empty and it is washed out with an alkaline solution.

Post-operative nursing care. The patient is received into bed recumbent with a pillow underneath his knees. The foot of the bed is elevated on 18-inch blocks, an electric cradle is put over the body, and a blood transfusion may be given if necessary.

The patient is carefully watched. His colour is noted, his pulse is taken half-hourly, his abdomen is watched for distension and the dressing for the oozing of any serum; it is also important to keep the binder firmly applied, the amount that the patient vomits should be carefully noted and reported. If a Ryle's tube has been left in, any fluid that collects is evacuated but as a rule there is no residue after about twenty-four hours and the tube is removed.

The condition of shock should be very carefully noted, and as the patient improves he is raised into a sitting position; he may be given one pillow each hour until he is sitting erect in Fowler's position.

One ounce of water is given every hour as soon as the patient is fit for it. Milk and water, four ounces every two hours, are given on the second day and thereafter the diet is increased as given in the table on p. 654.

The bowels require a certain amount of careful regulation. A turpentine enema will be given after the first twenty-four hours for the relief of flatulence if necessary. From the second day onwards, until the fourteenth, a small enema is given daily to evacuate the bowel, but after the fourteenth day the patient is given liquid paraffin and phenolphthalein twice daily, and the bowels are regulated in this manner.

The stitches are usually removed about the tenth day, and the patient may get up between the twelfth and fourteenth day, and if the condition has not been complicated he will normally leave hospital about the eighteenth day.

HERNIA

A hernia is a protrusion of an organ into the walls of the cavity in which it is contained. The term is most often applied to herniae of the abdominal cavity, which occur most frequently in one of three situations: (*a*) *Inguinal hernia*, through the inguinal canal, having its exit at the external abdominal ring just above the groin; (*b*) *Femoral*, which exits by means of the crural canal at a point below the groin, and (*c*) *Umbilical*, protruding at the side of the umbilicus, the type most commonly occurring in infants and in persons of weak abdominal musculature such as fat, middle-aged women.

It will be seen, therefore, that a hernia occurs at what is naturally a weak spot in some part of the abdominal wall. A *hernia consists of a sac*, or lining; in the instances given this is peritoneum—*the coverings of the sac*, i.e. the abdominal wall, and the *contents* which in this case will be omentum and fat, and occasionally a portion of gut.

The operation undertaken is radical repair of the hernia, the weakened parts being darned or patched with strips of fascia.

Post-operative nursing care. Many surgeons like a firm roller bandage applied to secure the dressing and to give some support. The patient is nursed in a recumbent position with one or two pillows, a knee pillow to support the thighs and an air ring to relieve pressure on the lower part of the back. The diet should be fluid at first, or very light solids, until the bowels have been opened. An aperient is usually given on the second night after operation; clips are removed on the fifth day and stitches on the tenth day; but, in cases where Michel's clips are the only suture used, alternate clips are taken out on the fifth, and the remainder removed on the sixth day.

The patient is usually allowed to get up about the fourteenth or fifteenth day and discharged from the hospital about the twenty-first day, except in the case of umbilical hernia in which the time of getting up and of discharge are both delayed for a further week.

HAEMORRHOIDS

Haemorrhoids, or piles, are varicose veins in the region of the rectum and anus. They are *external* when on the skin, and *internal* when on the mucosa of the lower part of the rectum. As in all cases of varicose veins there is possibly a congenital tendency to this condition, but predisposing causes of haemorrhoids are numerous and various, such as long hours of standing and walking, straining at stool with constipation, the presence of abdominal and pelvic tumours, and congestive heart disease and diseases of the liver. Any or all of these conditions may be the cause of congestion of blood in the haemorrhoidal veins and will predispose to their dilation.

Symptoms. The symptoms are bleeding on defecation and prolapse of the piles, which in time will become thrombosed and the parts affected ulcerated.

Treatment. In the *palliative treatment* constipation must be considered and treated and the prolapsed parts kept very clean, and astringent and soothing, and even anaesthetic applications employed for the relief of pain. *Injection treatment* is undertaken for suitable cases of internal piles. *Operation* is performed in other cases and in some where injection treatment has been unsuccessful.

Pre-operative treatment. In addition to the pre-operative treatment already described on p. 632, certain special measures have to be considered in the preparation of cases of haemorrhoids. If possible the patient should be in hospital 2 or 3 days before operation. Two days beforehand an aperient should be given followed by an enema; one day before the operation the enema should be repeated. Some surgeons order another rectal wash-out 12 hours before the operation, others do not. The *diet preparatory to operation* should consist of non-residue foods.

Post-operative nursing care. If the patient has had a general anaesthetic and not a spinal, he will be put back into bed recumbent, with one pillow under his head, and he should be given a knee pillow and an air ring. During the first 4 days the diet will consist of cool fluids, and in addition some opiate mixture will be given, such as tinct. opium 10 minims, twice a day in order to delay peristalsis and prevent the patient from having his bowels moved for several days. As soon as the bowels are opened he may have light diet such as fish.

The most important point in the care of these cases is the attention to the wound and dressing. The patient will return from the theatre with vaseline gauze packed around a large rubber tube about 4 inches long which has been placed into the ano-rectal passage; a piece of silk thread or fine string will be stitched into the distal end of this tube and this string will be arranged outside the dressing and kept in position by a piece of vaseline gauze. Unless the patient bleeds it is usual to leave this tube in for from 2 to 4 days. If the vaseline gauze becomes displaced before this time it may have to be renewed. Preparatory to removing the tube the patient is given 6 ounces of olive oil through the tube, the bed being elevated on blocks; the patient is given a fairly large dose of castor oil about the same time and if the bowels do not act within a reasonable time this is followed by a simple enema also administered through the tube. When the bowels act the tube comes out. In some cases the tube may come out earlier, and some surgeons like to replace it, while others order vaseline gauze to be packed into the cavity until the enema is given. Once the bowels have been opened the patient is allowed to get up to the bath twice a day, and after each bath the wound is syringed with eusol, vaseline gauze being packed into the cavity; this treatment is also carried out after every act of defecation. Subsequently the bowels are kept acting by an emulsion of liquid paraffin and phenolphthalein given as required.

The second great difficulty the nurse will probably encounter will be *retention of urine.* These patients are frequently distressed by the inability to pass urine and the nurse will have to use all her ingenuity by alteration of position in order to effect relief. In rare cases it will be found necessary to take the tube out while the patient passes urine, a fresh tube being replaced and the dressing attended to immediately afterwards. Catheterization should not be resorted to unless specially requested by the surgeon.

RESECTION OF COLON: COLOSTOMY: EXCISION OF RECTUM

Resection of colon in which a portion of gut is removed and an end to end anastomosis performed, is undertaken when there is a large amount of destruction of a part of this organ such as may occur in diverticulitis, in carcinoma and in rare cases of paralytic ileus. The *post-operative nursing care* is similar to that of any other acute abdominal condition and the special observations and precautions have all been described on pp. 639–53.

Colostomy. Colostomy is an opening into the colon by which its contents can be made to discharge on to the surface of the body. Left iliac colostomy is difficult to keep clean and is often complicated by inguinal hernia, therefore para medial colostomy is preferable; in this the colostomy is placed just to the left of the middle line below the umbilicus. This condition *may be made permanent* in cases of excision of the rectum, and in cases of inoperable growth. It is performed *as a temporary measure* before operations of abdomino-anal excision of rectum when the colon is anastomosed to the anus, thus retaining the sphincter. It is also performed as a temporary measure before operating on some removable growth, and therefore may precede or may be associated with resection of the colon, in such cases the colostomy is termed a 'safety valve', and is only maintained until healing occurs. A Paul's tube is inserted into the colon, the tube sloughs off in about five days as the wound heals, and secondary suture will be employed if necessary to assist healing of the wound. During the time the contents of the bowel are draining and until the wound is healed it should be irrigated with a mild antiseptic and kept very clean in order to promote healing. The surrounding skin should be protected with some form of grease.

When a colostomy is performed with intent to be more permanent in character, a portion of the gut is brought out on to the surface and kept in position by means of a glass rod, which is usually retained for about 10 days. After the operation the nurse should see that the patient is wearing a firm binder and, as the colon is stitched to the subcutaneous tissues, movement ought to be avoided. The stitches on each side of the colostomy should be protected with antiseptic and covered with elastoplast in order to prevent their being soiled with the discharge from the colostomy opening; it is possible to wash the elastoplast when soiled, but it should not be removed until the tenth day when the skin sutures will be taken out.

The colostomy may be opened at the time of operation, but some surgeons will leave this for 3 or 4 days. When the skin stitches are removed the skin may be washed with soap and water. The glass rod is now removed and usually replaced by a small piece of rubber tubing which will be kept in for a further period of 4 days. The skin will be again covered with elastoplast, and the easiest way to do this is to cut a window through which the colostomy will protrude, having the elastoplast adherent to the skin all round. Once the rod has been removed colostomy wash-outs commence, and these may be carried out by the use of an ordinary Higginson syringe with a catheter attached, the wash-out being given into the proximal end, at the same time each day, usually early in the morning in order to educate the bowel to be emptied at a convenient time each day. If the abdomen is distended at any time a flatus tube may be passed into the colon through the proximal opening. In cases of emergency colostomy an olive oil enema, given via the proximal opening, may be required to start the faeces flowing. In cases when the rectum is not closed or obliterated and will serve as an opening, a wash-out is given into the distal end of the colostomy and, the patient sitting on a bedpan, the wash-out will be returned through the anus. This measure is employed in order to keep the lower part of the bowel clean and free of mucus.

The elastoplast application already described will be used until the rubber tube which has replaced the glass rod is removed; this is taken away on the fourteenth day and afterwards the patient may be taken to the bath. At this period the patient is supplied with a belt. There are a variety of belts available, and it is a good plan to have one lined with jaconet and to have the part over the colostomy slightly stiffened in order to prevent friction. The patient is now taught how to put his belt on and take it off, and also to wash his colostomy out daily either by means of a Higginson's syringe with a catheter attached or by using a catheter and tubing and irrigation can.

Excision of rectum. This operation is only undertaken in the presence of inoperable growth involving the rectum. As a rule a colostomy is performed some time beforehand, at least 14 days—and longer than that if the condition of the patient is poor—in order to give time for improvement before such a large and serious operation is undertaken. The blood urea content is investigated and the urine very carefully tested. As the patient will suffer from a good deal of shock it is usual to give him a blood transfusion either before, during or after the operation.

The *usual preparation for operation* is carried out; presuming that the operation is to take place at ten o'clock next morning, the last food will be given at night, but the patient may have barley sugar after this. Early the next morning the colon will be washed out as usual, the surrounding skin painted with an antiseptic solution and the colostomy covered with oiled silk and strapping in order to seal it during the operation. In a female patient the vagina would be douched, and both male and female patients would be catheterized a short time before the operation and have a self-retaining catheter left in.

Post-operative nursing care. This is a large operation and as the patient will suffer serious shock he should be received back into bed in a recumbent position and have the foot of the bed elevated on 18-inch blocks. He may have been given a blood transfusion in the theatre and this may be repeated afterwards; otherwise it is usual to give fairly large quantities of subcutaneous saline—up to 2 pints. The patient is kept as warm as possible by the use of electric cradles. After 36 hours the foot of the bed is gradually lowered, being put on to 12-inch blocks first, then on to 6-inch blocks and finally lowered to the floor. As this patient must not be disturbed for anything during this period of grave post-operative shock through which he is passing, the catheter is left in for two days, or some form of suction bladder drainage is employed. The patient is nursed in the recumbent position with two pillows and an air ring. As soon as vomiting ceases he should be given fluids by mouth, as much as he can take, so that he may be hydrated by this means and then subcutaneous saline or other artificial provision of fluid may be omitted. As soon as the patient feels he would like it he may be given light diet and he should have as much fluid and food as he can take in order to effect improvement in his general condition as rapidly as possible.

Care of the dressing. The patient will have returned from the operating theatre with a roll of vaseline gauze and two corrugated rubber drainage tubes about 6 inches long inserted into the wound and incorporated in the dressing on each side. This drainage tubing will be removed about the third day, a little at a time and, as the dressing is very painful, morphia is often ordered to be given when it is disturbed. The cavity should be kept loosely filled with vaseline gauze—the tube may inadvertently be pulled out when the gauze is changed but it should be put back, freshly sterilized pieces being used. The tubing is now gradually shortened, and unless the stitches slough, which often happens, they should be taken out about the sixth or eighth day, and as soon as they are out an attempt should be made to keep the buttocks together by putting elastoplast across them in order to compress the anal region and facilitate healing. Once the original pack is out the cavity should be irrigated and repacked three times a day, or as often as is necessary to keep it clean. The bowels are acting regularly by means of the colostomy opening. As soon as the patient's condition will permit it, usually after the fourteenth day, he is taken to the bathroom in a wheel chair and sits in a warm bath for 10, 20 or 30 minutes in order to soak the dressing, which is then removed and the wound irrigated. As the wound becomes cleaner the vaseline gauze is replaced by an antiseptic dressing—such as one of the many aniline dyes—which will stimulate healing.

THYROIDECTOMY

The **pre-operative treatment** of patients for the operation of thyroidectomy is usually undertaken in a medical unit. The medical care of these cases has already been described in the section dealing with the disorders of the endocrine organs, on p. 443. It is sufficient here to state that the principles of treatment include an attempt to get the basal metabolic rate at the lowest level to which it can be brought; frequent tests are carried out and at the same time the patient is given graduated doses of Lugol's iodine. It is very important for the nurse to realize that the patient requires to be frequently reassured, that his co-operation is necessary for the success of the treatment, and that he should be brought to look upon the operation and the effect he will obtain from it without any fear. In many instances the patient is not informed of the actual day of operation but is informed that it will take place in a day or so; then, for example on the morning of the day of operation, after a good night's sleep the patient will be warned that it is to take place in an hour or two.

The type of anaesthetic used varies with the wishes of the surgeon: if gas and oxygen are employed the patient will have an early breakfast; if a local anaesthetic only is to be used the patient may have a cup of tea a couple of hours after breakfast and half a glass of water an hour before the operation.

Three-quarters of an hour beforehand, the patient is prepared for the theatre and placed on the stretcher on his bed, he passes urine and has all other points attended to (see p. 635). The pre-operative drug is then given—$\frac{1}{3}$ grain omnopon and $\frac{1}{150}$ scopolamine unless the operation is to be performed under a local anaesthetic when a larger dose of omnopon ($\frac{2}{3}$ grain) is given.

Post-operative nursing care. The position in which the patient is received in bed depends on whether he has had a local or a general anaesthetic: in the former case he may be placed in whatever position he likes, either having one pillow to support him or several pillows; if a general anaesthetic has been employed he will have to be nursed recumbent until he regains consciousness. The pulse must be taken and recorded every half hour for the first 12 hours. The respirations tend to slow down to as low as eight a minute—this must be very carefully watched and, if they get below twelve, an administration of oxygen containing carbon dioxide 7 per cent should be given by the nasal route until the respirations are increased in depth and frequency up to 18 a minute. The pulse should be carefully noted, as irregularity and rapidity may occur and any tachycardia should be reported. This should also be noted upon the chart.

Two of the most important points in the care of cases after thyroidectomy are to make them *swallow* a drink of water and *speak* as soon as possible as they are likely to be afflicted by fear of being unable to use the throat for these two purposes which if not rectified at the outset may become an obsession. The nurse will notice that when she gives them a drink it has to be carefully administered, since the patient will choke and splutter and cough, and she must encourage and reassure him, knowing that he can swallow, and she should give him small drinks at fairly frequent intervals until he can accomplish this feat with comparative ease.

Another important point to be remembered is that these patients perspire a great deal. This must be expected and warm dry clothing should be provided and warm towels for rubbing the patient down. The administration of fluid is another important point. On return to the ward they will frequently be given a rectal saline containing glucose up to 2 pints; this may be continued until the next morning, by which time the patient should be able to take drinks very freely and in this way to get sufficient fluid.

The complication most to be feared is bleeding. The pulse will be an indication of this and the nurse must be on the look-out for the symptoms of bleeding characterized by a blanched skin, a weak, rapid, thready, irregular pulse and shallow breathing. Bleeding from a superficial vessel will soak through the dressing and can be seen, and the dressing can be changed; but in some cases the bleeding may come from a vessel deep in the tissues of the neck and the patient may bleed seriously before this is discovered. An observant nurse should be able to notice the filling up of the tissues of the neck in the form of a swelling in the area of the gland.

The *dressing* of gauze and wool is maintained in position by means of a piece of strapping which is brought over crosswise from the back and crossed on each side of the breast; it maintains the dressing in position without applying pressure as would a circular bandage. In cases of vomiting the patient should be supplied with a jaconet bib long enough and wide enough to cover the whole of the operation area—this is tied round the neck by tapes attached to the jaconet, care being taken that it is not tied tightly.

Wound. On the first or second morning after the operation the dressing is taken down and the drainage tubes removed. The surgeon takes a great interest in the perfect adhesion of the margins of the wound in order to ensure an excellent cosmetic result. On the second day alternate clips or stitches are removed and the remainder are taken out on the third day. A little lanoline rubbed gently into the skin will help to render it soft and pliant.

The patient in a satisfactory case is usually allowed up about the seventh day, and should have a basal metabolic rate test carried out before discharge and as a rule goes home between the twelfth and fourteenth days.

OPERATIONS ON THE BREAST

Operations on the breast include opening an abscess, removal of adenoma, *simple amputation of the breast* when it, only, is removed, leaving muscles and glands intact, and *radical mastectomy* performed for carcinoma. In this case large skin flaps are turned back and the breast, fascia, muscles and lymphatic glands are removed including dissection of the axillary group of glands. The skin flaps are then turned over and sutured together; in some cases they will not meet and a large exposed area may be left. The surgeon may perform a skin-grafting operation at the time of operation or wait to perform it later; but he does not as a rule attempt to pull the edges together as this would result in tension, and sloughing of the flaps might occur.

After *simple amputation of the breast* one or two drainage tubes are put in at the lower border where drainage is likely to be free, and owing to the extensive removal of the tissue there will be a good deal of oozing during the first 48 hours. A large dressing is put on in order to absorb the exudate and discharge.

Pre-operative treatment. Routine pre-operative measures are carried out, but a very large area of skin should be prepared as the area of operation is extensive. In addition an area of skin on the outer aspect of one thigh should be prepared in case the surgeon wishes to perform a skin-grafting operation (see p. 718.)

Post-operative care. There are three main points to be considered in the post-operative nursing care of cases of *radical mastectomy*: the first is that shock will be very marked owing to the exposure of the large area and fairly extensive amount of bleeding, and the other two considerations are intelligent care of the dressing and re-education of the movements of the arm.

The patient will be received back to bed in a recumbent position, and should be supported by pillows.

Shock will be treated by external applications of warmth by electric cradle, electric blankets, or hot-water bottles. Many sisters provide small blankets to drape round the patient's shoulders and have the bedgown and bedjacket ready warming in a hot chamber to put on before the patient leaves the operating theatre. As a rule a rectal saline will be administered and repeated in 4 hours if required. It may not be required, as although these cases suffer from a good deal of initial shock they respond rapidly to treatment.

Dressing. From the outset the dressing should be carefully watched for bleeding and, if it comes through, it should be repacked; it should not be redressed during the first 12–24 hours unless the bleeding is more extensive than might reasonably be expected.

The dressing should be changed on the first day, and the nurse should move the rubber drainage tube slightly in order to prevent its adhering to the flaps; the flaps should be very carefully inspected to see if they are ballooning as the result of serum beneath them; if this occurs the nurse should carefully insert a pair of sinus forceps at the side of a stitch at the most dependent part of the incision near the medial line—the drainage tubes will usually have been inserted at the lower border of the incision on its lateral aspect. When attending to the dressing she should also inspect the edges of the wound for any sign of sloughing and should note whether there appears to be undue tension, as this will invariably result in sloughing.

On the second day the tube is usually removed. Throughout the whole of the post-operative period in her care of the dressing the nurse will make the observations described above and deal with them as they arise. As soon as possible she will encourage healing by the application of sulphathiazole powder. In an uncomplicated case continuous sutures would be removed about the seventh or eighth day, clips alternately on the fifth and sixth day, and tension stitches between the tenth and fourteenth days.

When radium is used special care is necessary, see p. 809.

Care of the arm. It is important for the nurse to see that the movements of abduction and external rotation of the arm are performed several times a day as these are the movements which are important to a woman in doing her hair, and fastening her clothes at the back. The patient may get up after the fourth day and she should be able to do her hair by the end of a week.

The *complications* which may arise are bronchitis, broncho-pneumonia, thrombosis and sepsis but the danger of these can be reduced by the administration of penicillin.

OPERATIONS ON THE GALLBLADDER

Inflammation of the gallbladder or cholecystitis has been described on p. 395. In surgical treatment the gallbladder may be opened and drained, *cholecystotomy*, or it may be removed, *cholecystectomy*. Before an operation is undertaken the function of the organ will be investigated by means of cholecystography.

Vitamin K which controls the prothrombin content of the blood and maintains it at the level required to give normal coagulation time is often given to cases of obstructive jaundice for several days before operation in order to prevent post-operative bleeding in jaundiced patients. *Kapilon* is the synthetic preparation recently produced by the Glaxo laboratories. The dose is from 1 c.c. to 2 c.c. by hypodermic injection for several days before and several days after operation.

In the **post-operative nursing care** the patient is propped up into Fowler's position as soon as he recovers from the anaesthetic in order to aid the action of the diaphragm and so prevent the complications of hypostatic pneumonia and abdominal distension; and also to facilitate drainage from the wound, and avoid any possibility of retention of bile in the abdominal cavity which might give rise to sepsis. Vomiting, which may last for some hours, and a fair amount of abdominal distension, are the discomforts which prove troublesome after the operation of cholecystectomy. Small drinks of hot water containing sodium bicarbonate may be sufficient to relieve vomiting, abdominal distension may be relieved by passing a flatus tube or it may need the administration of a carminative enema. An aperient should be given as soon as possible, within 24 to 36 hours after the operation, and when the bowels have acted the patient may be able to take light diet.

The dressing should be watched, a drainage tube or glove drain is inserted as there may be oozing from the liver and leakage of bile for a few days.

SURGICAL AMPUTATION OF A LIMB

Amputation is only employed when all attempts to save a limb in case of injury or disease have failed. A limb amputated is a deformity which may upset the balance of weight and give rise to deformity of the spine.

In the **post-operative care** of a patient with the leg amputated above the knee, a divided bed will be used (see p. 90). The bedclothing is so arranged that the stump can be seen. A tourniquet should be in readiness in case of bleeding and the nurses in the ward should know how to apply it. Bleeding is not very likely to occur, but should this happen the patient's life will be in immediate danger and unless those on duty can act he will bleed to death in a few minutes. The nurses should be warned of this possibility, warned not to be frightened and told exactly how to act if this emergency arises.

The stump will be supported by a sandbag covered by jaconet and a sterile towel, for the first few days after operation. There will be considerable oozing of serum, and a drainage tube or tubes will have been inserted. The gauze and wool should be changed as often as necessary. During the dressing of the stump it should be firmly held, as it will jump and this is distressing to the patient. Particular attention should be paid to the skin flaps, in order to observe whether serum is collecting beneath them and to effect its removal.

After the first few days the sandbag which is supporting the stump will be removed and it should then lie flat on the bed. It is important to see that the bed does not sink in the middle as the possibility of flexion occurring at the hip joint has to be remembered, because any flexional deformity would have to be corrected before the patient could use an artificial limb with comfort.

SKIN GRAFTING

Skin grafting is the transplanting of skin from one area to another in order to cover a part which is denuded of skin, either as the result of injury as in burns, or to reduce deformity such as for example may result from scarring. Skin grafting was introduced by Reverdin in 1869. It now forms a most important part of plastic surgery.

Types of Graft. The *pinch graft* which was Reverdin's original method consists in pinching up small pieces of skin, separating them by means of a knife and transferring them to a raw area. The pinch grafts vary in size from that of a ladybird to a postage stamp. They are dotted over the area to be covered.

The *Thiersch graft* consists of larger pieces of skin which may be thin or thick grafts according as the graft needs to be adapted to the surface on which it is to be placed. This form of graft is taken by means of a special razor.

Wolfe's graft. In this graft the whole thickness of skin is taken. It is dissected out, denuded of fat and subcutaneous tissue and applied to the raw surface for which it is intended. It may be stitched in position.

Dermatome graft is a term used to describe a graft taken by means of a special cutting instrument, a dermatome. By this means long strips of skin can be removed. These grafts are usually taken from the area of the abdomen or from the back.

Pedicle graft. This method is used when it is required specially to ensure that the graft retains a good blood supply. The skin is raised and sutured tubular fashion. It is left attached at each end and dressed without pressure and avoiding all tension. After a period of about two weeks, provided that all has gone well with the graft, one end of the pedicle is detached and implanted on to the area to be grafted. This part of the body is then fixed to the donor area until the graft has taken and is receiving a good blood supply. Then supposing, for example, the area to which this graft is to be applied is a scar; the scar is excised, the pedicle is detached from its second end, the tube-like structure is unrolled and spread out and laid on to the area to be grafted.

Preparation for skin grafting. Speaking generally only autogenous grafts are successful. If sometimes grafts from other individuals are considered, it is important that the donor and recipient shall be of the same blood group.

The donor area of skin and the area to be grafted receive the same preparation. The skin is cleansed with a weak solution of dettol, about 10 per cent, and then with saline. In the operating theatre the same solution of dettol is used and the skin is cleansed with ether in addition. When a mucous surface such as the nose is to be included in the area to be grafted a very weak solution of mercury is sometimes employed.

Dressing skin grafted areas. The *donor area* is dried with sterile swabs, covered with tulle gras over which a compress of saline is put.

This is firmly bandaged on and finally the bandage is either secured by some adhesive substance, or by strapping in order to ensure that the dressing remains absolutely immobile.

The *grafted area* is covered with tulle gras and saline compresses, or alternatively with cotton wool soaked in flavine and paraffin. This dressing is covered by gauze wrung out in saline and finally bandaged and firmly secured as in the case of the donor area. To render immobile the dressing applied to a skin grafted area is a most important nursing point.

Pressure. The surgeon will indicate what degree of pressure is required. In some cases when considerable pressure is needed a form of plasticine, known as *stent*, is employed. The graft laid over the specially cut and prepared piece of stent is applied to the area to be covered.

Chapter 46

Surgery of the Thorax including Nursing Care

Introduction—Thoracoplasty and post-operative nursing care—Lobectomy and pneumomectomy—Rib resection—For minor operations on the thorax *see pulmonary tuberculosis, p.* 504

In dealing with patients who have had operations performed on the thorax the nurse must consider whether the patient is suffering from pulmonary tuberculosis, septic infection or carcinoma, in order to be fully aware of the patient's general condition.

In all cases breathing exercises will be taught, and if the patient's condition permits these are taught before the operation is performed. This work is usually in the hands of an experienced physiotherapist but the nurse should be familiar with the procedure and encourage the patient to persevere. The physiotherapist may visit once or twice a day, but nurses are at the service of the patient day and night and expansion of the lungs, to be of value, must be practised frequently, 'little and often' should be the maxim.

A patient on whom thoracoplasty has been performed will need rest in bed for several months. But all other chest cases should get up as soon as possible because getting up and walking are exercises which demand expansion of the lungs. The clothes of these patients should not be sent home, they need them, and a wardrobe, not a locker, should be provided in which to keep them.

Modern methods of treatment by blood transfusion and fluid infusion lessen and in many cases avoid altogether any post-operative shock. A patient who has had pneumomectomy performed may be allowed to get up on the second day, have a bath on the fourth day and go out for walks at the end of a week.

This aspect of surgery is pioneer in treating the hospital ward as a hotel where the patient lives a normal life, getting up and pottering around, going out and coming in, resting and walking, eating and sleeping; in fact a place where everything has some therapeutic value tending to the desired end—the ultimate and effective reablement of the patient.

SURGERY OF THE THORAX

Thoracoplasty is removal of a number of ribs which result in collapse of the chest wall and consequently in collapse of the lung. It is performed in pulmonary tuberculosis, empyema and bronchiectasis. Before operation the patient should be as well as possible.

In order to obtain the best results, a highly skilled team of surgeons, physicians and nurses are required both in the operating theatre and in the recovery ward. Further, the patient should know the object and extent of the operation, and as the operation will be performed under a local anaesthetic he should be able to play his part by intelligent co-operation with the nurse and anaesthetist in attendance. The patient may have to be removed to a hospital for this operation, although many modern sanatoria are equipped for this purpose. If the patient can be in the environment he is used to, this is an advantage because he feels he is amongst trusted friends. Moreover the morale is usually high in a sanatorium where patients are confident of the success of the operation owing to experience in the success of it in others who have undergone the same operation.

The skin of the back requires very careful preparation, any acne or pustules should be healed before the operation. The patient is placed on his side on the operating table and comfortably steadied by sandbags. A large J-shaped incision is made extending between the spine and the scapula, the scapula is lifted off the chest wall and held firmly out of the way by suitable retractors.

As the operation will be performed in stages (usually 3 stages), the 3 upper ribs are generally removed at the first stage, then two to three weeks later, the next three or four ribs are removed and the remaining ones at a subsequent operation. The ribs to be excised are well exposed, and denuded of their periosteum. Special attention is paid to cutting through the ribs as near the vertebral ends as possible so that the pulmonary collapse finally produced may be as complete as possible. As the incision made is an extensive one, considerable bleeding occurs. Moreover very large muscles are incised and the loss of blood and muscle trauma results in considerable shock.

The surgeon works swiftly and skilfully. Bleeding points are sealed by cautery. The wound is sutured without drainage, but great care is exercised in excluding all serum from beneath the skin so that healing may take place without sepsis intervening. This is important as the original wound will have to be re-incised for the subsequent operations. The gauze and wool dressing is strapped in position by means of elastoplast but no turns of strapping or bandage may encircle the chest, as the movements of respiration must be encouraged and not impeded.

Post-operative care. The patient is put carefully back to bed supported by pillows and in such a position that the movements of the sound side of the chest are not interfered with. The position adopted depends a great deal on the general condition of the patient and also on the post-operative routine measures prescribed by the surgeon. The patient may be placed flat in bed with the foot raised on blocks until his pulse is satisfactory. To assist pulmonary drainage in cases where the patient finds expectoration a difficulty this position may be maintained for several days. Alternatively on returning from the theatre the patient may be propped up on pillows and placed on his affected side. Although he is suffering from a good deal of shock he will be quite able to follow any instructions given him and will be interested in the progress he makes. His position should be changed at frequent intervals as movement will help to stimulate coughing and expectoration. He may have been given a blood transfusion in the operating theatre. This will be repeated as required. It is essential that the patient should have plenty of fluid, he will be able to take some by mouth; the amount can be supplemented by the administration of fluid by other routes.

At least 5 to 6 pints of fluid must be administered daily by mouth, rectum, subcutaneous tissue or vein during the first few days. The patient may complain of nausea at first, but as soon as possible he should be given small drinks of water, tea, and fruit juice every 15 minutes. The amount he can take should be gradually increased. As soon as the patient wishes he may have solid food, this should be of high calorie value and have a high vitamin content. If the patient is nursed in his cubicle, this will be closed at first and the temperature of the room kept at about 68° to 70° F. For the first 24 to 48 hours or until he has recovered from shock the patient must be kept warm. He must not be subjected to draught or chilling. Ordinary sanatorium temperature cannot be considered safe until several days have elapsed. The pulse rate or volume should be watched and recorded every 15 minutes at first, and then every hour. The temperature should be taken and charted regularly. The amount of fluid given (by all routes) should be carefully recorded.

Drugs will be given to relieve pain but consideration must be made as to the effect of such drugs on the respirations and cough reflex. Pain and shock tend to diminish the cough reflex. Morphia further inhibits it. Small doses of sedative drugs given at regular intervals are recommended. The patient should be kept free from discomfort but the cough reflex should not be affected by the sedatives given. It is important that the patient should cough frequently, at least every hour.

As the result of removal of ribs the lung collapses and the walls of cavities in the lung which contained secretion are brought together. This results in the secretion being squeezed out and it must be coughed up, otherwise it will lodge in healthy bronchial tubes and cause fresh tuberculous lesions.

Difficulty in expectoration can be relieved by hot lemon or lime juice drinks or sipping hot sodium bicarbonate solution. It may also be stimulated by steam inhalations.

The amount of sputum should be charted by weight or volume. Rattling in the air tubes shows they want clearing and if the fluid secretion cannot be removed by effective coughing aided by posture the surgeon will extract the collection of fluid by means of a bronchoscope.

The patient must be encouraged to cough at regular intervals, at least every hour during the days immediately after the operation and the cough must result in the bringing up of sputum. Various measures have been devised to encourage a patient to cough. The nurse standing on the patient's sound side should get him to sit forward and placing one arm across the front of his chest give support with the flat of the hand to the lower part of the wound, at the same time she supports the back of the chest with her other hand. Thus supported the patient will cough. Or she may stand on the affected side with the flat of one hand over the lower part of the wound and the other hand on the front of the chest. She must never be content with feeble attempts at hawking but must see that coughing is effective. The patient should take a few deep breaths and then cough. The value of effective coughing cannot be over-emphasized for the reasons given above. At the end of a period spent in coughing the patient should rest. Oxygen is given if necessary to relieve respiratory distress. It is usually administered by mean of a B.L.B. mask (see p. 319). to ensure that the patient is given a fairly high concentration of the gas.

The wound will be dressed when required. As a rule it is carefully attended to the morning after the operation, though it may be necessary to change the dressing earlier than this. It is important to keep the wound edges in apposition and to press out, from beneath skin flaps and wound edges, any serum resting there. The skin is usually painted with some antiseptic. Iodine, alcohol or an aniline dye preparation may be used. After the first day or two the wound may not need to be disturbed until the stitches are removed in 7 to 10 days. The wound and stitch marks are then kept clean and free from scabs, because, as already mentioned, the original incision will be used again in performing the next stage of thoracoplasty in 2 or 3 weeks' time.

Complications which may occur and which pre- and post-operative care go far to prevent include local *sepsis* and *haematoma* which may cause the wound to break down.

Spread of tuberculous infection to adjacent bronchi has already been mentioned. *Scoliosis* may result but it is preventable.

As the result of removal of ribs the normal alignment of the trunk is interfered with and stability can only be obtained by re-education. This work is principally in the hands of an experienced physiotherapist but the nurse should make it her business to know the aims of treatment so that she may co-operate. It is important for example that the patient should learn to lie and sit upright, to have his head in a straight line with his trunk. The movement of the arm and shoulder girdle should be practised. A patient should be able to elevate his arm above his head as in arm stretching upwards, within a fraction of the movement possible on the sound side. Provided that these points are attended to and that the patient learns to lie, sit and walk with his head straight, shoulders squared and head in line with the trunk scoliosis will not occur. As the aim of treatment is to restore the function of the lungs as fully as possible *breathing exercises* are taught to encourage movement of the chest and expansion of the lungs. A clever physiotherapist can teach patients to expand different portions of the lung indicating the area to be expanded by placing the hand over the area upon which the patient is to concentrate. Localized breathing can be made an interesting occupation.

Pressure by means of weights and sandbags is applied to the parts of the chest from which the ribs have been removed, particularly the upper parts, over the apex and in the axilla, in order to ensure that collapse of the lung will be as complete as possible. New ribs grow from the periosteum which was stripped off the ribs removed at the time of operation. They will grow in a new position. The ribs of a patient who has had thoracoplasty performed can be described as lying in the position of a bucket handle which lies against the edge of the bucket placed on its side, and not, as in the normal chest, where the ribs correspond in position to the handle elevated from the side of the bucket.

After care. After thoracoplasty a patient requires a period of from three to six months' rest in bed. During this time breathing exercises and exercises which aim at maintaining good posture of the head and shoulders in relation to the trunk and in addition to general exercises for the whole body in order to make the patient breathe deeply, are taught. After a period of rest in bed the patient is allowed to get up and finally he is sent to a sanatorium for graduated exercise treatment until he is considered to be ready to take up some employment. He will spend approximately six months in the sanatorium.

A patient who has had thoracoplasty performed should keep in touch with his surgeon or hospital for about 2 years so that the condition of his chest and his general state of health may be observed.

Lobectomy is performed in bronchiectasis and in some cases of abscess of the lung. It is usually performed under a spinal anaesthetic. The chest is opened, a portion of rib is removed, and through this opening the diseased lobe is severed from its attachments and the stump sutured.

Before operation the patient is taught how to breathe and how to empty his chest of air. He has been subjected to a long course of postural drainage treatment in order to have the lung as free of pus as possible.

In order to make the pleural surfaces adhere together *poudrage* is carried out several weeks before operation. A pneumothorax is performed and a thorascope is passed, through which a special powder is blown on to the surface of the visceral pleura. Talc containing an antiseptic is employed, this is irritant to the lung and causes the two pleurae to adhere and by this means the lobes of the lung which are not removed at the operation are prevented from collapsing.

Post-operative care. Treatment for shock will usually be necessary and a blood transfusion may be required. But as soon as possible the patient should be propped up in bed as he must be encouraged to cough up secretion or pus.

Getting the patient up causes him to move and increases the need for deep breathing, it promotes expansion of the lungs. As soon as the general condition permits the patient should be helped out of bed, morning and evening, after the second day; he should get up to go to the lavatory as soon as possible, be taught general physical exercises and go out for walks in the fresh air.

X-ray examination is carried out to observe the rate of expansion of the remaining lobes of the lung which, if all goes well, will soon fill the chest cavity.

Complications which may arise include haemorrhage from the stump or from an intercostal vessel. Collapse of the lung may occur but the formation of adhesions between the pleura and the maintenance of intrapleural negative pressure aim at preventing this complication.

Pneumomectomy is removal of a lung which is performed for carcinoma and in some cases of bronchiectasis when the lung is very fibrous. The lung is collapsed before the operation by means of a pneumothorax partly to accustom the patient to breathing with one lung and thus minimise his post-operative discomfort. Before operation the patient should be in as good a general state of health as possible.

Post-operative care. Shock must be treated and a blood transfusion is usually needed. The patient should get up as soon as possible and have the same treatment as described above (see Lobectomy). The chest cavity will contain fluid at first, but as the wound is closed there is little danger of infection, and little by little fibrin will be found and the fluid replaced by it, will gradually be absorbed.

Rib resection is performed for the relief and drainage of empyema (see p. 674). From 1½ to 3 inches of rib are removed, the pleural cavity is opened, carefully inspected, pus and clots are removed, the cavity is irrigated and a flanged tube, such as Tudor Edwards's, is inserted and the wound is sutured.

Post-operative Care. In many instances this operation is performed under a local anaesthetic so that the patient is able to be propped up on pillows as soon as he returns to the ward. The first consideration is to maintain drainage of the empyema cavity. A tube, usually Tudor Edwards's tube which is a combined drainage and irrigation tube is employed. This tube is attached either to a simple underwater drainage bottle or a suction drainage apparatus. It is very important to see that the tube does not get kinked; it is equally important to ensure that no air enters the cavity. Dressings around the tube and over the wound should be maintained in position by pieces of elastoplast. The chest should not be encircled by any turns of bandage or binder.

The day after operation pleural irrigation will be started. No force may be employed, fluid either saline, boracic or Dakin's solution will be gently run in to the cavity by means of a tube and funnel. The small bore tube on Tudor Edwards's tube is employed for this so that the fluid returns through the larger tube. The empyema cavity will heal slowly as the lung expands slowly so that the drainage tube should not be omitted too soon. The depth of the cavity may be investigated by a fine gum elastic bougie and the tube shortened as necessary at intervals of about a week. Breathing exercises should be taught. Systemic administration of penicillin will help to combat sepsis.

The danger of empyema is that it may, even after operation and drainage, become chronic. To prevent this, drainage should be efficient and the daily irrigation of the cavity as complete as possible, breathing exercises will assist expansion of the lung.

A patient who has had an empyema for some time will be very toxic, he may be considerably wasted as he has had a grave toxaemia. He needs fresh air and good food, interest and recreation, as he needs encouragement in order to face the difficulties of life again.

Minor operations on the thorax (pneumothorax, pneumoperitoneum, phrenic crush and avulsion, and thoracoscopy) have been mentioned in chapter 35.

Chapter 47

Common Surgical Conditions of the Genito-Urinary Tract, including Points in the Preparation and Post-Operative Care

Surgical conditions of the genito-urinary tract: pyelitis, acute suppurative nephritis, stone in kidney, stone in bladder, enlargement of the prostate gland—Operations on the genito-urinary organs: nephrectomy, nephrostomy or nephrotomy, nephropexy, cystostomy or cystotomy, cystectomy, litholapaxy, prostatectomy, urethrotomy, amputation of penis—Decompression of the distended urinary bladder

Investigation of the genito-urinary tract includes:
Chemical examination of the urine;
Microscopic examination of the urine;
Bacteriological examination of the urine;
Examination of the urinary tract by direct X-ray; and
Examination of the urinary tract by pyelography.

These investigations have been described in the sections dealing with the examination of urine, and investigations and tests (see pp. 69 and 169).

SURGICAL CONDITIONS OF THE GENITO-URINARY TRACT

Surgical diseases of the kidney may be classified under three headings: (1) *injury to the organ*, which may cause serious haemorrhage and necessitate removal, (2) *congenital abnormalities*, the commonest of which is the horseshoe-shaped kidney in which the lower poles of the organ are united by a band of renal tissue passing across in front of the lumbar vertebrae, and (3) *inflammatory conditions of the kidney*. Nephritis, which is treated medically, has been described on p. 399. Apart from this condition surgical inflammation of the kidney may be either acute or chronic.

Pyelitis is acute inflammation of the kidney pelvis, and is usually due to the presence of *Bacillus coli*. There are a diversity of opinions as to how this organism reaches the kidney. Many surgeons think it is due to direct infection of the organ from the colon which lies in front of it and, as in many instances only one kidney is infected, it is thought that infection by means of the blood stream is comparatively rare. (For description of symptoms and treatment see Pyelitis, p. 403.)

Acute suppurative nephritis. This condition is quite distinct from the acute nephritis treated medically (see p. 399), and is due to organisms which may have reached the kidney from some septic focus, such as an infective skin lesion, especially carbuncle.

The *symptoms* are pain in the loin, and tenderness over the affected kidney accompanied by a rise of temperature. The pain may be very acute and may be mistaken for an acute attack of appendicitis. As the disease progresses pus forms, and will be found to be present in the urine.

A chronic inflammatory condition of the kidney may also occur, probably due to tuberculosis. The symptoms in these cases are similar, but less acute than those described above.

Stone in the kidney. A stone in a kidney is an accumulation of salts, normally present in urine, which have formed a concretion. It occurs most commonly when the urine is highly concentrated. The substances of which these stones are formed are *calcium oxylate*, which forms the majority, and *uric acid*, *urates* and *phosphates*. The stone begins to form in one of the tubules and, as it gets larger, it forces its way into the pelvis of the kidney, and may remain there, gradually increasing in size or, if it is very small, it may pass down the ureter and may even reach the bladder and be passed out in the urine.

The *complications* of stone in the kidney are (1) *blockage of the ureter*, which may cause renal colic (see below); (2) *hydronephrosis*, which is due to damming the urine back on to the kidneys which results in damage to the kidney substance. When a kidney is filled with urine the condition is termed hydronephrosis. If this stagnant urine becomes infected, which is very likely to happen, it gives rise to a kidney full of pus—*pyonephrosis*.

The *symptoms* of stone in the kidney vary—there may not be any at all, if the stone grows slowly, and does not move. On the other hand there may be *pain* in the loin, owing to irritation of the kidney substance by pressure or movement of a stone. When definite symptoms arise there is pain in the loin which is made worse by activity. *Haematuria* may be present, movement of the stone into the pelvis of the kidney and ureter gives rise to *renal colic*, characterized by attacks of acute pain in the loin, passing round to the side of the abdomen and shooting down to the groin. It is cramplike in character, causing the patient to roll about in agony. His skin becomes covered with cold sweat and he vomits. He has an uncontrollable desire to pass urine, and passes a few drops at a time every few minutes. This condition is described as *strangury*. An attack usually lasts for several hours, and it may subside or can generally be relieved by morphia.

A *complication* of a stone in the ureter is impaction, giving rise to hydronephrosis, because the urine is pent back on the kidney and, if infection occurs, the condition proceeds to one of pyonephrosis. The *treatment* is removal of the stone. A high acid content diet is considered useful in avoiding the formation of calcium oxylate stone.

Stone in the bladder. A stone may form in the bladder or it may form in the kidney and, passing into the bladder, lie there and increase in size. The symptoms are pain when jolted, and on passing urine. As the bladder empties during the act of micturition its walls contract on the stone, pressing it down against the most sensitive part of the bladder which is the urethral opening, and causing great pain. As the bladder fills again the pain is relieved. Stone in the bladder is usually accompanied by some haematuria which may be slight or severe.

Surgical treatment is removal of the stone, either by opening the bladder from above—suprapubic cystotomy—or by removing it via the urethra.

The position and size of the stone is previously investigated by cystoscopy (see p. 171).

Enlargement of the Prostate Gland occurs in elderly men. In many cases this enlargement is physiological; in others it may be due to carcinoma, but recent research into the relationship of *sex hormones* to the cause of cancer has led to the discovery that carcinoma of the prostate gland can be successfully treated by the oral administration of a synthetic preparation of oestrin—stilboestrol. The *history* obtained and the *symptoms* present vary. There may have been frequency of micturition for some time, urine dribbling away day and night, the bladder always containing some residual urine which may, and frequently does, result in cystitis. On the other hand, the first indication of prostatic enlargement may be acute retention of urine or an alarming attack of haematuria. In most cases there is some degree of renal inefficiency.

OPERATIONS ON THE GENITO-URINARY ORGANS

In *the preparation for operations on the kidney* the renal function is thoroughly investigated as described in the case of prostatectomy. It is important that the patient should have one healthy kidney before removal of the second kidney—which may be a diseased organ—is considered. The general preparation is as described for any other abdominal operation. It is important to prepare a large area of skin back and front. The following are operations most commonly performed.

Nephrectomy is removal of the kidney.

In the *post-operative nursing care* considerable pain and shock will need to be relieved. The *complications* which constitute the greatest danger in these cases are *secondary haemorrhage* and *suppression of urine*. The patient is put in Fowler's position as soon as possible. The dressing is carefully observed for bleeding. A drainage tube will usually have been inserted, and the dressing will be taken down after 24 hours and the flaps examined for the presence of fluid beneath them, particularly on the anterior aspect of the wound. The margins should be inspected to see that overlapping does not occur. The drainage tube will be removed in 2 or 3 days as the quantity of serous discharge lessens. The stitches are usually removed after 7 days.

The pulse should be observed every half-hour, as bleeding may occur. Blood may collect in the tissues, or it may move from the kidney to the bladder, and be passed in the urine. The urine should be measured and inspected for the amount of blood, which ought to decrease as the days go by. Until the urine is free from blood it is very important that the patient should lie quietly and not make any exertion. The administration of bland fluids in large quantities in order to maintain the activity of the renal tract is important. Many surgeons order sulphadiazine for the first 7 days. Patients get up after the tenth day and go home about the sixteenth day.

Nephrostomy or nephrotomy is opening into the kidney, usually performed for the removal of stone and in this case the term *nephrolithotomy* may alternatively be employed. Nephrostomy is also undertaken to drain an obstructed kidney. A tube is inserted to drain the cavity; the dressing is performed after 36–48 hours when the tube is turned to prevent it becoming adherent; this is repeated every day until the tube is removed.

When nephrostomy is performed with the object of *plastic repair of a kidney damaged by hydronephrosis* a tube is inserted through which the cavity will be irrigated until it is clean and the wound can be closed; a ureteric catheter is inserted for drainage purposes and when the surgeon considers the condition of the operation area permits, the sutures retaining this in position are cut, the catheter slips out and is dispensed with.

Nephropexy is stitching the kidney to the posterior abdominal wall which is very occasionally performed in cases of visceroptosis of the kidney

In addition to the operation for removal of the prostate gland operations may be undertaken for the removal of growths or stone from the bladder. The same preliminary investigation, preparation and after care are needed as in the case of prostatectomy (see below).

Cystostomy may be performed by the open or closed method. **Closed cystostomy** is rarely performed. It may be used for the removal of a large stone which cannot be crushed or evacuated.

Suprapubic cystostomy. The bladder is opened and drained by the insertion of a tube suprapubically or by a self-retaining catheter through a wound made in the bladder. The urine is drained away into a receptacle by the bed, the bladder is irrigated once or twice a day and in some cases continuous bladder irrigation and drainage is employed (see p. 145).

Post-operative nursing care. It is essential to endeavour to keep the suprapubic wound dry. There are a variety of methods employed including Hamilton-Irving's box and the nurse should be familiar with the management of drainage apparatus. The patient must be encouraged to take copious fluids to drink, the volume of fluid intake and urinary output should be carefully measured. Seventy to eighty ounces in the twenty-four hours would be a good urinary output. When the operation has been performed prior to prostatectomy the blood-urea and other renal efficiency tests will be performed at intervals and it will be observed that as the volume of urinary output improves the percentage of the blood-urea will approximate more to the normal.

Cystectomy is removal of the bladder. This operation is performed when there is a tumour, usually a malignant one, in the bladder.

The pre-operative treatment includes daily colonic washout, a low residue diet for several days and most surgeons use sulpha-therapy.

The operation is often performed in two or three stages. First the ureters are transplanted into the colon; in most instances the right ureter is transplanted first because it is the easiest, a period of 14 days elapses and the second is transplanted. A week later the bladder is removed.

The post-operative nursing care includes treatment for shock, if required, liberal administration of fluids, and observation of the urinary output. An intravenous continuous drip infusion of sodium sulphate 3·3 to 5 per cent is given in order to act as a diuretic; in addition it provides fluid and is continued for as long as is necessary. Blood transfusion is given as necessary to combat shock. A rectal tube is inserted for the first three days (after each transplantation). It is removed on the fourth day but the patient may have it in at night for a day or two longer. These patients get up as soon as possible, they may get out of bed to use a commode on the second day after transplantation. In some cases there is distension of the colon and this cannot be treated by the usual means, such as pituitrin, eserine and carminatives because anything which caused the muscle of the colon to contract might dislodge the transplanted ureter. To get the patient moving about, sitting on a commode to try to relieve himself, aided by plenty of fluids by mouth are simple but safe means of treatment. The next and greatest consideration is for the patient to learn to control the rectal sphincters. At first urine is passed every half-hour or so, later control may increase to three hours, but whatever the result may be, life holds a better and more comfortable future than would have been possible without the operation, as a growth in the bladder means either retention or incontinence with subsequent renal infection and uraemia.

Litholapaxy is crushing a stone in the bladder followed by evacuation, through the urethra, of the particles of crushed stone. A lithotrite is passed into the bladder by the urethra, as in passing a catheter; the stone is grasped between the blades and crushed, the particles being evacuated by means of a special instrument, Bigelow's evacuator, and the bladder is irrigated.

The *post-operative nursing care* includes observation of the character of the urine passed and the administration of copious bland fluids in order to flush the urinary system. Bladder irrigation and urinary antiseptics may be ordered.

Prostatectomy may be performed by various methods. The gland may be enucleated through an incision in the wall of the bladder, the approach may be made through the perineum or by the urethra. These three methods are termed *suprapubic*, *perineal* and *transurethral* resection respectively. More recently *retropubic prostatectomy* has been introduced (see below).

Pre-operative measures. Before prostatectomy is performed certain preliminary investigations are necessary including estimation of the blood pressure and blood-urea content, urea clearance and urea concentration tests, cystoscopy, examination of the teeth for sepsis, and investigation of the condition of the heart and lungs.

Whether the operation is performed in one or two stages, and whether treatment of the bladder is to be carried out before operation, depends on the presence of urinary infection and the degree of renal efficiency. In the two-stage operation suprapubic cystotomy is first performed and the bladder is drained by means of a self-retaining catheter, and bladder irrigation is carried out twice a day for about 10 days. Alternatively, bladder irrigation only may be utilized or continuous bladder irrigation and drainage employed (see also bladder drainage, p. 147).

General preparation. An aperient is given two mornings before operation and liquid paraffin three times a day; an enema is only given if required. The skin of the abdomen, penis, scrotum, the upper half of the thighs, and the buttocks and loins is prepared and a sterile dressing is bandaged on. Sulpha-therapy and/or penicillin is generally employed.

Amongst the patients the nurse will be called upon to take care of after the operation of prostatectomy some will have had *Freyer's* and some *Thompson-Walker's operations*, which are two-stage suprapubic methods entailing about six weeks' hospital care and prolonged convalescence.

The *post-operative nursing care* is similar to that of cystectomy (see p. 729). The bladder is drained through the suprapubic wound and irrigated either by the urethra or by the wound. Hamilton-Irving's box is usually applied. Shock, haemorrhage and renal failure are complications which may occur.

Other patients will have had *Harris's operation*, which is a more complicated procedure. The gland is enucleated through a suprapubic wound, and the prostatic bed is repaired which lessens the tendency to haemorrhage. The prostatic urethra is reconstructed, a whistle-tip catheter is passed and a silkworm gut stitch through the eye of the catheter is fixed to the anterior abdominal wall. The bladder is usually closed. Before the patient leaves the theatre some fluid is syringed in and out through the urethral catheter to make sure it is not blocked and to remove any clots which may have collected.

Millin's operation (*Retropubic Prostatectomy*) or some modification of it is the operation of choice at the present time.

The *pre-operative measures* are employed as described on p. 634. The operation may be performed in two stages or one stage. The retropubic incision is made transversely, the gland is enucleated with the finger, a urethral catheter is inserted for drainage and a corrugated rubber drain is placed in the wound. This is removed after about two days.

Post-operative care. The bladder drains into a bottle beside the bed. The patient is propped up in Fowler's position. He is given fluids for 12 hours and may then have light diet. He must drink many pints of fluid a day both before and after operation. An aperient is given on the second evening and liquid paraffin is given three times a day. An enema should never be given without the permission of the surgeon, as it may cause bleeding. Drainage from the bladder must be observed carefully, drainage must be maintained and the amount measured. If the catheter should appear blocked, 1 ounce of sodium citrate solution (2 per cent) may be passed gently into the bladder and withdrawn (the amount injected must always be recovered); this may be repeated, if it is not efficacious the condition must be reported to the surgeon.

It is very important that the bladder should not be distended, and if drainage cannot be re-established and the surgeon suspects that the bladder contains bloodclot he may inject 1 ounce of glycerine of pepsin which will dissolve the clot. After half an hour it may be possible to wash out the bladder, using a Canny-Ryall syringe and injecting and withdrawing 1 ounce of the sodium citrate solution until the fluid is clear.

The catheter is removed in three or four days. The patient may get up about the fourth day and may go home as soon as the wound is healed.

Urethrotomy is the cutting through of a dense mass of tissue in the urethra which is acting as a stricture, causing obstruction and retention of urine.

An instrument called a urethrotome is employed; it is a slender rod curved like a male catheter, having a thread at its tip on to which a filiform bougie can be screwed. A small groove on the upper or anterior aspect of the urethrotome carries a specially devised knife with a triangular shaped blade, which can be slipped along this groove and used to divide the stricture. It is very necessary to keep this knife sharp, and it should be oiled when put away and the instrument carefully cleaned.

Radical amputation of the penis is performed for carcinoma. The penis, scrotum and the inguinal glands are removed. The incision made is a transverse one on the lower part of the anterior abdominal wall.

Post-operative nursing care. An anterior drain is inserted and a urethral catheter is kept in for about six days. It is very important to watch the skin in the area of the incision as a large amount of tissue has been removed. The skin is unsupported and deprived of nourishment and unless care is taken to keep the parts firm, sloughing may occur.

Decompression of the distended urinary bladder by means of Kidd's inverted U-tube is one of the methods employed of gradually emptying a seriously distended bladder. A catheter is fixed into the bladder and connected by means of a glass tube to a length of rubber tubing which is attached to the shorter of the two limbs of the Kidd's tube. Rubber tubing from the longer limb carries urine syphoned from the bladder into a bottle at the bedside.

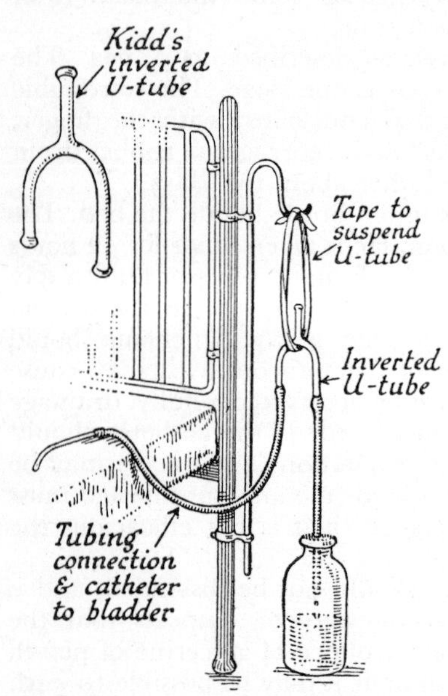

FIG. 268—KIDD'S U-TUBE SUSPENDED AT THE BEDSIDE FOR DECOMPRESSION OF URINARY BLADDER IN THE TREATMENT OF RETENTION.

The Kidd's tube is suspended at the bedside just high enough to permit a small quantity of urine to be syphoned out when the patient takes a deep breath; if it is too high no urine can escape, and if placed too low the contents of the bladder will be syphoned off too rapidly. When setting up the apparatus the correct level is determined by asking the patient to cough and when the correct level is found a little urine will escape. As the bladder is gradually emptied it will be necessary to lower the tube. The lower end of the tubing which conveys the urine into the bottle at the bedside should be above the fluid in this bottle. The amount of urine which is syphoned off must be carefully measured and a record should be kept of the fluid the patient takes. He should have plenty to drink.

The instruments required for some of the operations mentioned will be seen on pp. 681–4.

Chapter 48

Affections of the Ear, Nose and Throat—Harelip and Cleft Palate—Nursing Care

Examination of the ear—Syringing an ear—The insertion of drops—Affections of the ear: the presence of a foreign body, otitis media and mastoiditis—Affections of the nose—Affections of the throat—Tonsillectomy—Intubation—Tracheotomy—Laryngectomy—Harelip and cleft palate

The nurse will frequently be called upon to assist at the examination of the ear, nose and throat, and the conditions she will be expected to nurse in the ward include antrum puncture for drainage sinuses, operations on the nasal septum, removal of tonsils and adenoids, mastoidectomy and, less commonly, tracheotomy and laryngectomy.

The nursing of ear, nose and throat patients requires keen observation and great care, and a good deal of sympathy and thoughtfulness, as in many cases the subjects are children and conditions affecting the nose are particularly painful.

EXAMINATION OF PATIENTS

The articles needed for the examination of patients in this department are shown in fig. 242, p. 685. If the patient is an adult, two firm chairs are required, one for the surgeon and one for the patient who sits opposite him. A bell light has been shown in the list of apparatus, but a spot light is preferable where this is available. In holding a tiny child for examination he should be steadied (see fig. 241, p. 685). The nurse should learn to use a head mirror and should practise adjusting it; she should learn to look at the throat and be able to distinguish the different parts; she should use a speculum for examination of the ear and be able to distinguish the drum, and she should become familiar with investigation of the nasal cavities, using a nasal speculum for this purpose and being able to recognize the septum, and the inferior and middle turbinate bones. In examination of the nose or ear the head must be steady and the hand holding the speculum should be steadied against the patient's head so that if he moves it moves with him.

For a more extensive examination of the ear the articles shown in figs. 243 and 244, p. 686, may be required. These include a noise box, tuning fork and clapper to test hearing, and eustachian catheters, Politzer's bag and Seigel's speculum in case the surgeon wishes to test the patency of the eustachian tubes.

Laryngoscopy and **bronchoscopy** are performed when examination of the larynx, trachea and bronchi is to be undertaken. For *indirect laryngoscopy* some of the articles shown in fig. 245, p. 686, will be needed, including bell light and head mirror; laryngeal mirror and spirit lamp in which to warm the glass in order to prevent moisture from condensing upon it; local anaesthetic, tongue depressor and a cloth with which to hold the tongue forward and steady it.

In *direct laryngoscopy* the articles shown in fig. 245, p. 687, will be needed. The pharynx is cocainized, the mouth is held open, the tongue depressed and the laryngoscope passed as far as the opening of the larynx.

In **bronchoscopy** a larger instrument—the bronchoscope—is passed through the larynx for examination and inspection of the trachea and bronchi. (Both laryngoscope and bronchoscope carry an electric bulb which serves to illuminate the passage the surgeon is inspecting.)

Oesophagoscopy or examination of the oesophagus is performed by means of an oesophagoscope (see fig. 246, p. 688). This examination is undertaken when it is necessary to investigate the condition of the oesophagus in conditions of stricture or obstruction, or to determine the position of a foreign body or to obtain an estimation of the changes which may be occurring in disease of this organ.

TREATMENT OF THE EAR

Local cleansing treatment. The nurse may be asked to syringe the ear for the removal of either discharge or wax; or she may be asked to mop the ear; in both cases it is essential that after wet mopping or syringing the ear should be swabbed dry and quite free of fluid or discharge.

A discharging ear. In the care of any patient with a discharging ear, as in chronic otitis media, it is important to observe the type and amount of discharge—a mixture of pus and blood usually indicates some acute condition such as acute otitis media—a small quantity of thick pus may be coming from a boil in the meatus—a quantity of thin muco-purulent or thick purulent discharge frequently indicates some chronic condition such as chronic otitis media—and an offensive discharge may mean that there is some necrosed bone in the middle ear.

Patients with discharge should have the meatus cleaned several times a day, as careful *toilet of the canal* is essential if cure is to be effected. When *moist treatment* is ordered a gauze wick should be placed in the auditory canal and kept moist by frequent applications of the solution ordered, e.g. penicillin. Dry treatment means keeping the canal dry by careful swabbing and the insufflation of any powder prescribed.

In **syringing the ear** a special aural syringe (see fig. 247, p. 689) is employed, which can be used with one hand; the lotion used should be sterile and it should be warm, that is, about 99° F.; if it is cold or hot, it may cause the patient to feel dizzy. The patient may be seated on a chair or sitting up in bed, a receiver being held beneath the ear and the shoulders protected; the ear should then be inspected, the nurse using speculum, light and head mirror for this purpose—she should be able to see the drum and note the type and amount of discharge or of wax. She then takes hold of the pinna and pulls it in a direction upwards and backwards, and holding the syringe places the nozzle in the opening and empties its contents into the ear; the patient may move slightly, but the nurse follows these movements with care.

Very gentle syringing is necessary in order to remove discharge and emptying the syringe once may be found to be adequate; but for wax more force is necessary, and the stream of fluid should be directed up to the roof of the meatus—it will then pass upwards and inwards and run downwards and outwards along the floor of the canal. In syringing for the removal of wax a slightly jerky movement should be used. After syringing the ear the patient should be instructed to hold his head over to the side to empty the canal of fluid. The nurse should dry the meatus with wool, and for this purpose wisps of wool rolled up in the form of a stick, or a wooden stick dressed with wool, or aural dressing forceps may be employed.

To insert drops into the ear. The patient should lie on his side with the ear to be treated uppermost. The liquid may be drawn up into a pipette and the pipette held in a bowl of warm water for a moment or two just long enough to warm it slightly, and then applied to the ear and the contents gently dropped into the meatus. The patient should keep his head in position for from 5 to 10 minutes, and then turn his head over and shake out any fluid that may be left. The ear may then be syringed if ordered, or protected by a tiny piece of warm, sterile cotton wool placed gently in the canal.

Drops are frequently employed to soften discharge, and in this case peroxide of hydrogen is used, and this requires special mention as it is necessary to put in the drops several times at one sitting, emptying the drops off by turning the head over and repeating the process until the peroxide has ceased to bubble, the meatus being then dried in the ordinary way.

A mixture of glycerine and sodium bicarbonate is used to soften wax, glycerine and carbolic drops are frequently employed for the relief of pain and earache and spirit and saline for cleansing purposes.

AFFECTIONS OF THE EAR

Foreign body in the ear. An insect may get into the ear or a child may push a small bead or other little object in. An insect may be floated out by putting warm lotion into the ear, but if a solid foreign body is in the meatus the nurse should not attempt to deal with it as anything she does may probably push it farther in and render it more difficult for the doctor to remove later.

Infections of the Pinna. The pinna and the neighbouring regions of skin may be affected by eczematous or seborrhoeic conditions. These may become secondarily affected and in that case treatment with penicillin cream or powder will eradicate the infection. The underlying cause of the primary condition is then investigated and dealt with.

Furunculosis and inflammation of the auditory canal is usually due to staphylococcal infection. Systemic penicillin treatment may be necessary in severe cases. Local treatment consists in incision of any small boils that do not spontaneously rupture, then a gauze wick is placed in the canal which is kept moist by frequent application of penicillin solution. Later as the septic condition is cleared up, penicillin powder may be insufflated.

Otitis media. This condition may be acute or chronic, and is usually due to the spread of infection from the naso-pharynx by means of the eustachian tubes. The *symptoms* are pain, some degree of deafness due to blockage of the eustachian tube, a rise of temperature, and increase in pulse rate accompanied by headache and malaise. The causal organisms of acute otitis media are penicillin sensitive and immediate systemic treatment of penicillin is used when the patient is an adult but in children sulphonamide therapy is employed owing to the inconvenience of frequent penicillin injections.

When pus forms an abscess may arise behind the drum, and this causes the drum to bulge and it may burst, and the contents of the abscess be discharged; or the condition may be treated by making a small incision in order to make an outlet for the discharge, *myringotomy* (see fig. 248, p. 690). When this is carried out it is important to keep the ear as clean as possible by frequently mopping the meatus, and by the application of a penicillin wick. As healing occurs the discharge becomes less and insufflation of penicillin powder is used and the drum eventually heals.

In some cases infection of the middle ear passed to the mastoid antrum by the aditus, which is a short passage forming a communication between the middle ear and the antrum.

Acute Mastoiditis. The *most prominent symptoms* of this condition are pain and tenderness behind the ear, and there may, in addition, be thickening and swelling owing to the formation of an abscess under the periosteum in this region. A rise of temperature is variable but there is always notable quickening of the pulse rate.

The causal organisms are usually penicillin sensitive and generally a combination of systemic penicillin treatment and administration of sulphonamide is employed.

Operative treatment. The usual preparation for operation is carried out, an area of skin over the temporal bone behind the ear and down to the nape of the neck should be prepared. The meatus and the pinna should be very carefully cleansed.

In the *post-operative nursing care* the patient is received back to bed and is placed to lie on the affected side—when he comes round from the anaesthetic he will move if it is uncomfortable. Systemic chemotherapeutic treatment will be continued as long as is necessary, and in addition penicillin solution may be instilled into the packed wound every 3 or 4 hours in order to keep penicillin in contact with the walls of the cavity. A fine catheter drain is inserted through which the solution is instilled; the catheter is kept closed by a spigot.

In dressing a mastoidectomy wound the ear must be kept very clean, and strict asepsis observed. When removing a plug or packing, it should first be moistened and then very gently removed. When packing the wound ribbon gauze should be used and it should be inserted firmly into the bottom of the wound in order to ensure healing from the bottom upwards. As the wound is very often deep it is important to see that the edges do not curl under. This can be prevented by lifting them gently outwards with a pair of forceps and packing the gauze dressing firmly but gently beneath them so that they rest upon it.

Complications. Throughout the nursing care observation must be made for the possible onset of any symptoms that might indicate the presence of some complication. The most important things to observe are a rise of temperature and the occurrence of rigors, which would suggest the presence of some blood infection or *infection of one of the venous sinuses;* vomiting and headache might suggest the onset of an *extradural abscess;*

rigidity and stiffness of the neck might be the first signs of *meningitis*, and facial paralysis of the opposite side would suggest a *cerebral abscess* on the affected side. Other symptoms to be on the look-out for would be a marked increase in the pulse rate, the presence of squint, and the onset of drowsiness and stupor accompanied by an increase in the depth of respiration which would indicate an increase in the intracranial pressure.

Chronic otitis media is a longstanding condition, characterized by a discharging ear, which may be complicated by the presence of organisms insensitive to penicillin so that both factors have to be considered. Good results can often be obtained by local cleansing treatment as described on p. 735.

AFFECTIONS OF THE NOSE

Nose bleeding. Epistaxis may occur at any age. The bleeding is usually from the front and lower part of the septum, and can therefore be controlled by pinching the nose and applying pressure in an upward and backward direction towards the bleeding point. If the bleeding continues and is noticed to run down the throat it is coming from a point farther back and cannot be controlled by pinching the nose. The treatment in this case is to pack the nostrils with gauze and adrenalin, a piece of sorbo, or the finger of a rubber glove filled with wool or gauze. The latter is a favourite packing as when it is removed later it does not start the bleeding again.

Nasal obstruction. The commonest cause of obstruction is abnormality in structure, and this may be due to fracture of either the bridge, or the septum, or of both. A fall on the front of the nose pushes the soft part backwards and causes deformity of the septum—marked deviation or deflection may block both sides of the nose. Similar deformity may be due to mal-development of the septum. General swelling of the nasal mucous membrane will also give rise to obstruction, and the presence of nasal polypi is another cause.

For a deflected septum, the treatment is operative and submucous resection of septum is performed. The *preparation* includes cleansing the nose, mouth and nasopharynx by frequent mouth washes, gargles and nose sniffs a day or two before the operation. The routine general preparation is employed and just before the operation the nose is packed with a mixture of cocaine and adrenaline in order to prevent bleeding. The operation may be performed under a local or a general anaesthetic. When the septum is removed it is fairly common but not invariable practice to insert some form of splint on each side of the mucous membrane of it, in order to keep the layers together and prevent the formation of haematoma between them. These splints may be either gauze plugs, strips of green protective, or rubber fingerstalls filled with gauze or wool. They are usually kept in for 18–24 hours. In addition a post-nasal sponge is employed—this is a piece of marine sponge with tapes attached which is put into the nasopharynx and removed as soon as the patient begins to be restless or as soon as the cough reflex returns. It serves the purpose of preventing blood from trickling down the nasopharynx into the respiratory passages.

In the **post-operative nursing care** the routine treatment will vary a little with each surgeon. The patient cannot breathe through the nose and therefore it may be necessary to wedge the mouth open and apply tongue forceps if the patient is deeply anaesthetized. Most surgeons permit the patient to be nursed in bed in a sitting posture, and a few surgeons like the patient to get up in a chair as soon as possible. The principal considerations in the post-operative nursing care are prevention of bleeding and sepsis; the patient should be provided with a covered receptacle containing pieces of gauze which have been sterilized, and he uses these to remove any slight moisture from his nose. He may only use one piece of gauze once and must then discard it into the bowl provided for this purpose. In no circumstances may an ordinary handkerchief be used.

The splints of tubing packed inside the nose are usually taken out within 24 hours, and it is a good plan to have a set time for doing this, say 2 p.m., as this ensures that it shall not be forgotten. Their removal should be checked by a responsible person and the fact should be noted on the patient's chart. Six hours later, provided that there is no bleeding, nose sniffs may be commenced (see note below). There should be no attempt to clean the nose, and it will be found that the sniffs are sufficient for this purpose. If any hard clots are present in the nose they may be moistened with liquid paraffin and this will facilitate separation.

As a general rule the diet should consist of cold fluids and jellied foods for the two first days after operation, and then the patient may have ordinary light diet, but stimulants should be avoided. Patients who are kept in bed usually like to get up about the fourth day and go home after a week, but they should be instructed to move about very carefully as quick movements may make the nose bleed. They should be instructed that if this happens they must sit quietly in a chair and hold the nose tightly between the thumb and finger and apply clean handkerchiefs wrung out of tap water to the upper lip: if the bleeding does not stop by this treatment they should send for a doctor. For the first week or two after returning home they must avoid the danger of infection and should therefore avoid all dusty places and thickly populated places, such as cinemas, etc. They should also put a little piece of clean cotton wool in each nostril when going out of doors for the first 2 weeks.

Nose sniffs. Any mild antiseptic or an alkaline lotion may be used, such as saline, sodium bicarbonate solution, etc. A tall glass such as a tooth-glass should be employed and the patient should put his nose into the fluid until the opening of both nostrils is covered, and then sniff fluid up the nose, and hawk it through in the throat, and spit it out into a receiver. It should not be sniffed up to the top of the nose as this will cause headache.

To insert drops into the nose a nebulizer may be employed or the drops may be put in by means of a pipette. The patient should lie down with the head well back and the drops should be placed into the floor of the nose. The patient should maintain this position for a few minutes, and may then bring his head forward and shake any free fluid out of the nose, but he should not wipe his nose or blow it.

To **douche the nose,** the apparatus frequently employed is a Higginson's syringe, or rubber tubing and funnel, with a nasal nozzle attached. The head should be held well forward over a basin and the fluid injected with very slight force and allowed to flow gently up one nostril and gently down the other. It is important for the patient to breathe through his mouth and he should do this in a conspicuous manner in order to assure himself and the nurse that he is breathing.

Nose blowing. It is important that patients should be taught the correct manner of blowing the nose. Take hold of the nose through the handkerchief and press on one side only, then blow mucus down the other side into the handkerchief, turn the handkerchief and repeat the same procedure on the opposite side and repeat the action until the nostrils are clean.

Infection of the sinuses. The nose is so intimately associated with the sinuses of the face that nasal inflammation often leads to sinusitis. This condition is characterized by very severe pain and marked malaise and if the sinuses become seriously infected the general condition of the patient will be markedly disabled.

Antrum puncture. The articles required for this operation are shown in fig. 249, p. 691. The opening into the antrum is made near the floor of the nose about 1½ inches from the external opening. The antrum is opened and the pus which has collected in it drained out. After this operation the nurse will be required to douche the antrum, and as a rule the first douching is carried out 24 hours after the puncture and for the first day or two it may be found necessary to cocainize the nose before passing the cannula.

The apparatus used is a Higginson's syringe and a special antrum cannula (see fig. 249). These are sterilized. Saline, or some other mild fluid, is used. This is followed in suitable cases by instilling penicillin solution into the cavity. The patient sits up in bed or on a chair with his head forward over a bowl or receiver, the cannula being passed along the floor of the nose, its curved point turned outwards, and passed in a direction downwards and outwards into the opening made in the wall of the antrum. It is comparatively easy to pass it, and yet extraordinary how few people can do so with confidence, both patients and nurses seeming afraid—and yet if this cannula is taken in the hand and a half-circle made in a direction outwards and slightly downwards as it is passed, it easily slips into place. Once in place it will be felt to impinge on the wall of the antrum and the dull thud which can be felt by gently moving it is unmistakable. The cannula having been inserted, it is then attached to the syringe and the treatment carried out. It is a very good plan to allow the patient to hold the cannula, and it is important to teach him to pass it as he will be expected to continue his self-treatment when he leaves the hospital.

AFFECTIONS OF THE THROAT

As already stated, a nurse will be frequently called upon to examine a patient's throat and she will often be required to paint the throat. Various antiseptic and astringent throat paints will be employed, including glycerine, tannic acid and carbolic.

To **paint the throat** the following articles are needed: a head mirror, a good light, a tongue spatula which ought to be warmed—the rectangular metal tongue spatula shown in the illustration on p. 685 is a useful one—and a camelhair brush is usually employed for applying the paint—one with a curved handle is better than a straight one. A receptacle should be provided in which to put the quantity of paint that is to be used and a receiver for the used brush; a towel may also be required to protect the bed or the patient's clothing.

With a good light falling on the back of the throat the nurse inspects it and makes a mental note of the part she wishes to cover. She asks the patient to keep his tongue in the floor of the mouth and puts the tongue spatula on it taking care not to get it too far back as this causes the patient to gag. She then applies the paint, sweeping it well over the area of the fauces and tonsils—trying to avoid the soft palate—and applying it firmly with confidence and not tickling the patient.

Gargles. Lotions are frequently used for cleansing the throat, but to ensure this they must be retained fairly low down in the throat, and the air breathed through the fluid displaces it. As one sister aptly remarked, 'gargling is laughing through fluid'.

Antiseptic gargles such as glycothymolin are employed for cleansing; *astringents* such as solutions of tannic acid are used in the treatment of relaxed throat; *sedative* gargles such as aspirin are used in painful conditions including acute tonsillitis and after the operation of tonsillectomy. Gargles are employed hot or warm.

Tonsillitis. Inflammation of the tonsils is usually an acute condition; in *follicular tonsillitis* white patches appear on the edge of the tonsil; in *parenchymatous tonsillitis* the substance between the follicles is infected, and in *quinsy* the abscess lies beneath the tonsil causing it to extrude and pushing it across the throat.

The *symptoms* in all cases include redness and inflammation of the tonsils, with a yellow exudate oozing on to the surface; the condition is accompanied by a rise of temperature, rapid pulse rate and marked malaise, the tongue is usually very dirty and the breath offensive, swallowing is difficult and painful and the local lymphatic glands become swollen and tender.

Treatment. Success has attended the use of penicillin and/or sulphonamides. Rest in bed, a liberal fluid diet, a daily bowel action and a four-hourly record of temperature and pulse are important.

Local treatment employed may be frequent swabbing of the infected tonsils to remove the exudate, or gargling—when the patient can manage this—but when the throat is very inflamed gargles become useless, as the fluid does not pass far enough into the throat to have any effect. *Syringing* the throat is often found to be very comfortable, and it should be carried out with the patient lying on his side, his head over the edge of the bed and a receiver held beneath it; fluid is passed into the lower cheek, using a rubber catheter and Higginson's syringe. If quite gentle syringing is employed it is found to be very comforting and gives much relief.

The early *treatment of quinsy* by penicillin is effective. Only in rare instances will surgical treatment be necessary.

It is important for nurses to remember that tonsillitis may be associated with rheumatism; in most cases the organism of tonsillitis is a very virulent one, producing a very grave condition of toxaemia and necessitating a long convalescence, a change of air and the administration of good nourishing diet in order to increase the resistance and raise the general health of the patient.

Tonsillectomy. In patients who have complained of frequent sore throats and whose tonsils are enlarged and unhealthy, the operation of tonsillectomy is frequently undertaken.

In the *preparation* it is necessary to attend to the hygiene of the mouth for some days beforehand, the usual general preparation being also employed.

The post-operative care. Bleeding is the complication to be feared and this danger must be in the mind of the nurse from the moment she receives the patient back into bed until he is out of her care. The position in which the patient should lie until he comes round from the anaesthetic is on his side, the shoulders should be higher than the head, and the face should be seen, and be in such a position that any blood will run out of the nose and mouth and not down the throat. The mattress is tilted up behind the patient to prevent his turning over and lying flat. The bed is protected by a drawsheet folded in four and an anaesthetic cloth is under the patient's face—a kidney dish or receiver might be placed under the nose and mouth to receive fluid or blood as it runs out. It is important that the mouth should be kept open and this position maintained until the cough reflex is thoroughly well established. Whenever in charge of cases after tonsillectomy, nurses should see that the patient is not swallowing blood, for the act of swallowing in such a patient usually means that bleeding is quietly going on unobserved. (See figs. 251 and 252, p. 693.)

The throat will be very sore for some days after the operation and it is usual to employ aspirin gargles—5–10 grains in an ounce of water—before asking the patient to swallow fluid or food. As a rule it is employed three times a day and the nurse must find out whether the surgeon wishes the patient to swallow the aspirin or not.

The mouth and throat must be kept very clean and for this purpose antiseptic gargles of glycothymolin are employed three times a day after the three main meals. Any nourishing drinks given in between meals should be followed by a drink of water in order to cleanse the throat. The diet is usually fluid until the soreness disappears; milk should not be employed as this tends to form a layer over the throat; children will be found to be able to take jelly and ice-cream with comparative ease and pleasure.

As a rule children are kept in bed for 2 or 3 days and return to school after 10 days. In adults the shock of the operation is greater and they are kept in bed 5 or 6 days and ought to have a holiday and not return to work for a month.

Complications. The complication most to be feared is bleeding. If this happens the nurse should notify the doctor; he may order morphia, but he should see the patient again 15 minutes afterwards and, if the bleeding is not being arrested, he may wish to apply a tonsil clamp. The nurse should prepare the articles in fig. 253, p. 694. A tonsil clamp is never used by a nurse, but she should provide a small piece of gauze as shown in the illustration and larger pieces to guard the skin of the neck from injury by pressure of the external blade. Once the tonsil clamp has been applied the doctor will decide how long it should be left on; he may say 1 or 2 hours, for example, and he may leave it for the nurse to remove.

To remove a tonsil clamp it should be gently loosened, one ratchet at a time, until it ceases to exert pressure, and it may then be lifted off. If bleeding occurs again the doctor must be informed.

Other dangers occasionally met with are sepsis, earache and secondary haemorrhage. In many cases where complaint of earache is made after tonsillectomy, relief may be obtained by putting glycerine and carbolic drops into the ear, covering it with a pad of warm wool and bandaging it on. It is important to see that the patient is not spitting blood before he is allowed to get up, as this would indicate the onset of secondary haemorrhage. A rise of temperature usually indicates the onset of sepsis.

Advice to patients going home. After any operation on the throat the patient should be told to avoid vigorous movement as this may make the nose bleed. If this should happen he must be told to sit quietly in a chair and put a handkerchief soaked in cold water each side of his neck. If this does not stop the bleeding he should send for his doctor.

INTUBATION

Intubation of the larynx is performed by inserting a metal or vulcanite tube into it, the instruments used being O'Dwyer's intubation set, which consists of a set of tubes of various sizes, an intubator for introducing the tube, and a mouth gag; an extubator for removing the tube is also supplied although this is rarely used.

An intubation tube is hollow, and has a small lip at the upper end pierced in one place by a tiny hole through which a silk thread is passed. This is fastened to the outside of the cheek.

Intubation is valuable in obstruction of the larynx when it is not desirable to make an incision, and it is performed for many cases in which tracheotomy would formerly have been used.

In the **nursing care** of these cases the nurse should see the tube is not coughed out. She should have ready at hand a second tube, mouth gag and intubator, and also the instruments necessary for performing tracheotomy (see fig. 254, p. 695). If the tube becomes blocked the nurse should send for the doctor and remove the tube, either by pulling it out by the silk thread, or by exerting pressure on the tube. To do this a finger and thumb should be placed on each side of the trachea above the level of the thyroid cartilage; then, with the back of the head supported by the left hand, the tube is easily jerked out of the larynx by pressure of the right hand. In some hospitals nurses are taught to reinsert a tube, but this is not invariable.

The patient is usually nursed flat and may be fed with the nasal tube or by means of a spoon; in the latter case the head should be held well back and food of soft solid consistence passed to the back of the mouth on the spoon. In the case of children it is necessary to prevent the child from attempting to pull the tube out, and in most cases it will be found advisable to fix cardboard splints to the flexures of the elbows.

TRACHEOTOMY

This operation is in England more commonly performed than intubation, in the relief of laryngeal obstruction. The instruments required are: tracheotomy tube and pilot—the tube should be ready taped—scalpel, tracheal dilators, two double blunt hooks to act as retractors, and one sharp hook to steady the trachea, probe, sinus forceps, artery forceps, and dissecting forceps; scissors and a blunt dissector should also be supplied (see fig. 254, p. 695). Sterilized towels, swabs and gauze will be needed and a tracheotomy pillow or sandbag and mackintoshes. See also figs. 255–7, pp. 696–7.

The nurse should be prepared to assist the surgeon during the performance of tracheotomy as an emergency measure; there may not be time for the patient to have an anaesthetic; if a child, he should be rolled in a drawsheet and blanket, reaching from the nipple line to the iliac crest, the arms being pinioned to the sides of the body beneath the drawsheet which is securely pinned; the child is placed on his back on the table and a tracheotomy pillow or sandbag should be placed under the upper part of his shoulders—not under his head—the head should be tilted well back, and the occiput tucked well under, in order to bring the trachea or front of the neck prominently forward.

During the performance of the operation it is essential to keep the head and neck in a straight line, so that the trachea does not deviate to either side. One nurse standing at the head holds it, on either side, keeping it in position; a second nurse standing against the side of the table leans across the child's body, taking hold of the arms above the elbows in order to steady trunk and pelvis. It is important to prevent rotation of the pelvis.

The post-operative nursing care. The patient should be received back to a warm bed or cot, which should be elevated at the foot, in order to relieve shock and also to assist the gravitation of mucus from the respiratory tract to the opening of the tube. The air of the room should be warm, about 65° F., and in some cases it may be desirable to moisten it by the use of steam. A patient who has suffered from laryngeal obstruction may be very fatigued and tend to sleep; it is important that this sleep should not be disturbed.

In her nursing care of patients upon whom tracheotomy has been performed the most important point for the nurse to attend to is the maintenance of an adequate airway. The inner tube is removable, but it may become blocked, and whenever this happens the nurse should remove it, cleanse it with warm sodium bicarbonate solution, shake it free of moisture and reinsert it. In a well-fitting tracheotomy tube the inner tube is easily removable; at the same time care should be taken not to hurt the patient, and in performing this office the outer tube should be steadied while the inner tube is removed. For bedside tray see fig. 255, p. 696.

If removing the inner tube does not relieve the obstruction the nurse should send for the doctor and watch the child carefully in the meantime, and if his distress is very severe she must cut the tapes, remove the outer tube, insert the tracheal dilators and keep the trachea gently open until the doctor arrives. In using dilators the nurse should not open them too far—if she does so, she will tear the trachea; the blades should be gently held apart.

The length of time the tracheotomy tube is kept in depends entirely on the cause of its insertion. In a few cases there is difficulty in getting the patient to talk after removal of the tube—he seems afraid of his own voice—and another point of difficulty is that the patient fails to open his mouth when he coughs, as hitherto he has been coughing through the tracheotomy tube. To obviate the former difficulty it is advisable to get the patient used to the sound of his own voice before the tube is taken out by teaching him that if he places his finger over the opening of the tube he can speak.

After the tube is out he must be trained to open his mouth when he coughs.

If the tracheotomy tube is to be kept in permanently the metal tube will be replaced by a rubber one after the first few days and the patient will be taught to take this out, clean and reinsert it.

The *complication* most to be feared in the post-operative nursing care of tracheotomy is pneumonia, and it should be remembered that the patient is breathing the air of the room directly into his trachea; it is for this reason that the temperature of the room should be high, and the air moistened and filtered by means of a piece of gauze placed in front of the opening of the tube. In a few instances a little local suppuration may occur, but this is usually preventable, and sometimes there may be some local emphysema; when this happens the tissues of the neck will be seen to swell, and when the hand is placed on them a crackling sensation will be heard and felt; it is not usually severe enough to be serious, and the air will be absorbed after a few days.

LARYNGECTOMY

Either partial or complete removal of the larynx may be undertaken. It is usually performed when a growth is present in the upper part of the respiratory tract. In some cases preliminary tracheotomy will be performed, while in other cases the trachea is turned forwards and sewn to the skin and a tube is worn permanently.

The **post-operative nursing care** of these cases requires great patience, tact and observation. The procedure is a great strain on the patient's mental stability, as for some days he will be unable to speak and will find feeding very difficult. These patients are usually elderly people, and the disturbance of their routine mode of life becomes very distressing to them.

The patient should be nursed sitting upright, his chest should be carefully protected by a warm jacket and the skin on the front of his chest kept as dry as possible, as there is a good deal of leakage of moisture from the wound, making the skin wet and cold. It is important to keep the head very still, as movement delays healing. The patient should be provided with a pad and pencil on which to write his wishes, and a bell should be within reach at all times. He must be made to feel that there is someone within call, and that the moment he touches the bell he will be attended to.

The treatment of post-operative shock will be carried out as necessary, rest being very important, and if the patient is elderly it is advisable to give a fair amount of stimulant. Feeding will be a difficulty; in some cases the patient may be able to swallow fluid or soft solid, in other cases he will be fed by means of a tube passed through an opening in the neck into the oesophagus, which will be kept in position until the parts are healed. In many cases, when a patient begins to take food by mouth, there is a tendency for it to regurgitate through the wound on to the skin of the neck; the nurse standing by should cleanse it as it occurs, and gradually, as healing takes place, this difficulty will disappear.

The prognosis of such cases is always grave, and every possible means must be taken to obtain rest and sleep for the patient and to maintain a good resistance and tone of the body by the administration of as liberal and nourishing a diet as it is possible to give.

HARELIP AND CLEFT PALATE

In the development of the face, fusion of the necessary parts may be incomplete. The commonest deformities, due to arrest of development here, are harelip and cleft palate. The deformity may be combined; when this occurs the nose and mouth are one cavity and there is difficulty in feeding the infant with the inevitable result of wasting. Owing to the communication between the two cavities, nose and mouth, the mucous membrane of the nose soon becomes infected, which gives rise to chronic catarrh with a tendency to bronchitis and broncho-pneumonia. Infection of the middle ear may also be caused. Some babies with harelip and cleft palate are undersized and debilitated at birth; but even in cases of normal weight the difficulty of feeding readily gives rise to digestive disturbances early in life.

Harelip. The cleft is usually in the upper lip; it occurs to the side of the lip and may occur on one side, *unilateral*, or both sides, *bilateral* harelip. The condition may be *complete* when it extends into the nostril, or it may be *incomplete*, not involving the nostril.

The *treatment* is operative and it is usual to operate on harelip at the age of 2–3 months, repair of cleft palate is performed later. Before operating on harelip it is necessary to train the infant to take food from a special spoon (see fig. 269 below). Operation consists in repair of the edges of the division in the lip and in bringing the parts together with as little tension as possible. Fine ophthalmic silkworm gut is used for the skin. A general anaesthetic is given.

After operation two dangers have to be considered. (1) *Tension* which may be due to dragging together the sides of a wide gap, or to movement of the face muscles in crying. The use of Logan's bow as a 'tension bridge' is recommended (see fig. 266, p. 704 and fig. 269 below). This is worn for 2 to 3 weeks.

(2) *Sepsis.* Nasal discharge must not be allowed to flow over the wound, as it is irritating and delays healing. This can be prevented by keeping a little *loosely rolled cotton wool* in the nostrils which will absorb the discharge;

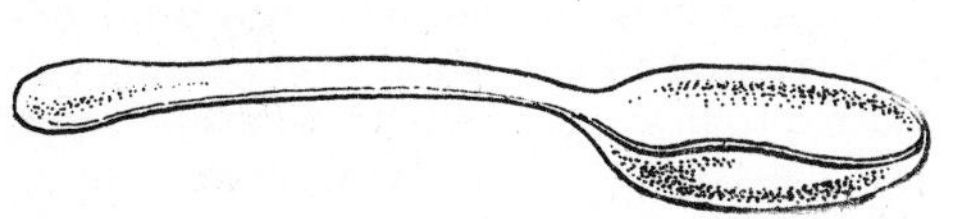

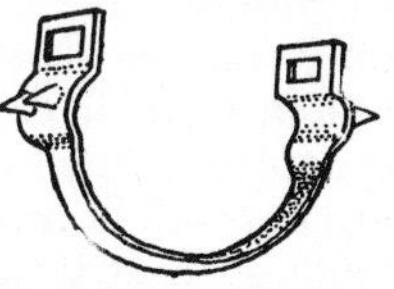

FIG. 269.—SPECIAL DEEP SPOON FOR FEEDING CLEFT PALATE AND HARELIP BABIES. Logan's bow (see also Fig. 266, p. 704).

this cotton wool must be changed immediately it is soaked and when discharge is profuse it will need changing frequently, but it is important, and is part of the intelligent nursing co-operation upon which a surgeon is so dependent.

The stitches may be swabbed with saline and weak peroxide and smeared with flavine 1–1,000 in paraffin which is both protective and antiseptic, or the area may be dusted with penicillin and sulphonamide powder. Stitches are removed on the sixth or seventh day and the infant is sent home wearing Logan's bow.

Feeding. It would be ideal to have these babies fed with expressed breast milk for the first few days and put to the breast as soon as possible, but in the majority of cases, owing to the deformity, breast feeding has proved difficult from the outset and most of the babies presented for treatment are being artificially fed.

The spoon shown in fig. 269 is an ordinary teaspoon compressed to trowel shape. It can be used in feeding both harelip and cleft palate cases. After each feeding it is important to give water so that the mouth is kept quite clean and no milk remains in it. To prevent the baby rubbing his face light cardboard splints may be bandaged on to the front of his elbows so that he cannot bend them.

Cleft palate. The palate forms the floor of the nose and the roof of the mouth. When it fails to unite the cleft may be partial or complete. A *bifid uvula* is fairly common; *the cleft may involve the soft palate* as well as the uvula or it may extend farther and *involve part or the whole of the hard palate.* It may be associated with harelip or occur independently of this.

The *treatment* is to repair the cleft by trimming the edges and bringing them together without tension. This operation is usually performed when the child is from 1½ to 3 years of age; by this time the mouth is large enough to permit of a reasonable amount of manipulation and the child old enough to be persuaded to be good and not cry.

During the years of infancy a child with cleft palate requires to be carefully fed as the cleft in the palate makes mouth and nose one cavity. For this purpose a special teat, Carmichael's teat, which has a flap that fills up the cleft in the roof of the mouth, may be used, or a teat with a large hole so that the feed runs easily, or the baby may be spoon fed. Breast milk may be expressed and used for feeding. Water must be given after each feeding. The nasal mucous membrane easily becomes infected, and infected adenoids and tonsils are comparatively common. It is inadvisable to operate if infection is present and this requires adequate treatment first.

Many surgeons remove the tonsils and adenoids before attempting repair of the cleft palate. Another consideration before operation on cleft palate can be undertaken is that the tiny child should be nursed in the surroundings and amongst those who will look after him after operation, long enough to get quite used to them, and be able to be happy and contented in their care. He should be trained to take fluid from the special spoon. In many cases infants admitted to hospital for cleft palate operation are not well nourished and should be given a liberal diet of soft nourishing foods so that weight and general condition may be improved. In some cases sedatives such as small doses of chloral or nepenthe will be given before operation in order to have the child in a quiet, sleepy state for a few days after operation.

Post-operative care. At first the child may have difficulty with his intake of air owing to closure of a large cleft between nose and mouth; he should be watched carefully and given a little oxygen if necessary; quite soon he will learn how to breathe. He should be propped up on several pillows or held upright in the arms.

As it is essential that his mouth be kept closed he must not be allowed to cry. He should sleep as much as possible, and when awake he must be kept amused but not made to laugh.

Some physicians continue the use of nepenthe or chloral or some other sedative for a few days; some also give a little atropine to inhibit secretion in the upper respiratory tract; this makes the child thirsty, but so long as he is content to sip fluid from a spoon he may have as much as he wishes. The fluids given at first ought to be water, lemonade with glucose and whey, avoiding milk and all tacky fluid. The object is to keep the mouth as clean as possible. There should not be any need to clean the mouth; it should never be opened for this purpose, but the child may be given sips of water frequently. The child must not touch his mouth with his hands and he may need to have his elbows splinted in order to restrain him.

A general anaesthetic is usually given when the stitches are removed.

Cases unsuitable for operation may have palliative measures by the insertion of an artificial plate to fill the opening.

The instruments required for some of the operations mentioned will be seen on pp. 701–703.

Chapter 49

Affections of the Eye and their Nursing Care

Examination of the eye—Local treatment—Affections of the lids: styes, cysts, blepharitis, lacrimal obstruction—Conjunctivitis: pink eye, purulent gonorrhoeal, and phlyctenular conjunctivitis—Affections of the cornea and iris: corneal ulcer, keratitis, arcus senilis, iritis—Affections of the lens: cataract, preparation and post-operative nursing—Glaucoma—Detached retina—Enucleation of eye

THE NURSING OF PATIENTS WITH DISEASE OF THE EYE

The care of eye conditions requires a nurse who is very much alive to her responsibilities and exceedingly interested in her patients. It needs very special people who should have had equally special training, and yet in the ward allocated to diseases of the eyes in a general hospital many changes will invariably be made in the junior nursing staff during any one period of 12 months; it is specially important therefore that both the ward sister and the staff nurses should be highly experienced.

One of the points that will strike the newcomer to such a ward may be the rigid adherence to conservative treatment in the preparation and post-operative care of patients, and the apparently exaggerated fussiness in attention to detail practised by surgeon and ward sister; but it will soon be realized how very necessary this all is and how often the success of the nursing of eye conditions depends on the very minutest attention to small detail, as well as on the most exquisite accuracy in carrying out instructions, and on careful observation.

A nurse can be of little use in making observations in conditions and diseases of the eye unless she is familiar with the anatomy and physiology of this organ and its appendages; and she must also take every opportunity of being present at the ward round of the surgeon and in the operating theatre, watching every detail as closely as she can, and following each step of an operation with such intelligence as is only possible if she has a sound knowledge of the anatomy of the parts which are being handled.

Imagination is valuable and so is common sense—for example, if an eye is to be operated on and there is nothing external to distinguish it, the affected side should be marked by blue pencil or a strip of adhesive strapping; if eyelashes are to be cut, common sense with imagination might help a nurse to foresee that, unless the precaution of smearing them with vaseline is taken, stray hairs will be likely to fall into the eye and irritate it.

Relaxation is essential, but it is impossible to relax if one expects to be hurt; the precaution of telling a patient exactly what is going to happen and the behaviour expected of him should always be taken, and then his co-operation may be expected. If the fingers of the nurse handling an eye are stiff and rigid they will hurt; gentleness is specially necessary in the nursing of eye conditions, and the hands of the nurse should also be comfortably warm, and she should take care to keep them soft and free from roughness and chapping.

Nurses must move quietly, and unless the ward has a rubber floor they should wear rubber heels on their shoes. In many instances both eyes of a patient will be bandaged, so that he is blindfolded; in approaching the bed of this patient the nurse should move quietly but not stealthily and should take the precaution of speaking gently before she touches the bed. When instructing a patient to move his eye he should be asked 'gently to close or open it', as the case may be, rather than to close or open gently. It is imperative the word gently should be emphasized, and that it should precede the direction to act. If the patient finds that keeping his eye open is difficult he must not use his hands for this, but the assistance of another nurse should be obtained.

EXAMINATION OF THE EYE

The articles provided for examination of the eye are shown in fig. 270, p. 753. The surgeon first inspects the eye in a general manner and notes the position and movements of the lids, the condition of the conjunctiva, the clearness or opacity of the sclera, the colour of the iris and the size and regularity of the pupils.

He likes the patient to be so placed that the light falls on the eye from above and from the opposite side to that on which he is working. He may evert the eyelids and examine the condition of the eye, and he tests the condition of the normal reflexes and the tension of the eyeball. He may wish to investigate any injury to the cornea by using fluorescein. He places a small drop on the margin of the cornea and allows it to run over it. An abrasion or an ulcerated area which is deprived of epithelium will stain green, but healthy parts are unaffected by the fluid.

When he wishes to illuminate the eye he will use a magnifying lens to direct the light on to the eye and a corneal loupe or lens or an ophthalmoscope in order to inspect the different parts of the eye.

If the surgeon wishes to have the pupil dilated before the examination is carried out he will order atropine or homatropine. The nurse should see that the pupils are adequately dilated before the time of examination. For a more extensive examination the surgeon may wish to cocainize the eye with a solution of 2 per cent or 4 per cent cocaine and he may need an eye speculum.

LOCAL TREATMENT OF THE EYE

To evert the eyelids. If possible have the patient seated, his head resting against the operator, who stands behind him. Tell the patient to look down, grasp the lashes of the upper lid and pull it gently down over the lower lid, then turn the upper lid outwards and upwards, at the same time exerting gentle pressure over the upper part of the lid with one finger of the free hand. Glass rods or other articles should not be used, as injury to the eye may be caused by undue pressure.

To remove foreign bodies. (*a*) *From the lower conjunctival sac*, pull down the lower lid and gently touch the foreign body with a fine camel's-hair brush, a small piece of dry cotton wool, or a clean cotton handkerchief; if in the upper sac, evert the upper lid and do the same. (*b*) *From the cornea*, if superficially placed the eye should be cocainized and the foreign body removed with a small pad. If embedded, it may be removed by a needle or spud. The eye must then be covered by a sterile pad and irrigated twice a day until the corneal wound has healed; and careful inspection should be made as an ulcer may result. The removal of metallic pieces which have penetrated the tissues should be assisted by the use of a magnet.

To dilate the pupil. These drugs are called *mydriatics*. Atropine in a one per cent watery solution is used, but atropine is also a *cycloplegic*, that is, it paralyses accommodation, and as it takes over a week for this effect to pass off, an alternative may be used when dilation for a short time only is required. Paredrine is a preparation which dilates the pupil, the effect passing off in an hour or so. Two per cent homatropine and cocaine can be counteracted by eserine.

To contract the pupil. These drugs are called *miotics*. Eserine in 0·5 per cent solution is used.

To induce local anaesthesia. One drop of 4 per cent cocaine, followed in two to three minutes by another drop will render the surface of the eye insensitive and permit a foreign body to be painlessly removed. For operative procedures the surgeon will order the amount of cocaine to be used.

To constrict the blood vessels adrenalin is used; its object is to contract the vessels and reduce bleeding. It is sometimes used in conjunction with cocaine.

To inhibit the growth of pathogenic organisms. Penicillin drops are instilled when the organism is sensitive to this drug, as in gonorrhoeal ophthalmia. Argyrol and protargol are silver preparations used for the same purpose.

To lubricate the eye. Bland oily drops may be instilled by means of a pipette, or dropped from the end of a glass rod into the lower conjunctival sac. When *ointment* is used a small quantity is taken on a glass rod and placed in the lower lid which is drawn down, the eye is closed and the glass rod drawn gently through leaving the ointment in the sac. Gently rubbing the upper lid will cause the ointment to be spread all over the eye.

To apply ointment to the lids. First clean away all crusts by bathing with sodium-bicarbonate solution and picking the crusts off with swabs and forceps, then gently rub the ointment into the margins of the lids by means of a dressed rod, trying to get it well into the roots of the lashes.

To insert lamellae. These are small gelatinous discs used for convenience instead of fluid. They contain drugs, such as atropine, cocaine or eserine, and are placed in the lower conjunctival sac where they dissolve.

To insert powder. Dress a glass rod with wool, dip this into the powder, open the eye as for irrigation (see below) and drop the powder on to the lower sac by vibrating the rod with the action used to shake the ash off a lighted cigarette. Close the eye for a few minutes to allow the powder to be dissolved by the conjunctival fluid.

To stain a corneal abrasion or ulcer. When any part of the cornea is deprived of epithelium this area will stain green with fluorescein. A little fluorescein is placed, by means of a glass rod, in the lower conjunctival sac, followed by some dilute saline solution. When excess fluid has been swabbed away the abraded area will be seen as a bright green patch. The method of cauterizing a corneal ulcer is given on p. 763.

To irrigate an eye. An undine should be used for irrigating an eye; the lotion should be warm, neither hot nor cold, it should always be tested on the back of the hand of the nurse before she uses it, and the undine should be held quite close to the eye and not at a distance above it. The patient may be lying on his back or seated in a chair, a receiver should be held closely against the side of his face to catch the lotion as it runs out of the eye. The patient is requested to look up and the lower conjunctival sac, held gently down by the forefinger of one hand, is irrigated, and then he is asked to look down whilst the upper one is similarly treated; lotion must not be poured directly on to the cornea as this would be irritating and possibly painful. When the treatment is over the eyelids should be carefully dried with small pieces of absorbent cotton wool. See fig. 271, and fig. 272, p. 753.

To apply heat to an eye. Hot applications are ordered when the eye is very congested and painful; these may be dry or moist. *Dry heat* is applied by means of an electric pad, so that the heat can be regulated. *Moist heat* is commonly applied by frequent bathing; a convenient method in common use is carried out by wrapping a pad of sterile wool on to the convex side of a wooden spoon (see fig. 272, p. 754); the patient is seated at a table—if in bed a bedtable is used—a basin of hot lotion is placed in front of him and he is taught to dip the padded spoon in this lotion, press some of the lotion out against the side of the bowl and then, carrying the steaming spoon to the vicinity of his eye, hold it against the closed eye as soon as he can bear the heat of it. This treatment is repeated for from ten to fifteen minutes every three or four hours.

Whenever an eye has been treated by an application of heat it should be protected from cold air for at least twenty minutes afterwards; if a patient wishes to move about immediately after the treatment he should have the eye covered by a warm pad and bandage.

To apply sulphate of copper (blue stone) to the lid. This treatment is ordered in cases of trachoma. The eye is cocainized, the upper lid everted, the granules of lymphoid tissue observed and touched with copper stick, which may also be rubbed gently upwards and downwards over the inner surface of the lid.

To paint the eyelids. Silver-nitrate solution 1 per cent, and weak solutions of argyrol and protargol are used for this purpose. The upper lid is everted and the paint applied to it by means of a dressed rod or orange stick. Excess solution may be mopped away with a swab of dry wool, or the eye may be irrigated with boracic lotion after painting.

The method of bandaging an eye is described on p. 247.

AFFECTIONS OF THE EYELIDS

A stye (hordeolus) is infection of a lash follicle; a small abscess forms and there may be considerable swelling of the surrounding tissues, because the skin covering the eyelid is loose and does not contain a layer of fat as does subcutaneous tissue elsewhere, consequently fluid collects rapidly in this region.

The *local treatment* is to apply hot moist dressings (see p. 751); the infected eyelash should be removed as soon as it becomes a little loose; the application of weak mercurial ointment to the margin of the affected lid will act as an antiseptic and, being greasy in character, will prevent the lids from being fastened together by the sticky exudate or discharge which is usually present.

It is necessary to investigate the cause of repeated styes; the condition may be due to some general constitutional disease or to debility; on the other hand the styes may be secondary to some uncorrected error of refraction, such as astigmatism.

Cysts of the eyelids or *meibomian cysts* are caused by abnormal development of the sebaceous glands secreting the fatty substance which is needed in order to keep the edges of the margins of the eyelids slightly greasy and so prevent the watery fluid from running out of the eyes. A meibomian cyst can be felt as a small swelling when the eyelid is taken and held between the finger and thumb of the examining hand. The eyelid is uncomfortable and painful, and sooner or later the cyst bursts. In severe cases the *treatment* is to incise the cyst in order to evacuate it and then to bathe the eye.

Blepharitis is inflammation of the margins of the eyelids; the eyes are red and sore, the margins ulcerated, the lids are inflamed and the lashes fall out, a sticky exudate forms and the red inflamed lids become glued together.

The *local treatment* consists in removing the crusts from the margins of the lids by bathing with an alkaline solution such as sodium bicarbonate, two teaspoonfuls to the pint of warm water; epilation of any remaining eyelashes is usually performed and the margins of the lids are smeared with weak mercurial ointment particularly at night in order to prevent their sticking together. Alternative local treatment is the application of penicillin.

The general health should be attended to, as blepharitis may be associated with ill health. The eyes should be tested for errors of refraction for the same reasons as in the case of persistent styes.

Ectropion is eversion of the eyelid which may occur when ulcers are numerous on the lids.

Epiphora is a flowing over of the conjunctival fluid on to the cheek; it may occur when the lids are everted, and also in lacrimal obstruction (q.v.); it also occurs whenever lacrimation is excessive as may result from any irritation of the conjunctiva.

Entropion is inversion of the lids; it most commonly occurs as the result of contraction following ulceration of the lids, and in such a case the eyelashes lie against, and irritate, the front of the eyeball.

Ptosis is drooping of the eyelids, usually of the upper one.

Lacrimal obstruction occurs as the result of narrowing of the tear ducts which is often brought about by slight catarrh of these extremely delicate structures; the congestion first obstructs the duct and is then followed by permanent thickening which maintains the obstruction. In persons with a tendency to this condition it is found to be made worse by

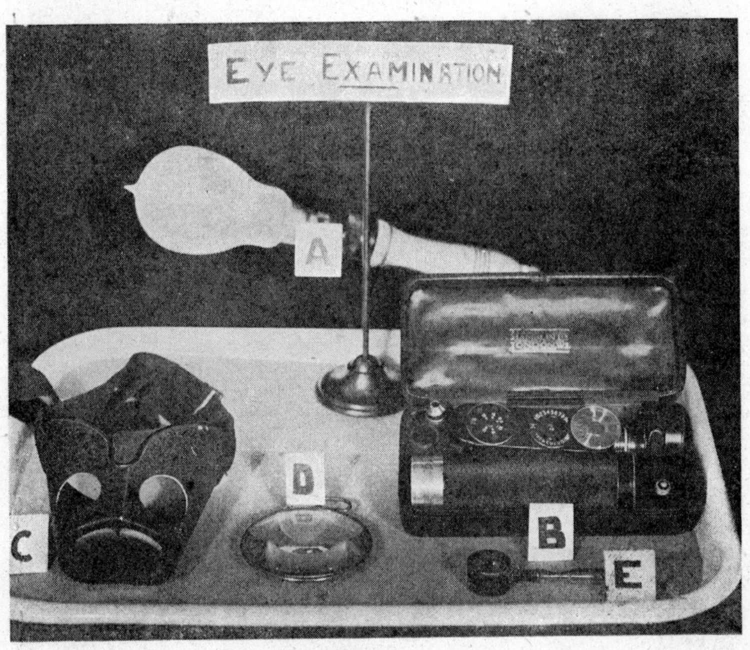

FIG. 270.—*see page* 749

The articles required for an examination of the eye include—(A) light, (B) ophthalmoscope, (C) binocular lens or loup, (D) single lens, (E) corneal lens or loup.

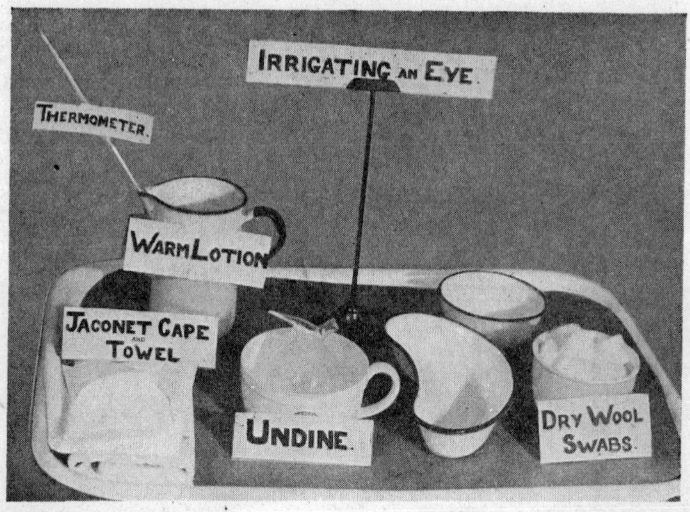

FIG. 271.—*see page* 752. The articles required for irrigating the eye by using an undine.

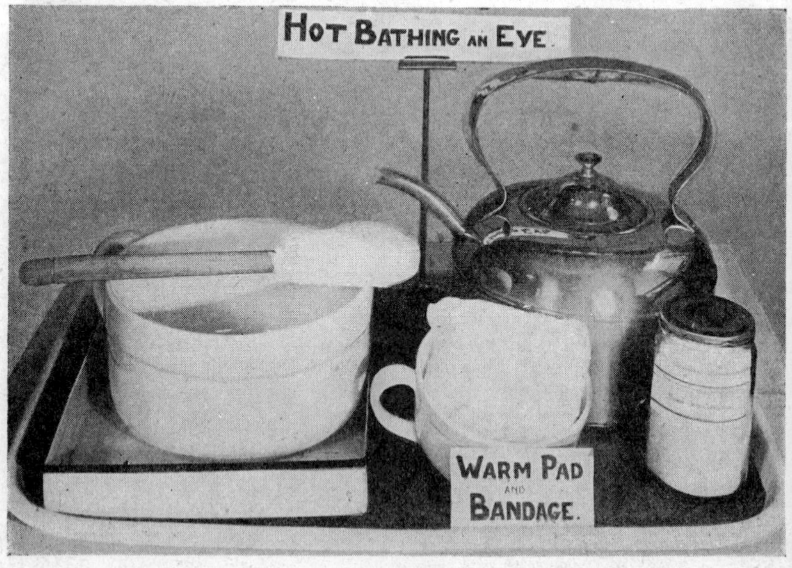

FIG. 272.—*see page* 752. The articles required for hot bathing the eye. The wooden spoon is padded on the curved side. A pad of warm wool is bandaged over the eye to prevent chilling after hot bathing.

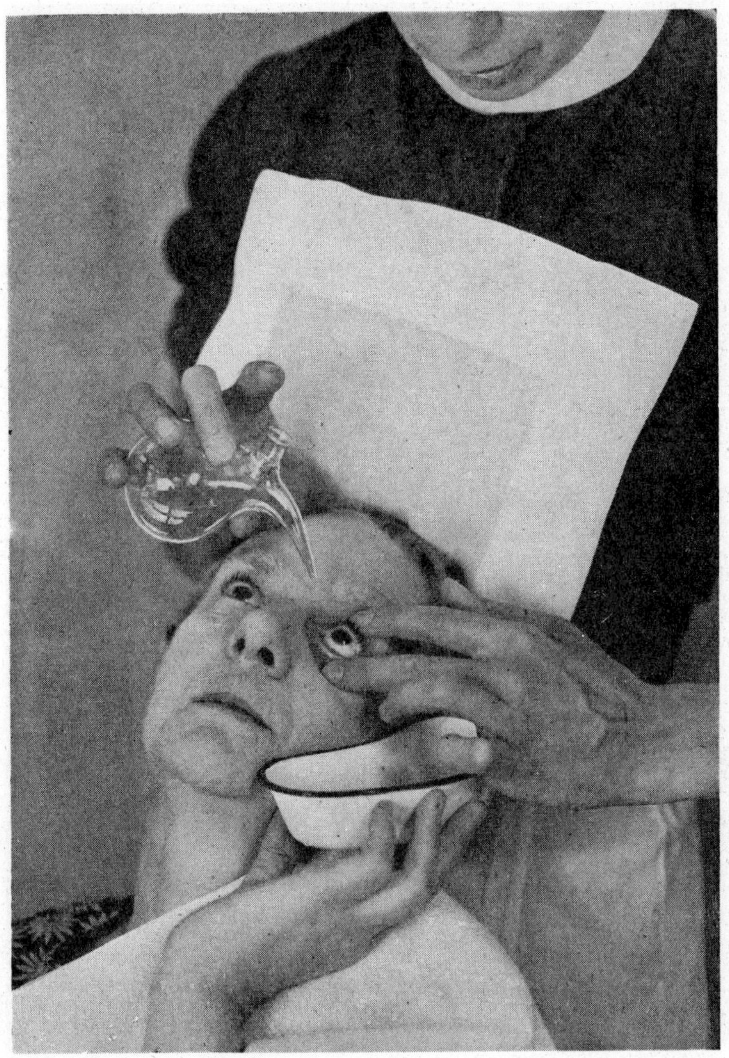

FIG. 273. IRRIGATING THE EYE.
The position adopted when irrigating the eye. The fluid from the undine is poured gently on to the lower conjunctival sac (*see page* 751).

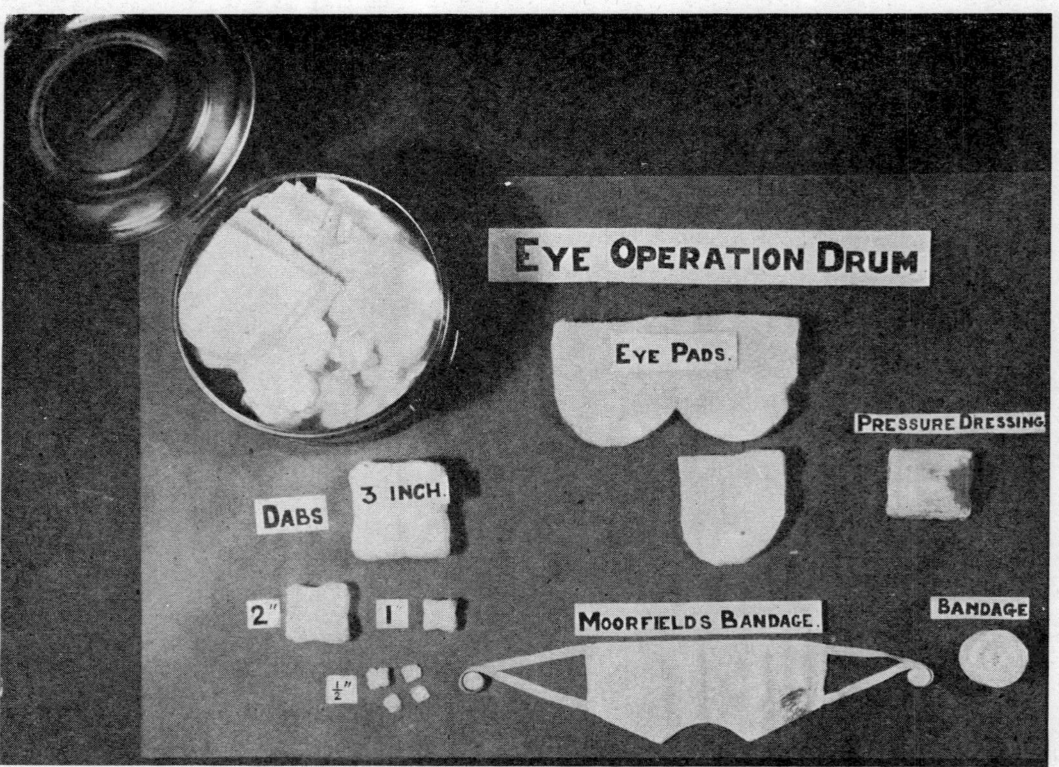

FIG. 274.
An eye operation drum contains a variety of minute swabs or dabs, ½-inch, 1-inch, 2-inch and 3-inch. Single and double eye pads are used as a covering dressing. A pressure dressing composed of graduated pieces of folded gauze, layer upon layer, until a cone-shaped pad is formed is used as a dressing after enucleation of the eye. The special bandages used are also sterilized.

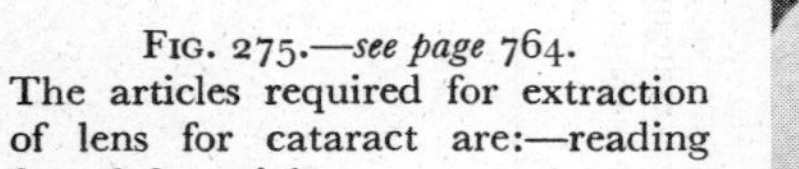

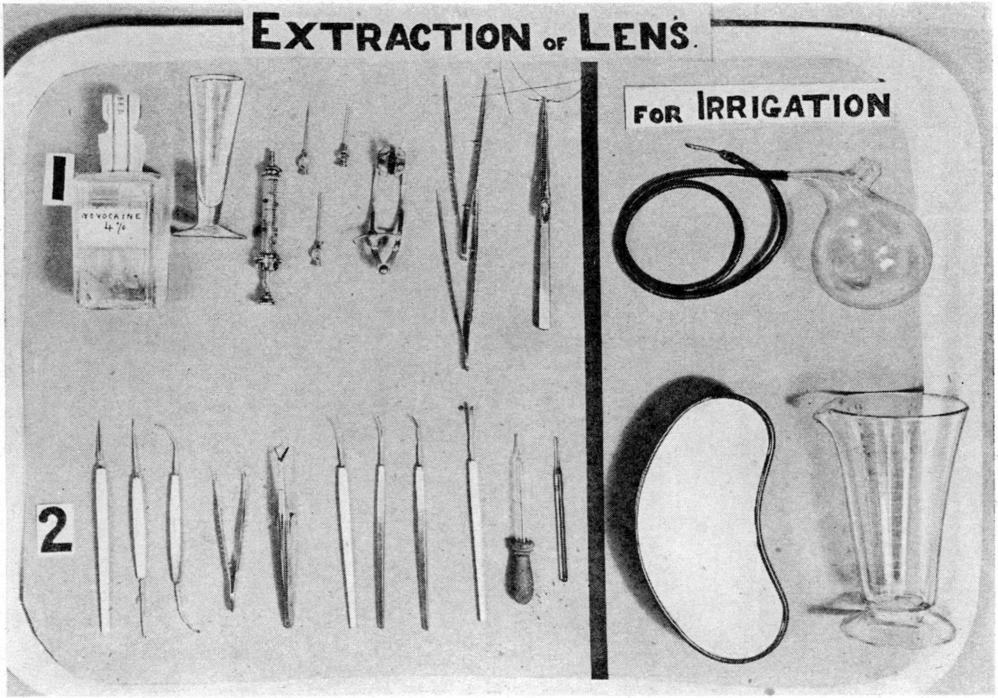

FIG. 275.—*see page* 764.
The articles required for extraction of lens for cataract are:—reading from left to right:—
(1) UPPER ROW. Novocaine, measure, syringe and needles, eye speculum, fixation forceps and needle-holder with needle and silk suture.
(2) LOWER ROW. Graefe's knife, curette and cystotome, cataract spoon, iris forceps, de Wecker's iris scissors, three iris repositors, curette, pipette and glass rod.
Articles for irrigation of the eye should also be provided.

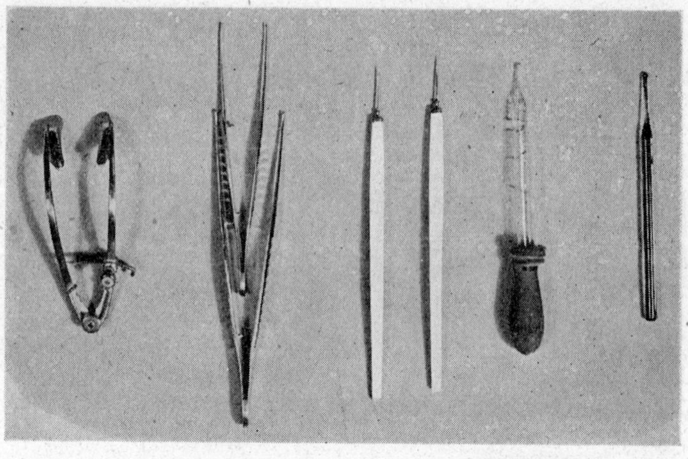

FIG. 276.—*see page* 764. NEEDLING OR DICISSION.
Reading from left to right:—Speculum, fixation forceps, Saunders's capsule needles, pipette and glass rod.

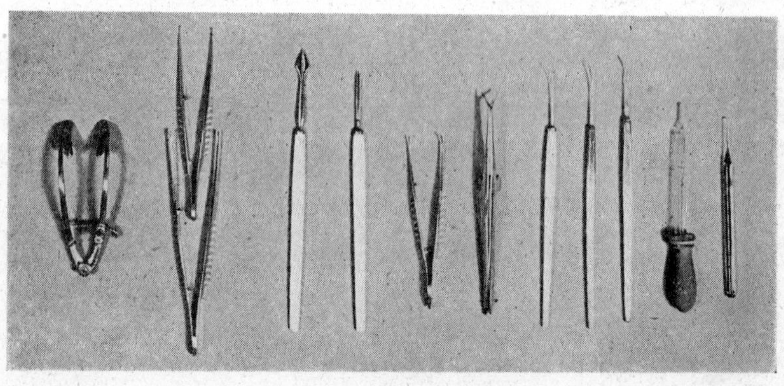

FIG. 277.—*see page* 764. IRIDECTOMY.
Reading from left to right:—Speculum, fixation forceps, keratome, Graefe's knife, iris forceps, de Wecker's iris scissors, iris repositors (3 sizes), pipette and glass rod.

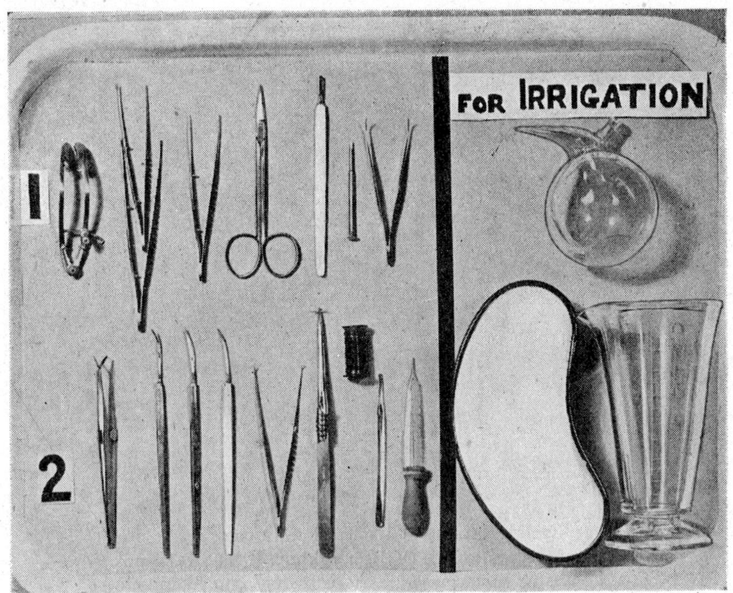

FIG. 278.—*see page* 767. TREPHINING FOR GLAUCOMA.

A tiny circular cutting instrument, a trephine, is used to make a small opening at the limbus in order to allow fluid to escape for the relief of glaucoma.

The articles required for trephining for glaucoma are—

(1) UPPER ROW. Speculum, three pairs fixation forceps (one pair plain), conjunctival scissors, splitting knife, trephine and iris forceps.

(2) LOWER ROW. de Wecker's iris scissors, three iris repositors, disk forceps, needle in needle-holder and spool of silk, glass rod and pipette. (In addition the articles required for irrigation of the eye should be provided.)

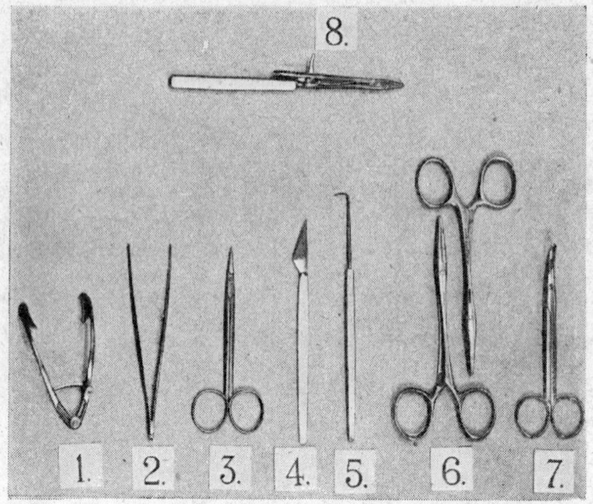

FIG. 279.—*see page* 768. ENUCLEATION OF EYE.
(1) Eyelid retractor, (2) fixation forceps, (3) Conjunctival scissors, (4) Beer's knife, (5) Strabismus hook, (6) Spencer-Wells's forceps, (7) curved muscle scissors, (8) needle holder.
In addition, black eye silk No. 0 or 1 and curved eye needles Nos. 3 and 4 will be required. Peroxide may be needed to swab the eye cavity and a pressure dressing as shown in Fig. 270.

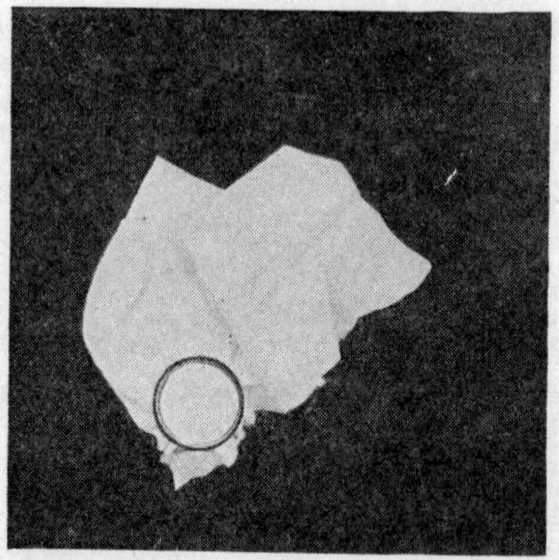

FIG. 280. KID DRUM used for testing the edges of all cutting instruments used in surgery of the eye.

exposure to cold winds and by any slight irritation. If the contents of an obstructed lacrimal sac become infected a *lacrimal abscess* or acute dacryocystitis occurs; this is seen as a small painful red swelling just below the inner canthus of the eye; if the swelling is pressed upon the contents can, unless the obstruction in the duct is complete, be pressed out of the sac along the ducts into the conjunctival sac; the eye can then be bathed to remove the pus so released.

The *treatment* of lacrimal obstruction is not very satisfactory because the canal is so tiny, but attempts are made to dilate it by passing a fine probe along the obstructed canal. In persistent cases the sac is incised and removed.

CONJUNCTIVITIS

Inflammation of the conjunctiva, or conjunctivitis, may be acute or chronic; it may also be catarrhal, as when it is due to some irritation or associated with a cold in the head; it may also be infective, in which case it is produced by a definite micro-organism.

Whatever the cause may be, the early symptoms of all forms of conjunctivitis are much the same; the patient complains that his eye feels gritty, he will often insist that he has a speck of dust or an eyelash in his eye, though this is not so; the eye feels hot, the conjunctiva looks red and injected and may later become congested. Other classical signs include extreme watering, swollen eyelids and photophobia.

Pink eye is a form of conjunctivitis which is due to a specific organism —usually the *Koch-Weeks bacillus*—and this form is infective, being rapidly spread by using the same towels, sponges, etc., and it quickly becomes epidemic among schoolchildren.

The ordinary signs of conjunctivitis are present with, in addition, a muco-purulent discharge, and for this reason it is sometimes described as *muco-purulent conjunctivitis*.

The *treatment* of the above forms of conjunctivitis may be local frequent penicillin applications or consist of frequent *irrigation* by means of weak antiseptic lotions (strong solution would injure the conjunctiva).

If the eye is very painful it will need rest, and for this purpose should be covered with a pad and bandage, but in no circumstances should eye-shades be employed, as these fit closely around the eye and bottle up any discharge which may be present, thus providing an ideal medium for the growth of organisms.

Purulent conjunctivitis. Any form of pus-producing organism may give rise to purulent conjunctivitis, a very serious form of which, because the causative organism attacks the cornea, is gonococcal conjunctivitis (see note below).

In the *treatment of purulent conjunctivitis* the measures already given are employed; there is a creamy purulent discharge from the eyes, the lids are markedly inflamed and swollen and there is a tendency for the pus to collect, under tension, within the eyelids.

In carrying out treatment for cases such as these the one additional point which requires attention is that irrigation must be sufficiently frequent to keep the eyes quite free of discharge; in severe cases almost constant irrigation will have to be employed, and it is therefore necessary that the lotion used should be bland and entirely non-irritating in character, such as either saline or boracic.

Gonorrhoeal conjunctivitis. This is a very serious form because the cornea is so easily abraded. *Ophthalmia neonatorum* is the term used to describe gonorrhoeal conjunctivitis when it occurs in the newly born, the baby being infected as he passes through an infected birth canal; several days later the signs of conjunctivitis appear, but fortunately babies have a good resistance to this type of organism so that in them the disease is much less severe than when it attacks adults.

Ophthalmia neonatorum is a notifiable condition and preventive treatment, whether necessary or not, is carried out at the birth of every child by putting one or two drops of a weak solution of silver nitrate, usually 1 per cent strength, into each eye.

In the **treatment and nursing of severe purulent ophthalmia,** such as gonorrhoeal, the chief care must be to prevent the collection of discharge over the cornea, as the gonococcus destroys the cornea and blindness would result. Irrigation is ordered to be carried out every 1 or 2 hours, and oftener if necessary. Should only one eye be affected the sound eye should be protected by means of a Buller's eye shield. The affected eye should never be covered.

As the pus in the eyes is under tension, and is very infectious, the nurse who is bathing or otherwise treating the eyes must take precautions to protect her own eyes; she should wear goggles, an overall and rubber gloves. In order to prevent spread of infection all the utensils used by or for the patient should be kept separate; all swabs and used dressings should either be burnt or put into 1–20 carbolic lotion at once, until they can be taken to the incinerator; all apparatus used for cleansing the eyes should be washed in carbolic lotion and boiled before they are used again.

Phlyctenular conjunctivitis is associated with generally poor hygienic conditions and malnutrition. The eyes water and there is photophobia (pain on exposure to light). Small yellow blobs are seen where the cornea joins the sclera (at the limbus). The condition may spread on to the cornea. The treatment consists in keeping the pupil dilated, irrigating the eye with saline and wearing dark glasses. The general health must be improved.

Penicillin is effective provided the treatment is sufficiently frequent. The eye is first irrigated with half-strength saline in order to remove pus. Then two drops of penicillin (2,000 units per c.c.) are instilled every minute for half an hour; at intervals of five minutes for the next half-hour, then at half-hourly intervals for three hours and hourly intervals for the following six hours and two-hourly for the next twelve hours. The result is that pus is suppressed and the inflammation gradually subsides.

AFFECTIONS OF THE CORNEA AND IRIS

Corneal ulcer may be due to local injury or inflammation, or it may be brought about by debility. The surface of the cornea is covered by epithelium, as is the skin; if a superficial abrasion occurs it will heal without leaving a scar; but, if the deeper layers of this structure are involved, scarring will result. The scar will be opaque and consequently sight will be impaired.

In corneal ulcer the eyes look red and inflamed and the ulcer appears as a greyish patch; the size of the ulcer is determined by the instillation of several drops of fluorescein which stains the affected area green but does not stain the healthy surface, so that the shape and size of the ulcer are clearly defined.

In treating cases of corneal ulcer it is important to try and discover the cause and then to direct treatment to the relief of this; the general health must be attended to, as when debility persists the ulcers tend to spread and become very difficult to cure. Penicillin sensitive organisms will be treated by local applications of penicillin. Sulphonamides are given.

Intractable cases will be cauterized, this is carried out as follows:

Application of pure carbolic to a corneal ulcer. The patient is placed in a position in which he is comfortable and can keep quite still, a good light is provided, the eye is cocainized with drops of 2 or 4 per cent cocaine, and one drop of fluorescein is then instilled to stain the ulcer. A blunt orange stick is dipped in pure carbolic and the ulcer is gently touched with this: a small piece of blotting paper is used as a mop on the eye at the margin of the ulcer to prevent the carbolic from touching the healthy part of it. Pure carbolic destroys the structure and will leave an opaque scar. It is very important for the eye of a case of corneal ulcer to be covered with a comfortable eye pad; the condition is very painful, even the slightest ray of light causing great pain and distress to the patient which is accompanied by profuse watering of the eye. The pupil is kept dilated by atropine, and irrigation and hot bathing may be employed.

Keratitis or interstitial keratitis is inflammation of the cornea, and it is characterised by a non-suppurative inflammation which results in considerable opacity and so interferes with sight. It is most commonly met with in congenital syphilis. Treatment consists in dilating the pupil and the wearing of dark glasses. Anti-syphilitic treatment (see p. 532) is necessary.

Arcus senilis is a degeneration of the cornea which occurs in some persons in old age; the cornea is composed of three layers—an outer, known as Bowman's membrane; an inner layer, Descemet's membrane; and an intermediate layer which is described as the substantia propria, and it is this latter which is affected in arcus senilis.

Iritis or inflammation of the iris is frequently associated with inflammation of the ciliary body and is then known as *irido-cyclitis*. It is due to disturbance of the general health, is sometimes associated with rheumatism and may follow influenza and may also be due to local sepsis.

The iris looks dull and inflamed, an exudate forms and this causes the iris to become adherent to the lens, unless prevented by proper treatment. The patient complains of pain, especially when light falls on the eye (photophobia).

Treatment. The main point in the treatment is to keep the pupil constantly and completely dilated so that there is no opportunity for adhesions to form between iris and lens. Hot bathing is employed (see p. 751). The general health should be attended to and the cause of the condition investigated and treated.

AFFECTIONS OF THE LENS

Cataract is opacity of the crystalline lens of the eye, the cornea remaining clear; such opacity interferes with vision and if the affected lens is removed there is a clear space provided for the passage of light into the eye, but the element which normally focuses objects is absent and therefore such a patient will be obliged to wear strong lenses (glasses) in front of the eyes to make up for the absence of the crystalline lens.

Cataract may be *congenital*, it may be caused by *injury*, it is *a complication of diabetes* owing to defective nutrition of the eye and, lastly and most commonly, it is the result of degenerative changes taking place in old age and is then described as *senile cataract.* The majority of the cases admitted for treatment will be old persons, a few will be very young children.

The *treatment for cataract in adults* is excision of the lens. In young children the lens is soft and the operation of *needling* or *discission* is carried out, the capsule of the lens being punctured, divided or incised by a sharp needle, permitting the aqueous humour which fills the anterior chamber of the eye to penetrate the lens, and this fluid dissolves the lens substance and washes it out of the capsule.

In middle-aged persons and old people the lens is hard so that the aqueous humour has no effect upon it and the more extensive operation has to be performed.

Excision of lens for cataract is carried out under a local anaesthetic; a knife is inserted at the margin of the cornea and taken across the anterior chamber of the eye and out at the other side, a slightly sawlike movement being adopted in cutting, and two-fifths of the cornea formed into a flap and the upper part lifted as one lifts the lid of a box; sufficient pressure is then made on the lower part of the eye beneath the lowest margin of the cornea and the lens is slipped out of its capsule as a pea is shelled from its pod; none of the vitreous humour is allowed to escape.

The operation of *iridectomy* is sometimes performed at this point, in order to lessen the danger of prolapse of the iris later on.

The raised flap of cornea is gently laid back in position but is not stitched, and the parts must be kept quite still during the days following this operation, so that healing can take place, and it is for this reason that the care described below in the post-operative nursing of cataract cases is carried out. Once a nurse has carefully followed the steps of this operation she must realize that any increase of intra-ocular pressure will tend to separate the margins of the injured cornea and that any sudden or great increase of pressure will cause the contents of the eye to prolapse through this wound.

Pre-operative treatment. The patient should if possible be in hospital a few days before the operation in order that certain investigations and observations may be carried out:

(1) Swabs of both eyes are taken to determine the presence of any micro-organisms which might contraindicate the operation since they would result in sepsis. A few staphylococci albi and diphtheroids are not considered serious, but staphylococci aurei would necessitate delay.

(2) It is important to investigate the condition of the patient's heart and lungs; he is elderly, and may have a cough or suffer from asthma, and as complete rest and freedom from movement is necessary after a cataract

operation the undue movement produced by coughing might be serious.

(3) The patient's mental condition should also be noted; elderly people are inclined to imagine all kinds of queer things, they will not be able to sleep at nights and in this case they are inclined to get fidgety and might want to remove their bandages after the operation.

(4) The bowels should be properly regulated so that the bowel is empty, the colon free from gas and the abdomen comfortable before the operation.

(5) It is usual to test the urine for the presence of albumin which might indicate some renal failure, and also for sugar and diacetic acid which would indicate that the patient was a diabetic subject.

(6) On the day before the operation it is desirable to keep the patient in bed in order to accustom him to lying on his back and to keep him quite still; he should practise the use of the bedpan lying down, learn to drink out of a feeding cup and be taught to turn over on to his side, that is, the unaffected side, to which he will be gently rolled in order to have his back rubbed and the drawsheet changed after the operation.

The patient will wear a double eye bandage after the operation and this should be carefully fitted the day before; he might be allowed to lie wearing this bandage for an hour or so in order to get used to the sounds of the ward when lying with his eyes covered. The double eye bandage having been carefully fitted will be sterilized along with the other necessary articles in the special eye-operation drum. Some surgeons supply a wire cage or shield to protect the operated eye, and when this is used it should be carefully fitted and the edges bound with cotton wool.

Immediate preparation. A local anaesthetic is given to adult patients for this operation because the effects of retching and vomiting would cause much movement and serious harm to the eye. The precaution of marking the eye which is to be operated on may be taken.

Some surgeons like the eyelashes cut, though others do not have this done. *To cut the eyelashes,* smear the scissors with vaseline so that the hairs will stick to the blades, the type of scissors used being similar to small curved embroidery scissors, and the convex edge being used against the eyelashes. If the eyelashes are very long it may be possible to steady them by grasping with the finger and thumb of one hand, otherwise the patient should be told exactly what is to be done and asked to keep very still and quiet.

The eye to be operated on should be prepared by having the pupil dilated, atropine being used for this; and it will be cocainized by a 4 per cent solution of cocaine. The surgeon will usually give quite definite orders as to how often he wishes cocaine to be instilled, the strength to be employed and the number of drops to be used at a time.

Post-operative nursing care. After the operation the patient is wheeled quietly back to bed, both eyes are bandaged, the idea of covering the sound eye being not so much to keep light out of it as because each movement would necessarily carry the affected eye with it, as movement of the eyes is bilateral.

The patient is placed gently in bed with one soft pillow, but if at all 'chesty' he may be propped up on several pillows, the main point being that the head should be kept quite still and not moved. He has not had a general anaesthetic and therefore he is instructed to keep quite still and then, 6–8 hours afterwards, with two nurses attending him he is gently turned to the unaffected side and his back is washed and rubbed. The lumbar region is apt to become very stiff and the nurse should take the opportunity of rubbing it well to stimulate the circulation and relieve the stiffness.

Diet. During the first 12 hours many surgeons prefer that their patients should have an all-fluid diet, drinking this from the feeder they have learned to use before the operation. As soon as they like they may have a light diet, such as crustless bread and butter and any other soft food, pounded fish and minced meat, anything, in fact, that they can manage to eat without having to bite and masticate it, as these movements, involving the temporal muscle, may cause movement of the eye. As the patient has both eyes bandaged, he must be fed.

Bowels. As the bowels have been carefully regulated before the operation, the giving of an aperient is usually delayed until the third morning and the patient should be warned not to worry about having his bowels opened as a small enema will be given if the aperient does not act. In having a bedpan the patient should not make any effort at all, he must be lifted on to it and taken off by two or three nurses, and if left at all he must be so placed that he is quite comfortable and can lie without discomfort, stress or strain.

Sleep and rest. It is very difficult to lie in one position and very boring to have both eyes bandaged and be unable to see what is going on, time is apt to drag and it is very necessary that the patient should have a really good night's sleep; in many instances the surgeon will order a sedative on the first night and repeat it on other nights if necessary.

Dressing. The surgeon will usually prefer to do the first dressing himself. The bandage is gently removed, the eye is bathed with warm boracic lotion. In swabbing the eye the movement should be performed by sweeping the lashes from underneath upwards in order efficiently to remove discharge—this is better than the usual method of swabbing the eye from within outwards. At the time of the first dressing the surgeon will carefully inspect the eye for any prolapse of the iris which would be seen as a little dark mass at the opening of the wound; atropine is instilled, either atropine ointment or atropine 1 per cent solution. The good eye is kept covered for the first 4 or 5 days, because it takes at least three days for healing to begin at the edges of the wound. After this time a single eye bandage is used for the affected eye. If the case progresses satisfactorily the affected eye will usually be uncovered after the seventh day, dark glasses being then worn during the day, but it is advisable to cover the eye with a pad and bandage at night.

For fear the patient should touch his eye during sleep it is usual to hobble the hands by tying them to the bedsides; considerable freedom should be allowed, but the bandage used should not be long enough to permit the patient to reach his face. In the case of elderly persons this may be found irksome and, if it is irritating, it is better that the hands should not be tied.

The patient usually gets up about the ninth or tenth day for a short time but should be warned not to stoop or bend down as the wound is usually feeble for the first few weeks. As a rule the patient goes home about the fourteenth day, taking with him atropine drops to be instilled at night and being advised to attend for examination a few weeks later for the provision of special glasses.

In some elderly persons where the capsule of the lens becomes thick and fibrous it may be opaque and interfere with vision. When this happens it is usual to make a hole through the capsule large enough for the patient to see through. This operation is called 'needling', but it is not the same as the discission described on p. 765.

Complications. *Post-operative mania* is probably the complication mostly to be feared in elderly persons, since if it does occur, and the patient becomes quite irrational, the whole effect of the operation is spoilt.

Prolapsed iris. The provision of absolute rest which has been insisted upon in the foregoing notes is essential in order that there should be no increase of intra-ocular pressure causing prolapse of the iris through the wound. It is to prevent this that iridectomy is often performed in the course of operations for cataract.

Sepsis may complicate an eye operation. This will result in conjunctivitis, delay in healing of the wound and reforming of the anterior chamber.

Iritis and *bleeding* may also occur, particularly in diabetic cases.

GLAUCOMA

Glaucoma is increase of tension in the eye, and it may be acute or chronic—the *chronic type* is most commonly met with, the history obtained being of gradually failing eyesight.

Acute glaucoma comes on suddenly, with acute pain and congestion, accompanied by marked malaise, vomiting and much distress. If the patient is able to give any account of himself at all he may remember that his sight has been failing and that he has been seeing haloes round the light at night.

The increasing tension in glaucoma is due to the fact that the fluid contained in the anterior chamber does not drain away as it should. This fluid usually drains into the general circulation by passing into a tiny vein at the side of the eye. When this is imperfectly carried out the shallow anterior chamber cannot increase in size and therefore pressure is directed backwards on to the optic disk, resulting in atrophy of the optic nerve and consequently loss of sight. The longer this pressure is allowed to remain the greater will be the interference with sight, and eyesight once lost cannot be regained by any medical or surgical method.

In the treatment of glaucoma the first thing that every nurse should realize is in the nature of a negative proposition—that atropine should never be employed. On the contrary the pupil must be kept contracted and for this purpose eserine is used.

In acute glaucoma the patient is admitted with the eye very injected and extremely painful. After the initial instillation of eserine, which aims at relieving the tension, hot eye bathings should be carried out, and leeches or other forms of counterirritation may be applied, just inside the outer aspect of the orbit. The patient should be kept as quiet as possible, the bowels should be well opened, and the administration of magnesium sulphate will probably help to relieve the tension. Light diet should be given.

When a very acute case is admitted, the surgeon will at once be informed and the operation of iridectomy will be carried out.

The surgical operative treatment for *chronic glaucoma* is to make a tiny opening at the margin of the limbus—that is, where the cornea joins the sclerotic coat of the eye—the eye is cocainized as described in the operation for cataract, a tiny incision is made on the surface of the eyeball in the conjunctiva under the upper lid, the flap is turned downwards to expose the limbus and trephining is performed at the margin, resulting in a tiny permanent perforation through which the fluid in the anterior chamber can drain away under the conjunctiva, and it is usually successful.

DETACHED RETINA

The retina, which is the innermost coat of the eye, rests on the choroid from which it receives nourishment, and if contact does not take place its nutrition is therefore impaired. *Detachment of the retina* is a very serious condition, as the main organ of sight atrophies and the detachment rapidly spreads until the whole organ is affected and if untreated the patient will become blind.

Treatment is operative. The eye is cocainized, the eyeball is then very carefully retracted, the conjunctiva removed to expose the sclerotic coat and heat is applied by means of a diathermy electrode; this results in adhesions between the sclera and the retina. Before the end of the operation the sclera is punctured by a diathermy needle and the fluid which has collected between the detached retina and the choroid coat is evacuated. In successful cases the retina then falls back into its original place and is retained there by the formation of permanent adhesions.

The *preparation of the patient* for this operation is similar to that described for cataract. The *post-operative nursing care* is also similar, except that for detached retina the position in which the patient is to be nursed depends on the site of the scleral punctures and will be specified by the surgeon, and both eyes are bandaged for 14 days. At the end of this time special opaque glasses with a small central opening (Loch-Brille) are worn on both eyes, and the patient is allowed to sit up and gradually to get up. Stooping, lifting and exertion are forbidden for several months.

ENUCLEATION OF EYE

Serious injury to the eye may necessitate enucleation of the eyeball.

The instruments required for some of the operations mentioned will be seen on pp. 757–60.

Chapter 50

Surgery of the Brain and Nursing Care

Degrees of unconsciousness—The nursing of an unconscious patient—Preparation for an operation on the brain and the post-operative nursing care

Before considering or attempting to nurse cases of brain surgery, it is important that a sound knowledge of the degrees of unconsciousness, their significance and appropriate treatment, with special reference to the dangers which threaten the life of a patient who is unconscious, should be studied carefully.

Degrees of unconsciousness. A *person who is asleep* is unconscious, but he will move and turn over if he is disturbed. A *stuporous patient* will not be affected by a slight touch, but he can be roused if roughly shaken and shouted at; a person who is in a deep state of stupor can be aroused by sustained pressure at the side of the bridge of the nose. A patient in *coma* cannot be roused.

It is very necessary for a nurse to be able to recognize when unconsciousness is becoming deeper, and this has already been referred to in the note on cerebral compression on p. 613 and in the care of a case of fracture of base of the skull on p. 611. The main points to be observed are—increasing depth of breathing; slowing and increase in volume of the pulse, fixation of the pupils together with absence of any reaction, disappearance of cough and swallowing reflexes. In nursing cases of injury or disease of the brain it is most important that accurate attention should be given to these points and that a written note should be made, with mention of the time, whenever any one of them is observed.

The **dangers of unconsciousness** which a nurse should do her best to prevent are—fatal pneumonia from food, fluid, and saliva trickling down into the trachea; hypostatic pneumonia and bedsores resulting from the patient's having been allowed to lie like a log.

Nursing care. An unconscious patient depends entirely for his well-being, and possibly also for his life, upon intelligent nursing care. *Ordinary routine nursing* measures will be employed to prevent bedsores and to keep the patient clean, his mouth and eyes requiring particular attention. His urine should be measured and tested at regular intervals, his bladder observed for fear lest retention of urine should occur, and his bowels kept regularly acting and his abdomen watched for distension.

Special nursing measures will be required in order to prevent occurrence of the complications mentioned above—inhalation and hypostatic pneumonia.

Feeding. When a normal person eats or drinks and some of the food or fluid enters the larynx or, as it is called, 'goes the wrong way', the subject splutters and coughs and his friends give him a good thump on the back in order to dislodge the particle and so relieve his distress. This, in the case of an unconscious patient, unfortunately will not do, since the cough reflex has been abolished and some of the fluid or food put into the mouth will therefore trickle slowly down into the trachea—to cause fatal pneumonia later.

Semiconscious patients who have a good swallowing reflex, and in whom the cough reflex is not abolished, may be fed in small amounts given from a spoon—a feeder should not be used. Many patients who are semiconscious will chew if food is put into the mouth, and when the nurse discovers this she should, in preference to fluids, give such a patient semisolid food such as jellies, thick ground rice puddings and porridge, which will cause him to move his jaws as in the act of chewing.

A patient in whom the swallowing reflex is absent must never have food or fluid put into his mouth, but should be fed by means of the nasal tube. The use of an oesophageal tube for feeding purposes is not recommended, because passing this rather large tube results in regurgitation of fluid around the tube in the pharynx and mouth; this fluid will then trickle into the trachea unless the precaution is taken of letting the patient lie on an inclined plane with his head low.

The fatal pneumonia already mentioned is not solely due to the injudicious introduction of fluid or food into the trachea; another danger is the patient's saliva. Various devices have been adopted to prevent saliva from trickling into the trachea, and one of the most efficient ways of accomplishing this is by the use of a suction apparatus—a catheter can be passed through the nose, with its end lying in the pharynx; negative pressure is then applied by means of a piece of tubing from the catheter connected to a tap, from which water is running. The patient is arranged on his side and the saliva which collects in his mouth and throat is sucked out by the negative pressure apparatus.

If a nurse has to deal with an unconscious patient who is making a lot of saliva she should—pending the arrival of a doctor—arrange pillows under the trunk of the patient as he lies prone and support his head, with the forehead resting on a pillow or sandbag. A basin put on the bed beneath the patient's mouth will catch the saliva as it runs out.

To *prevent hypostatic pneumonia* it is necessary to move the patient frequently, at least every hour and a half, and then not gently; he should be thoroughly disturbed; if he is semiconscious and can be made to cough this is excellent, but even when unconscious the nurse may notice that his breathing is slightly increased in depth by movement. When deeply unconscious he should be given inhalations of a mixture of oxygen 93 per cent and carbon dioxide 7 per cent at regular intervals. It is necessary to get good ventilation of the lungs if the danger of hypostatic pneumonia is to be obviated.

The patient should be propped up in a different position each time he is moved; sometimes he may be drawn up the bed and propped, as if sitting; at other times he may be placed first on one side and then on the other.

Prevention of deformity. Unconscious patients who are in bed for some time tend to get footdrop, and to help to prevent this it is advisable to use a low bedcradle over the feet to take the weight of the bedclothes—a footrest may also be used. The bedclothes should never be drawn tightly over a patient's feet when tucking them in.

Preparation of a patient for an operation for removal of a tumour of the brain. The routine general preparation of the patient is similar to that described on p. 632.

A patient admitted to hospital for an operation on the brain may be in a good or a poor general condition. He may, for example, have been in a state of stupor for some days, and having taken little fluid and food during this time it may be found that his mouth is dry, tongue dirty and teeth covered with sordes. His skin may be dry and he may be beginning to develop bedsores.

The surgeon will have to decide whether an operation is urgently needed or not. When possible it will be considered advisable to try and improve the patient's general condition first. The symptoms mentioned above will be relieved and the general condition improved by the liberal administration of fluids by mouth, when the patient can swallow, or alternatively by rectum or by means of the nasal tube.

It is very important for the surgeon to obtain all the information possible before operating on the brain, so nurses will be called upon to make careful observations and be prepared to give a detailed report on anything they observe which might have a bearing on the condition of the patient. Observation which might help the surgeon to judge the position of a tumour of the brain or the extent of injury to the brain would include the following:

Speech difficulties. A patient may be unable to express what he wishes to say. He may not understand what is said to him.

Loss of memory. This may be complete or incomplete. Loss of memory may be remote or immediate and it may cover only a certain definite period of time.

Hemianopia. In this condition the patient is unable to see as well on one side as on the other. He may not complain of this, but the nurse may notice that he only sees objects at one side of his bed.

Stupor. If a patient is in a state of stupor it is important to notice whether there is any increase in the depth or the degree of unconsciousness, as this would denote increasing intracranial pressure.

Changes in the character of the pulse and respirations. Any slowing of the pulse and increase in the depth of respiration are symptoms which may denote increasing pressure.

Alteration in the size of the pupil or any inequality of the pupils. Either of these symptoms should immediately be reported, as the onset of these may be an indication that operation is urgently necessary.

Fits and Convulsions. Any type of seizure the patient may have should be observed. With pad and pencil the nurse should write down the following particulars: the time the fit started, how it began, where jerking movements started and the order in which these progressed, how long the fit lasted, whether the patient lost consciousness during the fit and for how long he remained unconscious, how the fit terminated and the state of the patient after the fit, whether he wanted to sleep, complained of headache or whether he was restless and irritable.

Any complaints the patient makes. No detail is too small to be of importance and a nurse should note and report any complaint a patient may make.

Before operation an X-ray examination of the skull is made and in many cases ventriculography (see p. 167) is performed in order to discover whether there is any displacement of the fluid in the ventricles of the brain.

During the operation a careful record of the pulse, respiration and blood pressure is kept. An intravenous drip infusion of saline or blood is set up so that a blood transfusion can be given without delay should this become necessary. Operations on the brain often take a long time—from 6 to 8 hours—and the patient is not, as a rule, removed from the operating table until he has regained consciousness.

Post-operative nursing care. On return to bed the head should be kept low at first. The bed is protected by a mackintosh and towel. The side which has been operated on should be kept uppermost. The pulse and respirations should be noted frequently, every half hour at first, and later every two hours. The temperature should be taken at two-hourly intervals. Should the temperature rise to 102° F. all bedclothing, except a covering sheet, should be removed; if it rises to 103° F. the patient should be sponged with tepid or cold water.

It is important to watch the patient carefully for any signs of increasing intracranial pressure such as *slowing of the pulse, increase in the depth of respiration, drowsiness increasing to stupor*. These are probably due to pressure caused by blood clot which may occur during the first 24 hours after operation. It is essential to report any of these symptoms to the surgeon without delay and he will take immediate steps to remove the pressure because otherwise it may cause permanent injury to the brain.

When the mouth is dry the lips, tongue, gums and teeth should be kept very clean and moist, and it will be found that as the patient can take fluids, his mouth will become clean, moist and comfortable.

The *position in which the patient lies* should be changed every three hours; a patient who has had a cerebellar operation should not be placed on his back, but may be placed on either side; a patient who has had an operation on one side of his cerebrum can be placed on the opposite side, and on his back alternately.

The *patient may be given fluid*, sucking it from a swab placed in his mouth for the first few hours after operation, until he has ceased to vomit. As soon as his swallowing and cough reflexes have returned he may be given fluids to drink; a spoon should be used until the nurse is quite certain that these reflexes are acting normally. He may then be given small drinks from a feeding cup. On the second or third day the patient can usually be allowed to sit up in bed and may be given a fairly full diet.

The *bowels are opened* by means of an enema on the second day and magnesium sulphate is given regularly afterwards. It is the best aperient to use for cases of surgery of the brain, as it reduces intracranial pressure by removing fluid. Its use is commonly continued for months, not necessarily as an aperient but in order to effect the slight dehydration which is found to be necessary.

If sedatives are necessary mild analgesics such as aspirin and pyramidon are employed in preference to morphia which is likely to mask the symptoms of increasing intracranial pressure should these arise.

The *dressing* is usually performed on the second day, some of the stitches being taken out then, and it is repeated on the fourth day when the remainder of the stitches are removed. This is an advantage as, by taking the stitches out soon, stitch marks and wound scars are avoided—an important point on an exposed area such as the scalp and forehead.

The scalp should be kept clean, and this can be done by swabbing it with equal parts of methylated spirit and water; when the hair has grown brushing it will keep the scalp free from dandruff.

Getting up. Cases of surgery of the brain are allowed to get up at the end of the first week, and they are encouraged to mix freely with other patients. A certain degree of *euphoria* is present until the patient has completed his convalescence, and this is characterized by an attractive, obliging, very agreeable manner; with marked good temper which makes the patient a great favourite with others.

The patient needs encouragement and re-education so that he may be helped to take his place in society again; when he has completely recovered his normal temperament may not be nearly as attractive as the one associated with the slight euphoria present after his operation.

The instruments shown in fig. 235, p. 679, are some of those which are essential for decompression or trephining the skull. Surgery of the brain is a very specialized branch and many surgeons have designed their own instruments.

Chapter 51

Orthopaedic Nursing

Classification of deformities—The treatment and care of cases met with in an orthopaedic unit, including: Common congenital deformities—Flatfoot and other conditions of the feet—Deformities of the vertebral column—Prolapsed intervertebral disc—Deformities due to rickets, to diseases of the central nervous system and to contractures

The word orthopaedics is derived from Greek and means 'the straightening of children'. Orthopaedic surgery deals particularly with the parts of the body that are concerned with movement—the muscle, joints and bones of the trunk, back and limbs.

It includes in its practice manipulations, operations on the structures mentioned, massage and remedial exercises. It is employed in the correction of deformities, both congenital and acquired. The nurse who wishes to prepare herself for orthopaedic work should have a sound knowledge of the skeleton, the positions of the major groups of muscles and their action on joints, of the normal range of movement at joints and of its limitations. She should develop the habit of observation, and train herself to see errors of poise, balance and alignment. This can best be done by having an intimate knowledge of the normal poise of the body, in repose and during activity. She will then at once detect the irregularities which occur in abnormal conditions which if left untreated will result in deformity.

It is essential that a nurse should learn to be constructive in the criticism she may make regarding errors of balance and poise. When for example a parent can be brought to see that his child is stooping a little, or habitually standing in an attitude which is likely to cause deformity, and then helped to realize that seeing a special surgeon now need not mean that surgical intervention is necessary, but that only a surgeon who has specialized in orthopaedic work is competent to suggest that some special exercises might be taught which would correct the condition before it becomes more serious. The nurse, although she may recognize the condition, is not qualified to deal with it.

CLASSIFICATION OF DEFORMITIES

A classification of deformities, not confined to those which affect only the organs of locomotion—with which orthopaedics is solely concerned—is given below. A deformity is a deviation from the normal physical structure.

Congenital deformities arise before or at birth. The true cause is indiscoverable, but there are many theories as to possible causes. Examples are, *harelip, cleft palate*—these conditions are dealt with in ear, nose and throat surgery on p. 746.

Spina bifida. This is a gap in the posterior part of the bony arch of the neural canal. Through this gap the contents of the spinal canal protrude.

The complications are paralysis, infection and spinal meningitis. Treatment aims at closure of the opening when possible.

Mal-descent of testes. The testes are arrested in descent to the scrotum; they do not develop and are liable to inflammation.

Failure of development of the intestinal canal. Occlusion of the oesophagus is rare, and is practically untreatable. An *imperforate anus* may be present, and it is possible to operate successfully on this.

Congenital pyloric stenosis has been dealt with on p. 391. *Congenital clubfoot* and *congenital dislocation of the hip, congenital absence of a bone* in the upper or lower extremity, *supernumerary digits in hands and feet, webbed fingers or toes,* and *congenital amputation* of part of a limb may all be met with occasionally.

Torticollis is frequently classed as a congenital deformity, but it is more probably produced by injury at birth than as the result of a developmental defect.

Acquired deformities provide a twofold interest; the interest involved in discovering the cause of the deformity and the cure to be carried out combined with arrest of progress of the deformity.

The causes of acquired deformities are numerous and include *injury* to the skeleton as in fractures and dislocation, and injury to the soft parts, burns for example, when the injury sustained may result in deformity due to the contraction of scar tissue.

Disease of bones and joints. Arthritis, tuberculosis, osteomyelitis, tumours of bone, osteomalacia and rickets may all result in deformity of bone.

Diseases of the central nervous system, particularly infantile paralysis, may result in deformity.

Disease and weakness of muscle. Deformity produced by muscle weakness may be only postural, as occurs in many cases of flatfoot, lordosis, scoliosis and kyphosis. It may also be the result of disease of muscle.

Surgery may produce deformity. For example, amputation of a breast or of a limb, which may be necessary in order to remove a diseased organ, produces a definite deformity. The accidental division of a nerve in surgery will if the injury is irreparable, result in paralytic deformity. A ventral or incisional hernia, occurring in the region of an abdominal incision, is another example of deformity resulting from surgery.

THE TREATMENT OF DEFORMITY IS DIVIDED INTO PREVENTIVE AND CORRECTIVE TREATMENT

Prevention of deformities is necessary in the care of all surgical cases and especially in the case of burns and fractures. In the *treatment of fractures,* the aim is to *reduce the fracture* and place the broken bones in *correct alignment*; and then to fix them in this position by means of splinting and extension. Having performed this, and arranged to have the necessary fixation maintained until the fracture has healed, the next very important consideration is *to maintain the function* of the limb or part affected.

In the illustration attached for example the case is one of fracture of the femur; the limb is put up in a Thomas's knee splint, weights are planned to provide accurate balance in order to make it possible for the patient to use all his muscles all the time he is in bed. This patient was able to raise himself in bed on the first day, and to place himself on the bedpan; he could turn about from one side to the other in order to reach articles from his locker and bedside table at about the same time. See fig. 110, p. 237.

In the care of cases of burns very close consideration must be given during the healing stage to prevent any deformity from contractures. The position in which the patient is nursed and the pliability of the superficial structures must be constantly noted, in order to prevent either limitation of the normal range of movement or actual deformity.

The *prevention of rickets* by eradication of slums and overcrowding, and by the provision of welfare centres and adequate diet for all children, are factors of importance in the prevention of one of the most crippling of diseases.

DEFORMITIES OF THE FEET

Congenital clubfoot is one of the commonest of these deformities; as a rule it is seen in the form of *talipes equino-varus*, but it may be present in other forms of talipes. The four main varieties of foot deformity are:

Talipes equinus. The foot is plantar-flexed as in the position of standing on the toes.

Talipes calcaneus is exactly the opposite deformity; the heel has dropped, as in the position of standing on the heel.

Talipes varus. The front of the foot is turned inwards and the inner border elevated.

Talipes valgus is exactly opposite to talipes varus; the front part of the foot is turned outwards, and the outer border elevated.

Each of these deformities may occur alone, or two types may be associated. As mentioned above, the commonest congenital deformity of the foot is clubfoot or talipes equino-varus, in which the foot is plantar-flexed and inverted.

The **treatment of clubfoot** should commence as early as possible; a few days after birth the foot may be manipulated into the correct position and maintained by adhesive strapping. The nurse in charge of the infant should see that this strapping does not get wet and she should also notice that it does not become tight. As a rule it is allowed to remain on for a week and is then renewed and the manipulation of the foot and application of strapping is repeated so that as the foot grows it will improve in shape. In a slightly older child plaster of paris may be employed. A specially adapted shoe, designed to maintain correction of the deformity, is necessary when the infant begins to walk.

When the infant is not seen by a surgeon until he is about 2 years of age the simple manipulation just mentioned is not likely to be sufficient to correct the deformity which exists. At this age it is usual to correct the deformity by manipulation of the foot under a general anaesthetic and to put on plaster of paris in which the child may walk about. If the condition is not treated until the child is 4 or 5 years of age, operation on the soft parts may be necessary, combined with manipulation and overcorrection of the foot in plaster of paris.

In older children the deformity may be so marked that it is impossible for it to be corrected except by operation on the bones, and the removal of wedge-shaped pieces of bone is carried out in order to bring the foot into a normal position.

The *after care of cases of clubfoot* has to be continued until the child has grown up, since the tendency for the foot to revert to the old position of deformity is ever present. Constant supervision of the function of the muscles controlling the foot, the mobility of the joints of the foot and the provision of suitable footwear is essential if any degree of success is to be attained.

CONGENITAL DISLOCATION OF HIP

Congenital dislocation of the hip may be bilateral, or unilateral, when only one hip joint is affected. This condition may not be noticed until the infant begins to walk, when it is observed that he develops an awkward gait with marked lordosis and an ungainly limp. This is because the weight of the body pushes the head of the femur up on to the external surface of the ilium since the head is not adapted, as it should be, to the acetabulum (see fig. 285, p. 793).

Treatment. The aim of treatment is to obtain reduction of the dislocation without injury to the femoral head and it is now considered best to abduct fully the hips on an abduction frame (see fig. 281) and allow the dislocated femur or femora to descend gradually to the level of the acetabulum. The child is put on a double abduction frame with strapping extension on both legs and the hips are gradually abducted as widely as possible. This may take a week to 10 days, the child is left on the frame for 4 to 6 weeks and in that period of time the dislocation is usually reduced.

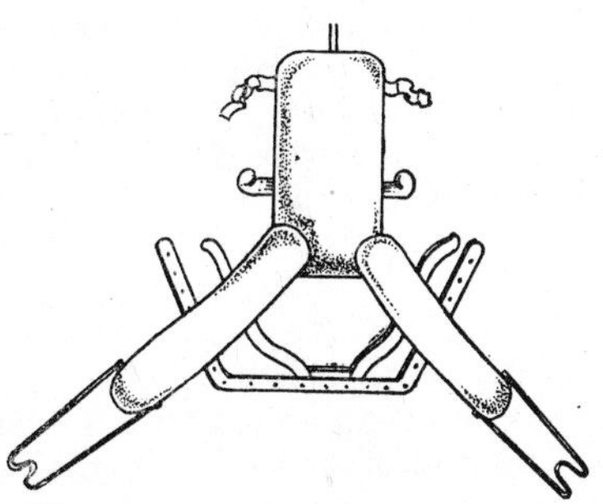

FIG. 281.—DOUBLE ABDUCTION FRAME.

The next step is to apply plaster of paris after the method employed by Mr. J. S. Batchelor. A general anaesthetic is given, the bandages and extensions are removed and the child is lifted from the frame. The affected femur is gently rotated, pressing it against the acetabular surface of the innominate bone, getting as much internal rotation as possible and maintaining good abduction. Plaster of paris is then applied. The limbs are first wrapped in splint wool and then plaster of paris bandages are applied,

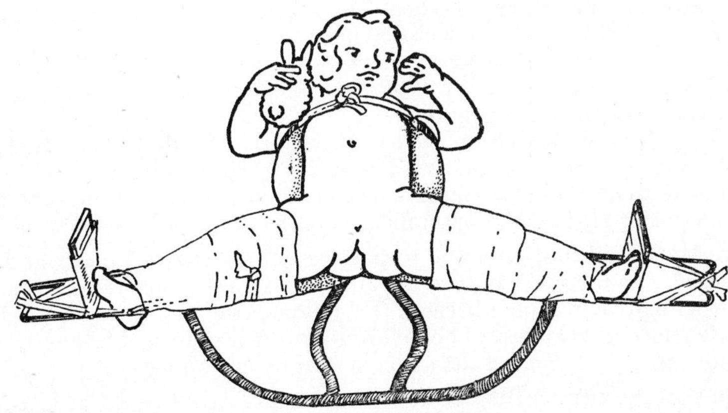

FIG. 282.—SHOWING CHILD WITH CONGENITAL DISLOCATION OF HIP FULLY ABDUCTED ON FRAME.

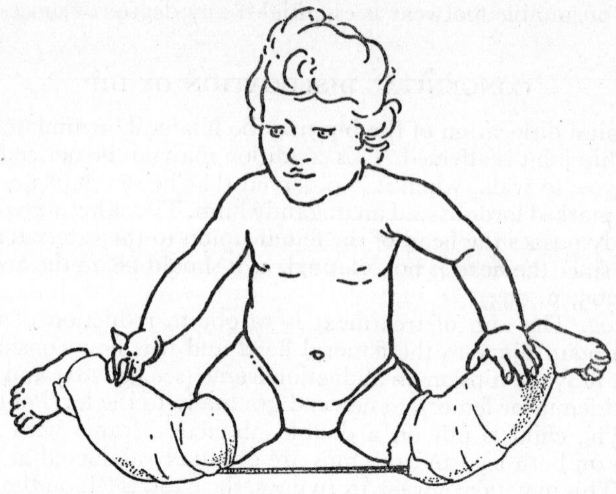

FIG. 283.—SHOWING CHILD IN PLASTER OF PARIS WITH LIMBS INTERNALLY ROTATED.

the knees being fixed at right angles, and a bar adjusted between the legs as above. This position is maintained for 12 to 18 months, the plaster being renewed as often as necessary. The child gets used to the position in a week or two and may sit up and crawl around, but he should not be allowed to bang his hips about for fear of causing injury which might result in osteoarthritis.

TORTICOLLIS

Torticollis is usually the result of some injury during birth which causes rupture of certain muscle fibres of sternocleido-mastoid with the result that contraction of the injured side occurs. This type of torticollis is painless; the head is flexed to one side and the face rotated to the opposite side. The contracted muscle is seen to stand out prominently.

The *treatment* is to divide the muscle either by subcutaneous tenotomy or by an open operation. The head should be kept in an overcorrected position until the divided structures have healed, to prevent their contracting again. This overcorrection may be maintained by sandbags at first, and afterwards by plaster of paris; or the head may be put in plaster of paris at the time of operation.

The plaster is worn for from 4 to 6 weeks and then cut down and the child taught to control the movements of his head by exercises performed in front of a mirror. The plaster splint may be worn in between the times devoted to exercise until the patient has sufficient control of the position of his head.

Paralytic torticollis is due to paralysis of the sternomastoid muscle of one side. As the result of this, the other, sound side, becomes shortened and eventually contracted because the action of the muscle is unopposed and therefore unbalanced. The deformity of torticollis in this case, is on the side opposite to that of the affected (paralysed) muscle.

Spasmodic torticollis occurs as the result of irritation of the muscles of one side of the neck. It is sometimes associated with rheumatism, but it may also arise in any painful condition of the neck.

FLATFOOT AND OTHER CONDITIONS ASSOCIATED WITH IT

Flatfoot may be congenital but it is much more often an acquired deformity and frequently postural in origin.

The foot is made up of a series of bony arches; the inner longitudinal arch and the anterior transverse metatarsal arch are those affected in flatfoot (see illustration). The changes in the structures occur in the following order—*The muscles which normally sustain the arches of the foot in position may be stretched and weakened*, and this may occur as the result of

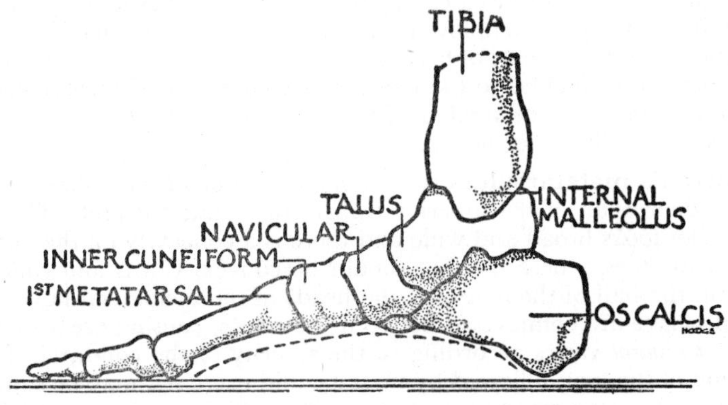

FIG. 284.—THE INTERNAL LONGITUDINAL ARCH.

illness, anaemia, and debility or owing to continued overstrain with fatigue, or as the result of slovenly habits in walking and standing. *The strain of the weight of the body then falls on the ligaments* binding the bones together and, as these are not sufficiently elastic to bear the extra strain for long, they stretch, and in time *the bony arch becomes depressed*; and when the condition has persisted for some time the foot becomes stiff and rigid.

The symptoms of flatfoot. The condition may be acute, subacute or chronic and the symptoms will vary with the condition present. *Acute flatfoot* is painful; the usual sites of pain are the dorsum, the inner side of the foot and the calf of the leg. The foot may be swollen, tender and hot. In some cases the pain is so severe that it involves the whole foot and the patient develops an awkward gait because he tries to walk on the outer aspect of his foot in order to get relief. Walking in this strained position causes the legs and back to ache.

Treatment. Rest is necessary whilst the foot is swollen and very painful. *Massage* and *exercises* are then ordered, to restore the tone to the muscles and enable them to raise and maintain the structure of the bony arch. *Manipulation*—when the foot is rigid it is manipulated in order to make all the joints supple and pliant, and this may be done under a general anaesthetic or without one, according to the amount of rigidity present and the wish of the patient.

Some surgeons advocate slight elevation of the inner side of the sole of the boot in order to assist inversion of the foot whilst the function of the muscles is being restored; others consider it better not to have any support.

Very rigid and spasmodic flatfoot is treated by forcible wrenching of the foot into inversion, and fixation in plaster of paris for several weeks in order to overcome the spasticity by prolonged stretching and rest. The foot is then treated by massage, and flatfoot exercises are employed to train the patient in the correct use of the foot.

Clawfoot or **pes cavus** is a hollow foot. There is exaggeration of the normal arch. The tendon of Achilles is usually contracted in clawfoot. This condition may be congenital or it may be acquired as the result of injury or because of slight paralysis of the dorsi-flexors of the ankle.

The *treatment* depends on the severity of the contracture of the structures in the sole of the foot. In slight cases manipulation is carried out to stretch these, though more severe cases may require operation. After manipulation of the foot, massage is employed and exercises given to teach the patient control of the movements of his foot.

The extensor tendons to the toes become contracted in severe cases of clawfoot, especially the tendon of the great toe. Tenotomy of the tight tendons is usually performed at the time the foot is manipulated.

Morton's metatarsalgia is a painful condition of the front of the foot due to depression of the anterior transverse metatarsal arch. The front of the foot looks broad and wide and there is a concavity on the dorsum, behind the toes, where the foot should be convex. Corns and callosities form on the ball of the foot over the heads of the metatarsal bones. The digital nerves are compressed between the bones, causing great pain.

The *treatment* varies according to the severity of the condition. Manipulation of the foot, followed by massage and exercises, may be sufficient to cure it. In some cases a metatarsal pad is worn in the shoe; it forms a little convexity and is placed behind the metatarsal heads and the patient is encouraged to employ gripping or clawing movements of his foot over this pad.

Very severe cases are treated by operation; the heads of some of the metatarsal bones are removed, but although this may relieve the pain it often results in an ungainly awkward gait, and it is a measure which the surgeon considers only as a last effort.

Hallux valgus is a deviation of the great toe, outward, either over or under the other toes, and this causes a bunion to form—an adventitious bursa under the skin over the joint which becomes inflamed and painful.

Unfortunately hallux valgus is a very common deformity of the foot; it may affect one or both feet and is due to the wearing of unsuitable shoes early in life. It is the duty of all persons who have charge of children and young people to see that their shoes are always long enough. A short shoe is one of the commonest causes of bunion.

The *treatment* is to manipulate the toe and if possible to teach the patient control of it in movements of abduction; this is rarely successful because the muscles which perform abduction are wasted and the amount of patience needed for success does not seem to be forthcoming. Operative treatment is to excise the base of the proximal phalanx of the great toe and any excresences on the head of the first metatarsal. After this operation the patient is kept in bed for a fortnight; then the stitches are removed and he is taught to walk, and to bear weight on the great toe; this is very important, otherwise he will develop an awkward ambling shuffling gait which will result in strain on the knee and hip.

Hallux rigidus is a condition allied to hallux valgus. The great toe is rigid in the attitude of plantar-flexion and cannot be dorsi-flexed, so that it is in the way in walking and subject to constant injury. It is a condition in which arthritis of the joint commonly occurs which is probably rheumatic in origin.

Hammer toe is often associated with hallux valgus; it may also be met in cases of flatfoot and clawfoot and it may be congenital. The proximal interphalangeal joint is dorsi-flexed and the distal one plantar-flexed. It may be treated by manipulation and tenotomy of the contracted tendons; in severe cases operative treatment is necessary.

DEFORMITIES OF THE VERTEBRAL COLUMN

Deformity of the vertebral column is usually postural in origin. Kyphosis may arise as the result of Pott's disease (see fig. 297, p. 796). Infantile paralysis by affecting the tone of the muscles of the trunk may give rise to any of the known deformities of the spine.

Scoliosis is a lateral curvature of the vertebral column. It may occur to either side and may involve the whole of the column or only part of it. A curve to one side, right or left, in one region of the column may be compensated by another curve, to left or right, in a region either above or below it. Figure 299, p. 797, shows a right dorsal left lumbar scoliosis.

Treatment is by means of massage and exercises; the manipulations which are used aim at stretching the muscles over the concavities, and stimulating those over the convexities to contract and shorten. The exercises employed are directed at obtaining expansion of the chest on the concave side by means of breathing exercises and by teaching side bending to the convex side in order to tone up and shorten the stretched muscles. In advanced cases, such as that shown in the illustration, correction of the bony deformity is attempted by stretching and manipulation of the vertebral column and thorax and a plaster of paris jacket is applied.

Kyphosis is a round back—a deformity in which the vertebral spines are directed convexly backwards. It may be localized, as occurs in Pott's disease when the bodies of the diseased vertebrae collapse and the spines form an acute angular curve, convex backwards.

Occasionally, a total backward curve is seen, due to osteochondritis, the patient being doubled up and unable to straighten himself. A less severe kyphosis is shown in fig. 302, p. 798. This one was due to bad habits of standing owing to debility—at first the normal physiological curve of the dorsal region became exaggerated, the condition then got worse and the back became rigid. This case was stretched on an Abbott's frame and treated in plaster of paris jackets, and given massage and exercises later.

Lordosis is a hollow back. Some degree of lordosis is seen in fig. 303, p. 798. This is compensatory to the kyphosis present in the case shown. Lordosis is due to the adoption of bad standing positions which may be due to weakness of the abdominal and gluteal muscles, or may occur as the result of some other deformity, as in the case shown.

It may be treated by exercises or by the application of plaster of paris, combined with exercises.

PROLAPSED INTERVERTEBRAL DISC

During recent years symptoms of persistent pain in the back, the inguinal region, and the region of the sciatic nerve have proved, in some instances, to be due to displacement backwards, into the spinal canal of the vertebral column, of an intervertebral disc.

The condition is determined by X-ray examination. The *treatment* may be either conservative or surgical. *Conservative treatment* consists of rest in bed on a firm mattress followed by graduated exercise, or rest in a plaster of paris spinal jacket which is put on with the trunk extended. The condition in about eighty per cent of patients responds to this method of treatment. Very few need surgical treatment. The *operation of hemi-laminectomy* is performed and the portion of the protruded disc, which is causing the pressure which results in pain, is removed.

DEFORMITIES DUE TO RICKETS

Rickets is a deficiency disease of which the early manifestations are described on p. 433. The deformities which arise in rickets are due, in some cases, to the bearing of weight on bones which are soft, and in other instances to enlargement of the epiphyses of the long bones. Examples of the latter are seen in the enlargement of the wrists and ankles, where two long bones lie together, and in the protuberances at the anterior ends of the ribs, described as the rickety rosary.

Deformities of the head. The head may be square, the eminences of the frontal bones being seen as enlarged bosses on the forehead, and it should be remembered that the fontanelles are late in closing in rickets.

Deformities of the trunk. The *chest* has a constricted appearance from side to side. The *enlargement of the anterior ends of the ribs* has been mentioned. The *sternum* may be projected forwards producing a 'pigeon breast'. The *lower ribs* are everted over the abdomen, which is usually large and distended. A *groove in the axillary line* is described as *Harrison's sulcus*.

The *spine* may appear flat; or it may present a long round back; or some degree of kypho-lordosis may be present. Scoliosis may arise in rickets and the pelvis may be deformed. In some cases the pelvis is flattened from before backwards, in other cases it is tri-radiate in shape. Either of these deformities may in female subjects result in difficulties in midwifery later.

Deformities of the limbs are commonest. *Bowlegs* may affect the tibia only or the whole of the lower limb may be bowed (as shown in fig. 305, p. 799). This is treated by manipulation in slight cases when the bones are still soft; but when the bones have hardened osteoclasis is performed, which consists of breaking the tibia over a wedge of wood. The limb is then put up in plaster of paris long enough for the break to heal—from 5 to 6 weeks—and the child then walks on the straightened legs.

Knock-knee or *genu valgum* is a deformity in which the knees are directed inwards towards one another (as shown in fig. 304, p. 799). In slight cases a knock-knee brace may be worn to correct the deformity and help the child to walk with his legs straight. Massage and exercises will help by teaching control of the movements of the knee. In severe cases osteotomy of the femur, just above the knee joint, is performed; the limb is put in plaster of paris for about 6 weeks, massage and exercises are then employed and the child walks.

Knock-knee may also arise as the result of abnormal overgrowth of the lower end of the femur at adolescence—the treatment of this being the same as when due to rickets.

Coxa vara is a varus deformity at the hip joint. In a varus deformity the part is always directed towards the middle line, in a valgus deformity it is directed away from this point.

In coxa vara the lower limbs are adducted towards the middle line; the pelvis looks wide and there is lordosis; the child walks with an awkward waddling gait.

The treatment is traction by means of extension if the bones are still soft; but if hardened the deformity is corrected by osteotomy of the femur, which is performed either across or just below the great trochanter of the femur, and followed by fixation in plaster of paris with the limb well abducted until the parts have healed.

Coxa vara may also be due to injury to the epiphyses at the upper extremity of the femur or to deformity resulting from fracture of the femur.

Deformities of the arm can occur in rickets though, as weight is not usually borne on the arms, these are rare. The bones of the forearm may be bowed if the child crawls.

DEFORMITIES DUE TO DISEASE OF THE CENTRAL NERVOUS SYSTEM (see also chapter 26).

Infantile paralysis is the cause of a large percentage of crippling deformity in this country. The condition is difficult to control, because, as well as loss of power of muscles over joint movement, there is lack of development of the affected limbs and consequent loss of balance. Therefore paralysis of the muscles of a lower limb may result in deformities of hip, knee and foot, and may affect the trunk as well, causing scoliosis.

In infantile paralysis the muscles are not primarily affected, as it is a disease of the central nervous system; the motor nerve cells in the anterior horns of the spinal cord are affected, many of them are destroyed and, as the result of this, communication between the voluntary muscles and the nervous system is lost; the muscles cannot contract, they are flail, and the deformities which arise are numerous.

The *symptoms* present during the acute stage of this disease are described on p. 411. As a rule the description of the symptoms of infantile paralysis is divided into a stage of onset, a stage during which the amount of paralysis which will accrue is seen, and a further stage when, as the result of this, deformities may arise. It is with the last stage that orthopaedic treatment deals.

The affected parts are examined from time to time in order to determine the damage which is present; some muscles or muscle fibres may be entirely devoid of nerve supply, while others will be only partially deprived. For a further period splinting is employed, in order to keep the affected muscles at rest; it is now advisable to adopt a position of greatest rest for the flail muscles rather than a neutral position. If for example the dorsi-flexors of the foot are flail, the foot may be splinted in slight dorsi-flexion so that these muscles are as relaxed as possible.

At the end of a given time the position is reviewed, some muscles may be found completely flail while others will have wholly or partially recovered.

To compensate for the muscles which are not acting, some mechanical device may have to be worn permanently; or an operation may be undertaken either to transplant healthy muscles to take the place of those not acting or arthrodesis of one or more joints may be performed so as to limit the movement possible at a joint and so stabilize the joint and improve its general usefulness.

One of the objects of early treatment is to prevent deformity. In the upper limb contractures and deformity occur at the shoulder, elbow, wrist and fingers; in the lower limb the hip, knee, ankle, foot and toes may be similarly affected. Other deformities which result from neglect in the treatment of infantile paralysis include wryneck, scoliosis, kyphosis and lordosis.

Spastic paraplegia is a disease which affects the control of the nervous impulses passing to the muscles; it is a condition which in its effects is exactly contrary to that caused by infantile paralysis. In spastic paralysis there is a functional increase of the nerve supply to the muscles, and the affected parts are rigid and spastic and the tendon reflexes exaggerated.

This condition may be seen in both children and adults—in children, when it appears early in life, due either to some congenital abnormality or to injury at birth, it is described as *Little's disease*. The condition may not be noticed until the infant begins to walk, when he will be found to make spastic erratic movements, appear very frightened, and clutch at his mother's skirts and at the furniture near him.

When the spasticity affects the lower half of the body—both lower limbs—it is called *paraplegia*; when one side only is affected, *hemiplegia* (see also p. 409); when only one limb is affected, *monoplegia*; and when limbs on both sides are affected—for example one arm and both legs—it is described as *diplegia*.

In the care of cases of spastic paralysis certain points have to be considered. The child is very likely to manifest some degree of mental deficiency; he may be irritable and ill-tempered, or else very placid, not moved by anything. In spastic paraplegia the typical scissor gait will be seen; the child will attempt to walk on his toes, with his knees flexed and his thighs so tightly adducted that one leg is thrown across the other in the movements of walking. When an arm is affected it will be held tightly to the side of the body, with the elbow and wrist flexed and the forearm pronated.

On examination the adductor muscles of the hip joint, the flexors of the thighs, and very often also the tendon of Achilles, will all be found tightly contracted.

The *surgical treatment most commonly* undertaken to correct the spasticity is division of some of the nerves passing to the muscles—*Stoeffel's operation.* Other measures include stretching the contracted muscles by splinting and division of the tightened tendons and strands of muscle fibres by tenotomy, or excision of them by open operation.

Stoeffel's operation is considered to be the most successful method, and the *post-operative care* is not difficult as subsequent stretching and splints are not necessary. The child should be trained to use his limbs quietly, slowly and rhythmically. He will need a lot of encouragement and should never be ridiculed or allowed to get tired.

When the patient is also mentally deficient he should be made to feel that he is wanted and should be encouraged to take part in the play of other children. Such children are often timid and easily frightened. They may have difficulty in eating and should be trained to use the ordinary feeding utensils and to eat nicely, not bolting their food; when there is incontinence of urine and faeces, attempts should be made to overcome this, by giving the child urinal and bedpan at regular and fairly frequent intervals in order to teach him proper control if possible.

Birth palsy is a term used to describe a state of paralysis produced by injury at birth. Any spastic paralysis may be due to this cause; the injury usually affects the upper motor neurones (see p. 408), so that the lesion results in spasticity. *Erb's palsy* is one type; it affects the muscles of the shoulder girdle resulting in adduction of arm and pronation of hand.

The *treatment* is on the same lines as described for spastic paralysis.

DEFORMITIES ARISING FROM CONTRACTURE OF THE SOFT STRUCTURES

In the notes on congenital deformities, and deformities due to paralysis, it has been suggested that any persistent mal-position at joints will give rise to anatomical changes which will eventually result in deformity. In the case of injuries where healing takes place by scarring and the formation of fibrous tissue, as in burns and injury to muscle, this danger must be constantly borne in mind.

The injuries arising as the result of infantile and spastic paralysis have been enumerated above. In addition two contractures which are specially designated may be mentioned:

Dupuytren's contracture occurs for the most part in middle-aged men, and more especially in those who follow such occupations as may cause constant friction on the palmar surface of the hand, as in the case of cobblers. Contracture of the fascia on the palm of the hand begins as a small fibrous band, the skin over this becomes puckered and the ring finger and sometimes the other fingers are drawn down in flexion.

The *treatment* is to excise the contracted fibrous structure by an open operation on the palm of the hand.

Volkmann's contracture occurs as the result of injury to the muscles of the anterior aspect of the forearm. The usual *history* is that in the treatment of an injury to the elbow the arm was put up in acute flexion of the elbow. This position may have interfered with the blood supply so that the muscles on the front of the elbow were deprived of nourishment; they become degenerated in consequence, fibrous tissue forms, and this contracts so that the fingers of the hand are contracted in flexion.

This condition is always preventable, but when it occurs it is usually in children, who may not complain of pain due to pressure. It is essential to watch with care for swelling of the fingers in any case of injury to the arm, forearm or elbow. If there is disappearance of the pulse at the wrist this indicates serious obstruction to the flow of blood into the fingers. In such a case the need for relief of pressure is urgent, and a nurse should get a doctor at once; if he cannot come, she should cut the bandages or the plaster of paris over the bend of the elbow, and keep the patient waiting and resting so that the position of the elbow is not interfered with until the surgeon can come, readjust the position of the arm and make a fresh application of plaster of paris.

Chapter 52

Surgical Tuberculosis

(See also Chapter 35)

Infection by the tubercle bacillus—Changes in the tissues—A tuberculous abscess—Tuberculosis of glands—Tuberculosis of bones and joints—Tuberculosis of the genito-urinary system

Tuberculosis is an infective disease caused by the tubercle bacillus which was discovered by Koch in 1882. The disease affects certain parts of the body, principally the lungs, bones, joints, meninges, lymphatic glands and the kidneys, prostate gland and testes.

The **tubercle bacillus** is a minute organism about 1/10,000 of an inch in length and can only be seen by the aid of a high-power microscope. It possesses a stout resistant capsule which makes the organism difficult to destroy by chemicals; but fortunately it is easily destroyed by exposure to heat—even quite moderate heat—and it has been found that exposure of infected articles to the sun's rays is sufficient to destroy the organism.

Infection is spread by means of discharges, secretions and excretions from the lesions of tuberculosis in infected persons. The disease is largely disseminated by means of sputum which becomes dried, and is carried by particles in the air, to be deposited on articles of food, or inhaled by persons breathing the infected air.

Another source of infection is dairy produce from infected cattle, in the forms of milk, butter and cheese; by this means bovine tuberculosis is spread, and children are frequently infected in this way. A rarer form of infection is by inoculation, which occurs when the abraded skin is infected, and may result in lupus.

Inhalation. When tubercle bacilli are inhaled the organisms may be arrested on the mucous surface of the pharynx and tonsils; from this area infection may be conveyed by means of blood and lymph to the local lymphatic glands in the neck. The organisms may enter the lungs, setting up pulmonary tuberculosis (see description of this disease on p. 504), or it may get into the lymph stream and be conveyed to the lymphatic glands in the thorax or be spread by means of the blood to distant parts of the body and infect the bones, joints or meninges.

Ingestion. When tubercle bacilli are taken in with food or fluid they may again become arrested by the tonsils; or, entering the stomach and intestine, may cause infection of the lining of the intestine (tuberculous enteritis). By means of the lymph they may reach the mesenteric glands in the abdomen, causing tabes mesenterica; and, from an infected gland the peritoneum may become infected and tuberculous peritonitis follow. Again, the organisms may enter the blood stream and be conveyed by it to cause disease in some distant part, such as in the bones, joints, lungs or meninges.

Changes in the tissues. As the result of infection by tubercle, the tissues are irritated and a certain amount of reaction occurs; this may give rise to proliferation of cells and destruction of some of the tissues. A very typical change is described in the formation of tubercles. A *tubercle* is a collection of cells which takes the form of a greyish mass large enough to be visible to the naked eye. It is composed of a little group of tubercle bacilli, surrounded by leucocytes, giant cells and epitheloid cells. This group of tubercle bacilli is antagonistic to the tissue in which it lies, and the subsequent changes which occur depend on whether the tissues are resistant and can overcome the activity of the organisms, or whether the organisms are sufficiently virulent to cause breakdown of the tissues, and spread of the disease.

Caseation. The tuberculous lesion now established usually extends farther by development of a number of tubercles and their coalescence into a large mass; the centre of this becomes dry and crumbling like crumbs of cheese—hence the term *caseation.* In this state the tubercle bacilli are still separated from the surrounding tissue and their destructive action is arrested; after this stage either healing will take place in the changes described as *fibrosis* and more rarely *calcification* (see note below); or the mass will soften and liquefy, indicating spread of the disease; the softened mass forms a *cold abscess*—a term used to describe a tuberculous abscess, which is subacute in character.

When *fibrosis* takes place a large number of fibrous tissue cells form, contraction and scarring occurs and the area invaded by disease germs is thus rendered innocuous; it ceases to function and becomes a sterile mass, functionally separated from the remainder of the organ in which it lies.

In *calcification,* lime salts become deposited in the fibrous tissue formed in the area of the tubercle and hardening takes place.

A **tuberculous abscess** is the result of the liquefaction into pus of the caseated tuberculous material. This collection of pus is not accompanied by the usual signs of inflammation—heat, redness and pain—and it is therefore called a 'cold abscess'. When mixed infection occurs and the tuberculous abscess is complicated by the presence of other pyogenic bacteria, such as staphylococci and streptococci, then the ordinary changes of inflammation occur.

A tuberculous abscess consists of a central liquefied mass, surrounded by an area which is caseated; if the disease is progressing, further liquefaction takes place in the walls around the pus and so the abscess increases in size.

Another interesting feature about a tuberculous abscess is that the direction in which it may spread is determined by the anatomical arrangement of the tissues in which it has formed, and to some extent by gravity. In the case of a *psoas abscess* for example, the tuberculous lesion is usually the dorsal vertebrae; the abscess collects in the psoas muscle because the pus tracks down along the side of the vertebral column and along the sheath of the psoas muscle until it comes to the surface just above Poupart's ligament at the groin.

As a tuberculous abscess reaches the surface fluctuation of the pus contained in it is noticed; if left untreated the abscess may open spontaneously, the cavity of the abscess will thus usually become infected by secondary organisms and a persistent sinus be left, so that healing is delayed or prevented.

The *treatment of a tuberculous abscess* depends on its size; in some cases, if left alone, and the general health of the patient is improved, it will disappear; if it increases in size and becomes superficial some surgeons advocate its evacuation, either by means of a hollow needle with which the contents can be aspirated, or by means of a small incision. The abscess cavity may be filled with bismuth and iodoform paste which is antagonistic to the action of bacteria, and so healing of the cavity may be stimulated. When the contents are thick and cannot be evacuated the cavity may be curetted, and the wound is packed and allowed to heal from the bottom.

In some cases applications of radium have been found of value in stimulating absorption of fluid and repair of the tissues in cases of glandular abscess.

TUBERCULOSIS OF GLANDS

Tuberculous disease of the lymphatic glands occurs with comparative frequency, especially in children and young people; the lymphatic glands in the neck are often affected, as they probably arrest the tubercle bacilli which get into the lymphatic stream when inhaled, or ingested with food. One gland or several glands may be infected; the glands swell and the patient may complain of a little stiffness of the neck due to interference with the action of the muscles in the neighbourhood of the enlarged gland, or the swelling may be the first indication. The ordinary changes described on p. 507 occur and, if liquefaction results, an abscess forms (see above).

The **treatment** varies according to the state of the condition when seen by physician or surgeon; at first the general care of a tuberculous person is applied; the child is allowed to be in the fresh air as much as possible, and is given a diet of high calorie value supplemented by cod-liver oil. (For details of the general care of tuberculosis see p. 512).

Swelling of the glands may be treated by radium or X-rays, and if an abscess occurs it may be aspirated or evacuated in some other way. Extensive disease of the glands may need excision of a group of them and of the adhesions which have occurred in the immediate neighbourhood.

TUBERCULOSIS OF BONES AND JOINTS

Tuberculosis of bone commences in the marrow or periosteum and is transmitted to the bone in the immediate neighbourhood, and in many instances the joint in the vicinity becomes infected. *Tuberculous periostitis* gives rise to a subacute swelling over the affected bone; *tuberculous osteomyelitis* is of very slow onset and may not be discovered until the bone is considerably affected and the inflammation has spread to the surface of it.

Tuberculous dactylitis is the occurrence of osteomyelitis in the bones of the hands and feet, the carpus, metacarpus, tarsus, metatarsus and phalanges; the fingers become spindle-shaped and swollen, abscesses arise and sinuses form.

Tuberculous disease of joints usually begins in the synovial membrane, or the marrow in the cancellous tissue of the ends of the bone. The synovial membrane is thickened, it becomes adherent to the hyaline cartilage covering the ends of the bones which enter into the formation of the joint affected; the cartilage becomes ulcerated and tuberculous infiltration of the cancellous tissue takes place, resulting in destruction which is described as *caries*. Extensive destruction of bone may so interfere with the function of the joint that a pathological dislocation occurs. A considerable amount of fluid collects in the joint causing the swelling which is often noticeable and by stretching the ligaments predisposes to a pathological dislocation.

Tuberculosis of the spine or Pott's disease begins at the front of the bodies of the vertebrae and which crumble as decay occurs giving rise to the deformity of kyphosis or angulation of the spine. The deformity present in an advanced case is shown in fig. 297, p. 796.

The *symptoms and signs* of joint tuberculosis may be classified as general and local. The patient may, however, exhibit a few constitutional symptoms.

A *typical history* often elicited is as follows—The mother might have noticed the child was slightly unwell, that he did not sleep at night or perspired during sleep, he may have exhibited some lack of appetite and lost a little weight.

As time went on, he refused to play and, if the lower limb was affected, began to walk with a slight limp; this may have been attributed to some blow or kick the child had received months or years previously. The mother might say that the child cries out in the night and, when she uncovers him, she observes that his hands are protecting the suspected joint as if to prevent pain. At this period the child may have a slight rise of temperature in the evening, the mother may notice that he is a little feverish and perspires a good deal during the night so that his bedclothes are wet in the morning.

On examining the limb, it might be found to be slightly wasted and the joint somewhat swollen. When asked to move the joint it will be noticed that the child guards it carefully and moves it slowly and deliberately, and that movement obviously causes some pain.

If the child has not been treated before this stage has been reached, he will develop a rigid joint, which in time will become fixed in a position of deformity; in the case of a knee, the joint will be flexed; the hip joint may be flexed and adducted.

Treatment. The general treatment for all cases of tuberculosis will be employed; the patient should be nursed in the open air if possible and given a liberal nourishing diet; he should be weighed regularly and will gain in weight if the treatment is successful.

The *local treatment* is rest in the first instance, and many cases recover as the result of carefully applied rest. If the joint is deformed as the result of muscular contraction, the deformity is carefully reduced, the limb immobilized on a splint aided, if necessary, by the application of extension.

In severe cases in which there is bony deformity operation may have to be undertaken to excise the diseased parts and so shorten the period of rest necessary.

In the nursing care of cases of joint tuberculosis the position of the limb obtained by the surgeon must be maintained; the nurse should see that the splint is kept in position and that any extension apparatus is in good working order and does not slip or move. She must realize that in order to maintain accurate immobilization of the joint she may have difficulty in moving the patient and all her nursing measures must be sacrificed, if necessary, to maintaining the degree of immobilization and rest the surgeon desires. She should tell him her difficulties, and he will show her how much she may move the patient without harm.

It is necessary to observe the patient carefully for improvement in his general condition, and to see whether the treatment which he is undergoing is resulting in improvement of sleep. The nurse should watch for crying or restlessness at night and be able to state whether or not this symptom is improving as it should, now that the diseased parts have been put at rest by immobilization. The fact that this symptom does not improve will show that the rest is not sufficient and the surgeon ought to to be informed of this.

TUBERCULOSIS OF THE GENITO-URINARY TRACT

Any part of the tract may be infected; in the majority of instances the kidney is the part first involved. The tubercle bacilli reach the kidney in the blood stream and usually one kidney becomes affected. The usual changes take place and the substance of the organ is destroyed, while an abscess may form giving rise to pyonephrosis.

Symptoms and signs. The first symptom complained of will be frequency of micturition. On examination the urine may contain blood, albumin or pus, and careful investigation should be made for the presence of tubercle bacilli. The urine should be measuresd as polyuria is sometimes present.

The patient may have a dull aching pain in the loin of the affected side, which is not relieved by rest. As time goes on there will be a rise of temperature in the evening, the patient will sweat at night, complain of loss of appetite and will lose weight. By this time he will present the characteristic appearance of one suffering from toxaemia due to tuberculosis.

The bladder will eventually become infected, cystitis will be present and the discomfort of the patient is greatly increased.

The **treatment of a tuberculous kidney** is to remove it, but the functioning of the other kidney must first be investigated, for fear lest it also is diseased. The existence of pulmonary tuberculosis or other lesions adds much to the gravity of the prognosis. (For the preparation and post-operative nursing of nephrectomy, see p. 729.)

Chapter 53

Rheumatic Affections of Joint and Muscle

Symptoms of arthritis—Treatment of rheumatoid arthritis—Gold therapy—Treatment of osteoarthritis—Muscular rheumatism (Acute rheumatism is described in chapter 34)

Arthritis deformans, rheumatoid arthritis, toxic arthritis, osteoarthritis and hypertrophic arthritis are a few of the titles used to describe one form of chronic joint affection or another. Arthritis is a disease which may occur at any age; in children it is known as Still's disease. In adults it may occur in either sex and unfortunately it attacks quite young persons, in young women the form known as *rheumatoid arthritis* which commences in the small joints of the hands and wrist is most prevalent; whilst men more often than women suffer from the type known as *osteo-arthritis* which may affect the joints of the fingers or commence in one of the large joints as in the shoulder, hip or knee. Rheumatic arthritis is a serious crippling disease which is responsible for a large percentage of the total disablement of workers in this country.

Of the *cause* little is known but many theories are put forward for consideration. Some consider the condition is due to infection either by *B. coli* or by one of the non-haemolytic strains of streptococcus. The infected focus may exist in the teeth, tonsils, cranial sinuses, gallbladder, appendix, colon or in the genito-urinary tract. In some a septic focus is found, in others if present it fails to be detected. A few suggest that the disease is due to an endocrine deficiency resulting in faulty metabolism, and adherents of this school of thought go so far as to describe the condition as 'non-infective'. Others again consider that rheumatic arthritis depends on some inherent familial tendency and that given suitable circumstances the disease will develop. *Predisposing factors* may include anything which lowers the resistance of the body, such as anxiety and worry, mental strain, sustained fatigue, and exposure to damp and cold.

Onset and Symptoms. In the majority of cases the onset is insidious but cases are known in which the disease began suddenly. The distribution is symmetrical. In *rheumatoid arthritis* the proximal interphalangeal joints of the fingers and the metacarpo-phalangeal joints are first affected, the knees, ankles, elbows, shoulders and hips becoming affected later; in some the spine is involved, in other cases it escapes.

The affected joints appear swollen and the fingers become fusiform in shape; the knuckles are prominent and enlarged and the wrist subluxated. There is a tendency for the fingers to deviate to the ulnar side as shown in fig. 288, p. 794. During the earliest phase of the disease there is often considerable tenderness, and movement causes severe pain; the skin over the joints is tense and glazed and the circulation is poor. Wasting of muscle is a feature of arthritis because movement is limited, the joints stiffen and are difficult and painful to move, and movement is accompanied by creaking and cracking. The grip of the hand gets weak. As the disease progresses fibrous adhesions form which cause further limitation

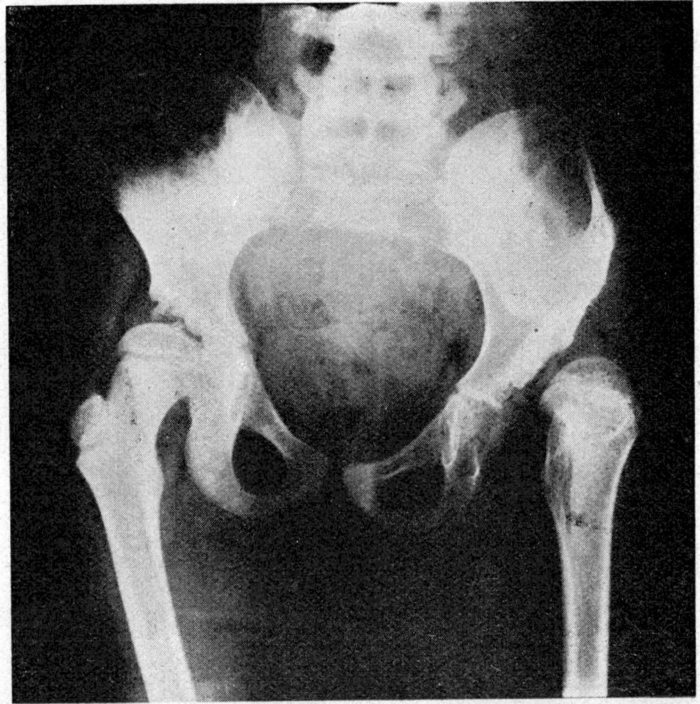

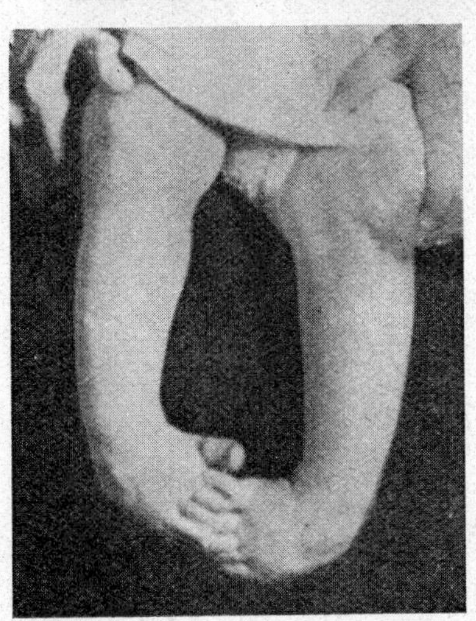

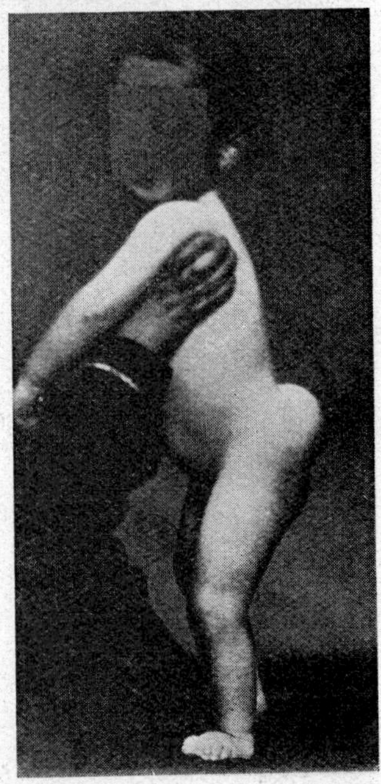

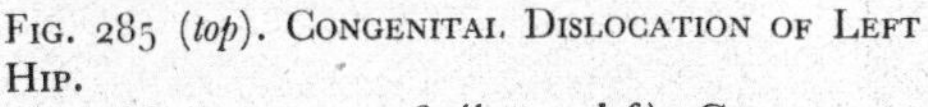

Fig. 285 (*top*). Congenital Dislocation of Left Hip.

Fig. 286.—*see page* 776 (*bottom left*). Congenital Clubfoot.

Fig. 287 (*bottom right*). Spina Bifida due to Congenital Malformation of the Spinal Column.

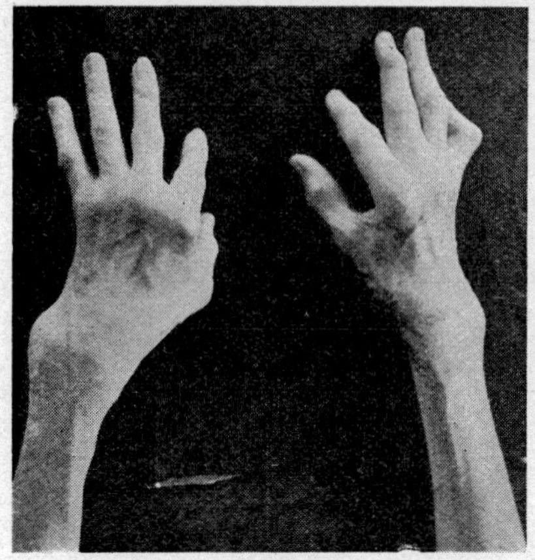

FIG. 288.

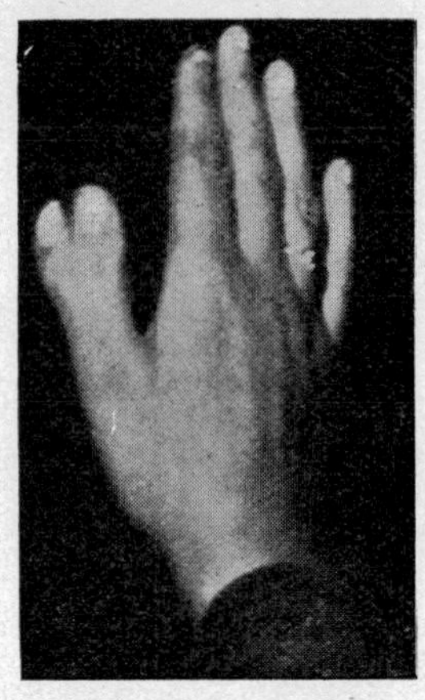

FIG. 290.

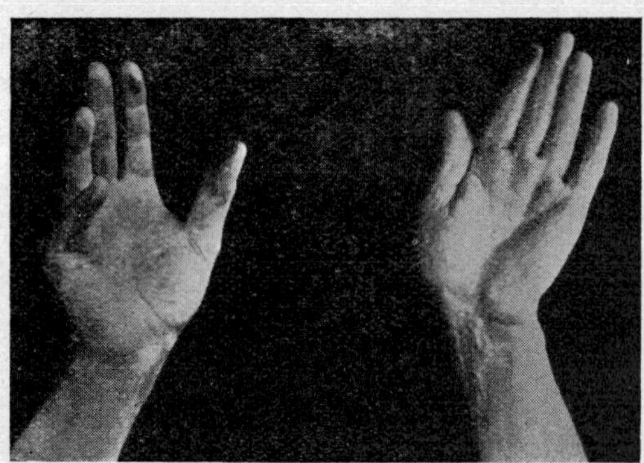

FIG. 289.

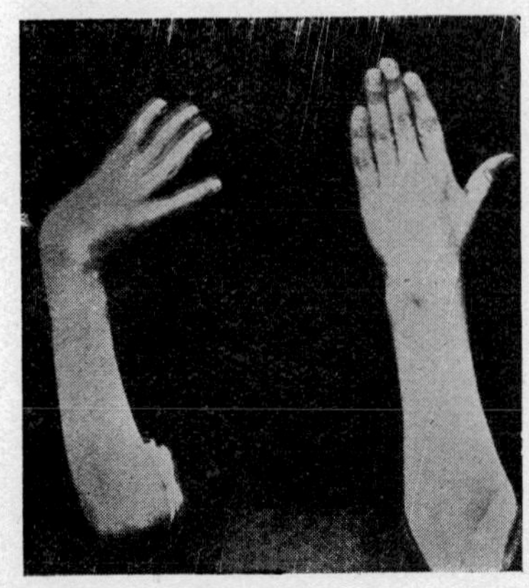

FIG. 291.

FIG. 288 (*see also Fig.* 300). DEFORMITY DUE TO RHEUMATOID ARTHRITIS.

FIG. 289. DUPYTREN'S CONTRACTIONS BEFORE AND AFTER TREATMENT.

FIG. 290. EXTRA DIGIT (CONGENITAL MALFORMATION OF THUMB).

FIG. 291. ULNAR DEVIATION OF HAND BEFORE AND AFTER TREATMENT.

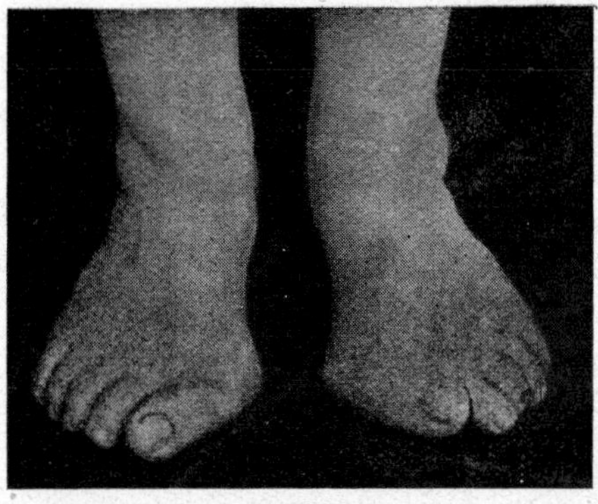

FIG. 292.—*see page* 780. HALLUX VALGUS.

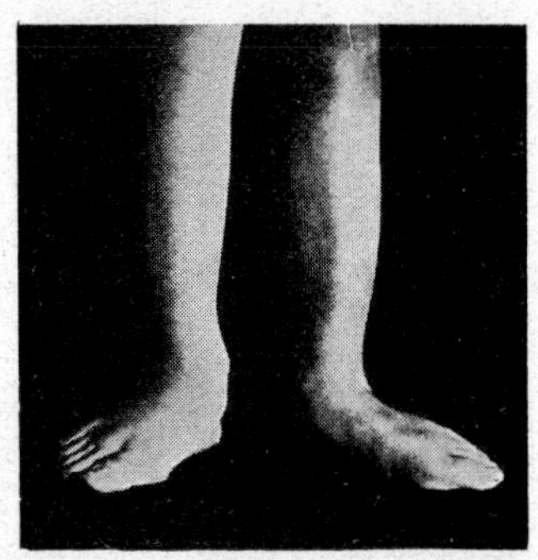

FIG. 293.—*see page* 779. FLATFOOT.

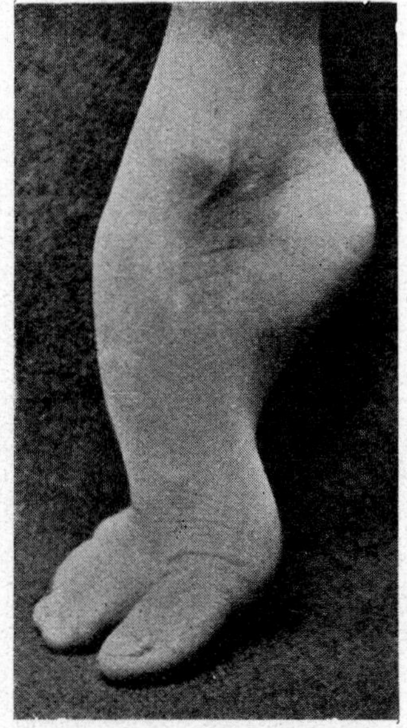

FIG. 294.—*see page* 776. TALIPES EQUINUS.

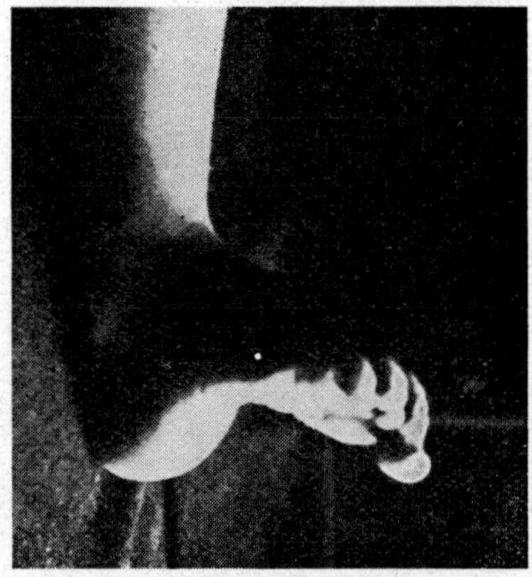

FIG. 295.—*see page* 780. PES CAVUS OR HOLLOW FOOT.

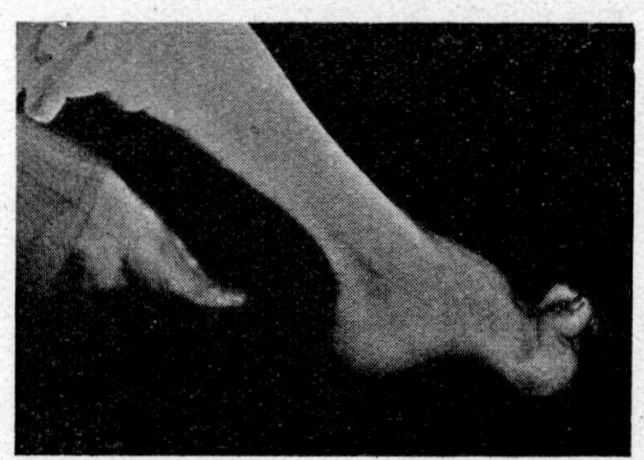

FIG. 296.—*see page* 780. CLAWFOOT.

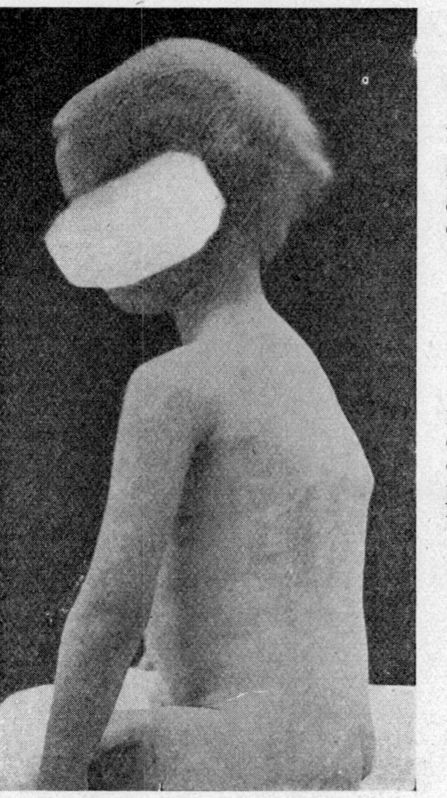

DEFORMITIES OF THE SPINE

FIG. 297 (*left*).—*see page* 790.

POTT'S DISEASE OF THE SPINE.

Kyphosis which occurs as the result of disease of the spine in the case of Pott's disease or spinal caries due to tuberculosis.

FIG. 298 (*right*).—*see page* 760.

POTT'S DISEASE OF THE SPINE.

Radiogram of spine showing collapse of two of the bodies of the vertebrae as the result of tuberculous disease of bone. This collapse produces the type of deformity seen in Fig. 297.

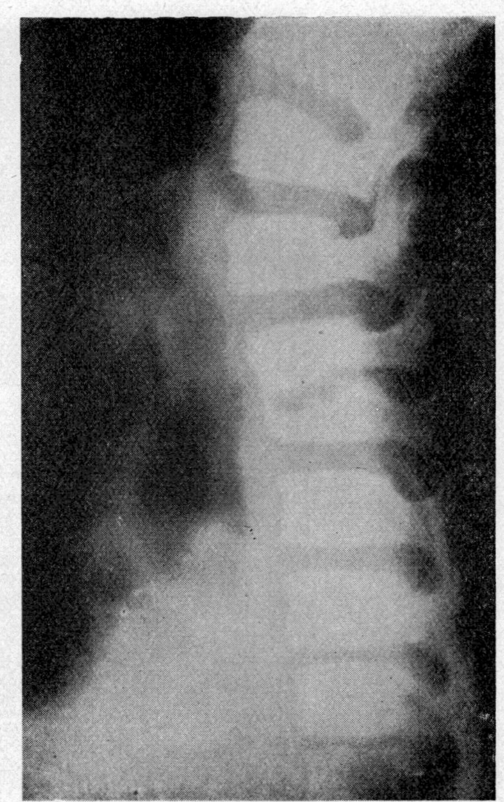

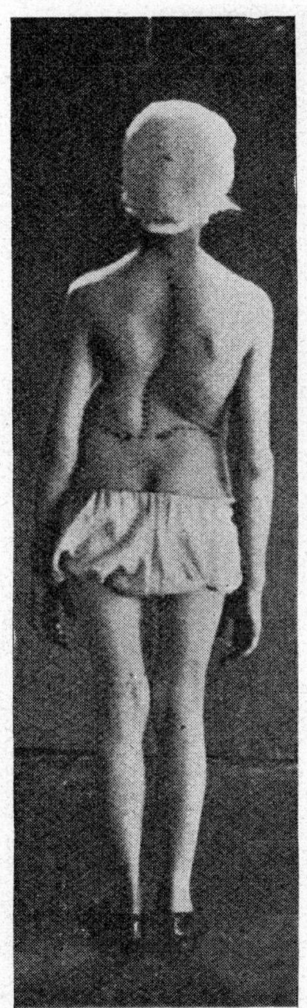

FIG. 299.—*see page* 781. SCOLIOSIS.
Lateral curvature of the spine. Fig. 293 shows right dorsal and left lumbar curves. The curve is named after the *convex* side. The opposite or *concave* side of the curve shows depression of the structures of the trunk.

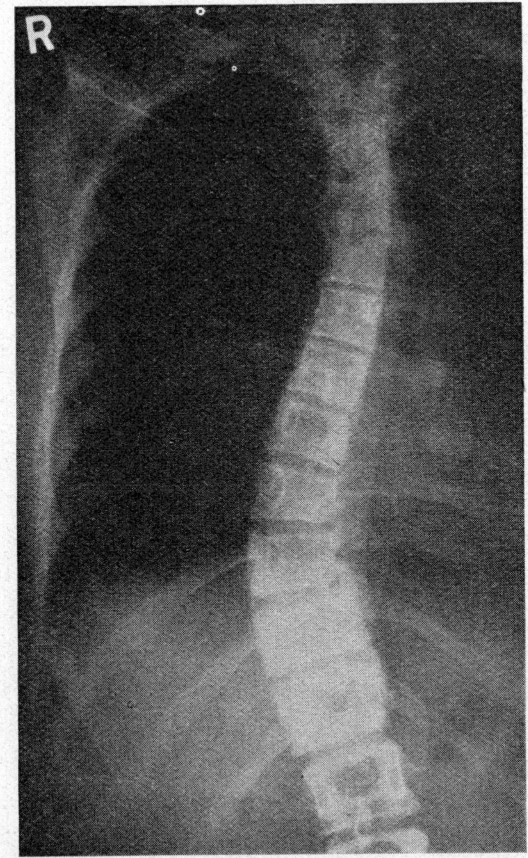

FIG. 300.—*see page* 781.
SCOLIOSIS.
Radiogram of spine showing the changes in position of the vertebrae which occur to produce deformity similar to that seen in Fig. 299.

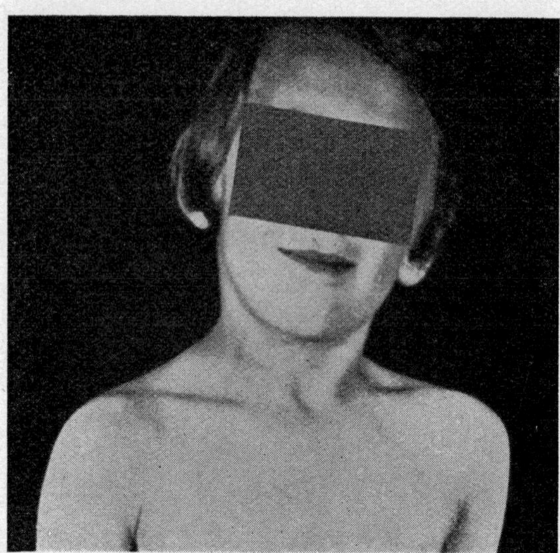

FIG. 301.—*see page* 778. TORTICOLLIS.

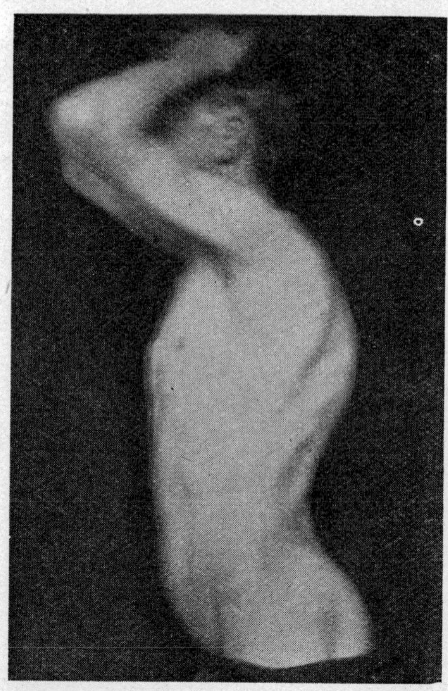

FIG. 302.—*see page* 781.
ROUND BACK OR KYPHOSIS.

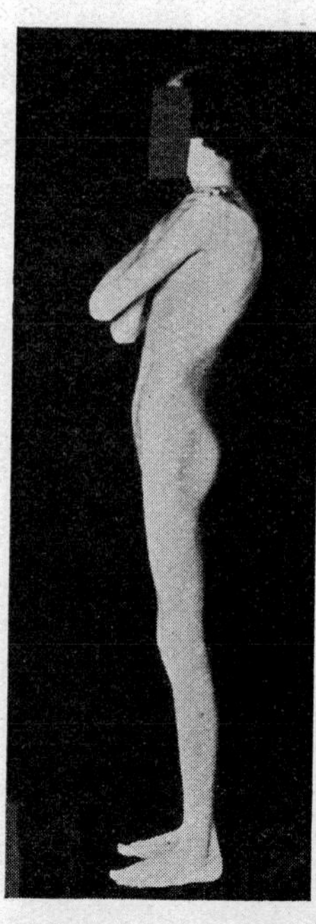

FIG. 303.—*see page* 781.
HOLLOW BACK OR LORDOSIS.

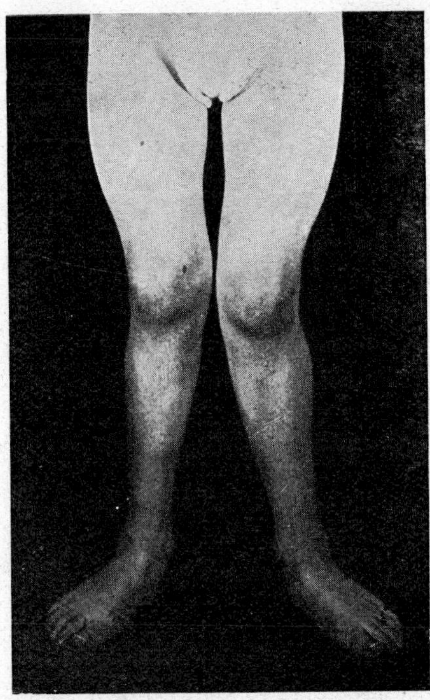

FIG. 304.
KNOCK KNEE IN AN ADOLESCENT DUE TO NEGLECTED RICKETS.

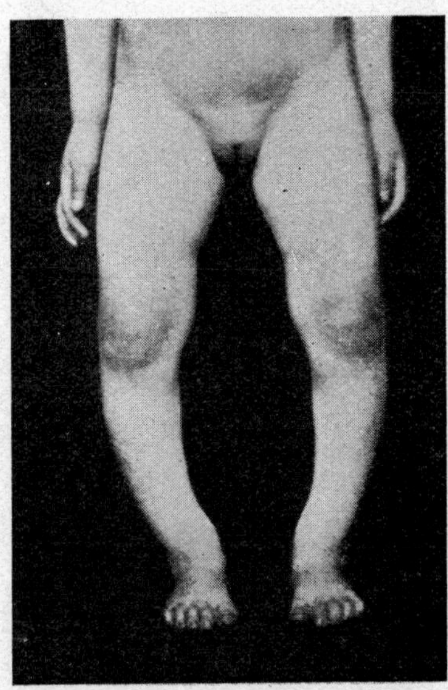

FIG. 305.
BOWLEGS IN A CHILD DUE TO NEGLECTED RICKETS.

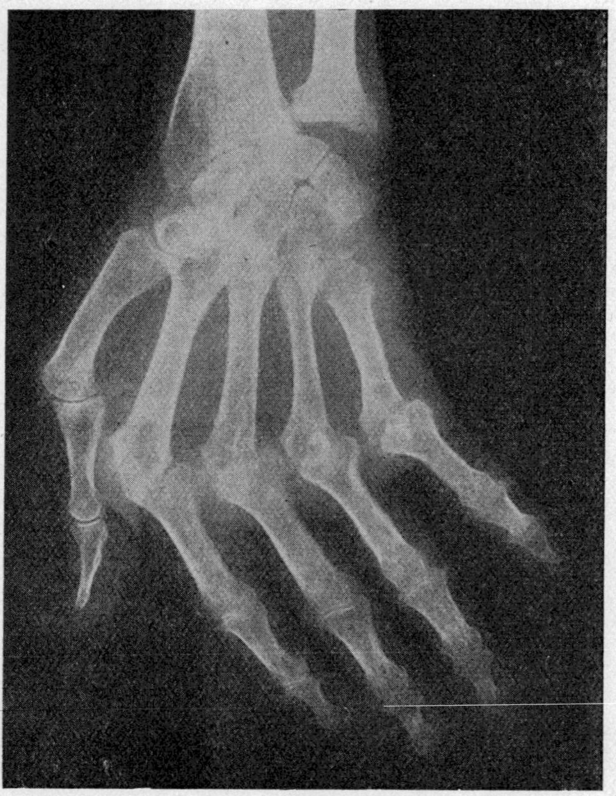

FIG. 306 (*left*). DEFORMITY OF THE BONES OF THE HAND DUE TO RHEUMATOID ARTHRITIS (*see also Fig.* 286).

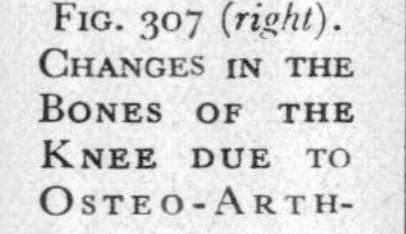

FIG. 307 (*right*). CHANGES IN THE BONES OF THE KNEE DUE TO OSTEO-ARTHRITIS.

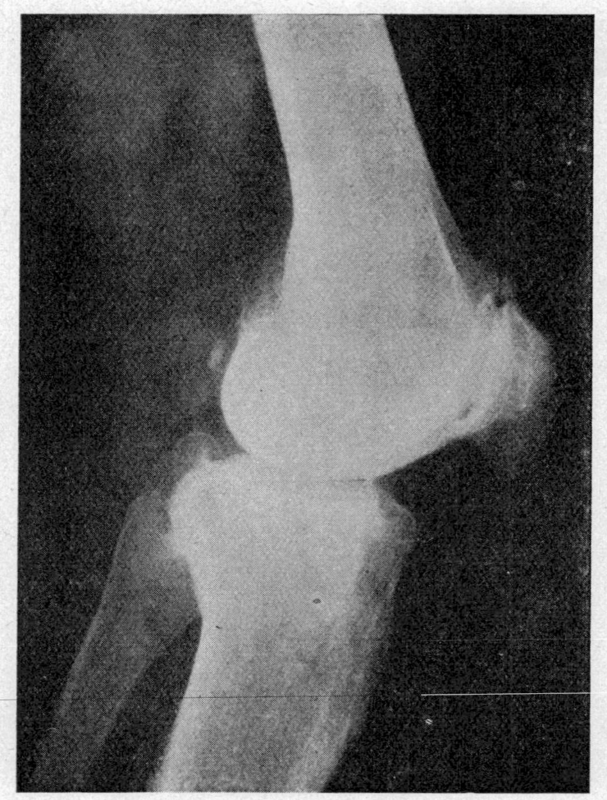

of movement, and in some severe and long-standing cases bony changes may result in ankylosis.

The disease seems to progress to a point, more or less advanced, where it becomes arrested, and one of the aims of treatment is to arrest the progress of the disease at the earliest possible moment, in order to preserve the function of the joints and prevent deformity.

Some *general symptoms* are present in most instances; there may be a rise in temperature, and anaemia, the patient often looks ill and loses weight, sweating of the skin is noticeable particularly of the palms of the hands. Pain and stiffness cause sleep to be interrupted and the patient gets very tired and exhausted.

TREATMENT OF RHEUMATOID ARTHRITIS

The *aims of treatment* are to effect arrest of the disease at the earliest possible moment, to relieve pain and to prevent deformity. As regards *general treatment*, rest in bed is advised, a nourishing diet is provided, any impairment of digestion should be investigated, the bowels should be kept acting regularly and anaemia and any endocrine deficiency noted and treated.

Sleep is essential and as the patient is often kept awake by pain and discomfort, immobilization of the affected joints at night may help, and the administration of some form of salicylate may relieve pain in joint and muscle. Sedatives are rarely ordered as there is a danger that the patient may learn to depend on them and develop the habit of taking sedatives.

Many drugs have been tried, some are palliative and others of little value; sera and vaccines have proved useful in some cases and protein-shock therapy has been successful in the later stages of the disease in others. The injection of gold salts has been found beneficial in selected cases.

Local treatment. During the acute phase of the disease when pain and tenderness are marked, immobilization of the affected joints is necessary. Very light *splints* only are advisable and these should be removable; bi-valved light plaster of paris splints are best. A splint which is removable enables the joint to be moved as soon as the acute phase is beginning to abate and at the same time it provides the immobilization necessary in the intervals between treatment.

Heat in some form or another is probably the most valuable local treatment. It may either be employed with the intention of producing a good skin reaction, as when vapour baths, brine baths, foam baths, anti-phlogistine, mud packs, paraffin wax, and radiant heat are used (paraffin wax bath is a valuable and comfortable form of treatment), or heat may be applied to penetrate the tissues, as when an electric current is employed by means of diathermy, inducto-thermy and short-wave currents.

Applications of heat are valuable in increasing the blood supply to the part treated and help to relieve pain; maintain the tone of the tissues; prevent wasting of muscle; and render the joints more supple and so facilitate movement. Heat may be used independently of any other form of treatment, or it may be employed before some form of manipulation such as massage and passive movement, and also before active exercise, as movement is easier and can be more comfortably performed when the blood supply to the part has been improved by inducing hyperaemia which is one of the effects of heat.

Massage and passive movement may be employed after the acute phase, gentle movements are given first, progressing as pain is relieved. The work must be very carefully graduated so that any reaction which would result in return of the acute symptoms is avoided.

Active movement is essential as soon as the acute pain is relieved in order to prevent rigidity and muscle wasting, and to maintain the function of the affected joints which so quickly get stiff if they are not moved. Active movement is more valuable than massage and passive movement and the patient should be encouraged to move his joints many times during the day in between the visits of the masseuse. He may be given small interesting recreations which necessitate fine movements of the fingers and hand, such as knitting, basket weaving, playing patience with small cards and so on.

Sometimes the visiting masseuse uses the faradic current as an adjunct to her work to stimulate the contraction of muscles, and the patient should take an interest in the contraction of individual muscles and innervate these as the current is applied, and then, at intervals during the day, voluntarily contract these, as by so doing he will improve the tone and power of the muscle.

Prevention of deformity is important, the means employed by splinting, the stretching of tendons which may be getting tight, and constantly performing movements of the affected joints have been indicated.

Forcible manipulation may be necessary in some cases. In those, for example, where fibrous contraction had occurred before the patient presented himself for treatment; and in cases where limitation of further increase in the restoration of function is reached. Some physicians recommend the very gradual breaking down of adhesions, others progress more rapidly. In either case it is essential that any manipulation performed is followed by massage and passive and active movement, otherwise adhesions will quickly form again and no good will result from the manipulation. The physician should be informed of any reaction which follows forcible manipulation, as he will wish to avoid producing an inflammatory state which could only result in the formation of adhesions.

GOLD THERAPY

Abour 25 years ago gold was first used in the treatment of pulmonary tuberculosis; it has since been employed in some forms of skin eruption and more recently in the treatment of *rheumatoid arthritis*. A number of gold preparations are obtainable, and most of them are administered by intra-muscular injection; gold is a heavy metal and tends to accumulate in the system, but in order to avoid this intervals are arranged between courses of treatment to allow time for the proper excretion of the gold salts. Gold is a dangerous treatment and the physician will explain the risks to the patient. Gold is contraindicated when there is disease of the heart, liver, or kidneys.

As a *preliminary to treatment* the general condition of the patient's health is examined, the function of the kidneys investigated, and a blood count made and the sedimentation rate of the red blood cells noted. Gold may be given either in large or in small doses; when the latter method, which is more usual, is adopted, a preparation such as *allochrysine* or Solganal B may be employed—this substance is usually given in doses of from 0·01 to 0·05 of a gramme, at intervals of from 5 to 7 days until the patient has had a gramme or a gramme and a half. An interval follows of from 8 to 12 weeks and if the patient is considered a suitable subject for gold, a further course or even two courses of treatment may follow.

Nursing observations are important, gold is a dangerous drug, and any nurse who did not know what untoward symptoms to watch for and the necessity of reporting these to the physician without delay, would be guilty of culpable neglect. *As soon as any untoward symptoms are observed gold must be withheld* until the physician has seen the patient and made his decision, and in the meantime the patient should be given copious fluids containing glucose.

Exfoliative dermatitis is the biggest danger and the most serious complication which may arise; when fully developed the skin will be inflamed and weeping and the patient in great pain, and in order to avoid this danger careful watch should be kept on the skin for any complaint of irritation, the slightest sign of redness and any tenderness, as either of these symptoms may indicate the onset of dermatitis. *Albuminuria* may be the first indication of failure of the kidneys; the urine should be tested daily in the case of a patient in hospital. Alteration in the character of the blood may arise and this might be indicated by purpuric spots or by rapid increasing anaemia. *Impairment of digestion*, characterized by loss of appetite, soreness of the mouth, a dirty tongue and diarrhoea should be carefully noted; the general condition of health should improve under treatment and *increased malaise*, feelings of fatigue, soreness of the throat, a rise of temperature and restlessness are all symptoms which should be noted at once.

The *good effects likely to arise* from injections of gold salts are relief of pain and improvement in the function of the affected joints; combined with improvement in the general health of the patient, which increases as the patient himself notes the improvement and becomes happy and optimistic about the future.

But a note of warning is again necessary. It is this: many patients suffering from rheumatoid arthritis have tried a number of cures which have been disappointing; perhaps the patient had heard of gold and has hoped it would be ordered for him, and anxious to persist with a treatment which he may have come to look upon as a last resort, he will desire to persist with it in spite of not feeling well, and he will try and hide his symptoms from the physician and nurse. When patients are attending an out-patient clinic for gold injections it is essential not only to question them about their general health on the lines already indicated, but also to scrutinize their appearance very carefully—the tongue, gums, mouth and throat should be examined, the temperature and pulse taken, the patient weighed, the urine tested and the skin inspected.

At the first appearance of symptoms the treatment should be stopped. Glucose, liver, calcium and vitamins B and C are given to improve the condition of the blood, and sometimes a physician will order these to be given to less robust patients before a course of treatment is commenced in order to lessen the probability of untoward symptoms developing.

A high calorie diet should be given which should be well balanced but the patient should not be allowed to put on excessive weight.

TREATMENT OF OSTEOARTHRITIS

Osteoarthritis, although it may affect the small joints of the fingers, is very often associated with the large joints such as hips, knees and shoulders. Patients with a tendency to osteoarthritis are inclined to obesity because the activity of their movements is limited. Very little can be done as regards treatment and this in the main is only palliative and corrective. The following points should be considered.

The affected joints should be rested. Local heat in the form of radiant heat, diathermy and paraffin wax baths increase hyperaemia. Massage and radiant heat are employed to relieve pain and increase movement. The joints should be put through the full range of movement of which they are capable but no strain should be imposed. Discomfort resulting from treatment should be of short duration; lasting discomfort means that the treatment has been too strenuous.

If the patient is overweight a weight-reducing diet should be given. Vitamins B and C are given as in rheumatoid arthritis. In some cases thyroideum gr. ½ to 1 two or three times a day is ordered. A Thomas's walking caliper may be ordered to take the weight off the knee joint when it is affected. In some cases operative measures are considered to improve existing deformity and aid joint movement or stabilize a weight-bearing joint.

MUSCULAR RHEUMATISM

(*Fibrositis*)

Inflammatory changes occurring in the muscles, fascia, tendons, ligaments and in the sheaths of nerve is often described as *muscular rheumatism*. Pain in the muscle is called *myalgia*.

The muscles most commonly affected are those of the neck, the trapezius and the sternomastoid muscle, which may result in spasmodic *torticollis* and *stiff neck*; the intercostal muscles when the pain is described as *pleurodynia*; the thick muscles and fascia of the lumbar region in the back in *lumbago*. In stiff neck the inflammation may spread to the brachial plexus of nerves giving rise to brachial neuritis; and in lumbago it may spread to the sheath of the sciatic nerve causing sciatica.

Fibrositis is thought to be due to bacterial infection and the source of this infection may be the teeth, tonsils, sinuses, gall-bladder and colon. Cold and physical strain are exciting causes which may precipitate an attack. An attack of lumbago may come on quite suddenly on stooping or on performing some violent movement.

Treatment when the pain is acute is by rest and applications of warmth, either superficial applications such as hot stupes, antiphlogistine, radiant heat, of which infra-red rays is one example; or heat may be applied by electricity in diathermy or short-wave therapy. In some cases the application of analgesic liniments may give relief, as A.B.C. liniment; and in lumbago the application of a belladonna plaster, and sometimes cupping the loins may relieve stiffness and pain. Aspirin will sometimes give relief from pain. When the pain is acute and can be located in the muscle an injection of ½ per cent novocain often gives immediate relief.

The patient should only stay in bed when the pain is too acute for him to move; otherwise it is better that he should get up and attempt to move about.

Chapter 54

The Nursing of Patients with Cancer

Common sites and early signs of cancer—Radium and X-ray treatment—General nursing care of patients—Protection of nursing staff

In many general hospitals nurses complete their training without having acquired very much knowledge of the care of patients with cancer; yet, if they are to be of general use to the community in the control of this disease, they ought to know something about its early signs and the commonest sites where it may arise.

Every nurse should be able to discuss with an inquiring patient the lines on which treatment of cancer is carried out and the great advantage to be derived from early treatment. She should be able to dispel much of the fear which leads so many sufferers to hide any symptoms they think may be due to cancer, and should encourage all patients to consult a specialist as soon as their suspicions are aroused.

The treatment of cancer can be divided into *radical* and *palliative* treatment; the record of cures resulting from early diagnosis and early treatment is most encouraging.

The **commonest sites** of cancer are the alimentary canal, the breast and the female organs of generation. In men the mouth is one of the sites most commonly affected, and the disease may begin in the lip, cheek or tongue. *Cancer of the lip* often commences between the centre and the angle; the neighbouring lymphatic glands soon becoming infected. *In the cheek* it may begin as a small wartlike growth. *In the tongue* it affects the anterior two-thirds, along the margin of the tongue, beginning as a small ulcer.

Cancer of the breast may begin as a small nodule palpable when the hand is placed flat on the breast, or by a slight discharge from the nipple. *Cancer of the uterus*, including the cervix, begins by bleeding between the periods, metrorrhagia, and in older women by post-menopausal bleeding.

Cancer of the oesophagus may arise at the junction of the pharynx and oesophagus, opposite the bifurcation of the trachea or near the cardiac end. The patient first complains of difficulty in swallowing solids.

Cancer of the stomach usually begins with vague symptoms of indigestion. *Cancer of the colon* most often arises at the flexures, particularly the sigmoid flexure and rectum. This form is often not noticed until the patient complains of bleeding from the bowel with discharge of mucus.

The **early signs of cancer** are very insidious. A rodent ulcer for example may begin as a small raised eminence on the skin, usually of the face and head, which after a time the patient notices does not heal, and is covered by an exudate, and then it may begin to spread. A man may notice he has a slightly thickened area on his lip, or a little ulcer on the tongue. A woman may discover a very small nodule in her breast; in some cases, the onset of Paget's disease of the nipple may cause slight discharge from the nipple. Irregular or profuse menstruation may be the first symptom of cancer of the uterus. Slight hoarseness may be the onset of carcinoma of the larynx. Sarcoma of bone may give rise to pain, which may be treated as rheumatism for months, with no suspicion of the presence of cancer.

The **diagnosis of cancer** is not easy because it so often begins in such a simple way, characterized only by some symptom which may be present in dozens of other conditions and diseases. For example many women think that profuse or irregular menstruation is to be expected at the menopause, though it cannot be too emphatically stated that this is not so, and that such symptoms ought to be reported to a gynaecologist without any delay.

Cancer of the rectum may be thought to be only haemorrhoids, and the sufferer may go on for months, thinking that his trouble is one of the minor discomforts associated with advancing years. A little hoarseness, due to cancer of the larynx, may be attributed to the onset of chronic bronchitis in a man of advancing years.

Nurses should know that whereas the diagnosis of cancer may be less difficult when the condition is far advanced, it is to the interest of the sufferer that he should recognize and report any symptoms of which he is suspicious as soon as he becomes aware of them. In many instances the condition may not be due to cancer; but, when the patient thinks or even fears it is, a correct diagnosis should be made, so that either the condition can be treated or his fears dispelled. No nurse should suggest that a patient may have cancer, she should merely advise consultation with a specialist, and point out that a less serious condition may easily become more serious unless treated early.

Treatment of cancer. The means at the disposal of the medical profession in the treatment of cancer are radium, X-rays and surgery, and the choice will depend on the individual judgement of the surgeon in each case.

RADIUM

Radium is a radioactive substance, made up of atoms and particles having a high velocity. The rays emitted are called *alpha*, *beta* and *gamma* rays. The latter have great power of penetration of tissue, and it is the gamma rays which are employed for therapeutic purposes. The rays emitted are similar to X-rays. Radium disintegrates slowly and presents a constant source of radioactivity; in practice, either radium is used, or radon, which is a gas given off from radium. It is collected in small tubes or seeds; it disintegrates in the course of a few days and is useful for out-patient work, as the patient may be sent home, wearing radon, which could not be done with radium.

The **effect of radium on the tissues** was first shown on workers who carried radium in the trouser pockets which resulted in inflammation and destruction of the tissues of the thigh. In therapeutic practice some tumours are found to be more sensitive to radium than others. The tissue cells are most vulnerable when they are rapidly dividing so that rapidly growing tumours are more susceptible.

The susceptibility of tissue to radium also depends to some extent on the presence of connective tissue, and on the blood supply. Cancer cells are killed by radium and the growth of connective tissue is stimulated; this results in the formation of fibrous tissue which will contract and so, by pressure and strangulation, further help to destroy the cancer cells. The blood-forming organs, particularly the marrow of long bones and the cells of the liver, are also very susceptible to the action of radium.

The problem with which the radiologist is faced is the provision of a correct dose of radium for every patient; the necessity of cutting out the alpha and beta rays, which are more destructive to healthy than to cancerous tissue; and the limitation of the application of gamma rays to the diseased area which he wishes to radiate. The nurse fortunately is not concerned with this problem, except in so far as she can help by maintaining any application in a given situation and removing it at the exact time that has been indicated.

The nurse, however, must be interested in the facts stated above that (1) the skin is more sensitive to radium than deeper structures; (2) the blood-forming organs are very susceptible to radium; (3) radium acts most effectively and easily on rapidly dividing cells, and the cells of sex glands divide more rapidly than any other glands in the body.

The **application of radium** is carefully calculated and regulated for each individual case, and the *gamma rays* are utilized. The *alpha rays* are very irritating to the tissues, but do not travel far and can be stopped by very slight protection; they will not go through a piece of paper. The *beta rays* are sometimes used in the treatment of warts, but for the radiation of tumours, means are taken to prevent their penetrating the tissues. They can be stopped by a layer of platinum of a given thickness.

The *gamma rays have a selective action on tumour cells*, especially when rapidly dividing; these will pass through several inches of lead and will penetrate fairly deeply into the tissues of the body. Radium is applied to the surface of the body on specially designed applicators; the radium is contained in platinum or gold screens. It is employed in needles of the same substance when interstitial radiation is employed; these needles are placed at regular intervals so as to obtain fairly even radiation. This form is used, for example, in the treatment of the tongue and breast. Silk thread is attached to each needle so that its position is known and it can be removed by pulling on this thread.

A large collection of radium is sometimes arranged as a *radium unit* or *bomb*. It may contain ½–2 grammes or more, and is used for application to the surface in order to irradiate a tumour at some distance from the surface. The size of the dose of radium employed has to be large enough to produce a superficial reactionary inflammation.

Radon consists of the emanations given off from radium, compressed by a special apparatus and enclosed in glass tubes known as radon *seeds*. By this means patients may be treated with radium in their own homes without danger to others from the radium, or danger of losing the radium. Radon gradually loses its potency and becomes inert in 5 or 6 days.

A **radium reaction** is accompanied by redness, irritation and pain. A few days after the application the skin will begin to tingle; the inflammation proceeds, and the reaction reaches its maximum within two weeks. At this time the skin is very red, covered with an exudate; it blisters and peels. A nurse in charge of a patient must keep the radiologist informed of the onset and progress of the reaction.

Treatment. Bland applications are essential. Parémanol, which contains olive oil and bismuth, is particularly smooth and comforting; alternatively lanoline may be used. In some cases penicillin cream may be ordered.

The systemic administration of penicillin is occasionally used to reduce the incidence of sepsis in some cases.

In addition to the local reaction described, *prolonged radiation produces a general reaction*, with symptoms of headache and giddiness—in some cases there is loss of appetite, nausea, vomiting and diarrhoea, and many other symptoms suggestive of malaise occur, and various nursing and medical measures are undertaken for the relief of these symptoms. The anaemia may require to be treated, and the diet should be very nutritious. Another point that requires consideration is the degree of toxaemia sometimes met with during the administration of radium.

Patients wearing radium should if possible be confined to bed, but in a few cases where bed is apt to be tiresome to the patient he is permitted to sit in a chair near his bed; in this case the chair ought to be marked by a special label so that everyone in the ward knows that the patient is undergoing treatment.

The nurse will be concerned not so much with the actual application, since this is carried out by radiologists, as with maintaining the radium in the position in which it has been placed, and with seeing that applicators do not slip, and so come in contact with healthy tissue. The applicator must be firm, and may require to be retained in position by the use of sandbags or bandages; and above all the patient must be comfortable, as otherwise he will not be able to keep still for long. Another very important point is that the patient should be warned not to touch the area that is being radiated, since his hand might receive injury. In cases where the breast is undergoing treatment it is a good plan to put a small pillow between the arm and the side of the patient's body, so that the arm does not come into contact with the application. The radium in use should be checked each time the nurse attends to the patient, and at least once or twice a day.

When an application of radium is made to the vagina or cervix it is most important to inspect the contents of bedpans for the presence of any of the gauze packing used, radium needles, or other forms of application.

When the mouth is being treated only liquid food can be given, and the mouth should be irrigated both before and after feeding. If swallowing is difficult or painful, aspirin gargles or spraying with a weak solution of cocaine before meals will give relief. When an application is made to the eye a good deal of discharge occurs, and the applicator has to be removed at fairly frequent intervals and the eye irrigated to render it free of discharge. The insertion of drops of liquid paraffin will relieve discomfort.

It is very important that nurses should realize that metallic substances cannot safely be used in cases undergoing treatment by radium and X-rays. Aperients such as calomel, which is a preparation of mercury, should be avoided; solutions of mercury may not be used in preparing the skin of the patient, the hands of operators, or appliances. Ointments containing any metallic substances, such as mercury and zinc, cannot be employed for treatment of the skin. Iodine also should never be used on surfaces which are to be irradiated since iodine alters the character of the reaction by rendering the skin more sensitive to the rays applied.

Protection of nursing staff. Prolonged working with radium will cause anaemia, and this is why nurses working in the radium wards have their blood count estimated at regular intervals. Recreation should be taken, as far as possible, in the open air and a good nourishing diet should be provided. In the case of young nurses it is inadvisable that they should be in attendance on patients wearing radium for more than two or three months at a time. But the nurse must exercise precautions and use the means supplied her for self-protection. She should be quick in her movements and remain near the bed as little as possible—this need not mean that she will neglect the patients but that she will use her common sense. For example, in attending a patient wearing radium on the left side, it would be advisable to attend to the patient from the right side of the bed. When obliged to handle radium, it should be taken to the bedside in the receptacles provided, which are leadlined.

X-RAY TREATMENT

As already stated, X-rays are like those of radium, and X-ray treatment is employed for similar purposes. The dose is very carefully calculated, a minimum dose being described as an erythema dose, and this is the amount necessary to cause reddening of the skin about ten days after exposure. The types of treatment employed are described as *superficial*, in which the less penetrating rays are used, and *deep therapy*, when rays are employed which penetrate farther; this form is used for the treatment of internal organs and deep-seated glands.

Preparation of a patient for X-ray treatment. All abdominal and pelvic conditions, e.g. carcinoma of cervix, carcinoma of testes and ovarian cases, should have an aperient the night before they are to undergo treatment. Any vegetable laxatives, cascara, rhubarb, or castor oil may be given, but no metallic purgative may be used, such as calomel.

Effect of X-ray treatment. The *general effect* on the patient may vary considerably; some will have more or less marked malaise; most cases complain of listlessness, disinclination for any exertion; others suffer from nausea and may or may not be sick. A few are sick—in some cases the patient will vomit immediately after treatment, in other cases a few hours later and some not until the following day. Diarrhoea may occur, and in cases where the cervix has been treated there may be frequency of micturition.

The nurse who receives a patient back to the ward, after X-ray treatment has been carried out, should observe the patient closely for the symptoms mentioned and note his pulse and colour. He should be spoiled a little and given a light meal immediately; if he feels sick and disinclined for food she should try to persuade him to have a lemon or orange drink containing glucose. If a patient is very sick, it may be impossible for him to take any other form of nourishment for some hours or so. But usually the sickness will abate and as soon as possible a liberal nourishing diet should be given. The general condition and appetite may be improved by iron and vitamins.

Local reaction. A local reaction in the form of reddening of the skin over the area exposed to X-rays may be expected in from two to three weeks, or may not appear for three or four weeks. In a few cases it may occur much earlier, even as soon as within the first 24 hours. This initial reddening is temporary, and will usually subside in a few days.

The *treatment applied to the skin* depends on the degree of reaction; it may be sufficient to dust the area with powder or it may require anointing with a bland ointment.

General nursing care. In both radium and X-ray treatment there is a tendency for physicians and nurses to concentrate on a special treatment the patient with cancer may be having, and to overlook the fact that he may be suffering marked malaise as the result of a general reaction or local discomfort so great as to deprive him of sleep. In the case of women undergoing irradiation of the cervix and uterus they will often be anticipating the next treatment with dread and fear.

On the whole, patients suffering from cancer are cheerful persons with whom it is a pleasure to deal; nevertheless they have much to make them worried and depressed and it is the first duty of nurses to preserve a cheerful, hopeful attitude, particularly in the nursing of the untreatable cases which are so difficult to handle, where in most cases it is only possible to alleviate symptoms and make them as comfortable as possible.

It is advisable to supply the patients with some form of interest—in some hospitals occupational therapy is employed which encourages the patient to make an effort and so exercise both his hands and his mind, and thus he is prevented from brooding over his condition.

Special treatment, necessary in certain instances, includes estimation of the basal metabolic rate in thyroid cases; the taking of a blood count after cases of leukaemia or other blood diseases have been treated; and washing the affected area of the head twice a day with soap and water, after ringworm has been treated. In this case all hair should have fallen out from the irradiated area by the eighteenth day.

Out-patient Treatment. Many patients, particularly when the disease is diagnosed early, can be treated by regular attendance at a centre. It will be noticed that the patients are very fit and well but they do need encouraging to maintain regular attendance over what may be a long period of four to six weeks' daily treatment five days a week.

After-care. A definite system of after-care is advisable and the need of this should be explained to patients; they should be warned of the necessity of following whatever advice the physician has given.

On going home the patient should be told to eat well, to keep out of the sun, to avoid exposure to keen cold wind and not to sit near a fire, as anything which will irritate a recently treated skin surface should be avoided. Patients who have had the mouth treated should be advised to continue using a simple mouth-wash before and after food.

Chapter 55

The Nursing of the Dying and the Care of the Dead

Death, the duties of doctor and nurse—The mental and physical state of a dying patient—Relief of distressing symptoms—Care of the body after death, last offices

Every nurse, sooner or later, will be present at the bedside of a dying patient for the first time. What does she think of death? A moment's reflection and she will remember that everyone must die, she will recollect that death is a bridge between time spent on earth and eternity. Death—this separation of the soul of a man from his material part or body—is dreaded by many as a terrible thing.

As a nurse tends to the comfort and wellbeing of a patient who is ill during his life, so she will be prepared to help him, to the best of her ability, in the important act of dying. A patient usually knows he is dying though he may not wish to speak of it, particularly to his relatives. But he may ask the doctor or the nurse; the doctor will have to decide whether the patient can bear the answer. It will depend on circumstances whether a direct answer will be given; but the doctor, alive to his responsibilities, must answer—though the answer will more often be conveyed by an increased note of sympathy and affection in his bearing, rather than by words.

When a doctor knows a patient is dying it is his duty to inform the relatives. The sorrowing relatives will be round the bedside of the dying patient; his death will leave a great blank in their lives, they will be obliged to reorganize their future plans without him and will attempt to console one another now.

The doctor, in hospital practice, does not linger at the bedside of the dying; his part is easy, his visit can be made one of activity. He will now order remedies which will help to make the last hours of the patient as comfortable as possible.

The nurse, who spends many hours with her patient, will feel his dying; it leaves a sense of loss; she has learnt to know him intimately, she has been indispensable to his needs and has grown attached to him whilst ministering to them. Her presence will help to console and comfort him now, and it will comfort his relatives also. A dying person is very lonely and, unless his relatives are present, consoling and comforting him, the nurse should go to his side from time to time, take hold of his hand, lay a hand on his forehead, thus manifesting her presence by her touch. A dying person is glad to feel the presence of someone he knows, it relieves his loneliness, and even though he appears to be unconscious and unperceiving, yet, when he does open his eyes he is helped by the presence of another.

Conversation which the dying person is not meant to hear should not take place at the bedside because, even though incapable of movement, even of smiling, or of speech, he may be able to hear and understand distinctly. He may also be acutely conscious of discomfort even when unable to give expression to his needs and will be very grateful when these are relieved, as, for example, by moistening his dry lips with water, wiping his nose, mopping his brow and straightening the hair which may be falling into his eyes; or by relieving his limbs of the weight of bedclothing or altering his position in bed so that cramp is relieved. Distension of the bladder may be prevented by giving the patient a bedpan or urinal; he may not have realized his need but will probably use it.

In other patients the mind wanders and memory may play tricks—at one moment the dying patient is back in the days of his childhood, holding imaginary conversations with persons of the past, the next moment he may be sensible of his immediate surroundings. The touch and the sound of the voice of the nurse may help to recall his wandering mind. When a patient is irrational, the nurse should try to humour him—her presence at the bedside lets him see he is cared for and may quieten him.

Dying people are apt to think of God and are grateful for the suggestion that a minister of religion of the denomination to which the patient belongs should be summoned. After the visit of the minister the nurse should try not to disturb the patient for fear of depriving him of his peace of soul.

In dealing with patients who are very ill and dying, whatever the belief or non-belief of the nurse may be, she must obtain for her patient what he, or his parents or guardians, would wish for him. When, for example, the patient belongs to a church in which the sacramental system exists, or is practised, it is important to send for the priest or administrator of the sacraments as soon as possible and whilst the patient is in full possession of his faculties. The priest should be informed if the patient is unconscious or unable to swallow.

The nurse will appreciate the deep consolation brought to the heart of her patient by reception of sacraments which to him are channels instituted by Christ through which His grace flows, and the essence of the spiritual help she can give lies in obtaining these for him without delay. Another more minor point she might consider would be to treat with respect any objects of piety which seem dear to the patient and to place these in his hands from time to time, as to him, on whose lips the words 'God be merciful to me, a sinner', will often be found, these objects act as a reminder of the mercy of God. An observant nurse will notice the fingers of the dying trace the outline of the object under his hand, indicating that though his lips may cease to move—as he becomes deprived of the power of speech—the desires of his heart continue to rise to God. She might point this out to the relatives to whom it will give great consolation.

The following symptoms and appearance are characteristic of dying: The face is pale and grey, the nose pinched and cold, the eyes glazed and sunken with the lids half closing over them and the ears are pale and cold or blue and shrivelled. The skin is clammy and covered with sweat. The pulse is weak, irregular and intermittent, the breathing is deep and noisy and stertorous, or it may be shallow and sighing in character. In most patients, as death approaches, breathing is of the Cheyne-Stokes type. The patient may lie quietly fingering the bedclothes or he may toss his arms about restlessly. As he gets weaker he is unable to support himself and he sinks very low in the bed as he slips from his pillows and the muscles of his legs relax so that they lie heavily on the bed.

The death rattle, stertorous breathing and breathing of the Cheyne-Stokes type are very distressing for the relatives to hear. The rattle is due to mucus in the bronchial tubes or to the trickling of saliva into the trachea, or it may be due to giving the patient fluid when he cannot swallow. As the patient gets weaker the amount of fluid given should be reduced; his mouth and lips should be moistened. As long as he can swallow he should be given sips of wine and water or brandy and water or champagne.

Salivation may be increased and the head should be held over to one side and inclined downwards so that saliva will run out of the mouth and not into the trachea. Atropine is often ordered to limit bronchial and salivary secretion and so prevent the unpleasant rattle due to breathing through fluid.

Stertorous breathing is due to obstruction of the respiratory passages by falling back of the tongue. The nurse can prevent this by keeping the tongue well forward, or by altering the position of the patient's head. If he is lying flat the head should be held over on to one side; when the patient is sitting up the head should be supported and not allowed to roll backwards. Cheyne-Stokes breathing occurs in most instances, particularly as the patient gets weaker. The administration of inhalations of carbon dioxide will do much to obviate this unpleasant symptom.

The mouth of a dying patient is usually open, and this naturally causes the tongue to be very dry. Smearing it with vaseline or liquid paraffin will do a great deal to keep it soft, moist and comfortable, for as long as possible. It should be smeared very often—every 15 or 20 minutes—to be of real value.

The nurse should have a dying patient propped up when possible as breathing is easier in this position; it may not be possible in a patient in deep coma. The head and arms should be supported and there should be a pillow beneath the knees in order to prevent his slipping down.

As the circulation continues to fail the skin becomes covered with sweat; this should be wiped off with warm towels and the patient's clothing changed when necessary. The feet get cold with a coldness hot-water bottles and hot blankets will not warm. This coldness is progressive, and creeps up the body to knees, thighs and trunk. It distresses the relatives but the patient does not feel cold; he will complain of being hot. Death is very near now and it is better to remove some of the bedclothes than to pile more on to him. But the nurse must consider the wish of the relatives, as they may not understand, and if they want to add more bedclothes she might suggest that a bedcradle should be inserted so that the patient will not have to bear the weight of them.

Dying patients feel the need for air and light, and here again the relatives might not understand if the nurse opened wide the window. They would think he might be chilled, but they will be grateful if they are asked to do something during these last hours, and if they will gently fan the air on each side of the patient's head, though not directly over his face, this will create a movement of air which will help to relieve his distress. Towards the end the sphincters relax and urine, and possibly faeces, may be involuntarily passed. The provision of pads of tow and wool, which can be changed frequently, will prevent soiling of the bed and keep it free from unpleasant odours.

The faculties are rapidly failing and the patient feels very lonely. He can now hear only what is said directly into his ear; he clings to the touch of those about him, lapses into a state of semiconsciousness, but from time to time will perhaps open his eyes and be content to see those he loves around him. He knows he is dying and he puts the hand of one friend into that of another, mutely saying—'be good to my mother', or, 'look after my child' as the Founder of Christianity said when He was dying. His lips may be moving as he utters the name of a loved one or, in prayer.

As the relatives, the nurse and perhaps the doctor, if he is a family friend, stand around the bed it can truly be said—'they also serve who only stand and wait'. Even if silent, their silence is active as the silence of the millions who keep the two minutes' silence at the cenotaphs of the world on Remembrance Sunday in November. They are helping their dying one as best they know how.

Pray for me, O my friends; a visitant
  Is knocking his dire summons at my door,
The like of whom, to scare me and to daunt,
  Has never, never come to me before;
'Tis death—O loving friends, your prayers!—'tis he! . . .
As though my very being had given way,
  As though I was no more a substance now,
And could fall back on nought to be my stay,
  (Help, loving Lord! Thou my sole Refuge, Thou,)

. . . . .

So pray for me, my friends, who have not strength to pray.

Dream of Gerontius.

If the patient is conscious and is opening his eyes from time to time the shade should be removed from the light and the curtains drawn back from the window. The dying person will try to face the light, as for him darkness is falling rapidly and, like a child, he fears the dark.

At the end, death is often very easy—it is like falling asleep. Many persons are quite oblivious of dying. Any convulsive movements which occur do not distress the patient and the nurse should tell the relatives—for their consolation—that he does not feel them. He has ceased to feel and is at peace. To some extent this accounts for the peaceful expression so often seen on the face of the dying and the recently dead. It is often a great consolation to the relatives and helps them to realize that for him life's struggle is over and reminds them that they can have confidence in his happiness.

As soon as the patient has breathed his last the nurse should gently close his eyes, if they are not already closed. She should then lead the relatives from the room, and in hospital should bring sister or the doctor to speak with them. She then returns to the sickroom in order to attend to the body. If possible she should have help as the body can be more easily and more reverently handled by two, as it is now a dead weight to move.

The bedclothing should be removed and one sheet left covering the body. All pillows, bolsters, air ring or water pillows should be taken out of the bed and if a large water bed has been used it should be emptied.

The body should be placed flat on the bed with the legs quite straight, and to prevent their falling apart they may be tied together with a piece of bandage or kept in position by means of sandbags; the feet should be supported by a sandbag to prevent footdrop. The hands and arms should be arranged according to the custom of the hospital—in many cases straight down by the sides of the body, unless the relatives wish them to be crossed on the breast. In private practice the relatives should be consulted on this point. Some means should be taken to prevent the jaw from dropping—it may be secured by means of a four-tailed jaw bandage or kept in position by placing a small pillow beneath the chin—one could be improvised by wrapping a wad of brown wool in a towel. Jewellery is usually removed from the body in hospital, but when private nursing the nurse must consult the relatives.

The bottom sheet should be drawn tight and the bed made quite tidy. The body is allowed to lie for an hour before the last offices are performed.

LAST OFFICES

The laying out of the dead should be reverently and quietly performed; all unnecessary talking must be avoided. The articles needed for this include: Warm water, soap and flannels, and towels to wash and dry the body; a hairbrush and comb, nailbrush and nail scissors. Moist swabs should be provided to cleanse the orifices and wool and forceps if they are to be plugged; fine forceps and small pieces of wool for nose and ears, larger forceps and a wad of white wool for the rectum and brown wool for the lower part of it. White wool is absorbent and will collect fluid, the brown wool being non-absorbent will prevent the fluid from running out. In some gynaecological cases the vagina should be packed tightly with gauze. If there is a wound, a clean dry surgical dressing should be supplied. In the case of a discharging wound, gauze packing should be inserted and a carbolic compress used to cover the wound, and wool, binder and needle and cotton to secure the dressing in position.

Either clean personal clothing should be provided or whatever dress the relatives wish used for the dead body. In hospital a shroud with tapes to fasten it and a label to attach to the body are usually employed.

If the body is verminous it will be necessary to supply a small tooth comb for the hair and swabs to pick the lice off the body; every particle must be removed as lice walk off the dead and will crawl on to other people, and this point must therefore be most carefully attended to.

Whenever possible two nurses should be supplied for the laying out of the dead; it is difficult for one to move the body and with two the office can therefore be more rapidly and more quietly and reverently carried out. The amount of washing necessary depends on the condition of the body, but it should be sponged and dried in all instances in order to remove moisture, though it need only be thoroughly soaped if the body is dirty. If the nails require to be cut this should be done quietly, particularly if the work is being done behind screens in the general ward of a hospital—the other patients know that the patient has died and they are following the movements of the nurses behind the screens however much they may be trying not to take any notice of them; therefore the more noiseless the work the less distress is given to others.

The hair should be brushed and combed and arranged as the patient liked it during his life, as this will be most pleasing to the relatives; the features should be set to look natural and the lips for example placed to look as if the mouth has just closed and not be set and hard. The face should look as if in peaceful sleep. It is usual to get a barber to shave the face of a man, so that it looks freshly groomed.

The shroud supplied in hospital is easy to adjust, the body is then tightly fastened up, mummy fashion, in a mortuary sheet stitched, not pinned, a label on which is written the name of the patient, the time of his death and the name of the ward is stitched on the front of it. In addition, in some hospitals, a label bearing the name of the patient is fastened round his ankle. These precautions are taken so that the undertaker shall not make a mistake when he comes to make funeral arrangements.

In a private house the nurse should arrange the patient lying on a clean white sheet, wearing the clothing provided, and cover the body with a sheet and perhaps a white quilt—turning the sheet over so as to give the impression that the patient is lying in bed. The head should be arranged on a fairly low pillow and the face covered with a linen or lace veil; this can be removed when the relatives are in the room but it prevents flies from settling on the face when no one is in attendance.

The nurse should inquire whether there is any object of piety the relatives would wish to be arranged in or about the hands of the dead person—they may prefer to attend to this point themselves, but will be grateful for the consideration of their feelings shown by this request.

Everything used for the last offices should be removed from the room as quickly as possible and the nurse should take pains to make the room neat, and pleasant to look upon. She should inquire whether the relatives would care for her to arrange flowers in it and, as she will remain in the house until after the funeral, she should be at hand to take in flowers as they come, and place them in the room or help to do so, but she must ask where the relatives would like them put and suggest that perhaps they would like to move them. If she shows that she realizes that those sent by the nearest and dearest ones would be liked nearest the bed or on the bed the relatives will be grateful for her understanding sympathy.

In the case of Hebrew patients who die, every nurse should know that the Jews do not like their dead handled by Christians and she must respect this. In some hospitals special Hebrew watchers are appointed; in others they are available and can be obtained as required. The nurse should be careful to ask the relatives what their wishes are; she may in some cases be asked to perform the last offices for them, in others she may be asked to help; but, in all cases, she should not touch the body after death without first ascertaining the wishes of the relatives or of those responsible.

Appendix I

Abbreviations of Instructions used in Prescriptions

Abbreviation	*Latin*	*English translation*
a.a.	ana	of each, to the desired amount
a.c.	ante cibum	before food
a.h.	alternis horis	every other hour
aeq.	aequales	of equal amounts
a.m.	ante meridiem	before noon
a.p.	ante prandium	before dinner
ad.lib.	ad libitum	at pleasure or, as liked
add.	adde	add
altern. d.	alternis diebus	every alternate day
altern. hor.	alternis horis	every alternate hour
ante	ante	before or, to precede
aq.	aqua	water
aq. bull.	aqua bulliens	boiling water
aq. cal.	aqua calida	cold water
b.	bis	twice
bib.	bibe	drink
bidi.	bidium	two days
b.i.d.	bis in dies	twice a day
c.	cum	with
c. aq.	cyathus aquae	a glass of water
c.m.	cras mane	tomorrow morning
c.n.	cras nocte	tomorrow night
c.v.	cras vespere	tomorrow evening
cib.	cibus	food
coch.	cochleare	spoonful
coch. amp.	cochleare amplum	a tablespoonful
coch. med.	,, medium	a desertspoonful
coch. parv.	,, parvum	a teaspoonful
cont. rem.	continuatur remedia	let the remedy be continued
d.	dies	day
d.d.	de die	daily
d. in p. ae.	divide in partes aequales	divide into equal parts
d. seq.	die sequente	on the following day
dim.	dimidius	half
det.	detur	let it be given
dil.	dilue	dilute
ex aq.	ex aqua	in water
garg.	gargarisma	a gargle
gutt.	gutta	a drop
gr.	granum	a grain
gm.	gramma	a gramme

Abbreviation	*Latin*	*English translation*
h.	hora	at the time of
h.d.	*hora decubitus	at bedtime
h.n.	hac nocte	this night
h.s.	*hora somni	at bedtime
inf.	infusum	an infusion
inj.	injectio	an injection
m.	misce	mix
m.	*mane	in the morning
m. et v.	*mane et vespere	morning and evening
m. et n.	*mane et nocte	morning and night
mist.	mistura	a mixture
n.	*nocte	by night or, at night
n.m.	*nocte maneque	night and morning
O	octarius	a pint
o. alt. hor.	omnibus alternis horis	every alternate hour
o.m.	omni mane	each morning
ol.	oleum	oil
p.c.	post cibum	after food
p.m.	post meridiem	the afternoon
prim. m.	*primo mane	first thing in the early morning
p.r.n.	pro re nata	as occasion arises, and the prescription is required
p.r.	per rectum	by the rectum
pulv.	pulvis	powder
p.v.	per vaginam	by the vagina
q.d. or q.i.d.	quater die / quater in die	four times a day during the 24 hours
q.l.	quantum libet	as much as you please
q.q.h.	quaque quarta hora	every four hours
q.s.	quantum sufficit	as much as is required
℞	recipe	take
rep.	*repetatur	let it be repeated
rep. sem.	repetatur semel	to be repeated once only
sem.	semel	once
s. (ss.)	semis	half or, a half
s.o.s.	sit-opus sit	as necessary or, if and when required.
stat.	statim	immediately
stat eff.	statu effervescentiae	give whilst effervescing
s.v.g.	spiritus vini gallici	brandy
t.	ter	three times
t.i.d.	ter in die	three times a day
t.d.s.	ter die sumendum	to be taken three times a day
tuss. urg.	tussi urgente	if the cough is troublesome
tinct.	tinctura	tincture
ung.	unguentum	ointment

* The instructions marked with an asterisk appear to provide for some measure of discretion. In most hospitals there is a known usage of these terms; and the custom in use at the hospital is understood and followed by all those concerned.

For example, *nocte* means at night. It does not mean this night (only) *hac nocte*, or tomorrow night *cras nocte*; it means at night or by night, not necessarily every night, but any night with the use of discretion. It is necessary therefore for nurses and others to make themselves familiar with the usage of the hospital or institution in which they may be working, and with the wishes of the doctor who is attending the patient when nursing an individual patient or engaged in district or visiting nursing.

Appendix

Table of Vitamins, Giving the Name, Source, Requirements

NAME	SOURCE	DEFICIENCY DISEASES
A Fat Soluble (Anti-xerophthalmic or anti-infective vitamin). *Carotene* is pro-vitamin A which is converted into vitamin A in the body.	Fishliver oils { halibut, cod Milk. Butter. Vitaminized margarine. Carrots. Green vegetables. Preparations of vitamin A (concentrated).	***Night Blindness.*** ***Xerosis,*** a condition of the mucous membranes which predisposes them to local infections. ***Xerophthalmia.***
B_1 **Aneurin** in this country; **Thiamin** in U.S.A. **Water soluble, also known as vitamin F** (anti-beri-beri or anti-neuritic vitamin). It is necessary for health as it is intimately concerned with cell metabolism.	Wheat germ. Wholemeal bread. Brewer's yeast. Egg yolk. Peas. Oatmeal. Fruits. Vegetables. Synthetic preparation—aneurin.	***Beri-beri*** (a form of polyneuritis) which occurs in the East where polished rice is the principal food taken by the natives. ***Polyneuritis*** due to toxic conditions.
B_2 **Complex, Water soluble, contains several constituents.** Riboflavin or lactoflavin, often called B_2 (concerned with cell metabolism and essential for health). Adermin or B_6 (pyridoxin in U.S.A.) Nicotinic Acid or B_7 the P.P. (pellagra-preventing) factor. Other factors include vitamin H or Biotin and Pantothenic acid and Folic acid.	Same foods as B_1 and Cheese. Liver. Meat.	***Pellagra*** which occurs chiefly in countries such as the Southern States of U.S.A. where the natives eat principally maize. ***Stomatitis*** particularly at the angles of the mouth. Soreness of mouth with thin shiny mucous membrane (Cheiliosis).
C Water soluble (Anti-scorbutic vitamin).	Fresh fruits. Orange and Lemon juice. Black currants. Tomato juice. Potatoes. Cabbage. Spinach. Salads. Rose hip syrup. Ascorbic acid.	***Scurvy*** (1) the infant becomes restless and sallow, and is liable to bronchial and skin infections. (2) If the condition is allowed to continue, Barlow's disease or 'scurvy rickets' develops with the typical symptoms described on p. 434.
D Fat soluble (Anti-rachitic vitamin). Promotes absorption of calcium and phosphate and therefore promotes bone calcification. By taking in *excess* hyper-vitaminosis may be caused, giving rise to increased density in bone, and pyrexia.	Fishliver oils { halibut., cod., tunny. Herring. Egg yolk. Butter. Synthetic vitamin (calciferol prepared by irradiation of ergosterol). Irradiation of the body by sunlight, natural or artificial, helps the formation of vitamin D in the skin.	***Rickets.*** Tooth caries. Osteomalacia in adults.
E Fat Soluble	Wheat germ. Green leaves such as lettuce.	By experiments on animals it is found that vitamin E promotes fertility. It is thought that vitamin E may prevent abortion in women, and a diet rich in vitamin E is recommended for expectant mothers. Synthetic preparations of it are given to women with a tendency to abortion.
K Fat Soluble (anti-haemorrhagic or 'Koagulation vitamin').	Green leaves. Pig's liver.	***Hypo-prothrombinaemia*** in which haemorrhagic disease is likely to occur in infants, and bleeding in post-operative obstructive jaundice because the blood loses the power of clotting, and clotting time is prolonged.
P Water Soluble	Lemon juice.	***Capillary fragility.***

II

and Diseases Produced by Deficiency, and Daily When Known

DAILY REQUIREMENTS	DIET PROVIDING APPROXIMATE DAILY REQUIREMENTS
Adults 3,000 I.U. minimum. Children 4,000 to 6,000 I.U. Pregnant Women 6,000 to 8,000 I.U.	Ordinary diet provided one pint of milk daily and a reasonable supply of butter or vitaminized margarine and good allowance of green vegetables are given. A pint of milk and one egg will provide about 2,000 I.U. of vitamin A. and 1,000 I.U. of carotene, but under existing dietary conditions this is not obtainable and about a pound of carrots should be eaten every week to provide sufficient vitamin A.
Adults 500 I.U. Children 400 I.U.	A good mixed diet containing wholemeal bread in place of white bread.
No international standard.	As B_1 and contained in cheese in addition.
Adults 50 to 100 mg. Children 50 to 150 mg. obtainable as ascorbic acid in tablets of 25 and 50 milligrammes. Babies 15 to 50 mg. Vitamin C is of great importance in raising the resistance in acute infections and in promoting the healing of wounds. Up to 300 mg. may be given. There is no danger of an overdose.	A diet containing a reasonable amount of green vegetable with the juice of an orange or lemon a day is adequate. In war-time either the specially prepared black currant purée or rose-hip syrup, or ascorbic acid 25 to 50 mg. daily should be added to the diet. Vitamin C should always be added to gastric diets and to the diet in most institutions, including hospitals.
Adults 300 to 500 I.U. Children 500 to 2,000 I.U. The British Association recommend 700 I.U. daily for babies. This is increased as the infant gets older to 1,500 I.U. As a curative dose in rickets, 3,000 to 5,000 I.U. is recommended. (10,000 I.U. daily would constitute an overdose.)	Children do not receive sufficient vitamin D in their diet and therefore always require fishliver oils or synthetic vitamin D added to the diet.
No international standard.	
No international standard.	A mixed diet. *Comment.* Before operation for the relief of obstructive jaundice the pro-thrombin level of the blood is determined and if deficiency is shown one of the proprietary preparations is given for several days either by mouth or by intramuscular injection.
No international standard.	

Appendix III

Questions Set in the Final General State Examinations February 1946 to February 1949

February 1946

MEDICINE AND MEDICAL NURSING TREATMENT

Time allowed 1½ hours. Three questions in all are to be answered.

Compulsory. 1. Give an account of the symptoms and treatment and nursing care of acute nephritis.

Compulsory. 2. State briefly what you know about:

(*a*) Rickets;
(*b*) Threadworms;
(*c*) Cheyne-Stokes respiration;
(*d*) Blood sedimentation rate;
(*e*) The uses of iron and its administration.

3. Describe an epileptic fit and its management. What drugs may be prescribed in the treatment of epilepsy?

4. Describe a case of exophthalmic goitre (thyrotoxicosis). State what you know about the treatment and nursing care of a patient suffering from this condition.

SURGERY AND GYNAECOLOGY AND SURGICAL AND GYNAECOLOGICAL NURSING TREATMENT

Time allowed 1½ hours. Three questions in all are to be answered.

Compulsory. 1. What is the difference between an innocent and a malignant tumour? Describe the nursing of a patient who has been operated on for carcinoma of the breast.

Compulsory. 2. What is meant by dysmenorrhoea? Give some of the causes of this condition, and mention briefly how they may be treated.

3. Mention five appliances or accessories commonly used in surgical practice, which are made of rubber, or its substitutes. Give a brief description of their use.

4. State what is meant by:

(*a*) Conjunctivitis;
(*b*) Iritis;
(*c*) Glaucoma;
(*d*) Cataract;
(*e*) Stye.

GENERAL NURSING

Time allowed 2½ hours. Five questions in all are to be answered.

Compulsory. 1. Enumerate the chief points to emphasize in a report by the night-nurse who has been in charge of the following patients during their first night in hospital:—

(*a*) A case of diabetes mellitus having insulin;
(*b*) A case of haematemesis;
(*c*) A case of asthma.

Compulsory. 2. Describe the preparation of a patient who is to undergo the operation of supra-pubic cystostomy for an enlarged prostate gland. Give reasons for the steps taken in the preparation.

Compulsory. 3. A patient is admitted with a fractured pelvis. Describe the general nursing care.

4. Explain how you would prepare and carry out the following treatments:—
   (*a*) A nasal douche;
   (*b*) Irrigation of an eye.

5. Describe the treatment and nursing care of a patient suffering from eczema.

6. Describe the post-operative care of an infant who has been operated upon for intussusception.

June 1946

MEDICINE AND MEDICAL NURSING TREATMENT

Time allowed 1½ hours. Three questions in all are to be answered.

Compulsory. 1. Describe an attack of acute bronchitis. What do you know of the causes of this condition and how may it be treated?

Compulsory. 2. State briefly what you know about:—
   (*a*) Koplik's spots;
   (*b*) Psoriasis;
   (*c*) Stomatitis;
   (*d*) Nikethamide (coramine);
   (*e*) Overdosage of insulin.

3. Describe the signs, symptoms and treatment of pernicious (Addison's) anaemia.

4. Describe a case of scabies and give a detailed account of its treatment.

SURGERY AND GYNAECOLOGY AND SURGICAL AND GYNAECOLOGICAL NURSING TREATMENT

Time allowed 1½ hours. Three questions in all are to be answered.

Compulsory. 1. What are the dangers and complications of a severe burn, extending from the middle of the back of the thigh to the ankle? What measures can be taken in order to prevent their occurrence?

Compulsory. 2. What is meant by an ectopic gestation? Describe the complications that may occur and how they may be dealt with.

3. What is the difference between a " suture " and a " ligature." How should the materials commonly used be sterilised?

4. State briefly what you know about:
   (*a*) Otorrhoea;
   (*b*) Adenoids;
   (*c*) Erysipelas;
   (*d*) Carbuncle;
   (*e*) Quinsy.

GENERAL NURSING

Time allowed 2½ hours. Five questions in all are to be answered.

Compulsory. 1. Describe the nursing care and medical treatment that may be ordered for a patient of fifty years of age suffering from congestive heart failure.

Compulsory. 2. A patient returns from the theatre to the ward at 4 p.m. after the operation of abdominal hysterectomy. Describe in detail the nursing care required by this patient during the next twenty-four hours.

Compulsory. 3. Enumerate the requirements for examination of the ear, nose and throat. In what cases may the ear be syringed? Describe exactly how this is done.

4. Describe in detail the nursing care of a patient suffering from influenzal broncho-pneumonia.

5. What nursing treatments might be ordered in a case of post-operative flatulent distension of the abdomen? Describe one of these treatments in detail.

6. What are the different methods by which penicillin may be given? What special care must be taken in the administration and storage of this drug?

October 1946

MEDICINE AND MEDICAL NURSING TREATMENT

Time allowed 1½ hours. Three questions in all are to be answered.

Compulsory. 1. Give an account of the complications, nursing care and treatment of lobar pneumonia.

Compulsory. 2. State briefly what you know about:

(*a*) The important complications of typhoid fever;
(*b*) Urticaria;
(*c*) Embolism;
(*d*) Leukaemia;
(*e*) The doses, methods of administration and uses of paraldehyde.

3. Describe the symptoms of an infant suffering from acute gastro-enteritis and give an account of the nursing and medical treatment.

4. Enumerate the conditions which may cause ascites. Describe the management and treatment of a case of ascites due to cardiac failure.

SURGERY AND GYNAECOLOGY AND SURGICAL AND GYNAECOLOGICAL NURSING TREATMENT

Time allowed 1½ hours. Three questions in all are to be answered.

Compulsory. 1. A patient has undergone an abdominal operation (under general anaesthesia), which is concluded at 3 p.m. From this time onward describe the duties of the nurse in charge of the patient in preventing, as far as possible, such complications as may occur.

Compulsory. 2. What are the dangers of salpingitis? Describe briefly the causes of this condition and its treatment.

3. What is meant by "haemorrhoids"? State briefly what you know of the causes of this condition, and how it may be treated.

4. State briefly what you know about:

(*a*) Varicose ulcer;
(*b*) "Sprain";
(*c*) Hallux valgus;
(*d*) Flat foot;
(*e*) Hammer toe.

GENERAL NURSING

Time allowed 2½ hours. Five questions in all are to be answered.

Compulsory. 1. A patient aged sixty is admitted to a ward with hemiplegia. What nursing care would you observe to prevent the development of complications?

Compulsory. 2. What *special* pre-operative treatment is required for a patient who is about to undergo (*a*) mastoidectomy; (*b*) cataract extraction; (*c*) perineorrhaphy.

Compulsory. 3. What are the duties of the nursing staff in a ward with regard to the care and economy in the use of (*a*) milk; (*b*) bread; (*c*) linen.

4. In the absence of immediate medical aid state how you would deal with the following emergencies: (*a*) a case of coal gas poisoning; (*b*) ruptured varicose veins; (*c*) a child who has swallowed ammonia.

5. What preparation would you make for a patient to have paracentesis thoracis (aspiration of pleural cavity) performed?

6. State why you would suspect that a child in a ward is about to develop measles?
How would you nurse such a patient and what precautions would you take to prevent the spread of infection?

February 1947

MEDICINE AND MEDICAL NURSING TREATMENT

Time allowed 1½ hours. Three questions in all are to be answered.

Compulsory. 1. Describe a case of acute rheumatic fever and give an account of the nursing and medical treatment of this condition. Enumerate the complications which might arise.

Compulsory. 2. State briefly what you know about:

(*a*) Quinsy;
(*b*) Congenital syphilis;
(*c*) Cirrhosis of the liver;
(*d*) Chloral hydrate;
(*e*) Mumps.

3. Give an account of the symptoms of uraemia. What may cause this condition and what treatment may be carried out?

4. What do you understand by coronary artery thrombosis? Give an account of the symptoms and the treatment which may be given for this condition.

SURGERY AND GYNAECOLOGY AND SURGICAL AND GYNAECOLOGICAL NURSING TREATMENT

Time allowed 1½ hours. Three questions in all are to be answered.

Compulsory. 1. What is a hernia? What are the common sites at which abdominal herniae may occur? What dangers may occur in a case of untreated hernia?

Compulsory. 2. Give examples of (*a*) an innocent tumour, and (*b*) a malignant tumour which may occur in the uterus.
Describe the nursing treatment of a patient who has had a hysterectomy.

3. What is an ulcer? Describe any case that you have seen of an ulcer of the leg; how may such a patient be treated?

4. State briefly what you know about:

(*a*) Incontinence of urine;
(*b*) Residual urine;
(*c*) Retention with overflow;
(*d*) Complications after the operation of circumcision;
(*e*) Intravenous pyelography.

GENERAL NURSING

Time allowed 2½ hours. Five questions in all are to be answered.

Compulsory. 1. A young adult suffering from diabetes mellitus is admitted to hospital for the first time. What are the nurse's duties in this case and what instructions should be given to the patient?

Compulsory. 2. Describe the nursing care and general management of a patient who has had colostomy performed. What instruction and advice should the patient be given before his discharge from hospital?

Compulsory. 3. For what reasons may a vaginal douche be ordered? Describe in detail the preparation for and the administration of a vaginal douche.

4. Describe the nursing care of a child who has had tracheotomy performed.

5. In the absence of the physician what can a nurse do to relieve the following:

(*a*) headache; (*b*) irritation of the skin in urticaria; (*c*) sleeplessness in an elderly patient; (*d*) hiccough; (*e*) wasp sting?

6. For what conditions may the following enemata be ordered:

(*a*) olive oil; (*b*) starch and opium; (*c*) magnesium sulphate? Describe the preparation and method of administration of one of these.

June 1947

MEDICINE AND MEDICAL NURSING TREATMENT

Time allowed 1½ hours.

NOTE.—You must answer THREE questions and not more than three.

1. Give an account of the symptoms, nursing care and treatment of cerebro-spinal fever (meningococcal meningitis). What other types of meningitis may occur?
2. Describe the method of taking the radial pulse. What are the common abnormalities which may occur and what conditions may cause them?
3. What do you understand by pulmonary embolism? Describe the nursing and treatment of a patient in whom this has occurred.
4. Give a brief description of the common causes of sore throat and describe the treatment of a case of acute tonsillitis.
5. What are the causes of haemoptysis? What should a nurse do in a severe case pending the arrival of a doctor?
6. State briefly what you know about:

(*a*) Hiccough;
(*b*) The complications of measles;
(*c*) Ryle's tube;
(*d*) Sodium salicylate;
(*e*) Atropine.

SURGERY AND GYNAECOLOGY AND SURGICAL AND GYNAECOLOGICAL NURSING TREATMENT

Time allowed $1\frac{1}{2}$ *hours.*

NOTE.—You must answer THREE questions and not more than three.

1. What is meant by "gangrene"? Give the common sites where this condition may occur. How can "senile gangrene" be treated and nursed?
2. Describe the difference between a malignant and a non-malignant tumour of the breast. Give the nursing treatment of a patient who has been operated on for carcinoma of the breast.
3. What is an "Ectopic Pregnancy"? What are the dangers of this condition, and how may they be treated?
4. What conditions following child-birth may require operation? Describe the treatment and nursing care of any one of these.
5. Describe the nursing care after an operation of tonsillectomy.
6. State briefly what you know about:
   (*a*) Cystitis;
   (*b*) Pyelitis;
   (*c*) Pyo-salpinx;
   (*d*) In-growing toe nail;
   (*e*) "Housemaid's knee" (pre-patellar bursitis).

GENERAL NURSING

Time allowed $2\frac{1}{2}$ *hours.*

NOTE.—You must answer FIVE questions and not more than five.

1. Describe the nursing care of a patient suffering from infective hepatitis (catarrhal jaundice).
2. A patient is admitted to hospital suffering from a perforated peptic ulcer. How would you prepare him for operation? Give reasons for the steps taken.
3. How would you prepare and administer a nasal feed to an unconscious patient?
4. Discuss the causation, prevention and treatment of bed sores.
5. Describe diets suitable for each of the following conditions, stating your reasons for the choice of food: (*a*) ulcerative colitis; (*b*) carcinoma of the oesophagus where gastrostomy has been performed; (*c*) acute nephritis.
6. A patient is admitted with a severe head injury. What observations would you make and what is the nursing care of the patient during the first twenty-four hours in hospital?
7. What is meant by dysmenorrhoea? What advice would you give to an adolescent regarding the rules of health during the menstrual period?
8. Describe in detail the method of giving a patient a "tepid sponge."

OCTOBER 1947

MEDICINE AND MEDICAL NURSING TREATMENT

Time allowed $1\frac{1}{2}$ *hours.*

NOTE.—You must answer THREE questions and not more than three.

1. What symptoms may be observed in a case of chronic heart failure? State briefly the treatment which may be given to relieve the patient.

2. Describe a case of chorea and give an account of the medical and nursing treatment of this condition.
3. Give an account of the symptoms, complications and treatment of scarlet fever.
4. What is meant by hemiplegia? Give a brief account of the causes of this condition and state how you would nurse a case during the early stages.
5. What is meant by the term melaena?
   Give a brief account of the causes of this condition and state how you would nurse a severe case.
6. State briefly what you know about:
   (*a*) Koplik's spots;
   (*b*) Bronchiectasis;
   (*c*) Cirrhosis of the liver;
   (*d*) Schick test;
   (*e*) Adrenaline.

SURGERY AND GYNAECOLOGY AND SURGICAL AND GYNAECOLOGICAL NURSING TREATMENT

Time allowed 1½ hours.

NOTE.—You must answer THREE questions and not more than three.

1. What are the complications of a severe burn or scald involving the face and front of the neck? How may such a patient be treated and nursed?
2. State briefly what you know about:
   (*a*) Colles' fracture;
   (*b*) Talipes equino-varus (club-foot);
   (*c*) Genu valgum (knock knee);
   (*d*) Pott's fracture;
   (*e*) Pott's disease (tuberculosis of the spine).
3. What are the causes of severe uterine haemorrhage? Describe the treatment and nursing care of any one of the conditions you mention.
4. What are the causes of uterine prolapse? How would a patient be treated and nursed after an operation for this condition?
5. Discuss the nursing care of a patient who has been operated on for the removal of a renal calculus.
6. What are the causes, symptoms and treatment of the following:
   (*a*) Corneal ulcer;
   (*b*) Conjunctivitis?

GENERAL NURSING

Time allowed 2½ hours.

NOTE.—You must answer FIVE questions and not more than five.

1. Give an account of the post-operative nursing treatment of a patient who has undergone the operation of partial gastrectomy.
2. Describe the nursing care of a patient with a fracture of the cervical region of the spine.
3. What are the contra-indications for breast feeding? What instructions would you give for the feeding of an infant of one month old when breast feeding has been discontinued?
4. Describe the general nursing care of a patient who has been ordered " complete rest."

5. What are the duties and responsibilities of the nurse in connection with drugs included in the Dangerous Drugs Act? Describe how and where you would give an intramuscular injection.
6. Enumerate the different types of catheter. State the uses and advantages of each kind you mention and the method of sterilization.
7. What preparation of the patient is necessary before the operation of haemorrhoidectomy?
   Describe the post-operative nursing care of the patient.
8. What instruments are required for the operation of dilatation and curettage? Describe in detail the after care of the patient.

FEBRUARY 1948

MEDICINE AND MEDICAL NURSING TREATMENT

Time allowed 1½ hours.

NOTE.—You must answer THREE questions and not more than three.

1. What do you understand by constipation? State what may give rise to this condition. Indicate briefly the treatment which may be adopted.
2. Give an account of the symptoms and treatment of acute poliomyelitis (infantile paralysis).
3. Describe an epileptic fit and state how you would deal with a patient who is having one. What treatment may be given to prevent attacks?
4. What are the common causes of insomnia? Describe what may be done to alleviate this condition.
5. Describe a case of thyrotoxicosis (exophthalmic goitre). State what you know about the treatment of this condition.
6. State briefly what you know about:
   (*a*) Laryngeal diphtheria;
   (*b*) Angina pectoris;
   (*c*) Blood urea;
   (*d*) Diamorphine (heroin);
   (*e*) Impetigo.

SURGERY AND GYNAECOLOGY AND SURGICAL AND GYNAECOLOGICAL NURSING TREATMENT

Time allowed 1½ hours.

NOTE.—You must answer THREE questions and not more than three.

1. For what reasons have you known fluids to be given by the intravenous route? What fluids can be given, and what are the dangers that may arise?
2. What is the difference between (*a*) an anal fistula and (*b*) an anal fissure? Describe the post-operative treatment of an anal fistula.
3. What is meant by the term haematoma? How would this condition be recognised after operation, and what treatment could be applied?
4. What do you understand by (*a*) cystocele and (*b*) rectocele? How may these conditions arise and how may they be treated?
5. What are the dangers of:

(a) A bead up one nostril;
(b) A bead in the ear;
(c) A severe blow on the eyeball;
(d) The swallowing of a needle;
(e) A cut on the finger?

Give briefly the treatment of each condition.

6. What is meant by "dislocation of the shoulder joint"? How may this condition be recognised? Describe briefly the treatment.

GENERAL NURSING

Time allowed 2½ hours.

NOTE.—You must answer FIVE questions and not more than five.

1. Give an account of the nursing care required for a patient suffering from acute nephritis.
2. A patient suffering from pulmonary tuberculosis is admitted to a general ward. What steps would you take to prevent the spread of infection? How would you deal with the complication of haemoptysis?
3. What nursing care and treatment may be carried out to prevent post-operative chest complications?
4. How would you nurse a patient after amputation through the thigh? What complications may arise?
5. What preparation should a nurse make for the following investigations: (a) vaginal examination; (b) rectal examination; (c) examination of the throat?
6. In the absence of a doctor, what would you do to relieve (a) a patient with a severe skin irritation; (b) a baby having a convulsion?
7. For what purposes are the following used: (a) a ring pessary; (b) uterine sound; (c) Playfair's probe? What advice would you give to a woman who is wearing a pessary?
8. What do you understand by the term "abortion"? Describe the nursing care of a patient who is suffering from a threatened abortion.

June 1948

MEDICINE AND MEDICAL NURSING TREATMENT

Time allowed 1½ hours.

NOTE.—You must answer THREE questions and not more than three.

1. What observations would you make on a comatose patient admitted to hospital? Indicate how they might be of assistance in arriving at the diagnosis.
2. Discuss the differences between suppression and retention of urine. Mention briefly the causes of these conditions and indicate the treatment which may be carried out.
3. Give an account of the symptoms, complications and treatment of measles.
4. What do you understand by auricular fibrillation? Describe the symptoms and treatment of this condition.
5. Describe the symptoms of ulcerative colitis and give an account of the nursing and treatment of this condition.

6. State briefly what you know about:
   (*a*) Leukæmia;
   (*b*) Coal gas poisoning;
   (*c*) Paralysis agitans (Parkinson's disease);
   (*d*) Thread worms;
   (*e*) Phenobarbitone (luminal).

SURGERY AND GYNAECOLOGY AND SURGICAL AND GYNAECOLOGICAL NURSING TREATMENT

Time allowed 1½ hours.

1. State the causes of intestinal obstruction. Give a description of any one case, its treatment and subsequent nursing.
2. How does an adenoma of the breast differ from a carcinoma? What is the difference in the treatment of these two conditions?
3. Give the causes of frequency of micturition in a middle-aged woman. Indicate what treatments may be carried out.
4. State briefly what you know about:
   (*a*) Menopause;
   (*b*) Amenorrhoea in young women;
   (*c*) Dilitation and curettage;
   (*d*) Pessaries;
   (*e*) Volsellum forceps.
5. What are the causes of infection of the maxillary antrum (of Highmore)? Describe the symptoms and how this condition may be treated.
6. How may a severe septic thumb be treated? What complications may occur?

GENERAL NURSING

Time allowed 2½ hours.

1. An old man is admitted to hospital suffering from apoplexy due to cerebral thrombosis. How would you nurse him?
2. What observations should be made and what records should be kept when nursing a patient with lobar pneumonia?
3. Give an account of the post-operative care of a patient after cholecystectomy.
4. A patient is admitted to hospital with burns extending from the buttocks to the ankles. How would you nurse him? Give one method of treatment.
5. A patient is suffering from an advanced stage of carcinoma of the uterus. What nursing care and treatment might be given to alleviate the symptoms?
6. What preparation is necessary for a patient before perineorrhaphy? Describe the post-operative nursing treatment.
7. Discuss the relative merits of the different methods of administering oxygen. What are the nurse's responsibilities regarding this treatment?
8. Discuss the different methods by which heat may be applied for the relief of pain.

OCTOBER 1948

MEDICAL AND NURSING TREATMENT

Time allowed 1½ hours.

1. Give an account of the causes of hæmoptysis. Describe the treatment and nursing care of a severe case.
2. Describe briefly the clinical manifestations of the various stages of syphilis.
3. What are the signs and symptoms of uræmia? Mention the causes of this condition and describe its treatment.
4. What is meant by 'the pulse'? State briefly what you know about the causes of:
   (*a*) a slow pulse;
   (*b*) a rapid pulse;
   (*c*) an irregular pulse.
5. Describe the symptoms of a gastric ulcer. Give a brief account of the treatment which may be employed. What complications may occur?
6. State briefly what you know about:
   (*a*) Mantoux test;
   (*b*) lumbago;
   (*c*) mitral stenosis;
   (*d*) bronchoscopy;
   (*e*) diuretics.

OCTOBER 1948

SURGERY AND GYNAECOLOGY AND SURGICAL AND GYNAECOLOGICAL NURSING TREATMENT

Time allowed 1½ hours.

1. In what circumstances may blood transfusion be given? Mention the complications which may result from this procedure and state how a nurse would recognise them.
2. Explain what is meant by a compound fracture. Indicate the treatment that may be given for a compound fracture of the tibia.
3. What is meant by hydronephrosis? Discuss the possible causes and mention the investigations which may be carried out to establish the diagnosis.
4. What complications may follow tonsillectomy? How may they be recognised and treated?
5. In what different ways may the uterus be affected by carcinoma? Discuss the treatment of these conditions.
6. State briefly what you know about:
   (*a*) cataract;
   (*b*) carbuncle;
   (*c*) flat feet;
   (*d*) scoliosis;
   (*e*) alveolar abscess.

October 1948

GENERAL NURSING

Time allowed 2½ hours.

1. What observations should be made on a patient who is having the following drugs:
   (*a*) a sulphanomide;
   (*b*) digitalis;
   (*c*) insulin?
2. How would you nurse a patient with bacillary (e.g., Sonne) dysentery? What precautions should be taken to prevent the spread of infection?
3. A patient is suffering from appendicitis and general peritonitis. Describe in detail the post-operative nursing care and treatment.
4. How would you prepare a patient for:
   (*a*) mastoidectomy;
   (*b*) hæmorrhoidectomy?
5. What complications may occur after the operation of colpo-perineorrhaphy? State what a nurse can do to prevent them.
6. Give an account of the nursing care of a patient during the first twenty-four hours after the operation of total hysterectomy.
7. How would you deal with the following emergencies:
   (*a*) a patient has a rigor;
   (*b*) a patient recovering from an anæsthetic becomes cyanosed;
   (*c*) a nurse in the ward splashes lysol in her eye?
8. What preparations would you make for a patient to have paracentesis abdominis performed? What nursing points have to be considered while this treatment is in progress?

February 1949

MEDICINE AND MEDICAL NURSING TREATMENT

Time allowed 1½ hours.

1. Describe an attack of bronchial asthma. State what you know about the causes and treatment of this condition.
2. Give an account of the symptoms and complications of diabetes mellitus. State how a case of diabetic coma would be treated.
3. What symptoms may be present in a case of early pulmonary tuberculosis? Discuss the treatment which may be employed in a patient who has one lung affected by the disease.
4. Describe the symptoms, complications and treatment of scarlet fever.
5. What conditions may cause the appearance of blood in the urine? How may this be recognised and what investigations might be carried out to ascertain the cause of the bleeding?
6. State briefly what you know about:
   (*a*) venesection;
   (*b*) quinsy;
   (*c*) infective hepatitis (catarrhal jaundice);
   (*d*) paraldehyde;
   (*e*) thioracil.

SURGERY AND GYNAECOLOGY AND SURGICAL AND GYNAECOLOGICAL NURSING TREATMENT

Time allowed 1½ hours.

1. What do you understand by:
   (*a*) post-operative pulmonary embolism;
   (*b*) post-operative pulmonary collapse?
   How are these conditions treated?
2. For what conditions is colostomy performed? Describe any one type of colostomy and its after-care.
3. What are the signs and symptoms of otitis media? Give an account of the treatment and complications.
4. A young man is admitted to hospital with suspected internal injuries following a street accident. What signs and symptoms may develop and what may be their significance?
5. What would lead you to suspect that a woman was suffering from a ruptured ectopic (tubal) pregnancy? What is the treatment of the condition?
6. For what purposes are the following performed:
   (*a*) bronchoscopy;
   (*b*) gastroscopy;
   (*c*) sigmoidoscopy?

GENERAL NURSING

Time allowed 2½ hours.

1. What would you consider to be unfavourable signs and symptoms when nursing patients with the following conditions:
   (*a*) lobar pneumonia;
   (*b*) acute nephritis?
   What may these signs indicate?
2. Describe the nursing care and treatment of a patient suffering from severe hæmatemesis.
3. How would you nurse a patient who has had a radical mastectomy for carcinoma of the breast?
4. What can a nurse do to relieve the following post-operative complications:
   (*a*) vomiting;
   (*b*) retention of urine;
   (*c*) flatulent distension?
5. Explain how a patient's eye is irrigated and how drops are instilled. Mention two drugs which affect the size of the pupil and indicate their use.
6. Describe how you would keep a record of the fluid intake and output of a patient over a period of twenty-four hours. Discuss the importance of these observations.
7. A patient recovering from the operation of colpo-perineorrhaphy has a severe vaginal hæmorrhage. What can a nurse do in this emergency in the absence of the surgeon?
8. Describe in detail how you would give an intramuscular injection. What are the dangers attached to this treatment and how are they avoided?

Index